A synopsis of

Anaesthesia

A synopsis of

Anaesthesia

R. S. *Atkinson* MA MB BChir FFARCS
Consultant Anaesthetist, Department of Anaesthetics
Southend-on-Sea Hospital

G. B. *Rushman* MB BS FFARCS
Consultant Anaesthetist, Department of Anaesthetics
Southend-on-Sea Hospital

and

J. *Alfred Lee* FFARCS Hon FFARCSI DA
Honorary Consulting Anaesthetist
Southend-on-Sea Hospital

Tenth edition

WRIGHT

1987 Bristol

Published under the Wright imprint by
IOP Publishing Limited, Techno House, Redcliffe Way, Bristol BS1 6NX, England.

By J. Alfred Lee

First Edition 1947
Second Edition 1950
Third Edition 1953
Reprinted with minor
  amendments 1955
Reprinted 1956
Reprinted 1957
Fourth Edition 1959
Reprinted 1960
Italian First Edition 1963

*By J. Alfred Lee
and R. S. Atkinson*

Fifth Edition 1964
Spanish Edition 1966
Sixth Edition 1968
Seventh Edition 1973
French Edition 1975
Portuguese Edition 1976
German Edition 1977

By R. S. Atkinson, G. B. Rushman and J. Alfred Lee

Eighth Edition 1977
Reprinted 1979
Ninth Edition 1982
Tenth Edition 1987

Greek Edition 1979
Polish Edition 1981
Spanish Second Edition 1981
Italian Second Edition 1986
German Second Edition 1986

British Library Cataloguing in Publication Data
Atkinson, R. S.
  A synopsis of anaesthesia. —10th ed.
  —(Synopsis series)
  1. Anesthesia
  I. Title II. Rushman, G. B. III. Lee, J.
  Alfred IV. Series
  617'.96   RD81
ISBN 0 7236 0807 5

Typeset by
Activity Ltd, Salisbury, Wiltshire

Printed in Great Britain by
The Bath Press, Lower Bristol Road, Bath BA2 3BL

To N. L., V. A. *and* G. R.

Among the experiments that may be tried on man, those that can only harm are forbidden; those that are innocent are permissible; those that are beneficial are obligatory—Claude Bernard (1813–1878)

A new scientific truth does not triumph because it convinces its opponents making them see the light, but rather because its opponents eventually die and a new generation grows up that is familiar with it.—Max Planck (1858–1947)

It is the duty of the anaesthetist to study the well-being of the patient as well as the convenience of the surgeon.

Eternal vigilance is the price of safety.

The duty of the anaesthetist towards his patient is to take care.

Primum non nocere—First of all, do no harm.

The proper dose of any drug is enough.—Dr J. H. Drysdale.

Knowledge is of two kinds; we know a subject ourselves or we know where we can get information about it.—Samuel Johnson (1709–1784).

When you breathe you inspire, when you do not you expire.

Worry enough, but not too much. — C. L. H.

Preface to the Tenth Edition

For this tenth edition the authors have felt it necessary to make substantial changes to the text. Most pages have been extensively revised and much material formerly included has been removed to make way for newer information and newer references. Many of the references excised can be found in previous editions. Nevertheless the overall size of the book has increased. We believe it is due to an increase in muscle rather than fat, to sturdiness and not to obesity.

The number of anaesthetic texts has proliferated in recent years, making it difficult and expensive for the young trainee to make a choice. In this volume it is hoped that he will be able to refer to most topics of current interest in a small book offered at a reasonable price. As in earlier editions, an effort has been made to provide references for further reading and we hope that these will continue to prove useful. Once again, in discussing techniques we have not forgotten those anaesthetists who work in underdeveloped areas and may not have access to all the recently introduced techniques now commonplace in our modern hospitals.

For this edition there has been a major re-organization of the text which is now divided into six parts. The first deals with History. As in former editions we make no apology for this, believing that a knowledge of the past can enable practitioners to understand the roots from which present practice derives. We are indebted to Professor Ole Secher for providing additional historical data and hope that the Synopsis of Anaesthesia will continue to be a valuable source of information for those interested in the history of our specialty. Basic Sciences, General Anaesthesia, Choice of Anaesthetic, Regional Techniques and Intensive Therapy form the five main divisions of the book. We thank former readers for helpful suggestions and have incorporated many of them. The new arrangement will make it easier for the anaesthetist faced with a problem of how to manage a case to look it up with a minimum of trouble. One enlarged section is the Dictionary of Rare Diseases presenting problems to the anaesthetist and this now occupies a chapter on its own.

The first edition, published in 1947, contained 254 pages and cost 12 shillings and sixpence (63p). The changes which have taken place in anaesthesia in 40 years are immense; most, but not all of them, for the better. What is certain is that the professional expertise of the anaesthetist has improved enormously in this time. The authors hope that the new edition will continue to be useful to trainee anaesthetists, examination candidates and experienced workers both at home and abroad who wish to keep their knowledge up to date.

RSA   GBR   JAL

From the Preface to the First Edition

This book is not designed to take the place of the larger textbooks of anaesthesia and analgesia. It is a summary of current teaching and practice, and it is hoped that it will serve the student, the resident anaesthetist, the practitioner and the candidate studying for the Diploma in Anaesthetics as a ready source of reference and a quick means of revision.

January 1947   JAL

Contents

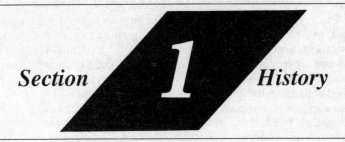

Section 1 History

Chapter 1   **_HISTORY OF ANAESTHESIA_**

Because of the enormous amount of current knowledge they have to absorb, young anaesthetists sometimes comment that they have no time to study the history of their subject, but a knowledge of its historical development is often necessary for a full understanding of the present situation. History has been crowded out so that the new generation tends to be ignorant of the achievements of its forebears and many discoveries are now incorporated into the textbooks without any reference to their originators. This we have endeavoured to correct. For the history of pain relief in surgery before 1846, *see* Smith W. D. A. Surgery without pain. *Anaesth. Intensive Care* 1986, **14**, and 186.

The development of anaesthesia since its introduction in 1846 has been erratic, long periods of stagnation being occasionally broken by improvements and advances.

Anaesthesia as we know it today was first used by W. T. G. Morton of Boston in the US who gave ether at the Massachusetts General Hospital on 16 October 1846 to Gilbert Abbott. C. W. Long of Georgia had given the same agent several times 4 years previously but failed to report his work so that this was unknown to Morton. Thus was Henry Hill Hickman's idea, that anaesthesia could be produced by the inhalation of gases and vapours, finally vindicated. Horace Wells, a colleague of Morton, had used nitrous oxide for the painless extraction of teeth quite successfully in 1844, but his public demonstration of this practice was a disastrous failure so that the gas was temporarily forgotten. The news of Morton's discovery soon spread throughout the civilized world, and on 19 December 1846 Francis Boott, a physician, born and trained in the US but working in London, received news of Morton's discovery and encouraged Mr Robinson, a dentist to give ether to a Miss Lonsdale for a dental extraction, Mr Robinson acting as dentist and anaesthetist. (On the same day, Dr Scott operated under ether at the Dumfries and Galloway Infirmary in Scotland.) So successful was this that Boott persuaded Robert Liston, the University of London's professor of surgery, to experiment with the new drug. It was tried out with considerable publicity and brilliant success for the amputation through the thigh of Frederick Churchill's leg at University College Hospital on 21 December 1846.

The technical difficulties associated with the administration of ether were partly overcome by the substitution of chloroform by James Young Simpson, professor of midwifery at Edinburgh University, in the following year. He poured drops of this newer agent on to gauze held near the face of the patient, so avoiding the use of the inhalers which were used for ether.

1

John Snow, a London physician, was the first to attempt some sort of scientific investigation into the new anaesthetic agents and the methods of their administration, and he devised several pieces of apparatus for delivering to the patient known percentage concentrations of anaesthetic vapour in an attempt to increase their safety. This work was undertaken because of the reports of deaths associated with anaesthesia. Different uses of the drugs and different methods of administration were adopted in different countries. Thus chloroform was used more frequently in Scotland, the greater part of Europe and in the southern states of America, while ether remained the favourite in England and in the northern states of America. There was much controversy as to which was the safer of the two drugs but eventually ether won the day. When in 1858 John Snow, who was England's leading physician anaesthetist, died, his place was taken by J. T. Clover, and partly due to the influence of these two pioneers, the administration of anaesthetics in the UK has always been in the hands of medical men and, as time has passed, in the hands of specialists in the subject.

Meanwhile, nitrous oxide still had its friends in the US, and in 1863 G. Q. Colton, who introduced it to Wells, embarked on a campaign of popularization of the gas. Its disadvantages were difficulty in administration and the asphyxia inseparable from its use. The latter was partly overcome by Edmund Andrews of Chicago who in 1868 gave it with 20% oxygen, and by Paul Bert of Paris who gave in under pressure 10 years later. The first major war in which anaesthetics were used was the Crimean War (1854–1855). It is an interesting fact, however, that even 25 years after Morton introduced the use of ether in surgery, operations were still being performed in the complete absence of any form of anaesthesia, even in European teaching hospitals (*Med. Times; Lond.* 1868, **2**, 9; and Pernick M. S. *A Calculus of Suffering*. New York: Columbia University Press, 1985).

During the next 40–50 years there were few significant changes in anaesthesia, but in the 1920s the pace of progress quickened. In the 1920s, ether and chloroform were the main agents used but ethyl chloride and nitrous oxide were often employed for induction. Simpson's open drop method was the most popular, while the first Boyle machine appeared in 1917. Before the 1930s the anaesthetist administered one or two volatile agents to produce unconsciousness, muscle relaxation and deafferentation. This gave place to various techniques of so-called balanced anaesthesia and so the amount of toxic drugs to which the patient was exposed was reduced and the hazard of general anaesthesia made less. Among other innovations were the popularization of endotracheal techniques by Ivan W. Magill and E. Stanley Rowbotham, the appearance of bromethol (Avertin), divinyl ether, cyclopropane and trichloroethylene, and the induction of anaesthesia by intravenous barbiturates in the early 1930s. Because of the difficulty of obtaining relaxation of the jaw and larynx with ether, blind nasotracheal intubation became increasingly used. Controlled respiration was used with cyclopropane so that when curare was first tried out by Harold Griffith in Montreal in 1942, the way to deal with hypoventilation and apnoea was well established, and soon intermittent positive-pressure ventilation became routine practice.

Local analgesia made its appearance in 1884 when Carl Koller of Vienna demonstrated the use of cocaine for topical analgesia in the eye. Infiltration and regional block followed from this. Spinal analgesia was first described by August Bier in Kiel in 1898 and extradural block by Fernand Cathelin and Jean Athanase

Sicard in Paris in 1901 and by Fidel Pagès of Madrid in 1921 and Achille Mario Dogliotti of Turin in 1931. The two world wars stimulated both surgery and anaesthesia, and following each, the number of doctors who continued their anaesthetic work, learnt under service conditions, into civilian life had a considerable influence on the development of the specialty.

Technical improvements were slowly accompanied by academic recognition, but not always by adequate financial rewards. The first examination for the Diploma in Anaesthetics was held in London in 1935 and the first chair in anaesthetics was created in Oxford (Macintosh R. R. (1897–) In: Rupreht J. et al. (ed.) *Anaesthesia; Essays on its History*. Berlin: Springer-Verlag, 1985, p. 352), with R. R. Macintosh as professor, 2 years later. Ralph Waters was appointed as the first professor of anaesthesia in a university in the US in 1933. In the UK the recognition of anaesthesia as a specialty with full equality with other medical and surgical specialties was secured in 1948 with the introduction of the National Health Service, and since then anaesthesia has not only kept pace with the rapid advances made in surgery, but has in many instances enabled these advances to be made. In recent decades the scope of the anaesthetist's work has widened and now takes in not only preoperative assessment and postoperative care, but supervision of intensive therapy units, pain clinics, and in many cases research and postgraduate education. An enormous development in the use of monitoring equipment, some of it highly sophisticated, has taken place in the last 20 years. Among those workers who remember clinical anaesthesia in the 1930s and early 1940s, few would disagree with the statement that what is known as 'modern anaesthesia' commenced with the introduction of the muscle relaxants. (*See also* Duncum B. *The Development of Inhalation Anaesthesia*. London: Oxford University Press 1947; and Rupreht J. et al. (ed.) *Anaesthesia; Essays on its History*. Berlin: Springer-Verlag, 1985.

While anaesthesia has advanced and anaesthetists have greatly improved the quality of their work, they have still a long way to go. Morbidity and mortality associated with anaesthesia are far from satisfactory; there are difficulties in attracting young doctors into the specialty; conditions of work are in need of great betterment; the satisfaction derived from the daily round of work is not always what it could be. We must strive in the future to give an even better and safer service of pain relief and care to our patients.

Following a joint congress of anaesthetists in London in 1951 of which Sir Ivan Magill was President, and a similar meeting in Paris the same year, it was decided to form a Federation of Societies of Anaesthesiologists and the first Congress of the new body was held in Scheveningen in Holland in 1955. Other similar congresses have been held in Toronto (1960), Sao Paulo (1964), London (1968), Kyoto (1972), Mexico City (1976), Hamburg (1980), and Manila (1984). It is proposed to hold the 9th congress in Washington in 1988. (*See also* van Lieburg M. J. In: Rupreht J. et al. (ed.) *Anaesthesia; Essays on its History*. Berlin: Springer-Verlag, 1985, p. 307; Organe G. *ibid*. p. 309; and Howat, D. D. C. *ibid*. p. 314.)

Among training courses arranged by the World Health Organization were those of the Anaesthesiology Centre in Copenhagen (1950–1973) and in Manila (under the guidance of Professor Quintin Gomez).[1]

Some outstanding Contributors to the Science and Art of Anaesthesia
Joseph Priestley (1733–1804)
Born in Fieldhead near Leeds, the son of a handloom worker, and brought up in a

strict Nonconformist Calvinistic atmosphere by an aunt. Educated at Batley Grammar School. Trained as a dissenting minister and took charge of Mill Hill Chapel in Leeds in 1773. He then became a schoolmaster and experimenter in chemistry, physics and electricity. He never gave up the phlogiston theory, unlike Lavoisier who discredited it and who was guillotined during the French Revolution. Next he spent seven years as librarian and companion to the second Earl of Shelbourne (1737–1805) at Bowood, and isolated or identified 'alkaline air' (NH_3), 'vitriolic acid air' (SO_2), 'dephlogisticated air' (O_2) in 1774, a gas given the name of oxygen by Lavoisier (1743–1797) and produced by heating mercuric oxide with a burning glass; 'dephlogisticated nitrous air' (N_2O) in 1773 and 'Nitrous acid air' (NO_2). (One of his teachers, Mathew Turner of Manchester, described the anaesthetic effects of ether in 1744.[2]) He also discovered methane and the absorption of carbon dioxide (fixed air) by green plants in the presence of sunshine with the formation of oxygen. By subjecting carbon dioxide to pressure in water he discovered 'soda water'. He was elected a Fellow of the Royal Society and became a Doctor of Laws of the University of Edinburgh. From the former institution he received a Copley Medal for a paper on 'The Different Kinds of Air'.[3] His discoveries led Thomas Beddoes (1760–1808) of Bristol to experiment with the therapeutic effects of these 'airs'. In 1780 he went to Birmingham to take charge of a Unitarian congregation, The New Meeting House, and in this city he became a member of the famous Lunar Society which brought him into contact with Erasmus Darwin (1731–1802), physician and grandfather of Charles (1809–1882), James Watt (1736–1818), scientist and inventor and William Murdoch (1757–1839), engineer and the inventor of gas lighting. He became a close friend of, and correspondent with Benjamin Franklin (1706–1790), American printer, inventor and diplomat. He was an opponent of political discrimination against Dissenters, and on the second anniversary of the fall of the Bastille (14 July 1789) his chapel, home, scientific apparatus, books and manuscripts were looted by a High Tory Royalist mob, forcing him to seek refuge in Hackney, near London. His left-wing political opinions still separated him from his scientific colleagues so that in 1794 he joined his sons in Northumberland, Pennsylvania. Here, he added farming to his other activities and soon became a leader of his new community. He died of oesophageal obstruction in 1804 at the age of 70. A statue to Priestley was unveiled in Birmingham by Thomas Henry Huxley in 1874 to mark the centenary of the discovery of oxygen. Hilaire Belloc (1870–1953), the poet, journalist and historian, was a great-grandson. (*See also* Smith W. D. A. *Under the Influence; A History of Nitrous Oxide and Oxygen Anaesthesia*. London: Macmillan, 1982; and McDowell D. G. *Anaesth. Intensive Care* 1982, **10**, 4.)

Humphry Davy (1778–1829)

Born in Cornwall, the son of a wood carver. Became apprenticed to J. B. Borlase, surgeon, of Penzance, in 1795. At the age of 17 he experimented with nitrous oxide and the effects of its inhalation. In 1798 Davy became superintendent of Thomas Beddoes's (1760–1808) Pneumatic Institute in Clifton, Bristol, for the treatment of pulmonary tuberculosis by inhalation of gases; other gases used were hydrogen, oxygen, 'water gas' and carbon dioxide. Humphry Davy published his book *Researches, Chemical and Philosophical; Chiefly Concerning Nitrous Oxide* (London: J. Johnson, 1800). 'On the day when the inflammation was most troublesome, I breathed three large doses of nitrous oxide. The pain always diminished after the first four or five respirations.'[5] In this, Davy suggested that nitrous oxide inhalations might be used to relieve the pain of surgical operations and named it 'laughing gas'. A nitrous oxide container was made by James Watt (1736–1819) in 1799 to assist this research.[6] The idea was not pursued by Humphry Davy or anyone else, except for its entertainment value, but his work was known to, and may have influenced, Gardner Quincy Colton (1814–1898) 44 years later. In later life, Davy became famous. He invented the miner's safety lamp, was created a baronet in 1818, and was elected President of the Royal Society in 1820. Among Davy's colleagues at Bristol was Dr Peter Mark Roget, FRS, famed for his *Thesaurus of English Words and Phrases* (1852). Davy prepared nitrous oxide by the method of Berthollet (1785) by heating ammonium nitrate. He was Faraday's teacher and was the first to describe sodium and potassium.

Henry Hill Hickman (1800–1830)[7]

Born 27 January 1800 at Lady Halton, Bromfield, in Shropshire. Medical education received in Edinburgh, but did not graduate there (MRCS, England, 1821). He settled in practice in Ludlow and later in Tenbury Wells in Worcestershire. He married in 1821. While at Shifnal, in Shropshire, his interest in gas therapy was aroused, as the village was the birthplace of Thomas Beddoes. Familiarizing himself with the pioneer work of Davy, Priestley and Michael Faraday (1791–1867), Hickman returned to Ludlow and commenced experiments on animals (controlled asphyxiation) in 1825. He was able to perform surgical operations painlessly on them, by causing them to inhale carbon dioxide. This was the first work on surgical anaesthesia induced by inhaling a gas. His results where published in a paper, 'A Letter on Suspended Animation' (Ironbridge, 1824), when W. T. G. Morton was a child of 5, but attracted no attention from scientific men in England. Even Sir Humphry Davy, who was approached by Hickman's friend, T. A. Knight, FRS,[8] showed no interest. Charles X of France (1752–1827) was appealed to in 1828,[8] and the French Academy of Medicine agreed to investigate Hickman's results, but nothing came of the matter. Baron Dominique Jean Larrey (1766–1842), one of Napoleon's surgeons, however, gave Hickman some encouragement. Hickman died prematurely, aged 29, at Tenbury Wells, and was buried in Bromfield churchyard, Shropshire, where, in 1930, a memorial was erected in the porch by the Anaesthetic Section of the Royal Society of Medicine, unveiled by Sir St Clair Thompson and dedicated by the Bishop of Hereford (*Br. Med. J.* 1930, 12 April). The first allusion to Hickman in recent times was in an article by C. J. S. Thompson in the *Br. Med. J.* 1912, **1**, 843.

Horace Wells (1815–1848)

Born in Hartford, Vermont. In 1844, on 10 December, Gardner Q. Colton (1814–1898), a travelling lecturer in chemistry, gave a demonstration of the effects of inhaling nitrous oxide at Hartford, Connecticut. Horace Wells, a local dentist, was present and noticed that a young shop assistant, Samuel Cooley, while under the influence of the gas, banged his shin and made it bleed, but stated afterwards that he experienced no pain. Wells persuaded Colton to try the gas during a dental extraction, and on the following day, 11 December 1844, the experiment was carried out with Colton as anaesthetist, John M. Riggs (1810–1885) as dentist and

Wells as patient. It was a big success. 'A new era in tooth pulling', according to Wells. Wells learnt from Colton the method of manufacture of nitrous oxide and used it in his dental practice on 15 patients. It was administered from an animal bladder through a wooden tube into the mouth, while the nostrils were compressed. Later he went to Boston to interest a larger audience in his discovery. He demonstrated the method to the students of Harvard Medical School, in the class of Dr John Collins Warren (1778–1856), but the patient complained of pain; the affair was a fiasco and Wells was hissed out of the room as a fraud. Morton and Charles T. Jackson (1805–1880) were present at this operation in January 1845. Wells returned to Hartford and continued to use the gas, but the introduction of ether gradually ousted nitrous oxide. In 1847 Wells published his letter 'A History of the Discovery of the Application of Nitrous Oxide Gas, Ether, and Other Vapours to Surgical Operations' (Hartford, Conn., 1847; also 'Classical File', *Surv. Anesthesiol.* 1958, **2**, 1). In 1847 he opened a dental office in New York City but soon afterwards Wells gave up dentistry, became a chloroform addict, travelled around the country with a troop of performing canaries, and was incarcerated in jail after bespattering a New York prostitute with sulphuric acid, while recovering from self-administered chloroform.[9] He commited suicide by cutting his femoral artery, aged 33.

Colton reintroduced the use of nitrous oxide in dentistry in 1863, at New Haven.

William Thomas Green Morton (1819–1868)[10]
Morton deserves the chief credit for the introduction of ether as an anaesthetic agent, although W. E. Clarke (1818–1878), of Rochester, New York, gave ether for a dental extraction in 1842, and Crawford Williamson Long (1815–1878) removed a tumour from the neck of James M. Venable quite painlessly, in Jefferson County, Georgia, a few months after Clarke's experiment. By the time (1849) that Long reported his work,[11] Morton's fame was well established. In science, the credit for a new discovery belongs to the man who convinces the world, not to the man to whom the idea first occurs. Morton convinced the world of the advantages of ether anaesthesia and the credit for this discovery is his.

Morton, born at Charlton, Worcester County, Massachusetts, started work at the age of 16 in a printing house; later went into business but was a failure. As a young man he suffered the pain of a surgical operation, in Cincinnati. He studied at the Baltimore College of Dental Surgery, set up in practice at Farmington, Connecticut, and later became a pupil and later a partner of Wells, at Hartford. He separated from Wells and, becoming a medical student in Boston at the Harvard Medical School, was present when Wells failed to satisfy the audience as to the efficiency of nitrous oxide. He never qualified in medicine, but received an honorary MD in 1852. Charles T. Jackson (1805–1880),[12] one of Morton's lecturers at Harvard, suggested that ether could be used as a surface analgesic in dentistry.[12] Morton, however, went further; he experimented on dogs to find out the effect of giving ether vapour by inhalation. Impressed with the results, he gave the vapour to Eben Frost for the removal of a tooth of 30 September 1846. The operation was painless. After gaining further experience, including the administration of 37 anaesthetics for Henry Bigelow, and while still a medical student, Morton gave a demonstration at the Massachusetts General Hospital on 16 October 1846, in what is now the 'Ether Dome', when Dr John Collins Warren (1778–1856) removed a tumour from the jaw of his patient, Gilbert Abbott, a printer and journalist (Vandam L. D. and Abbott J. A. *N. Engl. J. Med*. 1984, **311**, 991), without producing any pain. This success gained him the support of Warren and also of Henry Jacob Bigelow (1818–1890), surgeon and professor of materia medica. Oliver Wendell Holmes (1809–1897), professor of anatomy and physiology at Harvard Medical School, said:[13] 'This priceless gift to humanity went forth from the operating theatre of the Massachusetts General Hospital, and the man to whom the world owes it is Dr T. W. G. Morton.' Much wrangling occurred between Morton and Jackson as to who should be given credit for the discovery.[12] Morton three times petitioned the US Congress, and even obtained an interview with the President (Franklin Pierce, 1804–1869), but he was never in his lifetime officially recognized as the pioneer of ether anaesthesia. Time later vindicated his claim. He spent his later years farming at Needham, Massachusetts, and died of cerebral haemorrhage quite suddenly in Central Park, New York City, on 15 July 1868;[14] a disappointed man. The inscription on his tombstone in Mount Auburn Cemetry, Boston, composed by Henry J. Bigelow reads: 'Inventor and Revealer of Inhalation Anesthesia: Before Whom, in All Time, Surgery was Agony; By Whom, Pain in Surgery was Averted and Annulled; Since Whom, Science has Control of Pain'. His agent, which he tried to patent under the name Letheon, became widely used.

It was given in London and Paris in 1846. Robert Liston (1794–1847) was the first surgeon to operate under ether in England (Liston died of a ruptured aortic aneurysm 1 year after this operation); this was at University College Hospital on 21 December 1846, using Squire's inhaler when he amputated the leg of Frederick Churchill, a 36-year-old butler.[15] The apparatus was designed by Peter Squire, the Queen's chemist and druggist (who in 1804 founded the *Companion to the British Pharmacopoeia*, which later became *Martindale's Extra Pharmacopoeia*) as a modification of Dr Nooth's apparatus for the production of soda water. The actual anaesthetic was given by the designer's nephew, William Squire, a 21-year-old medical student.[16] When the leg had been painlessly amputated Liston said to the large audience: 'This Yankee dodge beats mesmerism hollow.' It was, however, probably given on 19 December in the Dumfries and Galloway Royal Infirmary by William Scott (1820–1887), surgeon and William Fraser (1819–1863), ship's surgeon (Baillie T. W. *From Boston to Dumfries*. Dumfries, 1966; and *Br. J. Anaesth*. 1965, **37**, 952). This followed a verbal report of Morton's successful use of the agent, carried by Fraser, who arrived in Liverpool from Boston on 16 December, as medical officer on the steamship *Arcadia*.

The name anaesthesia was suggested by Oliver Wendell Holmes. It also appeared in Bailey's *English Dictionary* in 1751.[17]

Ether became known in England through a letter written by Jacob Bigelow (1786–1865), Henry's (1818–1890) Father, to his friend. Dr Boott (1792–1863) American doctor practising in Gower Street, London,[18] who, with Mr J. Robinson (1813–1861), gave the first ether anaesthetic, a dental case, 2 days before Robert Liston's first use of it. Malgaigne was the first man to use ether in France, on 12 January 1847. News spread quickly to all parts of the civilized world. The first ether anaesthetic in Australia was administered by William Ross Pugh (1805–1897) (buried in Brighton and Preston cemetery, England) on 7 June 1847, at Launceston in Tasmania,[19] in Germany by Johan F. M. Heyfelder (1798–1869) of Erlangen, (*see* Heyfelder, *Die Versuche mit dem Schwefeläther*, Erlangen, 1847, reprinted Druckerei S. Kriegelstein Erlangen, 1974).

John Snow (1813–1858)

Born in York, 15 March, 1813, the eldest of 9 children of a farmer. After Morton, the first whole-time anaesthetist. Starting his medical studies in Newcastle, at the age of 14, as apprentice to Mr William Hardcastle, he was one of the eight medical students who entered the Newcastle-on-Tyne Medical School at its inception in 1832. Snow worked at the Newcastle Infirmary and became interested in the first cholera epidemic at Killingworth Colliery in 1831–1832. In 1833 he left Newcastle and worked for a time at Burnop Field near Newcastle, then at Pateley Bridge in Yorkshire and in 1836 he migrated to London, travelling on foot, and attended lectures at the Hunterian School of Anatomy in Great Windmill Street, founded by William Hunter (1718–1784), elder brother of John Hunter (1728–1792) and also at Westminster Hospital. He became a member of the Royal College of Surgeons of England in 1838 and also passed the examination of the Apothecaries Hall; became MD, London, in 1844, and was appointed lecturer (1844–1849) in forensic medicine at the Aldersgate School of Medicine just before its closure. Settled first at 54 Frith Street and then at 18 Sackville Street in London as a general practitioner. Here he lived for the remainder of his life. He became interested in ether soon after its introduction and quickly perceived that the common method of administration was faulty. To overcome this, he invented an ether inhaler in 1847 and adapted the face-piece of Dr Francis Sibson (1816–1876) of Nottingham. Later he invented his own. He was appointed anaesthetist to Out-patients at St George's Hospital, where his first anaesthetics (for dental extraction) were given, and in 1847 was promoted to the In-patient appointment. He also worked with Robert Liston (1794–1847) at University College Hospital and with Sir William Fergusson (1808–1877) at King's College Hospital. His health was poor and he suffered from phthisis and from nephritis, being treated for the kidney disease by Richard Bright (1789–1858). For many years he was a vegetarian and temperance advocate. He experimented with many substances to see if they possessed anaesthetic properties, trying many of them on himself.

Snow rapidly became the leading anaesthetist in London and wrote a book in 1847, *On the Inhalation of Ether in Surgical Operations* (reprinted in the *Br. J. Anaesth.* 1953, **25**, 53 et seq.). He did much useful work on the physiology of anaesthesia, and described five stages or degrees of anaesthesia. He emphasized the importance of knowing how deep to take the anaesthetized patient. He later abandoned ether for chloroform in adults, but was familiar with the dangers of the newer drug, believing it to cause primary cardiac failure consequent on the use of too strong a vapour. To overcome this danger he invented a percentage chloroform inhaler. For anaesthesia during labour, Snow poured a little chloroform on to a folded handkerchief but for surgical operations he preferred the greater accuracy provided by his inhaler. In Scotland, the 'open method' originated by Simpson was the usual method of both types of administration. He gave over 4000 chloroform anaesthetics without a death. In 1853 Snow originated the method of 'chloroform *à la reine*', when he acted as anaesthetist at the birth of Queen Victoria's (1819–1901) eighth child, Prince Leopold (1853–1884) (later Duke of Albany, who died of haemophilia), at the request of Sir James Clark, on 7 April and in 1857 at the birth of Princess Beatrice (1857–1944) on 17 April. These royal occasions made anaesthesia in midwifery morally respectable. He gave his royal patient 15-minim doses intermittently on a handkerchief, the administration lasting 53 minutes: it met with the Queen's warm approval: 'Dr Snow gave that blessed chloroform and the effect was soothing, quieting, and delightful beyond measure.' The birth of Leopold George Duncan Albert (1853–1884), later Duke of Albany, finally canonized 'that blessed chloroform'. Even the names of the Queen's attendants seemed to share the aura of purity which her royal participation had given to the subject: Mrs Lilly and Mrs Innocent the midwives, and of course Dr Snow.[20] Snow introduced amylene as an inhalation anaesthetic in 1856. His income never exceeded £1000 per annum although during the last 10 years of his life he gave an average of 450 anaesthetics a year. His last work, *On Chloroform and Other Anaesthetics*, was published posthumously in 1858, Snow having been seized with paralysis while at work on the manuscript and dying on 11 June 1858.

In his later years he proved that cholera is a water-borne disease, when he ordered the removal of the Broad Street (Golden Square) pump handle in 1854 in London and so terminated the third cholera epidemic (although this particular epidemic had commenced to wane before the actual removal of the handle!).[21] The theory of the mode of transmission of cholera was set out in the second edition of his book (first edition 1849, following the epidemic of 1848 in which over 5000 people died), *On the Mode of Communication of Cholera*, 2nd ed. (London: Churchill, 1855). Snow's theories were substantiated by William Budd (1811–1880) ('Malignant Cholera: Its Mode of Propagation, and its Prevention', *Lond. Med. Gaz.* 1849, **44**, 724). It was, however, many years before Snow's views were generally accepted, Max von Pettenkoffer (1818–1901) being a leading anti-contagionist until his suicide in 1901. It is interesting that the cholera vibrio had been described in 1854 by Picini of Florence,[22] 30 years before Koch's paper.[23] Near the site of the pump, in Broadwick Street, a public house has been named 'The John Snow' (although Snow was a teetotaller!). Snow's grave in Brompton Cemetery was restored in 1938 by anaesthetists from Britain and the United States. Benjamin Ward Richardson's (1828–1896) (*see Br. J. Anaesth.* 1955, **27**, 517) epitaph reads: 'In Brompton Cemetery there was laid to rest, at the age of forty-five, John Snow (1813–1858), exemplary citizen and useful physician. He demonstrated that cholera is communicated by contaminated water; and he made the art of anaesthesia a science.' The tombstone was destroyed by bombing in April 1941, but was restored in 1950 and unveiled on 6 July 1951.[24] Three of his case books with a record of his chloroform administrations 1848–1858 are in the possession of the Library of the Royal College of Physicians of London.[25]

(*See also*: 'John Snow; First Anaesthetist', *Bios*, 1936, **7**, 25; Keys T. E. 'John Snow; Anaesthetist', *J. Hist. Med. Allied Sci.* 1946, **1**, 551; *John Snow: Biography*, by Sir Benjamin Ward Richardson, reprinted in the *Br. J. Anaesth.* 1952, **24**, 267; 'Snow on the Water of London', *Mayo Clin. Proc.* 1974, **49**, 480; Lord Cohen of Birkenhead, 'John Snow—the Autumn Loiterer', *Proc. R. Soc. Med.* 1969, **62**, 99.)

James Young Simpson (1811–1870)[26]
Born at Bathgate, near Edinburgh. Qualified 1830; MD, 1832. Elected to Chair of Midwifery at Edinburgh, 1840, spending £500 on canvassing, etc. Started university career in atmosphere of hostility from his colleagues, but his ability as a lecturer soon attracted large classes of students. Simpson took an interest in a wide range of subjects, including leprosy, puerperal sepsis and hospital design. He put forward the method of haemostasis by acupressure to promote better wound healing. He made many contributions to the literature of archaeology, becoming

President of the Society of Antiquaries of Scotland in 1861. He was made one of Her Majesty's Physicians in Scotland in 1847 and was created baronet in 1866. He also received many foreign honours.

He is most famous for the introduction of chloroform in 1847.[27] (Davy, Faraday, Hickman, Wells, Morton, and Koller were all in their twenties when they made their discoveries: Simpson was a veteran of 36.) He was the first to use ether in obstetric practice on 19 January 1847, but wanted to find a better agent. Chloroform was discovered independently by Justus von Liebig (1813–1873), Darmstadt chemist, Soubeiran (1793–1858), Paris pharmacist, and Guthrie (1782–1848), American chemist, in 1831. Jean Baptiste Andre Dumas (1800–1848), Paris pharmacist, gave it its name and wrote the first full description of its physical and chemical properties. In 1847 Flourens showed that it had anaesthetic powers on animals.

David Waldie (1813–1889), a Liverpool chemist, suggested that Simpson should try chloroform as an anaesthetic vapour.[28] Simpson experimented on himself and his assistants, Matthews Duncan (1823–1890) and George Keith, on 4 November 1847 at Simpson's house, 52 Queen Street, Edinburgh. Four days later it was used clinically and a report was read to the Edinburgh Medical and Chirurgical Society on 10 November: 'Notice of a New Anaesthetic Agent as a Substitute for Sulphuric Ether in Surgery and Midwifery'. Simpson was harshly attacked more on moral than on theological grounds[29] (Genesis, ch. 3, verse 16) for using pain relief for women in labour, but following the administration of chloroform to Queen Victoria during the delivery of her eighth child (Prince Leopold) in 1853 by John Snow, the seal of respectability was set on the relief of pain in childbirth by anaesthetics. Although Simpson was the first obstetrician to employ ether for delivery (19 January 1847), he held that chloroform has the following advantages over ether: (1) Action more rapid, complete and persistent; (2) Smaller quantity required; (3) Pleasanter; (4) Cheaper. Chloroform was first given in London at St Bartholomew's Hospital on 20 November 1847 (though it had in fact been used at St Bartholomew's Hospital earlier in the year under the name of 'chloric ether' by Sir William Lawrence (1783–1867) and Holmes Coote at the suggestion of Michael Cudmore Furnell—before Simpson).[30] After the publication of Simpson's works chloroform temporarily displaced ether in most parts of the world. Simpson remained an enthusiastic salesman for chloroform anaesthesia.

From 1845 to his death in 1870, Simpson lived at No. 52 Queen Street, Edinburgh. The dining room has been preserved as 'The Discovery Room' and contains some of Simpson's furniture and possessions.[31] There is a memorial to Sir James Young Simpson in Westminster Abbey. He was buried in the family plot in Warriston Cemetery, Edinburgh.

In its day, chloroform was a superb anaesthetic, easy to administer, portable, capable of producing good abdominal relaxation and reasonably safe. Joseph Clover is reported to have given over 7000 administrations without a death. What other agent, excepting ether and nitrous oxide was in use for 100 years? It gave way to safer agents, but Simpson's achievement must not be forgotten, for it was meritorious

Joseph T. Clover (1825–1882)

After the death of Snow, Clover became the leading scientific anaesthetic investigator and practical anaesthetist in Britain. He was born in Aylesham,

Norfolk, and was educated at the Gray Friar's Priory School in Norwich and at University College Hospital in London (1844). Although it is unlikely[32] that Clover was present in the operating theatre at University College Hospital on 21 December 1846, when Robert Liston (1794–1847) amputated the leg of Frederick Churchill when ether was given by William Squire, a medical student, the first major operation performed under ether anaesthesia in England, he was interested in anaesthesia from its commencement. Joseph Lister (1827–1912) was a fellow student. Became house surgeon to James Syme (1799–1870) and later RMO at University College Hospital and took FRCS in 1850. He was the pioneer of the art of completely and immediately removing from the urinary bladder the calculus fragments produced by lithotrity and invented a bladder aspirator (the forerunner of Bigelow's evacuator (1878)). He also devised 'Clover's crutch', a simple but effective piece of apparatus for maintaining a patient in the lithotomy position. Worked as general practitioner in London (because of poor health!) (1853), later specializing in anaesthetics, thereby helping to fill the vacancy created by the early death of John Snow in 1858. Was appointed to staff of University College and Westminster Hospitals, and also worked at the London Dental Hospital. Was for many years the leading anaesthetist in London and attended many famous people, including the ex-Emperor Napoleon III of France at Chislehurst, in 1871, the Princess of Wales (later Queen Alexandra), Sir Robert Peel and Miss Florence Nightingale. In 1862 he invented a chloroform inhaler which enabled percentage mixtures of chloroform and air to be accurately measured and administered. It took the form of a large bag, slung over the back of the anaesthetist, and it contained 4·5% of chloroform vapour in air. Realizing the dangers of chloroform, Clover set to work to make the administration of ether more simple and easy. This he did by inducing anaesthesia with nitrous oxide, later adding ether to the gas.[33] Was co-opted on to Committee of Royal Medical and Chirurgical Society which advised the use of a mixture of chloroform and ether, because of the danger of chloroform alone (1864). In 1868 published a paper 'On the Administration of Nitrous Oxide', *Br. Med. J*, 1868, **2**, 491. In 1877 he described his portable regulating ether inhaler[34] which did much to make ether more popular at the expense of chloroform. Ombrédanne's inhaler from France was a slightly modified copy, using a pig's bladder instead of a rubber bag[35] (Louis Ombrédanne (French surgeon, 1871–1956). 'L'Anaesthésie par l'Éther', *Gazette des Hospit.* 1908, 1095). Another of Clover's achievements was his teaching that ether could be safely given over long periods with anaesthesia carried to adequate depth. He was never a man of robust constitution and died at the age of 57.[36,37] Eleven years before his death he was to claim that he had had no deaths in 11 000 administrations, 7000 of then using chloroform.[38] An eponymous lecture is given every two years in his honour, alternately with a similar lecture honouring the name of Frederick Hewitt, at the Royal College of Surgeons in London. He is buried in Brompton Cemetery, London, his grave (No. U 113122) being 200 yards from that of John Snow.[39]

Sir Frederick Hewitt (1857–1916)

Educated at Merchant Taylors' School, Christ's College, Cambridge, and St George's Hospital, London, where he was a distinguished student. Became an anaesthetist as defective eyesight prevented his becoming a consulting physician, and was appointed to Charing Cross Hospital in this capacity in 1884, the National Dental Hospital in 1885, and lecturer on anaesthesia at the London Hospital in

1886. In 1902 became physician anaesthetist to his old teaching hospital, St George's. He emphasized that nitrous oxide anaesthesia is possible without asphyxia and that chloroform is specially dangerous during induction. Hewitt modified Junker's chloroform bottle and redesigned Clover's inhaler, enlarging the bore of the central tube (as suggested by Wilson Smith)[40] and arranging for its rotation within the ether reservoir.[41] He devised a dental prop and also an airway (*Lancet*, 1908, **1**, 490), and wrote a popular textbook (1893) on anaesthesia (*Anaesthetics and their Administration*. London: Griffin), the fifth edition of which appeared in 1922. He strongly advocated better teaching of anaesthetics to medical students. A superb clinical anaesthetist, he was a tireless advocate for greater care to be taken in the administration of anaesthetics and constantly sought to improve conditions under which anaesthetics were given, and to protect the public against their use by unqualified persons. Hewitt invented the first practical machine for giving nitrous oxide and oxygen in fixed proportions in 1887 and the years following.[42] In 1911 he was knighted. Administered an anaesthetic to Edward VII for drainage of an appendix abscess on 27 June 1902,[43] two days before his coronation day (the ceremony took place on 9 August 1902). Sir Frederick Treves (1853–1916) was the surgeon. Hewitt died at Brighton of a gastric neoplasm. His grave lies in Brighton and Preston Cemetery.[44]

Sir William Macewen (1847–1924)

Born in Rothesay in the Isle of Bute, Scotland, on 22 June 1847 youngest of 12 children and son of a sea captain, just 7 months after Simpson's introduction of chloroform. A medical student in the University of Glasgow, he qualified in 1869 and proceeded to the MD degree 3 years later. While the Regius Professor of surgery, Joseph Lister, was developing his system of antiseptic surgery, Macewen became his dresser and this association with the great man had a profound effect on Macewen's subsequent professional development. Following resident appointments in the Royal Infirmary, he was appointed medical superintendent of the Belvidere Fever Hospital, where he had the harrowing experience of treating patients suffering from respiratory obstruction due to laryngeal diphtheria, an experience which led him to his great discovery of oral laryngeal intubation. Leaving the Fever Hospital he went into general practice and became a parochial medical officer but gradually his interests centred on surgery and he obtained appointments at both the Glasgow Royal Infirmary and Western Infirmary, culminating in his nomination to the chair as Regius Professor of surgery in the University of Glasgow in 1877, a post he was to fill with great distinction for the next 15 years. He was invited to become the first professor of surgery at the new Johns Hopkins Hospital in Baltimore, but refused it, the post going to William Stewart Halsted. On the accession of King Edward VII in 1902, he was knighted. Macewen became president of the British Medical Association in 1922 and of the International College of Surgeons when it met in London the following year. A tall, handsome, impressive personality who tolerated fools badly, and went his own way.

His numerous surgical contributions included the diagnosis and treatment of cerebral abscess, surgery of the brain, the spine, chest and bones. He was an early exponent of aseptic surgery in which sterilization of instruments and dressings was carried out by heat.

He was the pioneer of oral and nasal tracheal intubation as an alternative to tracheotomy, performing the manoeuvre by touch in the conscious patient. He first used rubber and gum elastic catheters in the treatment of laryngeal diphtheria, later metal and 'flexometallic tubes' during operations on the base of the tongue and pharynx in 1878.[45] A sponge was packed round the superior laryngeal aperture and chloroform and air administered through the tube, thus protecting the lungs from contamination.

In addition to his great technical advances. Macewen paid constant attention to teaching his students the rudiments of safe anaesthesia, a form of tuition uncommon at that time. He remained a great believer in chloroform anaesthesia. He became a Surgeon Rear-Admiral and Consultant to the Royal Navy in Scotland in 1914.

(*See also* Keys, T. E. *Anesth. Analg. Curr. Res*. 1974, **53**, 537; James C. D. T. *Anaesthesia*, 1974, **29**, 743; Bowman A. K. *The Life and Teaching of Sir William Macewan*. London & Edinburgh: Wm Hodge, 1942; and Wakeley C. (ed.) *Great Teachers of Surgery in the Past*. Bristol: Wright, 1969.)

Carl Koller (1857–1944)

Carl Koller was the first medical man to make use of and to publicize the analgesic properties of cocaine (which had been known for 25 years) to prevent the pain of a surgical operation. This he did in September 1884 in Vienna where he was a 27-year-old trainee ophthalmologist. He was born in 1857 in Schüttenhofen, then in Bohemia, a part of the Austro-Hungarian empire, the son of a Jewish business man who lacked strict religious convictions. He was educated in Vienna, thought of studying the law, served for two years as a conscript in the imperial army and finally enrolled as a medical student in the University of Vienna. While still an undergraduate he published the results of some highly regarded experimental pathological investigations into the embryology of the mesoderm of the chick. He qualified as a doctor in 1882 at the age of 25 and became a member of the department of ophthalmology in the Allegemeine Krankenhaus whose director was Professor Arlt (1812–1887).

Koller soon began to share with his professor considerable dissatisfaction with the standard of the anaesthetists and of the conditions of anaesthesia they produced; restlessness during the operation and cough and vomiting afterwards. He began to realize that this problem would only be solved if he could find some drug which, when instilled into the conjunctival sac would abolish pain. With this end in view he tried morphine and other sedative drugs, but of course without success. So the turbulent general anaesthetics continued.

In the summer of 1884, Sigmund Freud (1856–1939) a friend and contemporary who was working in a junior capacity in the neurology department of the hospital and who was later to achieve world fame as the originator of psychoanalysis, was busy investigating what was then a fairly new drug, cocaine, which had reached Europe from South America in the middle 1850s. It was an alkaloid extracted from the bush erythroxylon coca which grew in Bolivia and Peru and was well known to the local Indians as a euphoriant and stimulant. Freud's studies led him to believe that it might be a remedy for morphine addiction as well as a tonic for his psychoneurotic patients. He wrote a monograph entitled 'Ueber Coca' in August 1884. He knew that it deadened mucous membranes but was not clear as to its effects on muscular contraction, and asked Koller to do some experiments to elucidate the problem. Freud then went on holiday while Koller set to work with cocaine. He started by applying some to his own tongue[46] and was immediately struck, as others had been before him, by its strange power to deaden all sensation. In a flash he realized that this might be the agent he had been looking for to act as a local analgesic in his eye operations. He quickly set about investigating its analgesic effects in the experimental pathology laboratory on animals, then on himself on his friends and lastly on his patients. He satisfied himself that not only did it work but that it worked extremely well, and lost no time in making his discovery public. He wrote a short preliminary report[46] and asked his friend Dr Josef Brettauer to read it for him at the forthcoming meeting of the German Ophthalmological Society to be held in Heidelberg, which Koller himself was not able to attend. Brettauer's paper caused a sensation and this was reinforced when, after a lecture, he gave a clinical demonstration of the use of two per cent cocaine solution in the out-patient clinic. The date was 15 September 1884. The following month Koller read two fuller papers before the Imperial Medical Society. Freud, whose interest in surgical anaesthesia was minimal, made no claim to the discovery.

News of the event soon spread throughout Europe and the US and Koller became a notable figure. But not notable enough for him to secure a senior post in the academic department of eye surgery to which he aspired and to which he was reasonably entitled. So he moved off from Vienna and joined the eye clinic in Utrecht where he pursued his postgraduate studies under Professor Donders (1818–1889) and his son-in-law, H. Snellen (1834–1908) and where he remained for two years. Koller was, however, a restless and somewhat awkward man and decided to try his luck once more in Vienna, but he found the going hard. His prospects were not enhanced by his involvement in a duel, fought with sabres, against a fellow reserve medical officer because of a personal quarrel. So, although Koller wounded his opponent and won the day, the illegality of duelling placed him in a difficult professional position and had an adverse effect on his advancement. Once again he decided to leave Vienna, this time for New York where he arrived in 1888 and where he spent the remainder of his active life. He soon built up a thriving hospital and private practice and established a solid reputation as a first-class ophthalmic surgeon. He took no further part in the development of local analgesia, leaving that to others. As time passed he achieved something of the fame his discovery as a young man rightly earned for him and he was awarded gold medals, scrolls and commendations from various academic bodies in Europe and America. Some controversy arose about this great discovery, but Carl Koller was its true begetter. He died in 1944 aged 86.[47]

William Stewart Halsted (1852–1922)
For anaesthetists, Halsted's claim to fame is his early experiments with the new local analgesic solutions of cocaine. He originated nerve-block or regional analgesia and showed that a reduction in the circulation of a part of the body, as by an Esmarch bandage, would prolong the effects of local analgesia. He demonstrated that for skin analgesia, intradermal injection—'the distension method'—was superior to subcutaneous injection.

His ancestors came from Britain in the seventeenth century and he was born into a substantial family in New York City. He was educated at Yale College where his athletic prowess surpassed his academic abilities. Deciding to study medicine, he entered the College of Physicians and Surgeons in New York in 1874 and graduated 3 years later. While a resident at Roosevelt Hospital, New York, in

1878 he became friendly with William H. Welch (1850–1934), later to become the first professor of pathology in the US and the world-famous dean of American medicine. The next 2 years were spent in postgraduate studies in Austria and in Germany, where he visited the clinics of Theodore Billroth (1829–1924) and Anton Woefler (1850–1917) in Vienna, Ernst von Bergmann (1836–1907) in Würzburg, Carl Thiersch (1822–1895) in Leipzig, Richard von Volkmann (1830–1889) in Halle and J. F. A. von Esmarch (1823–1908) in Kiel. When he returned home he entered surgical practice in New York City. He achieved considerable success and developed into a bold extroverted and original surgeon. Halsted was one of the first to recognize the importance of the discovery of cocaine and, with some of his colleagues, commenced to experiment with the new drug on themselves, not realizing its grave addictive properties. The results of their work were soon published (Hall R. S. *New York Med. J.* 1884, **40**, 643; Halsted W. S. *New York Med. J.* 1885, **42**, 294). Halsted was the first surgeon to block the nerves of the face, the brachial plexus, the internal pudendal and posterior tibial nerves. In 1886, his uncontrolled addiction to cocaine led to his admission to a psychiatric hospital. He seems to have exchanged the craving for cocaine for the craving for morphine, possibly as a result of therapy, and remained, off and on, a morphine addict for the rest of his life.

On discharge from hospital his personality was seen to have changed and he now appeared as a slow, meticulous and rather morose man who gave great attention to the smallest detail of what occupied him. He found his way back to Welch's laboratory at the new Johns Hopkins Hospital in Baltimore in 1887 where he aspired to become surgeon-in-chief, but Sir William Macewen (1847–1924) was offered the post (although he never took it up). Eventually in 1889 Halsted was appointed the first professor of surgery in the Johns Hopkins University and chief surgeon to the hospital. During the next 30 years of his life he made his clinic world famous and became one of the founding fathers of twentieth-century surgery, becoming mentor, guide, philosopher and friend to countless young colleagues, over fifty of whom eventually occupied chairs of surgery in American hospitals. His early enthusiasm for regional analgesia waned and in later life he always preferred to operate on unconscious patients. He died following a second operation for gallstones and obstructive jaundice.[48]

Among his contributions to surgery were his radical operation for the removal of the whole breast with its lymphatic drainage for the relief of breast cancer (1890).[49] In 1890 he introduced the use of rubber gloves into surgery, an idea borrowed from his colleague W. H. Welch the pathologist (in an effort to prevent skin irritation from antiseptic solutions affecting the hands of his operating-room sister, who was later to become his wife).

(*See also* MacCallum W. G. *William Stewart Halsted.* Baltimore: The Johns Hopkins Press, 1930; Boise M. 'Halsted as an anesthetist knew him', *Surgery*, 1952, **32**, 498; Halsted Centenary Meeting. *Proc. R. Soc. Med.* 1952, **45**, 555; Olch P. D. *Anesthesiology*, 1975, **42**, 479; letter from W. S. Halsted to Sir William Osler in Fulton J. *Harvey Cushing; A Biography*, Oxford: Blackwell, 1946, p. 142; 'William Stewart Halsted and the Germanic influence on training and education programs in surgery', *Surg. Gynecol. Obstet.* 1978, **147**, 602; *Bull. N.Y. Acad. Med.* 1984, **60**, 176; Matas, Rudolf, *Am. J. Surg.* 1934, **25**, 195, and 362; Matas R. *Bull. Johns Hopkins Hosp*, 1925, **36**, 1; Matas R. *Arch. Surg.* 1925, **10**, 293 and Boulton T. B. 'Classical File' *Surv. Anesthesiol.* 1984, **28**, 150.

August Karl Gustav Bier (1861–1949)

Bier was born in Helsen in Waldeck in Germany in 1861 and graduated in 1889 at Kiel where he later became assistant to the professor of surgery, von Esmarch. While there he supervised the transition from antiseptic to aseptic techniques in the operating theatres, following the teachings of von Bergmann (1836–1907) and Curt Schimmelbusch (1860–1895) of Berlin. He became familiar with the work of a medical colleague at Kiel, Heinrich Irenaeus Quincke (1842–1922), who established lumbar puncture as a safe investigation in routine neurological examination (Quincke H. I. 'Die Lumbalpunktur des Hydrocephalis', *Berlin Klin. Wochenschr.* 1891, **25**, 809). In 1898 he gave the first deliberate spinal anaesthetic[50] and to prove his faith in the method allowed his assistant, Dr Hildebrandt, to inject into his own theca 2 ml of 1% cocaine solution. Leaving Kiel, Bier became professor of surgery successively at Griefswald, Bonn, and as successor to Ernst von Bergmann at Berlin, and in the capital he was to spend the greater part of his professional life. In addition to his discovery of spinal analgesia, he invented the method of treating chronic inflammation by the method of passive hyperaemia with Esmarch's (1823–1908) bandage (1892)[51] and pioneered intravenous procaine analgesia (1908)[52] while holding the chair of surgery at Bonn (*see* Chapter 17 for a modern description of this technique). He was one of the great figures of German surgery, as teacher, lecturer and operator (Hon. FRCS (Eng.), 1913). Introduced the 'tin helmet' into the German army in the First World War. In later life he came to hold unorthodox ideas, advocated physical education, callisthenics, etc. and deviated from the views of his colleagues. He died, aged 88, at Sauer in the German Democratic Republic in 1949.

Heinrich Friedrich Wilhelm Braun (1862–1934)

Braun has been called 'the father of local analgesia' and he coined the term 'conduction anaesthesia'. He was born in Rawitch in Poland in 1862, and although intending to become a musician, he graduated in medicine in 1887 in Dresden, and after a period as assistant to Karl Thiersch (1822–1895) in Leipzig and Richard von Volkmann (1830–1889) in Halle, whose niece he married in 1888, became director of the Deaconess Hospital in Leipzig where his interest in local analgesia was developed, having been stimulated by Max Oberst (1849–1925) of Halle. In 1902 he introduced the use of adrenaline in local analgesic solutions of cocaine,[53] and in 1905 became the pioneer of the new drug procaine.[54] In this year also appeared the first edition of his classic textbook, *Local Anaesthesia*; the eighth edition was published in 1933. He preferred conduction (nerve) block to Schleich's infiltration. Braun was appointed to direct the new hospital at Zwickau in 1906, and here he passed the remainder of his professional life. He introduced dental local analgesia into Germany. He described the anterior approach to the coeliac plexus (anterior splanchnic block) and was the inventor of the Braun splint. He was also interested in general anaesthetics but realized their danger and devised an apparatus for the safe administration of chloroform and ether vapour.[87] Was president of the German Surgical Society in 1924 and retired in 1928 (*see also* Röse W. *Anesteziol. Reanimatol.* 1982, **1**, 3). He died in 1934, aged 72.

Arthur Läwen (1876–1958)

Läwen was born in 1876 in Waldheim in Saxony, and qualified at Leipzig in

1900. He became in Leipzig a pupil of Heinrich Braun and later of Friedrich Trendelenburg (1844–1924) and Erwin Payr (1871–1976) of Griefswald. He held senior posts at Leipzig and Marburg and was appointed professor of surgery at Königsberg in East Prussia where his chief work was done. In 1912 he employed curare to reduce the amount of ether needed for relaxation, in an attempt to reduce the incidence of postoperative pulmonary complications which were then thought to be due to ether vapour.[55] This work was interrupted by the First World War. Läwen was the first to describe paravertebral conduction anaesthesia, and in 1910 he was the first to show that extradural analgesia was a safe and practical form of pain relief in pelvic and abdominal surgery. For this he used large volumes of 1·5 or 2% procaine solution with sodium bicarbonate, injected through the sacral hiatus.[56] He did a great deal to popularize local analgesia, tracheal intubation and artificial respiration. After 1945 he became a refugee from East Germany, having lost his sons, his possessions and his university chair during the war. He died in 1958, aged 82.

Gaston Labat (1877–1934)

Born in the Seychelles and graduated at Montpellier. Took up the study of medicine at the age of 37 in 1914 after running a successful pharmacy in Mauritius. Became anaesthetist to Victor Pauchet (1869–1936), surgeon to the St Michael Hospital in Paris, and was co-author with Pauchet of the later editions of the latter's book *L'Anaesthésie Régionale* (Paris: Doin, 1921; *see also* Macintosh R. R. *Region. Anesth.* 1978, **1**, 2 and Lee, J. Alfred, *Region. Anesth.* 1985, **10**, 99). Was invited to the Mayo Clinic in 1920 and became special lecturer on regional anaesthesia there. Wrote his classic book *Regional Anesthesia; Its Technique and Clinical Application* in 1922. Subsequently became clinical professor of surgery (anesthesia) at New York University and worked at the Bellevue Hospital. Founded American Society of Regional Anesthesia in 1923. Died in October 1934 in New York. A third (posthumous) edition of his book was published in 1967, edited by J. Adriani, and a fourth in 1985.

His book, outstanding in its time, had a great influence on the development and acceptance of regional analgesia. In 1922 its main readers were surgeons. Only in later years was regional analgesia practised by anaesthetists.

Arthur E. Guedel (1883–1956)

Born in Cambridge City, Indiana, and received his medical education at the Indiana School of Medicine, Indianapolis, qualifying in 1908. Lost three fingers of his right hand, aged 13, but nevertheless became a skilled pianist. Started as a general practitioner/anaesthetist. Lecturer on anaesthesia in the University of Indianapolis (1920–1928), during which time he was a practising anaesthetist in that city. Gave anaesthetics in France during the First World War (1917–1919) and made notes on which his book is based. Later moved to Los Angeles, where he became associate clinical professor of anesthesiology at the University of Southern California School of Medicine. A leading pioneer of American anaesthesia, and like most of his contemporaries in the specialty he was self-taught.

He made many contributions to his chosen specialty, including an early description of the self-administration of nitrous oxide and air for obstetrics and minor surgery (*Indianap. Med. J.* October 1911);[57] a description of the anaesthetic properties of divinyl ether; reintroduction, with R. M. Waters, of a cuffed tracheal tube,[58] a systemization of the signs of inhalation anaesthesia (*Curr. Res. Anesth.* May 1920; *Inhalation Anesthesia, A Fundamental Guide.* New York: Macmillan, 1937); a pharyngeal airway;[59] the introduction of controlled respiration using ether, with Treweek (*Curr. Res. Anesth. Analg.* December 1934); and a classic description of the clinical use of cyclopropane (*Anesthesiology*, 1940, **1**, 1). He received the Hickman Medal from the Royal Society of Medicine in 1941, the first worker outside the UK to do so, and the Distinguished Service Award of the American Society of Anesthesiologists in 1951. There is a Guedel Memorial Anesthesia Centre in San Francisco, together with an eponymous lecture established in his honour by the University of California Medical Center in Los Angeles.

(*See also* Waters R. M. 'Eminent Anaesthetists: A. E. Guedel', *Br. J. Anaesth.* 1952, **24**, 292; Neff, W. B. In: Volpitto P. P. and Vandam L. D. (ed.) *The Genesis of Contemporary American Anesthesiology*, Springfield Ill.: Thomas; and Calverley R. K. In: *Anaesthesia; Essays on its History*. (Rupreht J. et al. ed.) Berlin: Springer-Verlag, 1985, p. 18.)

Henry Edmund Gaskin Boyle (1875–1941)

Born in Barbados and qualified at St Bartholomew's Hospital, London, in 1901, where as a student he was president of the Abernethian Society. Became casualty officer in Bristol and then returned to St Bartholomew's as junior resident anaesthetist, rising in due course to become head of the department. About 1912, became interested in nitrous oxide and oxygen anaesthesia and in 1917 got Coxeter, the instrument maker, to copy James Tayloe Gwathmey's (1855–1943) gas–oxygen machine which became the first 'Boyle' apparatus (Boyle H. E. G. *Br. Med. J.* 1917, **2**, 653). He introduced gas–oxygen into France for use in anaesthetizing wounded soldiers in the First World War and for this received the decoration of OBE. After the war he visited the US and brought back with him Davis's gag[60] which he introduced to British throat surgeons. He was an early user of Magill's endotracheal techniques and was elected FRCS and DA in 1935; was one of the original pair of examiners for the latter diploma. A founder member of the Association of Anaesthetists of Great Britain and Ireland in 1932.

In 1907 wrote the first edition of his textbook *Practical Anaesthetics*, the third edition of which was prepared by his junior colleague C. Langton Hewer. Boyle was a 'character' and was universally known as 'Cockie'.

His anaesthetic machine, modified in every particular, is used in most British hospitals today.[61]

(*See also* Hadfield C. F.[61] 'Eminent Anaesthetists: H. E. G. Boyle', *Br. J. Anaesth.* 1950, **22**, 107).

Ralph Milton Waters (1883–1979)

Born in North Bloomfield, Ohio, of Anglo-Scottish descent. Became a student at Western Reserve University in Cleveland in 1903 and after taking an arts degree became MD in 1912. Settled in general practice in Sioux City in Iowa, married and remained there for 5 years. Gradually became interested in anaesthesia and the basic sciences so that by 1916 anaesthesia came to occupy much of his time and he decided to specialize; an unusual step to take at the time. He opened a private clinic as a commercial venture with an operating room and facilities for minor surgery, where he gave the anaesthetics, one of the first 'day-stay' clinics in the US. In 1923, he acquired an anaesthetic practice in Kansas City where he remained for 3 years. He hurt his back, lifting an overweight patient, and as a result had to spend 6 months in a brace. On recovery he visited John S. Lundy (1884–1973), chief anaesthetist at the Mayo Clinic, and on his way home stopped off with friends at Madison. Here he met Chauncey Leake (1896–1978) the pharmacologist, and Erwin Schmidt, professor of surgery, and as a result he was invited in 1927 to take charge of anaesthesia at the new Hospital of the State of Wisconsin at Madison which opened in 1924. He became in turn assistant professor, associate professor and in 1933 full professor of anaesthesia with clinical charge of anaesthesia in the university hospitals. This was the first such post in the US. He had a long and distinguished career and his clinic became one of the leading centres of anaesthesia in the world. He visited Europe and the UK in 1936 and was awarded the Hickman Medal by the Royal Society of Medicine in London in 1938. He retired in 1949 and was succeeded by Alexander MacKay and then by Sidney Orth in 1952. His pupils included Drs Rovenstine, Gillespie, Hingson, Lucien Morris, Gordh, Apgar, Neff and many others (*see also* Morris L. E. In: (Rupreht J. ed.) *Anaesthesia; Essays on its History*. Berlin: Springer-Verlag, 1985, p. 32 and Gordh T. *ibid*. p. 36).

His contributions to the growing specialty were numerous and important and he wrote more than a hundred papers. Among the more noteworthy are the following: insistence on proper training programmes for young anaesthetists; encouragement on careful note keeping during anaesthesia by means of 'punch-cards'; the introduction of cyclopropane into anaesthetic practice;[62] the development of the to-and-fro carbon dioxide absorption system;[63] a re-evaluation of chloroform;[64] pioneering use of thiopentone in 1934;[65] endobronchial intubation.[66]

He exercised a great influence on anaesthesia in the US and in the UK during 1930–1950 and trained many anaesthetists who later occupied important posts in universities in the US and in Europe. He was one of the most important founding fathers of anaesthesia as we know it today. He received numerous medals, citations and honours from academic bodies throughout the world and lived to enjoy 30 years of retirement, latterly growing citrus fruit in Florida, where he died in Orlando on 19 December 1979.

Sir Ivan Magill (1888–1986)

Ivan Whiteside Magill was born in Larne, Northern Ireland, then with what is now the Republic, an integral part of the UK. His birth in 1888 took place 42 years after Morton's first use of ether and just two years after the discovery of local analgesia, using cocaine. He attended the local grammar school and then became a medical student at Queen's University, Belfast, qualifying in 1913. He became a house surgeon at the Stanley Hospital in Liverpool and with the outbreak of the 1914–1918 War, joined the RAMC and served with the Irish Guards at the battle of Loos. When peace came again, Magill was posted to the Queen's Hospital in Sidcup, Kent. With a young colleague, Stanley Rowbotham (1890–1979), neither of whom was at that time an experienced anaesthetist, they soon found themselves responsible for giving anaesthetics for reconstructive operations on the face and jaws in wounded soldiers, under the care of Harold Gillies, later to become a world famous pioneer of plastic surgery. Here after trial and error, they became among the first workers to develop tracheal intubation, first using two narrow gum-elastic tubes, one afferent and the other efferent, for the insufflation of ether vapour under slight positive pressure, and then employing a single wider bore rubber tube for spontaneous breathing. They were also among the first to develop the technique of nasotracheal intubation by the so-called blind method. These Magill tubes eventually became indispensable to all anaesthetists. While their methods earned for them the support and approval of the surgeons with whom they worked, many other surgeons discouraged the use of intubation partly because of the possibility of tissue damage and partly due to conservatism. It took many years before intubation was accepted into the general employment of anaesthetists. Those who learnt how to perform blind intubation soon realized its great advantages, especially the fact that it would enable a patient to be taken to the level of anaesthesia necessary for a laparotomy very quickly with ether, then the commonly used agent, thus reducing the time for induction. In addition, intubation provided a clear airway, prevented laryngeal spasm and enabled the lungs to be protected against foreign material.

When the work at the unit in Sidcup decreased, Magill decided to devote his professional life to the administration of anaesthetics and was soon elected to the staffs of various hospitals in London. Eventually he chose the Westminster Hospital and the Brompton Hospital for Diseases of the Chest as his main bases, while, in addition, his skill and his personality enabled him to acquire a large private practice in London and beyond. He was a man of great practical ingenuity and over the years originated or developed many new pieces of equipment and refinements of technique for the safety of his patients and the convenience of his surgeons. Among these must be mentioned a laryngoscope and laryngeal forceps, and the 'Magill attachment' a simple combination of a breathing tube, reservoir bag and expiratory valve, used for spontaneous respiration, which featured on all anaesthetic machines in the UK for over 50 years. He developed methods of administering anaesthetics in thoracic surgery employing endobronchial tubes and bronchus blockers for the control of pulmonary secretions, and these techniques for the production of one-lung anaesthesia greatly contributed to the development of thoracic surgery in the 1920s and 1930s.

He took a leading part in organizing the Association of Anaesthetists of Great Britain and Ireland in 1932; in instituting an examination for the Diploma in Anaesthetics, the first such examination in 1935; and in persuading the Royal College of Surgeons of England to found a Faculty of Anaesthetists in 1947. His great experience and his reputation as a safe and skilled clinical anaesthetist resulted in his being asked to employ his abilities on a large number of very distinguished patients, including many members of the British and other royal families when they required surgical treatment. He received a very large number of honours and medals including a knighthood (the KCVO) awarded personally by the Queen in 1960, the FRCS (Eng), the honorary FFA RCS, the DSc of his old University, the Henry Hill Hickman Medal from the Royal Society of Medicine, and many others. For 50 years he was the doyen of British anaesthetists and his name was known world-wide. Tracheal intubation is the *sine qua non* of safe anaesthesia in many operations and it was largely due to Ivan Magill and his colleague Stanley Rowbotham, 60 years ago, who popularized it.

In the 1920s when Ivan Magill's career began, anaesthesia was a little regarded specialty and those who practised it exclusively attracted little esteem from their colleagues. He lived to see it achieve parity with other specialties, a change in which he took a leading part because of his firm character and common sense, his pre-eminence in clinical anaesthesia and his international reputation. (*See also* Bowes J. B. and Zorab J. S. M. in: *Anaesthesia; Essays on its History*. (Rupreht J. et al. ed.) Berlin: Springer-Verlag, 1985, p. 13.)

Helmut Weese (1897–1954)

Helmut Weese deserves an honoured place in the history of anaesthesia as the first man to make intravenous induction a safe and practical procedure. He was born in Munich into a family originating from the German part of Poland, and the son of a lecturer in the history of art. When he was nine, the family moved to Berne where his father became a privatdozent at the University. Switzerland had a great influence on his development. He decided to study medicine and attended the Universities of Berne, Zurich and Munich where he qualified. His first post was in internal medicine under von Romberg, and then he changed to pharmacology in 1925 and worked with W. Straub. He did well in the new discipline and in his own turn became privatdozent. He paid particular attention to the study of digitalis, wrote a book on it and as a result, became well known both inside and outside Germany to physicians as well as to pharmacologists. When in 1928, F. Eicholtz who had previously described the effects of bromethol (Avertin) moved to Konigsberg and then to Heidelberg, Weese followed him as director of pharmacology at the Farbwerk Bayer at Wuppertal-Elberfeld, and as lecturer at the University of Cologne. He was appointed professor there in 1936. Following the debacle of 1945 he took charge, in addition, of the department of pharmacology at Dusseldorf. He was no purely academic scientist and always strove to direct his energies to the relief of his fellow men. In 1931, Kropp and Taub synthesized a new barbiturate, hexobarbitone, later to become known as Evipan. He saw that this might be the long-awaited short-acting and safe agent for induction of anaesthesia, and at once set about investigating it both in the laboratory and personally in the operating theatre. He was soon able to show that it fulfilled his expectations and in 1932 he published his results, thus becoming the undisputed creator of practical clinical modern intravenous anaesthesia. He won recognition at the International Congress of Anesthesia at New York in 1938, during which he was elected as an honorary member.

During the Second World War, Weese, who was consultant pharmacologist to the armed forces, investigated the possibility of producing a synthetic plasma volume expander, and as a result, polyvinyl pyrrolidone (Periston, polyvidone) became available and saved many lives. He also devoted time to investigating the application of phenothiazines to clinical anaesthesia, following the stimulus of the Frenchmen, Laborit and Huguenard. With Hans Killian he wrote a book on anaesthesia, *Die Narkose*. Weese practised both anaesthesia and pharmacology and was honoured by members of both specialties. He used his considerable influence to advance the status of anaesthesia in postwar Germany.

He died following a fall from a chair in his laboratory, an unusual event in a man well used to climbing in the high Alps (*see also* Obituary: Killian, Hans. *Der Anaesthesist*, 1954, Band 3; Heft 2. 97. Translation, Dr Heinrich Niehoff).

John Silas Lundy (1894–1973)

Dr Lundy of the Mayo Clinic, Rochester, Minn., had a great influence on our specialty, particularly as the pioneer of the use of thiopentone (Pentothal sodium). He was born in Seattle, Washington, the son of a doctor. He took an arts degree in 1917 and qualified in medicine from the Rush Medical College in

Chicago two years later. After serving as a resident in Chicago hospitals he returned to his birthplace and entered general practice. In April 1924 he was invited to become head of the Department of Anesthesiology at the Mayo Clinic and this he directed for the next 28 years although his connection with the Clinic did not end until 1959. He became professor in the Mayo Graduate School of Medicine in 1934 and was one of the founders of the American Board of Anesthesiology. He was a prolific writer, and this together with the worldwide reputation of the Mayo Clinic where he worked, soon carried his name throughout the US and Europe. He established the first laboratory of gross anatomy to be used at the Clinic and this was important for his teaching of the techniques of regional analgesia which had been stimulated there by Gaston Labat. In 1925 he developed the theory and practice of 'balanced anesthesia'[67] and although Waters of Madison used thiopentone before he did, Lundy used it on 18 June 1934 and continued throughout his professional life to advocate its use. It is largely due to his efforts that intravenous induction spread so widely. In 1942 he opened the first post-anaesthesia observation room in the world at St Mary's Hospital, Rochester. In 1935 he established the first blood bank in the US at Rochester. Dr Lundy was the author of the textbook *Clinical Anesthesia* published in 1942, one of the first authoritative volumes dealing with the so-called 'modern anaesthesia'. He received many medals, awards and honours from academic bodies throughout the world. He retired first to Chicago and later to Seattle where he continued to practise anaesthesia (*see also* Corssen G. In: (Rupreht J. et al. ed.) *Anaesthesia; Essays on its History*. Berlin: Springer-Verlag, 1985, p. 42).

Harold Randall Griffith (1896–1985)
On 23 January 1942 Harold Griffith, assisted by his resident Enid Johnson, injected Intocostrin intravenously, a preparation containing curare, to aid muscle relaxation in a 150-lb male patient undergoing interval appendicectomy under cyclopropane anaesthesia at the Homeopathic Hospital (later the Queen Elizabeth Hospital) in Montreal. This was an outstanding event of supreme importance in the development of modern anaesthesia.[68]

Harold Griffith was born near Montreal on 25 July 1894, obtained the BA (Magill) in 1914 and the MD CM in 1922. In this year he also married. The following year he obtained the MD in homeopathic medicine from the Hahnemann Medical College in Philadelphia. Before graduating in medicine he served with distinction as a stretcher-bearer in the Canadian Army and was awarded the Military Medal for bravery in the 1914–1918 war. An interest in anaesthesia developed early in his career and after a time he became chief anaesthetist at the Montreal Homeopathic Hospital where his father had been medical director and his brother, surgeon-in-chief, and here he spent his active professional life until his retirement in 1966. Before the days of relaxants he developed an expertise in tracheal intubation and, along with Dr Ralph Waters of Madison, became a world expert on the use of the then new agent cyclopropane. As anaesthesia advanced he became involved in its academic side and was appointed professor of anaesthesia and chairman of the department at Magill University. He held high office in the International Anesthesia Research Society and was a founder member of the World Ferderation of Societies of Anesthesiology and president of its first Congress held in Holland in 1955 and at its second congress held in Toronto in 1959 he was elected permanent Founder-President.

Dr Griffith was a much loved man of modest disposition who was known to his younger colleagues as 'Uncle Harold'. In later life he received many honours and distinctions including the Hickman Medal from the Royal Society of Medicine in London in 1956, and he was the only non-US citizen to receive the Distinguished Service Award from the American Society of Anesthesiology.

The sample of Intocostrin was handed to him in 1942 by Dr Lewis Wright of the pharmaceutical firm of E. R. Squibb. They were aware of the muscle relaxing 'shock-absorbing' effects of curare when used to control the muscular spasms associated with ECT,[69] while his familiarity with the treatment of respiratory depression by controlled breathing following his very frequent use of cyclopropane, enabled him to deal with the same complication which might be associated with curare, and presented to him no problems.

Harold Griffith died aged 90 of Parkinson's disease on 7 May 1985.[70]

(*See also* Seldon T. H.)[88]

Christopher Langton Hewer (1896–1986)

He worked at St Bartholomew's Hospital, London from 1918 until 1961, first as student and junior colleague of Boyle (with whom he wrote the 3rd edition of *Practical Anaesthetics* in 1923), latterly as senior anaesthetist. He was largely responsible for the introduction of trichloroethylene into clinical anaesthesia in 1941. He is remembered for the influence he exerted on the development of anaesthesia during the greatest period of its growth, by his writings. He was author and later editor of *Recent Advances in Anaesthesia and Analgesia* from 1932 until 1982, and was editor of the journal *Anaesthesia* for the first 20 years of its publication from 1946 until 1966. He was the recipient of many honours in the UK.

(*See* Boulton T. B. *Anaesthesia* 1986, **41**, 469.)

(*See also* Orth S. In: Volpitto, P. P. and Vandam L. D. (ed.) *The Genesis of Contemporary American Anesthesiology*. Springfield, Ill: Thomas, 1982; Morris Lucien In: Rupreht J. et al. (ed.) *Anaesthesia; Essays on its History*. Berlin: Springer-Verlag, 1985, p. 32; Gordh T. *ibid*, p. 36; Steinhaus J. E. *ibid*, p. 198.)

The Corporate Organization of Anaesthesia in Britain[71]

The Society of Anaesthetists was founded in 1893 by J. F. W. M. Silk (1878–1943) of King's College Hospital, and forty anaesthetists joined it. First president, Woodhouse Braine with Silk as Honorary Secretary and Dudley W. Buxton (1855–1931) of University College Hospital, as Treasurer. Published first volume of Transactions in 1898. In 1908 was incorporated into the Anaesthetic Section of the new Royal Society of Medicine. The first society of anaesthetists in the world which had as its object the discussion of problems of anaesthesia and the advancement of the science and art of the subject. The Scottish Society of Anaesthetists dates from 1914.

The Association of Anaesthetists of Great Britain and Ireland was founded in 1932 to perform functions which could not be performed by the Anaesthetic Section of the Royal Society of Medicine. These were (and are): 'To promote the development and study of anaesthetics and their administration and the recognition of the administration of anaesthetics as a specialized branch of medicine. To co-ordinate the efforts and activities of anaesthetists. To represent anaesthetists and to promote their interests. To promote the establishment of diplomas and degrees in anaesthesia. To encourage and promote co-operation and friendship between anaesthetists. And to do all such lawful things as may be incidental or conducive to the attainment of such objects'. The first president was Henry Featherstone (1894–1967) of Birmingham with W. Howard Jones of Charing Cross Hospital as Secretary and Z. Mennell (1876–1959) of St Thomas' Hospital, London (*see also* Hunter A. R. *Anaesthesia*, 1983, **38**, 1214) as Treasurer. At this time there were only fifty specialist anaesthetists in the whole of the UK. (For a description of the 'Arms' of the Association, *see* Boulton T. B. 'Arms and the Anaesthetist', *Anaesthesia*, 1974, **29**, 627).

The Faculty of Anaesthetists of the Royal College of Surgeons of England was created in 1948 at the request of the Association of Anaesthetists. The Fellowship (FFA RCS) was proposed in 1946 and the first examinations held in 1953. A. D. Marston (1891–1962) of Guy's Hospital was the first dean.

For the present position of the organization of anaesthesia in Britain *see* Fitch W. (ed.) *Handbook of British Anaesthesia 1980/81*, published by *British Journal of Anaesthesia*.

The National Health Service came into operation in Britain in 1948.

The Faculty of Anaesthetists of the Royal College of Surgeons in Ireland was founded in 1959, the first examination for its fellowship taking place in 1961. Early history of the Association of Anaesthetists of Great Britain and Ireland *see* Editorial, Helliwell P. J. *Anaesthesia*, 1982, **37**, 394 and 913, and the first anaesthetic society of the UK *see* Dinnick O. P. *Progress in Anaesthesiology*, Amsterdam: Excerpta Medica, 1970, p. 181; Ellis R. H. The introduction of ether anaesthesia to Great Britain *Anaesthesia*, 1977, **31**, **766** and **32**, 197.

For a history of anaesthesia in the Scandinavian countries, *see Acta Anaesth. Scand*. 1975, **13**, 317 and Introduction of anaesthesia to Denmark. Secher, Ole. *Progress in Anaesthesiology*. Proc. 4th World Congr. Anaesth. Amsterdam: Excerpta Medica, 1970.

For the history of World Federation of Societies of Anesthesiologists, *see* Griffith H. R. *Anesth. Analg. Curr. Res*. 1963, **42**, 389; *Indian J. Anaesth*, 1970, **18**, 145; Zorab J. *Anaesthesia*, 1976, **31**, 285; Boulton T. B. *Anaesthesia* 1976, **31**, 1103.

Development of anaesthesia in the US, *see* Waters R. M. *J. Hist. Med. Allied Sci*. 1946, **1**, 595; and Eckenhoff J. E. *Anesthesiology* 1978, **49**, 272.

Introduction of anaesthesia into France (by Jobert de Lamballe and J. F. Malgaigne at the Hôpital St Louis, Paris), *see* Neveu R. *J. Hist. Med. Allied Sci*. 1946, **1**, 607.

Introduction of anaesthesia into Germany (by Heyfelder of Erlangen), *see* Frankel W. K. *J. Hist. Med. Allied Sci*. 1946, **1**, 612; Whitacre R. J. and Dumitra J. H. M. *J. Hist. Med. Allied Sci*. 1946, **1**, 618.

First anaesthetic in New Zealand (for dental extraction) given by Mr Marriott with Dr J. P. Fitzgerald as surgeon, *see* Newson A. J. *Anaesth. Intensive Care*, 1975, **3**, 204; first anaesthetic (ether) given in Ireland, at the Richmond Hospital, by John MacDonnell in Dublin and first anaesthetic in Australia given by Dr Wm Russ Pugh of Tasmania on 7 June 1847 (Wilson G. C. M. *Anaesth. Intensive Care*, 1985, **13**, 71). For historical details of the Australian Society of Anaesthetists, *see* Maxwell D. C. *Anaesth. Intensive Care* 1985, **13**, 89.

Walser H. H. The introduction of ether anaesthesia into the German-speaking areas in the year 1847. *Schweizerischen Gessellschaft fur Geschichte der Medicin and Naturwissenschaften*, 1957, Band 21, 1–55; Kok O. V. S. History of anaesthesia in the republic of S. Africa. *Progress in Anaesthesiol*. Proc. 4th World

Congress Anaes. Amsterdam: Excerpta Medica, 1970, 167; Matsuki A. A chronology of the very early history of inhalation anaesthesia in Canada. *Can. Anaesth. Soc. J*, 1974, **21**, 92, Anaesthesia in Argentine. Cooper I. *Br. Med. Bull*. 1946, **4**, 147.

Review of history of anaesthesia in Australia, *see* Wilson G. E. M. *Anaesth. Intensive Care*, 1972. **1**, 9; *Anaesthesia; Essays on its History*. Rupreht J. et al. (ed.) Berlin: Springer-Verlag, 1985. Other countries with page numbers— Czechoslovakia; Dworacek B. and Keszler H. 41; Italy; Pantaleoni M. 113; Ecuador, Pinto O. M. 115; Japan, Yamamura H. 165; China, Shieh Yung, 136; Yugoslavia, Darinka Sobin, 139; Nigeria, Sodipo J. O. A. 141; Ukraine (USSR) Treshchinsky A. I. 153; Holland, Vermeulen-Cranch D. 156; Thailand, Tupavong S. 154; Lebanon, Haddad F. S. 60; Spain, Franco A., Ginesta M. V. et al. 48; Hungary, Forgacs I. and Varga P. 45; USSR Damir E. 28.

For a list of some of the earliest books dealing with anaesthesia, *see* Secher O. *Anaesthesia* 1985, **40**, 385.

Interesting and Important Dates in the History of Medicine and Anaesthesia

1516 Curare, South American arrow poison, described by Peter Martyr Angherius.

1518 Foundation of the College of Physicians in London.

1540 Valerius Cordus (1515–1544) synthesized sweet oil of vitriol (ether), possibly aided by Theophratus Bombast von Hohenheim, named Paracelsus (1493–1541).
United Company of Barber Surgeons given Royal Charter by Henry VIII.

1543 Andreas Vesalius (1514–1564) of Basel, Louvain and Padua published his revolutionary book on anatomy *De Humani Corporis Fabrica*. Professor of surgery and anatomy at Padua, where he replaced moribund mediaeval scholarship by detached scientific observation.
Publication of *The Revolutions of the Heavenly Spheres* by Copernicus.

1628 Wm Harvey (1578–1657) of London, (pupil of Galileo (1564–1642) of Padua and contemporary of Francis Bacon (1561–1626), English philosopher, and of Descartes (1596–1660), French philosopher), described the circulation of the blood: *De Motu Cordis*. Frankfurt: Fitzeri.

1662 Robert Boyle (1627–1691) enunciated his law of the relationship of the volume and pressure of a gas.

1665 First intravenous injection of a drug (tincture of opium) into an animal (a dog) by Sir Christopher Wren (1633–1723) and Robert Boyle (1627–1691) using a bladder attached to a sharpened quill.
Richard Lower (1631–1691) transfused blood from one animal to another.

1707 Sir John Floyer (1649–1734) of Lichfield, the first physician to time the pulse during his clinical examination of patients.

1730 August Siegmund Frobenius, a German chemist, living in London, named 'sweet oil of vitriol' ether.

1733 Stephen Hales (1677–1761) inserted tubes into the arteries and veins of animals; the first experiments in direct measurement of blood pressure. (Clark-Kennedy, A. E., *Br. Med. J.* 1977, **2**, 1656).

1742 Anders Celsius (1701–1744) of Sweden described his system of thermometry, which has displaced the 'centigrade' scale.

1751 'Anaesthesia' defined in Bailey's *English Dictionary* as 'a defect of sensation' (Gillies J. quoted by Beecher H. K. *Anesthesiology*, 1968, **29**, 1068).

1754 Carbon dioxide ('fixed air') discovered by J. B. von Helmont (1577–1644), Belgian physician, and isolated by Joseph Black (1728–1799).

1761 Joseph Leopold Auenbrugger (1722–1809) in Vienna described percussion of the chest.

1768 Wm Heberden (1710–1801), of London, described angina of effort (*Med. Trans. Coll. Phys. Lond.* 1768, **2**, 59).

1771 Discovery of oxygen by Joseph Priestley (1733–1804) and Carl Wilhelm Scheele (1742–1786) of Uppsala, independently.

1772 Priestley discovered nitrous oxide.

1777 Antoine Lavoisier (1743–1794) of Paris, scientist and tax collector, named the 'new air' of Priestley 'oxygen' and demolished the 'phlogiston' theory which supposed that only substances containing 'phlogiston' would burn and in so doing would lose their 'phlogiston'.

1788 J. A. C. Charles (1746–1823) of France formulated his law of the pressure/temperature relationship of a gas.
Chas. Kite of Gravesend first used tracheal tubes in resuscitation of the drowned.

1794 Thomas Beddoes (1760–1808) founded the Pneumatic Institute in Bristol for the treatment of pulmonary tuberculosis and experimented with the therapeutic inhalation of gases and vapours. Humphry Davy (1773–1829) appointed superintendent in 1798.

1800 Discovery of analgesic properties of nitrous oxide by Davy who named it 'laughing gas'.
Royal College of Surgeons of England given Royal Charter by George III (1738–1820).

1806 Isolation of morphine from opium by Friedrich Wilhelm Adam Sertürner (1783–1841), a Paderborn pharmacist.

1807 Baron Larrey (1766–1842) performed painless amputations, using ice, on the battlefield of Preuss Eylan.
Seishu Hanaoka (1760–1835) of Hirayama, Japan used a mixture of alkaloids, mainly scopolamine and atropine ('tsusensan') in Oct. 1807 for the first time, to give pain relief to a 60-year-old woman for the removal of a breast cancer (*Anesthesiology* 1970, **33**, 476).

1811 Charles Bell (1774–1842) of Edinburgh published his *Idea of a New Anatomy of the Brain* in which he differentiated motor nerves and sensory nerves.

1816 René Laënnec (1781–1826) of Paris invented stethoscope (*stethos* = the chest; *skopeein* = to explore).[72] The binaural stethoscope introduced by Camman in 1855.

1818 Michael Faraday (1779–1867) is said to have discovered narcotic action of ether vapour.

1822 François Magendie (1783–1855) of Paris proved in humans that while anterior spinal roots are motor, posterior roots are sensory: 'insensible' and 'sensible' nerves.

1824 Henry Hill Hickman (1800–1830) of Ludlow, England carried out operations on animals under carbon dioxide, with freedom from pain, thus establishing the principle of inhalation anaesthesia.

1831 Chloroform discovered independently by von Liebig (1830–1873) in Darmstadt, Germany, Guthrie (1782–1848) in New York and Soubeiran (1793–1858) in France.

Atropine prepared from *Atropa belladonna*, by Mein a German pharmacist (*Ann. Pharmacie*, 1833, **6**, 67) and by P. L. Geiger (1785–1836) professor of pharmacy of Heidelberg and Hesse.

1832 Thomas Aitchison Latta used intravenous saline in the treatment of circulatory collapse in cholera (not in surgical shock).

1833 Marshall Hall (1790–1857), English physician, introduced the concept of reflex action. Thomas Graham (1805–1869), a Scottish chemist, published *On the Law of the Diffusion of Gases*.

1834 Jean-Baptiste Dumas (1800–1884) in Paris described chemical composition of, and gave name to, chloroform.

1842 Ether given by W. E. Clarke (1818–1878) of Rochester, New York, for dental extraction, and by Crawford W. Long (1815–1878) on 30 March in Jefferson, Georgia (the patient, John Venable), in the US (*see* Young H. (1870–1945), *A Surgeon's Autobiography*. New York: Harcourt Brace, 1940, p. 69).
Marie Jean Pierre Flourens (1794–1867), Paris physiologist, first isolated respiratory centre in medulla.

1843 Royal Charter given by Queen Victoria (1819–1901) to Royal College of Surgeons of England. Establishment of FRCS (England) diploma.

1844 Horace Wells (1815–1848), dentist, of Hartford Connecticut, introduced nitrous oxide inhalation to produce anaesthesia during dental extraction.
Francis Rynd (1801–1861), surgeon, of Dublin invented hypodermic trocar.

1846 Wm T. G. Morton (1819–1868), Boston dentist, successfully demonstrated the anaesthetic properties of ether, 16 October.* The word 'anaesthesia' was suggested by Oliver Wendell-Holmes (1809–1894), Boston academic and writer, for Morton's 'etherization'.
Tooth extracted and ether given by a dentist, Mr Robinson in London, 19 December. Dr Francis Boott (1792–1863) in attendance at 52 Gower Street (now Bonham Carter House, London).[15]
(Letters of Boott to *Lancet* reprinted in 'Classical File', *Surv. Anesthesiol.*, 1957, **1**, 65).
First surgical operation performed in England under ether anaesthesia by Robert Liston (1794–1847), 21 December, when Frederick Churchill underwent amputation through the thigh and William Squire gave the anaesthetic at University College Hospital (North London Hospital).

1847 Marie Jean Pierre Flourens (1794–1867), French physiologist, described anaesthetic properties of chloroform and ethyl chloride vapour in animals.
James Y. Simpson (1811–1870) on 8 November introduced chloroform into clinical work, to ease pains of labour in Edinburgh.
John Snow (1813–1858), London practitioner, published his book, *On the Inhalation of Ether in Surgical Operations*, the first scientific description of its clinical uses, physical and pharmacological properties.
Deaths from ether reported from Grantham and Colchester.[73]

1848 Hannah Greener, aged 15, died from chloroform administered by Dr Meggison, 28 January—the first recorded case—at Winlayton, Co. Durham, 11 weeks after its introduction into medicine (*see* Snow, *On*

*The operation was on Gilbert Abbott (1825–1855) a not very robust printer/editor, for a congenital vascular malformation of the floor of the mouth and tongue, the surgeon being Dr J. C. Warren. The patient remained 7 weeks in hospital (Eavey R. D. *N. Engl. J. Med.* 1983, **309**, 990).

Chloroform and Other Anaesthetics, reprinted in *Br. J. Anaesth.* 1955, **27**, 501; 'Classical File', *Surv. Anesthesiol.* 1973, **17**, 381; report of coroner's inquest reprinted in *Surv. Anesthesiol.* 1959, **3**, 137 and Annotation, *Lancet*, 1848, **1**, 161 (reprinted in 'Classical File', *Surv. Anesthesiol.* 1959, **3**, Feb.)

Johan Heyfelder (1798–1869) of Erlangen first used ethyl chloride in humans and first to use ether in Germany (in 1847).

1849 First anaesthetic death in a London teaching hospital—chloroform—10 October—St Thomas's Hospital.[74]

1850 Wm Gairdner (1824–1907) of Glasgow differentiated between postoperative pneumonia and pulmonary collapse, the latter due to bronchial obstruction.

1853 John Snow, London physician and anaesthetist, gave chloroform analgesia on 7 April to Queen Victoria (1819–1901) at birth of Prince Leopold (1853–1881), later Duke of Albany, hence 'chloroform *à la reine*'. Sir Charles Locock (1799–1875) was the accoucheur.

Invention of hypodermic syringe and needle by Alexander Wood (1817–1874) of Edinburgh.

1855 Friedrich Gaedicke of Germany isolated cocaine from coca plant.

Indirect laryngoscopy described by Manuel Garcia (1805–1906), a Spanish singing teacher working in London.

Foundation of the British Medical Association which developed from Sir Charles Hastings' Worcester Medical and Surgical Society.

1857 Claude Bernard (1813–1878), physiologist of Paris, showed that curare acts on the myoneural junction.[75]

1858 Publication of John Snow's book, *On Chloroform and Other Anaesthetics*. General Medical Council established in the UK to supervise medical registration, education and professional conduct.

1859 First examination for the MRCP (London) held.

Charles Darwin (1809–1882) published *The Origin of Species by Natural Selection*.

1860 Albert Nieman (1834–1861) purified the alkaloid which Gaedicke had isolated from coca leaves. He named it cocaine.

1861 I. P. Semmelweiss (1818–1865), a Hungarian obstetrician, demonstrated that puerperal fever is both infectious and contagious, in Vienna.

1862 Thos. Skinner, a Liverpool obstetrician, introduced his domette-covered, wire-framed mask, frequently imitated since (e.g. by Curt Schimmelbusch (1860–1895), of Berlin, in 1890).

Clover's chloroform inhaler.

1863 Gardner Quincy Colton (1817–1898) popularized the use of nitrous oxide in dentistry, neglected since Horace Well's discovery in 1844.

Louis Pasteur (1822–1895) showed that micro-organisms cause fermentation, which led Lister to his discovery of antisepsis in 1865.

1864 Report of Chloroform Committee of Royal Medical and Chirurgical Society, which confirmed chloroform's position as first favourite although ether was shown to be safer.

Johan Nepomuk von Nussbaum (1829–1890), surgeon of Munich gave morphine preoperatively to prolong the action of chloroform.

1865 Professor J. Lister (1827–1912) of Glasgow treated by means of carbolic acid the compound fracture of James Greenlees's leg—the birth of antiseptic surgery (12 August) in Glasgow (*Lancet*, 1867, **1**, 326; **2**, 353).

1867 Ferdinand Edelberg Junker (von Laugegg) (1828–1902), Austrian surgeon working in London described his chloroform insufflation apparatus.

1868 Edmund Andrews (1824–1904) surgeon, of Chicago combined oxygen with nitrous oxide. (*See* 'Classical File', *Surv. Anesthesiol.* 1963, **7**, 74.) Thomas Wiltberger Evans (1823–1897), American dentist working in Paris, who had learnt about nitrous oxide administration from Colton in 1867, introduced it to London dentists. In the following year, nitrous oxide was supplied in cylinders in compressed form commercially 4 years before US manufacturers put it on the market. Supplies of nitrous oxide may well have been obtainable in London in 1856 from the Medical Pneumatic Appliance Co. (Barth).
C. A. Wunderlich (1815–1877) of Leipzig published his work on medical thermometry, *Temperature in Diseases; A Manual of Medical Thermometry*. London: New Sydenham Society, 1868. He found fever a disease and left it a symptom (Garrison).

1869 Nasal N_2O inhaler used (independently) by Joseph Thomas Clover (1825–1882) and Alfred Coleman (1828–1902), London dentist.

1870 Gustav Simon (1827–1913) of Heidelberg performed the first nephrectomy.

1871 Friedrich Trendelenburg (1844–1924) surgeon from Rostock, gave anaesthetics via a tracheostomy wound, and used in 1869 a cuffed tracheostomy tube (*Arch. Klin. Chir.* 1871, **12**, 112).

1872 Antisalivary effects of atropine described by R. P. H. Heidenhain (1834–1897), Breslau (Wroclaw) physician.
In England, use of ether became much more frequent following the visit of B. Joy Jeffries, an ophthalmic surgeon of Boston, Massachusetts, USA. He 'sold' the American method of ether administration to British surgeons and anaesthetists, a method involving forcing ether on to the patient who was, if necessary, held down during induction. Previously in Britain, chloroform was used almost exclusively.
Pierre-Cyprien Oré (1828–1889) of Bordeaux produced general anaesthesia with intravenous chloral hydrate in animals and 2 years later applied the method in man (*C. R. Acad. Sci. Paris*, 1874, 515, 651).
Clover introduced his nitrous-oxide–ether sequence at BMA Annual Meeting at Norwich.

1874 Forné, French naval surgeon, gave chloral hydrate by mouth to produce sleep before chloroform anaesthesia.

1875 Richard Caton (1842–1926) of Liverpool demonstrated the presence of electric currents in the brain and so was the pioneer of electro-encephalography.

1876 Hyperventilation (which produced hypocapnia) with air shown to have analgesic effects by Bonwill W. G. A. *Phil. J. Dent. Science*, 1876, **3**, 37 (*see* 'Classical File', *Surv. Anesthesiol.* 1964, **8**, 348).

1877 Joseph Clover introduced his portable regulating ether inhaler.

1880 W. Macewen (1848–1924), Glasgow surgeon, introduced tracheal intubation by mouth (Macewen W. *Br. Med. J.* 1880, **2**, 122).

1881 Stanislaw Klikovich (1853–1910), of St Petersburg, surgeon, used nitrous oxide and oxygen to ease labour pains (*Arch. Gynaek.* **18**, 81),[76] a technique later employed by Frederick Hewitt in 1887.

Frederick Trendelenburg (1844–1924), professor of surgery at Rostock (afterwards at Bonn and Leipzig), introduced the head-down tilt with pelvic elevation, for abdominal surgery.

First successful partial gastrectomy performed by Theodore Billroth (1829–1894) at Allgemeine Krankenhaus on 29 January on Therese Heller, in Vienna.[77]

First successful gastrojejunostomy performed: A. Woelfler (1850–1917).[78]

1882 Synthesis of cyclopropane by August von Freund (1835–1892), Viennese chemist.

Robert Koch (1843–1910), Berlin physician, described the tubercle bacillus.

1884 Koller, Vienna ophthalmologist, demonstrated local analgesic properties of cocaine on the cornea (in a paper read by Joseph Brettauer) (1835–1905) of Trieste, at Ophthalmological Congress at Heidelberg.

W. Stewart Halsted (1852–1922) and Richard John Hall, in New York, did the first nerve block with cocaine: the nerve, the mandibular.

Rickman J. Godlee (1849–1925), Lister's nephew and biographer, performed the first operation for the removal of a cerebral tumour.[79]

1885 J. L. Corning (1855–1923), New York neurologist, produced analgesia by the accidental subarachnoid injection of cocaine.

Medical Defence Union founded in London.

1886 Ernst von Bergmann (1836–1907), Berlin surgeon, introduced heat sterilization, the beginning of aseptic surgery.

1887 Sir Frederick Hewitt (1857–1916), London anaesthetist, invented the first practical gas and oxygen machine.

1888 First Hyderabad Chloroform Commission.

1889 Second Hyderabad Chloroform Commission. Reports stated that chloroform is never a cardiac depressant and that breathing stops before the heart. This is now known to be untrue.

1890 P. Vera Redard of Geneva introduced the ethyl chloride spray for local analgesia.

W. Stewart Halsted (1852–1922), professor of surgery at the Johns Hopkins Hospital, Baltimore, introduced rubber gloves for surgery.

Paul Reclus (1847–1914), Paris surgeon, advocated infiltration analgesia with cocaine.

1891 Lumbar puncture demonstrated to be a practical clinical procedure by H. I. Quincke (1842–1922) of Kiel in Germany and by Essex Wynter (1860–1945), a physician, in England at the Middlesex Hospital.

1892 The term 'Nerve blocking' introduced by Francois-Frank (*Arch. Physiol. Normal Path.* 1892, **24**, 562).

Heinrich Braun introduced the term 'conduction anaesthesia'.

Karl Ludwig Schleich (1859–1922) of Berlin introduced infiltration analgesia.

1893 London Society of Anaesthetists founded by F. W. Silk of King's College Hospital, London, with Woodhouse Brain as its first president. Other early presidents were G. Hewlett Bailey (1896–1898); Dudley W. Buxton (1897–1898); F. W. Silk (1899–1900) (see Dinnick O. P. *Progress in Anaesthesiology*, Proc. 4th WFSA London, 1970. Amsterdam: Excerpta

Medica, 1970). It became the Anaesthetic Section of the Royal Society of Medicine in 1908.

1894 Ernest Amory Codman (1869–1940) and Harvey Cushing (1869–1939) in Baltimore advocated use of anaesthetic record charts. Later, 1901, blood-pressure readings, taken with a Riva-Rocci instrument, were added to these charts. (Scipione Riva-Rocci (1863–1937) of Padua).

1895 X-rays discovered on 8 November by Wilhelm Konrad v. Roentgen (1845–1923) of Würzburg, Nobel prizeman, 1901 (1st award).

1898 August Bier (1861–1949), surgeon of Kiel, induced first successful clinical spinal analgesia.
Theodore Tuffier (1857–1929) of Paris developed and popularized spinal analgesia.
Transactions of the Society of Anaesthetists founded in 1893, published fairly frequently from this date.

1899 Rudolf Matas (1865–1957), New Orleans surgeon, adapted the technique of artificial respiration with bellows (the Fell–O'Dwyer technique) to thoracic surgery.[80]

1900 Karl Landsteiner (1868–1943) of the University of Vienna, later of the Rockefeller Institute, New York City, Nobel prizeman, 1930, described ABO blood groups.

1901 Extradural caudal injection introduced by Sicard (1872–1929) and Cathelin (1873–1945) both of Paris, independently.
First awards of Nobel prizes established by Alfred Bernhard Nobel 1832–96, Swedish chemist and inventor of dynamite.
Franz Kuhn of Kassel published his work on tracheal intubation (*see* Sweeney B. *Anaesthesia* 1985, **40**, 1000).

1902 Heinrich Braun (1862–1934), Leipzig surgeon, added adrenaline to cocaine solution to prolong its effect and retard its absorption.
A. G. Vernon Harcourt (1834–1919), FRS, reader in chemistry at Christ Church, Oxford, described his chloroform inhaler in which the concentration of vapour could be measured and its volume regulated, e.g. 2% at temperatures between 16 and 18 °C.
E. H. Embley, anaesthetist of Melbourne, Australia described death due to vagal inhibition of the heart during chloroform anaesthesia.[81]

1903 Barbitone (veronal) synthesized by Emil Fischer (1852–1919), Berlin chemist and Nobel prizeman, 1902, and von Mering (1849–1908) of Munich. This was the first barbiturate.
Willhelm Einthoven (1860–1927) of Leiden, Holland, applied the principles of the string galvanometer to ECG recording and for this was awarded the Nobel prize for medicine in 1924.[82]

1904 Ernest Fourneau (1872–1949) of Paris synthesized stovaine.
Procaine synthesized by Alfred Einhorn (1856–1917), Munich chemist.

1905 The first society of anaesthetists founded in the US by G. A. F. Erdmann, the Long Island Society of Anesthetists, later (1911) combined with a group from Manhattan to form the New York Society of Anesthetists; in 1935 the organization became national and in 1936 was named the American Society of Anesthetists Inc. In 1945 the title was changed to the American Society of Anesthesiologists Inc., at the suggestion of Paul Wood (1897–1963), New York anaesthetist, the name 'anesthesiology' having been coined by Seifert in 1902.

Procaine used by Heinrich Braun (1862–1934).

1907 Arthur E. Barker (1850–1916), surgeon, of University College Hospital, London, made use of the curves of the vertebral column in spinal analgesia and introduced hyperbaric solutions. The pioneer of spinal analgesia in Britain.[83]

Foundation of the Royal Society of Medicine in London.

Chevalier Jackson (1865–1958), of Philadelphia, described his work on laryngoscopy.

1908 Massive collapse of the lungs described by Wm Pasteur, English physician (1856–1943).[84]

Louis Ombrédanne (1871–1956), Parisian surgeon, described his ether–air inhaler.

Bier described intravenous procaine local analgesia.

George Washington Crile (1864–1943), of Cleveland, Ohio, surgeon, described his theory of 'anociassociation' (*Am. Surg.* 1908, **47**, 864).

The Society of Anaesthetists became the Anaesthetic Section of the Royal Society of Medicine.

1909 S. J. Meltzer (1851–1920) and J. Auer (1875–1948), of the Rockefeller Institute NY used tracheal insufflation anaesthesia in animals.

First Nobel prize awarded to a surgeon Theodore Kocher of Berne (1841–1907) for his work on the treatment of goitre.

1910 C. A. Elsberg (1871–1948), New York surgeon, applied Meltzer and Auer's technique to man (tracheal intubation).

Elmer Ira McKesson (1881–1935) of Toledo, Ohio, anaesthetist and inventor, introduced the first on-demand intermittent-flow gas and oxygen machine, with percentage calibration of the two gases (*Surg. Gynecol. Obstet.* 1911, **13**, 456; *see also* Waters R. M. *J. Hist. Med. Allied Sci.* 1946, **1**, 595).

Arthur Läwen (1876–1958) of Königsberg showed that extradural analgesia via the sacral route was a useful and practical method of analgesia.

1911 Goodman Levy (1856–1954) proved that chloroform can cause death (from ventricular fibrillation) in light anaesthesia.

A. E. Guedel (1883–1956) working in Indianapolis, reported on the technique of self-administration of nitrous oxide in obstetrics (*Indianap. Med. J.* 1911, **14**, 476).

Commencement of the National Insurance Act in the UK with its 'panel' of general practitioners.

Robert Kelly of Liverpool (1879–1944) was first to use insufflation tracheal anaesthesia in England (*Br. J. Surg.* 1911, **1**, 90).

1912 Walter Meredith Boothby (1880–1953), of Rochester, Minn. and Frederic Jay Cotton (1869–1938), Boston surgeon, introduced a sight feed gas and oxygen flow-meter.

A. Läwen (1876–1958), Königsberg surgeon, used curare to produce relaxation.

J. B. Herrick (1861–1954), Chicago physician, described the features of acute coronary thrombosis (*JAMA* 1912, **59**, 2015).

1913 Danis was first to describe trans-sacral analgesia.

James Tayloe Gwathmey (1865–1944) of New York introduced rectal oil-ether and in the following year published his classic textbook *Anesthesia*. New York: Appleton.

1914 Albert Hustin of Belgium (1882–1907) was first to use citrate in blood transfusion.

Anesthetic supplements to the *American Journal of Surgery* commenced publication, quarterly—the first official regularly published literature devoted to the specialty, edited by Frank Hoeffer McMechan (1879–1939). Terminated in the US 1926.

1915 Use of carbon dioxide absorption in animals by Dennis Jackson of St Louis, later of Cincinnati (*J. Lab. Clin. Med.* 1915, **1**, 1).

1916 Sir F. E. Shipway (1875–1968) of Guy's Hospital, London, introduced his warm ether insufflation apparatus (*Lancet*, **1**, 70).

1917 Edmund Boyle (1875–1941) of St Bartholomew's Hospital, London, described his portable N_2O and O_2 apparatus.

Avertin described by Fritz Eicholtz (1889–1968), pharmacologist, of Heidelberg.

1919 The American Association of Anesthetists founded by James T. Gwathmey and Frank McMechan (1879–1939).

1920 Guedel's first paper on signs of anaesthesia. These supplanted Snow's signs.

Ivan Whiteside Magill (1888–1986) and E. Stanley Rowbotham of London (1890–1979) developed endotracheal anaesthesia.

1921 Extradural lumbar analgesia described by Pagés (1886–1923) of Spain.

1922 *Current Researches in Anesthesia and Analgesia* appeared in August. Founded and edited by Dr. F. H. McMechan and sponsored by the National Anesthetic Research Society in the US. In 1957 changed its name to *Anesthesia and Analgesia Current Researches*; the first journal to appear regularly in the world exclusively devoted to anaesthesia.

Labat's (1877–1934) *Regional Anesthesia* published.

1923 Carbon dioxide absorption used in man, by Ralph Milton Waters.

British Journal of Anaesthesia appeared.

1924 Howard Wilcox Haggard (1891–1959) of Yale University published his classic papers on 'The Absorption, Distribution and Elimination of Ether' (*J. Biol. Chem.* 1924, **59**, 737 et seq.; reprinted in 'Classical File', *Surv. Anesthesiol.* 1957, **1**, 629; *see also Anesth. Anal.* 1975, **54**, 654).

1926 Concept of 'balanced anaesthesia' put forward by J. S. Lundy (1894–1972) of the Mayo Clinic (*Minn. Med.* 1926, **9**, 399).

Otto Butzengeiger of Wuppertal-Elberfeld, used tribromethyl alcohol (Avertin) (*Dtsch. Med. Wochenschr.* 1927, **53**, 712).

For the first time there was a Section of Anaesthetics at the annual scientific meeting of the British Medical Association.

1927 Ocherblad and Dillon of Kansas City, used ephedrine in spinal analgesia to prevent hypotension.

Pernocton used in Germany by R. Bumm. The first barbiturate routinely used for induction of anaesthesia.

1928 Lucas and Henderson in Toronto proved that cyclopropane had anaesthetic properties.

I. W. Magill popularized blind nasal intubation.

1929 Alexander Fleming (1881–1955) of St Mary's Hospital, London, Nobel prizeman, 1945, discovered that the mould *Penicillium notatum* secreted an anti-staphylococcal substance.[85] This discovery was later developed.[86]

1930 Introduction of circle method of carbon dioxide absorption by Brian Sword (1889–1956) of New Haven, Conn.

1931 Achille Mario D. Dogliotti (1897–1966) of Turin, reintroduced extradural analgesia in Italy, and 4 years later founded the Italian Society of Anaesthetists.

Foundation of the Liverpool Society of Anaesthetists, the oldest provincial society in the UK.

1932 Helmut Weese (1897–1954), Scharpff and Rheinoff were the first to use hexobarbitone (Evipan) (*Dtsch. Med. Wochenschr.* 1932, **2**, 1205) synthesized by Kropp and Taub.

Christopher Langton Hewer's (1896–1986) *Recent Advances in Anaesthesia* appeared. 14th (Jubilee) edition 1982 (*see* Hewer, C. Langton, in edition 14).

Foundation of the Association of Anaesthetists of Great Britain and Ireland; the first president, Henry Featherstone (1894–1976) of Birmingham.

1933 A. Evarts Graham (1883–1957) of St Louis performed the first successful pneumonectomy for cancer.

Ralph Waters (1883–1979) appointed professor and chairman of the new Department of Anesthesia in the University of Wisconsin at Madison: the first such appointment in the USA. (Thomas Drysdale Buchanan was appointed clinical professor of Anesthesiology at the College of Physicians and Surgeons of Colombia, New York, a non-university appointment in 1918).

Polyethylene (polythene) synthesized by R. O. Gibson and E. W. Fawcett in the UK. Manufacture commenced in 1939 by Imperial Chemical Industries.

1934 Ralph Waters and associates from Madison, Wisconsin, reported on the clinical use of cyclopropane where it was first administered on 9 October 1930.

J. S. Lundy anaesthetist of the Mayo Clinic popularised thiopentone.

Australian Society of Anaesthetists formed.

1935 Commencement of the intravenous drip (Marriott H. L. and Kekwick A. *Lancet* 1935, **1**, 977).

Gerhardt Domagk (1895–1967) (*Dtsch. Med. Wochenschr* 1935, **61**, 250). Nobel prizeman 1939, of Germany, introduced the first 'sulpha' drug for the control of haemolytic streptococcal infections.

First examination for DA held. H. E. G. Boyle and C. W. Morris, the first examiners.

1936 Successful treatment of puerperal fever with sulphanilamide, by Colebrook C. L. and Kenny M. *Lancet* 1936, **1**, 1279.

1937 R. R. Macintosh (1897–) appointed Nuffield Professor of Anaesthesia in the University of Oxford, the first chair of anaesthesia in Europe.

American Board of Anesthesiology established.

Guedel's *Inhalation Anesthesia* published.

1938 Positive-pressure respirator used in surgery by Crafoord, surgeon, (1899–1984)—the spiropulsator of Frenckner in Stockholm.

1939 Pethidine synthesized by Schaumann and Eisleb at Hoechst Farbwerke, Germany.

1940 The journal *Anesthesiology* first published.

Development of controlled breathing by Guedel and by Michael Nosworthy (1902–1980) of St Thomas' Hospital, London.

Karl Landsteiner (1888–1943) and Alexander Wiener of the Rockefeller Institute, New York City, isolated the Rh factor in blood.

Preparation of an active and concentrated form of penicillin described (Chain E. B. et al. *Lancet* 1940, **2**, 226).

Penicillin given on 15 October at Colombia-Presbyterian Hospital, New York to a patient by Dr Aaron Alston.

1941 Trichloroethylene advocated by Langton Hewer and Charles Frederick Hadfield (1875–1965).

1942 Harold Randall Griffith (1894–1985) and G. Enid Johnson of Montreal used curare in anaesthesia.

1943 Macintosh described his curved laryngoscope in Oxford.

The first electronic computer was designed in the USA by Eckert and Mauchley to calculate artillery firing tables (electronic numerical integrator and computer—ENIAC). It weighed 30 tons and contained 18 000 thermionic valves. Created at the University of Pennsylvania.

1946 Centenary celebrations of anaesthesia (*see* Bourne W. *Anesthesiology*, 1948, **9**, 239, 358; *J. Hist. Med. Allied Sci.* 1946, **1**, No. 4, October).

The journal *Anaesthesia* appeared.

1947 First clinical use of lignocaine (Xylocaine) by Torsten Gordh (1907–) of Stockholm.

1948 Faculty of Anaesthetists established by the Council of the Royal College of Surgeons of England; A. D. Marston (1891–1962), of Guy's Hospital, London, the first dean.

First use of hypotensive anaesthesia by H. W. C. Griffiths and John Gillies (1895–1976) in Edinburgh using high spinal analgesia.

Commencement of the two-part Diploma in Anaesthetic examination.

National Health Insurance started in the UK (July).

Invention of the transistor in the US.

1949 Penta- and hexamethonium described by W. D. M. Paton and Eleanor Zaimis (1915–1983).

Short-acting muscle relaxants described by Daniel Bovet (who was the first to prepare antihistamines) and used clinically 2 years later in Italy and Sweden.

Cortisone used at the Mayo Clinic (Hench P. S. et al. *Proc. Staff Meet. Mayo Clin.* 1949, **24**, 181).

1950 Induced hypothermia in cardiac surgery described by Wilfred Gordon Bigelow, surgeon, and his colleagues from Toronto.

Scandinavian Society of Anaesthetists formed. Their first Congress held in Oslo.

1951 C. W. Suckling of Manchester synthesized halothane.

1952 Faculty of Anaesthetists of the Royal Australasian College of Surgeons founded; D. Renton, the first dean. First examination for fellowship held in 1956.

Use of IPPV with bag and tracheal tube in Copenhagen polio epidemic. (Lassen H. C. A. *Lancet*, 1953, **1**, 37; Ibsen B. *Proc. R. Soc. Med.* 1954, **47**, 72).

1953 First examination for Fellowship in Faculty of Anaesthetists of the Royal College of Surgeons of England in London.

First successful open-heart operation performed by John J. Gibbon at Thomas Jefferson Medical School, Philadelphia, using Gibbon extracorporeal bypass apparatus 6 May.

1954 Canadian Anaesthetists' Society Journal first published.
1955 Vibierg Olof Björk and Carl Gunnar Engström, surgeons, described IPPV for the treatment of postoperative respiratory failure.
World Federation of Societies of Anaesthesiologists formed. First Congress in Scheveningen, Holland.
1956 Michael Johnstone of the Manchester Royal Infirmary used halothane clinically.
1957 *Survey of Anesthesiology* and *Acta Anaesthesiologica Scandinavica* first published.
1959 Faculty of Anaesthetists established by the Royal College of Surgeons in Ireland. T. Gilmartin, the first dean.
Neurolept analgesia reported by De Castro and Paul Mundeleer.
1962 First European Congress of Anaesthesiology in Vienna.
First Asian–Australasian Congress of Anaesthesiologists held in Manila.
1966 Ketamine used clinically by Corssen and Domino in the USA.
Enflurane used by Virtue of Denver and his colleagues.
1970 Intensive Care Society founded in the UK. Society for Critical Care Medicine founded in the US.
1971 Isoflurane first used.
1982 First Meeting of the European Society of Regional Anaesthesia (ESRA) held in Edinburgh.
First International Symposium on the History of Anaesthesia held in Rotterdam.
See also Davison M. H. Armstrong, *The Evolution of Anaesthesia*. Altrincham: J. Sherratt and Son, 1965; Duncum, Barbara, *The Development of Inhalation Anaesthesia*. London: Oxford University Press, 1947; Faulconer A. Jr and Keys T. E. *Foundations of Anesthesiology*. Springfield, Ill.: Thomas, 1965; Thomas K. Bryn, *The Development of Anaesthetic Apparatus*. Oxford: Blackwell, 1975; Keys T. E. *The History of Surgical Anesthesia*. New York: Dover Pubs. Inc. 1963; Bryce-Smith R., Mitchell J. V. and Parkhouse J. *The Nuffield Department of Anaesthetics, 1937–62*. London: Oxford University Press, 1963; Smith W. D. A. *Under the Influence; a History of Nitrous Oxide and Oxygen Anaesthesia*. London: Macmillan, 1982; *Genesis of Contemporary American Anesthesia*. Volpitto P. P. and Vandam L. D. (ed.) Springfield, Ill.: Thomas, 1982; *Essays on the first 100 Years of Anaesthesia*, Sykes W. D. Vol. 1 and 2. 1961/2 and Vol. 3 (ed. Ellis R. H.) London & Edinburgh: Churchill Livingstone, 1982; Anaesthesia and analgesia. Centenary of anaesthesia. *Br. Med. Bull.* 1946, **4**, 81; *Bibliography on the History of Anaesthesia*. Secher Ole. Copenhagen: Rigshospitalet, 1984; and Secher O. History of the modern development of the inhalation anaesthetics. *Acta Anaesth. Scand.* 1982, **26**, 269; *Anaesthesia; Essays on its History*, Rupreht J. et al. (ed.) Berlin: Springer-Verlag, 1985.

References

1. Secher O. In: *Anaesthesia; Essays on its History* (Rupreht J. et al. ed.) Berlin: Springer-Verlag, 1985, p. 321.
2. Fuller J. F. *Anesthesiology* 1947, **8**, 464.
3. *See* 'Classical File', *Surv. Anesthesiol.* 1976, **20**, 283.

4. *See also* Cartwright F. F. *The English Pioneers of Anaesthesia*, Bristol: Wright, 1952; and Bryn-Thomas K. *Anaesthesia* 1978, **33**, 903.
5. Excerpts reprinted in *Surv. Anesthesiol.* 1968, **12**, 92; also facsimile reproduction, London: Butterworths, 1972.
6. Cartwright F. F. *Proc. 4th World Cong. Anaesth.* 1968, 203.
7. *See also* Cartwright F. F. *The English Pioneers of Anaesthesia*, Bristol: Wright, 1952; Smith W. D. A. *Br. J. Anaesth.* 1966, **38**, 58; 1970, **42**, 347, 445; 1978, **50**, 623, 853.
8. Reprinted in 'Classical File', *Surv. Anesthesiol.* 1966, **10**, 92.
9. *Boston Med. Surg. J.* 1848, **38**, 25.
10. *See also* MacQuitty B. *The Battle for Oblivion*. London: Harrap, 1969.
11. Long C. W. *South. Med. J.* 1849, N.S.5, 705 (reprinted in 'Classical File', *Surv. Anesthesiol.* 1960, **4**, 120).
12. Gould A. B. In: *Anaesthesia; Essays in its History* (Rupreht J. et al. ed.) Berlin: Springer-Verlag, 1985, 384.
13. Holmes O. W. *Br. Med. J.* 1902, **2**, 1368.
14. Thomas, K. Bryn, *Anaesthesia* 1968, **23**, 676.
15. Dawkins R. J. Massey, *Anaesthesia* 1947, **2**, 51.
16. Zuck D. *Br. J. Anaesth.* 1978, **50**, 393; Squire W. *Lancet* 1888, **2**, 1220.
17. *See* Miller A. H. *Boston Med. Surg. J.* 1927, **197**, 1218; Miller A. H. *Anesthesiology* 1947, **8**, 471 (reprinted in 'Classical File', *Surv. Anesthesiol.* 1972, **16**, 193); also Straton J. *Br. Med. J.* 1972, **3**, 181.
18. Ellis R. H., *Anaesthesia* 1976, **31**, 766; Ellis R. H. *Anaesthesia* 1977, **32**, 1973.
19. Wilson G. *Proc. 4th World Cong. Anaesth.* 1968, 174, *See also* Annotation, *Boston Med. Surg. J.* 21 October 1846; Bigelow H. J. *Boston Med. Surg. J.* 18 November 1846; Annotation, *Lond. Med. Gaz.* 18 December 1846; Annotation, *Lancet* 26 December 1846.
20. Longford E. *Victoria, R. I.* London: Weidenfeld and Nicolson, 1964, p. 234.
21. Winterton W. R. *Hist. Med.* 1980, **8**, 11; Schoenberg B. S. et al. *Mayo Clinic Proc.* 1974, **49**, 680.
22. Picini F. *Osservazioni microscopische e deduction patologische sul cholera asiatica.* Firenze, 1854.
23. Koch R. Ueber die cholera bakterien. *Dtsch. Med. Wochenschr*, 1884, **10**, 725.
24. *Anaesthesia* 1952, **7**, 192.
25. Atkinson R. S. *Proc. 4th World Cong. Anaesth. (London).* 1968, 197.
26. *See also* Shepherd J. A. *Simpson and Syme of Edinburgh.* Edinburgh and London: Livingstone, 1969; Simpson, Myrtle, *Simpson the Obstetrician*. London: Gollancz, 1972.
27. Simpson J. Y. *Lond. Med. Gaz.* 1847, n.s., **5**, 934; *Lancet* 1847, **2**, 549 (reprinted in 'Classical File', *Surv. Anesthesiol.* 1961, **5**, 93).
28. Waldie D. *The True Story of the Introduction of Chloroform into Anaesthetics.* Edinburgh: Linlithgow, 1870.
29. Farr A. D. *Anaesthesia* 1980, **35**, 896.
30. Sykes W. S. *Essays on the First Hundred Years of Anaesthesia*, Edinburgh and London: Livingstone, 1961, Vol. II, p. 168; Coote H. *Lancet* 1847, **2**, 571.
31. Atkinson R. S. *Simpson and Chloroform.* London: Priory Press, 1973; and Atkinson R. S. *Anaesthesia* 1973, **28**, 302.
32. Thomas K. Bryn, *Anaesthesia* 1971, **27**, 436.
33. Clover J. T. *Br. Med. J.* 1876, **2**, 75 (reprinted in 'Classical File', *Surv. Anesthesiol.* 1964, **8**, 87).
34. Clover J. T. *Br. Med. J.* 1877, **1**, 69; Atkinson R. S. and Boulton T. B. *Anaesthesia* 1977, **32**, 1033.
35. Elliott C. J. R. *Anaesthesia* 1979, **34**, 681, Brown A. G. *Anaesthesia* 1979, **34**, 681, Weisser Ch. *Anaesthesist* 1983, **32**, 52.
36. Lee J. Alfred, *Ann. R. Coll. Surg.* 1960, **26**, 280.
37. Wylie W. D. *Ann. R. Coll. Surg.*, 1975, **56**, 171.
38. Clover J. T. *Br. Med. J.* 1871, **2**, 33.
39. *See* Calverley R. In: *Anaesthesia; Essays on its History* (Rupreht J. et al. ed.) Berlin: Springer-Verlag, 1985, 18.
40. Wilson-Smith T. *Lancet* 1898, **1**, 1005.
41. Hewitt F. W. *Anaesthetics and their Administration.* London: Macmillan, 1901, pp. 277–8.
42. Hewitt F. W. *Anaesthetics and their Administration.* London: Macmillan, 1901, p. 209.
43. *See* Edwards G. *Ann. R. Coll. Surg.* 1951, **8**, 233.
44. Binning R. *Anaesthesia* 1978, **33**, 55.

45. Macewen W. *Glas. Med. J.* 1879, **2**, 72; *Br. Med. J.* 1880, **2**, 122; *Lancet* 1980, **2**, 906.
46. Koller C. *Klin. Mbl. Augen.* 1884, **22**, 60; *Wien. Med. Wochenschr.* 1884, **34**, 1276, 1309 (translated in 'Classical File', *Surv. Anesthesiol.* 1965, **9**, 288).
47. *See also* Koller C. *JAMA* 1928, **90**, 1742 and *JAMA* 1941, **117**, 1284; Koller-Becker H. *Psychoanal. Q.* 1963, **32**, 509; Liljestrand G. *Acta Physiol. Scand.* 1967 (Suppl. 299), **3**, 30; Wyklicky H. and Skopec M. In: *Regional Anaesthesia, 1884–1984*, ed. Scott D. B. et al., 1984, Sodertalje, Production ICM AB; McAuley J. F. *Br. Dent. J.* 1985, **158**, 339.
48. Glen F. and Dillon L. D. *Surg. Gynecol. Obstet.* 1980, **151**, 518.
49. Halsted W. S. *Johns Hopkins Hosp. Rep.* 1890, **2**, 255.
50. Bier A. *Dt. Z. Chir.* 1899, **51**, 361 (translated in *Surv. Anesthesiol.* 1962, **6**, 352).
51. Bier A. *Zbl. Chir.* 1892, **19**, 57.
52. Bier A. *Verh. Dtsch. Ges. Chir.* 1908, **37**, 204.
53. Braun H. *Arch. Klin. Chir.* 1902, **69**, 541.
54. Braun H. *Dtsch. Med. Wochenschr.* 1905, **31**, 1667.
55. Läwen A. *Beitr. Klin. Chir.* 1912, **80**, 168.
56. Läwen A. *Zbl. Chirurg.* 1910, **37**, 708; *Dtsch. Zeit. Chir.* 1911, **108**, 11.
57. Reprinted in 'Classical File', *Surv. Anesthesiol.* 1979, **23**, 340.
58. Guedel A. E. and Waters R. S. *Curr. Res. Anesth. Analg.* 1928, **7**, 238.
59. Guedel A. E. *JAMA* 1933, **103**, 1862.
60. G. Davis was anaesthetist to Harvey Cushing at the Johns Hopkins Hospital.
61. Watt O. M. *Anaesthesia* 1968, **23**, 103.
62. Stiles J. A. et al. *Curr. Res. Anesth. Analg.* 1934, **13**, 56.
63. Waters R. M. *Curr. Res. Anesth. Analg.* 1924, **3**, 20.
64. Waters R. M. (ed.) *Chloroform; A Study after 100 Years*. Madison: University of Wisconsin Press, 1951.
65. Pratt T. W. et al. *Am. J. Surg.* 1936, **31**, 464.
66. Gale J. W. and Waters R. M. *J. Thorac. Surg.* 1932, **1**, 432.
    (*See also* Macintosh R. R. *Anaesthesia* 1970, **24**, 4; *Anesth. Analg. Curr. Res.* 1957, **36**, 81; *Anaesthesia* 1957, **12**, 497).
67. Lundy J. S. *Minn. Med.* 1926, **9**, 399.
68. Betcher A. M. *Anesth. Analg. Curr. Res.* 1977, **56**, 303.
69. Bennett A. E. et al. *JAMA* 1940, **114**, 322.
70. Griffith H. R. and Johnson E. *Anesthesiology* 1942, **3**, 418–20; Gillies D. M. M. *Can. Anaesth. Soc. J.* 1985, **32**, 570; 'Classical File' *Surv. Anesthesiol.* 1985, **29**, 358.
71. Dinnick O. P. *Proc. 4th World Cong. Anaesth. (London)*. 1968, 181.
72. Bishop P. J. *J. R. Soc. Med.* 1980, **73**, 448.
73. Nunn R. *Lond. Med. Gaz.* 1847, **39** (4, n.s.), 414; Annotation, *Lancet* 1847, **1**, 340.
74. Wylie W. D. *Ann. R. Coll. Surg.* 1975, **56**, 171.
75. Lee J. A. *Anaesthesia* 1978, **33**, 741.
76. Richards W. et al. *Anaesthesia* 1976, **31**, 933.
77. Billroth T. *Wien. Med. Wochenschr.* 1881, **31**, 161; Obituary, *Surg. Gynecol. Obst.* 1979, **148**, 252; Mann R. J. *Mayo Clin. Proc.* 1974, **49**, 132.
78. Woelfler A. *Zbl. f. Chirurg.* 1881, **8**, 705.
79. Bennett H. and Godlee R. J. *Lancet* 1884, **2**, 1090.
80. Matas R. *Ann. Surg.* 1899, **29**, 426.
81. Reprinted in 'Classical File', *Surv. Anesthesiol.* 1965, **9**, 511, 634, from *Br. Med. J.* 1902, **1**, 817, 885, 951. *See also* Wilson G. C. M. *Anaesth. Intensive Care* 1972, **1**, 9.
82. Einthoven W. *Arch. Ges. Physiol.* 1903, **99**, 472.
83. Lee J. A. *Anaesthesia* 1979, **34**, 885.
84. Lee J. A. *Anaesthesia* 1978, **33**, 362.
85. Fleming A. *Br. J. Exp. Pathol.* 1929, **10**, 226.
86. Chain E. et al. *Lancet* 1940, **2**, 226.
87. Röse W. In: *Regional Anaesthesia, 1884–1984*. Centennial Meeting of Regional Anaesthesia. Ed Scott D. B. et al., 1984, Sodertalje, Production ICM AB.
88. Seldon T. H. *Anesth. Analg. (Cleve.)* 1986, **65**, 1051.

Section **2** Basic Sciences

Chapter 2   **NOTES ON PHYSIOLOGY**

The Neuroendocrine System

The Stress Response
An interlinked set of reflexes basically designed to preserve life during injury and illness. The afferent side of these reflexes is frequently neural, e.g. pain sensation, and the efferent side frequently endocrine. The stimuli which alert it include physical pain, heat, cold, exposure of viscera to air or handling, toxaemia, fear, allergic reactions.

The response is the immediate secretion of catecholamines, adrenaline and noradrenaline, which generate the 'fear, fight and flight' reaction. (*a*) The central excitatory state is alerted, alarm is felt; (*b*) The pupils dilate; (*c*) The bronchi dilate; (*d*) Cardiac rate and output increase; (*e*) Blood flow is diverted to muscles; (*f*) Muscle tone increases; (*g*) The blood clotting cascade accelerates; (*h*) Metabolism moves into energy mobilization.

Other endocrine changes include:
1. Aldosterone secretion causing retention of sodium.
2. ADH secretion causing retention of water.
3. Insulin secretion, making glucose available for energy.
4. Immune mechanisms are mainly suppressed. e.g. operative stress reduces phagocytosis and T lymphocyte reactivity. However, both catecholamine release and ether anaesthesia may induce leucocytosis.
5. Secretion of renin, glucagon, growth hormone and somatomedin.
6. Steroid secretion.

Neurotransmitters
Characteristics of genuine neurotransmitters:
1. Synthesized in the nerve terminal.
2. Degraded in the nerve terminal.
3. There is a specific enzyme for this degradation.
4. There is a specific mechanism for their uptake at the nerve terminal.
5. The relevant receptor can be stimulated in vitro by the neurotransmitter.
A. Acetylcholine acts in at least four different ways:
1. At the skeletal neuromuscular junction where quanta of this transmitter are released in response to motor nerve stimuli. This causes depolarization of the cell membranes of the skeletal muscle fibre. Blocked by: (*a*) non-depolarizing relaxants; (*b*) its effects are thwarted by depolarizing relaxants which hold the

muscles in a depolarized state and therefore unable to react to acetylcholine; (c) toxins, e.g. botulinus, aminoglycoside antibiotics; (d) hypocalcaemia.

2. At parasympathetic nerve endings (muscarinic) causing smooth muscle activity in the gut, urinary tract and bronchi, secretion of digestive glands, bradycardia and miosis. Blocked by atropine, hyoscine, glycopyrrolate and other anticholinergic drugs.

3. At sympathetic ganglia including the adrenal medulla (nicotinic action) and sympathetic nerve endings to sweat glands. Blocked by ganglion blockers, e.g. trimetaphan at the ganglia and by atropine and hyoscine at the sweat glands.

4. In the brain and spinal cord. Blocked to some extent by large doses of atropine and hyoscine (the central anticholinergic syndrome), an effect which may be relieved by physostigmine.

B. Adrenaline and noradrenaline act at sympathetic nerve endings:

At α-receptors they cause skin and splanchnic vasoconstriction, and uterine contraction. Blocked by phenoxybenzamine and other α-blockers, α_2-adrenergic neurones cause inhibition of noradrenaline release.

At β_1-receptors, they cause cardiac stimulation, tremor and panic. At β_2-receptors they cause vaso- and bronchodilatation. Practolol is a β_1-blocker, propranolol is a mixed β_1- and β_2-blocker. These transmitters also act in the brain and spinal cord. They are destroyed in the blood by catechol-*o*-methyl transferase, and in the tissues by monoamine oxidase.

C. Dopamine acts on dopamine receptors in the brainstem to stabilize skeletal muscle control, and in the renal and mesenteric arteries causing vasodilatation, resulting in sodium excretion. In the hypothalamus it inhibits the release of prolactin and other hormones from the pituitary gland. In the heart it stimulates β_1-receptors, shortening the pre-ejection phase and increasing output. In large doses it also stimulates α_1-receptors. It does not cross the blood–brain barrier except in its laevorotatory form. Dopamine also acts as a transmitter in the spinal cord. In the medulla it is involved with vomiting and blood pressure control. It is rapidly metabolized in the blood by dopamine β-hydroxylase to noradrenaline. At D_1-receptors there is weak blockade by butyrophenones. At D_2-receptors, e.g. in the anterior pituitary, it may be blocked by butyrophenones, e.g. haloperidol, some phenothiazines, metoclopramide and domperidone. When it is acting at α-and β-receptors (usually in larger doses) these actions may be blocked by α- and β-blockers respectively. *See also* Chapter 19.

D. Substance P may be the neurotransmitter on the pain pathway in the substantia gelatinosa of the dorsal horn of the spinal cord. Substance P and GABA (spinal cord transmitters) are inhibited by baclofen, producing analgesia.[1]

E. Endorphins and encephalins[2] stimulate specific receptors in the substantia gelatinosa and brainstem to regulate pain reception and appreciation. They produce hyporesponsiveness to environmental stimuli, and are subdivided into: opiomelanocortins, e.g. β-endorphin; proenkephalins, e.g. methionine enkephalin; and dynorphins, e.g. leucine enkephalin.

Endorphin receptors are divided into μ-receptors (stimulated by morphine and blocked by naloxone), further divided into μ_1-receptors (analgesia), and μ_2-receptors (respiratory depression, pupillary constriction, constipation, addiction).

There are also κ-receptors, stimulated by dynorphin (analgesia), Δ receptors, stimulated by methionine enkephalin, and sigma receptors (dysphoria and cerebral arterial spasm). There is enormous species variation and data from one species cannot be extrapolated to another.

F. 5-hydroxytryptamine[3] is an inhibitory transmitter in the brain and spinal cord where sympathetic outflow from the vasomotor centre is conducted. It may be a transmitter at the dorsal horn cell in the mechanism of the central control of pain.
G. Glycine may also be a central inhibitory transmitter.
H. Gamma-aminobutyric acid (GABA)[4] is a spinal inhibitory transmitter which opens the cell membrane chloride channel, thereby stabilizing the membrane at its resting potential. It may be involved in Ia muscle afferents and inhibition of pain transmission.
I. S-Glutamate is a spinal excitatory transmitter.
J. Somatostatin, cholecystokinin and vasoactive intestinal polypeptide have also been proposed as dorsal horn transmitters.[5]
K. Peptides. Powerful coronary vasoconstrictors stimulate peptidergic receptors.
Slow synaptic transmission is seen in sympathetic ganglia, the inhibitory form mediated by dopamine and the excitatory form by acetylcholine. This slow transmission involves many more steps than the simple fast transmission of synapses and nerve endings.

Functions of the Medulla Oblongata
1. Transmission of impulses between cerebrum and spinal cord.
2. Control of automatic functions, e.g. respiration, circulation, balance, digestion.
3. Control of sleep and wakefulness (reticular formation).
4. Origin of some cranial nerves.
Brainstem death, *see* Chapter 39.

The Cell

Cellular Components
1. The cell membrane. This is a phospholipid bi-layer with the functions of physical separation of the cell contents from the milieu, and electrical insulation, important in cells whose function depends on depolarization. They maintain a membrane potential. A sodium pump mechanism constantly removes sodium from the inside of the cell. There are channels in the membrane, selectively permeable to various ions (*see below*).
2. Cytoplasm. This is the general area of the cytoplasm in which aqueous reactions take place.
3. Mitochondria are organelles within the cytoplasm loaded with enzymes for a host of various aerobic reactions. They operate at a Po_2 of $0.27-0.67$ kPa (2–5 mmHg). (Erythrocytes do not have them, so their metabolism is anaerobic.)
4. The sarcomere—a specialized structure in skeletal muscle, upon which actin and myosin contract.
5. The sarcoplasmic reticulum—a system of channels relating membrane to deeper structures.
6. The nucleus—the organizing centre of the cell and also initiating the process of cell division and reproduction. Its chromosome content defines the physical characteristics of the individual. Not all cells have nuclei, e.g. erythrocytes.
7. The reticular endothelium.
8. Inclusion bodies—substances produced by the cell and localized at various loci; also particles ingested by cells.

9. Cell membrane channels. These are proteins which become permeable in response to a variety of influences. They are frequently proteins, e.g. porin.

Sodium channels are voltage sensitive and open in response to depolarization of the cell membrane, thus propagating the wave of depolarization across the entire cell membrane, e.g. in nerve axons and muscle fibres. The sodium channel closes during the action potential. The sodium channel is specifically blocked by tetrodotoxin and reversibly blocked by lignocaine.

Potassium channels are also opened by the depolarization action potential, with a slower time course than sodium. The resultant outflow of potassium leads to repolarization and closure of the potassium channel. The Nernst equation describes the relationship between membrane potential (around 70 mV) and the ionic permeabilities of sodium and potassium.

$$Vm = \frac{RT}{F} \log.e \frac{[K^+]out}{[K^+]in}$$

where $[K^+]out$, the extracellular potassium concentration is normally 3·5–5·5 mmol/l; $[K^+]in$, the intracellular potassium concentration, is normally 120–150 mmol/l; R = the gas constant; T = absolute temperature; F = the Faraday constant.

$$\frac{RT}{F} = 61·5 @ 37°C.$$

Calcium channels (Vassalle, 1979) are of interest to the anaesthetist; in the heart, during contraction, calcium enters the cell transported by calmodulin and moves from the sarcoplasmic reticulum to the myofibrils, maintaining the contraction phase. They conduct slowly, giving a longer depolarization plateau. Calcium channels have also been noted in cortical dendrites in the central nervous system. Calcium channels may be reversibly blocked by verapamil, causing slower contraction rate, slower A–V conduction, reduced myocardial contractility and reduced myocardial vascular tone. Also reversibly blocked by halothane, enflurane and isoflurane. β-blockers slow calcium passage at these channels; isoprenaline opens them. Nifedipine reversibly blocks these channels at the sarcoplasmic reticulum with an effect mainly on the arterioles. (*See also* Chapter 19.)

Chloride channels. In the spinal cord these channels are opened by gamma-aminobutyric acid. The resultant chloride flux stabilizes the cell membrane acting as an inhibitor of depolarization.

Acetylcholine-sensitive channels are found at the neuromuscular junction, are glycoproteins and make the membrane permeable to sodium and potassium at the same time. Blocked by non-depolarizing relaxants (*See* Chapter 14.)

Cellular Respiration
Energy production takes place in mitochondria with metabolism of glucose to water and carbon dioxide

$$C_6H_{12}O_6 + 6O_2 \rightarrow 6CO_2 + 6H_2O + energy \text{ (approx. 33 high-energy bonds)}$$

There are two phases in this reaction.

1. Anaerobic phase: glucose → pyruvate (+ approx. 3 high-energy bonds)

2. Aerobic phase: pyruvate $\rightarrow$ CO_2 + H_2O (+ approx. 30 high-energy bonds)

Hypoxia (PaO_2 < 4 kPa, 30 mmHg) prevents aerobic metabolism of pyruvate, which is instead converted to lactate. The normal blood lactate/pyruvate ratio of 10 thus rises to 40 or more. Other anaerobic metabolites of pyruvate are also affected, e.g. the 3-hydroxybutyrate/acetoacetate ratio rises from 2·7 to 10 or 15 in lactic acidosis. This is an indicator of mitochondrial hypoxia. (*Note:* lactic acidosis also occurs in alcohol intoxication, liver disease, and after fructose, sorbitol and xylitol infusion.)

Muscle Tone

This is the ongoing action of a muscle or group of muscles with the purpose of controlling or preserving some position. It is produced by the gamma loop reflex, in which the muscle stretch is perceived by the muscle spindle receptors, relayed by sensory nerve fibres to the spinal cord, activating the anterior horn cells which in turn stimulate the muscle fibres (seen in the knee-jerk reflex). This simple system is controlled and modified by: (*a*) the gamma efferent nerves which sensitize the muscle spindle receptors. They are controlled from the cerebellum, the cortex, and sensation coming from eyes, ears, joints, skin, tendons, and other muscle groups (e.g. in the opposite limb); (*b*) catecholamines, increasing muscle tone; (*c*) hypoxia, hypotension and anaesthesia, reducing muscle tone; (*d*) hypocalcaemia, alkalosis, tetanus and strychnine, increasing muscle tone.

Sleep

Sleep is a recurrent state of unconsciousness associated with a decreased reponse to external stimuli, from which the patient can readily be aroused.

Two opposing states of sleep are described (Aserinsky E. and Kleitman N. *Science* 1953, **118**, 273; Dement, W. C. and Kleitman N. *Electroencephalogr. Clin. Neurophysiol.* 1957, **34**, 823).

1. Non-rapid eye movement (NREM) sleep where the EEG shows slow waves with bursts of 12–14 Hz spindles and K complexes. Heart and respiration rates are slow, motor tone is reduced. Non-REM sleep has four stages, each lasting 60–90 min, followed by REM sleep lasting 30–60 min. The cycle is repetitive with great variation between individuals.

2. REM sleep when there is a low-voltage EEG pattern with marked muscular relaxation, a rise in the heart and respiration rates, an increase in cerebral blood flow and tumescence of the penis. Dreams occur during REM sleep and this type is necessary for psychic well-being. It is inhibited by barbiturates, amphetamines, imipramine and mono-amine oxidase inhibitors, mood-enhancing drugs, but not by some benzodiazepines, e.g., flurazepam 15–30 mg (Dalmane) and reserpine.

Sleep Abnormalities

Hypersomnia with periodic apnoea includes primary alveolar hypoventilation (Ondine's curse, *see* Chapter 18) and the Pickwickian syndrome. Sleep apnoea with hypopnoea, periodic breathing and oxygen desaturation occurs in normal subjects, almost all of whom are males.[8] More frequent as age advances and in obesity; aggravated by premedication and after anaesthesia.

Pickwickian Syndrome:[6] nocturnal apnoea attacks with loss of sleep, causing day-time tiredness. Due to partial respiratory obstruction associated with obesity, micrognathia, macroglossia in acromegaly, vocal cord paralysis, and enlarged tonsils. May lead to cor pulmonale.[7] May be associated with chronic hypercapnia.

Cerebral Function Monitor
Gives an integrated and simplified version of the EEG in which the level of cortical electrical activity is displayed as recurring upward strokes of a pen on paper. The length of the strokes is related to the sum of cortical activity at that instant. As anaesthesia deepens, for example, the strokes become shorter and the baseline from which they arise is depressed towards a zero potential.

Action of Anaesthetic Agents on the Brain Cells[9]

Theories of Action of Anaesthetic Agents[10]
In clinical concentrations, there is no block of transmission in peripheral nerve fibres. Action is on specialized areas, such as synapses, and possibly on fine unmyelinated terminals. It is possible also that specialized areas of the cell membrane exist which are sensitive to hormones and other chemical agents.

Over the years various attempts have been made to account for the action of anaesthetic agents. Some of the most important theories are:

1. That anaesthetics interfere with intracellular oxidation, possibly by influencing enzyme action (Quastel[11] 1932).

2. That anaesthetic agents are readily absorbed by lipids, hence brain cells are specially susceptible to their action (H. H. Meyer (1853–1939) of Vienna[12] and C. E. Overton (1865–1933) of Zurich).[13] There is a positive correlation between narcotic activity and oil/gas partition coefficient.

3. That anaesthetics cause changes in cell metabolism of a physicochemical nature, e.g. precipitation of colloids (Claude Bernard (1813–1878) of Paris),[14] changes in surface tension, changes in permeability of cell membranes, changes in viscosity, etc.

4. That anaesthetics act by changing electric polarity of cells of the nervous system. Both ether and chloroform reduce the frequency and voltage of action potentials. The brain usually is electronegative to the rest of the organism, but under anaesthesia it becomes more positive.

5. The inert gas effect. Ferguson[15] (1939) postulated that the narcotic potency of inert gases and vapours were inversely proportional to their vapour pressure, provided that they are chemically unreactive. This is roughly true for the common anaesthetic agents, though it does not explain how the brain cells are affected.

6. The hydrate microcrystal theory of anaesthesia by non-hydrogen-bonding agents.[16] This involves primarily the interaction of the molecules of the anaesthetic agent with water molecules in the brain, rather than with molecules of lipids. It is suggested that the anaesthetic molecule acts as a centre about which water molecules form crystals or clones. The crystals might hinder the passage of ions through the cell membrane to impede polarization.

7. The multi-site expansion hypothesis.[17]

None of these theories is wholly satisfactory. Minimum alveolar concentrations (MAC) of anaesthetic agents correlate better with lipid solubility than with hydrate dissociation pressures.[18]

See also Koblin D. D. and Eger E. I. *N. Engl. J. Med.* 1979, **301**, 1222; Richards C. D. in *Topical Reviews in Anaesthesia* (Norman J. and Whitwam J. ed.). Wright: Bristol, 1980; Ueda I. and Kamaya H. *Anesth. Analg.* 1984, **63**, 929; Norman J. *Br. J. Anaesth.* 1983, **55**, 189; Wardley-Smith B., and Halsey M. J. in *Anaesthesia Review, 2.* (Kaufman L. ed.) Edinburgh: Churchill Livingstone, 1983, Ch. 6.

Cerebral Blood Flow
See Chapter 26.

The Cerebrospinal Fluid[19]
The term 'cerebrospinal fluid' was first used by the French physiologist F. Magendie (1783–1855).[20]

CSF pressure. Intracranial pressure is 100–150 mm H_2O above atmospheric. It is closely related to venous rather than arterial pressure. The source of this pressure is the secretory pressure of the choroid plexuses. The CSF pressure has to be sufficient to overcome the flow resistance of the microtubules of the arachnoid villi. Intracranial pressure oscillates with the arterial pulse and also varies with respiration. Pressure falls in inspiration and rises in expiration, and larger changes are produced by coughing, abdominal compression, etc., which cause rises in pressure transmitted from the thorax via the jugular and vertebral veins to the intracranial veins. More prolonged elevation of pressure can be caused by faulty positioning on the operating table, though in time compensation occurs due to increased absorption of CSF. The CSF pressure falls with elevation of the head, but not below atmospheric. It is raised by obstructing the jugular veins, so causing increased intracranial venous pressure (Queckenstedt's test (Hans Queckenstedt, 1876–1918, of Rostock)),[21] and by injections of glucose into the theca (*see* Chapter 26). About 500 ml can be secreted in 24 h if there is a free leak from the subarachnoid space. Changes in the osmotic pressure of the blood affect cerebrospinal fluid pressure.

Source. From the choroid arterial plexuses of the third, fourth and lateral ventricles, by either secretion or ultrafiltration about 0·5 ml/min.

It contains protein derived partly by filtration of serum, partly from brain interstitial fluid and brain cells, and partly from cells in the theca. These proteins can be studied by electrophoresis as to both quality and quantity and this may aid diagnosis of neurological disease.[22]

Removal. Into the venous sinuses of the brain via the arachnoidal villi, and into the lymph stream via the Pacchionian bodies (described by Antonius Pacchioni in 1705). When injected into the subarachnoid space, local analgesic drugs are absorbed into the bloodstream. (*See also* Plum F. and Siejo B. *Anesthesiology* 1975, **47**, 788.)

Physical characteristics. Clear and colourless with slight opalescence due to globulin. Sp. gr. at 37 °C is 1003–1009 (average 1004·5).[23] The viscosity averages 1·006 centipoise[23] the same as normal saline. The density is more dependent on the temperature and on the contained sodium, chloride and carbon dioxide than on the contained protein which is increased in diabetes, uraemia and old age. Poor in cellular elements, five or less/mm^3 (lymphocytes); an increase of cells indicates meningeal irritation. Quantity, 100–160 ml (average 135 ml). Volume of spinal cerebrospinal fluid about 75 ml, 15 ml of which is below T5. P_{CO_2} is 50 mmHg and sodium bicarbonate concentration is about 22 mmol/l.

Chemical characteristics. Protein low, 24–40 mg/100 ml. Sugar, 45–80 mg %
(2·5–4·4 mmol/l); sodium chloride, 7·5 g/l (sodium, 135–147 mmol/l;
chloride, 115–135 mmol/l); urea, 10–30 mg/100 ml (1·75–5·0 mmol/l);
bicarbonate, 24 mmol/l. Antibodies, enzymes, etc., not found in cerebrospinal
fluid, hence great risks of infection.

After spinal analgesia both albumin and globulin increase. Alkalinity and sugar
content lower, magnesium content higher, than in blood.

Functions

1. It is a fluid cushion to protect the brain and spinal cord from trauma.

2. By its absorption and formation, according to need, it regulates the volume
of the cranial contents.

3. It has a function in the metabolic exchanges of nervous tissue and may take
the place of lymph.

Non-inflammatory overproduction—liquorrhoea—is seen in cases of nasal
sinus infection, in otitis, at high altitudes (hypoxia) and after concussion and
lumbar puncture, and elevated $Paco_2$.

The opposite condition is aliquorrhoea and may occur spontaneously in
dehydration, or after lumbar puncture.

Circulation of Cerebrospinal Fluid

Fluid which is formed by the choroid plexuses in the lateral ventricles passes
through, on each side, the foramen of Monro (Alexander Monro (secundus), of
Edinburgh 1733–1817) to join that formed by choroid plexuses in the third
ventricle; thence through aqueduct of Sylvius (1616–1672) to the fourth
ventricle. Fluid leaves this for the subarachnoid space through the central
foramen of Magendie (Francois Magendie, 1783–1855, Parisian physiologist) and
the lateral foramina of Luschka (Hubert von Luschka, 1820–1875, German
anatomist), Key (Ernst A. H. Key, 1832–1901, of Stockholm) and Retzius
(Anders Adolf Retzius, 1842–1919, Stockholm anatomist) and reaches the
cisterna magna. It bathes the whole of the central nervous system and is absorbed
into the venous sinuses through the arachnoidal villi. This circulation takes no part
in spinal analgesia. There is evidence that cerebrospinal fluid passes along spinal
nerves in interaxonal channels within the subperineural space in both centrifugal
and centripetal directions and that the entire central nervous system is surrounded
by a membrane similar to and continuous with the pia-arachnoid.[24]

Ordinary doses of analgesic drugs injected into the spinal subarachnoid space
do not reach the fourth ventricle, which contains in its floor the centres for the
heart and for respiration.

(*See also* O'Connell J. E. A. *Proc. R. Soc. Med.* 1970, **63**, 507; Shantha T. R.
and Evans J. A. *Anesthesiology*, 1972, **37**, 543; Fisher R. G. *Proc. Staff Meet.
Mayo Clin.* 1975, **50**, 482; Bryce-Smith R. *Proc. R. Soc. Med.* 1976, **69**, 75.)

Identification of Fluid following a suspected Dural Tap

1. Temperature. CSF is warm when it falls on to the skin.

2. It forms a cloudy precipitate when it falls into 2·5 per cent thiopentone
solution.[25]

3. The glucose contained in CSF will turn a test strip containing glucose
oxidase, blue.[26]

Local analgesic solution, saline and water all give negative results.

The Blood–brain Barrier

Term coined by Ehrlich (Paul Ehrlich, 1854–1915, of Steglitz and Frankfurt) in 1885. The barrier prevents the uptake of some substances by the brain, as compared with other organs. There is no single membrane or anatomical structure which can be defined as the actual barrier.

Anaesthetic agents. Inhalation agents, thiobarbiturates, local analgesic drugs, etc., freely cross the barrier. When muscle relaxants are given intravenously they are found in the cerebrospinal fluid in extremely low concentration. Physostigmine crosses the blood–brain barrier, neostigmine does not. Atropine and hyoscine cross it more readily than glycopyrronium.

Varieties of Nerve Fibre

There are three main types of nerve fibre:[27]

A Fibres. All medullated somatic nerve fibres of various diameter (1–20 μ). Rate of conduction rapid. Skeletal motor fibres, touch, proprioceptor and some pain and thermal fibres. A fibres may be subdivided into α (70–120 m/s), β (50–70 m/s), γ (30–50 m/s) and δ (less than 30 m/s). α are largest and most rapidly conducting, δ fibres smallest and slowest conducting. The larger fibres develop more current at each node to stimulate the next node. The smallest fibres are most easily affected by drugs. Local analgesic agents block some of the larger fibres before all of the smaller fibres. But if the concentration of local analgesic is kept low enough, all the small fibres will be blocked without affecting the larger fibres. Local analgesics block fibres in the order: C fibres, δ fibres, γ fibres, β fibres, α fibres, and recovery occurs in the reverse order.[28]

B Fibres. Medullated autonomic fibres, i.e. preganglionic fibres, e.g. white rami. Diameter 1–3 μ. Conduction velocity 50–70 m/s.

C Fibres. Non-medullated fibres, both somatic and autonomic. All postganglionic sympathetic motor fibres (grey rami) and some preganglionic. Some afferents convey pain and heat sensation. Diameter less than 1 μ. Visceral afferents are C fibres. Compression blocks A fibres before C fibres, while local analgesics block C fibres before A fibres.

Pain is carried in C fibres and δ fibres. The former conduct at 2 m/s, the latter at up to 40 m/s. The difference in velocity gives rise to the 'dual' appreciation of certain painful stimuli.

Afferent fibres have been classified[29] as: Ia and b, from muscles and tendons (60–120 m/s.); II, all other afferent myelinated fibres with conduction velocity greater than 30, somatic and autonomic; III, all afferent myelinated fibres with conduction velocity less than 30 m/s, somatic and autonomic; IV, all unmyelinated afferent fibres travelling in dorsal roots.

Anoxia lowers threshold of pain fibres. Stimulation of C fibres may cause a fall in blood pressure.

The smaller the fibre the slower the conduction rate, and the more easily will local analgesic drugs produce a block. There is, however, some evidence that large fast conducting fibres are more, not less, susceptible to conduction block by local analgesics than are smaller, slower-conducting fibres.[30] Cold slows the rate of impulse conduction.

The Gate Control Theory of Pain[31]

This theory attempts to correlate physiological and psychological data. A schematic diagram (*Fig. 2.1*) assists in the understanding of the theory. It is

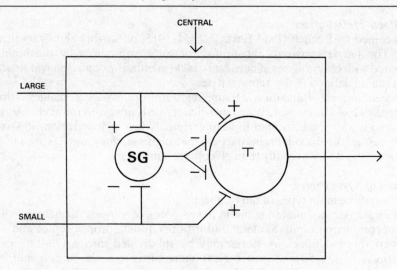

Fig. 2.1. The gate control theory of pain. T, target cells; SG, cells of substantia gelatinosa.

postulated that both large fibres and small fibres act on target cells, the first central transmission cells and also on cells in the substantia gelatinosa. Some substantia gelatinosa (SG) cells have an inhibiting effect on the target cells (T) and so act as a modulator or 'gate' to the onward transmission of the pain impulses. The large fibres stimulate the SG cells and thus close the gate. Central control from the midbrain is also operative, acting on the inhibitory SG cells. Thus prior conditioning (emotions, memory, etc.) can modify the system by opening or closing the 'gate'. The theory, however, does not explain all the known facts.[32]

A careful distinction should be drawn between conscious feeling of pain and motor reaction to a painful stimulus. The integrity of the cerebral cortex is necessary for the full appreciation of pain. Motor reactions to painful stimuli may occur in decorticate animals and in lightly anaesthetized man.

Prostaglandins E_1 and E_2 sensitize the body to pain and histamine, especially in inflammation, acting peripherally. This can be reduced locally by aspirin, indomethacin and diflunisal. Other prostaglandins act centrally to sensitize the body to pain. Paracetamol crosses the blood–brain barrier and reduces this activity. There is synergism between the actions of aspirin and paracetamol. Opiates reduce appreciation of pain by occupying central encephalin receptors. Acupuncture may promote encephalin secretion.

Autonomic Nervous System

The autonomic nervous system is important to the anaesthetist on several counts:

1. Its role in the physiology of the cardiovascular system, with maintenance of cardiac output and arterial pressure.

2. The adrenergic and cholinergic effects of many anaesthetic agents.

3. The specific blocking effects of certain drugs.

4. The ability of the anaesthetist to block certain autonomic pathways with local analgesic agents.

History[33]
For History, *see* the 9th edition of this Synopsis, page 43.

Anatomy
All efferent fibres from the central nervous system other than those supplying skeletal muscle are autonomic. These fibres make synaptic connections with the cell bodies of peripheral neurons, and these synapses are usually collected into ganglia from which postganglionic fibres, generally unmyelinated, are distributed to effector organs.

Autonomic transmission controls smooth muscle in vessels and viscera, specialized muscle in the heart and uterus, the secretion of salivary, mucous and eccrine sweat glands, together with the activity of the medulla of the adrenals.

Anatomically the sympathetic outflow extends from the first thoracic to the second or third lumbar segments of the cord. In each segment the connector cells in the intermediolateral horn send off fibres which leave with the anterior nerve roots. The fibres travel across the subarachnoid and extradural spaces, form part of the mixed spinal nerve and the anterior primary ramus, and then as *white rami* join the corresponding paravertebral ganglion of the sympathetic chain. Here they may end, synapsing with an excitor cell and being continued as a postganglionic fibre, or may pass, uninterrupted, through the ganglion to synapse with an excitor cell in a collateral ganglion (abdomen) or other paravertebral ganglion (e.g. superior cervical ganglion). In the thoracic region each white ramus measures about 1 cm in length; this increases to 2–3 cm in the lumbar region.

Craniosacral Outflow (Parasympathetic)
Parasympathetic nerve fibres come from the midbrain, the medulla and the sacral cord. Axons of these cells which are preganglionic and medullated, connect with ganglion cells very near the organs they innervate and from these, postganglionic fibres arise which are non-medullated; hence the midbrain (or tectal), bulbar and sacral outflows. Tectal fibres come from the Westphal–Erdinger nucleus of the 3rd nerve in the floor of the cerebral aqueduct, and go to the ciliary ganglion from which postganglionic fibres then proceed as the short ciliary nerves to the sphincter pupillae and ciliary muscles, controlling the size of the pupil and the canal of Schlemm. Bulbar outflow leave in the 7th, 9th and 10th nerves, the 7th and 9th being responsible for secretion of saliva; the 10th nerve wanders into the abdomen and provides inhibitory fibres for thoracic and abdominal visceral muscles and secretions.

The vagus is important to the anaesthetist, as it is not blocked by spinal analgesia. Stimulation of the vagal nerve endings, e.g. in the stomach during gastrectomy, results in discomfort to a conscious patient, an effect removed by the infiltration of a local analgesic into the paraoesophageal tissues near the cardia.

Sacral fibres leave the cord with the 2nd, 3rd, sometimes 4th, sacral nerves. They leave in the cauda equina, and after the anterior sacral rami have passed through the anterior sacral foramina the white rami are given off. As pelvic nerves or nervi erigentes, one on each side, they do not pass through the sacral sympathetic chain, but run direct to the hypogastric ganglia and thence to the pelvic viscera. Their postganglionic or excitor fibres are given off from cells in the walls of the genitalia, bladder and rectum. They cause contraction of the hollow viscera, relaxation of sphincters and vasodilatation. In addition, visceral afferents travel with these nerves.

Sympathetic chain. This is composed of three cervical, eleven thoracic, four lumbar and four sacral ganglia. The chain receives white rami from T1 to L2, while from it every one of the spinal nerves receives a grey ramus communicans, which is composed of excitor or postganglionic fibres. The grey rami carry pilomotor and vasomotor impulses, and secretory impulses to the sweat glands. They reach their destinations via spinal nerves and blood vessels.

Distribution of Vasoconstrictor Fibres

Head. Preganglionic fibres from the 1st, 2nd and 3rd thoracic segments are distributed to the stellate and superior cervical ganglia, thence to (1) The vertebral nerve, a plexus surrounding the vertebral and basilar arteries. (2) The internal carotid, external carotid, and middle meningeal arteries. (3) The cervical plexus. (4) The last four cranial nerves.

Parasympathetic. Vasodilator nerves leave the brain with the 7th nerve and, at geniculate ganglion, enter the greater superficial petrosal nerve from which fibres travel with the internal carotid artery and its branches.

Arm. Preganglionic fibres arise in lateral horn cells of 2nd to 7th thoracic segments (some authorities say T3 to T7; others, T5 to T9), ascend in the sympathetic trunk to the middle cervical, stellate and 2nd and 3rd thoracic ganglia, via the axillary artery and brachial plexus and thence to vessels of arm. There may be a small grey ramus, the nerve of Kuntz (1879–1957),[34] coming from the 2nd thoracic sympathetic ganglion direct to the lowest trunk of the brachial plexus, via the 1st thoracic nerve, so by-passing the stellate ganglion. A similar nerve described by Kirgis and Kuntz connects the 2nd and 3rd thoracic nerves. Hence to block all vasoconstrictors of arm there must be block of the 2nd and 3rd thoracic ganglia. If the stellate ganglion alone is blocked, Kuntz's nerve is missed; if brachial plexus alone is blocked, fibres going to the axillary artery escape.

Thoracic and abdominal wall. Preganglionic fibres arise in lateral horn of corresponding segment of cord and are distributed to spinal nerves as grey rami.

Leg. Preganglionic fibres arise in lateral horn cells of T10 to L2, pass out with anterior roots and white rami to corresponding ganglia, and descend in sympathetic chain to synapse with cells in L1–3 ganglia for upper part of limb, and with cells in L4 and L5 ganglia for lower part of limb. The third lumbar ganglion is of practical importance as it sends a grey ramus to the 4th lumbar nerve and hence to the inner side of the foot via the femoral and saphenous nerves.

Blocking of the 2nd and 3rd ganglia interrupts sympathetic impulses to whole of limb. Blocking of the 1st lumbar ganglion on each side will cause temporary impotence; extirpation will produce permanent sterility in the male.

Thorax. Preganglionic fibres from T1 to T6, passing in sympathetic chain to upper five thoracic ganglia and lower, middle and upper cervical ganglia, where they synapse. Postganglionic fibres are the three cardiac nerves from the cervical ganglia to the cardiac plexus, which also receives postganglionic fibres direct from the upper five or six thoracic sympathetic ganglia. The efferent fibres to the lungs come from T2 to T6 or T7 and synapse in the stellate and upper thoracic ganglia from which fibres pass to the posterior pulmonary plexus. The oesophagus derives its nerve supply from T4 to T6.

Visceral Afferent Fibres carrying pain from the heart and aorta (T1–T5) accompany the cervical and thoracic cardiac nerves and enter the cord via the white rami of the upper five thoracic nerves, to have their cell stations in the corresponding posterior root ganglia.

Abdomen. Preganglionic fibres from T5 to L2. These pass through the ganglia of the sympathetic chain to form the three splanchnic nerves. Synapse occurs in the coeliac (solar) plexus, from which postganglionic fibres reach the viscera with the arteries.

Afferent Side of the Autonomic System

There are afferent autonomic pathways carrying painful impulses from the viscera and probably from the limbs,[35] with cell stations in the posterior root ganglia of the spinal nerves. They are similar to somatic afferent fibres—are not divided into pre-and postganglionic neurons. They travel with autonomic nerves. All the fibres enter the cord between T1 and L3, except those from the bladder, rectum, prostate, cervix uteri and lower colon, which pass to the cord via nervi erigentes. For details of the nerve supply of the uterus *see* Chapter 27.

(*See also* Newman P. P. *Visceral Afferent Function of the Nervous System*. London: Arnold, 1974; and for anatomy *see* Johnson R. H. and Spalding J. M. K. *Disorders of the Autonomic Nervous System*. Oxford: Blackwell, 1974.)

Physiology of Autonomic System

The thoracico-lumbar outflow, the sympathetic, produces widespread diffuse effects. It activates the body for defence and is catabolic.

The craniosacral outflow, the parasympathetic, produces localized effects and is anabolic. When an organ is innervated by both systems they are synergistic in effect.

The cranial parasympathetic supplies the heart and the gut with its outgrowths; it is motor and secretory to the alimentary canal and constrictor to the pupil (3rd cranial nerve via ciliary ganglion and short ciliary nerves). The sacral parasympathetic is a mechanism for emptying, i.e. motor for bladder, rectum and erection of penis. The sacral sympathetic, on the other hand, causes contraction of the smooth muscle in the bladder neck, prostate and seminal vesicles; inhibition of peristalsis in the lower colon; contraction of internal anal sphincter; and vasoconstriction.

Functions of sympathetic system. (1) Inhibitory fibres to smooth muscle of alimentary canal and constrictor fibres to the sphincters; (2) Vasoconstrictor fibres to vessels of skin and splanchnic area; (3) Vasodilator fibres to muscle and coronary vessels; (4) Accelerator and augmentor fibres to the heart (chronotropic and inotropic); (5) Secretory fibres to sweat glands; (6) Pilomotor fibres; (7) Dilator fibres to bronchial tree; (8) Dilator fibres to the pupil; (9) Secretory fibres to the adrenal gland (medulla); (10) Inhibitory fibres to bladder wall and constrictor fibres to internal urinary sphincter; fibres to other pelvic viscera.

The Heart

The Electrocardiogram

Augustus Desirè Waller (1856–1922), head of the Physiology Department at St Mary's Hospital, London, first recorded, in 1887, the electric current which precedes muscular contraction of the heart.[36] He was one of the first two physicians appointed to the National Heart Hospital, London. Development of the string galvanometer (Einthoven, the Leyden physiologist (1860–1927), in 1903)[37] led to clinical and experimental studies of the electrocardiogram. Sir

Thomas Lewis (1881–1945) of University College Hospital, London, published his pioneering book in 1911, *The Mechanism and Graphic Reproduction of the Heart Beat*. The cathode-ray oscillograph was first used in ECG by Dock in 1929.[38] Auricular flutter was first described in 1910 by Wm Adam Jolly (1877–1939) and Wm Thos Ritchie (1873–1945), both of London,[39] auricular fibrillation, by Sir James Mackenzie (1853–1925) of Burnley and London in 1908,[40] pulsus alternans by Ludwig Traube (1818–1876) of Berlin in 1872[41] and gallop rhythm by Pierre C. E. Potain (1825–1901) of Paris 3 years later. Other pioneers of ECG were H. B. Williams in the USA and Karl Frederik Wenkebach (1864–1970) in Vienna.

For historical development of electrocardiography, *see* Howell J. D. *Bull. Hist. Med.* 1984, **58**, 83, and Comroe J. H. and Dripps R. D. *Science* 1976, **192**, 115.

Pioneers of the use of ECG in anaesthesia have included J. B. Heard and A. E. Strauss,[42] E. B. Krumbhaar,[43] and Michael Johnstone.[44]

The Standard Leads

Bipolar recordings measure the differences in electrical potential produced by the heart beat at two separate points of the body:

Lead I: Between right and left arms.

Lead II: Between right arm and left leg.

Lead III: Between left arm and left leg.

Unipolar recordings are made when one electrode remains at zero potential and the other measures electrical potential produced by the heart beat:

aVL, from the left arm.

aVR, from the right arm.

aVF, from the left leg.

The series of waves obtained are arbitrarily designated as the P wave, the QRS complex, the T wave and the U wave.

P Wave: Does not normally exceed 0·11 s. Represents the depolarization wave of the auricle.

P–R Segment: Represents the delay in transmission at the AV node.

P–R Interval: From beginning of P wave to beginning of QRS complex. Normal upper limit of duration 0·20 s.

QRS Complex: The depolarization complex of the ventricular muscle. Does not normally exceed 0·10 s.

S–T Segment: Represents the depolarized state, or the duration of the excited state of the ventricles.

T Wave: Ventricular repolarization.

U Wave: An 'after-potential' wave, usually of low amplitude.

Precordial Leads

The unipolar chest lead is placed in various positions over the chest wall:

V_1, fourth right interspace at margin of sternum.

V_2, fourth left interspace at margin of sternum.

V_3, midway between V_2 and V_4.

V_4, fifth left interspace at midclavicular line.

V_5, left anterior axillary line in horizontal line from V_4.

V_6, left mid-axillary line in same horizontal line.

Chest Leads

Introduced in 1932[45] these are popular in coronary care and intensive therapy units since they can be attached to the patient with little disturbance. The exact position is seldom important since they are used as monitors for abnormal rhythm rather than for accurate diagnosis. Unipolar limb leads were described by Goldberger.[46]

Interpretation of ECG
(1) Rate; (2) Rhythm; (3) Specific abnormalities. The common abnormalities encountered are ectopic beats, acute ischaemia, atrial fibrillation, asystole and ventricular strain, tachycardia or fibrillation.

The Cardiac Output (*see also* Chapter 41)
Determined by:

1. The Venous Return (Ventricular Preload)
Venous filling of the heart during diastole depends on the following: (*a*) The venous tone, controlled by vasomotor nerves, and chemical factors such as anaesthetics, blood oxygen and carbon dioxide tension, and amount of adrenaline and noradrenaline in the blood; (*b*) Negative pressure in the thorax during inspiration; (*c*) Contraction of the diaphragm causing descent and squeezing out of blood from the abdomen towards the heart; (*d*) Tone of the arterioles, capillaries, etc., which may contain much or little blood; (*e*) Gravity; (*f*) Muscular activity (muscle pump). The effect of venous return on cardiac output is summed up by Starling's (1866–1927) law of the heart.[47] 'The more the myocardial fibres are stretched during diastole, the more forcibly they will contract during subsequent systole, and therefore more blood will be expelled.'

2. Myocardial Contractility
This is defined in terms of the relationship between the velocity of shortening of the muscle fibres and the tension they develop. These are interrelated and are important because of the work and power the myocardium will produce. Work = force × distance. Power = force × velocity. More than 80% of the work of the left ventricle is expended in generating pressure of blood in the aorta and only a small fraction to produce forward movement of the mass of blood ejected at each systole (about 70 ml). Contractility is affected by: (*a*) The sympathetic nervous system. Increase in activity or in circulating catecholamines increases contractility; (*b*) Positive inotropic drugs, e.g. sympathomimetic agents, digitalis; (*c*) Negative inotropic drugs, e.g. quinidine, lignocaine, thiopentone, halothane; (*d*) Physiological depressants, e.g. hypoxia, hypercapnia, acidaemia; (*e*) Ventricular integrity; an abnormal area due to disease such as ischaemia or myopathy.
Assessment of myocardial contractility
   1. Clinical. Adequacy of perfusion and organ function. Peripheral and pulmonary oedema, jugular venous pressure, blood pressure.
   2. Cardiac output measurement (*see* Chapter 41).
   3. Left ventricular pressure/volume/flow/time measurement. The basic parameters are: (A) *Force of contraction* (relates to pressure generated); (B) *Length* (distance of shortening of muscle fibre, related to volume); (C) *Velocity* (rate of change of length of pressure). Various measurements give views of these parameters, but no one measurement gives a total description of contractility (inotropy): (*a*) *Starling's law of the heart*—states that the force of contraction of a

muscle fibre is directly proportional to its resting length (within limits);[47] (b) *Left ventricular change of pressure with time.* (LV dP/dT) Improved by: increase in preload, increase in afterload, and increase in heart rate. The maximum rate of change, LV dP/dTmax, is the relevant measurement. From a simple intraventricular pressure measurement with time, the derivative dP/dT with time gives the time taken to reach dP/dTmax from the start of the contraction phase. The shorter this time, the better the inotropy; (c) *Non-invasive analysis of the pre-ejection period* (PEP). The total active electromechlical time (TAEMT) is from the Q wave of the ECG to the closure of the aortic valve (first deflection of the second heart sound on the phonocardiograph). If the actual ejection time is subtracted from this, the difference is the pre-ejection period which correlates very well with other measures of inotropy. The actual ejection time is measured with a force transducer over the carotid artery; (d) *Circumferential velocity of shortening* (V_{CF}). Measured by echocardiography, in two dimensions. The trans-oesophageal route has been used.[48] It varies directly with heart rate and inversely with afterload; (e) The *ejection fraction* (normally 60–75%). This is the percentage of the diastolic content of the left ventricle that is ejected in systole.

3. The Cardiac Rate
Slowed by vagus action, speeded by sympathetic action. The heart rate may be less than 40 in 25% of normal healthy students while asleep. The mechanisms of bradycardia evoked by various reflexes act only during expiration. Bradycardia due to nasopharyngeal stimulation or pressure on the eyeball can be corrected by increasing the frequency and amplitude of IPPV or of voluntary respiration.[49] (*See also* Rawlinson A. L. et al. *Anaesthesia* 1979, **34**, 534.)

4. The Arterial Blood Pressure and Total Peripheral Resistance
These influence the output of the heart directly (through effect on venous return and venous pressure) and reflexly. *Ventricular after-load* is the ventricular wall tension developed during systolic ejection. It is frequently and usefully equated with peripheral arterial resistance. *Preload* is the left ventricular end-diastolic pressure (LVEDP). An increase in the preload always increases myocardial oxygen demand while reducing oxygen supply.

For management of blood viscosity *see* Dodds A. J. *Br. J. Clin. Equip.* 1979, **4**, 224.

5. Effect of Anaesthetic Drugs on the Myocardium (see Chapter 10)
The sarcomere, the basic intracellular unit of work production from ATP hydrolysis, has the following structure:

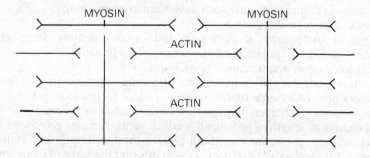

The sarcolemma is continuous with the cell membrane and is rich in calcium channels. The sarcoplasmic reticulum connects the sarcolemma more intimately with the contractile elements. Upon depolarization, calcium channels open and calcium ions enter the cytoplasm, binding with the troponin/tropomyosin complexes between actin and myosin, initiating cross-linking between these two proteins with forcible shortening of the sarcomere.

Arterial Blood Pressure
The blood pressure is the pressure of blood on the arterial walls, the systolic blood pressure, normally 120 mmHg, being the maximal pressure during propulsion of blood, the diastolic pressure, normally 80 mmHg, is the minimal pressure occurring at the end of diastole. The difference between them is the pulse pressure. Depends on: (1) Cardiac output; (2) Peripheral resistance. These are regulated reflexly by baroreceptors of the carotid sinus and aortic arch. The cardiac rate/pressure product correlates poorly with myocardial oxygen consumption during anaesthesia in patients with coronary disease.[50] Mean arterial pressure is diastolic plus roughly one third of the pulse pressure. It has recently undergone a revival of interest, and is usually displayed on automatic oscillotonometers.

Venous Pressure
Venous pressure depends on venous tone and blood volume and can easily be measured by simple water manometer (*see* Chapter 41). Central venous pressure in the great veins is normally 2–8 mmHg (3–10 cm H_2O) and peripheral venous pressure some 8 mmHg higher than this. CVP is raised by the Trendelenburg tilt, fluid infusions, IPPV, coughing, vomiting, straining, heart failure, the Valsalva manoeuvre[51] and catecholamines. It is lowered by sitting and standing upright, hypovolaemia, tachycardia and reduction of venous tone by unconsciousness, thiopentone, ganglion blockers, histamine, nitrites and nitroprusside. The central venous pressure is a measure of the competence of the right heart and the ability of the right ventricle to deal with venous return. Its measurement enables a distinction to be made between blood loss (low CVP) and heart failure (high CVP). It is especially indicated in old age, when large volumes of blood or fluid are being given, in patients with compromised cardiac function, in multiple injury and when a phaeochromocytoma is being removed.

Blood Volume
The normal blood volume may be taken as 85 ml/kg or 7·7% of body weight.[52] These values should be reduced by 10% in the short obese subject and in the elderly patient.[53] Otherwise it can be obtained from formulae, depending on height and weight,[54] or from nomograms. About half the total blood volume is contained by the systemic venous system.

Coronary Circulation
The normal coronary flow is about 250 ml/min or 5% of the resting cardiac output. The volume of oxygen consumed by the myocardium at rest is 40 ml/min or 15% of total body oxygen consumption. Blood flow through the coronary arteries is continuous throughout the cardiac cycle, about two-thirds occurring in diastole. The coronary sinus drains 90% of the blood from the left ventricle. Blood from the right ventricle drains into the cardiac veins of Adam Christian Thebesius (1686–1732), German physician.

Vagal stimulation has no direct effect on the coronary circulation. Sympathetic stimulation may have a slight vasoconstrictor effect. Increased coronary flow during sympathetic stimulation is a result of increased cardiac work. Coronary flow increases if cardiac output increases, and as a result of exercise. Angiotensin and vasopressin have a vasoconstrictor action. Adrenaline has a slight β-stimulating dilator effect. Other dilators include xanthine derivatives, papaverine, atebrine, ephedrine, amyl nitrite, sodium nitrite and nitroglycerin.

Cerebral Circulation
See Chapter 26.

Cardiac Product (Double Product, Rate-pressure Product)
This is an approximate but useful clinical concept. It is the product of systolic blood pressure and pulse rate and gives a rough indication of cardiac work load, useful for predicting angina levels in those with coronary artery stenosis. 20 000 is a reasonable upper limit in normal adults, 15 000 being more appropriate for patients with cardiac disease.

Pulmonary Circulation
The principal function of the pulmonary circulation is gas exchange. Flow of blood through the lungs approximates to that of the systemic circulation. Pulmonary arterial pressure is about one-sixth of systemic value. The pulmonary blood volume is of the order of 500 ml, about 20% of which constitutes a large capillary volume.

Pulmonary vascular pressures are affected by: (1) Posture. Since the pressure is lower than the systemic it is affected by gravity, so that there are differences between the apex and the base of the lung in the erect position. (2) Exercise results in increased pulmonary blood flow and moderate rise of pressure in the supine, but not in the erect position. Thus in the erect posture there is relatively more air flow at the apex of the lung and relatively more blood flow at the base of the lung. Carried to an unreal extreme, there would be air flow into unperfused alveoli at the apex (dead space), and blood flow to unventilated alveoli at the lung bases (shunting without oxygenation). These concepts of dead space and shunt actually occur to a smaller extent than at the above extremes. Normally the lung shows a mixture of positions between these two extremes. However, fully oxygenated blood flowing from ventilated alveoli cannot fully compensate for desaturated blood flowing from closed alveoli into the pulmonary veins. The resulting mixture of blood will only be partly oxygenated. Thus, shunting has a more severe effect on oxygen uptake. Shunting occurs in pneumonia, Mendelsson's syndrome, pneumonitis, ARDS, one-lung anaesthesia. Hypoxic pulmonary vasoconstriction in the shunted area does, however, tend to reduce the shunt. Hypoxic pulmonary vasoconstriction acts both globally and locally in the lungs and shuts down the blood flow to collapsed or unventilated areas, reducing shunt. It may be mediated by 'slow-reacting substance'.[55] The effect of shunting of blood on CO_2 elimination is less severe because the normally ventilated and perfused alveoli in other parts of the lung can compensate for the shunted areas thanks to the smooth slope of the CO_2 solubility curve in blood.

The 'shunt equation' for calculating pulmonary shunt from oxygen content of blood and alveoli is:

$$\frac{Qs}{Qt} = \frac{Cco_2 - Cao_2}{Cco_2 - Cvo_2}$$

where Qs is the shunted blood, Qt is the total pulmonary blood flow, Cco_2 is the alveolar capillary oxygen content, Cao_2 is the arterial oxygen content and Cvo_2 is the mixed venous oxygen content. Cco_2 is measured via the end-tidal alveolar oxygen content.

Total dead space is derived from the Bohr equation:

$$\frac{Vd}{Ve} = \frac{Paco_2 - Peco_2}{Paco_2}$$

where Vd = dead space, Ve = expired volume, $Paco_2$ = arterial CO_2 tension, and $Peco_2$ = mixed expired CO_2 tension.

A pulmonary shunt reduces the rate of gas uptake more with an insoluble agent, pulmonary dead space reduces the rate of gas uptake more with a soluble agent;[56] Capillary blood flow may be blocked by arteriolar constriction, embolus, or excessive alveolar pressure. Blockage to air flow may be caused by mucus or bronchoconstriction. (3) Intra-alveolar pressure changes up to about 8 mmHg cause an equal change in pulmonary arterial pressure. It rises during a Valsalva manoeuvre;[57] (4) Hypoxia. This results in rise of pulmonary arterial pressure. This autoregulation greatly reduces the amount of blood shunted in underventilated parts of the lung (the bases in the erect posture, the dependent lung in the lateral posture, blocked alveoli, and the clamped lung in one-lung anaesthesia; (5) Acidaemia due to respiratory or metabolic acidosis causes a rise in pulmonary arterial pressure; (6) Disease: (*a*) Mitral stenosis and incompetence, (*b*) Chronic lung disease, (*c*) Pulmonary embolus, (*d*) Left-to-right shunts as in patent ductus arteriosus. At alveolar level the capillaries are autoregulated by the local alveolar oxygen tension, closing when it falls. This effect is blocked by atropine. For Swan-Ganz catheters *see* Chapter 41.

The Respiratory System

The respiratory system exists for exchange of gases between blood and the environment. It is important to the anaesthetist since a large number of anaesthetic drugs are given by inhalation. The anaesthetist is also responsible for adequate oxygenation of the patient[58] both during and immediately after the operation. Since the normal mechanism of ventilation is disturbed during clinical anaesthesia, knowledge of the anatomy and physiology of respiration is essential to the anaesthetist.

Anatomy

Larynx
The organ of voice, the sphincter between the pharynx and trachea. It extends from the root of the tongue to the trachea (*Fig. 2.2*). It is opposite the 3rd, 4th, 5th and 6th cervical vertebrae; higher in children and in females. The average length is 44 mm in males, 36 mm in females; transverse diameter 43 mm in males, 41 mm in females; its anteroposterior diameter averages 36 mm in males and 26 mm in females. It is covered by the depressor muscles of the hyoid bone, by

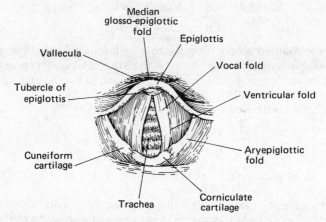

Fig. 2.2 A laryngoscopic view of the interior of the larynx.
(*From 'Gray's Anatomy', by kind permission of Professor T. B. Johnston.*)

the thyroid gland and by the cricothyroid muscles. Composed of the following cartilages, joined together by ligaments; thyroid, cricoid, two arytenoid, two corniculate (Santorini), two cuneiform (Wrisberg) and the epiglottis.

The cavity of the larynx extends from the superior laryngeal aperture to the lower border of the cricoid cartilage, when it is continuous with the trachea. The *piriform fossa* is a recess, on each side, bounded by the aryepiglottic fold medially and the thyroid cartilage and thyrohyoid membrane laterally. Beneath its mucosa lie twigs of the internal laryngeal nerve, which are blocked when local analgesic solutions are applied to this area. The depression between the dorsum of the tongue and the epiglottis is divided into two valleculae by the glosso-epiglottic fold. The epiglottis is not essential for swallowing, breathing, or phonation.

The entrance to the larynx or superior laryngeal aperture is wider in front than behind, and slopes downwards and backwards. Bounded anteriorly by the epiglottis; laterally by the aryepiglottic folds containing the two small nodules on each side, cuneiform anteriorly and the corniculate posteriorly; posteriorly by the arytenoids. This view is seen by laryngoscope. The vestibule of the larynx is the superior part of the cavity of the larynx and extends from the aryepiglottic folds to the vestibular (ventricular) folds. Each of the latter is a ridge formed by the vestibular ligament and extends from the angle of the thyroid cartilage anteriorly, backwards along the side cavity of the larynx to the cuneiform cartilage. The vestibular folds are the false cords, the space between them is the rima vestibuli, while a depression on the side-wall of the larynx between the vestibular fold and the vocal fold (false and true cords) is the saccule of the larynx.

The vocal cords (folds) stretch from the thyroid cartilage anteriorly, to the arytenoid cartilage of the corresponding side posteriorly. The space between the cords is the glottis. It is bounded in front by the intermembranous part of the cords—the vocal folds: behind, by the intercartilaginous part. The glottis is the narrowest part of the larynx in adults and measures about 2·5 cm from front to back: less in females. In children, the narrowest part is found just below the cords at the cricoid ring. The shape and width of the glottis vary with phonation and respiration and the tone of the muscles controlling it. When these are in spasm, the glottis is obliterated.

Muscles. The extrinsic muscles are the thyrohyoid and the sternothyroid and the inferior constrictor of the pharynx. The first elevates, the second depresses the larynx, while the third constricts the pharynx.

The intrinsic muscles: Those which open and close the glottis: (1) The posterior (open) and lateral crico-arytenoids (close); (2) The interarytenoid.

Those controlling the tension of the cords: (1) The cricothyroids are tensors of the cords; (2) The posterior crico-arytenoids; (3) The thyroarytenoids are relaxers of the cords; (4) The vocales.

Those controlling the inlet of the larynx: (1) The aryepiglottics; (2) The thyroepiglottics. In laryngeal spasm both the true and the false cords are adducted.

The lowest part of the larynx extends from the vocal folds or cords to the cricoid cartilage. The mucosa of the upper part of the larynx is lined by squamous cells like the oropharynx; the part above the cords by ciliated epithelium; the cords are covered by a thin layer of mucosa, closely adherent to them, white in colour. The lower larynx is lined by ciliated epithelium with mucous glands and goblet cells.

Nerve supply from the vagus. (For anatomy of vagus nerve, *see* Chapter 31.) *The superior laryngeal branch* of the vagus arises near the base of the skull and divides into the *internal laryngeal nerve*, the sensory nerve of the larynx, down to the level of the vocal cords and the *external laryngeal nerve* which supplies the cricothyroid muscle and the inferior constrictor of the pharynx, the division taking place slightly below and anterior to the greater cornu of the hyoid bone. The external laryngeal nerve may be injured during the ligation of the superior thyroid vessels, during thyroidectomy, such injury causing temporary huskiness of voice. The *recurrent laryngeal branch* supplies the remaining intrinsic muscles and the mucosa below the cords.[59] It carries abductor and adductor fibres, but if it is injured abductor paralysis is greater than adductor paralysis. With bilateral recurrent laryngeal nerve paralysis, there is respiratory difficulty as the cords lie together, and speech is difficult with a valve-like obstruction and inspiratory stridor. The inferior surface of the epiglottis gets its nerve supply from the internal laryngeal. The sensory supply from the larynx ascends in the internal and recurrent laryngeal nerves to the nucleus solitarius in the medulla.

1. Incomplete paralysis of a recurrent laryngeal nerve may cause paralysis of abductor before that of adductor muscles and results in respiratory distress from adduction of cords when bilateral.

2. Complete paralysis of recurrent nerve inactivates both abductor and adductor muscles. The tensing action of the cricothyroid muscles maintains cords in adduction.

3. Paralysis of both recurrent and superior laryngeal nerves together produces the cadaveric position. The cadaveric position, also seen when relaxants have had a full effect, is characterized by the cords being midway between abduction and adduction; they are not under tension due to cricothyroid paralysis. Paralysis of one cord may be symptomless. Paralysis of both is serious and may require surgery, *see* Chapter 24.

Topical analgesia of the larynx may, by paralysing twigs from the external laryngeal nerves going to the cricothyroids, cause both an alteration in the appearance of the cords and an alteration in the voice.

Movements of Larynx.[60] During inspiration, cords abduct. On expiration they return nearly to the midline. On phonation they actually touch.

Arteries are the laryngeal branches of the superior and inferior thyroid arteries. They accompany the nerves.

Trachea

Length about 10–11 cm. It commences at the level of the 6th cervical vertebra and ends by dividing into the two bronchi at the carina, level of the 5th thoracic vertebra. Anteriorly, this corresponds with the junction of the body and manubrium sterni—the angle of Louis. In children, carina is on a level with 3rd costal cartilage. The diameter of the trachea is about 1·5–2 cm; much smaller in the child, e.g. 3 mm during first year of life, and thereafter the diameter in mm corresponds to the age in years.

Abnormal narrowing of the trachea in its middle third, making it difficult to introduce a tube of adequate size, has been reported.[61] Abnormal dilatation of the trachea has also been described in a patient with chronic bronchial infection, treated by tracheostomy and insertion of a cuffed tube.[62] High tracheal bifurcation and deformity may cause problems during intubation.[63]

Tracheostomy should be done below the first tracheal ring, to avoid stenosis.

Blood supply. Upper two-thirds are supplied by the inferior thyroid artery, lower one-third by the bronchial arteries. The arteries run circumferentially and there are few anastomoses in the long axis of the trachea.

For diagram of bronchial tree, *see* Chapter 29.

Right Bronchus

Shorter and more in line with the trachea than the left bronchus; enters the right lung opposite the 5th thoracic vertebra; greater in diameter than left bronchus— hence a long tube or a foreign body passes more easily into it than into the left bronchus. The main upper lobe bronchus, given off within 2 cm of the commencement, arises above the right pulmonary artery and was accordingly called the eparterial bronchus. The opening is on a level with the carina. The right bronchus leaves the trachea at an angle of 25° from the vertical.

Left Bronchus

Narrower, but longer, than the right. Length before dividing into upper and lower lobe bronchi, 5 cm. The aorta arches over it and it enters the left lung opposite the 6th thoracic vertebra. It leaves the trachea at an angle of about 45° from the vertical. In children under 3 years, the right and left main bronchi branch from the trachea at equal angles.

Bronchial Tree

This subdivides progressively, the terminal bronchioles being the last twigs. Air is carried by these twigs to the 'leaves' of the tree, where active interchange of gases is carried on. The respiratory unit is composed of respiratory bronchioles, alveolar ducts and sacs, and pulmonary alveoli. These, together, form a primary lobule. Air in the alveoli is separated from blood in the capillaries by two thin layers of cells, the capillary and alveolar walls. Estimated area of respiratory epithelium—55 m^2 or over twenty-five times the skin area.

Elastic tissue is plentiful right down to the alveoli. Recoil of the lung during expiration is probably due to this tissue.

Muscular fibres surround the air ducts, stopping at the end of the respiratory bronchioles. When strongly contracted they have a sphincter-like action: they also produce a peristaltic movement, to remove irritating foreign matter. This peristaltic action is depressed by morphine.

Bronchial arteries from the thoracic aorta (one for the right, two for the left lung) supply as far as the end of the respiratory bronchioles. Distal to this, blood supply is from the pulmonary artery. There is a communication between the bronchial arteries and the pulmonary veins. The bronchial vessels are more under neural control than the pulmonary vessels.

Nerve supply. Each vagus passes to the back of the hilum and is joined by branches of the sympathetic, from the 2nd to the 4th or 5th thoracic sympathetic ganglia, and also from the inferior and middle cervical ganglia, forming the anterior and posterior pulmonary plexuses. From there, fibres go to the main bronchi and the pulmonary artery, and their branches.

Motor nerves are from the vagus (constriction) and the sympathetic (dilatation). Afferent impulses pass along the vagus.

Lining mucosa is of ciliated epithelium. The cilia have a wave-like motion resembling a cornfield in a breeze. The direction is upwards towards the mouth. The respiratory bronchioles are devoid of cilia, but above this level they are plentiful and act most efficiently. They are not under nervous control. Action depressed by general anaesthetics.

Nomenclature[64]
The right lung
A. *The Right Upper Lobe*. (1) The apical bronchus and segment; (2) The posterior bronchus and segment; (3) The anterior bronchus and segment.

B. *The Middle Lobe*. (4) The lateral bronchus and segment; (5) The medial bronchus and segment.

C. *The Lower Lobe*. (6) The apical bronchus and segment; (7) The medial basal (cardiac) bronchus and segment; (8) The anterior basal bronchus and segment; (9) The lateral basal bronchus and segment; (10) The posterior basal bronchus and segment.

The left lung
A. *The Left Upper Lobe*. Upper division bronchus: (1) The apical bronchus and segment; (2) The posterior bronchus and segment; (3) The anterior bronchus and segment. The lingula (lower division) bronchus; (4) The superior bronchus and segment; (5) The inferior bronchus and segment.

B. *The Left Lower Lobe*. (6) The apical bronchus and segment; (8) The anterior basal bronchus and segment; (9) The lateral basal bronchus and segment; (10) The posterior basal bronchus and segment.

The absence of a medial basal (cardiac) segment involves omission of segment (7) in left lung.

Lungs
Each lung is invaginated from the hilum into the closed sac of the pleura. If the thorax is laid open on both sides, a pressure of 7 mmHg in the trachea is necessary to keep the lungs from collapsing. The right lung has three lobes, the left lung two.

If the free flow of air into and out of the lungs is obstructed, the intrapulmonary pressures will be increased beyond the normal range (from −40 mm to +40 mmHg) so that blood will be compressed from the atria and great veins into the venous system, producing venous oozing—true engorgement with blue venous blood.

Handling of bioactive materials by the lungs. The lungs have an important non-respiratory function involving the metabolism of many active substances, in the same way as the liver. There is a substantial pulmonary clearance of the catecholamines, adrenaline, noradrenaline and dopamine, in critically ill patients.[65] These activities may be influenced by lung disease or by a raised or lowered Pa_{O_2}.[66]

Other non-respiratory functions of the lung include filtration of blood, and phagocytosis by macrophages.

Tracheal Mucus
See Richardson P. S. and Peatfield A. C. *J. R. Soc. Med.* 1980, **73**, 123.

Surfactant
The alveoli are lined with a monomolecular layer of lipoprotein—the pulmonary surfactant. This produces a marked reduction in surface tension, and so helps to keep the alveoli open. It is greatly reduced in the lungs of babies with respiratory distress syndrome, and after cardiopulmonary bypass. It may be reduced in pulmonary oedema, oxygen poisoning and after prolonged artificial ventilation with large tidal volumes.

Physiology of Respiration[67]

Respiration
Defined as the gaseous interchange between an organism and its environment. Oxygen is absorbed and carbon dioxide excreted. External respiration takes place between the alveoli and the capillaries; internal respiration occurs in the tissue cells.

Symbols used in Respiratory Physiology[68]
1. *Gases*
    Primary Symbols (large capitals): V = gas volume; P = gas pressure; F = fractional concentration in a dry gas phase; f = respiratory frequency (breaths per unit time); D = diffusing capacity; R = respiratory exchange ratio. C = concentration of a gas; F = fractional concentration in the dry gas phase; p = partial pressure (gas); Q = volume of blood; S = saturation of haemoglobin with either CO_2 or O_2. A dash above any symbol indicates a mean value: e.g. $\bar{P}$ = mean gas pressure. A dot above any symbol indicates a time derivative: e.g. $\dot{V}$ = gas volume per unit time.
    Secondary Symbols (small capital letters): I = inspired gas; E = expired gas; A = alveolar gas; T = tidal gas; D dead space gas; B = barometric.
    STPD = 0°C, 760 mmHg, dry, BTPS = body temperature and pressure, saturated with water vapour. ATPS = = ambient temperature and pressure, saturated with water vapour.
2. *Blood*
    Primary Symbols (large capitals): Q = volume of blood; C = concentration of gas in blood phase; S = percentage saturation of Hb with O_2 or CO.
    Secondary Symbols (small letters): a = arterial blood; v = venous blood; c = pulmonary capillary blood.

3. *Lung volumes.* VC = vital capacity; IC = inspiratory capacity; IRV = inspiratory reserve volume; ERV = expiratory reserve volume; FRC = functional residual capacity; RV = residual volume; TLC = total lung capacity; CV = closing volume.

Examples of use of symbols. P_{AO_2} = alveolar O_2 tension. D_{O_2} = diffusing capacity for oxygen. $\dot{Q}_C$ = blood flow through pulmonary capillaries per min. V_{O_2} = O_2 consumption per min. F_{IO_2} = fractional inspired oxygen concentration P_B = barometric pressure. Ca_{O_2} = ml O_2 in 100 ml arterial blood.

Exchange of Gases on Lungs

Diffusion is aided by differences in pressure or tension. As inspired air is sucked into the alveoli, it mixes with air already there and so its oxygen becomes diluted, its carbon dioxide increased and water vapour added. It is the partial pressure of the oxygen (13·5 kPa) which drives it into the blood across the pulmonary epithelium and the walls of the pulmonary capillaries as the pressure of oxygen in these capillaries is about 5·3 kPa. Transfer of oxygen from alveoli to blood depends on: (1) The pressure gradient; (2) The rate of pulmonary blood flow; (3) The solubility coefficient. Equilibrium may not be reached if (1) is affected by high altitude or (2) is affected by heavy exercise. It is also affected by changes in ventilation-perfusion ratios and by incomplete diffusion of inspired air within the terminal airways.

P_{ACO_2} is primarily determined by alveolar ventilation and is nearly independent of blood flow.

Air in the alveoli is 98% saturated with water vapour (tension of 6 kPa).

Table 2.1 shows the partial pressures of gases in the lungs and blood.

Table 2.1. Partial pressures of gases in lungs and blood

	Inspired air	Expired air	Alveolar air	Arterial blood	Venous blood
Oxygen					
Tension in kPa	20·0	15·0	13·5	13·3	5·3
Volumes per cent	20·9	16·0	15·0	19·8	15·2
Carbon dioxide					
Tension in kPa	0·04	3·75	5·3	5·3	5·7
Volumes per cent	0·04	4·5	5·6	50·0	55·0
Nitrogen					
Tension in kPa	78·0	75·0	74·0	74·0	74·0
Volumes per cent	79·0	75·8	75·0	0·83	0·83
Water vapour					
Tension in kPa	0·6	6·0	6·0		
Volumes per cent	0·6	6·0	6·0		

Alveolar Oxygen Concentration

Factors influencing this include: (1) Dry barometric pressures. Other factors remaining constant, P_{AO_2} is directly proportional to barometric pressure. With increasing altitude it would theoretically become zero at 19 km, where the actual barometric pressure equals the saturated water-vapour pressure at body temperature. Under hyperbaric conditions the same considerations apply so that P_{AO_2} at 2 atmospheres (absolute) is approximately doubled; (2) Ventilation. The relationship between P_{AO_2} and alveolar ventilation is hyperbolic. As ventilation increases P_{AO_2} rises towards (but never reaches) the P_{O_2} of the inspired gases. At very low levels of alveolar ventilation, small changes may produce considerable variation of P_{AO_2}; (3) Oxygen consumption. This is important under some circumstances. For example, in a patient shivering the oxygen consumption may rise to 500 ml/min, and hypoxia may result; (4) Cardiac output. Fall in cardiac output means that less oxygen is removed from alveolar gas. But there is also increased oxygen extraction from tissues, so that the P_{O_2} of blood returning to the lungs falls. Alveolar P_{O_2} is likely to remain unchanged, except in the short term. (5) Inspired oxygen concentration. P_{AO_2} will vary according to changes in inspired concentration; (6) The third gas or Fink effect.

Alveolar/Arterial Po₂ Difference

Alveolar/Arterial P_{O_2} Difference
Normally a few mmHg only. Increases where there are abnormal ventilation-perfusion relationships. Factors influencing the magnitude of the difference include: (1) The magnitude of venous admixture; (2) Actual P_{AO_2}; (3) Cardiac output; (4) Temperature, pH and base excess of the blood; (5) Haemoglobin concentration; (6) Alveolar ventilation; (7) The state of the alveolar membrane. Compensation by increasing the inspired oxygen concentration is effective up to a point.

Table 2.2

Per cent shunt	Per cent inspired O_2 to restore normal P_{AO_2}
10	30
20	57
30	97
40	Not possible to restore to normal
50	Changes in inspired concentration have almost no effect on P_{AO_2}

Shunts in excess of 30% may be seen in congenital cardiac disease, lung trauma, fat embolism, pneumonia and gross obesity.

Exchange of Gases in Blood

Again, gas passes from a zone of high to a zone of low pressure, or, in other words, the pressure gradients enable oxygen to diffuse inwards from alveolar air to capillary blood; and carbon dioxide to diffuse in the reverse direction. The diffusion coefficient of carbon dioxide (500) is greater than that of oxygen (25–45), i.e. it diffuses twenty times as readily, so this compensates for the lower pressure gradient of this gas as compared with that of oxygen.

In whole blood 0·3 vol % of oxygen is carried in simple solution.

In whole blood 2·5 vol % of carbon dioxide are carried in simple solution.

In arterial blood 19·8 vol % of oxygen are carried, the greater part combined with haemoglobin.

In arterial blood 40–55 vol % of carbon dioxide are carried, the greater part as bicarbonate.

1 g of haemoglobin carries 1·34 ml of oxygen when fully saturated.[69]

15 g of haemoglobin (the normal amount in 100 ml of blood) carry 20 ml oxygen. The tissues require about 250 ml of oxygen each minute—the basal oxygen consumption.

For measurement of oxygen tension, invasive and non-invasive, *see* Chapter 41.

Oxygen Carriage in Blood

The oxygen dissociation curve of haemoglobin (Barcroft, 1872–1947, and Poulton, 1883–1939),[70] worked out for temperature of 37 °C and CO_2 tension of 40 mmHg, and plasma pH of 7·40, shows the relation between the partial pressure of oxygen (abscissae) and the percentage saturation of the haemoglobin (ordinates) (*Fig. 2.3*). It shows that at 13·5 kPa partial pressure (i.e. partial pressure of O_2 in alveoli) haemoglobin is 97% saturated, whereas at 9·3 kPa haemoglobin saturation is still 90%. Normally, oxygen in arterial blood is at a tension of 13·3 kPa, at which haemoglobin is 97% saturated and the oxygen content is 19·8 vol%, 0·3 ml of this being dissolved in plasma. Venous blood has an oxygen tension of 5·3 kPa and its oxygen content is 15 vol%. The Pao_2 falls with increasing age. There is loss of respiratory response to hypoxia with anaesthesia.

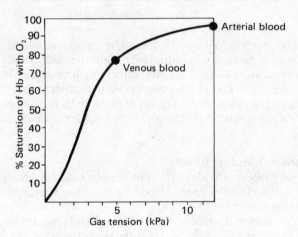

Fig. 2.3 The oxygen dissociation curve of haemoglobin.

Oxygen Flux
See Chapter 36.

P50

This is the oxygen tension needed to provide 50% saturation of haemoglobin. Its value is an expression of shift of the dissociation curve to left or right. The dissociation curve may be altered by changes in the pH, 'the Christian Bohr (1855–1911), Copenhagen physiologist, effect';[71] it is shifted to the right in anaemia and acidaemia and to the left in alkalaemia. Carbon dioxide increase causes a flattening of the curve to the right. An increase in temperature has a similar effect, while in hypothermia the curve is shifted to the left. Shift of the curve is influenced by the concentration of 2,3-diphosphoglycerate (2,3-DPG) in the red cells, a decrease displacing it to the left, an increase to the right. This concentration may be affected by storage, general anaesthesia, chronic hypoxaemia or massive transfusions. 2,3-DPG described in 1925.[72] An increase improves tissue oxygenation and a decrease may cause tissue hypoxia. An increase reduces the affinity of haemoglobin for oxygen, and vice versa.

Table 2.3 assumes an Hb concentration of 15 g/100 ml and a cardiac output of 5 litre/min. The 'available' scale allows for the fact that many tissues cannot tolerate a capillary Po_2 below about 2 to 2·5 kPa and cannot extract the last 20% of oxygen.

Table 2.3. Oxygen saturation and oxygen flux[73]

Per cent saturation	O_2 content (ml/litre)	O_2 supply (ml/min)	Available O_2 (ml/min)
100	200	1000	800
80	160	800	600
60	120	600	400
40	80	400	200
20	40	200	0

Stored Blood

The oxygen and carbon dioxide dissociation curves in blood stored in an acid-citrate-dextrose medium are shifted to the left, the extent being related to the duration of storage, the 'Valtis-Kennedy' effect. Such changes with depletion of 2,3-diphosphoglycerate (DPG) are progressive with storage and the effect lasts several hours after transfusion. As a result of these shifts the blood of an anaemic patient may for a few hours after transfusion be unable to release as much oxygen as it did before.[74]

Carriage of Carbon Dioxide in Blood

Total amount of carbon dioxide carried in venous blood is about 50–60 vol %. Venous blood contains 5–10% more carbon dioxide than arterial blood, its carbon dioxide combining power being greater.

The tension of carbon dioxide in arterial blood and alveolar air is 5·3 kPa. In venous blood at rest it is 5·7 kPa. Carbon dioxide output, about 200 ml/min, at rest.

Carbon dioxide is carried in blood in three forms:

1. As dissolved carbon dioxide in plasma—from 3 to 5%. It is very rapidly exchangeable. The partial pressure of carbon dioxide in mixed venous blood is 5·7 kPa and is greater than that in the alveoli, which is 5·3 kPa, so the gas passes from the blood to the alveoli and is exhaled.

2. As carbamino compounds formed by the combination of carbon dioxide with NH_2 groups from haemoglobin in the red cells—called carbamino-haemoglobin or carbhaemoglobin. Carbon dioxide also combines on a small scale with plasma proteins. Reduced haemoglobin can take up more carbon dioxide in this way than oxyhaemoglobin. The formation and dissociation of carbamino compounds is a rapid process. About 2–10% of the total blood carbon dioxide is carried in this way, the amount depending on the degree of oxygenation of haemoglobin.

3. As bicarbonate, chiefly of sodium and potassium. Mainly in plasma and very slowly exchangeable. It is of importance in acidosis, alkalosis and acclimatization.

In addition to transporting CO_2, sodium bicarbonate also acts as the alkali reserve, neutralizing strong acids which may enter the bloodstream. The pH of plasma depends on the ratio of H_2CO_3 to bicarbonate. Breathing thus assists in the pH control of the blood.

Regulation of Respiration

Rhythmical breathing is controlled by cells in the respiratory centre in the floor of the fourth ventricle (C. J. J. Legallois (1770–1814) in 1812[75] and Marie Jean Pierre Flourens (1794–1867), French physiologist). There would appear to be three main parts of the respiratory centre: (1) A medullary centre capable of initiating and maintaining sequences of respiration, though not of normal character; (2) An apneustic centre in the middle and lower pons, which if unopposed tends to produce inspiratory spasm or apneustic breathing; (3) A pneumotaxic centre in the upper third of the pons that restrains the apneustic centre periodically. While essentially automatic, the centre may be influenced from many sources: (1) From changes in carbon dioxide tension in the blood.[76] The respiratory centre is normally set to maintain the Pa_{CO_2} at 5·3 kPa. When the Pa_{CO_2} falls below 4–4·5 kPa, respiratory drive from the centre usually ceases, leading to apnoea. The effect of Pa_{CO_2} on the respiratory centre is modified by the cerebrospinal bicarbonate concentration, changes in which form the basis of acclimatization. The respiratory centre takes about 30 s to respond to a change in Pa_{CO_2}; (2) By changes in body temperature. (3) By Hering–Breuer reflexes[77] (Hering, 1834–1918; Joseph Breuer, 1842–1925, Viennese general practitioner and psychiatrist); (4) By carotid-body reflexes, largely oxygen lack. Oxygen lack shown to stimulate respiration by John Scott Haldane (1860–1936), Oxford physiologist, in 1905;[78] (5) By proprioceptive impulses from intrathoracic structures and from muscles and joints throughout the body, the so-called ergoreceptors, so that respiration can fit in with exercise and movement, etc.; (6) By reflexes which modify rhythm during talking, swallowing and inhaling strong anaesthetic vapours (glossopharyngeal and vagus nerves); (7) Reflexes from the hypothalamus and cerebral cortex; (8) The will and emotional states; (9) Pain.

Carotid and Aortic Reflexes and Respiration

Pressoreceptors are present in the carotid sinus (described by H. E. Hering (1866–1948) in 1923.[79] They are also present in the aortic arch. Stimulation of the nerve endings (stretch receptors) in the outer wall of the sinus and aorta inhibits respiration (Corneille Heymans, 1892–1968, Belgian physiologist).[80] Pressoreceptors are also present in the great veins, right auricle and pulmonary artery, and increased pressure here may stimulate respiration. Such reflexes may be involved in the dyspnoea of heart failure and pulmonary embolism.

There is evidence that pressoreceptors, when stimulated by low blood pressure, can produce reflex bronchial dilatation.[81]

Peripheral chemoreceptors are present in the carotid body[82] and the aortic bodies.[83] Their main function is to prevent hypoxia by stimulating respiration when arterial Po_2 falls. Thus hypoxia directly depresses the respiratory centre, but secondarily stimulates it via this reflex. Stimulation only occurs if plasma oxygen tension is reduced, not blood-oxygen content (as in anaemia). Chemoreceptors are important when the respiratory centre is depressed, as in severe chronic bronchitis, with hypercapnia, $Paco_2$ greater than 10 kPa, when the resulting hypoxia stimulates respiration reflexly. If at such times oxygen in excess is given, the sole remaining stimulant to breathing is removed and hypopnoea may follow with its resulting hypercapnia. Some patients have a diminished hypoxic drive (possibly including those with the Pickwickian syndrome). Oral medroxy-progesterone restores the hypoxic drive to normal. (*See also* Leitch A. G. *Lancet* 1981, **1**, 428.)

Central chemoreceptors are present close to the ventrolateral surface of the medulla near the respiratory centre and sense the cerebral gaseous environment. These receptors respond to changes in pH and Pco_2 in the cerebrospinal fluid. Such changes are not necessarily the same, nor do they occur at the same rate, as in the blood. The pH of the CSF is maintained at normal values by alteration of bicarbonate concentration. The CSF pH can be maintained at normal values during chronic respiratory and metabolic acidosis.

Lung Function

The spirometer was invented in 1846 (Hutchinson, 1811–1861).[84] The first measurement of blood gases was made in 1837.[85] Analysis of respiratory gases by Haldane (1860–1936) in 1896.[86]

Routine tests of lung function[87] are: (*a*) Exercise tolerance; (*b*) Lung volumes; (*c*) Blood gas tensions.

1. *Tidal volume* (V_T). The volume of gas inspired or expired during each respiratory cycle (400–500 ml). The effective tidal volume is the air which reaches the alveoli (the tidal volume less the dead space ($V_T - V_D$)).

2. *Inspiratory reserve volume* (IRV). The maximal amount of gas that can be inspired from the normal end-inspiratory position (3000 ml).

3. *Expiratory reserve volume* (ERV). The maximum amount of gas that can be expired from the end-expiratory position (average 1200 ml).

4. *Residual volume* (RV). The volume of gas remaining in the lungs at the end of a maximal expiration (average 1200 ml).

5. *Total lung capacity* (TLC). Formerly total lung volume. The amount of gas contained in the lung at the end of a maximal inspiration (average 6000 ml). The sum of (1) to (4) above.

6. *Vital capacity* (VC). The maximal volume of gas that can be expelled from the lungs by forceful effort following a maximal inspiration (average 4800 ml). The sum of (1) to (3) above. The concept of measuring the FEV as a fraction of the VC was introduced in 1951.[88]

7. *Inspiratory capacity* (IC). The maximal volume of gas that can be inspired from the resting expiratory level (average 3600 ml). The sum of (1) and (2) above.

8. *Functional residual capacity* (FRC). Formerly functional residual air. The volume of gas remaining in the lungs at the resting expiratory level. The sum of (3) and (4) above. Varies according to posture. About 3500 ml in the upright position, but only 2500 ml in the supine position due to higher position of the diaphragm and weight of the viscera. It is decreased during and after anaesthesia by about 16%, the cause not yet being certain.[89]

9. *The vital spirogram.* The patient expires and inspires maximally into a specially designed spirometer. The tracing obtained in the vital spirogram has characteristics from which lung function can be deduced.

10. *Forced expiratory volume* (FEV). There is a close correlation between the expiratory curve of the vital spirogram and the maximal breathing capacity. The

volume exhaled in a given unit of time, usually 1 sec. from the start of expiration, is recorded, and this volume known as the $FEV_{1.0}$ gives an indirect measure of the MBC and is easier to obtain in ill patients. A normal individual can expire 83% of his vital capacity in 1 sec. Where there is an obstruction to air flow (emphysema) the $FEV_{1.0}$ is reduced to a much greater degree than the vital capacity. Where there is no resistance to air flow (restricted chest movement) the $FEV_{1.0}$ shows a proportional reduction to that of the VC. These measurements can now be made easily and rapidly using a dry spirometer, the Vitalograph. $FEV_{1.0}$ first described by Ehrner.[90]

This is a simpler test than the MBC and is more applicable to the conditions of the pre- and postoperative periods.

11. Peak expiratory flow rate. This is the steepest part of the spirometer trace of a forced vital capacity estimation. It may be conveniently measured by using the Wright peak flow-meter.[91] The peak flow rate is usually four to five times the MBC. A small whistle, which can be carried in the pocket, has also been designed for the measurement of maximum expiratory flow rate.[92]

12. Capnograph (alveolar air analysis) (*see* p. Chapter 41). The air in contact with the pulmonary capillaries, which therefore carries out gaseous interchange with the blood. Expired air is a mixture of alveolar air and dead space air. The air in the lower part of the trachea at the end of expiration is for all practical purposes identical with the alveolar air.

13. Dead space volume (V_D).

a. Anatomical Dead Space. Extends from the nostrils and mouth down to, but not including, the alveoli (about 2 ml/kg body weight).[93] Reduced by tracheostomy and by endotracheal intubation by about 80 ml. Increased by: (1) sitting up, (2) extending the neck, (3) advancing age.

$$\text{Anatomical dead space} = \text{tidal volume} \left(\frac{\text{end-exp. } CO_2 \text{ conc.} - \text{mixed exp. } CO_2 \text{ conc}}{\text{end-exp. } CO_2 \text{ conc.} - \text{inspired } CO_2 \text{ conc.}} \right).$$

b. Physiological Dead Space. A dynamic volume, this denotes all air not available for respiratory exchange, as when alveoli have no capillary blood flow or when alveoli become distended. It may therefore be greater than anatomical dead space. Physiological dead space cannot be measured directly, but a value can be derived using the Bohr equation (modified by Enghoff[94]):

$$\text{Physiological dead space} = V_T \left(\frac{Pa_{CO_2} - P_E{CO_2}}{Pa_{CO_2}} \right)$$

where V_T = tidal volume, Pa_{CO_2} = tension of CO_2 in arterial blood, and $P_E{CO_2}$ = tension of CO_2 in expired air.

The physiological dead space and dead space/tidal volume ratio (V_D/V_T) increase (1) when anaesthesia is induced, (2) when ventilation is controlled, (3) with short inspiratory period, (4) with increased end-expiratory pressure.

c. Extra dead space produced by anaesthetic apparatus, face-masks, breathing tubes, etc.

Dead space takes no part in the actual respiratory exchange. Rapid shallow breathing is therefore less efficient than slower deeper respiration for the same minute volume. The nearer the tidal volume approaches the dead space volume, the less real respiratory exchange occurs. In normal patients V_D/V_T is less than 30% (i.e. ventilation is more than 70% efficient). With lung disease the V_D/V_T

may be increased to 60–70%. The *effective tidal volume* is the tidal air minus the dead space.

Factors affecting dead space include: (1) Tidal volume and respiratory rate; (2) The pattern of respiration; (3) Lung volume; (4) Pulmonary blood flow; (5) Body position; (6) Alveolar P_{CO_2}; (7) Changes in bronchomotor tone; (8) Tracheal intubation; (9) General anaesthesia; (10) Hypotension.[95] (*See* 'Deadspace; invasive and non-invasive.' Editorial. Fletcher, R. *Br. J. Anaesth.* 1985, **57**, 245.)

14. Minute volume. The volume of air breathed each minute. 5–8 litres/min.

15. Alveolar ventilation ($\dot{V}_A$). This is the effective tidal volume × rate of respiration. Average values are 2·0–2·5 litres/min/m^2 body surface area.

16. Compliance. The volume change produced by each unit pressure increase, expressed as litre/cm water pressure. Normal values for a healthy young man are pulmonary compliance (C_L) 0·2 litre/cm water, chest wall compliance (C_{CW}) 0·2 litre/cm water, with a total compliance of 0·1 litre/cm water.[96] With an open chest, compliance is due to the lungs alone. Lung compliance depends on the lung volume into which the inspired gas is distributed and on the elasticity of the lung tissues. Compliance (in litres/cm H_2O) equals 0·05 × functional residual capacity and is therefore less in the child.

Static and Dynamic Compliance. Static compliance is measured at zero air flow after the preceding inflow of air has been sufficiently slow for distribution within the lung to be solely in accord with regional elasticity. Dynamic compliance is measured at zero air flow, but when the inflow has been rapid so that dynamic factors have influenced the distribution. These concepts are important in emphysema, when static compliance may be raised due to breakdown of septa, while dynamic compliance is reduced due to airway resistance.

Elastance is the reciprocal of compliance and measures the increase in airway pressure for a given increase in volume. Average elastance is 10 cm of water/litre of air inhaled.

17. Mean mechanical resistance. The amount of pressure necessary to obtain a certain flow rate. Expressed as cm of water/litre/second. Normal value from 0·6 to 2·4 cm of water/litre/sec. About half occurs in the upper, and half in the lower airways. In emphysema there is high resistance and low compliance. Airway resistance is increased in asthma and in a wide variety of disorders where there is airway obstruction, measured in the body plethysmograph.

18. The work of breathing. This can be found by measuring the total pressure required to force a known volume of air into the thorax. Normal value is 0·5 kg.m/min, but may be increased five-or tenfold in the presence of heart or lung disease. The normal metabolic cost of breathing is about 0·5–1·0 ml O_2/litre of ventilation at rest. With hyperventilation this may increase to 3–4 ml O_2/litre.

19. Diffusion. May be impaired as a secondary factor in disease, or it may occur specifically as 'alveolar capillary block' which has been found present in some cases of Boeck's sarcoid of the lung, beryllium granulomatosis, asbestosis, pulmonary scleroderma, alveolar cell carcinoma, sulphur dioxide poisoning, certain metastatic lung lesions and pulmonary oedema. The test requires the use of gas which is considerably more soluble in blood than in the alveolar capillary membranes. Apart from oxygen, only carbon monoxide fulfils this criterion because of its combination with haemoglobin. The rate of carbon monoxide uptake is limited by diffusion, and the uptake is measured after adding 0·2% CO to inspired air.

Pulmonary diffusing capacity for CO

$$= \frac{\text{ml CO transferred from alveolar gas to blood per min}}{\text{mean alveolar CO pressure} - \text{mean capillary CO pressure}}$$

Normal values range from 17 to 25 ml/min/mmHg.

20. *Ventilation–perfusion relationships*. During normal spontaneous respiration in the healthy subject, there are some variations in the ventilation–perfusion ratio between different parts of the lung. These variations account for the differences in oxygen tension between alveolar gas and arterial blood. The balance is upset to a greater degree in the diseased lung. In emphysema, for example, some distended alveoli may be underperfused (increased dead space effect) and some underventilated alveoli may receive normal perfusion (venous admixture effect). The result is a rise of P_{CO_2} and a fall of P_{O_2} of the arterial blood. Temporary changes in ventilation–perfusion relationships may occur during controlled respiration in anaesthesia and also in the postoperative phase.

21. *Maximal breathing capacity (MBC)*. The maximum volume of air that can be breathed per minute. Usually measured for 15 s and expressed as flow per min. Average values 120 litres/min. May be only 25 litres/min in emphysema. A disadvantage is that it is difficult for ill or postoperative patients to carry out the test. Equals $35 \times FEV_{1.0}$.

22. *Match test*. Success or failure to blow out a lighted paper match held 15 cm from a patient's wide open mouth. It is essential that the lips are not allowed to come together. Patients who can perform this test should maintain adequate ventilation after thoracic or abdominal surgery. Patients who cannot extinguish the match require further investigation before operation.

23. *Auscultation over the trachea during a forced expiration*. Breath sounds audible for more than 6 s denote airway obstruction. If the time is less than 5 s airway obstruction is most unlikely. A simple test requiring no complicated apparatus.

24. *Closing volume of the lungs (CV)*. The lung volume below which there is a detectable failure of ventilation in the dependent parts of the lung, caused by airway narrowing due to gravitational forces and reduction in overall volume.

When the FRC is less than the closing volume there will be regional hypoventilation in dependent areas of the lungs, a shunt and increased alveolar/arterial P_{O_2} difference.

The closing volume can be measured using a bolus of marker gas, such as radioactive xenon, argon or helium, which is introduced at the mouth after maximal expiration. After a full inspiration, the subject exhales his vital capacity slowly. Expired volume and marker gas concentrations are measured. The onset of 'closure' is indicated by a sharp rise in concentration over the second half of the vital capacity. Expiration must be slow (less than 0·5 litre/s) as with higher rates dynamic airway narrowing rather than closure may become significant.

In normal subjects CV increases with age to approach the FRC. At the age of 65 years (upright position) or 44 years (supine position) CV begins to encroach on tidal volume.[97] CV is increased in smokers, despite normal readings with other lung function tests.

Airways closure, most likely due to loss of tissue elasticity, results in air trapping and alterations in ventilation–perfusion relationships (V̇/Q̇). This may be the principal cause of the normal inverse relationship between age and P_{aO_2}.

CV rises with increasing age, with obesity, with the supine as opposed to the erect posture and with anaesthesia, whether respiration is spontaneous or controlled. Positive end expiratory pressure (PEEP) is thought to be valuable during IPPV in certain clinical situations because it increases the FRC above the CV of the lungs.

References

1. Corli O. *Minerva Anestesiol.* 1984, **50**, 401.
2. Hughes J. *Br. Med. Bull.* 1983, **39**, 17.
3. Light A. R. et al. *Somatosensory Res.* 1983, **1**, 33.
4. Curtis D. R et al. *Brain Res.* 1977, **130**, 360.
5. Hokfelt, T. et al. in: *Brain Stem Control of Spinal Mechanisms* (Sjolund B. and Bjoiklund J., ed.). Amsterdam: Elsevier.
6. Gastaut H. et al. *Brain Res.* 1966, **1**, 167; Burwell C. S. et al. *Am. J. Med.* 1956, **21**, 211.
7. Thompson P. J. and Sawicka E. *Br. Med. J.* 1982, **285**, 648; Annotation, *Br. Med. J.* 1982, **285**, 528.
8. Block J. *New Engl. J. Med.* 1979, **300**, 513.
9. *See also* Robson J. G. *Proc. R. Soc. Med.* 1971, **64**, 211.
10. Burney J. P. *Anaesthesia* 1981, **36**, 1027.
11. Quastel J. H. and Wheatley A. H. M. *Proc. R. Soc. Med.* 1932, **112**, 60. Reprinted in 'Classical File', *Surv. Anesthesiol.* 1959, **3**, October.
12. Meyer H. H. *Arch. Exp. Path. Pharmak.* 1899, **42**, 109.
13. Overton C. E. *Studien über Narkose.* Jena: G. Fischer, 1901.
14. Bernard C. *Leçons sur les Anaesthésiques et sur l'Asphyxie.* Paris: Baillière, 1875.
15. Ferguson J. *Proc. R. Soc.* B 1939. **127**, 387.
16. Pauling L. *Science* 1961, **134**, 15; *Anesth. Analg.* 1964. **43**, 1 (reprinted in 'Classical File', *Surv. Anesthesiol.* 1970. **14**, 194).
17. Editorial, *Anesthesiology* 1977, **47**, 1: Halsey M. J. and Wardley-Smith B. *Br. J. Anaesth.* 1978, **50**, 1091; Wardley-Smith B and Halsey M. J. *Br. J. Anaesth.* 1979, **51**, 619; Wardley-Smith B. and Halsey M. J. *Br. J. Anaesth.* 1985, **57**, 1248.
18. Eger E. I. et al. *Anesthesiology* 1969, **30**, 129.
19. Cerebrospinal fluid, a term first used by F. Magendie (1783–1825) in 1825 (Magendie F. J. *Physiol. Exp. Path.* 1825, **5**, 27).
20. Magendie F. *J. Physiol. Exp. Pathol.* 1825, **5**, 27 and 1827, **7**, 1.
21. Queckenstedt H. H. G. *Dt. Z. NervHeilk.* 1916, **55**, 325.
22. Thompson E. J. and Johnson M. H. *Br. J. Hosp. Med.* 1982, **28**, 600.
23. Bryce-Smith R. *Proc. R. Soc. Med.* 1976, **69**, 75.
24. Steer J. L. and Horney F. D. *Can. Med. Ass. J.* 1968, **98**, 71.
25. Clatterberg J. *Anesthesiology* 1977, **46**, 309.
26. Berry A. *Anaesthesia* 1958, **13**, 100.
27. Erlanger J. and Gasser H. S. *Am. J. Physiol.* 1924, **70**, 624; 1929, **88**, 581 (reprinted in 'Classical File', *Surv. Anesthesiol.* 1970, **14**, 471). (For this research on neurophysiology Erlanger and Gasser were awarded the Nobel Prize in 1944.) *See also* Whitwam J. G. *Anaesthesia* 1976, **31**, 494.
28. Nathan P. W. and Sears T. A. *J. Physiol. (Lond.)* 1961, **157**, 565; **164**, 375; *Anaesthesia* 1963, **18**, 467.
29. Whitwam J. G. *Anaesthesia* 1976, **31**, 494.
30. Gissen A. et al. *Anesthesiology* 1980, **53**, 467; Annotation, *Anesthesiology* 1980, **53**, 443.
31. Melzack R. and Wall P. D. *Science* 1965, **150**, 971 (reprinted in 'Classical File', *Surv. Anesthesiol.* 1972, **16**, 583).
32. Annotation, *Br. Med. J.* 1978, **2**, 586.
33. Leake C. D. *Anesthesiology* 1968, **29**, 623; Feldberg W. S. *Fifty Years On.* University of Liverpool Press, 1982.
34. Kuntz A. *The Autonomic Nervous System*, 2nd ed. Philadelphia: Lea & Febiger, 1934.
35. de Jong R. H. and Cullen S. C. *Anesthesiology* 1963, **24**, 628.
36. Waller A. D. *J. Physiol. (Lond.)* 1887, **8**, 229; Besteman E. and Creese M. *Br. Heart J.* 1979, **42**, 61.
37. Einthoven Willem *Pflugers Arch.* 1903, **99**, 472 (translated in *Cardiac Classics* (Willius F. A. and Keys T. E., ed). St Louis: Mosby, 1941, Vol. 2, p. 722); *Lancet* 1912, **1**, 853.

38. Dock W. *Proc. Soc. Exp. Biol. Med.* 1929, **24**, 566.
39. Jolly W. A. and Ritchie W. R. *Heart* 1910, **2**, 177.
40. Mackenzie J. *Diseases of the Heart*. London: Oxford University Press, 1908.
41. Traube L. *Berlin Klin. Wochenschr.* 1872, **9**, 1, 185, 221.
42. Heard J. B. and Strauss A. E. *Am. J. Med. Sci.* 1918, **155**, 238.
43. Krumbhaar E. B. *Am. J. Med. Sci.* 1918, **155**,
44. Johnstone M. MD Thesis, University of Belfast, 1948.
45. Wolferth C. C. and Wood F. C. *Am. J. Med. Sci.* 1932, **183**, 30; Wilson F. M. et al. *Am. Heart J.* 1934, **9**, 447.
46. Goldberger E. *Am. Heart J.* 1942, **23**, 483.
47. Starling E. H. *The Linacre Lecture on the Law of the Heart*, given at Cambridge, 1915. London: Longmans, Green & Co., 1918.
48. Beaupre P. N. et al. *Anesthesiology* 1983, **59**, A59.
49. Brodsky M. et al. *Am. J. Cardiol.* 1977, **39**, 390.
50. Moffitt E. A., Sethna D. H. et al. *Can. Anaesth. Soc. J.* 1983, **31**, 5.
51. Valsalva, Antonia Maria (1666–1723) *De aure humana tractatus*. Bononiae: Typ. C. Pisarii, 1704.
52. Scholar H. *Am. Heart J.* 1965, **69**, 701.
53. Albert S. N. *Blood Volume*. Springfield, Ill.: Thomas, 1963.
54. Nadler, S. B., Hidalgo J. V. and Bloch T. *Surgery* 1962, **51**, 224.
55. Ahmed T. and Oliver W. *Am. Rev. Resp. Dis.* 1983, **127**, 566.
56. Stoetling R. K. and Longnecker D. E. *Anesthesiology* 1972, **36**, 352.
57. Rawlinson, W. A. L. *Anaesthesia* 1979, **34**, 534.
58. Patient is from *pati*, Latin, to suffer or to bear.
59. *See also* Rustad W. H. *The Recurrent Laryngeal Nerves in Thyroid Surgery*. Springfield: Thomas, 1956, 1978.
60. *See also* Fink B. R. and Demarest R. J. *Laryngeal Biomechanics*. Cambridge, Mass.: Harvard University Press, 1978.
61. Stewart S. and Pinkerton H. H. *Br. J. Anaesth.* 1955, **27**, 492.
62. Robbie D. S. and Feldman S. A. *Br. J. Anaesth.* 1963, **35**, 771.
63. Hall R. M. *Anaesthesia* 1979, **34**, 503.
64. *Thorax* 1950, **5**, 3, 222.
65. Russell W. J. *Anaesth. Intensive Care* 1982, **10**, 319.
66. Fishman A. P. and Pietra G. G. *N. Engl. J. Med.* 1974, **291**, 884, 1953.
67. *See also* Nunn J. F. *Applied Respiratory Physiology*. London: Butterworths, 2nd ed. 1977.
68. Comroe J. H. et al. *The Lung*, 2nd ed. Chicago: Year Book Publishers Inc, 1962: Pappenheimer I. R. et al. *Fed. Proc.* 1950, **9**, 602.
69. Hüfner C. G. von *Arch. Anat. Physiol.* 1894, p. 130.
70. Barcroft J. and Poulton E. P. *J. Physiol.* 1913, **46**, 4; *Respiratory Function of the Blood*. Cambridge: Cambridge University Press, 1914; and Harken A. H. *Surg. Gynecol. Obstet.*, 1977, **144**, 935.
71. Bohr C. *Skand. Arch. Physiol.* 1904, **16**, 402.
72. Greenwald G. *J. Biol. Chem.* 1925, **63**, 339; MacDonald R., *Anaesthesia* 1977, **32**, 544.
73. Sykes M. K., McNicol M. W. and Campbell E. J. M. *Respiratory Failure*, 2nd ed. Oxford: Blackwell, 1976, p. 64.
74. Valtis D. J. and Kennedy A. C. *Lancet* 1954, **1**, 119.
75. Legallois J. J. C. *Expérience sur le Principe de la Vie*. Paris, 1812.
76. Haldane J. S. and Priestley J. G. *J. Physiol. (Lond.)* 1905, **32**, 225.
77. Hering E. and Breuer J. *Akad. Wiss. Wien.* 1868, **57**, 672 (reprinted in 'Classical File', *Surv. Anesthesiol.* 1971, **15**, 595); and **58**, 909; *see also* Lee J. A. *Anaesthesia* 1968, **23**, 683.
78. Haldane J. S. *J. Physiol. (Lond.)* 1905, **32**, 225.
79. Hering H. E. *Münch. Med. Wochenschr.* 1923, **70**, 1287.
80. Heymans C. *Le Sinus carotidien et les autres Zones vasosensibles réflexogènes*. Presse Université de France, 1929. (This work earned Heymans the Nobel Prize in 1938.)
81. Daly M. de B. and Schweitzer A. *J. Physiol. (Lond.)* 1951, **113**, 442; Daly M. de B. and Angell James J. F. *Lancet* 1979, **1**, 764.
82. Heymans C. et al. *Archs Int. Pharmacodyn. Thér.* 1930, **39**, 400 (first described by H. W. L. Taube in 1743).
83. Heymans J. F. and Heymans C. *Archs Int. Pharmacodyn. Thér.* 1926, **32**, 9.
84. Hutchinson J. *Med. Chir. Trans.* 1846, **29**, 137.
85. Magnus H. G. *Ann. Physiol. Chem. (Leipzig)* 1837, **17**, 583.
86. Haldane J. S. *J. Physiol. (Lond.)* 1896, **13** 419.

87. *See also* Clarke S. *Br. J. Hosp. Med.* 1976, **15**, 137; Webb A. and MacCochrane G. *Hospital Update*, 1978, **4**, 339.
88. Gaensler E. A. *Am. Rev. Tuberc. Pulm. Dis.* 1951, **64**, 256.
89. Hewlett A. M. et al. *Br. J. Anaesth.* 1974, **46**, 486.
90. Ehrner C. *Acta Med. Scand.* 1960, **167**, suppl. 353.
91. Wright B. M. and McKerrow C. B. *Br. Med. J.* 1959, **2**, 1041: Wright B. M. *Br. Med. J.* 1978, **2**, 1627.
92. de Bono E. F. *Lancet* 1963, **2**, 1146.
93. Radford E. P. *J. Appl Physiol.* 1955, **7**, 451.
94. Enghoff H. *Förhandl.* 1938, **44**, 191.
95. Eckenhoff J. E. et al. *Br. J. Anaesth.* 1963, **35**, 750.
96. Comroe J. H. et al. *The Lung*, 2nd ed. Chicago: Year Book Publishers Inc., 1962.
97. Leblanc P. et al. *J. Appl. Physiol.* 1970, **28**, 448.

Chapter 3	# ACID–BASE AND ELECTROLYTE BALANCE

Hydrogen Ion Concentration and pH

Hydrogen ion concentration and pH described by S. P. L. Sorensen (1868–1939), Copenhagen physiologist. pH expresses hydrogen ion concentration as its negative logarithm to the base 10. Normal range for arterial blood, pH 7·36–7·44. Normal hydrogen ion concentration can be taken as 36–44 nanomoles (nmol)/litre. The range compatible with life is 20–160 nanomoles (nmol)/litre. Hydrogen ions do not exist free in water, but as $(H_3O)^+$. Electrometric methods of determination measure ionic activity and not concentration.

pH units	Hydrogen ions in nmol/litre
7·0	100
7·2	63
7·4	40
7·6	25
7·8	16
8·0	10

Acidaemia and Alkalaemia

In acidaemia, the hydrogen ion concentration is above, in alkalaemia below, the normal range.

Acidosis and Alkalosis

Acidosis is a condition which would tend to cause acidaemia if uncorrected. Alkalosis tends to cause alkalaemia if uncorrected.

Metabolic or Non-respiratory Acidosis and Alkalosis

This refers to acid–base disturbances due to any substance other than carbon dioxide. Acidosis means acid excess or base deficit (a deficiency of plasma bicarbonate). Alkalosis means base excess or acid deficit.

Metabolic Acidosis

This may occur: (1) In diabetic ketosis, due to β-hydroxybutyric acid; (2) in renal failure; (3) In starvation; (4) In infantile diarrhoea; (5) In salicylate poisoning; (6) After severe muscular exercise; (7) During rewarming after hypothermia; (8) During cardiopulmonary bypass causing tissue hypoxia; (9) During ether anaesthesia if lactate metabolism is depressed (Cushing's disease, parenteral steroid therapy, cirrhosis of the liver, in infancy); (10) In association with respiratory alkalosis; (11) Associated with hypoxia; (12) Shock. Inadequate tissue perfusion may result in anaerobic metabolism; (13) Prolonged intestinal obstruction; (14) Occlusion of large vessels; (15) Following cardiac arrest.

Clinical signs: (1) Gasping respiration; (2) Cold blue hands and feet; (3) Clouding of consciousness; (4) Hyperkalaemic effects on ECG.

Clinical effects: (1) CNS—depression of all functions including vasomotor and respiratory; (2) Cardiac—depression, dysrhythmias; (3) Respiration—depression, hypoxia; (4) Blood clotting—retarded; (5) Hepatic—reduced function; (6) Electrolyte balance—hyperkalaemia, lactate/pyruvate ratio increased.

The body compensates by increased pulmonary ventilation to remove CO_2 and by increased renal excretion of hydrogen ions. Treatment may include infusion of sodium bicarbonate intravenously, as well as treatment of the primary condition causing acidosis.

Sodium bicarbonate may be given: (*a*) as a 2·74% solution. This has twice the osmolarity of plasma and contains 166 mmol in 500 ml. Average dose 200 ml, which provides 1 mmol/kg in a 60-kg man; (*b*) As an 8·4% solution, which contains 1 mmol in each ml. Average dose about 50–150 ml. Clinical metabolic acidosis increases the bicarbonate space above the theoretical 33% of body volume.[2]

$$\text{Dose (in mmol)} = \frac{\text{base deficit} \times \text{body weight (in kg)}}{3}.$$

Metabolic Alkalosis

This may occur following ingestion of large amounts of bicarbonate or citrate, and in pyloric stenosis or use of nasogastric tube in ileus, with loss of acid. The body compensates by underventilation and increased renal bicarbonate excretion. Hypokalaemia occurs with excessive renal potassium and chloride loss (*see below*).

Treatment. Alkalosis is much more difficult to treat than acidosis.

1. Expectant, and correction of the primary cause. Potassium and chloride deficits are replaced with i.v. potassium chloride up to 150 mmol/day.

2. Rarely, oral administration of ammonium chloride, 10 g.

3. More commonly, i.v. ammonium chloride. It is safe and effective and is given over a 1-hour period:

$$\text{Dose (in mmol)} = \frac{\text{base excess} \times \text{body weight (in kg)}}{3}.$$

Buffer Base

Bicarbonate is the most important blood buffer in the consideration of acid–base balance. It can be measured, but the concentration is influenced by $P\text{CO}_2$, so that this factor must be excluded in determination of metabolic acid–base state.

Base Excess
This is the surplus of fixed acid or base in mmol/litre of blood. It is the amount of acid or base in mmol/litre required for titration back to pH 7·40 at P_{CO_2} of 5·3 kPa at a temperature of 38 °C. By convention an acid surplus (base deficit) is referred to as a negative base excess.

Standard Bicarbonate
This is the concentration in plasma at a P_{CO_2} of 5·3 kPa, with haemoglobin fully saturated, at 38 °C. No information is obtained about respiratory acid–base balance. Normally 24 mmol/l.

The Bicarbonate Buffer System
Carbonic acid exists in a state of equilibrium with hydrogen ions and bicarbonate ions:

$$H^+ + HCO_3^- \rightleftharpoons H_2CO_3.$$

The Law of Mass Action states that, when such a reaction has reached equilibrium, the product of the concentrations of the reagents on one side of the equation is proportional to the product of the concentrations of reagents on the other side of the equation:

$$[H^+][HCO_3^-] = K \times [H_2CO_3],$$

where K is a constant, which may be rewritten:

$$[H^+] = K \times \frac{[H_2CO_3]}{[HCO_3^-]}.$$

The carbonic acid in the equation can be replaced by P_{CO_2} if the solubility factor is known. If the units of measurements are defined, the value of K can be calculated.

The equation can then be written in a form which is more useful for clinical work:

$$pH \text{ or } [H^+] = 180 \frac{P_{CO_2} \text{ in kPa}}{[HCO_3^-]}.$$

Henderson–Hasselbalch Equation[3]
Hasselbalch (1874–1962, Copenhagen biochemist) expressed Henderson's (1878–1942, Boston physiologist) equation for hydrogen ion activity of the blood in logarithmic form. This classic equation links the same factors, expressed in logarithmic notation:

$$pH = pK + \log \frac{[HCO_3^-]}{[H_2CO_3]}.$$

As before, carbonic acid can be expressed in terms of P_{CO_2}:

$$pH = pK + \log \frac{[HCO_3^-]}{0·03 P_{CO_2}}.$$

pK varies with temperature and pH. An average figure at 38 °C is 6·1. The solubility factor of carbon dioxide in plasma is taken as 0·03 mmol/litre per mmHg. Total carbon dioxide content of plasma is expressed as $[HCO_3^-]$ + $0.03\,P_{CO_2}$.

Correction for temperature change. There is a rise of pH as the temperature of the blood falls due to changes in the degree of ionization of the protein elements. The usual correction factor is that pH rises by 0.0147 of a unit for each °C fall in temperature.[4]

Nowadays, however, the hydrogen ion concentration is measured and expressed directly, in nanomoles/litre, the normal value for arterial blood being 40 nmol/litre.

Other Buffers

Haemoglobin is the most important buffer after the bicarbonate system. Reduced haemoglobin is a stronger base than oxyhaemoglobin. Plasma proteins also act as buffers, but their capacity in mmol/litre in the blood is only one-third of that of haemoglobin.

The relationships can also be expressed graphically. When any two factors are used as co-ordinates, iso-lines can be constructed for the third.

Respiratory Acidosis and Alkalosis

Related to changes in carbon dioxide tension in arterial blood (P_{a,CO_2}). (Carbon dioxide forms the 'respiratory acid', carbonic acid.) Normal range is 4.6–5.9 kPa. Respiratory acidosis occurs at higher tensions.

Hypercapnia (Hypercarbia) ὑπὲρ (hyper), over + καπνός (kapnos), (smoke)

The ill effects of CO_2 excess were first emphasized by Waters (in the context of anaesthesia).[5]

Causes in Anaesthetic Practice: (1) Gross impairment of ventilation due to respiratory obstruction, profound narcosis, or relaxants; (2) Severe bilateral lung disease, perhaps complicated by thoracotomy; (3) Accidental administration of carbon dioxide; (4) Faulty carbon dioxide absorption. Defective soda lime in faulty system; (5) The technique of apnoeic insufflation oxygenation; (6) Hyperpyrexia.

Mild hypercapnia, up to P_{a,CO_2} 10.5 kPa, commonly causes dysrhythmias during anaesthesia. As the P_{a,CO_2} rises towards 25 kPa, narcosis deepens into coma. Over 25 kPa profound narcosis and respiratory failure resembling curarization occur.

Supercarbia, over 50 kPa, is associated with a zone of acute tolerance in animals, when respiration is possible again.

Effects of Hypercapnia

1. Central nervous system. (*a*) Increased cerebral blood flow, and thus cerebral volume; (*b*) Rise of cerebrospinal fluid pressure; (*c*) Progressive narcosis; (*d*) Inert gas effect.

In patients with chronic hypercapnia, e.g. in emphysema, a relatively high P_{CO_2} may be compatible with mental alertness.

2. Autonomic nervous system. (*a*) Sympathetic activation with a rise of circulating catecholamines; but with reduced sensitivity of the end organs to these catecholamines. Sweating. (*b*) Parasympathetic activation (though in general this is overshadowed by the sympathetic effect).

3. Respiratory system. (*a*) Carbon dioxide provides a most powerful stimulus to respiration, at the respiratory centre; (*b*) Severe hypercapnia produces respiratory failure; (*c*) Bohr effect:[6] more oxygen is released from combination with haemoglobin at the same oxygen tension in the presence of hypercapnia; oxygen is more readily liberated in the tissues but less is taken up in the lungs; the dissociation curve is shifted to the right.

4. *Cardiovascular system.* (*a*) Cardiac output, and force of contraction of the heart is increased due to direct effect of CO_2 on the heart, reflex sympathetic stimulation, and to greatly increased circulating catecholamines; (*b*) Tachycardia, due to catecholamine release; (*c*) Dysrhythmias: dysrhythmia CO_2 thresholds are described during cyclopropane and halothane anaesthesia; (*d*) Peripheral resistance; a central vasomotor effect leads to vasoconstriction; a peripheral effect in the capillaries leads to dilatation; the central effect is abolished by sympathetic block; (*e*) Blood pressure: rises in the absence of anaesthesia; during anaesthesia there is no absolute rule, and hypertension, normotension or hypotension may occur.

5. *Biochemical.* (*a*) pH changes: respiratory acidosis; (*b*) Compensatory metabolic alkalosis: secretion of acid urine with retention of bicarbonate and sodium; (*c*) Electrolytes: rise of serum potassium. Of the order of 0·5 mmol/litre at P_{CO_2} = 20 kPa; a further rise may take place in sudden withdrawal of carbon dioxide, causing cardiovascular changes which may be serious; (*d*) Rise of plasma 15-hydroxycorticosteroids.

6. *Effects on action of drugs.* (*a*) Changes of pH affect the ionization of many drugs thereby altering the concentration of the active fraction; (*b*) Changes of pH affect the fraction of some drugs which is bound to protein (e.g. respiratory acidosis increases the dosage requirements of thiopentone); (*c*) Tubocurarine, and probably pancuronium, potentiated in hypercapnia; other relaxants are antagonized.

Carbon Dioxide Withdrawal

Sudden fall of P_{CO_2} following a period of hypercapnia may itself produce untoward effects:

1. Hypotension. Sudden reversal of hypercapnia may produce the Brown and Miller effect of acute circulatory depression.[7] Not pronounced unless there has been moderate or severe hypercapnia for some time. More frequently seen after cyclopropane anaesthesia. Mechanism not established.

2. Dysrhythmia. It would appear that an immediate and sudden release of potassium from heart muscle and liver occurs to produce hyperkalaemia and dysrhythmia. This is followed by excessive excretion of potassium and hypokalaemia. Shift of the oxygen haemoglobin dissociation curve impedes oxygen exchange at tissue level. Another contributory factor might be hypoxia—when marked hypercapnia is terminated by ventilation with air (diffusion hypoxia).

Rapid lowering of the chronic hypercapnia in respiratory failure can lead to convulsions and death, unless the alkalaemia produced is corrected.

While every care should be taken to avoid hypercapnia, mild degrees of this condition may not be as serious as was once thought.

Recovery from severe respiratory acidosis may be associated with hypophosphataemia so that repeated serum phosphate estimations may need to be monitored.[8]

Respiratory Alkalosis (Hypocapnia)

This is caused by hyperventilation which produces hypocapnia and rise of blood pH. IPPV under clinical conditions may reduce the Pco_2 from a normal of 5·3 kPa to half of this value.

Effects of Respiratory Alkalosis
1. *Central nervous system.* (a) Reduction in cerebral blood flow,[9] and shrinkage of brain; (b) Reduction in cerebral oxygen tension; (c) Clouding of consciousness and analgesia, due to depression of the reticular formation. The threshold to pain may be increased by up to three times, as evidenced by a study in volunteers in whom the pH rose from normal to 7·7.[10] Voluntary hyperventilation to lessen the pain of surgery was described by Bonwill in 1876.[11]
2. *Cardiovascular system.* (a) Fall of blood pressure and cardiac output; (b) Vasoconstriction; (c) May protect the heart against the effect of atropine and neostigmine though it is more important to prevent hypoxia than to produce hypocapnia.
3. *Changes in the blood.* (a) Increase of circulating red cells; (b) Loss of plasma water from the circulation; (c) Fall of plasma sodium; (d) Small fall of plasma potassium; (e) Fall in ionized calcium, but slight increase in total plasma calcium; (f) Hinders the liberation of oxygen from oxyhaemoglobin; (g) Shift to the left of the oxygen dissociation curve.
4. *Fetus.* There is some evidence that hyperventilation during anaesthesia for Caesarean section carries some risk to the fetus. Fetal asphyxia is more likely if the Pco_2 falls below 2·2 kPa. There is a fall in fetal oxygen associated with maternal hyperventilation. The clinical importance of these observations is debatable, but in the light of present knowledge it is probably best to avoid hyperventilation during anaesthesia in obstetrics. There is some evidence that pH is the important factor rather than Pco_2 and that it causes intraplacental shunting in lambs.
5. *Tetany.* Not commonly associated with clinical anaesthesia.
6. Subsequent period of obligatory hypoventilation.
7. For effects on muscle relaxants *see* Chapter 14.

Active and Passive Hyperventilation
Active respiratory effort increases the metabolism of the muscles resulting in increased carbon dioxide production. There is a minute volume of about 60 litres/min where the increase in ventilation would be offset by the increased CO_2 production.

Advantages of Hyperventilation Techniques in Anaesthesia
Note: In ordinary British practice, IPPV during operations often reduces the $Paco_2$ down to 3 kPa (20–25 mmHg).
   1. Full oxygenation is maintained by adequately aerating the lungs.
   2. A mild respiratory alkalosis is generally held to be safer than a respiratory acidosis.
   3. The respiratory alkalosis itself contributes to the anaesthetic state. Smaller doses of anaesthetic drugs are required: (a) A reduction in the dose of intravenous barbiturates; (b) A reduction in analgesic agents; (c) A reduction in the dose of tubocurarine and an increase in potency. These effects are probably due to the production of general analgesia and the depression of other cerebral functions, e.g. a decrease in the frequency of discharge from the reticular activating system.

They are due not to a decrease in cerebral blood flow and tissue hypoxia but to changes in the P_{CO_2} and pH values. Inhalation of pure oxygen and removal of vasoconstriction in the retinal vessels (and so presumably in the cerebral vessels) do not decrease analgesia.

4. Moderate hyperventilation causes no significant increase in metabolic acidosis or in tissue hypoxia.

5. Cardiac effects of neostigmine minimized.

6. Hypocapnia is important during the production of induced hypotension.

7. Incidence of peripheral atelectasis reduced.

The analgesic effect of hyperventilatory hypocapnia is discussed by Geddes and Gray.[12]

Disadvantages of Hyperventilation in Anaesthesia

1. In unskilled hands, undesirable sequelae may follow due to faulty technique, e.g. hypotension.

2. Where cerebral perfusion is borderline (e.g. in cardiopulmonary bypass) cerebral vasoconstriction may be undesirable.

3. In obstetrics. Possible adverse effects on the fetus (*see* Chapter 27).

4. In patients with P_{CO_2} of less than 3·5 kPa due to hyperventilation (not uncommon after a period of hyperventilation), there is evidence of postoperative prolongation of reaction time lasting 3–6 days.[13] Carbon dioxide produced in metabolism may be needed to replenish body stores so that little is excreted in the first hour after cessation of hyperventilation.

5. Disadvantages of hypocapnia include: (i) Increase in lactate/pyruvate ratio in blood; (ii) Increase in lactate/pyruvate ratio in CSF; (iii) Fall in pH of CSF (all are signs of inadequate cerebral perfusion); (iv) Reduction of cardiac output; (v) Depletion of extracellular potassium.

If a relaxant is adequately reversed, respiration will start even in the presence of hypocapnia, always provided that the respiratory centre is not depressed (e.g. by narcotic analgesics) and that the peripheral receptors in the upper respiratory tract are not inactivated by local analgesic sprays or ointments.[14] The $P_{a_{CO_2}}$ may need to be restored back up to normal levels to restart respiration. Inhalation of 5% CO_2 will achieve this.

See also Norman J. *Br. J. Anaesth*. 1978, **50**, 45.

Electrolyte Balance

Flame photometry pioneered in 1947.[15] Ion selective electrodes described in 1963.[16]

1. Sodium

Total amount of sodium in the adult body is about 105 g; about one-third of this is in bone. Basic need of body is 1–2 g/day, but as much as 15 g may be taken with food, the excess being excreted in the urine (normal, 5 g/litre). Normal serum levels are 132–142 mmol/litre of sodium and 98–106 mmol/litre of chloride.

(*See also* Barton I. K. and Mansell M. A. *Br. J. Hosp. Med*. 1984, **32**, 8.)

Sodium Depletion

Causes. Usually occurs when salt is lost but fluid intake is normal as in vomiting, diarrhoea, intestinal fistulae or drainage, intestinal obstruction, etc.

Symptoms. Lassitude, apathy, weakness, anorexia, vomiting, peripheral circulatory failure. Urine normal in amount. The 'sick-cell syndrome' with loss of sodium into the intracellular space leads to similar symptoms (*see below*). Finally, coma and collapse.

Results

1. A loss of total osmotic pressure of extracellular fluid leading to excretion of water by the kidney and thus to decreased extracellular fluid volume with secondary or extracellular dehydration. Later follows a fall in serum chlorides with a low value for urinary chlorides. There may be a rise in blood urea.

2. There is a disturbance of acid–base balance if the loss of chloride and sodium ions is disproportionate. With continued loss of gastric juice there is hypochloraemia with the production of alkalosis as the freed sodium combines with carbonic acid. On the other hand, with continued loss of fluid from the gut distal to the pylorus, there is a greater loss of sodium ions, with resulting acidosis.

Diagnosis. On the clinical signs and symptoms. On the serum electrolyte estimation.

Treatment. Twice normal saline i.v. (1·8%).

Sodium Retention

This may occur with water retention, as in oedema, or as sodium retention alone, *hypernatraemia*. This is usually accompanied by hyperchloraemia. May be due to: (1) *Excessive intake* as in over-infusion, excessive oral intake, or use of sodium-containing medicines in babies; (2) *Inability to excrete* as in primary hyperaldosteronism, Cushing's syndrome, excessive steroid therapy, or essential (encephalogenic) hypernatraemia with some neurological lesions. Effects are: mild oedema, confusion, apathy, leading to coma. Treated by withholding sodium and giving frusemide or chlorothiazide.

The 'Sick-cell Syndrome'

There is evidence that in some pathological conditions the integrity of the cell membrane is diminished and intracellular metabolic processes are disturbed. This means that the 'sodium pump' mechanism is inefficient; water and sodium pass into the cells with resultant fall of serum sodium. Hyponatraemia occurs without loss of total body sodium. Potassium ions leak out of the cells. Treatment advocated includes administration of insulin and glucose in an effort to drive potassium into cells and reverse the ionic exchange, while measures must be taken also to improve perfusion and oxygenation of tissues and combat infection.

2. Potassium[17]

Most of the body potassium is found within the cells and only about 2% is in the extracellular compartment. Total average values may be taken as 3200 mmol for a 70-kg man. The average dietary intake of a normal healthy adult is 40–120 mmol (3–9 g)/24 h. Normal serum levels are 3·5–5·0 mmol/litre. Normal intracellular concentration is 135–150 mmol/litre. Daily urine loss is about 50–75 mmol.

(*See also* Allison S. P. *Br. J. Hosp. Med.* 1984, **32**, 19.)

Potassium Depletion

Causes. (*a*) Excessive loss from the gastrointestinal tract, vomiting, diarrhoea, *biliary fistula, etc.; (b)* Excessive loss in the urine if diuresis is marked; *(c)* Absence of normal potassium intake especially in the presence of excessive loss; *(d)* In cirrhosis of the liver; *(e)* In congestive heart failure; *(f)* May occur when patients are receiving intravenous glucose and saline drips for long periods; *(g)* Adrenal hyperactivity, whether pathological or therapeutic (intensive steroid therapy): *(h)* Insulinoma; *(i)* Familial periodic paralysis; *(j)* Myasthenia gravis; *(k)* Diabetic ketosis; *(l)* Renal tubular disease; *(m)* Ulcerative colitis. Alkalosis is a common cause of hypokalaemia as the ion moves from the serum into the cells, and gives a similar clinical picture.

Results. A clinical picture of lethargy, apathy, anorexia and nausea related to disordered function of the three types of muscle; *(a)* Smooth muscle—causing constipation, distension and ileus; *(b)* Skeletal muscle—causing hypotonia, weakness and paralysis; *(c)* Cardiac muscle—causing hypotension, dysrhythmia and arrest.

Diagnosis. Suspicion should arise when there is excessive fluid loss from urinary or gastrointestinal tracts, particularly when potassium intake is low or absent. It may be a factor in prolonged paralytic ileus or metabolic alkalosis not responding to normal treatment. Diagnosis is confirmed by: *(a)* Plasma potassium estimation, though this can sometimes be normal in the presence of intracellular depletion; *(b)* ECG changes: depression of ST segment, lowering, widening or inversion of T waves, prolongation of PR and QT interval, appearance of U waves—these are a reflection of intracellular potassium deficiency; *(c)* Response to treatment.

Management of Hypokalaemia. There is definite evidence of complications when the serum potassium is below 3·0 mmol/litre.[18] In the previously fit adult patient, this represents a deficit of 200 mmol which in anaesthesia and intensive care may be replaced intravenously using up to 200 mmol of potassium chloride diluted in 500–1000 ml of 5% dextrose over 4–8 h. Clinical judgement should be exercised before active treatment.

Proposed surgery may have to be delayed if the serum potassium is below 3·0 mmol/litre, because of the risk of cardiac dysrhythmias, potentiation of digitalis, muscle weakness, inability to reverse relaxants, myopathy and renal failure.[18] In those suspected of having whole-body potassium deficiency[19] e.g. the elderly, patients with alkalosis, on long-term IPPV and those who have received diuretics, intravenous potassium treatment is started at a serum potassium level of 3·5–4 mmol/litre, and may require to be continued for several days with ECG monitoring.

The correction of hypokalaemia contributes to the correction of concurrent metabolic alkalosis and vice versa.

Hyperkalaemia

This is dangerous, chiefly because of its effects on the heart. Causes: *(a)* Over-zealous intravenous replacement therapy, or when urine output is depressed or absent; *(b)* Administration of suxamethonium causes an acute rise in serum potassium. This occurs within 1–7 min of injection and is of the order of 0·5 mmol/litre in normal patients or 1·8 mmol/litre in patients with trauma and burns. Pretreatment with curare decreases the effect after suxamethonium (but not after decamethonium); *(c)* Muscle injury—may be late. *(d)* Muscle-wasting diseases and abnormalities, e.g. myopathies, motor neuron lesions, muscular dystrophy, denervation and spinal cord transection and tetanus; *(e)* In metabolic acidosis; (*f*) Acute renal failure; (*g*) Potassium sparing diuretics; (*h*) Adrenal insufficiency. Toxic manifestations may occur at concentrations above 7 mmol/litre, when the ECG shows a tall peaked T wave with a narrow base, diminished amplitude of R wave, absence of P wave, widening of QRS and finally a diphasic QRST. Ventricular fibrillation may supervene. Stored blood may contain 25 mmol/litre (*see* Chapter 42).

Treatment. (*a*) Administration of glucose and insulin, which causes shift of potassium ions into cells; (*b*) Bicarbonate infusion 150–300 mmol has a similar effect; (*c*) Calcium salts can be given because calcium ions oppose the action of potassium ions on the heart; (*d*) Long-term treatment includes diet, resonium cation exchange, peritoneal- and haemodialysis.

3. Calcium[20]

The serum-ionized calcium concentration may be important in certain patients. Normal range 2·1–2·6 mmol/litre. The level may be abnormal as a result of: (*a*) Changes in ventilation affecting $Paco_2$ (hyperventilation lowers serum ionized calcium); (*b*) Transfusion with citrated blood. This is seldom important in the healthy individual as the small changes, 0·1–0·2 mmol/litre, last only for minutes.[21] When there is a disorder of citrate metabolism (*see* Chapter 42) administration of calcium may be indicated; (*c*) In some patients with prolonged electrolyte problems, as in the presence of losses through fistulae, etc. during long-term intravenous therapy, calcium may become low and require correction. Calcium gluconate ionizes well in solution.[22]

An electrode for measurement of calcium ions has been described.[23]

(*See also* Drop L. J. *Anesth. Analg.* 1985, **64**, 432.)

4. Magnesium[24]

Serum-magnesium levels may fall after prolonged intravenous therapy in ill patients with electrolyte losses. Magnesium is important in various enzyme systems in cellular metabolism. Clinical signs associated with low magnesium include tremors, twitching, tetany, muscular weakness, confusion and hallucinations. It may be given as magnesium chloride, 2 mmol/kg in 4 hours. Normal values, 1·5–2·5 mmol/litre.

5. Zinc

It is suspected that lack of zinc may be a factor in delayed healing after prolonged severe illness with electrolyte imbalance. It may be given orally in cases of doubt.

6. Phosphate

Hypophosphataemia[25] exists when the serum phosphate is below 1 mmol/litre. Signs: Confusion, disorientation, dysarthria, paraesthesia, coma. The oxygen-dissociation curve shifts to the left, the erythrocyte P50 is below 25, there is poor oxygen transport with hypoxia, lactic acidosis and pulmonary oedema. There is also poor leucocyte function. The condition is seen mainly during i.v. feeding when fats and phosphate are not provided. The maintenance requirement is at least 10 mmol per day in the adult, given as sodium phosphate, orally or intravenously.

(*See also* Worthley L. I. G. *Anaesth. Intensive Care* 1977, **5**, 326; Davidson G. M. *Anaesth. Intensive Care* 1977, **5**, 333; Fisher M. M. *Anaesth. Intensive Care* 1977, **5**, 339; Waterwillata S. M. *Br. J. Med.* 1984, **32**, 8.)

References

1. p = Potenz or power; pH (Sorensen S. P. L., *C. R. Trav. Lat. Carlsberg* 1909, **8**, 1).
2. Adrogue H. J., Brensilver J. et al. *J. Clin. Invest.* 1983, **71**, 867.
3. Henderson L. J. *Am. J. Physiol.* 1908, **21**, 173; **21**, 427; Hasselbalch K. A. *Biochem. Z.* 1916, **78**, 112 (*see also* 'Classical File', *Surv. Anesthesiol.* 1964, **8**, 486, 607).
4. Rosenthal T. B. *J. Biol. Chem.* 1948, **173**, 25; Severinghaus J. W. *J. Appl. Physiol.* 1966, **21**, 1108.
5. Waters R. M. *New Orl. Med. Surg. J.* 1937, **90**, 219; *Can. Med. Assoc. J.* 1938, **38**, 240.
6. Bohr C., Hasselbalch K. and Krogh A. *Arch. Physiol. Scand.* 1904, **16**, 402.
7. Brown E. B. and Miller F. *Am. J. Physiol.* 1952, **169**, 56.
8. Storm T. L. *Br. Med. J.* 1984, **289**, 456.
9. Kety S. S. and Schmidt C. F. *J. Clin. Invest.* 1946, **25**, 107.
10. Robinson J. S. and Gray T. C. *Br. J. Anaesth.* 1961, **33**, 62.
11. Bonwill W. G. A. *Penna J. Dent. Science* 1876, **3**, 57 (reprinted in 'Classical File', *Surv. Anesthesiol.* 1964, **8**, 377).
12. Geddes I. C. and Gray T. C. *Lancet* 1959, **2**, 4.
13. Wollman S. B. and Orkin L. R. *Br. J. Anaesth.* 1968, **40**, 920.
14. Utting J. E. and Gray T. C. *Br. J. Anaesth.* 1962, **34**, 785.
15. Hald P. M. *J. Biol. Chem.* 1947, **167**, 499.
16. Friedman S. M., Wong S-L. et al. *J. Appl. Physiol.* 1963, **18**, 950.
17. Stockigt J. R. *Anaesth. Intensive Crae* 1977, **5**, 317.
18. Descamps C. et al. *Br. Med. J.* 1977, **1**, 272; Greenblatt D. J. et al. *Am. Heart J.* 1977, **94**, 6; Lowe J. et al. *Br. Med. J.* 1979, **2**, 360.
19. Morgan D. B. et al. *Postgrad Med. J.* 1978, **54**, 72.
20. Thomas D. W. *Anaesth. Intensive Care* 1977, **5**, 361; Stevenson J. C. *Br. J. Hosp. Med.* 1984, **32**, 71.
21. Hinkle J. E. and Cooperman L. H. *Br. J. Anaesth.* 1971, **43**, 1108.
22. Heining M. P. D., Band D. M. et al. *Anaesthesia* 1984, **39**, 1079.
23. Moore E. W. *J. Clin. Invest.* 1970, **49**, 318; Paymaster N. J. *Br. J. Anaesth.* 1975, **47**, 85.
24. Sawyer R. B. et al. *Archs Surg.* 1970, **100**, 343; Paymaster N. J. *Ann. R. Coll. Surg.* 1976, **58**, 315; Brenton D. P., Girdin T. E. et al. *Br. J. Hosp. Med.* 1984, **32**, 60.
25. Juan D. *Surg. Gynecol. Obstet.* 1981, **153**, 589.

Chapter 4   **NOTES ON PHARMACOLOGY**

Pharmacokinetics

Pharmacokinetics embraces the absorption, metabolism, excretion, distribution and protein binding of drugs (what the body does to a drug).

Drug Absorption
The routes of drug administration are:

Oral
An easy, painless and reliable route. Drug absorption may be affected by the functional efficiency of the gastrointestinal tract, concomitant administration of other drugs or food (e.g. metoclopramide may accelerate drug absorption) and the effect of the liver in metabolizing the absorbed drug (the 'first-pass' effect). For example, some 75% of absorbed propranolol is destroyed on its first pass through the portal system of the liver. However, some drugs are completely or

largely metabolized in the gastrointestinal tract and others are unpalatable. Some retrieval of administered drug may be possible with emetics.

Sublingual
Useful for drugs like buprenorphine and nitrates. Absorption depends on the ability and co-operation of the patient.

Inhalation
Reliable, usually swift. Retrieval of agents is usually possible. Speed of uptake and elimination is somewhat dependent on lung function and presence of other inhaled agents, e.g. 'second gas effect'.

Injection (intradermal, subcutaneous, intramuscular and intraperitoneal)
An accurate dose will be reliably absorbed but may be slow, e.g. digoxin by intramuscular injection. In obese patients it is difficult to be sure whether an injection is subcutaneous or intramuscular. There may be damage to other structures, e.g. sciatic nerve. There may be pain, e.g. penicillin injections. Retrieval is not possible. Intramuscular absorption may be severely delayed in shock, e.g. morphine.

Intravenous
Accurate, swift and certain. Retrieval is not possible. An ideal route for anaesthetic induction agents.

Rectal
Useful for sedatives and premedicants, e.g. diazepam, morphine, paraldehyde. The patient may not retain the drug long enough for absorption.

Transcutaneous
Slow but reliable and painless. Useful for long-acting coronary vasodilators, lignocaine and hyoscine, and glyceryl trinitrate.

Drug Elimination

Exhalation
The common and efficient route for inhalation agents and some other drugs, e.g. alcohol and paraldehyde.

Excretion
   1. Via the bile, e.g. some antibiotics, radiographic contrast media, alcuronium, tubocurarine, pancuronium, glycopyrronium. Active secretion of drugs or conjugates with a molecular weight above 400. Biliary excretion is saturable and can be inhibited.
   2. Via the urine. Through filtration at the glomerulus if the drug is not protein-bound.
   Through active secretion at the proximal tubule, e.g. acidic drugs are secreted by a specific transport mechanism. The same applies to basic drugs, but they do not usually interfere with the transport of acidic drugs and vice versa.
   Probenecid inhibits penicillin secretion and thiazides inhibit urate secretion (these are acidic compounds). Basic drugs cleared at the proximal renal tubule

include dopamine, lignocaine, morphine and neostigmine. Distal tubular diffusion of non-ionized forms of weak acids and bases leads to excretion of basic drugs, e.g. tertiary amines, and reabsorption of probenecid in acidic conditions. The diffusion of other drugs, e.g. barbiturates and salicylates, may be facilitated by alkaline urine.

3. Via the gastrointestinal tract, e.g. fentanyl. This drug may be absorbed lower down in the small intestine.

4. Via milk and saliva, e.g. narcotic and hypnotic drugs.

Metabolism
Phase 1 metabolism is oxidation-reduction or hydrolysis, mainly in the liver, catalysed by mixed function oxidase cytochrome P450.
Oxidation—halothane (to trifluoracetic acid), thiopentone (to pentobarbitone), alcohol, dopamine.
Reduction, e.g. reductive dehalogenation of halothane; chloral hydrate to trichloroethane.
Hydrolysis—pethidine, lignocaine and (in the plasma) suxamethonium to succinate and choline; acetylcholine to acetate and choline.

Phase 2 reactions are synthetic or conjugation reactions and they enhance water solubility. Glucuronide conjugation is te method for morphine, salicylates and bilirubin, among many others. Sulphate conjugation is employed, e.g. with isoprenaline and paracetamol. Acetate conjugation is the final phase for isoniazid, para-amino benzoic acid (PABA) and some sulphonamides.

Amino acid conjugation occurs, e.g. salicylic acid with glycine or glutamine. Glycine conjugation of bromsulphthalein is used as a test of hepatic function. Methylation is employed, e.g. with adrenaline.

Enzyme inducers enhance the rate and extent of metabolism of drugs. Many of these inducers are drugs themselves, causing increased synthesis and reduced elimination of enzymes, of both phase 1 and 2 reactions. Barbiturates and 3-methylcholanthrene are classic inducers. Other enzyme inducers are: hypoxia, analgesics, e.g. phenylbutazone, antibiotics, e.g. rifampicin (and isoniazid in the rapid acetylators), anticonvulsants, e.g. phenytoin, inhalation anaesthetics (but they inhibit their own metabolism when in anaesthetic concentrations), steroids, alcohol, anticoagulants and hundreds of other drugs.

Enzyme inhibitors, conversely, may prolong the action of drugs, e.g. plasma cholinesterase inhibitors (neostigmine, procaine, propanidid, ecothiopate) extend the action of acetylcholine and suxamethonium.

Hepatic enzyme inhibitors include phenylbutazone and isoniazid, monoamine oxidase inhibitors, cimetidine, amiodarone and toxic doses of alcohol.

Saturation of a metabolic pathway by a large dose of a drug may prevent its metabolism, e.g. phenytoin, inhalation anaesthetics, thiopentone and diazepam. Hepatic disease may also prolong and potentiate the action of drugs, e.g. opioids.

Drug Distribution
One- two- and three-compartment models have been devised.
One-compartment model, e.g. neostigmine and inhalation agents. There is a simple mono-exponential decline of plasma concentration after a bolus injection. The plasma half-life is the time in minutes taken for the plasma concentration of the drug to be halved. The decline of concentration of drug with time,

dx/dt = −kX, where X is the amount of the drug in the body at time t and k is the elimination rate constant.

Two-compartment model, e.g. phenoperidine and alcuronium. There is a bi-exponential decline in the plasma level of the drug, an initial rapid distribution phase, the α phase, with a distribution half-life $T_{\frac{1}{2}\alpha}$ followed by a slower elimination phase, the β phase with an elimination half-life $T_{\frac{1}{2}\beta}$. Distribution is assumed to be from a central compartment, e.g. blood, to a peripheral compartment, e.g. extravascular space, with rate constants governing transfer of drug in each direction.

$$\text{The elimination half-life, } T_{\frac{1}{2}\beta} = \frac{L_n 2 \times V_D}{CL}$$

where L_n is the total body clearance, V_D is the total apparent volume of distribution.

The two-compartment model describes the distribution of very many drugs.

Three-compartment model, e.g. some non-depolarizing muscle relaxants, assume a central compartment and two different peripheral compartments, with a tri-exponential decline in drug concentration in the central compartment.

Hysteresis loops occur when the concentration of a drug is plotted against its effect, and the relationship is different on decreasing the concentration of the drug from what it was on increasing it. Blood gas abnormalities may alter the pharmacokinetics of many drugs.

Binding of Drugs affects distribution, usually retarding it. Binding occurs with plasma proteins, e.g. tubocurarine, and fat, e.g. thiopentone.

Distribution volume (V_β) is the volume of water into which a drug disperses after administration, and is calculated from the measured dilution with an allowance for the elimination which has already occurred during this measurement.

Total volume of distribution at steady state (Vd_{ss}) is the same volume of water into which a drug disperses, measured by its dilution when as much drug is being administered as is being eliminated. (It is the mass of drug in the body divided by the plasma concentration of that drug.) If this volume is the same as plasma volume, this suggests that the drug remains in the vascular space. If smaller than the plasma volume, plasma protein binding is suggested. If larger than the whole body water, this implies much binding in the fat or tissue proteins.

'First order' or linear kinetics is when the elimination or distribution of a drug is proportional to its concentration. The 'rate constant' is the rate of this decline.

'Zero order' or non-linear kinetics is when the rate of elimination or distribution of a drug is not proportional to its concentration.

Clearance is the volume of blood or plasma from which a drug is removed in unit time.

$$\text{Clearance} = \frac{\text{Kel} \times [D]}{[D]} \text{ or } \frac{0 \cdot 693}{\text{elimination half-life}}$$

where [D] is the concentration of the drug and Kel is the elimination constant.

Pharmacodynamics

Pharmacodynamics concerns drug action—what a drug does to the body. The relationship between dose and response is frequently hyperbolic and lends itself to mathematical analysis. Drug action may be due to:

1. *Chemical properties*, e.g. chelating agents and antacids.

2. *Enzyme inhibition*, e.g. aspirin, neostigmine, penicillin and monoamine oxidase inhibitors.

3. *Receptor action* in which receptors are specific for certain drugs or groups of drugs with a high affinity for small concentrations of agonists and a variable degree of reversibility in response to changes in the concentration of the drug. The fraction of the receptors occupied,

$$f = \frac{[D]}{K_d + [D]} \, ,$$

where [D] is the concentration of the drug, and K_d is the dissociation constant for the receptors.

Receptor action may make use of 'second messengers', e.g. cyclic adenosine monophosphate at β-receptors, cyclic guanosine monophosphate at α-receptors, and calcium ions. A drug which produces a response at a receptor site is called an agonist.

Agonists and Antagonists
Agonists have both receptor affinity and intrinsic activity. Competitive antagonists have receptor affinity but no intrinsic activity. Non-competitive antagonists (e.g. high-dose phenoxybenzamine), have exceptionally strong receptor affinity and no intrinsic activity. Partial agonists have considerable receptor affinity, some intrinsic activity, and thus may produce antagonist or agonist effects, depending on the situation. In low dose they frequently show agonist effects. In higher dose, partial agonists show their own agonist effects and antagonize any other agonist which may be present. Common examples are the antagonists known as β-blockers, some of which (e.g. propranolol) have minimal agonist or 'intrinsic sympathomimetic' activity. Other β-blockers have strong partial agonist activity (e.g. pindolol). Likewise, among the opioids, there is a whole range of action from pure agonists, e.g. pethidine and fentanyl, through partial agonists, e.g. nalorphine (mild) and buprenorphine (strong partial agonist), to the (almost) pure antagonist, e.g. naloxone. The situation with opioids is complicated because some drugs are agonists at one type of receptor, while being antagonists at another type of receptor! For example nalbuphine and buprenorphine are μ agonists and kappa antagonists.

Efficacy is the maximum ceiling effect of a drug.

Potency is the dose required to produce a certain effect, and enables comparative *dose equivalence* of different drugs to be assessed.

Optimality is the dose of a drug which gives the best therapeutic effect without too many side-effects.

Chemotherapeutic index or ratio is the mean lethal dose divided by the mean effective dose, i.e. LD_{50}/ED_{50} or kill dose/cure dose.

Drug desensitization is decreasing response to a drug e.g. due to repeated exposure to it. It may be acute or chronic, as repeated exposure to adrenergic bronchodilators. It is characterized by receptors entering a desensitized state.

Tachyphylaxis is a decreasing response to a drug due to exhaustion of a transmitter, e.g. in the use of ephedrine.

Tolerance is decreasing response to a drug due to other causes.

very helpful!

Drug Interactions

1. Pharmacokinetic interactions modify the concentration of a drug at its site of action by affecting its absorption, excretion, metabolism or protein binding.

2. Pharmacodynamic interactions may be simply additive, synergistic or potentiating. Conversely they may be antagonistic.

3. Pharmaceutical interactions occur outside the body, resulting in precipitation, binding or inactivation of drugs.

Chapter 5   *NOTES ON PHYSICS*[1]

Laws of gases

The kinetic theory of gases postulates that the molecules of a gas in an enclosed space are constantly moving and so are constantly bumping into each other and into the walls of the enclosing space. These bumpings give rise to the pressure or tension of the gas in the space. The greater the number of molecules the greater will be the tension. Temperature increases movement and so increases tension.

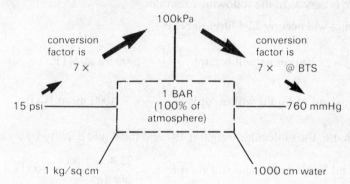

Fig. 5.1. Equivalent pressures in different units (a rough approximation). For exact values *see* Appendix.

Boyle's Law

(1662; Robert Boyle, 1627–1691, English chemist). The volume of a gas varies inversely with the pressure it is subjected to, the temperature remaining constant.

Charles's Law

(1787; Jacques Alexander César Charles, 1746–1823, French physiologist). At constant pressure, the volume of a gas is proportional to its absolute temperature.

Dalton's Law of Partial Pressure

(1801; John Dalton, 1766–1844, Manchester chemist). The pressure of a gas in a physical mixture of gases equals the pressure which that quantity of gas would produce were it alone. Thus the total pressure of a mixture of gases equals the sum of the partial pressures of the individual gases. The partial pressure of a gas in a mixture is proportional to its percentage by volume in the mixture.

If a liquid is exposed to a gas at a given pressure and equilibrium is established, the pressure of the gas in the liquid will equal the pressure of the gas in contact with it.

Henry's Law of Solution of Gases

(1803; William Henry, 1744–1836, English chemist).[2] With temperature remaining constant, the volume of gas going into solution in a given liquid is proportional to the partial pressure of the gas.

Graham's Law of Diffusion of Gases

(1831; Thomas Graham, 1805–1869, Scottish physician and chemist). The rate of diffusion of a gas varies inversely as the square root of its density. Important in the theory of flow-meters (*see* Chapter 9).

Avogadro's Law

(1811; Amadeo Avogadro, 1776–1856, Italian physicist). Equal volumes of a gas under standard conditions of temperature and pressure contain equal numbers of molecules. One gramme molecule of a gas occupies 22·4 litres at NTP. (*Note:* NTP is 760 mmHg and 273 °Absolute). This law is used in the calculation of the amount of a volatile liquid needed to make a known percentage vapour in air. Provided the molecular weight (x) is known and the density (y) of the liquid, calculation is easy as in the following example:

x grammes will occupy 22·4 litres at NTP.

$$1 \text{ gramme will occupy } \frac{22 \cdot 4}{x} \times 1000 \text{ ml at NTP.}$$

$$1 \text{ ml of liquid will occupy } \frac{22 \cdot 4 \times y}{x} \times 1000 \text{ ml at NTP.}$$

For halothane, the molecular weight is 197 and the liquid density 1·86.

$$1 \text{ ml liquid halothane will therefore } = \frac{22 \cdot 4 \times 1 \cdot 86}{197} \times 1000 \text{ ml}$$

$$\simeq 221 \text{ ml at NTP.}$$

It is then a matter of simple proportion to make a known percentage of vapour in air, bearing in mind that a concentration greater than the saturated vapour pressure cannot exist. Also, the pressure gauge on a cylinder acts as a content gauge above the critical temperature.

Ostwald's Solubility Coefficient

(1894; Wilhelm Ostwald, 1853–1932, Russian–German physical chemist. Nobel prizeman, 1909). The volume of a gas which dissolves in unit volume of solvent, measured under the conditions of temperature and pressure at which solution takes place.

Critical pressure. Pressure required to liquefy a gas at its critical temperature.

Critical temperature. Temperature to which a gas must be cooled before it can be liquefied by pressure.

Pseudocritical temperature. Temperature at which gas mixtures separate into component parts, e.g. Entonox.

Vapour pressure. Pressure exerted by molecules of a gas escaping from a liquid. The saturated vapour pressure of a volatile anaesthetic agent is important in consideration of those systems which depend on dilution of a saturated vapour (e.g. copper kettle, Halox vaporizer). Saturated vapour pressure varies with temperature. *The boiling point of a liquid* is that temperature at which the saturated vapour pressure equals atmospheric pressure.

Specific gravity of a gas. This is the ratio of the weight of a unit volume to a similar volume of air (regarded as 1), under the same conditions of temperature and pressure. Specific gravities of gases used by anaesthetists: Halothane vapour, 6·8; Trichloroethylene vapour, 4·5; Chloroform vapour, 4·12; Diethyl ether vapour, 2·6; Ethyl chloride, 2·28; Divinyl ether vapour, 2·2; Nitrous oxide, 1·53; Carbon dioxide, 1·5; Cyclopropane, 1·46; Oxygen, 1·1; Air, 1; Ethylene, 0·97; Nitrogen, 0·96; Water vapour, 0·6; Helium, 0·13.

Partition coefficient of a gas between two or more immiscible solvents is the ratio of the volumes dissolved in each at the temperature and pressure at which the solution takes place. Solvents may be liquids or solids (e.g. rubber). Solubility of gases in rubber may affect the initial speed of build up of concentration in a closed circuit.

Osmotic Pressure

This is the pressure required to prevent migration of a solvent across a semi-permeable membrane into a solution of a certain strength. Strength of solution is measured in terms of osmolarity (the number of osmoles/litre of solution, e.g. plasma) or osmolality (the number of osmoles/kg of solvent). For dilute solutions in water, these are of course nearly equal, and in clinical practice they are often used interchangeably.

If 1 mole of a compound which will not dissociate is dissolved in 22·4 litres of water, it will exert an osmotic pressure of one atmosphere (760 mmHg or 101·3 kPa). An osmole represents the amount of substance which exerts an osmotic pressure of 22·4 atmospheres when dissolved in 1 litre of water.

An osmole is the molecular weight of a substance in grams divided by the number of freely moving particles each molecule liberates in solution. A milliosmole is 1/1000 of an osmole. The osmolarity and osmolality of solutions are measured by the degree to which the freezing point is depressed. A solution of strength of 1000 mosmol/litre depresses the freezing point 1·86 °C. The freezing point of human plasma is −0·54 °C and the osmolarity 290 mosmol/litre. Its osmotic pressure is 7·3 atm.

Fluid Flow

Laminar Flow Through Tubes

Poiseuille's (1799–1868) Law:[3] In laminar flow through tubes, the flow rate is directly proportional to the perfusion pressure, but proportional to the fourth power of the diameter, that is,

$$Q \propto \frac{\pi(P_1 - P_2)r^4}{8\mu l},$$

where Q = flow rate, P_1 and P_2 are the pressures at each end of the tube, r = radius of the tube, μ = viscosity of the fluid, l = length of the tube.

Turbulent Flow Through Tubes

When flow rate through a tube exceeds a critical velocity (a critical Reynolds number),[4] turbulent flow occurs. Turbulence may be facilitated by irregularities and corners in the tube. Conversion from laminar to turbulent flow approximately halves the flow for a given pressure.

$$\text{Critical velocity} \propto \frac{2000 \times \text{viscosity}}{\text{diameter} \times \text{density}}.$$

Flow Through Orifices

The ideal orifice is one whose diameter greatly exceeds its length.

$$Q \propto r^2 \sqrt{(P/D)},$$

where Q = flow rate, P = pressure difference across orifice, D = density of fluid, r = radius of orifice. At low flows, the gas passing the bobbin of a rotameter is in laminar flow, and the viscosity is important. At high flows, the annular aperture around the bobbin resembles an orifice, and the density is important.

The Venturi Principle

Described in 1797. (Giovanni Battista Venturi, 1746–1822, Italian physicist). When a fluid flows through a tube of varying diameter, the pressure is lowest at the point of maximum velocity, because pressure energy is converted to kinetic energy at this point. With suitable flow and a 'venturi' cone-shaped tube, negative pressure can easily be produced. The injector replaces the smooth construction of a venturi tube with a nozzle through which fluid is injected at high velocity. Surrounding fluids are thus sucked in with the main stream.

The Bernoulli Law (Daniel Bernoulli, 1700–1782). His hydrodynamic theorem states that the lateral pressure exerted by a liquid is least where velocity is greatest. Examples of clinical application are: (1) Suction apparatus; (2) Entrainment of air or oxygen, in oxygen therapy; (3) Jet venturi bronchoscopy (Sander's injector).

Measurement of Flow

(1) Rotameter (e.g. anaesthetic flow-meters); (2) Pneumotachograph; (3) Thermal dilution; (4) Electromagnetic; (5) Mechanical (e.g. Wright's respirometer); (6) Bubble flow-meter; (7) Doppler principle.

Heat

One calorie raises the temperature of 1 g of water by 1 °C. The specific heat is the amount of heat required to raise 1 g of a substance through 1 °C.

Heat may be transferred by conduction, convection, radiation, evaporation or addition or subtraction of warm or cold fluids from a body.

The latent heat of vaporization is the quantity of heat required to change 1 g of a substance from liquid to vapour without change of temperature.

The latent heat of melting is the quantity of heat required to change 1 g of a substance from solid to liquid without change of temperature.

For temperature measurement *see* Chapter 41.

Electricity

Current (amps) is analogous to flow and is measured by a galvanometer. One coulomb is the quantity of electricity when 1 amp flows at a point in a conductor for 1 sec.

Voltage is analogous to pressure difference. Two points in an electric circuit have a potential difference of 1 volt if 1 joule of energy is released when 1 coulomb of electricity passes between the points.

Resistance to flow of electricity is measured in *ohms*. *Ohm's Law* (1827) states that 'The ratio of the potential difference between the ends of a conductor to the current flowing in it is always constant, provided that the physical conditions of the conductor such as temperature remain constant', that is,

$$\frac{E}{i} = R,$$

where E = potential difference in volts, i = current in amps, R = resistance in ohms.

Electric *power* is measured in watts. *Watts* = volts × amps.

Resistances in series are additive, i.e. $R = R_1 + R_2 + R_3 + R_4$, etc.

Resistances placed in parallel reduce the overall resistance, that is,

$$\frac{1}{R} = \frac{1}{R_1} + \frac{1}{R_2} + \frac{1}{R_3} \text{ etc.}$$

Static electricity is the charge produced by the contact of two dissimilar materials. It produces sparks of intense heat when it discharges by contact with a conductor.

A *resistor* is a device which limits flow of electric current and can be used to partition potential in a circuit.

A *capacitor* is a store for electric charge with valuable time constants in its function.

A *transistor* is an infinitely variable and controllable switching device, allowing enormous and accurate amplification of a signal.

A *transducer* is a device which converts one form of energy to another.

Surgical Diathermy[16]

Diathermy is a radiofrequency power oscillation with the patient in the circuit, producing intense heat at the small electrode, which the surgeon uses in the wound, and only slight warmth in the area of the 'earth-plate'. It uses electrical apparatus which may cause explosions, burns or electrocution, or may interfere with the action of monitoring apparatus[5] and cardiac pacemakers. Spark-gap sets give 350 kHz (coagulation) and 450 kHz (cutting). Valve and transistor sets produce bursts of megahertz oscillation at varying intervals (50 Hz–50 kHz). Poor contact of the earth-plate with skin may cause electrical burns. One method is to place the plate under the bare buttocks. A broken earth-plate lead may cause the patient to earth himself to a point on the operating table, etc. and thus acquire a burn. A sparking earth-plate lead may ignite a spirit or ether-based skin preparation. Accidental placement of the diathermy electrode on the wrong part of the patient, or on the surgeon or assistant may cause a burn; diathermy in the mouth has caused a tracheal tube to ignite. Opening a colostomy with diathermy has caused an explosion![6] (*See also* Watson A. B. and Loughman L. *Anaesth. Intensive Care* 1978, **6**, 310; Mitchell J. P. *Ann. R. Coll. Surg.* 1979, **61**, 287). First used by Harvey Cushing in neurosurgery.[17]

Electrocution

Mains frequency (50 Hz) is particularly effective in producing ventricular fibrillation. Dry skin resistance may be 5 megohms, which can be reduced to 500 ohms by wet electrode jelly; 1 milliamp (mA) AC or 5 mA DC gives a tingling feeling in the skin; 15 mA AC or 75 mA DC causes muscle paralysis; 70 mA AC or 300 mA DC causes ventricular fibrillation. (This current need only flow for less than 20 ms). 0·5 mA causes ventricular fibrillation if applied direct to the ventricle.[7]

DC with an open circuit flowing into skin can cause destruction of tissue giving a 'punched-out' open sore.

Safety Precautions

The patient should be isolated from earth if possible. The current between any electrode and earth should not be more than 10 μA (for ECG, etc.). Diathermy should make an audible noise when activated, and the electrode sheathed when not in use. Earth-free solid-state diathermy sets are preferred. Battery-powered sets are also preferred. With any monitoring or diathermy equipment, leakage current between mains supply and patient circuit must not exceed 0·1 mA; if it does, the mains should be automatically isolated with an alarm. Equipment should be properly wired in the mains plug—in Europe, brown = live conductor, blue = neutral conductor, green/yellow = earth continuity conductor.

Catheters should be filled with dextrose, not saline, and needle electrodes avoided where possible.

To prevent interference with cardiac pacemakers, place the diathermy electrode as far from the pacemaker as possible, make sure that transvenous leads cannot short on to wet towels, etc.

Monitor interference can be reduced by keeping patient impedance relatively low, keeping the source of the interference as far from the monitor as possible, screening the monitor and earthing the screen, using twisted leads in high-voltage lines, and rearranging the position of the monitor. (*See also* the excellent *Hospital Technical Memoranda.* HTM1—Antistatic precautions, rubber plastic and fabrics; HTM2—Antistatic precautions, flooring in anaesthetizing areas; HTM4—Colour codes of flexible cables and cords; HTM8—Safety code for electromedical apparatus; HTM15—Patient–nurse call systems; HTM16—Fire precautions. *Also*, Stevens A. J. in *Preparation for Anaesthesia* (Stevens A. J., ed.). Tunbridge Wells; Pitman Medical, 1980.)

Radiation

The Curies, Marie (1867–1934) and Pierre (1859–1906), isolated radium in 1898.[8] Wilhelm von Roentgen (1845–1923, Würzburg physicist) discovered the X ray.[9]

A *rad* (Roentgen absorbed dose) is the quantity of ionizing radiation which produces an energy absorption of 100 erg/g.

A *Curie* is a measure of radioactivity and equals $3·7 \times 10^{10}$ disintegrations/second.

The *Grey* equals 1 J per kg = 100 rad.

Fires and Explosions[10]

The vapours of certain volatile anaesthetic agents, and some gases, form flammable mixtures with air or oxygen. Nitrous oxide also supports combustion. Mixtures which correspond exactly with the chemical equation, so that combustion is complete, are said to be *stoichiometric*. The most powerful deflagrations occur when the concentrations of reactants approach stoichiometric values. There are limits of flammability, when the mixture becomes too weak, or the oxygen content too low.

Detonations or explosions are usually associated with a high oxygen content in the mixture, and are produced by an exothermic chemical reaction.

Table 5.1, published by the US Bureau of Mines, shows the limits of flammability of anaesthetics.

Table 5.1. Flammability of anaesthetics

	In air (%)	In oxygen (%)	In nitrous oxide (%)	Density (air = 1)
Ethylene	3·05–28·6	2·90–79·9	1·9–40·7	0·97
Cyclopropane	2·40–10·3	2·48–60·0	1·6–30·3	1·45
Ethyl chloride	4·00–14·8	4·05–67·2	2·1–32·8	2·23
Divinyl ether	1·70–27·0	1·85–85·5	1·4–24·8	2·42
Diethyl ether	1·85–36·5	2·10–82·0	1·5–24·2	2·56

Before an explosion can occur, a source of heat sufficient to raise a liquid to its flash point, or a vapour to its ignition temperature, is required. This is called the 'activation energy'.

Ether

Mixtures of nitrous oxide, oxygen and ether are always explosive and more dangerous than ether and oxygen alone. Pure ether vapour will not explode. Ether in air burns slowly, the flame being unlikely to travel to the patient's air passages.

If the administration of ether is discontinued 5 min before a possible source of ignition is exhibited, the patient's exhalations are unlikely to burn or explode provided an open circuit is used after the ether is discontinued.[11] Further anaesthesia can be maintained with a non-explosive agent. Open ether (without added oxygen) has never been known to cause injury to a patient from ignition or explosion.

The storage of diethyl ether for long periods at high ambient temperatures or with exposure to light can cause the formation of ether peroxides to an extent that spontaneous combustion can occur.

Cyclopropane

This is very explosive when mixed with oxygen, and can be ignited by a spark of less energy than that required to explode an ether–oxygen mixture.

Trichloroethylene

This is not flammable in air under operating theatre conditions. A vapour strength of or over 10% in air enriched with oxygen is flammable, but such a strength should never be used when it is considered that a vaporizing bottle of a Boyle machine with the plunger up is unlikely to deliver a concentration greater than 1·5%

Halothane

Is non-flammable and non-explosive. The halothane–ether azeotrope is non-flammable up to a concentration of 7·25% in oxygen. While such concentrations may arise in anaesthetic systems during induction, lower concentrations are generally required during maintenance.

Methoxyflurane, Enflurane and Isoflurane

Non-flammable and non-explosive at room temperature in either air or oxygen at normal concentrations.

Oxygen

If oxygen under pressure comes into contact with oil or grease, ignition may occur. Thus no oil must be used on valves, etc. The same applies to nitrous oxide and oil or grease.

Sources of Ignition

Heat. From open flames or fires; from hot surfaces or wires; from overheating electric bulbs, e.g. on endoscopes; from thermocautery. Pipes, lighters, cigarettes. The minimal temperature which will ignite an explosive anaesthetic mixture is stated to be 180 °C (335 °F).

Electric current. (*a*) Normal; (*b*) Faulty.

1. *Normal.* Diathermy which comes next in order of importance after static electricity as a cause of explosions; electric cautery; sparks from motors; sparks from X-ray machines; sparks from switches, etc.

2. *Faulty.* Short-circuits in electrical apparatus; faulty wires and cables; breaking of bulbs.

All portable electrical apparatus should be fitted with explosion-proof switches and three-wire flex, the earth wire being connected to the outer casing of the apparatus and to the earth point in a wall plug. The plug should incorporate a locking device making it impossible to remove the plug while the current is switched on.

Static electricity. The way to banish this danger is to arrange for static charges to be carried away to earth, and the conducting floor should be the common connection through which all objects in a theatre are intercoupled. A good conducting floor should have an electrical resistance between 25 000 and 500 000 ohms when measured between two electrodes placed 1 m apart, at any point on the floor. Floor conductivity having been attained, it becomes necessary for all equipment and personnel to be brought into electrical continuity with it.

One obvious way of preventing the development of static electricity would be to eliminate non-conductors and, wherever possible, conducting materials should be used.

The following items are all charge producers and non-conductors: rubber mattresses, plastic sheet material, plastic caps, plastic pillow covers, woollen blankets, woollen suits, rayon, terylene and nylon garments and hosiery, rubber stool tops, painted stool tops, rubber gloves, non-conductive castors on tables and trolleys, non-conductive rubber stool tips, interior non-conducting parts of anaesthetic machines. The following are both charge producers and insulators: non-conductive floors, non-conductive shoes, non-conductive rubber tyres, non-conductive rubber tubes of anaesthetic machines, tubes of some scavenging devices and anaesthetic masks. Undergarments are not included in the list as they do not add to a person's electrostatic charge when covered with a cotton gown.

Spontaneous ignition. This may occur if oil or grease is allowed to react with nitrous oxide or oxygen under pressure, e.g. when escaping from a cylinder. This absolutely contra-indicates the use of lubricants on reducing valves and gas cylinders.

Explosions can arise from ignition of such gases as hydrogen, methane and sulphuretted hydrogen arising from the stomach or bowel from fermentation.

Compression. Sudden severe compression of a combustible mixture may raise the temperature to ignition point, e.g. in diesel engines.

Recommendations for Prevention[12]

1. Explosive anaesthetics should not be used when the following potentially dangerous pieces of apparatus are employed: diathermy, cautery, X-rays, electric motors, electric and gas heating equipment.

2. Electric wiring and apparatus should be inspected frequently by an electrician, even though their function is not impaired. All electrical apparatus should have a third wire for positive grounding, or else the 'no-earth' system may be employed.[13]

3. Foot switches must be flame-proof, as ether vapour falls towards the floor. The zone of risk has previously been defined unnecessarily widely, and it has now been shown that this is restricted to a radius of only some 25 cm around and below anaesthetic apparatus.[14]

4. In all rooms where explosive anaesthetics may be used, a conducting floor should be provided. This includes X-ray rooms, where the risk of electric shock from the high potentials used is remote, but not recovery areas. Swabbing theatre floor with 4% calcium chloride solution is said to increase its electrical conductivity while damp sheets have the same effect. Wax polish must not be allowed on conducting floors.

5. Conducting rubber or vinyl thermoplastic products having antistatic properties should be used for tyres of trolleys, tables, stool tops, etc. The resistance of antistatic material should be between 10 megohms and 50 000 ohms/cm. It should be used for breathing tubes, face-masks, reservoir bags. The conductivity of antistatic rubber is attributed to microscopic chains of carbon particles. Resistance does increase gradually with time, and periodical checks are necessary. Where antistatic rubber is not available, the risk can be reduced if the rubber is wetted internally and externally before use. Non-conducting mattresses, rubber sheeting, aprons, etc. can be made reaonsbly safe if they are completely enclosed in a close-fitting cover of such antistatic material as cotton, linen or viscose rayon. All personnel should wear either conducting rubber or leather footwear, each shoe having a resistance between 0·1 and 1 megohm (if less than 0·1 megohm there is a danger of accidental electrocution should contact with electrical mains occur); cotton blankets and sheets should replace woollen articles in the theatre suite, and should not be allowed to become too dry. When a patient comes to the theatre covered by woollen blankets, they should never be removed

quickly and should be taken out of the theatre suite before the patient is anaesthetized. Woollen stockings should not be rapidly pulled off. It is possible that if all theatre suites were equipped with antistatic rubber exclusively and if all woollen blankets were prohibited, explosions from static electricity, the commonest cause of anaesthetic explosions, would almost disappear.

6. The relative humidity of the atmosphere should not be allowed to fall below 50%. Static sparks are more frequent when the air is dry and the barometric pressure high. Humidity of the atmosphere will not prevent explosions taking place in the anaesthetic apparatus.

7. When diathermy is applied to the bladder, hydrogen is given off and may ignite inside the bladder. Prolonged use of diathermy may cause a strong positive charge on the patient, which may lead to spark formation unless he is adequately earthed. If the diathermy electrode is actually touching the tissues or the haemostat before the current is switched on, arcing is minimized.

8. When there is the risk of an explosion, avoid the use of flammable agents.

9. See that fire-fighting equipment is available and in good order.

10. Dilution of cyclopropane–oxygen mixtures with nitrogen or helium to prevent the chance of explosion.[15]

11. Lasers in or near the airway may ignite vapours and rubber or plastic equipment.

12. The stomach may be a reservoir of flammable gases (as distinct from gases due to fermentation). Gases may be flammable up to 45 min after administration is stopped.

13. Rooms where explosive anaesthetics are used should ideally have 5–10 air changes per hour. Air inlets should be at least 2 m above floor level and air outlets at floor level.

This vast question is excellently discussed in a brochure published by the US Bureau of Mines (Report of Investigation 4833) entitled *Static Electricity in Hospital Operating Suites: Direct and Related Hazards and Pertinent Remedies*, by P. G. Guest, V. W. Sikora and B. Lewis. Pittsburgh, Pa, USA, 1952. (*See also* Vickers M. D. *Anaesthesia* 1970, **25**, 482).

References

1. *See also* Duffin J. *Physics for Anaesthetists*, Springfield, Ill.: Thomas, 1976; Macintosh R. R., Mushin W. W. and Epstein H. G., *Physics for the Anaesthetist*, 3rd ed. Oxford: Blackwell 1987.
2. Henry W. *Phil. Trans. R. Soc.* 1803, **93**, 29.
3. Poiseuille J. L. M. *C. R. Acad. Sci. Paris* 1840, **11**, 1041; Hagen A. *Ann. Phys. Leipzig* 1839, **46**, 423.
4. Reynolds O. *Phil. Trans.* 1883, **174**, 935.
5. Dobbie A. K. *Biomed. Eng.* 1969, **4**, 206.
6. Barrkman M. F. *Br. Med. J.* 1965, **1**, 1594.
7. Whalen R. E. and Starmer C. F. *Mod. Concepts Cardiovasc. Dis.* 1967, **36**, 7; Titel J. H. and el-Etr M. *Anesthesiology* 1968, **29**, 845; Klomp A. M. and Lucas J. H. M. *Med. Biol. Eng.* 1972, **1**, 135.
8. Curie M. and Curie P. *C. R. Acad. Sci. Paris* 1898, **127**, 175, 1215.
9. von Roentgen W. C. *S. B. d. Phys. Med. Ges. zu Würzb* 1895, 132.
10. *See Report of a Working Party on Anaesthetic Explosions, including Safety Code for Equipment and Installations* (Anaesthetic members: Drs Marston, Low, Morton and Galley), London: HMSO, 1956. Also Macintosh R. R., Mushin W. W. and Epstein H. G. *Physics for the Anaesthetist*, 3rd ed. Oxford: Blackwell, 1987. Also Hill D. W. *Physics Applied to Anaesthesia*, 4th ed. London: Butterworths, 1980.
11. Vickers M. D. *Anaesthesia* 1965, **20**, 315.

12. *See also* article in *Hospitals*, the journal of the American Hospitals Association, December 1949.
13. Hill D. W. *Electronic Techniques in Anaesthesia and Surgery*, 2nd ed. London: Butterworths, 1973.
14. Vickers M. D. *Anaesthesia* 1970, **25**, 482.
15. Bourne J. G. *Nitrous Oxide in Dentistry*. London: Lloyd-Luke, 1960, Chap. X; Corcoran J. W. and Hingson R. A. *Dent. Dig.* 1955, **61**, 303.
16. Nagelschmidt F. *Münch. Med. Wochenschr.* 1909, **56**, 2575.
17. Cushing H. and Bovie W. T. *Surg. Gynecol. Obstet.* 1928, **47**, 751; Goldwyn R. M. *Ann. Plast. Surg.* 1979, **2**, 135.

Section 3 — General Anaesthesia

Chapter 6 — THE UPTAKE OF ANAESTHETIC GASES AND VAPOURS[1]

The general laws governing diffusion, solubility and the relations of volume, pressure and temperature apply to the anaesthetic gases and vapours. Uptake by the body can be divided into two phases:

The pulmonary phase. Inhalation of gas or vapour to build up a significant alveolar concentration and diffusion across the pulmonary membrane to reach pulmonary and hence arterial blood.

The circulatory phase. Transfer to the brain and other organs by the circulation. The brain concentration must ultimately be proportional to the partial pressure of vapour in the alveolar air. We can therefore speak of the *minimal alveolar concentration* of an anaesthetic agent which will produce general anaesthesia[2] (*see* p. 105). Strictly speaking, tension rather than concentration is the important factor. It has been pointed out that minimal alveolar concentration (MAC) will vary with altitude, whereas minimal alveolar pressure (MAP) would be reasonably constant.[3]

The Pulmonary Phase

Diffusion across the pulmonary membrane is rarely a limiting factor when the lungs are healthy. In general, arterial tension will equate with alveolar tension. We may consider some of the factors which regulate alveolar tension:

Inhaled concentration. The inspired concentration (or tension) of the anaesthetic agent eventually determines the alveolar tension, the tension in arterial blood and the degree of body saturation, but not until a state of equilibrium has been attained. Increasing the inspired concentration will speed up the rate of induction, provided that breath holding, laryngospasm or coughing is not caused.

Alveolar ventilation. The anaesthetic agent in inspired gases is immediately diluted by the functional residual air. It takes many breaths in and out before the concentration in alveolar air comes to approximate to inspired concentration. In a non-rebreathing system equilibration takes about 3 min in a healthy subject. Equilibration is hastened by increasing alveolar ventilation. Induction is therefore speeded by taking deeper breaths and slowed down when there is rebreathing, respiratory depression or respiratory obstruction, even in one lung or part of a lung.

Blood/gas partition coefficient. The partition coefficient of a substance is the ratio, at equilibrium, of its concentration on the two sides of a diffusing membrane or interface. Alveolar concentration of anaesthetic agent does not in fact reach the inspired concentration because of the constant diffusion of molecules from the alveoli to the pulmonary blood. The solubility of the agent in blood is important. Approximate figures for the coefficient are:[4]

	Blood/gas
Cyclopropane	0·46
Nitrous oxide	0·47
Isoflurane	1·4
Enflurane	1·9
Halothane	3·6
Chloroform	8·4
Trichloroethylene	9·0
Diethyl ether	12·1

When blood solubility is high, alveolar concentration does not equilibrate with inhaled concentration. Induction is slow because alveolar tension, and hence arterial tension, remains low. It may be speeded by increasing alveolar ventilation.

When blood solubility is low, alveolar concentration soon equilibrates with inhaled concentration. Induction is rapid and is not materially affected by taking deeper breaths once the initial equilibration has occurred.

In other words, in the presence of a low blood/gas partition coefficient, a change in inhaled concentration is soon reflected as a change in arterial tension. When the coefficient is high the mechanism is 'buffered' so that changes in inhaled concentration are not rapidly reflected in the arterial blood. *This coefficient is the most important physical characteristic in determination of the clinical potency of a drug.*

Partial pressure of anaesthetic agent in blood returning to the lungs. The tension in mixed venous blood, and hence in pulmonary arterial blood, depends on the redistribution of the agent in the circulatory phase. A high tension in pulmonary arterial blood will raise alveolar concentration. This occurs when redistribution to other tissues is slowed (e.g. in shock) and as total body saturation occurs.

Pulmonary blood flow. Pulmonary blood flow carries away the anaesthetic agent from the lungs. It is equivalent to cardiac output, except in some cases of congenital heart disease, pulmonary haemangioma, etc.

The alveolar membrane. In health this is not a limiting factor. Disease, such as pulmonary oedema or pulmonary fibrosis, may interfere with diffusion across the membrane.

Ventilation–perfusion relationships. Gross disturbances may delay the uptake of anaesthetic agents.

The second gas effect. The uptake of one agent may be accelerated if given in association with a high concentration of another agent (e.g. halothane and nitrous oxide). The rapid absorption of the second gas has the effect of increasing the alveolar concentration of the first agent.

The concentration effect. The uptake of a vapour from the alveolus reduces the remaining vapour concentration in the alveolus, more at low concentrations than at high ones. (At 100% initial alveolar concentration, uptake from the alveolus would produce no change in residual alveolar concentration.) Thus absorption increases more at higher concentrations.

The effect of anaesthetic apparatus. Both the volume of the system, and the solubility of vapours in rubber components and soda lime, buffer the rise of initial concentration, especially in low-flow closed systems.

The Circulatory Phase

Cardiac output. Under basal conditions about 70% of the cardiac output goes to the brain, heart, liver and kidney, which comprise about 7% of the total body weight. About 14% of the cardiac output goes to the brain which comprises about 2·2% of the total body weight. During induction, therefore, a relatively high proportion of the inspired gas goes to the brain.

Cerebral blood flow. Cerebral blood flow is maintained even in shock states up to the moribund stage (BP less than 40 mmHg) and takes a greater proportion of cardiac output, increasing the effect of inhaled anaesthetics. Addition of CO_2 to inspired gases may speed induction by increasing cerebral blood flow (as well as tidal exchange). Many of these factors also apply to the uptake and distribution of intravenous anaesthetic agents.

Secondary saturation of body tissues.[5] The brain receives initially a high proportion of anaesthetic agent. But as time goes on there is a redistribution of the agent as it comes into equilibrium with the body tissues as a whole. Relatively large amounts of anaesthetic agent must be given during induction because of the recirculation of the agent to tissues other than the brain. As these depots becomes saturated, smaller amounts of anaesthetic are required to maintain anaesthesia (law of diminishing resistance of Gill[6]). The rate of saturation of the non-nervous tissues depends on:

1. The tissue blood flow. *The vessel-rich group* includes heart, kidney, liver and endocrine glands which, with the brain, receive 75% of the cardiac output. *Muscles and skin* less than 20% of the cardiac output under resting conditions. There is a *vessel-poor group* of tissues including bone, ligament and cartilage which makes up a quarter of the body mass but has little influence on redistribution. *Fatty tissues* have a perfusion similar to muscles at rest but a far greater capacity for uptake of anaesthetic agents. This may slow induction and emergence in obese subjects.

2. The tissue/blood partition coefficient for the anaesthetic agent which varies but little between the different body tissues with the exception of fat.

3. Time constants. These depend on the above two factors. The time constant is the time taken for the tissue to become equilibrated. It is short when perfusion is high and lengthened when solubility is great. Average values include: for nitrous oxide 1·3 min in the vessel-rich group, 30 min in muscle and 100 min in fat; for halothane the respective figures are 3·3, 106 and 2720 min.[7]

Recovery from Anaesthesia

Recovery is the period from the surgical procedure until the end of the effects of the anaesthetic agents used.

Emergence from inhalation anaesthesia involves all the factors mentioned concerning the uptake of the anaesthetic agent. It is in fact a re-equilibration of the body with atmospheric air.

Recovery is more rapid when secondary saturation of the body tissues has not had time to occur. Tension of the agent in the arterial blood and brain falls rapidly because equilibration is occurring both with alveolar air and body tissues. For example, a child given an inhalation induction in the anaesthetic room will rapidly lighten if allowed to breathe room air during transfer to the operating theatre (primary saturation) but recovery is slow after more prolonged anaesthesia. Hyperventilation aids elimination of gases and vapours and hypoventilation vice versa. Recovery from anaesthesia can be monitored by the cerebral function monitor. The central cholinergic syndrome may impede recovery of consciousness and can be controlled by physostigmine. 1–2 mg i.v. Some aspects of mental ability may be impaired for up to 48 hours after anaesthesia, especially if an inhalation has been used.[8] There is often divergence between subjective and objective estimates of recovery. Delayed recovery from general anaesthesia may occasionally be due to an occult meningioma, so this must be excluded.[9]

(*See also* Carson I. W. 'Recovery from Anaesthesia', *Proc. R. Soc. Med.* 1975, **68**, 108; Symposium on Recovery from Anaesthesia, *J. R. Soc. Med.* 1979, **72**, 270 et seq.; Herbert M., Healy T. E. J. et al. *Br. Med. J.* 1983, **286**, 1539; *Postanaesthetic Recovery*. Eltringham R. J., Durkin M. and Andrews S. ed. Heidelberg: Springer-Verlag, 1984.)

Metabolism of Volatile Anaesthetic Agents

Volatile agents are rapidly removed from the body via the lungs, and little evidence of metabolism can be demonstrated following short exposures. When the administration is long enough for the agent to be present in the body tissues in significant amounts due to redistribution, metabolism may be significant.

Experiments with radioactive labelling show that many inhalation agents do undergo some degradation, including diethyl ether about 2–3% of dose, chloroform, trichloroethylene, halothane up to 20% of dose and methoxyflurane, 50% of administered dose.

Metabolism is thought to occur in microsomes, and many of the reactions involved require nicotinamide adenine dinucleotide phosphate (NADPH), the cofactor responsible for hydrogen-ion transfer. Metabolism is not an important factor in the patient's recovery of consciousness following anaesthesia. But it does indicate biochemical reactivity, and this has important implications in consideration of the mode of action of anaesthetic drugs and their toxicology.

Metabolism, especially of halothane, may be far greater when there has been enzyme induction from any cause.

Trichloroethylene
Metabolism occurs. Important in industrial toxicology. Urinary metabolites identified are trichloroethanol, trichloroacetic acid, monochloroacetic acid and inorganic chloride. 1,2-dichloroethylene has been found in the expired air.

Halothane
Products of biotransformation appear in the urine for up to 13 days following 75 min anaesthesia. There is an oxidation and a reductive mechanism. Products of the latter are more likely to be incriminated in halothane hepatotoxicity.

Methoxyflurane
The major metabolic pathway appears to be dechlorination and oxidation to methoxydifluoroacetic acid, which is excreted by the kidney. A smaller

proportion undergoes cleavage of the ether linkage to produce CO_2, fluoride ion and dichloroacetic acid. It is considered that a dose of more than $2 \cdot 0 \times MAC$ hours may be dangerous because of the amount of fluoride ion (toxic to the kidney) produced.

Enflurane
There is significant biotransformation with the production of fluoride ions, but these are excreted rapidly and do not present the same hazard as in the case of methoxyflurane.

Isoflurane[10]
There is no significant biotransformation in man.

Potency

The potency of an anaesthetic drug is related to the concentration in the blood necessary to produce anaesthesia, and also to those physical and pharmacological characteristics which assist or prevent the achievement of this concentration during inhalation anaesthesia. It may also be considered that certain drugs have a selective action and reduce the reflex response to surgical stimuli without having a comparable effect on the brain as a whole.

Minimal Alveolar Concentration (MAC)
The minimal alveolar concentration of an anaesthetic agent to produce lack of reflex response to skin incision in 50% of subjects. Studies in man give the following results (vol%): methoxyflurane, $0 \cdot 16$; halothane, $0 \cdot 765$; diethyl ether, $1 \cdot 92$; enflurane $1 \cdot 9$; cyclopropane, $9 \cdot 2$; nitrous oxide, 101. Minimum blood concentration (MBC) is another expression of potency. Another measure of potency is the AD_{95} (anaesthetic dose 95) or MAC_{95} which is the alveolar concentration of the agent to produce lack of reflex response to surgery in 95% of subjects (one standard deviation). This figure is much more relevant to clinical anaesthesia and values are approximately $1 \cdot 5$ times those for MAC_{50} (*see above*). When mixtures of agents are used their separate MAC fractions are simply additive in producing the total anaesthetic effect on the subject.

Physical Factors
1. *The saturated vapour pressure.* When this is low, it is not possible to make a high concentration available for inhalation. Thus, although methoxyflurane is the most potent agent in terms of minimal alveolar concentration necessary to produce anaesthesia, its low saturated vapour pressure means that induction is slow.
2. *Blood/gas partition coefficient.* When this is low, changes in inhaled concentration are quickly reflected as changes in alveolar and hence blood concentration. Anaesthesia can be deepened quickly and the agent is clinically potent.

Pharmacology
Alveolar equilibration is delayed when an irritant agent produces breath-holding or laryngospasm, or when it produces marked respiratory depression.

Clinical Applications

Factors which Increase the Speed of Induction of Inhalation Anaesthesia
1. Inhaled concentration of gas or vapour.
2. Carbon dioxide: (*a*) By increasing ventilation during early phase of equilibration, true for all anaesthetic agents. (*b*) By increasing ventilation with those agents where equilibration with alveolar concentration is delayed due to high solubility in the blood (ether). (*c*) By increasing cerebral blood flow, all agents. (Usually up to 5% administered.)
3. Hyperventilation, voluntary or controlled: (*a*) By increasing ventilation as in 2(*a*) and 2(*b*) above. (*b*) By altering pH of blood so that the bound fraction of thiopentone is mobilized.
4. Presence of poor circulation to the non-vital organs. Shock, dehydration, old age, wasting of body tissues.
5. High gas flow systems aid in speed of equilibration of alveolar gases with the anaesthetic mixture. Thus non-rebreathing methods allow for faster induction than low flow systems.
6. Uptake and elimination of anaesthetic agents is more rapid in infants than in adults, because of the relatively larger cardiac output and alveolar ventilation, and smaller functional residual capacity per unit of body weight.

Factors which Decrease the Speed of Induction
1. Respiratory obstruction, laryngospasm, bronchial secretions.
2. Reduction of effective ventilation, breath-holding, coughing. In the presence of ventilation/perfusion inequalities, e.g. severe emphysema or obesity.
3. Respiratory depression: (*a*) Due to premedication. (*b*) Due to use of intravenous barbiturates for induction of anaesthesia. (*c*) Due to the inhalation agent itself.
4. Increased circulation to non-vital organs. In anxiety, thyrotoxicosis, obesity, in children and young persons. Where the muscle mass is large, in robust subjects.
   (*See also* Eger E. I. *Anesthetic Uptake and Action.* Baltimore: Williams & Wilkins, 1974.)

References

1. *See also* Kety S. S. *Anesthesiology* 1950, **11**, 517; Eger E. I. *Anesthetic Uptake and Action.* Baltimore: Williams & Wilkins, 1974.
2. Merkel G. and Eger E. I. *Anesthesiology* 1963, **24**, 346 (reprinted in 'Classical File', *Surv. Anesthesiol.* 1974, **18**, 594); Eger E. I. et al. *Anesthesiology* 1956, **26**, 271.
3. Fink B. R. *Anesthesiology* 1971, **34**, 403.
4. Gregory G. A. and Eger E. I. *Fed. Proc.* 1968, **27**, 205.
5. McKesson E. I. *Can. Med. Assoc. J.* 1921, **11**, 130 (reprinted in 'Classical File', *Surv. Anesthesiol.* 1968, **12**, 435).
6. Gill R. *The Chloroform Problem.* Edinburgh and London: Blackwood, 1906, Vol. 2.
7. Eger E. I. *Anesthetic Uptake and Action.* Baltimore: Williams & Wilkins, 1974.
8. Herbert M., Healy T. E. J. et al. *Br. Med. J.* 1983, **286**, 1539.
9. Fraser A. C. L. and Goat V. A. *Anaesthesia* 1983, **38**, 128.
10. Holaday D. A. et al. *Anesthesiology* 1975, **43**, 325.

| Chapter 7 | **PREANAESTHETIC ASSESSMENT** |

The Preoperative Visit

The patient about to undergo an operation should receive a visit from an anaesthetist. In addition to taking an anaesthetic history, doing the relevant physical examination, and writing up the drugs for premedication, the anaesthetist should allow the patient to ask questions, state his anxieties, and be informed as to the likely plan of campaign leading up to the actual anaesthetic.

The Anaesthetic Outpatient Clinic[1]

The incidence of medical disease in the surgical outpatient is high,[2] so that it is advantageous to see patients in the outpatient clinic as soon as their names are placed on the waiting list for surgical operation. The patient should be referred to the clinic either routinely or: (1) When the operation is likely to be severe; (2) When special techniques (e.g. controlled hypotension) are envisaged; (3) In the presence of systemic disease which is likely to add to the risk of operation. In the clinic a full history and examination can be undertaken and special investigations ordered. Treatment can be instituted as an outpatient to render the patient as fit as possible by the time he is admitted to hospital. When necessary, the patient can be followed up by repeated attendances at the clinic. Time of bed occupancy may thus be reduced.

Attention should be given to the following points in the history:

1. Previous illnesses, operations and anaesthetics. Complications of previous administrations may be avoided on this occasion.

2. Drug therapy, e.g. corticosteroids, insulin, hypotensive drugs, calcium antagonists, tranquillizers, digitalis, mono-amine oxidase inhibitors, tricyclic antidepressants, anticoagulants, barbiturates, diuretics. Drug allergies.

3. Symptoms referable to the respiratory system. Respiratory reserve, cough, sputum, bronchospasm, ability to expel secretions. Smoking habits.

4. Cardiovascular system. Exercise tolerance. Anginal pain. Decompensation. Untreated hypertension is associated with increased risk to the surgical patient.[3]

5. Tendency to vomiting. This may affect the choice of anaesthetic drugs and techniques so as to reduce the likelihood of postoperative nausea and vomiting.

6. Pregnancy. Non-urgent surgery should be postponed if early pregnancy is suspected and menstrual history can often identify women at risk.

7. Alcohol intake.[4] The alcoholic patient may suffer from cirrhosis of the liver, cardiac myopathy, diminished adrenocortical response to stress, electrolyte imbalance, hypoglycaemia, bone marrow depression, neuropathy and psychosis. The anaesthetist should look for signs and symptoms appropriate to these complications as well as to the alcohol withdrawal syndrome. Perioperative infusion of alcohol, 8% in saline, has been suggested in such cases.

Preoperative assessment is often less thorough than it might be and there is sometimes insufficient consultation between the operating surgeon and the anaesthetist.[5]

The patient should be given a full clinical examination, bearing in mind:

1. Signs of respiratory disease.[23] Respiratory pattern and character, type of operation, presence of added sounds on auscultation, localizing signs, mediastinal shift, finger clubbing, cyanosis. (For assessment of respiratory function *see* Rigg J. R. A. and Jones N. L. *Br. J. Anaesth.* 1978, **50**, 3.)

2. Signs of heart disease.[6] Serious heart disease is almost always associated with obvious symptoms and signs, e.g. angina of effort. A diastolic murmur is unequivocal evidence of heart disease. A systolic murmur with no interval between the murmur and the second heart sound is likely to be associated with organic disease. Presence of a thrill indicates organic disease.[7] Acute myocardial ischaemia may be present without obvious symptoms; the silent coronary. The blood pressure above which hypertension is significant is probably 140/95. Note should be made of cardiac rhythm. Signs of cardiac failure should be sought for: raised jugular venous pressure, hepatic enlargement, oedema; cardiac enlargement should be noted. The risks of surgery and anaesthesia in patients with congestive cardiac failure are very high. Patients with cardiac prostheses are likely to be on anticoagulant therapy and this should not be reversed without good reason. Anaesthesia in a patient with a heart transplant presents special problems due to treatment with immunosuppressive drugs and denervation of the heart.[8]

3. The airway. Teeth, loose teeth, porcelain caps, crowns, jaws, neck. Intubation hazards.

4. The state of nutrition, malnutrition or obesity.

5. Colour. Cyanosis or pallor.

6. Examination of the nervous system, particularly where spinal or extradural block is envisaged.

7. Examination of the urine for sugar and albumin. Albustix is a good screening test for albuminuria but the reading correlates more with albumin than with total protein in the urine. The strips are impregnated with tetrabromophenol, buffered with citrate to a pH of 3·5. Protein binds the dye, causing a shift in the transformation range of the indicator.

8. Assessment of the psychological state of the patient. Calm, apprehensive, unstable, etc.

9. The state of the veins.

10. Racial characteristics.

Simple tests which can be carried out in the clinic include:

1. The breath-holding test of Sabrasez.[9] The resting patient takes a full inspiration and holds his breath. A time of 25 s or longer may be taken as normal. A time of 15 s or less indicates a lack of cardiorespiratory reserve.

2. The forced expiratory volume and vital capacity can be readily measured.

3. The Wright Peak Flow-meter can be used to measure peak expiratory flow rate.

Special investigations may be ordered where indicated. They may include:

1. Haemoglobin and blood groups. Sickledex tests for appropriate racial groups.

2. Blood urea and serum electrolytes. Other biochemical screening tests are sometimes justified. Random blood sugar estimation above 11 mmol (200 mg %) is almost diagnostic of diabetes mellitus.

3. Chest radiograph. Routine chest X-ray may reveal pulmonary disease or may be useful as a baseline for postoperative care. It does, however, carry a small risk of radiation damage and routine films may be reserved for those over 30 years of age[10] (or over 50); those with acute pulmonary symptoms; with possible

metastases, or with chronic cardiopulmonary disease, who have not had a chest X-ray within the past 12 months; immigrants not previously examined and following trauma. In the presence of heart disease, X-ray provides evidence of enlargement of the chambers and of pulmonary oedema. Routine chest radiography of patients not being operated on for chest or heart conditions is of doubtful value.[11] Other workers disagree.[12] If an X-ray is necessary it should be taken in the supine A-P position so that it can be compared with the postoperative radiograph which may have to be done in this position.[13]

4. Electrocardiogram. An abnormal ECG is associated with an increased operative risk.[14]

In certain cases it may be desirable to refer the patient to other departments for advice (e.g. cardiology).

Assessment of Physical Status (PS)

The American Society of Anesthesiologists classified patients into a number of grades according to their general condition. There were originally seven grades, but the classification has been amended by the 1962 House of Delegates of the Society[15] as follows: (1) A normal healthy patient; (2) A patient with a mild systemic disease; (3) A patient with a severe systemic disease that limits activity, but is not incapacitating; (4) A patient with an incapacitating systemic disease that is a constant threat to life; (5) A moribund patient not expected to survive 24 hours with or without an operation. In the event of emergency operation, precede the number with an E.

The system (which has now been revised)[16] has been criticized in that different anaesthetists do not always agree about the classification,[17] so that comparisons of different surveys may not always be meaningful.

Risk (See also Chapter 22)

Physical status is not synonymous with risk.[18] There have been attempts to analyse the relationship of physical status to risk,[19] and in a study eight significant correlates have been found between data obtained at preoperative examination and life-threatening or fatal cardiac complications.[20] These are: (1) A preoperative third heart sound or jugular vein distension; (2) Myocardial infarction during the previous 6 months; (3) More than five premature ventricular beats/min at any time; (4) Dysrhythmia, other than sinus rhythm or premature atrial beats on ECG; (5) Site of operation (intraperitoneal, thoracic or aortic); (6) Emergency operation; (7) Significant aortic valvular stenosis; (8) Poor medical condition (including abnormal blood gas values and biochemistry). A scoring system has been suggested to aid evaluation.

Risk factors have been related to the severity of liver disease, and a scoring system, taking into account the grade of encephalopathy, ascites, serum bilirubin, serum albumin, and prothrombin time has been described.[21]

Treatment

Some forms of treatment may be instituted before operation.

Dental treatment. Refer the patient to the dental surgeon.

Treatment of anaemia.[22] Valuable time can be saved by treating anaemia before admission. Oral iron is effective in most cases of simple anaemia.

Respiratory disease.[23] No patient should undergo a non-urgent operation while he is suffering from an acute infection of the upper respiratory tract. There are, however, some exceptions to this in the case of classic acute coryza when the operation is superficial and postponement is inconvenient. But operations which cause pain on coughing such as laparotomy, perineal repair or haemorrhoidectomy, should usually be postponed. Chronic chest disease is more difficult to control, but much can be done.

Smoking should be stopped 4–6 weeks before operation to reduce postoperative pulmonary morbidity. Stopping for 12–24 hours benefits the cardiovascular system by reducing the need for carbon monoxide and nicotine elimination; stopping for a few days will benefit ciliary activity; stopping for 1–2 weeks will reduce sputum volume. If stopping smoking increases the risk of deep vein thrombosis, this can be prevented by anticoagulants.[24] Smokers exhibit a variety of pulmonary disorders including airway obstruction and reduced lung compliance, diminished peak flow rate, increase in functional residual capacity, diminished diffusing capacity and reduced surfactant. Those who smoke one or more packets of cigarettes daily have chronic bronchitis. Elevated carboxyhaemoglobin levels are also found. There is statistical proof that in abdominal operations postoperative chest complications are six times more frequent in smokers than in non-smokers.[25] There is also evidence that smoking may interfere with wound healing, especially in plastic surgery.[26]

Obstructive airways disease. If the patient gives a history of chronic winter cough which improves during the warm weather, he should, if possible, have his operation postponed until he is at his best. Chemotherapy, penicillin, postural drainage, etc. may be suggested in suitable cases. Breathing exercises should be started in the clinic and should be conducted if possible by the same personnel who will later be met in the ward after operation, though they do not necessarily improve respiratory function. Group therapy has a place here, and classes of patients can be put through a suitable drill with advantage both to their physique and their morale.

Asthma of the extrinsic variety is usually associated with hypersensitivity to an allergen and seldom causes problems during anaesthesia provided the patient is in remission. Patients with obstructive airways disease who suffer from intrinsic asthma have some bronchospasm on most days and this can be aggravated by general anaesthesia and tracheal intubation. Bronchodilator drugs may be useful. Some patients with asthma have been treated with steroids and so may have adrenal suppression.

Pleural effusion. Large effusions may prevent lung expansion and should be tapped preoperatively.

Pneumothorax is also associated with lung collapse with the risk of increase in size if nitrous oxide is used. Drainage is indicated before operation. (*See also* Rigg J. R. A. and Hones N. L. *Br. J. Anaesth.* 1978, **50**, 3.)

Estimation of the ventilatory reserve can be aided by estimating the peak flow rate and the FEV. Blood-gas values may be required in handicapped patients. (*See also* Blery C. et al. *Effective Health Care* 1983, **1**, 111; Holdcraft A. *Ann. R. Coll. Surg.* 1980, **62**, 382.)

Hypertension. When possible this should be treated before operation as the risks to the patient are greater when the condition is untreated.[27] This is true whether the anticipated technique is one of general anaesthesia or extradural blockade.[28] Medication should not be withdrawn preoperatively.

Atrial fibrillation. When the ventricular rate is rapid, this should be treated with digitalis.

Complete heart block. Cardiac pacing should if possible be instituted before operation.

Malnutrition. In appropriate cases high-protein diets, vitamins, etc. can be ordered. Intravenous feeding is justified preoperatively in certain patients, e.g. those with carcinoma of the oesophagus.

Obesity.[29] This is the enemy of both surgeon and anaesthetist. Treated properly by a 1000-calorie diet excellent results may be obtained, even in the few weeks at the anaesthetist's disposal. Walking for 1 hour expends 300 calories. It is important to give the patient a diet sheet he can readily understand, to explain to him the purpose of the diet, and for him to attend the outpatient clinic at regular (fortnightly) intervals for weight check and for interview so that the anaesthetist can give appropriate encouragement or scolding. (*See also* Chapter 22.)

Psychological factors.[30] Occasionally patients are terrified of anaesthesia, or they may fear a particular anaesthetic technique (face-mask, spinal anaesthesia). A little time spent in discussion with these patients is invaluable and may in fact bring some patients into hospital who would otherwise default. It should rarely be necessary to force an unwelcome technique on a patient.

Diabetes. See Chapter 22.

One other advantage of the thorough preoperative investigation of the patient is the assurance and confidence that the anaesthetist feels, should medicolegal proceedings be instituted by the patient after operation. 'It is the fate of those who toil at the lower employments of life, to be exposed to censure without hope of praise; to be disgraced by miscarriage or punished for neglect, where success would have been without applause, and diligence without reward' (Dr Samuel Johnson).[31] Among these unhappy mortals is the administrator of anaesthetics, and he must cover himself in every way possible.

Fit for Anaesthetic

This is a vague concept but usually implies that the patient who is not unduly old, lives a normal life, is free from serious signs and symptoms of disease, is not receiving drug treatment for abnormalities, has reasonable exercise tolerance for his age, is not unduly overweight and appears emotionally stable.

The physician should be asked 'Is there any way in which this patient can be improved?' not 'Is he fit for operation?' That is a decision for the anaesthetist. However, the advice of the physician concerning diagnosis and treatment may be sought.

Preoperative Preparation

The patient should be seen in the ward a day or two before his operation takes place. This enables the anaesthetist to make contact with his patient and enables the patient to make enquiries and to state his anxieties. The anaesthetist then has an opportunity to check the notes made in the outpatient clinic and to look for any recent change in the patient's condition. If the patient has not been seen before, a more detailed history, including that of drug medication, must be taken, and appropriate examination made. At this visit the anaesthetist should check laboratory findings and if necessary order cross-matching of blood. Sedation and preoperative medication may then be prescribed.

Preoperative preparation in special cases is discussed in Chapters 22–29.

The Day of Operation

Food and drink should be withheld during the 6 hours preceding operation. It is often wise to order nothing by mouth on the day of operation, but excessive starvation and dehydration are to be avoided, especially in infants, who may suffer dangerous hypoglycaemia.[32] Morphine premedication delays gastric emptying time, but diazepam, 10 mg does not.[33] Gastric emptying time is decreased after both atropine and glycopyrronium.[34]

Lipstick, nail varnish and other cosmetics should be removed before the patient comes to theatre so that the anaesthetist can readily appreciate cyanosis, etc.

Dentures, artificial limbs, artificial eyes, contact lenses, etc. should be removed before the journey to the theatre. Hearing aids may often be retained by the patient so that communication can be maintained.

The patient should not come to theatre with a full bladder.

It is wise to tie an identification label around his wrist or neck. This should state the name and case record number. Where indicated the side or number of digit should be marked on the patient's skin with indelible ink.

Since 1 January 1970 in the UK a minor who has reached the age of 16 may consent to surgical, medical or dental treatment on his own behalf and parental consent is no longer necessary.

Emergency cases should be delayed if possible to allow the stomach to empty as gastric emptying may be considerably delayed after accidents, in labour and in the anxious patient. Resuscitative measures, such as intravenous infusion, may be required to improve the patient's condition. (*See also* Chapters 35 and 42.)

Legal Responsibilities of the Anaesthetist (*see also* Chapter 18).
See also Havard J. D. J. *Anaesthesia* 1977, **32**, 25. For practice in the US *see* Dripps R. D., Eckenhoff J. E. and Vandam L. D. *Introduction to Anesthesia—The Principles of Safe Practice*, 5th ed. Philadelphia: Saunders, 1977, Ch. 5.

The Effects of Drug Therapy[35]

The majority of drug interactions can be explained as follows:
1. Potentiation, additive or synergistic effect, e.g. barbiturates and alcohol.
2. Enzymatic inhibition by one drug preventing normal metabolism of another, e.g. mono-amine oxidase inhibitors and pethidine.
3. Enzyme induction. Stimulation of enzyme systems by one drug leading to an increased rate of metabolism of another. It is thought that phenobarbitone stimulates metabolism of anticoagulants so that dosage of the latter must be increased and a dangerous situation may arise if phenobarbitone is withdrawn. Other examples are barbiturates and diphenylhydantoin, and griseofulvin and digitoxin. Enzyme induction may also occur as the result of the stress of surgery and anaesthesia and severe illness.
4. Displacement of one drug from plasma or tissue protein by another. For example, phenylbutazone may displace a coumarin anticoagulant which has an enhanced effect with danger of bleeding.
5. Electrolyte imbalance. Loss of potassium induced by thiazide diuretics may cause abnormal reactions to digoxin and muscle relaxants.
6. Influence of drug on urinary pH may affect excretion of drugs.
7. Interference with other renal mechanisms affecting drug excretion.

Other examples of drug interaction include: phenelzine interacts with phenylephrine, causing hypertension; insulin interacts with propranolol causing hypoglycaemia; prednisone interacts with butobarbitone causing reduction of steroid effect; mono-amine oxidase inhibitors interact with tyramine present in red wine, cheese, yoghurt, broad beans and meat extract, causing hypertensive crises.

Drug interaction may be specially dangerous in patients on treatment with anticoagulants, antidiabetics, digoxin, cytotoxic agents and mono-amine oxidase inhibitors.

In cases of doubt concerning this problem, the best sedative is diazepam; the best analgesic, paracetamol; the best soporific, temazepam.

Drugs Affecting Sympathetic Responses

Hypotensive agents produce their effects by a reduction in peripheral vascular tone. The hypotensive effect may be augmented by general anaesthesia, especially when this is combined with sudden change of position, head-up tilt, use of ganglion-blocking drugs, sudden haemorrhage, etc. Care should be exercised in the use of spinal or extradural techniques.

Adrenergic α-receptor blockers. Phenoxybenzamine and phentolamine are powerful blocking agents and too potent for use in the treatment of essential hypertension. There is no antagonist available and side-effects are common, so that these drugs are not used in antihypertensive therapy.

Adrenergic β-receptor blockers. These agents prevent inotropic and chronotropic cardiac responses and diminish the reflex cardiovascular responses to laryngoscopy and tracheal intubation. Sudden withdrawal may be dangerous. Patients should be maintained on therapy when presenting for anaesthesia. Halothane, isoflurane[36] and nitrous oxide can be used. Enflurane,[37] trichloroethylene and methoxyflurane may be best avoided. Hypoxia and hypercapnia may cause cardiac depression.

Adrenergic β-receptor stimulants. β-stimulants[38] (e.g. adrenaline and isoprenaline) may cause ventricular dysrhythmias if halogenated agents are used, especially in the presence of hypoxia or hypercapnia. The anaesthetist may treat these with β-blocking agents in small doses, bearing in mind the possibility of increased vagal tone and bronchospasm. Felypressin is an alternative to adrenaline and does not stimulate the heart (for use with local analgesics).

Diuretics. Most diuretics potentiate the more effective hypotensive agents, though their action is not understood.

Tricyclic antidepressants. These inhibit the metabolism of catecholamines. May result in dysrhythmias. There is evidence that imipramine potentiates the cardiovascular effects of these agents used in local analgesics. They reduce the hypotensive effects of guanethidine.

Ganglion-blocking drugs. These produce hypotension by ganglionic blockade.

Guanethidine (Ismelin). An antihypertensive agent with a prolonged effect. May cause diarrhoea and postural hypotension. Has been used to produce regional intravenous sympathetic block for intractable pain in a limb with autonomic dysfunction. Causes depletion of noradrenaline from the sites associated with adrenergic nerve function but also blocks transmission before significant depletion has occurred.

Rauwolfia compounds. Named in honour of Leonard Rauwolf, a physician and botanist of the sixteenth century: reserpine was the first of the modern tranquillizers, described in 1952 by R. W. Wilkins of Boston: traditional Indian drug. Reserpine causes a depletion of the stores of catecholamines of the body, including the brain (adrenaline, noradrenaline and 5-hydroxytryptamine). Effects last for 2 weeks after cessation of therapy. Side-effects include nasal congestion, increased salivation, weight gain and mental depression.

Methyldopa (Aldomet, Dopamet). An inhibitor of the enzyme decarboxylase which is necessary in the biosynthesis of adrenaline and noradrenaline. It also depletes the noradrenaline stores. Side-effects include nasal congestion, mental depression, abdominal colic and diarrhoea.

Mono-amine oxidase inhibitors. (*See* Chapter 19.)

Significance of Antihypertensive Therapy on the Conduct of Anaesthesia
1. Threat to circulatory homeostasis. Sympathetic blockade is likely to interfere with the normal compensatory mechanisms of the cardiovascular system which are called into play during anaesthesia.
2. The response to pressor amines may be altered. This will depend upon the nature of the sympathetic block and on the mechanism of the pressor itself (direct or via noradrenaline release). Mono-amine oxidase inhibitors preserve noradrenaline stores and may dangerously potentiate the indirect vasopressors, and care is necessary with adrenaline and noradrenaline. β-adrenergic blockers do not affect pressor action.

Cessation of Drug Treatment
The activity of the drug ceases:
1. Within 24 hours. Ganglion-blocking agents, bethanidine (Esbatal), mecamylamine (Inversine), bretylium, adrenergic α- and β-blockers.
2. Prolonged action. Recommended period to allow for normal function: methyldopa, 7 days; guanethidine, 10 days; reserpine, 14 days; mono-amine oxidase inhibitors, 14–21 days; tricyclic antidepressants, several weeks.

Disadvantages of Withdrawal
(1) Possibility of renal damage if diastolic pressure rises; (2) Possible precipitation of cardiac failure or cerebrovascular accident; (3) Inconvenience to the patient and the hospital; (4) The patient presents for anaesthesia in a state of hypertension, and there may be added systolic peaks as a result of intubation, hypoxia, etc. Studies indicate that the non-treated hypertensive patient presents a significant risk in association with anaesthesia and surgery as compared with those whose blood-pressure has been controlled by drug therapy.

The Patient Maintained on Hypotensive Drugs
Opinion now tends to favour keeping patients on antihypertensive medication. The safety factor is the knowledge that these drugs have been given and their pharmacology is known.

There have been no conclusive demonstrations that any particular anaesthetic technique is contra-indicated, apart from the reaction between mono-amine oxidase inhibitors and pethidine. The patient should be observed carefully during anaesthesia. Bradycardia, due to unopposed vagal action, should be treated with atropine or gallamine. Blood loss requires careful replacement. Intravenous fluids are probably preferable to pressor drugs, and if the latter are used, careful selection is necessary. Hypercapnia should be prevented.

The pressor drug of choice in the patient treated with reserpine, guanethidine or methyldopa is one of the group methoxamine, phenylephrine, metaraminol;

atropine should be given if associated with bradycardia. Extreme caution should be used if any pressor agent is given to a patient receiving mono-amine oxidase inhibitors, especially methylamphetamine.

Patients receiving β-blocking drugs should not have the medication discontinued. There is evidence that halothane is a safe agent in these circumstances.[39]

Calcium antagonists. See Chapter 19.

Antibiotics
There is convincing evidence that large parenteral doses of neomycin, streptomycin and dihydrostreptomycin can cause a neuromuscular block, which is potentiated by ether or depolarizing muscle relaxants. Other antibiotics which may cause a similar effect include kanamycin, tobramycin, polymyxin B, biomycin, bacitracin and colistin. Clinical reports of prolonged apnoea have been associated with the administration of a large dose of antibiotic into the peritoneal or pleural cavity towards the end of an operation with ether or relaxant anaesthesia. The effect may not become apparent until the patient has returned to the ward. Use of depolarizing muscle relaxants does not obviate this danger since there has been a report of this syndrome when suxamethonium had been used as the relaxant,[40] presumably due to the onset of dual block.

Psychotropic Drugs
All psychotropic drugs may produce sedation and occasionally excitement and restlessness. Extrapyramidal effects (Parkinsonism, akathesia, dystonia, dyskinesia) can occur, especially with butyrophenones. Dystonia may respond dramatically to injection of anti-Parkinson drugs such as benztropine, 1–2 mg i.v. Grand mal epilepsy can be precipitated by tricyclic antidepressants, lithium and major tranquillizers, as well as by abrupt withdrawal of benzodiazepines. Major tranquillizers and tricyclic antidepressants have anticholinergic side-effects. Tricyclic antidepressants block the re-uptake of mono-amines into adrenergic nerve terminals so that circulating catecholamines are increased. Sinus tachycardia and ventricular dysrhythmias can occur. Sudden withdrawal of tricyclic antidepressant therapy can lead to malaise, fatigue, muscle pains, vomiting and diarrhoea. The effects of mono-amine oxidase inhibitor therapy may last up to 3 weeks after withdrawal. Adrenaline is best avoided in patients on treatment with tricyclic antidepressants.

Mono-amine Oxidase Inhibitors
These include phenelzine, iproniazid, tranylcypromine and isocarboxazid. They should be discontinued 2–3 weeks before elective surgery. The mode of action of this group of drugs is imperfectly understood and cannot be explained solely in terms of mono-amine oxidase inhibition. They are used in psychiatry in the treatment of depressive states. Reactions to pethidine, fentanyl and phenoperidine and morphine have been reported in patients taking these drugs and deaths have occurred. They include severe depression, coma, muscle twitching, hypotension, ataxia, ocular palsies, cerebral excitement and Cheyne–Stokes respiration and may be due to liver dysfunction, though relief has been obtained following administration of 25 mg of prednisolone hemisuccinate or chlorpromazine. Only a small proportion of patients receiving treatment show adverse reactions. It has been suggested that a test dose of 5 mg pethidine should be given intravenously and the effect on blood pressure and pulse rate observed. This is

followed by test doses of 10 mg and 20 mg. If the patient has a stable blood pressure and pulse, and is not comatose or cyanosed, the administration of pethidine is probably safe. Severe hypertensive effects and even death may occur when pressor drugs are given to patients on treatments with this group of drugs, but may be counteracted by phentolamine. The effects of these drugs may last for 14 days. Hypotension, should it occur, may yield to hydrocortisone. For postoperative analgesia in patients receiving mono-amine oxidase inhibitors, a combination of chlorpromazine and codeine has been used without ill effect.

Phenothiazine Derivatives
These cause peripheral vasodilatation and a fall in blood pressure in some subjects, which may become severe during anaesthesia. Narcotics are potentiated. Other side-effects include liver dysfunction, anti-analgesia and pseudo-Parkinsonism.

Disulphiram (Antabuse)
Blocks the normal metabolism of alcohol causing an accumulation of acetaldehyde which is responsible for the 'disulphiram reaction'. Used in the treatment of alcoholics. There may be a synergistic depressant effect with thiopentone.

Lithium Carbonate and Anaesthesia
(*See* Mogelnik S. and Ominsky A. J. *Anesth. Analg.* 1977, **56**, 462.) Lithium should be stopped 48–72 h before a relaxant is given.[41] It potentiates the non-depolarizing group of relaxants.

Levodopa
This is converted, chiefly in the basal ganglia, to dopamine, producing α-, β- and dopaminergic stimulation. There is a slight risk of tachycardia and ventricular dysrhythmias when cyclopropane and halothane are used, so it may be stopped on the day of operation only. Levodopa inhibits prolactin secretion and stimulates growth hormone production, which may make diabetic patients more liable to hyperglycaemia. The danger of stopping levodopa for longer than the day of operation is the reappearance of severe Parkinsonism, dysphagia and the risk of aspiration pneumonia. Butyrophenones antagonize the action of levodopa on dopaminergic receptors in the brain and should be used with caution.

Steroid Therapy
See Chapter 22.

Insulin
See Chapter 22.

The Contraceptive Pill
After major surgery, the relative risk of deep venous thrombosis in women taking oestrogen-containing combined oral contraceptive pills is about 2 : 1, compared with non-users.[42] Anaesthesia and the combined pill have additive effects as both reduce the activity of anti-thrombin III.[43] The risk is greatest following hypotensive anaesthesia and major abdominal, orthopaedic and cancer operations.

Oestrogen-containing pills should, if possible, be discontinued 4 weeks before elective surgery and started again at the first period following an interval of 2 weeks after the operation providing that the patient is fully mobile. Should this not be possible because of unexpected surgery or other cause, prophylactic low dose heparin should be considered.[43] The risk increases with age, obesity, cigarette smoking, diabetes, hypertension and familial hyperlipidaemia. The risks associated with minor surgery or day-stay operations followed by full mobilization are not great so that oral contraceptives need not be discontinued unless the surgery is on the legs such as ligation of varicose veins. The progesterone only pill need not be discontinued before elective surgery.[44]

References

1. *See also* Lee J. A. *Anaesthesia* 1949, **4**, 169; Green R. A. and Howat D. D. C. *Anaesthesia* 1952, **7**, 40; Lee J. A., Thorne T. C., Atkinson R. S. et al. *Br. J. Anaesth.* 1975. **47**, 1117; Frost E. A. *Anesth. Analg.* 1976, **55**, 307; Atkinson R. S. in: *Preparation for Anaesthesia* (Stevens A. J., ed.). *Clin. Anesthesiol.* 1986, **4**, 445; Norman J. *Br. Med. J.* 1980, **1**, 1507.
2. Kyei-Mensah K. and Thornton J. A. *Br. J. Anaesth.* 1974, **46**, 570.
3. Foëx P. and Prys-Roberts C. *Br. J. Anaesth.* 1974, **46**, 575; Prys-Roberts C. in: *Medicine for Anaesthetists* (Vickers M. D., ed.). Oxford: Blackwell, 1977; *Anaesthesia and the Patient with Heart Disease* (Brown B. R., ed.). Philadelphia: Davis, 1980.
4. Edwards R. *Br. Med. J.* 1985, **291**, 423.
5. Lunn J. N. and Mushin W. W. *Mortality associated with Anaesthesia* London: Nuffield Provincial Hospitals Trust, 1982; Curran J. and Chmielewski A. T. *Br. Med. J.* 1985, **291**, 391.
6. Foëx P. *Br. J. Anaesth.* 1978, **50**, 15.
7. Fleming P. R. *Br. J. Anaesth.* 1974, **46**, 555.
8. Kanter S. F. and Samuels S. I. *Anesthesiology* 1977, **46**, 65.
9. Sabrasez *Bordeaux Med. J.* 1902.
10. Rees A. M. et al. *Br. Med. J.* 1976, **1**, 1332; Loder R. E. *Anaesthesia* 1978, **33**, 969.
11. National Study by R. Coll. Radiol. *Lancet* 1979, **2**, 83; Loder R. E. and Richardson H. J. *Lancet* 1954, **1**, 1117; Denham M. and Thakker R. et al. *Br. Med. J.* 1984, **288**, 1726.
12. Tornebrandt K. and Fletcher R. *Anaesthesia* 1982, **37**, 901.
13. Kubota Y. *Anaesthesia* 1983, **38**, 165.
14. Chamberlain D. A. and Edmonds-Seal J. *Br. Med. J.* 1964, **2**, 784; Iyer V. S. et al. *Anaesthesia* 1972, **27**, 41.
15. *Anesthesiology* 1963, **24**, 111; Owens W. D. et al. *Anesthesiology* 1978, **49**, 239; Editorial, *Anesthesiology* 1978, **49**, 233.
16. Keats A. S. *Anesthesiology* 1979, **51**, 179.
17. Owens W. D. et al. *Anesthesiology* 1978, **49**, 239.
18. Keats A. S. *Anesthesiology* 1978, **49**, 233.
19. Vacanti C. J. et al. *Anesth. Analg.* 1970, **49**, 564; Lewin I. et al. *Ann. Surg.* 1971, **174**, 217.
20. Goldman L. et al. *N. Engl. J. Med.* 1977, **297**, 845.
21. Pugh R. N. H., Murray-Lyon L. M. et al. *Br. J. Surg.* 1973, **60**, 646.
22. Gillies I. D. S. *Br. J. Anaesth.* 1974, **46**, 589.
23. *See also* Milledge J. S. in: *Preparation for Anaesthesia* (Stevens A. J., ed.).*Clin. Anesthiol.* 1986, **4**, 687.
24. Pearce A. C. and Jones R. M. *Anesthesiology* 1984, **61**, 576; Cole P. and Saloojee Y. *Br. Med. J.* 1985, **291**, 142.
25. Morton H. J. V. *Lancet* 1944, **1**, 368.
26. Nolan J., Jenkins R. A. et al. *Plast. Reconstr. Surg.* 1985, **75**, 544; Rees T. D., Liverett D. M. et al. *Plast. Reconstr. Surg.* 1984, **73**, 911.
27. Foëx P. and Prys-Roberts C. *Br. J. Anaesth.* 1974, **46**, 575; Prys-Roberts C. *Br. J. Anaesth.* 1984, **56**, 711.
28. Dagnino J. and Prys-Roberts C. *Br. J. Anaesth.* 1984, **56**, 1065
29. *See also* Fisher A. et al. *Anaesthesia* 1975, **30**, 633.
30. *See also* Maxwell H. in: *Preparation for Anaesthesia* (Stevens A. J., ed.). *Clin. Anesthesiol.* 1986, **4**, 473.
31. Mann G. V. *N. Engl. J. Med.* 1974, **291**, 178, 276; Smith L. H. Jr. *The Obese Patient.* Philadelphia and London: Saunders, 1976; Johnson S. Preface to *The Dictionary of the English Language* 1755.
32. Fry E. N. S. and Ibrahim A. A. *Anaesthesia* 1976, **31**, 552.

33. Todd J. G. and Nimmo W. S. *Br. J. Anaesth.* 1983, **55**, 1189.
34. Clark J. M. and Seager S. J. *Br. J. Anaesth.* 1983, **55**, 1195.
35. Baker A. B. in: *Preparation for Anaesthesia* (Stevens A. J., ed.). *Clin. Anesthesiol.* 1986, **4**, 631.
36. Horan B. F. et al. *Br. J. Anaesth.* 1977, **49**, 187.
37. Horan B. F. et al. *Br. J. Anaesth.* 1976, **48**, 817.
38. *See also Prescriber's Journal* 1980, **20**, 14.
39. Roberts J. G. *Br. J. Anaesth.* 1976, **48**, 315.
40. Foldes F. F. et al. *JAMA* 1963, **183**, 672.
41. *Drug Ther. Bull.* 1981, **19**, 21.
42. Stadel B. V. *N. Engl. J. Med.* 1981, **305**, 612 and 672.
43. Sagar S., Stamatakis J. D. et al. *Lancet* 1976, **2**, 509.
44. Guillebaud J. *Br. Med. J.* 1985, **291**, 498; *British National Formulary* 1985, **10**, 260.

Chapter 8	**THE PHARMACOLOGY[1] OF DRUGS USED FOR PREOPERATIVE AND POSTOPERATIVE MEDICATION**

'Empirical procedures, firmly entrenched in the habits of good doctors, seem to have a vigour and life, not to say immortality of their own' (H. K. Beecher).

History of Premedication

In pre-anaesthetic days, both wine and opium were given to mitigate the terrors of surgery. The word itself first appeared in print in an article by the American editor-anaesthetist Frank Hoeffer McMechan (1873–1930) in 1920[2] and in an annotation in the *Lancet*.[3] The technique was employed only infrequently during the 50 years following the introduction of anaesthesia. It was recommended by Bellamy Gardner[4] and Dudley Buxton[5] (1855–1931) of University College Hospital in the UK, and rules determining whether or not 'preliminary medication' should be used were published in 1911 in the USA,[6] while in 1914 it was stated that 'preliminary medication' was employed in 59% of hospitals in the USA.[7]

Morphine, the first alkaloid to be isolated from a crude drug, was discovered by F. W. A. Sertürner (1783–1841), pharmacist of Paderborn, in 1806. It was used before anaesthesia to prevent anxiety by Bruno of Turin in 1850[8] and by the Munich surgeon J. N. von Nussbaum (1829–1890) to reduce the amount of anaesthetic needed, in 1864.[9] In 1869, Claude Bernard (1813–1878), professor of physiology at the Sorbonne, used morphine in animals before anaesthesia[10] and this led some of his pupils (e.g. Guibert[11] of St Brieuc) to use it clinically in an effort to reduce the amount of chloroform needed to ensure deep anaesthesia.[12] (*See also* report in *Medical Times, London*,[13] and Aubert of Lyons.[14]) As the combination of morphine and anaesthesia caused hypoventilation resulting in a rigid abdomen, it failed to become a popular method, although in intracranial surgery, Sir Victor Horsley (1857–1916) pioneer neurosurgeon, used it to reduce bleeding in 1886.[15]

The somewhat mutually antagonistic effects of morphine and atropine were pointed out by Benjamin Bell,[16] by John Harley[17] and by the French physiologist, Brown Séquard (1817–1894), Claude Bernard's successor in Paris. The report of the Second Hyderabad Chloroform Commission in 1889–1890 recommended the use of morphine before chloroform as an aid to anaesthesia, not to reduce anxiety. Chloral hydrate given to produce sleep and sedation before operation in 1874 by Forné.[18]

Atropine isolated by Louis Nicolas Vaquelin, Paris pharmacist (1763–1829) in 1809 and recognized as an alkaloid by Rudolf Brandes (1795–1842) in 1819.[19] Purified form, described by Mein in 1831, was shown to have an inhibitory effect on salivary secretions by R. H. P. Heidenhain of Breslau (1834–1897), a German physician, in 1872.[20] First used as a bronchodilator in 1836,[21] Albert von Bezold and Bloebaum of Würzburg (1836–1868) demonstrated in 1867 that it could block the cardio-inhibitory effects sometimes seen after chloroform, and this was confirmed by A. J. F. Dastre[22] (1814–1917), Paris physiologist, in 1878, E. A. Schafer (1850–1919) and F. R. Fraser (1841–1920) both of Edinburgh.[23] Franz Pitha (1810–1875), a surgeon from Vienna, gave 20 gr. of extract of belladonna as an enema to quell an anaesthetic-resistant patient in 1861.[24] Twenty-two years later, E. H. Embley, a Melbourne anaesthetist, showed experimentally once again[25] that the occasional cardiac arrest caused by chloroform was due to a vagal effect and could be prevented by section of both vagi or by full atropinization. This observation led clinicians to give it for the same purpose, although the doses they used did not cause complete vagal block. Thus atropine was employed for some time before chloroform anaesthesia. As ether gradually displaced chloroform it was found that atropine was beneficial for its drying effect on salivary secretions.[26]

Hyoscine, isolated in 1871, was originally used as a mixture of laevo- and dextro- alkaloids, and achieved a reputation for unreliability. When it was discovered that only the laevo form was pharmacologically active, this was prepared and sold in Germany under the name of Scopolamine, where it soon became widely used. A pioneer in the UK was Dudley Wilmot Buxton.[27] In 1903, Schneiderlin used it with morphine to treat acute mania and as a full anaesthetic[28] (just as years later, bromethol (Avertin) was first used to produce full anaesthesia). Later this combination became popular for preoperative medication.

Papaveretum was prepared in 1909 by Hermann Sahli (1856–1933) of Berne and was marketed in Germany as Pantopon. Later, as Omnopon it became popular in the UK.[29] Aspirin introduced into medicine in 1899 by Dreser.

Pethidine, synthesized in 1939 by Schaumann and Eisleb in Germany during a search for an atropine substitute,[30] was first used in premedication by Schlungbaum[31] and in the USA in 1943.[32]

The term 'hypodermic' was first used in 1859.[33] Morphine introduced under the skin using a vaccination lancet, by G. V. Lafargue of St Emilion in 1836.[34]

(*See also* Duncum Barbara M. *The Development of Inhalation Anaesthesia*. London: Oxford University Press, 1947; Shearer W. *Br. J. Anaesth.* 1960, **32**, 554; 1961, **33**, 219).

Premedication

This term was first used in the 1920s. A preoperative visit by the anaesthetist with an explanation of the anaesthetic procedure, and perhaps a booklet describing how things will go, reassures the patient and relieves anxiety. Its purpose is the administration of drugs to facilitate the induction and maintenance of and the recovery from anaesthesia. At the present time the intramuscular injection of doses of sedative and a drying agent, which has been customary for decades, is being questioned as it is realized that: (1) Anxiety is not always relieved: drowsiness does not necessarily abolish apprehension; (2) Some patients have in fact little anxiety concerning the induction of anaesthesia. It is held by some that opioids are too toxic to warrant their present popularity.[35] Drying agents are not always required and may have undesirable side-effects. The need for routine administration of anticholinergic drugs before anaesthesia needs reconsideration.

Reasons for Administration

A. Reduction of fear and anxiety before anaesthesia and operation.

B. Reduction of secretion of saliva.

C. Prevention of undesirable reflexes, e.g. cardiac dysrhythmia due to: (*a*) Drugs such as volatile agents and suxamethonium; or (*b*) Afferent impulses from, for example, the upper respiratory tract, the eye, abdominal and thoracic viscera; postoperative vomiting.

D. As part of the anaesthetic technique, e.g. narcotic analgesics reduce the tachypnoea of trichloroethylene and the extrapyramidal movements sometimes seen after the intravenous injection of methohexitone or thiopentone; they also provide analgesia. Also to reduce the possibility of awareness during very light anaesthesia.

E. To produce amnesia. This may be retrograde (loss of memory for events prior to drug administration) or anterograde (following drug administration). The incidence of amnesia is low with routine opiate premedication. Hyoscine causes amnesia in a small but significant group of patients. Opiate–diazepam combination results in greater anterograde amnesia, but diazepam–hyoscine combinations are most effective, though only resulting in partial amnesia in about 25% of patients. Amnesia is more likely to occur when drugs are administered intravenously rather than intramuscularly. Good amnesia can be achieved with pethidine 100 mg, diazepam 10 mg and hyoscine 0·4 mg intravenously, but such a mixture is too depressant for routine use.[36] Oral lorazepam 2·5–5 mg is associated with a high incidence of amnesia.

Drugs Used

These may include:

1. *Sedatives*. e.g. barbiturates, benzodiazepines, phenothiazines, etc. Patients in hot climates are more sensitive to sedative premedication than those living in temperate zones, due to their reduced BMR.

2. *Narcotic Analgesics*. Opium and its derivatives, pethidine, methadone. Narcotic analgesics may be derived from opium, e.g. morphine and codeine; they may be semisynthetic and obtained by chemical alteration of the morphine molecule, e.g. diamorphine (heroin); or they may be entirely synthetic e.g. pethidine, fentanyl, alfentanyl, sufentanyl, lofentanyl, pentazocine, phenoperidine, etc. Some anaesthetists regard narcotic premedication as undesirable. It is now considered both humane and safe to administer an opioid analgesic to a patient with undiagnosed pain, by cautious and repeated intravenous injections. Should diagnostic problems arise, naloxone can be given 'to bring the pain back'.[37]

3. *Neuroleptic Agents* such as dehydrobenzperidol (droperidol).

4. *Anticholinergic Agents*. Atropine, hyoscine and glycopyrronium. A dose of 1·5–3 mg of atropine is probably necessary to block the cardiac vagus completely although half of this will inhibit salivary secretion.

Sedative action is helped by the oral administration of a suitable hipnotic the night before operation. Examples are temazepam 5–10 mg, flurazepam (Dalmane) 15–30 mg, nitrazepam (Mogadon) 5–10 mg, promethazine (Phenergan) 50 mg and pentobarbitone (Nembutal) 100–200 mg.

Sedative premedication does not lessen the need for kind, sympathetic care for patients at a time of great stress. For depressed patients, amitriptyline 25–50 mg is suitable given by mouth at bedtime.

In many hospitals, non-anaesthetic junior staff have a rather poor knowledge of the use of drugs employed by anaesthetists.[38]

Postoperative Pain

Pain relief is necessary for: (1) Humanitarian and (2) Therapeutic reasons. Pain causes peripheral vasoconstriction, and reduces FRC and sputum clearance. About 70% of patients in all human trials get pain relief from inert placebos.

Severity of pain depends on: (1) The site of operation (in a report of a large series of operations, postoperative analgesia was required in 74% of thoracic cases; 63% of upper abdominal cases; 51% of lower abdominal cases; 23% of body-wall operations).[39] (2) Age, (3) Sex, (4) Premedication employed, (5) Anaesthetic agents used, (6) Psychological factors.

Abdominal and thoracic wounds result in grunting, inefficient respiration with the production of hypoxia. Areas of spontaneous atelectasis may arise with regional underventilation, perfusion inequality and shunting of venous blood. FRC is reduced. The normal periodic deep breaths are inhibited by pain so that its relief undoubtedly aids respiration.

The relief of postoperative pain is often very badly managed.[40]

In war injuries, infusion of pentazocine relieves pain efficiently, but in the presence of hypotension or respiratory depression, ketamine is superior.[41]

Methods of Pain Relief

1. *Simple analgesics*, e.g. aspirin, diflunisal (Dolobid) indomethacin, phenyl-butazone, indoprofen. They relieve some skeletal pain, as well as headache. These should not be given over long periods of time because of the risk of papillary necrosis and interstitial nephritis or liver damage. A suppository, aspirin 1 g is effective.[42] Aspirin is also an antiplatelet agent, its antithrombotic activity being thought due to its effect on thromboxane A2 synthesis together with the reduction of the formation of prostacyclin.

Paracetamol is an active metabolite of phenacetin; it is analgesic and antipyretic, although not anti-inflammatory. It inhibits prostaglandin synthesis within the central nervous system. It does not cause gastric irritation and is relatively non-toxic in therapeutic doses, but 5 g may be enough to cause centrilobular hepatic necrosis. Codeine may be combined with simple analgesics.

2. *Non-steroidal anti-inflammatory drugs (NSAIDs)*:
   1. Modify the nociceptive responses caused by bradykinin.
   2. Inhibit synthesis of prostaglandin E.
   3. Have direct analgesic effect on the higher centres.
   4. Reduce stickiness of blood platelets.

5. May cause hypothrombinaemia in large doses.
6. Lowers body temperature in pyrexia, in low dosage.
7. Lowers blood sugar in low dosage; reverse effect in high dosage.
8. May cause acid–base imbalance and acidosis.

Indomethacin can be given per rectum for postoperative pain relief[43] and indoprofen has also been recommended.[44] Indomethacin can also be given i.v. for pain relief after operation.[45]

3. *Opiates or opioids* can be arranged in a long series depending on their affinities for opium receptors, ranging from pure agonists (morphine, pethidine, diamorphine, methadone), through partial agonists (phenazocine, codeine) and partial antagonists (pentazocine, nalorphine, levallorphan), to the pure antagonists (naloxone).

Oral opioids. Morphine and diamorphine, given in water or chloroform water without any additions, give good analgesia; with diamorphine the analgesia comes on quicker but is of shorter duration. An anti-emetic may be required should the patient require more than 20 mg of morphine.[46] The Brompton cocktail is now outdated as oral cocaine does not relieve chronic pain. A tablet of morphine containing 10 mg of base, placed and kept between the upper lip and the upper gum will control pain as efficiently as the same dose given intramuscularly.[47]

Opioids influence the emotional aspects of pain, such as anxiety and fear, rather than reducing the actual pain threshold, so making intolerable pain, tolerable. Specific opiate receptors probably exist in both the brain and in the spinal cord. Encephalins are present in the brain and in the gastrointestinal tract; they may be formed in the adrenal medulla and are neurotransmitters. They are like natural opioids. Beta-endorphin is a potent opioid, more stable and potent than the enkaphalins.[48] The side-effects of nausea and vomiting can be distressing.

4. *Opioids by injection.* Morphine 10 mg, heroin 5 mg, pethidine 100 mg or buprenorphine 0·3 mg can be given intramuscularly, although in reduced dosage in children, the elderly and the unfit.

A continuous intravenous drip of morphine or other narcotic analgesic can be given until pain is relieved, and then the dose titrated against the pain. Infusions of fentanyl efficiently relieve postoperative pain.[54] Such infusions need not be followed by either psychological dependence or physical sequelae[53] (*see also* patient-controlled analgesia; the Cardiff Palliator[50] and the Janssen on-demand infusion of dilute fentanyl[51]). This gives good pain relief at a lower dosage than intramuscular injection.

Efficient postoperative pain relief can be provided by a continuous subcutaneous drip infusion powered by a syringe pump.[52] Continuous subcutaneous pethidine for routine postoperative analgesia (2 mg/h) after a loading dose, has proved successful and reasonably free from side-effects.[58] Morphine (1·5–2 mg/h) has been given too, with good results.[60]

It has been reported that the opioid requirements of patients receiving high doses of corticosteroids is less than normal in the control of postoperative pain.[49]

The sale of opium was unrestricted in the UK until the Pharmacy Act of 1868.

Anxiety due to depression can be relieved by amitriptyline 25–50 mg at night.

5. *Extradural injections of narcotic analgesics* (*see* Chapter 32).

6. *Blockade of pain afferents by regional techniques,*[55] e.g. postoperative high extradural analgesia,[187] intercostal nerve block,[56] subcutaneous bupivacaine after herniorrhaphy.[57] A continuous lignocaine drip (2 mg/min) has been used

with success and absence of signs of toxicity.[59] For paravertebral and sacral block, *See* chapters 31 and 32.

7. *Inhalation of analgesic gases and vapours*, e.g. nitrous oxide and oxygen or air; trichloroethylene or methoxyflurane and air.

8. *Transcutaneous electrostimulation.*[61]

9. *Cryoanalgesia* of individual nerves may be used (Wood G. J. et al. *Anaesthesia* 1981, **36**, 603; Evans P. J. D. et al. *Br. J. Anaesth*, 1981, **53**, 1121).

(*See also* Symposium on Post-operative Pain. *Br. J. Anaesth*, 1967, **39** (September); Annotation. *Br. Med. J.* 1978, **2**, 517; Utting J. E. and Smith J. M. *Anaesthesia* 1979, **34**, 332; Dodson, M. E. *Ann. R. Coll. Surg.* 1982, **64**, 325.) When possible analgesics after operation should be given as a continuous intravenous injection or infusion, if adequate facilities are available.

Morphine (from the Greek, Morpheus, god of dreams, son of Somnos, god of sleep.)

Opium is derived from the Greek word for 'juice'. Has been in use as opium for over 2000 years and is still the best available analgesic (first used by Theophrastus in the third century B.C.). ('Among the remedies which it has pleased Almighty God to give to man to relieve his sufferings, none is so universal and so efficacious as opium'—Thomas Sydenham 1627–1682), London physician, 1680, who introduced tincture of opium (laudanum) into England, and still true in 1987.) Opium comes from the dried latex from unripe capsules of the poppy head.

Morphine isolated from opium by F. W. A. Sertürner (1783–1841) of Paderborn in 1806.[62] Morphine salts are not destroyed by boiling.

One of over 25 alkaloids[63] contained in opium (*Papaver somniferum*), but only morphine, codeine and papaverine have wide clinical use. Concentration of morphine in opium is 9–17%.

Summary of actions of morphine. (1) *Central nervous system.* (*a*) Depresses awareness, anxiety, pain sensation and respiration; (*b*) Stimulates vomiting centre; secretion of antidiuretic hormone; Edinger–Westphal nucleus causing small pupils; (2) *Smooth muscle.* (*a*) Depresses vascular tone and peristalsis; (*b*) Stimulates bronchoconstriction, bowel sphincters, biliary spasm, Fallopian spasm, erectores pilorum; (3) *Addiction.* Both psychological and physical. Patients may develop both tolerance (or tachyphylaxis) and dependence (or addiction). In addicts, withdrawal symptoms come on in about 8 hours after the last dose and are very distressing. They include agitation, severe abdominal cramps, diarrhoea and lacrimation ('cold turkey'). Relieved by further doses of morphine or methadone; (4) *Other.* Stimulates secretion of catecholamines.

Pharmacology. Morphine is a direct metabolic depressant. Its chief effects are on the central nervous system, the respiratory system and the bowel. Chemical structure determined in 1925 and was synthesized by Gates and Tschudi (1952).[64] Like codeine, it is related to phenanthrene and piperidine, this group of drugs being good analgesics and poor relaxers of smooth muscle. Papaverine is related to benzyl isoquinoline and like its congeners is a poor analgesic but a good relaxant of smooth muscle. Morphine may release histamine and 5-hydroxytryptamine from the tissues (sometimes there is a skin weal following preoperative injection of the drug). Taken by mouth is useful when given 4-hourly in doses up to 100 mg for chronic pain.[65] Given into the rectum as a suppository (30 mg), pain is relieved.

Central Nervous System. It raises the pain threshold, elevates mood, and usually causes euphoria with agreeable drowsiness. More effective against dull, continuous, than against sharp, intermittent pain. Morphine relieves visceral pain more efficiently than bone and muscle pain, which responds to aspirin, etc. Analgesia more efficient if given before onset of pain than if given to relieve existing pain. With high enough dosage analgesia adequate for the performance of surgical operations can be obtained but only at the expense of severe respiratory depression. A drug of addiction. Very rarely, restlessness and delirium follow its injection (as in the horse and cat) and dysphoria follows. Depresses respiratory centre. Spinal cord reflexes sometimes exaggerated. Parasympathetic tone may be increased due to the anticholinesterase effect of morphine. The cerebrospinal fluid pressure is increased because of the raised P_{CO_2}. Intravenous injection causes a more rapid but less prolonged effect than intramuscular injection. Reduces time of paradoxical sleep (REM).

Effect on the Eye. It constricts the pupil by a central not a peripheral action, stimulating the pupillary fibres of the Edinger–Westphal nucleus, the oculomotor nerve being the efferent pathway. Atropine can counteract this miosis. Intraocular tension reduced in both normal and glaucomatous eyes.

Respiratory System. The sensitivity of the respiratory centre to changes in Pa_{CO_2} is diminished. Respiratory rate, rather than tidal volume, decreased. Arterial and alveolar P_{CO_2} not usually much raised. Breathing may become periodic (Cheyne–Stokes)[66] or irregular (Biot). Atropine does not reverse the respiratory depressant effects of morphine. There may be bronchoconstriction due to histamine release, and this is worse in asthmatic patients. Maximal respiratory depression comes on 30 min after intramuscular injection, sooner after i.v. injection. Depresses the cough reflex.

Gastrointestinal Tract. Morphine constricts the sphincters of the gut. The movements of the stomach are reduced, while the pylorus is contracted. Given i.m., gastric emptying time increased, less when given orally.[67] The tone of the muscles of the small and large intestines is increased, but peristalsis is reduced, and so constipation results from a state of spastic immobility of the bowel. The effects of morphine on the alimentary canal after injection are local and not central. Atropine and propantheline bromide, 15–30 mg, antagonize this action, neostigmine increases it. It has been reported that a tablet of morphine tartrate, 13·3 mg placed between the upper lip and the gum, will provide analgesia, as efficient as that after an intramuscular injection of the same dose.[68]

Nausea and vomiting are due to stimulation of the medullary chemoreceptor trigger zone and not due to direct stimulation of the vomiting centres. This is seen most strongly with the allied drug, apomorphine. Vomiting after morphine depends partly on the movements of the body and the position of the patient; it sensitizes the vomiting centre to vestibular movements. Ambulation after morphine will cause more nausea than quiet bed-rest. Certain phenothiazines, antihistamines, droperidol and other drugs may act as anti-emetics.

Morphine produces a contraction of the muscle at the lower end of the common bile duct (sphincter of Oddi), and so raises the bile pressure in the bile ducts by preventing emptying. Atropine does not fully antagonize this action, but nitroglycerin, nalorphine, levallorphan, adrenaline, aminophylline and amyl nitrite do. Naloxone antagonizes most side-effects.

Urinary Tract. The tone and peristalsis of the ureters and other smooth muscle, e.g. of the hollow viscera, bladder sphincter, etc., are increased, an action antagonized by atropine. The tone of the Fallopian tubes is increased and spasm potentiated. The tone of the detrusor muscle and of the vesical sphincter is increased and may hinder micturition. Urinary output decreased from stimulation of secretion of antidiuretic hormone.

Little or no influence on uterus during labour. Crosses placental barrier and depresses fetal respiration.

Cardiovascular System. Not greatly altered by clinical doses of morphine, e.g. 10 mg, but if this is doubled, effects may be serious in handicapped patients. There is sometimes a slight fall in pulse rate and blood pressure, especially if the drug is given intravenously. Vascular collapse may follow if a morphinized patient suddenly sits up or is moved. There is vasodilatation of skin vessels, especially in the head and neck (the blush area). Morphine decreases vascular resistance and increases forearm blood flow.[69] Skin weals may also be seen when morphine is applied to scarified skin, e.g. sometimes following an injection. Sweating may be stimulated.

Patients in shock should be given their morphine intravenously, so that it does not accumulate unabsorbed in the ischaemic tissues, only to produce a massive effect when absorption occurs with improvement in the circulation. Only small doses needed.

Morphine sometimes causes itching, especially of the nose. It may occasionally cause anaphylactoid and allergic reactions, ranging from slight syncope to anaphylactic shock with bronchial asthma due to histamine release. Useful in the management of paroxysmal nocturnal dyspnoea (cardiac asthma).

Endocrine System. Posterior pituitary and adrenal medulla stimulated, so antidiuretic hormone and blood catecholamine levels increased. May cause rise in blood sugar.

Pharmacokinetics. Elimination about 3 hours. Biotransformation is by conjugation with glycuronic acid in the liver, followed by excretion in the bile and by the kidneys. Deficient renal excretion may cause accumulation and respiratory depression.[70]

It appears in breast milk, saliva and sweat.

Advantages and disadvantages of morphine as premedication. Advantages. (1) Relieves anxiety and produces tranquillity; (2) Reduces amount of anaesthetic needed; (3) Helps to prevent tachypnoea, e.g. with trichloroethylene; (4) Provides analgesia; (5) Facilitates controlled ventilation when this is desired; (6) Reduces the incidence of awareness during nitrous-oxide–oxygen relaxant anaesthesia.

Disadvantages. (1) May produce postoperative vomiting, constipation and ileus; (2) Causes respiratory depression and so may retard induction of inhalation anaesthesia; (3) It interferes with pupil signs of depth of anaesthesia; when morphine is combined with atropine or hyoscine its miotic action usually proves stronger than their mydriatic effect; (4) It is habit forming; tolerance follows repeated doses and addiction can occur; abstinence symptoms are seen when addicts are suddenly deprived of their drug; (5) It may delay resumption of spontaneous respiration.

Special care is necessary. (1) In infants under 6 months, the aged, feeble and debilitated; (2) In patients with a raised P_{CO_2}, suprarenal insufficiency, myasthenia, myotonia, hypothyroidism, asthma, raised intracranial pressure, respiratory depression, liver disease, acute alcoholism, diverticulitis and labour; (3) In some patients taking mono-amine oxidase inhibitors; (4) In patients who are to breathe spontaneously because of the respiratory depression which may result; (5) In the period immediately following general anaesthesia.

Morphine kills by causing respiratory arrest.

Dose. The hydrochloride, sulphate and tartrate are used, while the dose in adults in usually 0·15 mg/kg or 10–15 mg in fit adults. Given 90 min before anaesthesia, so that peak of respiratory depression is passed before induction commences.

(*See also* Twycross R. G. *J. Med. Ethics* 1975, **1**, 10.)

Codeine Phosphate, BP (codeine is derived from the Greek name for 'poppy-head').
This is methyl morphine and together with morphine and papaverine forms the chief alkaloidal derivative of opium. It was isolated in 1832 by Pierre Jean Robiquet (1780–1840).[71]

It depresses respiration less, causes less constipation and vomiting than morphine. Its analgesic effect is one-tenth that of morphine and it fails to produce progressive sedation with increasing doses. Less likely to cause addiction than morphine. Most of drug is excreted unchanged by kidneys. The usual dosage is 15–50 mg of the phosphate by mouth. Increasing the total dose above 60 mg does not increase analgesia. Used as a cough suppressant and to treat mild pain. Codeine may release histamine in children.[72]

Dihydrocodeine Tartrate (DF118) (Paracodin, Paramol)
This drug in 20–30 mg doses is a very powerful analgesic, remarkably free from unpleasant side-effects such as nausea and respiratory depression. Duration of pain relief after hypodermic injection is about 4 hours. Put up in ampoules of 50 mg in 1 ml the solution has a pH of 3·2, so that it should be diluted before intravenous injection. Also in 30-mg tablets. It releases histamine. When 30 mg are taken by mouth it tends to cause nausea and vertigo in women and constipation in men. Sometimes relieves both cough and the severe chronic pain of cancer. Intravenous injection of 25 mg or more after dental extraction *increases* pain, although the pains of labour, skeletal origin or laparotomy are relieved.[73]

Diamorphine Hydrochloride, BP (Heroin)
This is the diacetyl ester of morphine and is the most likely of the opium derivatives to become a drug of addiction, because of the euphoria it creates. Introduced into medicine in 1898 by H. Dreser (1860–1924). In the US and in Australia its use is proscribed. Should be freshly prepared from powder. It depresses the respiratory centre and the cough reflex more than morphine and is twice as efficient as an analgesic. Diamorphine 5 mg has a quicker onset of activity, more marked sedation and fewer emetic sequelae than morphine 10 mg. An excellent postoperative analgesic although its effect does not last as long as that of morphine. In coronary occlusion, 5 mg i.v. cause little cardiovascular depression or vomiting, if given slowly. Useful by mouth in the treatment of chronic pain in doses up to 30 mg.[74]

Excretion is chiefly by the kidneys after conversion to morphine in the body.
The usual dose is 2·5–5 mg of the hydrochloride.

Table 8.1. Narcotic analgesics (with doses in mg)

Alkaloids of opium
　Morphine (10)
　Codeine (30)
　Papaveretum (15)
Semisynthetic alkaloids
　Diamorphine (5)
　Dihydrocodeine (D.F. 118) (50)
　Dihydromorphinone (Dilaudid) (2)
Synthetic agents
　Benzomorphinans and morphinans
　　Levorphanol (Dromoran) (2)
　　Pentazocine (Fortral, Talwin) (30)
Piperidine derivatives
　Pethidine (Mepiridine, Demerol) (100)
　Phenoperidine (Operidine) (2)
　Fentanyl (Sublimaze) (0·05–0·2)
　Alfentanil (Rapifen) (0·25–0·5)
　Sufentanil (0·005–0·01)
　Lofentanil (0·005)
Diphenylheptane derivatives
　Methadone (Physeptone) (10)
　Dextromoramide (Palfium) (5)
Mixed agonist-antagonists
　Pentazocine (30)
　Buprenorphine (0·3)
　Butorphanol (2)

Papaveretum, BPC (Omnopon, Pantopon, Alopon, Opoidine)
Introduced in 1909 by Sahli[75] (1856–1933) of Berne. These are mixtures of purified opium alkaloids in the proportion found in nature. Papaveretum contains the hydrochlorides of the alkaloids of opium as follows: anhydrous morphine 47·5–52·2%, anhydrous codeine 2·5–5%, narcotine 16–22%, papaverine 2·5–7%.[76] Clinically 20 mg papaveretum equals 13·3 mg morphine sulphate, and its properties are not entirely due to its morphine content. The papaverine content is phamacologically inert. There is no evidence that papaveretum causes fewer unpleasant side-effects than morphine. Dosage, 10–20 mg. Premedication in children: 0·2 mg/kg. (*See also* Chapter 28.)

Papaverine, BP
Isolated by Georg Franz Merck (1825–1895) of Darmstadt in 1848 from opium.[77] Related to isoquinoline and is different in constitution and action from morphine. Possesses an antispasmodic action but does not suppress intestinal peristalsis. Relieves spasm in arteries. Has almost no effect on the central nervous system, on respiration or on mood, and causes no euphoria. Dose up to 30 mg intravenously, very slowly; orally, 120–250 mg.

Pethidine Hydrochloride, BP (Demerol, meperidine hydrochloride USP, isonipecaine, Dolatin, Dolantal, Dolosal, Pantalgin)
The hydrochloride of the ethyl ester of 1-methyl-4-phenyl-piperidine-4-carboxylic acid. Intravenous dose 5–25 mg repeated as necessary.

Pharmacodynamics

1. Has a morphine-like action on pain, about one-eighth to one-tenth as powerful as morphine. Duration of analgesia shorter than that of morphine. Relieves most types of pain, especially those associated with plain muscle spasm—except biliary colic. Depresses respiratory centre and cough reflex. Is a local analgesic. No effect on ciliary body or iris. Raises the CSF pressure. Can cause addiction.

2. Has a direct papaverine-like effect on the smooth muscle of the bronchioles, intestine, ureters and arteries. In dilute solution is a vasodilator after intravenous injection. May cause hypotension. Will often relieve bronchial spasm. It causes spasm of the sphincter of Oddi, an effect counteracted by amyl nitrite and naloxone (not by atropine or papaverine). Reduces tone and amplitude of contraction of ureters. Does not lead to constipation.

3. Has an atropine-like effect on cholinergic nerve-endings.

4. May release histamine from tissues.

5. Side-effects may include sweating, hypotension, vertigo and limb tingling. Postoperative nausea is similar to that following morphine, but comes on earlier. These are worse after intravenous than after intramuscular injection. Like morphine, pethidine may cause hypotension if the head of the patient is raised, or with sudden movement. May increase the incidence of postoperative nausea and vomiting, an effect reduced by its combination with atropine or hyoscine. Because of its circulatory depressant effects it is probably not the ideal drug for the relief of pain in myocardial infarction. Phenobarbitone enhances the production of toxic metabolites of pethidine. These two drugs should not be given together.[78]

Uses. Can be given intravenously, or intramuscularly when effect comes on in 15 min, is at its height in 90 min and lasts up to 2 h.

1. For premedication (dose 25–100 mg).

2. For postoperative analgesia 50–100 mg i.m., by mouth or infusion.

3. For analgesia during intravenous barbiturate, gas and oxygen anaesthesia with or without a relaxant (dose 10 mg i.v., repeated as necessary).

4. For the reduction of tachypnoea during anaesthesia (10–20 mg i.v.).

5. For the relief of pain in labour (75–100 mg i.m.).

It forms a precipitate with thiopentone solution.

Pharmacokinetics. Pethidine is metabolized at the rate of 17%/h. The biological half-life is 3–4 h in man.[79] Destroyed in body to extent of 80%, probably by hydrolysis in liver, disease of which may retard its destruction. About 5–10% is excreted unchanged by the kidneys. One metabolite, norpethidine, may cause convulsions or hallucinations if pethidine is given in large doses or with mono-amine oxidase inhibitors. Five per cent excreted in the urine and 64% plasma protein bound.

Pethidine in labour. See Chapter 27.

Precautions. The administration of pethidine to patients under the influence of mono-amine oxidase inhibitors may cause alarming reactions and even death. There may be restlessness, hypertension, convulsions and coma (sometimes reversed by acidifying the urine) with absent tendon jerks and an extensor plantar response; hypotension may also be seen. The reaction is said to be due to interference with the microsomes in liver cells which detoxicate pethidine. When the reaction does occur treatment with 25 mg prednisolone or chlorpromazine is worth trying but not all patients are at risk.

There are with pethidine, as with other powerful drugs, two types of sensitivity.

In the first the patient shows signs of overdosage following average amounts given, e.g. vasodilatation and hypotension. In the second the patient shows an abnormal reaction to the administration of the drug. Dose should be reduced in old age, in renal and liver disease.

Phenoperidine (Operidine) (*see* Chapter 13)

Fentanyl (Sublimaze, Fentanest, Lepantal) (*see* Chapter 13)

Alfentanil (Rapifen) (*see* Chapter 13)

Lofentanil
Twenty times more potent than fentanyl, 6000 times more than morphine. Long duration of action attributed to persistent occupation of receptor sites.

Pentazocine (Fortral, Talwin)
The N-allyl derivative of phenazocine first described by Archer in 1962[80] and by Keats and Telford in 1964.[81] A narcotic analgesic derived from benzmorphinan. Analgesic potency of 30 mg equal to morphine 10 mg and pethidine 75–100 mg. Respiratory depression equal to that of morphine and pethidine in equipotent doses but causes less vomiting than either. Stated to be non-addictive by WHO Expert Committee on Dependence-producing Drugs, 1966, 1969 and 1970. Not subject to control under the Misuse of Drugs (Sch. 2.3) Regulations. Does not result in euphoria. Chemically incompatible with diazepam, soluble barbiturates and sodium bicarbonate. Raises rather than lowers blood pressure and has a positive inotropic effect on the myocardium (β-receptor stimulation). This is due to the dextro-isomer.[82] Does not influence pupil size or intraocular tension. Crosses the placental barrier less easily than pethidine.[83] Should not be given to narcotic addicts as it may produce withdrawal symptoms. A very weak narcotic antagonist, one-fiftieth the activity of nalorphine. Has been used at the end of operation to reverse the respiratory depressant effects of fentanyl, while at the same time giving prolonged postoperative analgesia—'sequential anaesthesia'.[84] Hallucinations may follow its use but may be controlled by nalorphine[85] or diazepam. Skin rashes may follow parenteral injection.[86] Most of it is metabolized in the liver and partly excreted in the urine. Is active orally (adult dose 50 mg).
Uses   (1) For premedication it has no advantages over other opioids; (2) To potentiate barbiturate, gas–oxygen anaesthesia; (3) As the analgesic agent in neurolept anaesthesia; (4) For postoperative pain relief, 25–30 mg i.m. or by mouth; (5) For the relief of pain in labour; should not be given in the first trimester of pregnancy; has been approved by the English National Board for Midwifery for use by midwives; labour not retarded by 35–40 mg; (6) Small doses intravenously may be useful for the relief of pain in cases of head injury.
    Prepared in 1- and 2-ml ampoules (30 mg/ml).

Dextropropoxyphene
May cause dependence and, taken with alcohol, respiratory depression. Distalgesic is made up of 32·5 mg with paracetamol 325 mg. Overdose will result in liver toxicity and respiratory depression.

Dextromoramide Acid Tartrate, BP (Palfium)
A morphine-like analgesic but twice as potent. Dose 5-mg tablet or 5–10 mg by intramuscular injection. Relatively non-soporific. Can be given by mouth.

Methadone Hydrochloride, BP (Physeptone, Amidone, Dolophine, Miadone, Adanon, Butalgin)
This is a powerful analgesic, with a half-life up to 90 h. Causes less sedation and has a more prolonged action than morphine. Has been used to wean addicts from morphine and for easing the pain in chronic conditions. (*See also* Bullingham, R. E. S. *Br. J. Hosp. Med.* 1981, **5**, 59; and Gourlay G. K. et al. *Anaesth. Intensive Care*, 1981, **9**, 183.) Dosage 5–10 mg.

Levorphanol Tartrate, BP (Dromoran, laevo-morphinan tartrate, Levorphan, Methorphan)[87]
Dosage by mouth, 1·5–2 mg; in severe pain 4 mg. By injection 1–5 mg.

The most efficient drugs by mouth in the treatment of severe pain are methadone, dextromoramide and levorphanol. The last has the longest duration of action.

Piritramide (Dipidolor)[88]
Hypnotic effect greater than that after morphine or pethidine but causes less hypotension, nausea and vomiting. Useful in treatment of postoperative pain and as a supplement to gas–oxygen-relaxant anaesthesia. Dose for postoperative pain, 20 mg, i.m. repeated.

Buprenorphine (Temgesic)[91]
A synthetic analgesic of high potency and long action. A thebaine derivative, related in structure to morphine. Exhibits both agonist and antagonist action. Thirty-five times as potent as morphine, half as potent as fentanyl. Duration of action up to 10 h.[92] A single dose may therefore last through the night hours. The plasma buprenorphine concentration falls to low levels within 1 hour of administration and the long duration of action may result from the slow dissociation constant of the drug–receptor complex.[93] Buprenorphine can be given sublingually for postoperative pain (200 µg). For a speedy action this can be preceded by a parenteral dose. In patients with urinary obstruction, buprenorphine may accentuate this.[94] A dose of 0·3 mg relieves the pain of ureteral colic.[95] (*See also* Bullingham, R. E. S., O'Sullivan G. et al. *Anaesthesia* 1984, **39**, 329; Derbyshire D. R., Vater M. et al. *Anaesthesia* 1984, **39**, 324.) Commercially available in solution, 0·3 mg/ml. Dose 0·2–0·4 mg. Can be given sublingually (dose 0·2 mg[96]). Not reversed by naloxone but respiratory depression may be treated by doxapram. Has also been used as a supplement to nitrous oxide in surgical operations[97] and i.v. for postoperative pain.[98]

Nalbuphine Hydrochloride (Nubain)
Has been used for perioperative analgesia. Has less effect on delay of coordinated bowel motility than morphine.[99] Dose 10–20 mg.

Meptazinol (Meptid)
Used for perioperative analgesia. Dose by mouth 200 mg, repeated. Intramuscularly, 75–100 mg.

Other analgesic drugs include: *Butorphanol*.[89] Synthetic analgesic with benzomorphan nucleus, structurally related to pentazocine. Five times as potent as morphine, twenty times as potent as pentazocine. Dose 1–2 mg. *Oxypertine*.[90] Recommended for premedication by mouth. Dose 20 mg.

For discussion of the different opioid receptors, *see* Martin W. R. et al. *Br. J. Clin. Pharmacol.* 1979, **7**, 273S–279S.

(*See also* 'Synthetic opiate analgesics', Bullingham R. E. S. *Br. J. Hosp. Med.* 1981, **25**, 59.)

The Misuse of Drugs Act 1971[100]

Came into force 1 July 1973 in the UK. (*See* British National Formulary.)

Schedule 1
No records need be kept or entries made in a register of controlled drugs.

Schedule 2
Listed drugs: Class A. Opium, morphine, diamorphine, fentanyl, alfentanyl, cocaine, methadone, pethidine, dextromoramide, dipipanone, hydrocodone, hydromorphone, levanorphanol, oxycodone, phenazocine and piritramide. Phencyclidine, lycergide, together with Class B drugs when given by injection.
Class B. This includes oral amphetamines, codeine, cannabis resin, ethylmorphine, phenmetrazine and pholcodine, most barbiturates used by anaesthetists.
Class C. Benzphetamine, chlorphentamine and pipradol.

Records of Schedule 2 drugs must be kept in a special register and signed in the doctor's own handwriting.

'A sister or acting sister for the time being in charge of a theatre may, when acting in her capacity as such, supply any drug in Schedule 2 to any person who may lawfully have that drug in his possession provided that the drug is used in that theatre in accordance with the prescription of a doctor or dentist.' A record of administration should be made in the patient's casenotes.

Schedule 3
No need for records in the register.

Specific Narcotic Antagonists

These are usually the *n*-allyl derivatives of narcotic analgesics. The more potent the narcotic, the smaller the dose of its allyl derivative necessary to antagonize narcotic-induced respiratory depression. Main difference between narcotics and their antagonists is that the latter do not: (1) Cause euphoria; (2) Lead to addiction. They may cause signs of withdrawal in narcotic addicts. Probable mode of action is competition at receptor sites on cell surfaces. The antagonists counteract the analgesia produced by morphine, levorphan, pethidine and oxymorphone although less so with morphine.

Specific antagonism to narcotics was first described in 1915 by Pohl.[101]

Naloxone (Narcan)
This is *n*-allyl noroxymorphone and is derived from the potent oxymorphone

which is ten times as strong as morphine. It was synthesized in 1972.[102] It is a more effective antagonist of narcotic-induced respiratory depression than either nalorphine or levallorphan and antagonizes the respiratory depression caused by pentazocine and dextropropoxyphene. Duration of effect may be less than the narcotic it is designed to antagonize, so that repeat dosage may be necessary. It relaxes spasm of the sphincter of Oddi induced by narcotic analgesics. With careful titration of dosage, analgesia is not reversed. Naloxone, unlike the other drugs, has no intrinsic agonist activity. Can be used in the treatment of opioid-induced respiratory depression and in midwifery to reverse fetal respiratory depression due to opiates. It also prevents the impairment of psychomotor performance due to low levels of alcohol.[103] Naloxone reverses respiratory depression but not the analgesia of intrathecal morphine.[104] Naloxone may raise blood pressure in septic shock, suggesting that endorphins may contribute to this hypotension.[105] Naloxone has caused acute pulmonary oedema in a previously fit patient, so it is to be used with care.[106] Has also caused dysrhythmia and even sudden death.[107] Can be given i.m. for a more prolonged effect. A very expensive drug. Pharmacokinetics. Half-life 20 min. Metabolized in the liver. Dose 0·1–0·4 mg i.v. repeated. In neonates 0·01 mg/kg.

Levallorphan Tartrate, BP, USP (Lorfan)

It is the *n*-allyl derivative of laevomorphinan (laevo-dromoran) to which it bears a similar relationship as does nalorphine to morphine. Levallorphan was synthesized in 1950 by Schneider and Hellerbach[108] and used as an antidote to respiratory depression by Fromherz and Pellmond two years later.[109]

Suggested dosage to reverse the respiratory depressant effects 0·5–1 mg, i.v. repeated at 3–5 min intervals, 0·25–0·5 mg into the umbilical vein. *Pethilorfan* contains pethidine and levallorphan 100 to 1·25 (80:1).

Narcotic-induced Controlled Apnoea

A technique introduced by Francis Foldes[110] in which a narcotic analgesic, such as pethidine, fentanyl or phenoperidine, is given intravenously in incremental doses sufficient to cause, along with hyperventilation, apnoea. Useful in the intensive therapy unit as a means of producing apnoea before IPPV.

The Benzodiazepines

Diazepam, BP (Valium, Diazemuls, Atensine)

Diazepam has been used by mouth as a tranquillizer in the nervous patient awaiting surgery, 10–20 mg, and i.m. as part of premedication; 10 mg is more effective as a sedative if given by mouth than if given i.m.[111] *See* Chapter 13 for further details.

Nitrazepam, BP (Mogadon, Remnos)

Nitrazepam is allied to diazepam and is a safe and efficient hypnotic; 5 mg being equipotent with butobarbitone 100 mg. It does not induce microsomal activity and thus has no influence on the metabolism of other drugs.[112] It may, however, be contra-indicated in severe chronic obstructive airways disease, as it has been shown to produce a fall in ventilatory capacity and a worsening of ventilatory failure in such patients. The ageing brain becomes sensitive to it.[113] Dose 5–10 mg.

Flurazepam (Dalmane)
A useful hypnotic, without effect on REM sleep (15–30 mg).

Lorazepam (Ativan)[114]
Oral lorazepam 1·0–5·0 mg is a reliable effective sedative when given preoperatively. It has a duration of action of at least 4 hours and there is appreciable anterograde amnesia. Can be given i.m. or i.v. in dose of 4 mg. More effective given sublingually than when injected i.m. in premedication.[115] Useful premedicant agent before regional analgesia, e.g. central neural blockade.[116] Abolishes the vasoconstriction which accompanies fear[117] and attenuates the psychic sequelae of ketamine.[118] Lorazepam reduces anxiety preoperatively more effectively than papaveretum.[119] (*See also* Chapter 13).

Flunitrazepam (Rohypnol)
Flunitrazepam 1 mg by mouth, has been recommended for premedication and as more effective than diazepam 10 mg or lorazepam 2·5 mg.[120]

Temazepam (Euhypnos; Normison)
Short acting. Dose 10–30 mg. Useful for night sedation or for premedication in day-stay surgery.[121] Temazepam is suitable for premedication in elderly patients undergoing minor surgery.[122] (*See also* Oswald I. *Br. Med. J.* 1979, **1**, 1167.)

Midazolam (Hypnovel)
Midazolam is a water-soluble preparation which combines fast onset of sedation, rapid recovery, good amnesia, minimal irritation of veins, and no risk of secondary sedation as it has no clinically significant metabolites. Supplied in ampoules containing 10 mg in either 2 or 5 ml. Useful before fibreoptic gastroscopy. No pain on injection and good anterograde amnesia. Dose 5–7·5 mg i.v.[123] Useful for night sedation before surgery (15 mg) or as premedication.[124] It is a useful induction agent in a dose of 0·3 mg/kg in the elderly.[125]

Haloperidol[126] *and Droperidol*
These drugs have been used in premedication, since they produce mental detachment and are anti-emetic. Large doses may cause extrapyramidal disturbances. They are often combined with phenoperidine or fentanyl. (*See* Chapter 13).

Barbiturates and Other Drugs

For history of barbiturates, *see* Dundee J. W. and McIlroy P. D. A. *Anaesthesia* 1982, **37**, 726.

The parent molecule was described in 1882 by Conrad Guthzeit and synthesized by Adolf Bayer (1835–1917) of Ghent, later of Munich, who did not recognize its soporific properties. It was introduced into medicine by Emil Fischer (1852–1919) Nobel prizeman in chemistry, 1902, of Berlin (who was one of the first to use barbiturates to take his own life), and J. F. von Mering of Halle (1849–1908), the first Nobel Prizewinner in medicine (1901), in 1903[127] as barbitone (diethyl barbituric acid) and Veronal (sodium barbiturate), after the Italian town; pheno-[128] and allobarbitone followed in 1912.

Summary of Actions of Barbiturates
Barbiturates directly depress synaptic transmission by producing membrane

stabilization. In large doses the drugs depress dehydrogenase enzymes involved in glucose oxidation. The myocardial depression is due to membrane-stabilizing effects. In uraemia there may be a decrease in protein binding of thiopentone, and so an enhanced effect.

Actions: (1) Hypnotic; (2) Anticonvulsant; (3) Depression of respiration; (4) Depression of vascular tone; (5) Depression of myocardium; (6) Depression of urine secretion (stimulation of antidiuretic hormone secretion); (7) Depression of muscle tone; (8) Depression of reflexes; (9) Depression of body temperature; (10) Depression of intracranial and intra-ocular pressure; (11) Anti-analgesic in subhypnotic doses; (12) Reduces REM sleep; (13) Habituation.

Pharmacokinetics. Phenobarbitone is bound to plasma proteins only slightly; pentobarbitone is partly bound; thiopentone and methohexitone, highly bound and about 200 times more lipid-soluble than phenobarbitone. Solutions of thiopentone may remain stable for up to 2 weeks but must be discarded should cloudiness appear.

The medium-acting barbiturates form useful preanaesthetic sedatives. Contraindicated in porphyria.

They cause alteration in binding and in the rate of metabolism of other drugs (enzyme induction), e.g. coumarins, and may reduce their effects.

As preanaesthetic sedatives, barbiturates are administered by mouth or by the rectum.

Pentobarbitone Sodium, BP (Nembutal)
It is sodium ethyl-methyl-butyl-barbiturate. Can be given per rectum to children 0·5 mg/kg of body weight. The adult dose is 100–200 mg given at bedtime or 2 h before operation by mouth. This and other similar barbiturates are used less frequently than formerly.

Quinalbarbitone Sodium, BP (Seconal)
Action is shorter, more intense and more rapid in onset than that of pentobarbitone. Usually given by mouth. Usual adult dose 100–200 mg.

Butobarbitone Sodium, BP (Soneryl, Neonal, sodium butyethyl-barbiturate)
Adult dose 100–200 mg by mouth.

Amylobarbitone, BP (Amytal)
Is sodium ethyl-isoamyl-barbiturate. The adult dose in 200 mg.

The Signs of Acute Barbiturate Overdosage
Alcohol potentiates barbiturate toxicity. Depression of the central nervous system; depression of respiration; depression of reflex activity; depression of the cardiovascular system is a late result. For treatment *see* Chapter 40.

Barbiturates are less commonly prescribed than formerly owing to the risks of suicide. They are, however, efficient hypnotics.

Paraldehyde, BP, USP
Introduced into medicine in 1882 by Vincenzo Cervello (1854–1914).[129] A useful hynoptic in doses of 4–8 ml. Its stench is its chief disadvantage. It does not depress the heart. Can be given i.m. (10 ml) when it is a useful sedative for the

control of disturbed patients and anticonvulsant or per rectum for premedication. Intravenous injection of 2 ml will often cause an explosive cough.

Chlormethiazole (Heminevrin)
Useful as a hypnotic for confused patients and in the treatment of both eclampsia and status epilepticus and as a 0·08% infusion as a hypnotic during regional analgesia. Allied chemically to thiamin (vitamin B_1).

Chloral Hydrate, BP ($CCl_3.CH(OH)_2$)
A needlessly neglected hypnotic synthesized by Liebig of Darmstadt (1803–1873) in 1832 and introduced in 1869 by Liebreich (1839–1908),[130] a Berlin physician (who also introduced hydrated wool fat into dermatology), and hence (apart from alcohol) the oldest. Hypnotic dose is 0·6–2 g suitably diluted. Also as trichloro-ethyl phosphate, the phosphoric ester of trichlorethanol. Dose: 1–2 g (Triclofos, Tricloryl).

Phenothiazine Derivatives
These have been given as sedatives before operation in various doses and in diverse combinations. They are also likely to reduce the incidence of vomiting. A dose of 25–50 mg chlorpromazine intramuscularly has been advocated, but may cause a fall in blood pressure. Promethazine 50 mg with or without pethidine has been used with considerable satisfaction. Patients with alcoholic liver disease are very sensitive to phenothiazines. *Trimeprazine tartrate* (Vallergan) is another valuable member of this group of drugs; available as a syrup for oral administration to children. (*See* Chapter 28.)

Anti-analgesics
Anti-analgesic effects may follow the administration of small doses of barbiturates.[131] These may be seen immediately after the injection of subnarcotic doses, or at a later stage as the effective concentration of the drug falls. (Experience with light levels of methohexitone anaesthesia in the dental chair do not bear this out however.) A similar effect may be present with halothane in low concentration (0·5%), with promethazine and with hyoscine.

Anticholinergic Agents[132]

Atropine Sulphate, BP
History. (From Atropos, the oldest of the Three Fates who severed the threads of life, which were spun by Clotho and mixed, those of good and evil fortune, by Lachesis). The alkaloid of the *Atropa belladonna* or deadly nightshade. Atropine was first suggested by E. A. Sharpey-Schaffer (1850–1935) Edinburgh physiologist in 1880 to reduce vagal tone during chloroform anaesthesia, and advocated by Dudley Buxton (1855–1935), London anaesthetist, 35 years later to inhibit secretions during ether anaesthesia. (*See* also Kessel J. *Anaesth. Intensive Care*, 1974, **2**, 77.) Not used in premedication before 1890, although it was given, as the extract, per rectum, in 1861 to control patients resistant to chloroform.[133]

The atropine group of alkaloids are esters formed by the union of an aromatic derivative of benzyl alcohol, tropic acid, with organic bases—tropine (atropine) and scopine (hyoscine). The tropic acid is the active radical. Atropine is the racemic mixture of dextro- and laevohyoscyamine, the laevo form being the more active; hyoscine is laevorotatory. First synthesized by Richard Willstaetter (1872–1942) in 1896 and again by Robert Robinson in 1917. The routine use of atropine has been questioned since irritant agents such as ether are seldom used in the UK today and adverse consequences have not resulted from its omission. Nevertheless, a majority of anaesthetists in the UK often quite unnecessarily still use atropine to reduce secretions and vagal tone.[134] Probably better given i.v. if and when necessary. Today it is usually prepared from the plant *Duboisia myoporoides*.

Uses. (1) To reduce secretions of saliva, especially in children and when ether is used; (2) To depress the cardiac vagus, especially in patients on digitalis; (3) When more than one dose of suxamethonium may be used; (4) To protect against muscarinic effects of anticholinergic drugs given to reverse the effects of non-depolarizing relaxants; (5) To counteract bradycardia in high spinal block, and so raise blood pressure; (6) To reverse the bradycardia due to suxamethonium, β-blocking agents, halothane and cyclopropane; (7) As a cycloplegic, and to depress the oculocardiac reflex in ophthalmic operations.

Action on autonomic nerves. It has a blocking action on effector organs of structures supplied by the postganglionic cholinergic nerves, e.g. smooth muscles and secretory glands, acting on the effector cells, i.e. it competes with acetylcholine at the sites of its muscarinic activity. It has no effect on either production or destruction of acetylcholine. Complete vagal block requires a dose of 3 mg. It is a parasympatholytic anticholinergic drug.

Action on central nervous system. It stimulates the medulla and higher centres, and directly stimulates the respiratory centre sufficiently to counteract the depressing effect of morphine. Occasionally, restlessness and delirium are seen. In the elderly, prolonged sedation may result; this may be treated by physostigmine 1–2 mg i.v.[135] The peak of its effect is 1 hour after hypodermic injection, wearing off rapidly.

Effects on eye. There is paralysis of the sphincter of the iris resulting in dilated pupils although a dose of 0·5 mg intramuscularly does not greatly influence accommodation or size of pupil.[136] (The sphincter muscle is innervated from the third cranial nerve via the ciliary ganglion and short ciliary nerves.) Used as drops, 1% atropine does not appreciably raise the intraocular pressure in normal eyes. There is no contraindication to the use of intramuscular or intravenous atropine in a patient with glaucoma, even of the narrow-angle type, since significant dilatation of the pupil does not occur. Topical atropine is, however, contraindicated. Mongols may show sensitivity to atropine, especially when applied topically to the eye; a dose of hyoscine is perhaps better for injection.

Effects on respiratory system. Sweat, bronchial and salivary glands are paralysed, while bronchial muscle is relaxed, causing a slight increase in the anatomical and physiological dead space, possibly causing some fall in Pao_2. Acts as a bronchodilator: reduces excessive bronchial secretion, although bronchorrhoea may be of two types, one being reduced by atropine, the other by prednisone.[137] Intramuscular injection 1 hour before anaesthesia suppresses salivation more efficiently than intravenous injection immediately before induction.

Action on circulatory system. Rate of heart sometimes slowed at first (the Bezold–Jarisch reflex), due to action on the sino-auricular node, but this effect is not seen after intravenous injection of clinical doses. It may occur after hypodermic injection or after intravenous injection of small amounts such as 0·05 mg. Later, rate is quickened by peripheral vagal paralysis and its effect on the SA pace-maker. This tachycardia, by shortening diastole, may decrease coronary filling time and increase myocardial oxygen consumption. It may also increase cardiac output. Thus it should be used with care in patients with coronary disease. This increase in heart rate is not marked in infants and senile patients. Reflexes involving vagal stimulation, e.g. from the eye or larynx, and hence cardiac slowing and syncope, may be prevented by atropine. In cases of gross tachycardia, e.g. in thyrotoxicosis, hyperpyrexia or heart disease, atropine is better avoided. Both atropine and hyoscine may cause dysrhythmias. Some cases of asystole can be reversed by atropine.[138]

It has been shown:[139] (*a*) In patients not premedicated with atropine or hyoscine, doses less than 0·5 mg i.v. may cause a slow pulse; more than 0·5 mg i.v. causes quickening, with or without preliminary slowing, depending on the rate of injection; (*b*) In patients premedicated with atropine or hyoscine, subsequent intravenous injection causes tachycardia, whatever the rate of injection. Atropine premedication also tends to prevent the dysrhythmias (A–V dissociation; A and V extrasystoles; multifocal ventricular tachycardia) sometimes seen after intravenous injection of atropine. Gallamine does not alter the basic effects of atropine on the heart rate.

Atropine, given intravenously, may increase the incidence of dysrhythmias with or without halothane and cyclopropane, and transiently in unanaesthetized man.

Atropine sometimes causes dilatation of the vessels of the face and a scarlatiniform rash.

Blood pressure not affected unless heart rate is slowed by vagal overactivity, when atropine raises it.

Action on alimentary canal. The tone and peristalsis of the gut and urinary tract are decreased. Like hyoscine and glycopyrronium it lowers the opening pressure of the cardiac sphincter of the stomach and hence increases the chances of regurgitation.[140] Metoclopramide has the opposite effect.[141] It is anti-emetic.

Effect on the fetus.[142] Atropine passes the placenta rapidly (as a tertiary amine) to reach the fetal circulation. It has been used as a test of placental insufficiency and in the diagnosis of fetal hypoxia. Atropine administered as premedication to the mother may protect the fetus and newborn from vagal reflexes occurring during birth and resuscitation.[143]

Pharmacokinetics. Plasma half-life 2–3 hours, 50% is protein bound. Elimination is slow in children under 2 and in the elderly.[144] Excretion is partly by the kidneys, another part being destroyed in the body, with the formation of tropine and tropic acid. Must be used carefully in thyrotoxicosis because of action on heart rate and on BMR.

Dosage. Usual dose, 0·5–1 mg i.m. (in children 0·015 mg/kg) 1–1½ h before operation. Before neostigmine, 1–2 mg.

If atropine is given in a dose of 2 mg by mouth (or hyoscine 1 mg), 90 min before operation, it acts as well as 0·5 mg hypodermically.[145]

Given in adequate dosage of 1–1·5 mg intravenously, atropine blocks the muscarinic action of neostigmine on the heart, gut and salivary glands. Its cardiac effects come on more rapidly than its antisalivary effects. Atropine has a wide therapeutic ratio and doses up to 200 mg have been used in psychiatry.[146]

Inhibition of sweating may lead to increase in temperature. It may therefore be avoided in pyrexial children.

Milk secretion is not affected, although the drug may be excreted into the milk.

Acts as a local analgesic, being half as potent as procaine. Atropine methonitrate can be given by nebulizer.

It inhibits the muscarinic but not the nicotinic effects of acetylcholine. It raises the basal metabolic rate. Like morphine, may produce a skin weal after subcutaneous injection.

Effects of atropine on the eye, heart and salivary glands less marked in negroes than in white people.[147]

The toxic effects (the anticholinergic syndrome) can be blocked by physostigmine (*see* p. 139).

Hyoscine Hydrobromide, BP (Scopolamine)

History. The name 'scopolamine' is derived from *Scopolia carniolica*, the plant from which it was first isolated and named after Johannes Antonius Scopoli (1723–1788), a physician from Carniola, a province in Slovenia.[148]

The laevo-rotatory alkaloid is employed. Derived from *Hyoscyamus niger* (henbane). Isolated in 1873.[149] Used, together with morphine, before anaesthesia in 1900 by Schneiderlinn.[150] It is a better drying agent than atropine. Was used to produce amnesia in labour (twilight sleep).[151] Crosses the blood–brain barrier, as a tertiary amine.

Actions similar to atropine. Chief difference is that hyoscine is a depressant of the central nervous system, causing drowsiness, sleep, and amnesia in some patients. Occasionally it produces restlessness and excitement which can be relieved by physostigmine, especially in old patients and those with unrelieved pain. It decreases the intensity and duration of analgesia produced by opiates, pethidine and methadone. It should not be the sole premedicant before methohexitone as it fails to prevent muscular movements.

It is a mild respiratory stimulant, while its action on the iris, the salivary, sweat and bronchial glands is stronger than that of atropine. Has a beneficial effect on motion sickness. Tachycardia may occur, as after atropine. After a dose of hyoscine sufficient to cause tachycardia, a secondary bradycardia may develop and last up to 3 h. Action on heart, intestine and bronchioles is weaker than that of atropine.

Adult dose, 0·3–0·6 mg. For paediatric dosage, *see* Chapter 28.

Combination of hyoscine 0·4 mg with pethidine 100 mg or papaveretum 20 mg forms a useful sedative before operation in fit patients: in the handicapped, dose should be reduced.

Hyoscine Butylbromide (Buscopan)

A useful drying agent given i.v. immediately before induction of anaesthesia. It increases heart rate and reduces secretions, but its action is rather short. Like propanthelene bromide, it inhibits peristalsis during gastroscopy. Can be absorbed from skin, e.g. posterior to the pinna.[152] Dose 10–20 mg.

Glycopyrronium Bromide(Robinul, glycopyrrolate)

Synthesized by Franko and Lunsford[153] and first used in anaesthesia by Boawright C. F., Newell R. C. et al.[154] A quaternary ammonium compound with anticholinergic properties. It does not readily cross the placental or blood–brain[155] barriers, and does not cause central anticholinergic effects. It has been suggested as an alternative to atropine[156] but is considerably more expensive. Like atropine and hyoscine it reduces the tone of the lower oesophageal sphincter and so may contribute to regurgitation of gastric contents[157] (the opposite effect to metoclopramide).[158] It suppresses gastric secretion better than atropine or hyoscine, but results in less tachycardia and dysrhythmia. It efficiently dries up salivary secretions being five times more potent than atropine and longer lasting.[159] For ECT with methohexitone, atropine and glycopyrronium are identical in drying secretions, but the latter drug does not cause tachycardia.[160] Both drugs are satisfactory when used prior to suxamethonium in preventing bradycardia. Dose: Premedication i.m. (adult) 0·2–0·4 mg; (child) 10 µg/kg. Intravenous use to protect against bradycardia (adult) 0·2 mg or 4–5 µg/kg, (child) 5–10 µg/kg. The full dose of 0·9 mg does not cause significant changes in heart rate.[161] In clinical doses it does not affect the pupil size.[162] Not anti-emetic.

(*See* Mirakhur R. K. *Br. J. Anaesth.* 1979, **51**, 671; Mirakhur R. K. and Dundee J. W. *Anaesthesia*, 1983, **38**, 1195.)

Advantages and Disadvantages of Atropine and Hyoscine in Premedication
Advantages

1. Inhibit secretion which might interfere with airway or be aspirated into chest. An intramuscular injection of 0·5 mg reaches its maximum effect in 30–45 min and lasts 2–3 h. The same dose intravenously acts in 1 min and lasts about 30 min.

2. Hyoscine produces sedation and amnesia.

3. Atropine depresses vagal nerve endings in the heart and is useful when agents are employed which stimulate these, e.g. halothane, causing bradycardia.

4. They reduce the bradycardia and salivation caused by suxamethonium.

5. They reduce the postoperative nausea and vomiting caused by opioids.

Both atropine and hyoscine (dose 2 mg and 1 mg respectively) can be given by mouth to prevent salivation.[163] To avoid the double unpleasantness of an injection and a dry mouth, atropine can often be given intravenously just before induction of anaesthesia.

Disadvantages

1. Interfere with pupil reactions.

2. May cause thick tenacious mucus formation, which is removed from the bronchial tree only with difficulty.

3. May produce tachycardia.

4. May inhibit sweating and so cause pyrexia.

5. Hyoscine may cause restlessness, especially in the aged.

6. Atropine may cause hypoxaemia by increasing the pulmonary dead space.[164]

7. May cause unpleasant drying of the mouth.

In a large series of patients anaesthetized without anticholinergic premedication, only 2% developed 'troublesome' secretions.[165] It may be undesirable in patients with thyrotoxicosis, children with pyrexia and when induced hypotension is to be used.

The Central Anticholinergic Syndrome

Patients, especially elderly ones, may, after treatment with anticholinergic drugs, show excitement, drowsiness or even coma. They may also suffer from thought impairment, disturbances of recent memory, hallucinations, ataxia or behavioural abnormalities. Physostigmine salicylate, an anticholinergic drug with a tertiary amine, allowing it to cross the blood–brain barrier (neostigmine has a quaternary amine which prevents this), has been recommended as treatment.[166] Dose: 2 mg i.v. given cautiously, and repeated if necessary. The drug has also been used in the treatment of depressant effects on the central nervous system of ketamine,[167] tricyclics, phenothiazines, droperidol and even halothane.[168] In clinical doses it does not adequately reverse neuromuscular block,[169] while its cholinergic effects are minimal.

Rectal–basal Narcosis

Basal narcosis is deep premedication increased to the stage of unconsciousness.
History. Nicolai Ivanovitch Pirogoff (1810–1881) of St Petersburg, and Marc Deputy of Paris[170] gave ether into the rectum in 1847,[171] Oscar Wanscher (1874–1906) of Copenhagen revived it in 1882, and Daniel Mollière (1848–1890) of Lyons used it again in 1884. Reports by J. H. Cunningham (1877–1960) and Frank Lahey (1880–1953) of Boston followed in 1905. J. T. Gwathmey (1863–1944) of New York City introduced rectal oil-ether in 1913.[172]

Butzengeiger and Fritz Eicholtz (1888–1968) (head of pharmacological section of Bayer Products at Wuppertal-Elberfeld) used Avertin in 1927.[173] Edgar Stanley Rowbotham of London (1890–1979) used paraldehyde in oil in 1928.[174] Joseph Blomfield (d. 1948) and Sir Francis Shipway (1875–1968)[175] used Avertin in England in 1928.[176] (*See also* Edwards G. *Proc. R. Soc. Med.* 1945, **39**, 71.) Rectal use of thiopentone was first described in 1939,[177] methohexitone in 1963[178] and diazepam in 1981.

Bromethol, BP (Avertin, Tribromethanol)
This is tribromethyl alcohol, CBr_3CH_2OH. It was synthesized by Willstaetter and Duisberg in 1923 and is occasionally used for basal narcosis.

Presentation
Sold dissolved in amylene hydrate so that 1 ml of the solution contains 1 g of bromethol. The solution may decompose if exposed to light and heat above 70 °C or if left to stand when dissolved in water.

Dosage and Administration
The dosage is 80–120 mg/kg body weight. Children tolerate it well and need full doses.

It is given in 2·5% solution in distilled water.

The patient falls asleep in 10–15 min without any stage of excitement. Constant supervision by a skilled person is required to prevent respiratory obstruction consequent to the muscular atony.

Advantages
A pleasant method of losing consciousness.

Disadvantages
Expert nursing required, before and after operation.

Uses
Rarely used today.

1. Thyrotoxicosis. Was, in former times, used as premedication before thyroidectomy.

2. Has been used prior to ophthalmic operations, because intra-ocular tension is decreased and the conjunctival vessels are constricted.

3. In eclampsia.

Has also been used in the treatment of tetanus, strychnine poisoning and the delirium of acute alcoholism.

Paraldehyde (CH₃CHO)₃

Paraldehyde was discovered by Weidenbusch in 1829. It was introduced as a sedative into medicine by the Italian physician Vincenzo Cervello (1854–1918) of Palermo in 1882.[179]

Edgar Stanley Rowbotham (1890–1979) in London was the first, in 1928, to use paraldehyde in oil per rectum to produce basal narcosis.[180] Harold Sington used it for children in the following year,[181] while in 1932 Rosenfield and Davidoff gave it per rectum to obstetrical patients; seldom used today.

Thiopentone, BP[182] (Pentothal, Intraval)
See Chapter 13.

In a rectal dose of 22 mg/kg it gives good results and causes no significant respiratory or cardiovascular depression.[183]

Methohexitone
It has been given into the rectum with good results. Dosage 15 mg/kg.[178]

Diazepam
Can be used (0·4–0·5 mg/kg) in a small amount of solution per rectum as premedication in children.[184]

Rectal Ketamine
Has been used in children for premedication. Dose 4–10 mg/kg in 1–5% solution,[185] usefully combined with diazepam 0·4 mg/kg and for children undergoing multiple sessions of radiotherapy.[186]

For fuller information about basal narcosis, *see* earlier editions of this *Synopsis*.

References

1. The study of the effects of changes in the chemical environment of living material: from the Greek, 'pharmacos', a harmful item to be cast out, and 'logos', the word. The study of pharmacokinetics (first use of the word in 1953) is the study of drug distribution and elimination, or more accurately, a study of the mathematical and quantitative analysis of drug and drug metabolite levels in the body. Pharmacodynamics is the study of the relationship between the amount of drug at the site of action and the observed pharmacological response.
2. McMechan F. H. *Am. J. Surg.* 1920, Quarterly suppl. 34, 123.
3. *Lancet* 1928, **2**, 1252.
4. Bellamy Gardner H. *Br. Med. J.* 1910, **2**, 766.
5. Buxton W. D. *Proc. R. Soc. Med.* 1908–1909, **2**, 60.
6. Collins C. U. *JAMA* 1911, 26 March.
7. Gwathmey J. T. *Anesthesia*. New York and London: D. Appleton & Co., 1914, p. 847.

8. Quoted by Dogliotti A. M. *Anesthesia*. Chicago: S. B. Debour, 1939, p. 20.
9. von Nussbaum J. N. *Med. Times, Lond.* 1865, **1**, 259.
10. Bernard C. *Bull. Gen. de Thérap*, 1868, **77**, 241; Annotation, *Lancet* 1969, **2**, 789; Lee J. A. *Anaesthesia* 1978, **33**, 733.
11. Guibert C. R. *Acad. Sci. Paris* 1872, **74**, 815.
12. Labbé C. and Goujon E. *C. R. Acad. Sci. Paris* 1870, **74**, 815.
13. *Med. Times Lond.* 1872, **1**, 359.
14. Aubert P. *C. R. Soc. Biol. Paris* 1883, **5**, 242.
15. Horsley V. *Br. Med. J.* 1886, **2**, 670.
16. Bell B. *Edin. Med. J.* 1858–1859, n.s. **4**, 1.
17. Harley J. *Br. Med. J.* 1874, **2**, 518.
18. Lannelongue, *Bull Soc. Chir. Paris* 1874, **3**, 619.
19. Trease G. E. *Pharmacy in History*. London: Baillière, 1964.
20. Heidenhain R. H. P. *Arch. Ges. Physiol*, 1872, **5**, 309.
21. Sigmond G. G. *Lancet* 1836, **2**, 392.
22. Dastre J. A. F. *C. R. Acad. Sci. Paris* 1878, **86**, 1303.
23. Schafer E. A. *Br. Med. J.* 1880, **2**, 620, 715.
24. *Med. Times. Lond.* 1861, **2**, 121.
25. Embley E. H. *Br. Med. J.* 1902, **1**, 817.
26. Buxton D. W. *Proc. R. Soc. Med.* 1911, **4**, 53; Ebstein E. *Practitioner* 1873, **11**, 461.
27. Buxton D. W. *Proc. R. Soc. Med.* 1908/9, **2** (Sect. Anaesth.), 60.
28. Schneiderlin C. H. *Münch. Med. Wochenschr.* 1903, **1**, 137.
29. Leipoldt C. L. *Lancet* 1911, **1**, 368; Kerri Szanto M. *Can. Anaesth. Soc. J.* 1974, **23**, 239.
30. Schaumann O. and Eisleb O. *Dtsch. Med. Wochenschr.* 1939, **65**, 967.
31. Schlungbaum H. *Med. Klin.* 1939, **35**, 1259.
32. Rovenstine E. A. and Battermann R. I. *Anesthesiology* 1943, **4**, 126.
33. Hunter C. *Br. Med. J.* 1859, 19.
34. Lafargue G. V. *C. R. Acad. Sci. Paris* 1836, **2**, 397.
35. Dundee J. W., Loan W. B. and Morrison J. D. *Br. J. Anaesth.* 1970, **42**, 54.
36. Pandit S. K., Dundee J. W. and Keilty S. R. *Anaesthesia* 1971, **26**, 421.
37. Angell J. C. *The Acute Abdomen for the Man on the Spot*, 3rd ed. Tunbridge Wells, Pitman, 1978.
38. Carnie J. and Johnson R. A. *Anaesthesia* 1985, **40**, 1114.
39. Loan W. B. and Dundee J. W. *Practitioner* 1967, **198**, 759.
40. Cartwright P. D. *Ann. R. Coll. Surg.* 1985, **67**, 13.
41. Bion J. F. *Anaesthesia* 1984, **39**, 560.
42. Canto J. et al. *Acta Anaesthiol. Scand.* 1981, **25**, 25.
43. Keenan D. J. M., Cave K. et al. *Br. Med. J.* 1984, **288**, 240.
44. Rigamonti G., Zanella E. et al. *Br. J. Anaesth.* 1983, **55**, 513.
45. Mattila M. A. H., Ahlstrom-Bengs E. et al. *Br. Med. J.* 1983, **287**, 1026.
46. Hillier E. H. *Br. Med. J.* 1983, **287**, 701.
47. Bell M. D. D., Murray G. R. et al. *Lancet* 1985, **1**, 71.
48. See Editorial *Br. Med. J.* 1984, **288**, 259.
49. Korman B. and McKay R. J. *Anesth. Intensive Care* 1985, **13**, 395.
50. Chakravarty K. et al. *Br. Med. J.* 1979, **2**, 895.
51. White D. C. et al. *Br. Med. J.* 1979, **2**, 116.
52. Waldmann C. S., Eason J. R. et al. *Anaesthesia* 1984, **39**, 768.
53. Morgan R. J. M. *Anaesthesia* 1983, **38**, 492.
54. Nimmo W. S. and Todd J. G. *Br. J. Anaesth.* 1985, **57**, 250.
55. Edmonds-Seal J. et al. *J. R. Soc. Med.* 1980, **73**, 111.
56. Nunn J. F. and Slavin G. *Br. J. Anaesth.* 1980, **52**, 253.
57. Hashemi K. and Middleton M. D. *Ann. R. Coll. Surg.* 1983, **65**, 38.
58. Davenport H. T., Al-Khudairi D. et al. *Ann. R. Coll. Surg.* 1985, **67**, 379.
59. Cassuto J., Wallin G. et al. *Anesth. Analg. (Cleve.)* 1985, **64**, 971.
60. Goudie T. A., Allan M. W. B. et al. *Anaesthesia* 1985, **40**, 1086.
61. Baker S. B. C. et al. *Can. Anaesth. Soc. J.* 1980, **27**, 150.
62. Sertürner F. W. A. J. *Pharm. für Aertze und Apoth. Chem. Leipzig*, 1806, **14**, 47.
63. Alkaloid = like alkali, a term first used by K. F. W. Meissner (1792–1853) of Halle, Germany.
64. Gates M. and Tschudi G. *J. Am. Chem. Soc.* 1952, **74**, 1109.
65. Twycross R. G. *Br. Med. J.* 1975, **4**, 212.
66. Cheyne J. (1777–1836) *Dubl. Hosp. Rep.* 1818, **2**, 216 and Stokes Wm. (1804–1878) *The Diseases of the Heart and Aorta*. Dublin: Hodge & Smith, 1854.

67. Park G. R. *Anaesthesia* 1984, **39**, 645.
68. Bell M. D., Murray G. R. et al. *Lancet* 1985, **1**, 71.
69. Samuel I. D. et al. *Br. J. Anaesth.* 1977, **49**, 927.
70. McQuay H. and Moore A. *Lancet* 1984, **2**, 284.
71. Robiquet P. J. *Analls Chim. Phys.* 1832, **51**, 225.
72. Shanahan E. C., Marshall A. G. et al. *Anaesthesia* 1983, **38**, 40.
73. Seymour A. *Lancet* 1982, **1**, 1425.
74. Twycross R. G. *Br. Med. J.* 1975, **4**, 212.
75. Sahli H. *Ther. Mh. (Halbruch.)* 1909, **23**, 1.
76. Martindale in: *The Extra Pharmacopoeia* (Wade A. ed.), 1977, 27th ed. London: The Pharmaceutical Press, p. 976.
77. Merck G. F. *Ann. Phys. Chem. (Leipzig)*, 1848, **66**, 125.
78. Stambough J. E. et al. *Lancet* 1977, **1**, 398.
79. Mather L. E. et al. *Clin. Pharmacol. Ther.* 1975, **17**, 21.
80. Archer S. et al. *Science* 1962, **137**, 541.
81. Keats A. S. and Telford J. J. *J. Pharmacol. Exp. Ther.* 1964, **143**, 157.
82. Appleyard T. N. *Proc. R. Soc. Med.* 1975, **68**, 770.
83. Moore J. et al. *Br. J. Anaesth.* 1973, **45** (Suppl.), 798.
84. Rifit K. *Br. J. Anaesth.* 1972, **44**, 175.
85. Jago R. H. et al. *Anaesthesia* 1977, **32**, 904.
86. Sandoval R. G. and Wang R. H. *N. Engl. Med. J.* 1969, **280**, 1391.
87. Morrison J. D. et al. *Br. Med. J.* 1971, **2**, 287; Dundee J. W., Brown S. S. and McDowell S. A. *Anaesthesia* 1969, **24**, 52.
88. Janssen P. A. J. *J. Pharm. Pharmac.* 1961, **13**, 513; Saarne A. *Acta Anaesthesiol. Scand.* 1969, **13**, 11; Kay B. *Br. J. Anaesth.* 1971, **43**, 1167; Tunstall M. E. and Ogg T. W. *Anaesthesia* 1974, **29**, 728.
89. Dobkin A. B. et al. *Can. Anaesth. Soc. J.* 1976, **23**, 596.
90. Davie I. T. and Slawson K. B. *Br. J. Anaesth.* 1976, **48**, 913.
91. Lewis J. W. et al. *J. Med. Chem.* 1973, **16**, 12; Dobkin A. B. *Can. Anaesth. Soc. J.* 1977, **24**, 186; Dobkin A. B. et al. *Can. Anaesth. Soc. J.* 1977, **24**, 195; Downing J. W. et al. *Br. J. Anaesth.* 1977, **49**, 251; Hovell B. C. *Br. J. Anaesth.* 1977, **49**, 913.
92. Kay B. *Br. J. Anaesth.* 1978, **50**, 605.
93. McQuay H. J. et al. *Br. J. Anaesth.* 1980, **52**, 1013.
94. Murray K. *Br. Med. J.* 1983, **286**, 761.
95. Finlay I. G. et al. *Br. Med. J.* 1982, **284**, 1830.
96. Edge W. E. et al. *Anaesthesia* 1979, **34**, 463.
97. Kay B. *Br. J. Anaesth.* 1980, **52**, 453.
98. Budd K. *Anaesthesia* 1981, **36**, 900.
99. Shah M., Rosen M. et al. *Br. J. Anaesth.* 1984, **56**, 1235.
100. Singer G. E. *Health Trends* 1979, **11**, 32; Editorial *Anaesthesia*, 1980, **35**, 153.
101. Pohl J. *Z. Exp. Path Ther.* 1915, **17**, 370.
102. Blumberg H. and Drayton H. D. *Naloxone and Related Compounds* (Kosterlitz H. W. et al. ed.). London: Macmillan, 1972.
103. Jeffcote W. C. et al. *Lancet* 1979, **2**, 688.
104. Jones R. D. M. and Jones J. A. *Br. Med. J.* 1980, **2**, 646.
105. Peters W. P. et al. *Lancet* 1981, **1**, 529; Annotation, *Lancet* 1981, **1**, 538.
106. Taff R. H. *Anesthesiology* 1983, **59**, 576.
107. Dhamce M. S. and Ghandi S. K. *Anaesthesia* 1982, **37**, 342.
108. Schneider O. and Hellerbach J. *Helv. Chem. Acta* 1950, **33**, 1437.
109. Fromherz K. and Pellmond B. *Experientia* 1952, **8**, 394.
110. Foldes F. F. *Am. J. Med. Sci.* 1957, **233**, 1.
111. Assaf R. A. E., Dundee J. W. and Gamble J. A. S. *Anaesthesia* 1975, **30**, 152.
112. Stevenson I. H. et al. *Br. Med. J.* 1972, **4**, 322.
113. Castleden C. M. et al. *Br. Med. J.* 1977, **1**, 10.
114. Dundee J. W. et al. *Br. J. Anaesth.* 1977, **49**, 1047; Dundee J. W. et al. *Anaesthesia* 1978, **33**, 15.
115. Gale G. D., Galloon S. et al. *Br. J. Anaesth.* 1983, **55**, 761.
116. Russell W. J. *Anaesthesia* 1983, **38**, 1062.
117. Johnstone M. *Anaesthesia* 1976, **31**, 873.
118. Dundee J. W. and Lilburn J. K. *Anaesthesia* 1978, **33**, 312.
119. Wassenaar W. et al. *Br. J. Anaesth.* 1977, **49**, 605.
120. Male C. G. et al. *Br. J. Anaesth.* 1980, **52**, 429; Clarke R. S. J. *Br. J. Anaesth.* 1980, **52**, 437.
121. Beechey A. P. C. et al. *Anaesthesia* 1981, **36**, 10.

122. Clark G, Erwin D. et al. *Anaesthesia* 1982, **37**, 421; Greenwood B. K. and Beadshaw E. C. *Br. J. Anaesth*. 1983, **55**, 933.
123. Mcateer E. J., Dixon J. et al. *Anaesthesia* 1984, **39**, 1177; Whitwam J. G., Al-Khudari B. et al. *Br. J. Anaesth*. 1983, **55**, 77.
124. Kanto J. *Anaesthesia* 1982, **37**, 924.
125. Dundee J. W., Halliday N. J. et al. *Anaesthesia* 1985, **40**, 441.
126. Saarne A. *Acta Anaesth. Scand*. 1963, **7**, 21.
127. Fischer E. and von Mering J. F. *Ther. d. Gegenw*. 1903, **44**, 97.
128. Hauptmann, A. *Münch. Med. Wochenschr*. 1912, **59**, 1907.
129. Cervello V. *Arch. Ital. Biol*. 1884, **6**, 113.
130. Liebrich M. E. O. *Das Chloralhydrat, ein neues Hypnoticum und Anästheticum*. Berlin, Müller, 1869.
131. Clutton-Brock J. *Anaesthesia* 1960, **15**, 71; Dundee J. W. *Br. J. Anaesth*. 1960, **32**, 407.
132. Mirakhur R. K. *Br. J. Anaesth*. 1979, **51**, 671.
133. Pithra J. *Medical Times, Lond*. 1861, **2**, 121.
134. Mirakhur R. K. et al. *Anaesthesia* 1978, **33**, 133.
135. Smith D. S. et al. *Anesthesiology* 1979, **51**, 343.
136. Cozanitis D. A. *Anaesthesia* 1975, **34**, 236.
137. Lopez-Vidriero M. T. et al. *Thorax*. 1975, **30**, 543.
138. Laing G. S. and Redmond A. D. *J. R. Soc. Med*. 1982, **75**, 568.
139. Thomas E. T. *Anaesthesia* 1965, **20**, 340.
140. Mirakhur R. K. et al. *Anaesthesia* 1979, **34**, 453.
141. Brock-Utne J. G. et al. *Anaesthesia* 1976, **31**, 1186.
142. Kivalo I. and Saarikoski S. *Br. J. Anaesth*. 1977, **49**, 1017.
143. Gregory G. A. *Anesthesiology* 1975, **43**, 225.
144. Virtanen R., Kants J. et al. *Acta Anaesthesiol. Scand*. 1982, **26**, 297.
145. Sington H. *Proc. R. Soc. Med*. 1926, **19**, 1; Mirakhur R. K. *Br. J. Anaesth*. 1978, **50**, 591.
146. Miller J. J. et al. *J. Clin. Exp. Psychiat*. 1958, **19**, 312; McKenzie A. L. and Piggott J. F. G. *Br. J. Anaesth*. 1971, **43**, 1088.
147. Garde J. F. et al. *Anesth. Analg*. 1978, **57**, 572.
148. Soban D. *Progress in Anaesthesiology*. Amsterdam: Excerpta Medica Foundation, 1970, p. 193.
149. Ladenburg A. *Ann. Chem. Pharmac*. 1881, **206**, 274.
150. Schneiderlinn J. *Aertz. Mitt. a. Baden* 1900, **54**, 104.
151. Gauss C. J. *Arch. Gynaek*. 1906, **78**, 579.
152. Walt R. P. et al. *Br. Med. J*. 1982, **284**, 1736.
153. Franko B. V. and Lunsford C. D. *J. Med. Pharm. Chem*. 1960, **11**, 523.
154. Boawright C. F., Newell R. C. et al. *Am. Acad. Ophthal. Otolaryngol*. 1970, **74**, 1139.
155. Proakis A. G. and Harris G. B. *Anesthesiology* 1978, **48**, 339.
156. Ramamurthy S. et al. *Anesth. Analg*. 1971, **50**, 732; Mirakhur R. K. et al. *Br. J. Anaesth*. 1978, **33**, 906.
157. Brock-Utne J. G. et al. *Can. Anaesth. Soc. J*. 1978, **25**, 144.
158. Brock-Utne J. G. *Anaesthesia* 1976, **31**, 1186.
159. Mirakhur R. K. and Dundee J. W. *J. R. Soc. Med*. 1980, **73**, 727.
160. Greenan J., Dewer M. et al. *J. R. Soc. Med*. 1983, **76**, 309.
161. Salem M. G. and Ahearn R. S. *J. R. Soc. Med*. 1986, **79**, 19.
162. Cozanitis D. A. et al. *Anaesthesia* 1979, **34**, 236.
163. Mirakhur R. K. *Br. J. Anaesth*. 1978, **50**, 591.
164. Tomlin P. J., Conway C. M. and Payne J. P. *Lancet* 1964, **1**, 14.
165. Leighton K. M. and Sanders H. N. *Can. Anaesth. Soc. J*. 1976, **23**, 563.
166. Longo V. G. *Pharm. Rev*. 1966, **18**, 965; Rupreht J. and Dworack B. *Acta Anesth. Belge*. 1976, **27**, 45.
167. Greene L. T. *Anesth. Analg*. 1971, **50**, 222.
168. Hill G. E. et al. *Can. Anaesth. Soc. J*. 1977, **24**, 707.
169. Baraka A. *Br. J. Anaesth*. 1978, **50**, 1075.
170. Dupuy M. *C. R. Acad. Sci. Paris* April 1847; Mirakhur R. K. et al. *Anaesthesia* 1978, **33**, 133.
171. Pirogoff N. I. *C. R. Acad. Sci. Paris* 1847, **74**, 789; Secher O. *Anaesthesia* 1986, **41**, 829.
172. Gwathmey J. T. *Anesthesia*. London and New York: Appleton, 1914, p. 433.
173. Butzengeiger O. *Dtsch. Med. Wochenschr*. 1927, **53**, 712; Eicholtz F. *Dtsch. Med. Wochenschr*. 1927, **53**, 710 (translated in 'Classical File', *Surv. Anesthesiol*. 1979, **23**, 68).
174. Rowbotham E. S. *Proc. R. Soc. Med*. 1928, **22**, 653.
175. Shipway F. *Br. Med. J*. 1930, **7**, 114.
176. Blomfield J. and Shipway F. E. *Lancet* 1929, **2**, 546.

177. Weinstein M. L. *Curr. Res. Anesth. Analg.* 1939, **18**, 221.
178. Stetson J. B. *Br. J. Anaesth.* 1963, **35**, 811; Budd D. C., Dornette W. H. L. and Wright S. P. *Anesth. Analg. Curr. Res.* 1965, **44**, 222.
179. Cervello V. *Arch. per le Sci. méd.* 1882, **6**, 177.
180. Rowbotham E. S. *Proc. R. Soc. Med.* 1928, **22**, 653.
181. Sington H. *Proc. R. Soc. Med.* 1929, **22**, 1197.
182. Weinstein M. L. *Curr. Res. Anesth. Analg.* 1939, **18**, 221.
183. Magure H. T. et al. *Can. Anesth. Soc. J.* 1979, **26**, 29.
184. Mattila M. A. K., Ruoppl M. K. et al. *Br. J. Anaesth.* 1981, **53**, 1269.
185. Saint-Maurice C. et al. *Br. J. Anaesth.* 1979, **51**, 573.
186. Stevens R. W. and Hain W. R. *Anaesthesia* 1982, **37**, 1089.
187. Spence A. A. and Smith G. *Anaesthesia* 1979, **34**, 320.

Chapter 9	ANAESTHETIC EQUIPMENT

Anaesthetic Machines

Apparatus for Administration of Inhalation Anaesthesia

For the origins of the plenum system of vaporization of volatile agents, *see* Boulton T. B. Classical File; *Surv. Anesthesiol.* 1985, **29**, 191. The Junker's Inhaler (Junker F. A. 1828–1901) *Med. Times & Gaz.* 1867, **2**, 590; and ibid, 1868, **1**, 171) using air blown over chloroform with a hand pump, was an early example. It was founded on B. W. Richarson's ether spray, used for the production of analgesia by the use of cold. Dates of introduction of some machines: Frederick Hewitt (1857–1916) of London, 1898; Charles Teter of Cleveland 1902; Elmer Isaac McKesson (1881–1935) of Toledo, physiologist, anaesthetist and manufacturer, 1910; Walter R. Boothby (1880–1953) of the Mayo Clinic, 1910; Frederick J. Cotton (1869–1938) of Boston, 1910; James Tayloe Gwathmey (1863–1944) of New York, 1914; Karl Connell (1873–1941) New York anaesthetist, 1911; Richard von Forregger (1873–1960), New York manufacturer, 1914; Henry Edmund Gaskin Boyle (1875–1941) London anaesthetist, 1917. The majority work on the 'plenum system', the incoming gases and vapours being at a higher pressure than atmospheric. A few are arranged on the 'draw-over' system in which the patient's inspirations pick up anaesthetic vapour.

Plenum Machines

The Boyle machine.[1] Gases are delivered from the cylinders or pipelines, each via a reducing valve which reduces the pressure to the flow-meters where flow is controlled by a needle valve. Two or more vaporizers are usually provided and increasing amounts of the gases can be diverted through them. Gases then pass into a Magill attachment (Mapleson-A) or alternative system.

The original Boyle machine of 1917 was an adaptation of the American Gwathmey apparatus.[2] It was built by the firm, Coxeters, under the personal direction of Lord George Wellesley (a great grandson of the first Duke of Wellington). In its original form it housed two nitrous oxide and two oxygen cylinders in a wooden box and used a water-sight flow-meter and an ether vaporizer. It had a pressure gauge on the oxygen cylinders, fine-adjustment reducing valves and a spirit flame to warm these and prevent obstruction of gas flow from freezing of water vapour, an impurity in early gas supplies. A Cattlin bag, a three-way stopcock and a face-mask completed the apparatus. A portable form was designed for use with the British Army in France. Subsequent modifications were:

1920. Addition of vaporizing bottle to flow-meters.
1926. Addition of second vaporizing bottle and bypass controls.
1927. Addition of third water-sight feed tube for carbon dioxide.
1930. Addition of plunger device.
1933. Dry bobbin type of flow-meter displaced water-sight feed.
1937. Rotameters displaced dry bobbin flow-meters.

The modern Boyle's apparatus bears little resemblance to the original model. For a description of the modern machine *see* Ward C. S. *Anaesthetic Equipment*, 2nd ed. London: Baillière, 1985; Henville J. D. Recent developments in anaesthetic machines and ventilators, in *Anaesthetic Review—1* (Kaufman L. ed.) London: Churchill Livingstone, 1982.

Cylinders
The pressure inside a full nitrous oxide cylinder is $50\,kPa \times 100$ ($750\,lb/in^2$), and the gas is liquefied. Full oxygen cylinders contain the compressed gas at $120\,kPa \times 100$ ($139 \cdot 20\,kg/cm^2$; $1950\,lb/in^2$). Cylinders are made of molybdenum steel. They are checked at intervals by the manufacturer for defects by subjecting them to tests: (1) *Tensile test*: this is carried out on at least 1 out of every 100 cylinders manufactured. Strips are cut and stretched—the 'yield point' should not be less than 15 tons/in²; (2) *Flattening, impact* and *bend tests*, also carried out on at least 1 out of every 100 cylinders made; (3) *Hydraulic* or *pressure test*: usually a water-jacket test. The filling ratio of a cylinder is the ratio of weight of gas in the cylinder to weight of water the cylinder could hold. Nitrous oxide cylinders are filled to a filling ratio of $0 \cdot 75$. Great care is taken that the gas is free from water vapour, otherwise when the cylinder is opened, temperature falls and water vapour would freeze and block the exit valve. Cylinder outlet valves use the pin-index system so arranged that it is impossible to connect cylinders to wrong yokes or flow-meters.

Piped Gas Supplies[3]
In large hopsitals oxygen, nitrous oxide, Entonox (oxygen and nitrous oxide mixture in equal volumes) compressed air and vacuum may be supplied by pipe-lines. Banks of supply cylinders may be housed in a well-ventilated room constructed of fireproof material, and provision is made for automatic switching to the reserve bank when the running bank is near exhaustion. A system of warning lights is incorporated to indicate the need for replenishment of the used bank.

Liquid Oxygen Supply[4]
This is the most economical method for supplying oxygen to large installations. It is stored in a thermally insulated vessel at a pressure of about $1200\,kPa$ and at a temperature lower than the critical temperature which is $-119\,°C$. Evaporation requires heat. Fresh supplies of liquid oxygen are pumped from a tanker into a storage vessel which rests on a weighing balance so that a dial measures the mass of liquid. Reserve banks of oxygen cylinders are kept in case of failure of supply. Liquid oxygen plants are housed away from main buildings because of the fire hazard.

Accidents have occurred due to the wrong connection of pipe-lines to anaesthetic apparatus. It is now recommended that the union between hoses and the anaesthetic machine should be permanent.[5] Hoses are colour coded and when repairs are necessary a complete hose assembly should be provided. Accidents are likely to occur when unauthorized repairs are carried out. A 'permit to work' system[6] requires in the UK a certificate in six parts to be signed as appropriate and is used when the action of one group of workers could directly or indirectly expose others to hazard. Three levels of hazard are identified: High, when work involves cutting an in-service pipe-line, with danger of cross-connection or pollution: Medium, work on a terminal unit where more than one gas is supplied, with danger of cross-connection; Low, where only one gas is involved.

Testing the Anaesthetic Apparatus[7]
A single hose test has been recommended as a result of a Committee of Enquiry appointed by the Kensington and Chelsea and Westminster Area Health Authority (1977) following an accidental cross-connection. The tests have been criticized and the following procedure has been recommended.

At the start the apparatus is disconnected from all piped medical gases and the oxygen and nitrous oxide cylinders turned off.

1. Check that full cylinders are properly attached to their yokes and all turned off.

2. Open the O_2 and N_2O flow-meter valves 2–3 full turns and ensure all others closed. No flow occurs.

3. Turn on O_2 cylinder. Check O_2 gauge for adequate content. O_2 flow-meter should register a flow—adjust to test flow 4 litres/min. *If any N_2O flow registers, reject machine.*

4. Turn on N_2O cylinder and check that N_2O meter registers a flow. *If O_2 flow changes, reject machine.*

5. Set the O_2 failure device in operation if not automatic.

6. Turn off O_2 cylinder. Check that O_2 bobbin falls completely to bottom of tube. Check that O_2 failure device works. *If O_2 flow-meter registers any flow when N_2O only turned on, reject machine.*

7. Insert O_2 pipe-line probe into supply connection. This cancels operation of O_2 failure alarm. Apply tug test. Check the O_2 flow-meter. Set at 4 litres/min.

8. Turn off N_2O cylinder. *If O_2 bobbin demonstrates any fall when N_2O turned off, reject machine.*

9. Insert N_2O probe into pipe-line connection. Apply tug test. *If any change in position of O_2 bobbin, reject machine.*

10. Complete check by occluding machine outlet and ensure that pressure relief valve on back bar is operative (where fitted).

The whistle discriminator[8] enables the nature of a gas issuing from a pipeline to be determined. With nitrous oxide the note falls one and a half tones from the oxygen note.[9]

Reducing Valves
Reducing valves were first used in association with the oxygen–hydrogen blow lamp in 1816 and the 'lime-light' of 1826. These allow delicate control of gas flows. Without them constant adjustments are necessary to maintain constant flows, due to temperature and pressure falls within the cylinder. The classic

reducing valve is the Adams valve (named after an employee of Messrs Coxeter, the manufacturers) which reduces to 40–75 kPa but which has been superseded by the Medishield S.60M. A toggle mechanism occludes the orifice when pressure rises. The Medishield S valve reduces to 810 kPa and the M valve to 405 kPa. The McKesson valve to 465 kPa. In the US regulating valves vary from these values.

Flow Restrictors
Pipe-line gas supplies at 405 kPa are commonly transferred to the flow-meters without interposition of a reducing valve. Sudden pressure surges are prevented by the use of a flow restrictor which is a constriction in the low-pressure circuit upstream to the flow-meter. The fine-adjustment control would require recalibration if the pipe-line pressure changed markedly. Flow restrictors are also used downstream of vaporizers to prevent back-pressure effects.

Flow-meters
Theory
Flow rate through a tube is proportional to the square root of the pressure difference. With a given pressure difference across an orifice, flow rate of gas is proportional to the square of the diameter of the orifice. Flow rate along a tube depends on the viscosity of a gas. Flow rate through an orifice depends on density and varies as the reciprocal of the square root of the density.

Types of Flow-meter
These may be divided into variable orifice and fixed orifice types.
Variable-orifice Meters (or fixed-pressure difference):
 1. *The rotameter*. The type used today in most modern machines. This is an accurate meter with an error of ±2%. As a gas-measuring device it was patented in Germany in 1908 by Karl Küppers of Aachen, and used in anaesthesia by Maximilian Neu,[10] an obstetrician gynaecologist of Heidelburg, in 1910; Magill suggested its use independently in 1932 and used it a few years later. R. Salt developed it further in 1937. Gas is led to the base of a finely wrought glass tube, slightly smaller on cross-section at bottom than at top. A light metal float rides the gas jet and notches in its edge cause it to rotate. Height of top of float gives rate of flow, the gas escaping between the rim of the metal float and the walls of the glass tube. The glass tubes must be vertical. The calibrating of the glass tubes must take into effect both the density and the viscosity of the gases passing through them. Viscosity is important at low flows as gas flow round the float approximates to tubular flow (diameter of orifice less than length), but density is important at high flows (diameter of orifice greater than length). Consequently a rotameter calibrated for carbon dioxide will not read true for cyclopropane, because although their densities are similar (44:42) their viscosities are different (1:0·6). The rotameter turned full on gives a higher flow of oxygen than the emergency button.[11]
 2. *The Heidbrink meter*. A black inverted float is free to rise within a metal tube with a varying taper. The upper end projects into a glass tube. It is accurate for low flows and also accommodates high flows.
 3. *Connell meter*. A pair of stainless-steel balls move within a tapered glass tube on an inclined plane.
Fixed-orifice Meters (or variable-pressure difference). Pressure differentials across an orifice vary with changes in flow. Pressure varies as the square of flow rate.

1. *Pressure gauge meter*. The pressure build-up proximal to the constriction is measured utilizing a Bourdon pressure gauge which is then calibrated for flow.

2. *Water depression meter*. Pressure on two sides of the fixed orifice is measured by means of a water manometer.

Inaccuracies and Dangers[12]

1. Static electricity can cause as much as 35% inaccuracy. It can cause sticking of the bobbin, especially when low flows are used.

2. Damage to flow-meter tubes with consequent leak may result in delivery of a hypoxic mixture.[13] It would be safer to place the oxygen flow-meter last in the flow-meter bank except for the confusion that might arise in the transitional period. An ingenious solution is to transpose the position of bank and vaporizers. Gas flows from right to left, oxygen retains its familiar position within the rotameter bank, and the oxygen flow-meter is downstream in relation to the other flow-meters.

3. A defect in the top sealing washer of a rotameter can cause fatal deprivation of oxygen.[14]

4. The small bobbin of a cyclopropane or carbon dioxide flow-meter can become jammed at the top of the tube so that the anaesthetist is unaware that gas is flowing.

5. Some ventilators (e.g. Manley, Barnet) can exert a back pressure so that as much as 7% more gas flows than indicated.[15]

Effect of Barometric Pressure

Flow-meters are calibrated for use at sea level. They become inaccurate at high altitudes or in hyperbaric chambers.

Flow-meters also become inaccurate when a restriction at the outlet causes a pressure build-up. This may occur when some humidifiers, nebulizers, etc. are in use. Flow is then greater than indicated with variable-orifice-type flow-meters. In the fixed-orifice type a large flow may be indicated even when there is complete occlusion of the outlet. These inaccuracies can be corrected by placing the control valve distal to the orifice. In the pressure-compensated flow-meter, pressure in the flow-meter itself is the same as that in the supply line. The flow-meter is calibrated in terms of litres the gas will occupy after discharge to atmospheric pressure.

Vaporizers

Standard machines are supplied with vaporizing chambers for volatile liquids. Both variable bypass (tec-type) and measured-flow (kettle-type) vaporizers when fully turned off can leak anaesthetic vapours into the circuit.[16]

A wide variety of vaporizers is now available. In general they are designed for use with a particular agent (*see* Chapter 10) or in a particular situation (*see* Chapter 30).

In modern practice it is often thought desirable to administer known concentrations of vapour of volatile agents. In the simple vaporizers the concentration at any tap setting will vary according to ambient temperature, rate of evaporation and the degree of insulation to prevent heat-loss. Efforts can be made to overcome these factors.

1. Automatic variation of the port with temperature. The use of bimetallic bars or a thermosensitive capsule.

2. The use of an apparatus such as the 'copper kettle' to provide a saturated vapour which can be diluted to obtain the desired concentration.

3. To maintain the liquid at constant temperature. The use of a waterbath helps to prevent heat loss.

Oxygen Failure Warning Devices

The ideal warning device should: (1) Not depend on the pressure of any gas other than the oxygen itself; (2) An alarm system should not utilize battery or mains power; (3) The signal should be audible and of sufficient length, volume and character; (4) There should be a warning of impending failure, and a further warning that failure has occurred; (5) When it comes into operation; (*a*) other gases should cease to flow, (*b*) the breathing system should open to the atmosphere, (*c*) inspired oxygen concentration should be at least equal to that of air, and build-up of carbon dioxide should not occur; (6) It should be impossible to resume anaesthesia until the oxygen supply has been restored.

The 'Bosun' Visual Audible Warning Device emits a reed-type whistle and switches on a red light supplied by a dry battery, when oxygen pressure falls. The audible signal, however, fails unless the nitrous oxide pressure is present, and regular maintenance of battery and bulb is necessary. The apparatus is useful but not infallible.

Attention has been drawn to a danger when certain artificial ventilators (e.g. Manley) are used with the 'Bosun' device. To overcome this the whistle must be set to blow at 3 lb/in^2 instead of the usual 1·5 lb/in^2.

Modern devices approach the ideal requirements. A fail-safe device which can be fitted to the Boyle model M fulfils the desirable criteria and requires no servicing other than the usual maintenance every 3–6 months.

Pressure Relief Valves

Apparatus working with gases supplied at pipe-line pressure must be protected against possible damage should the outlet become obstructed. Flow restrictors (p. 148) are satisfactory only as a means of smoothing surges of pressure. Pressure relief valves may take the form of combined non-return and pressure relief valves and are usually fitted at the end of the back bar, downstream from the vaporizers. They are set to operate at about 30 kPa (305 cm H$_2$O).

Pressure Limiting Valves

These are desirable to prevent damage to the patients' airways. They should have a much lower opening pressure (e.g. 4 kPa) than when pressure relief valves are used to prevent apparatus damage. Such valves are not found on the majority of anaesthetic machines. They cannot be used in simple series with a pressure relief valve or they will never be activated. The rubber reservoir bag distends with pressure increase and seldom reaches pressures above 5 kPa[17] (though plastic disposable bags used in the USA can develop high pressures[18]). A pressure limiting reservoir bag used in conjunction with a pressure limiting valve has been described.[19]

Expiratory Valves

These are one-way, spring-loaded valves. They should have minimal resistance to expiration and during spontaneous breathing should always be fully opened, as their setting determines the mean pressure in the anaesthetic circuit and in the patient's respiratory tract. Their opening pressure must, however, be greater than the collapsing pressure of the reservoir bag or the bag will not act as a reservoir. The amount of carbon dioxide rebreathed depends more on the provision of a plentiful flow of gases to the patient than on the tension of the expiratory valve. Some workers remove the spring to reduce expiratory resistance to a miminum. Heidbrink-type expiratory valves should be sterilized by autoclaving as antiseptic solutions may produce corrosion, stickiness and consequent increased resistance to opening pressure.[20]

(*See also* Wright B. M. *Lancet* 1979, **1**, 854.)

Reservoir Bags

These are usually made of antistatic rubber and should be large enough to supply the patient's inspiratory volume. They also act as an excellent visual monitor of spontaneous respiration. (*See also above* 'Pressure Limiting Valves'.) In paediatric anaesthesia a smaller bag gives a better indication of tidal excursion.

(For assessment of expiratory valves and reservoir bags, *see* Mostafa S. M. and Hall I. D. *Anaesthesia* 1985, **40**, 55.)

Face Masks

These should be of simple construction, easy to clean and sterilize, hard wearing, anti-static and cheap. They should provide a good fit with the patient's face and add minimal dead space. Tests show that the increased dead space of a face mask may be considerable (78–198 ml) and this may equal or exceed the anatomical dead space of an average adult. In children and infants it is possible for the mask and attachments to double or treble the dead space. The face mask connectors also add to the dead space (Ruben valve: 9 ml; angle connection and expiratory valve: 28–30 ml).[21] A disposable face mask is available. An airtight seal between a face mask and the edentulous patient can often be improved by retention of dentures.

Intermittent-flow Apparatus

Mainly used in the dental surgery but now being superseded by continuous flow systems. The pressure setting will provide continuous flow (actual flow-rate not indicated), or flow during inspiration only. Provided there is an airtight fit between mask (or tube) and patient, the demand system operates to supply the patient's requirements. A reservoir bag, though provided, is not necessary.

The McKesson Machine. Designed and first manufactured in 1910 by Dr E. I. McKesson (1881–1935),[22] a pioneer anaesthetist of Toledo, Ohio, USA.[23] He classified the signs of anaesthesia with nitrous oxide and oxygen, and introduced the method of secondary saturation. His description of fractional rebreathing appeared in 1915.[24] The McKesson apparatus has separate controls for percentage of oxygen in the mixture with nitrous oxide, and for control of pressure.

The Walton machine (named after an employee of the manufacturing company). Has been made in five models. The first appeared in 1925, the Walton Mark V in 1958. The Walton V incoporates a safety device; should the oxygen cylinder empty, unobserved, the flow of nitrous oxide is cut off and the system opened to the atmosphere, activating a whistle as air is drawn in.

These machines are used in dentistry, often in association with the Goldman vaporizer. They must be regularly serviced. There is an increasing tendency to use continuous-flow machines in outpatient departments and the dental surgery.

Entonox Apparatus. The premixed gases are supplied from the cylinder via a two-stage valve. The first stage is a simple reducing valve which decreases pressure to about 1350 kPa (200 lb/in^2). The second incorporates a tilting valve which opens to the negative pressure of inspiration but is closed when the positive pressure of expiration pushes down a sensing diaphragm. Little inspiratory effort is needed to produce a high flow rate. Gas cannot flow when pressure in the cylinder falls below 1350 kPa (200 lb/in^2) so that a proportion of gas is wasted. This is a safety factor should separation of the premixed gases have occurred since residual gas is likely then to be rich in nitrous oxide. The apparatus is compact and portable, weighing 6·1 kg with a full 500-litre cylinder.

Premixed gases can also be used with a calibrated flow-meter and the Magill circuit.

Gas Delivery Systems

Semi-closed Methods

These methods may allow some degree of rebreathing and may or may not be used in conjunction with carbon dioxide absorption. If the Magill attachment (Mapleson System A) is used[25] effective carbon dioxide elimination requires spontaneous respiration, an expiratory valve of minimal resistance and a total gas flow greater than the alveolar ventilation (roughly 70% of the respiratory minute volume[26]) of the patient.[27] There is no rebreathing if the fresh gas supply is more than 5 litres/min. for a 70-kg patient.[28] Studies of the effect of fresh gas flows lower than alveolar ventilation indicate that with mild rebreathing the system acts as simple added dead space, but with gross rebreathing the entire system acts as a mixing device.[29] Variations in tidal volume can be significant. Mapleson has made a theoretical study of several variations of the Magill attachment. He classifies them as shown in *Fig. 9.1*.

System A is the most satisfactory with spontaneous respiration. A flow of about 5 litres/min is required (in young healthy patients) to flush carbon dioxide from the system. *In assisted or controlled respiration* the expiratory valve must be tightened. It opens only during the inspiratory phase, and all the expired gases are returned to the circuit. System D can be used for controlled respiration. Measurements of end-tidal carbon dioxide and minute volume support the view that the Magill system is efficient with regard to carbon dioxide disposal in both spontaneous[31] and controlled[32] ventilation with gas flows of 5–6 litres/min.[33]

The advancing cone front of laminar flow[34] may explain how some hypoventilating patients, breathing spontaneously under anaesthesia with small tidal volumes (e.g. 100 ml), may ventilate reasonably well. The gas in the centre of a tube may reach the end of the tube preferentially. This only occurs with laminar flow.

The closed-circuit apparatus can be used for the semi-closed technique, if excess gases are allowed to escape through an expiratory valve. High gas flows are not then necessary, since carbon dioxide is removed in the soda-lime canister provided that the patient's respiratory excursion is adequate. With controlled ventilation, however, the method may not be economical unless unidirectional valves are placed one in each limb of the Y connection to the patient, and the blow-off positioned immediately downstream from the valve in the expiratory limbs. Without these precautions fresh gases are likely to be blown off before

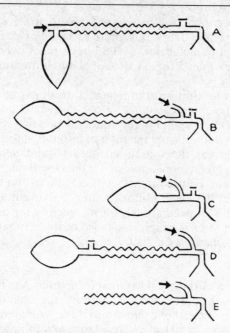

Fig. 9.1. The five semi-closed anaesthetic systems. (*By courtesy of William W. Mapleson and the 'British Journal of Anaesthesia'*)

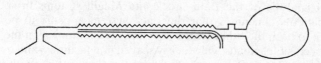

Fig. 9.2. The Bain System

reaching the patient. Care must, however, be taken that the valves are in phase with those of the circle absorber.

The Bain Co-axial System[35]

The principle was first used by R. R. Macintosh and E. A. Pask during the Second World War for experiments on the buoyant qualities of life-jackets (the Mae West) worn by unconscious subjects.[36] The system is a modification of the Mapleson D system in which the fresh gases enter the system by means of a narrow-bore inflow tube which lies within the lumen of the exhalation limb to terminate close to the patient end (*Fig. 9.2*). The system carries a single tube to the patient. It is light in weight and can be used in all age groups. It is adaptable to all types of anaesthetic procedures and can be used with spontaneous respiration and IPPV. It is useful for head and neck operations. The Penlon co-axial system is a modification in which the inner tube is made of anti-static material while the outer tube is transparent to facilitate inspection. The Penlon co-axial valve is used to fit the system to the outlet of the anaesthetic apparatus. Hazard can occur if the inner tube becomes broken or dislodged as considerable dead space may then occur.[37] Scavenging of expired gases is facilitated. With IPPV a fresh gas flow of 70 ml/kg (5 litres/min for a man of 70 kg) produces normocapnia, and

100 ml/kg mild hypocapnia.[38] Pa_{CO_2} is related to fresh gas flow in patients weighing more than 40 kg. Below this, more carbon dioxide is produced per unit of body weight and a minimal flow of 3·5 litre/min has been recommended for patients weighing less than 50 kg. A flow of about 3 litre/min is used with small children and infants.

With spontaneous respiration recommended fresh gas flow rates have varied from three times the minute volume[39] to between 90 and 160 ml/kg.[40] The differences probably depend on the respiratory depression caused by premedication, the depth of anaesthesia and the ratio of inspiration to expiration.[41] In view of the very wasteful gas flows required during spontaneous respiration, the Mapleson A system is then more appropriate than the Bain.[42]

The Bain system can be used in association with several types of mechanical ventilator[43] including the Cape Minor, Manley Servovent and Pulmovent, and Bird. Useful for IPPV in paediatrics. Not satisfactory for use with intermittent flow machines because of the high resistance of the inspiratory tube. (*See also* Baraka A. *Anaesth. Intensive Care* 1977, **5**, 172.)

The Lack System[44]
This is a modification of the Magill system (Mapleson A). The patient breathes through both tubes—the outer tube is inspiratory, the inner expiratory; the valve is situated near the anaesthetic apparatus. The commercial version has an inspiratory limb capacity of 500 ml and resistance to respiration is acceptable. The Lack system, unlike the Bain, does not readily permit the use of mechanical ventilators. It can be easily adapted for use with scavenging systems.

A careful analysis of the Bain, Lack and Magill systems in spontaneously breathing patients concludes that the Lack system appears to be superior in performance to both the other two. It is relatively economical in the use of fresh gas, has an accessible exhaust valve, easy scavenging facilities, and benefits in the provision of humidity.[45] Recommended fresh gas flows for use with spontaneous respiration were: Lack, 58, Mapleson A, 80, Bain, 173 ml/kg/min. These flows should be increased by about 10% for each degree Centigrade above 37 °C.[46]

The Hafnia Systems[47]
These are modifications of Mapleson A, B, C and D systems, using suction directly from the system to prevent atmospheric pollution. The expiratory valve is replaced by a suction port and an ejector flow-meter.

The Preferential Flow System (PFS)
With spontaneous respiration, the fresh gas flow is similar to that when a Magill system is used, but the resistance to expiration is less.[48]

The Burchett and Bennett Co-axial Breathing System[49]
This combines the benefits of the Mapleson A, D and E systems.

The Humphrey System
This combines the Mapleson A, D and E principles.[50]

Non-rebreathing Valves[51]
Advantages are: (1) No possibility of rebreathing provided the dead space of the valve itself is small; (2) Can be used for spontaneous or controlled respiration;

(3) Can be used to measure minute volume, if the flow-meters are accurate. *Disadvantages* are: (1) Wasteful; (2) Variations of minute volume during spontaneous respiration require frequent adjustment of the flow-meters to prevent collapse or distension of the reservoir bag; (3) Valves may stick; (4) Some valves are noisy.

Some *examples* of non-rebreathing valves:

1. The Ruben valve.[52] A bobbin moves against a spring to act as a unidirectional valve and an outlet valve prevents admission of atmospheric air. Dead space 9 ml. Low resistance. The resuscitation version has no outlet valve so that a patient breathing spontaneously will inhale air from the atmosphere.

2. The Ambu valves. The bobbin of the Ruben valve is replaced by one or two silicone rubber flaps. The valve can be dismantled easily for cleaning and sterilization. It is possible to reassemble the valve incorrectly with consequent risk of hypoxia. It can be used with a self-inflating bag. The valve with one flap is only suitable for IPPV. The valve with two rubber flaps is suitable for IPPV or spontaneous respiration. It has a very low dead space.

The ideal valve should have no forward leak, no back leak, low resistance, minimal dead space, minimal opening pressure without sticking, light weight, transparency, easy cleaning and sterilizing, reliability and durability, and a single expiratory port for collecting and measuring exhaled air.

The T-piece Technique[53] (Ayre) (Chapter 28)

Advocated primarily for use in infants and young children. In order to prevent dilution of inspired gases with air on the one hand, or rebreathing with carbon dioxide accumulation on the other hand, it is recommended that the total fresh gas flow should be about twice the minute volume of the patient, and the volume of the reservoir tube equal to about a third of the tidal volume.

For adults, the technique has been recommended in anaesthesia for neuro-surgery. A fresh gas inflow of 12–15 litres/min, with a reservoir tube of 150 ml will usually suffice. Gases can be scavenged.[54]

Variations of the T-piece technique to avoid expiratory resistance include the use of a Y-piece, the provision of a hole in the adaptor of the tracheal tube, lifting up the diaphragm of the expiratory valve with a safety-pin. The use of a reservoir bag on the open end for IPPV.[55]

The main advantage of the T-piece technique is the absence of resistance to expiration, a factor of crucial importance in small children.

Insufflation Techniques

Tracheal insufflation via a small catheter used by Elsberg of New York in 1910 and by Magill and C. Langton Hewer, of London[56] and later shown to be reasonably efficient in avoiding hypercapnia.[57] The development of inhalation tracheal anaesthesia with a wide-bore (Magill) tube for both inspiration and expiration supplanted this technique.

Pharyngeal insufflation of an anaesthetic mixture can be carried out using the Boyle–Davis gag, the mouth hook, the side-tube of a pharyngeal airway, or a catheter inserted down a pharyngeal airway. It is a useful method in children (e.g. in tonsillectomy or minor operations near the mouth) if tracheal intubation is not desired.

Tracheal insufflation with a high flow rate of oxygen is used to maintain oxygenation in the apnoeic patient. Oxygen reaches the alveoli by diffusion, but hypercapnia occurs (*see* Chapter 29).

Draw-over Methods
Ambient air drawn over a volatile agent by the patient's own inspirations was used by Morton in 1846, John Snow, Goodman Levy and P. J. Flagg. Stimulated by the needs of anaesthetists during the Second World War, Sir Robert Macintosh and his team in Oxford connected accurately-calibrated vaporizers to hand bellows so that such relatively simple apparatus could be used for IPPV with ether and air. It has been suggested that such methods should find a place in modern anaesthesia in all environments, using a volatile agent.[58]

Air, enriched if necessary by oxygen, is drawn over the surface of a volatile liquid or liquids. Inspiration of the patient is the motive force. Vaporization may be helped by the use of a gauze wick. Examples are the EMO Inhaler, Marrett's apparatus[59] and the inhalers designed for the self-administration of trichloroethylene and air. Draw-over inhalers can be used for IPPV if a suitable bellows is incorporated (*see* Chapter 30).

(*See also* the Ether-Pac and the Fluo-Pac draw-over vaporizers (Borland C. W., Herbert P. et al. *Anaesthesia* 1983, **38**, 852).)

Rebreathing with Carbon Dioxide Absorption

History
Introduced by John Snow in 1850,[60] used by Franz Kuhn (1866–1929), of Kassel, in 1906 in Germany.[61] A closed-circuit system for use by coal miners was described by Theodore Schwann (1810–1882), known for his nerve cells, and professor in the University of Liege, in 1877.[62] Revised by Dennis Jackson (1878–1930) of Cincinnati in 1915 for work on animals (after working on problems of ventilation in submarines, during the First World War);[63] used by Waters of Sioux City, Iowa, later of Madison, in 1920 in clinical anaesthesia, and the first reports appeared in 1924.[64] The circle or two-phase system was devised by Brian Sword (1889–1956) of North Carolina,[65] in 1926. W. B. Primrose (1892–1977), of Glasgow, used caustic soda solution as an absorber in 1931,[66] while Dräger patented an apparatus with a closed system in 1926. (*See also* Waters R. M. *Anesthesiology* 1943, **4**, 596; and Patterson R. W. in: *Anaesthesia; Essays on its History* (Rupreht J. and van Lieburg M. J., ed.) Berlin: Springer-Verlag, 1985 p. 74 and p. 167.)

The Closed System
Founded on principle that if sufficient oxygen is added to supply body's basal needs and carbon dioxide is absorbed, the same mixture of gases can be used repeatedly as it is exhaled unchanged. Basal oxygen varies between 200 and 400 ml/min, so that closed-system anaesthesia can only be used with a machine capable of delivering accurately measured small volumes of gases. The system may be completely closed as when cyclopropane is being used, or it may have a leak, which provides economy in gases and vapour, together with adequate removal of carbon dioxide from the system.

The vaporizer may be outside the breathing circuit (VOC) in the fresh gas supply line and the circuit may be to-and-fro or circle. The vaporizer may be inside the breathing circuit (VIC) when the patient's inspirations or expirations go through the vaporizer.[67]

The true closed system has no functioning expiratory valve, the fresh gas flow equalling oxygen consumption. Nitrogen will remain within the breathing system in significant amounts unless a period of high flow is used initially to aid its elimination. The new volatile agents are not easy to use in such a system unless special types of vaporizer are employed, the injection of calculated amounts of liquid being the easiest option.

Soda-lime

Used to absorb the carbon dioxide. A mixture of 90% calcium hydroxide with 5% sodium hydroxide and 1% potassium hydroxide, with silicates to prevent powdering. It is essential for effective absorption that moisture (14–19%) be incorporated within the granule. The hydroxides combine with carbon dioxide in the presence of water to form carbonates. Wilson soda-lime,[68] the type used in anaesthesia, is specially prepared; its granules are size 4–8 mesh to minimize resistance to breathing and to allow plenty of surface for absorption (4 mesh is 4 quarter-inch openings per inch; 8 mesh 8 eighth-inch openings per inch). Air space in the charged canister should equal the patient's tidal volume. Nearly half the volume in a properly packed canister consists of intergranular space. The chemical change involved in absorption results in heat production, the heat of neutralization. The end-products of the reaction are water and the carbonate of the respective metals. It can absorb about 20% of its own weight of CO_2. Storing soda-lime in its container does not interfere with its efficiency.

Durasorb is an improved soda-lime with a prolonged effective life which does not overheat. Its pink colour turns to white when it becomes inactive.

Baralyme (barium hydroxide lime, USP) is 80% calcium hydroxide with 20% barium octohydrate. It is said to be less caustic, and to produce less heat than soda-lime. No silica is necessary to produce hardness. It contains mimoza Z and ethyl violet as indicator; the pink granules change to purple when exhausted. Used in space craft.

The highest permissible concentration of carbon dioxide in an anaesthetic system is 0·2%. It is therefore most important to see that the soda-lime is fresh and that tidal exchange is adequate for efficient ventilation. There is a tendency for gases to flow so that more absorption takes place in the soda-lime in contact with the walls of the canister than in the middle. The canister must be tightly packed to prevent channelling.

Signs of exhaustion of soda-lime. (1) Rise in blood pressure followed eventually by a fall; (2) Rise in pulse rate; (3) Deepening of spontaneous respiration; (4) Increased oozing from wound and perhaps sweating; (5) Increase in the temperature of the canister.

Some brands change colour when exhausted, but this is not a reliable sign. The 1-lb canister will last about 6 h intermittently, 2 h continuously. In practice it is unwise to wait until the so-called signs of exhaustion of the soda-lime appear. Fresh absorbent should always be used if there is any doubt as to its efficiency.

Temperature during absorption. Nearly all from the heat of the chemical reaction of neutralization which is exothermic.

The temperature within the canister may reach 60 °C in that part of the canister where active absorption is occurring. Palpation of the canister jacket may yield little information about the temperature of the interior.

Advantages
(1) Economy in use of gases; (2) Less pollution of theatre atmosphere.

Disadvantages
(1) Tight fit of mask, tube, etc. to patient may cause trauma; (2) Alkaline dust may pass to patient; (3) Resistance to breathing and dead space are relatively high; (4) Increased carbon dioxide content of inspired gas, as absorption is far from perfect; (5) Dilution of gases in reservoir bag by nitrogen which in the early part of the administration may be removed from the system by emptying the bag on several occasions; (6) Volatile agents (e.g. halothane, isoflurane and enflurane) may be adsorbed to soda-lime initially, so that inspired concentration falls.

Apparatus
1. The Waters 'to-and-fro' single-phase system (*Fig. 9.3*).[69] Gases pass through the canister during both inspiration and expiration. Fresh gases are led to the patient close to the mask. Waters's canister was designed after much experimenting as to shape and size; it measures 12 cm long by 8 cm in diameter, and holds 1 lb of soda-lime. The air space between granules averages 400 ml. To obtain maximal efficiency, the tidal exchange should approximate the air space of the charged canister. If the tidal volume is greater than the air space the gases may pass through too rapidly for efficient absorption. If it is less than the air space, as when a large canister is used on a child, or when breathing is depressed, the soda-lime in the front of the canister becomes exhausted as the gases come into intimate contact with this part only and the result is an increase in dead space. In such circumstances a smaller canister should be used. It is heavy and rather awkward to use, but is cheap and and can easily be sterilized. Plastic models are available. Resistance to breathing 2–3 cm water. In the to-and-fro system the pressure in the face-piece varies from $+0.75$ cm H_2O to -0.75 cm H_2O.

2. The circle or two-phase system (Brian Sword).[70] An inspiratory and expiratory tube are used, with flap valves to ensure a one-way flow of gases;

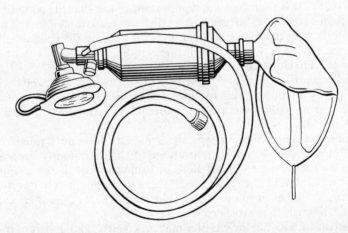

Fig. 9.3. The Waters 'to-and-fro' carbon dioxide absorber. (British Oxygen Company Ltd.)

breathing is thus divided into two phases and dead space is minimized. Efficiency is lost if the tidal volume is greater than the air space between granules. The soda-lime can be by-passed and the canister can be easily removed for recharging. For proper functioning there must be a valve between reservoir bag and patient on both inspiratory and expiratory limbs. Fresh gases must not enter between expiratory valve and patient. A pop-off valve must not be placed between patient and inspiratory valve.[71]

Circle and to-and-fro absorbers are equally efficient if properly designed, although resistance to respiration is nearly twice as great in the circle as in the Waters system because of the corrugated tubing. Adsorption of the vapour of volatile agents, e.g. halothane and enflurane, by rubber and soda-lime may reduce the economy of the system for expensive drugs.

Circle absorption and fresh gas flow.[72] At higher flows the system behaves like a semi-closed system and soda-lime is unnecessary. With basal flows, rebreathing is total and expired carbon dioxide is removed by soda-lime. With fresh gas flows between 1 and 4 litres/min the arrangement of the various components within the circle system assumes some importance. With spontaneous respiration the expiratory valve near the face-piece should be used; with controlled ventilation it should be located in the expiratory limb before the reservoir bag. When using halothane it has been shown that the flow-rate need not exceed 3 litres/min after the first 10 min in order to achieve inspired concentrations close to the delivered concentration.

The fresh gas flow-rates required for rebreathing systems has been studied using a mathematical model.[73] With a flow-rate of 7 litres/min, nitrogen elimination is complete in 5 min for practical purposes. With the flow reduced to 500 ml/min, the nitrogen concentration in the system is still 20% after 1 h. With an inflow of 500 ml/min Entonox F_{IO_2} falls to dangerously low levels, but at 1000 ml/min F_{IO_2} remains at about 40% (assuming an oxygen consumption of 225 ml/min).[74] A low flow regime of 1000 ml/min nitrous oxide and 600 ml/min oxygen will provide an F_{IO_2} between 35 and 25% over a range of oxygen consumption between 150 and 300 ml/min. Nitrous oxide uptake declines exponentially from 462 ml/min to 110 ml/min after 2 hours.

Some workers, using halothane and oxygen alone, have suggested that the presence of some nitrogen might act as a 'scaffold' to prevent peripheral lung collapse during quiet respiration.[75]

Mechanical Dead Space

Mechanical dead space is the addition to dead space which is produced by the anaesthetic apparatus.

Mechanical dead space in Waters's absorber is space between the face and the wire gauze of the canister. With a large mask, this may be 200 ml. Dead space may increase during use as the granules nearest to the patient become exhausted. A simple nylon pot-scourer should be inserted after the canister has been filled and shaken down as tightly as possible. Its presence ensures that the canister is packed tight, so that gases cannot pass around instead of through the soda-lime when the canister is in a horizontal position. Mechanical dead space in a circle absorber is space between face and beginning of double corrugated tubing.

Cope's modification of Waters's absorber is designed to minimize dead space when anaesthetizing children.

(*See also* Boulton T. B. *Anaesthesia* 1979, **34**, 605.)

Scavenging Systems[76]

Collection of effluent gases from anaesthetic systems requires the use of a collecting valve and the use of tubing to duct the waste to atmosphere. Scavenging systems may be classified as: (1) *Passive*. The total flow resistance should not exceed 50 kPa (0·5 cm H_2O) at 30 litres/min and copper pipes of 28–35 mm outer diameter are thought to be satisfactory. The discharge point should avoid wind pressures. A T-termination with a downward right-angle bend at each end is preferred, placed above a flat roof; (2) *Assisted passive*. The extract duct of a non-circulatory theatre ventilation system can be used instead of an exterior discharge point; (3) *Active scavenging*. The patient should be protected from negative pressures greater than 100 Pa (1 cm H_2O). There should be a reservoir which should take the form of an open T-piece or a reservoir bag in order to protect the patient from subatmospheric pressures. Piped suction[77] has been used and this may be combined with the use of activated charcoal[78] to remove anaesthetic vapours.

The Papworth block[79] has been recommended as a convenient link between the collecting and the scavenging system. It incorporates a safety valve opening at 500 Pa (5 cm H_2O) and a reservoir bag to absorb peak pressures. The latter also acts as a monitor of the system.

The Cardiff Aldasorber[80] contains activated charcoal which removes anaesthetic vapours but not nitrous oxide. Its duration of active use is gauged by the gain in weight due to adsorbed agent.

Portable Apparatus

1. Open Drop Administration

Introduced by Sir J. Y. Simpson for use with chloroform in 1847. He used a folded handkerchief. Today, the Schimmelbusch (1860–1895) (Berlin surgeon and pioneer of aseptic surgery) mask (*Fig. 9.4*) is employed,[81] which is a modification of Skinner's wire frame of 1862[82] (Liverpool general practitioner and obstetrician). The Esmarch mask (1884, J. F. A. v. Esmarch (1823–1908)), was popular in Europe. Plenty of air can be inhaled through the gap between the mask

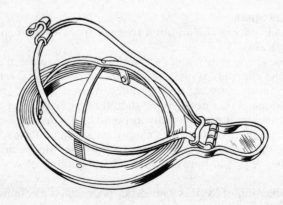

Fig. 9.4. Schimmelbusch mask.[83]

and the face. Useful for giving chloroform, ethyl chloride and diethyl ether. Used by Lawson Tait (1845–1899), of Birmingham, from 1873 onwards, it was employed by Prince of Chicago, for use with ether, in 1895. S. Griffith Davis, of Baltimore, further popularized the method in the early 1900s. H. Bellamy Gardner[84] of Charing Cross Hospital was a leading British exponent of the method.

2. The EMO Inhaler (Epstein–Macintosh–Oxford) (*Fig. 9.5*)[85]

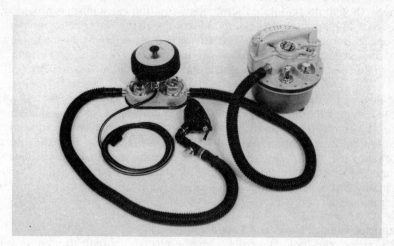

Fig. 9.5. EMO ether inhaler. (Penlon Ltd. Abingdon, Berkshire.)

Height 24 cm, diameter 23 cm, weight 6·5 kg when the water compartment is full. This has replaced the time-honoured and very useful Oxford Vaporizer[86] and, like it, was developed in the Nuffield Department of Anaesthetics in the University of Oxford. It will deliver a predetermined concentration of ether vapour in air, the accuracy of which is greatest at high concentrations and high tidal volumes.[87] It is only suitable for plenum use (continuous flow) if the carrier gas is greater than 10 l/min.[88] There is an automatic thermocompensator bellows mechanism. A water compartment of approximately 1200 ml volume acts as a heat buffer. It is usually employed as a 'draw-over' apparatus, but if combined with an Oxford Inflating Bellows,[89] can be used for IPPV. Rebreathing is prevented by the use of unidirectional valves. Hyperventilation can be employed to maintain satisfactory alveolar ventilation. The apparatus is useful in countries where nitrous oxide is not readily available or when portability is important. Ether and air can be used combined with a small dose of thiopentone or halothane for induction, and with a muscle relaxant and controlled respiration for major intra-abdominal or intrathoracic surgery. For light anaesthesia with spontaneous respiration the patient should breathe ether in concentrations gradually increasing to 15%, after which it may be reduced to about 7% for maintenance. During induction considerable falls in oxygen tension occur even though the respiratory minute volume is adequate, so that oxygen supplements and/or IPPV are necessary. For controlled respiration, induction with thiopentone and non-depolarizing muscle relaxant, intubation and controlled respiration with

12% ether in air reducing to 2–3% is very satisfactory. The ether concentration is reduced when the pupils no longer react to light, or should nodal rhythm (if ECG facilities are available) occur. Explosions have not been described during the administration of ether and air even when diathermy has been used.

3. The OMV[90]

This (the Oxford Miniature Vaporizer) can be calibrated for halothane, trichloroethylene, methoxyflurane or chloroform. Vaporization is from a stainless-steel wick and there is a permanent water jacket to limit temperature changes, though no elaborate thermocompensation mechanism is provided. Can be used (with halothane) to smooth induction with the EMO Ether inhaler.

(*See also* Boulton T. B. in: *Recent Advances in Anaesthesia*, 11th ed. (Hewer C. Langton, ed.). London: Churchill Livingstone, 1972, Ch. 6; Farman J. V. *Anaesthesia and the E.M.O. System*. London: English Universities Press, 1973.)

Open drop methods do not deserve the disdain they usually receive: *Advantages* are: (1) Immediate safety; (2) Cheapness; (3) Portability; (4) Ease of administration; (5) Minimal dead space. *Disadvantages* are: (1) Uneven anaesthesia due to variations in concentration of vapour; (2) Risk of fire, except with chloroform and halothane; (3) Wastefulness; (4) Atmosphere of theatre becomes laden with vapour; (5) Risk of damage to eyes or skin of patient from anaesthetic liquid; (6) Fall in oxygen concentration under the mask (easily remedied by trickling oxygen under the mask via small catheter).

Monitoring Inhaled Gases and Vapours

1. Oxygen; the fuel cell analyser can be placed in circuit to monitor inhaled oxygen tension.
2. Carbon dioxide; the capnograph gives an immediate indication of carbon dioxide concentration in anaesthetic systems. It depends on infra-red absorption.
3. Volatile agents; halothane concentrations up to 3% can be measured by the Drager Narkotest. The Engström Emma measures inhaled concentration of many volatile agents.

Artificial Ventilators

See Chapter 15.

Accidents Associated with Equipment

Accidental disconnection is an ever-present hazard, most serious if gaseous exchange relies upon IPPV. Constant vigilance is required.[91] Ill-fitting tapers should be discarded. Minor leaks may have serious consequences and adequate tests are required to detect them.[92]

(*See also* Cooper J. B., Newbower R. S. et al. *Anesthesiology* 1978, **49**, 399; Craig J. and Wilson M. E. *Anaesthesia* 1981, **36**, 933; Cundy J. and Baldock G. J. *Anaesthesia* 1982, **37**, 161; Shaw A., Davis P. D. et al. *Anaesthesia* 1982, **37**, 201; Spurring P. W. and Small L. F. G. *Anaesthesia* 1983, **38**, 683; Neufeld P. D. et al. *Can. Anaesth. Soc. J.* 1983, **30**, 646; Heath M. L. *Anaesthesia* 1984, **39**, 57; Wilson M. E. in: *Recent Advances in Anaesthesia and Analgesia—15* (Atkinson R. S. and Adams A. P., ed.) Edinburgh: Churchill Livingstone, 1985.)

Maintaining the Airway

To maintain a patent airway in an anaesthetized patient it is usually necessary to displace the mandible anteriorly (holding up the jaw) by pressure just superior to the angle of the mandible. Considerable force may be required and both skill and experience are necessary for success. The patient may complain of pain afterwards. If this method fails, a pharyngeal airway may have to be inserted, but this may cause coughing in light anaesthesia. Airway obstruction is usually due to the tongue but the epiglottis may be responsible.[93]

Many airways have been designed but today most anaesthetists use the Guedel pharyngeal airway in rubber or plastic.[94] In some instances use of a rubber or plastic nasopharyngeal airway is appropriate.

Tracheal Tubes and Connections

See Chapter 12.

See 'Equipment Design and Standardisation' Thompson P. W. *Ann. R. Coll. Surg.* 1983, **65**, 14, and for the history of the development of standards in the development of anaesthetic equipment Rendell-Baker J. in: *Anaesthesia; Essays on its History*. (Rupreht J. and van Lieburg M. J., ed.). Berlin: Springer-Verlag, 1985, p. 159; Ward C. S. *Anaesthetic Equipment*. 2nd ed. Eastbourne: Ballière Saunders, 1985.

References

1. Boyle H. E. G. *Br. Med. J.* 1917, **2**, 653; Hadfield C. F. *Br. J. Anaesth.* 1950, **22**, 107; Hewer C. Langton *Anaesthesia* 1967, **22**, 357; Obituary of Boyle, *Anaesthesia* 1967, **22**, 710; Watt O. M. *Anaesthesia* 1968, **23**, 103; Bryn Thomas K. *The Development of Anaesthetic Apparatus*. Oxford: Blackwell, 1975; Hewer C. L. *Anaesthesia* 1977, **32**, 908.
2. Gwathmey J. T. *Anesthesia*. New York: Appleton, 1914, p. 174.
3. *Health Technical Memorandum* No. 22 (and Supplement). London: DHSS, 1977.
4. Bancroft M. L. et al. *Anesthesiology* 1980, **52**, 504.
5. *Health Equipment Information* 1975, **61**, 38, 75.
6. *See also* Bushman J. A. *Br. J. Clin. Equip.* 1977, **2**, 190; *Hospital Technical Memorandum* No. 22 (HTM 22, DHSS, 1972); Elton V. *Health and Safety Executive* 1976, **29**, 4.
7. Adams A. P. and Henville J. D. in: *Recent Advances in Anaesthesia and Analgesia*—13 (Hewer C. L. and Atkinson R. S., ed.). Edinburgh: Churchill Livingstone, 1979, Ch. 2; Spurring P. W. et al. *Br. J. Anaesth.* 1978, **50**, 641; Craig J. and Wilson M. E. *Anaesthesia* 1981, **36**, 933.
8. Wright B. M. *Lancet* 1977, **2**, 1008.
9. Footerman D. S. *Anaesthesia* 1983, **38**, 672.
10. Neu M. *Münch. Med. Wochenschr.* 1910, **57**, 1873.
11. Venn P. J. H. *Anaesthesia* 1983, **38**, 703.
12. Thompson P. W. in: *Recent Advances in Anaesthesia and Analgesia*—12 (Hewer C. L. and Atkinson R. S., ed.). Edinburgh: Churchill Livingstone, 1976, Ch. 9.
13. Adams A. P. *Br. J. Hosp. Med.* April 1969, Suppl. 35; Ganendran A. *Br. J. Anaesth.* 1973, **45**, 1165; Rendell-Baker L. *Anesth. Analg.* 1976, **55**, 26.
14. Gupta B. L. and Varshneya A. K. *Br. J. Anaesth.* 1975, **47**, 805.
15. Conway C. M. *Proc. R. Soc. Med.* 1974, **67**, 1087.
16. Cook T. L. et al. *Anesth. Analg.* 1977, **65**, 793.
17. Johnstone R. E. and Smith T. C. *Anesthesiology* 1973, **38**, 192.
18. Parmley J. B. et al. *Anesth. Analg.* 1972, **51**, 888.
19. Newton N. I. and Adams A. P. *Anaesthesia* 1978, **33**, 689.
20. Mostafa S. M. *Br. J. Anaesth.*, 1980, **52**, 223.
21. Clarke A. D. *Br. J. Anaesth.* 1958, **30**, 176.

22. *See also* Waters R. M. *J. Hist. Med.* 1942, **1**, 595.
23. McKesson E. I. *Surg. Gynecol. Obstet.* 1911, **13**, 456.
24. McKesson E. I. *Am. J. Surg.* (Anesth. Suppl.) 1915, **29**, 51.
25. Magill I. W. *Proc. R. Soc. Med.* 1929, **22**, 83 and 1967, **60**, 16.
26. Conway C. M. et al. *Br. J. Anaesth.* 1976, **48**, 447.
27. Kain M. L. and Nunn J. F. *Anesthesiology* 1968, **29**, 964.
28. Ungerer M. J. *Can. Anaesth. Soc. J.* 1978, **25**, 122.
29. Conway C. M. *Proc. R. Soc. Med.* 1974, **67**, 1087.
30. Mapleson W. W. *Br. J. Anaesth.* 1954, **26**, 323.
31. Kain M. L. and Nunn J. F. *Proc. R. Soc. Med.* 1967, **60**, 749; Norman J., Adams A. P. and Sykes M. K. *Anaesthesia* 1968, **23**, 75.
32. Marshall M. and Henderson G. A. *Br. J. Anaesth.* 1968, **40**, 265; Baraka A. *Br. J. Anaesth.* 1969, **41**, 527.
33. *See also* review article Pollard B. and Gibb D. B. *Anaesth. Intensive Care* 1977, **5**, 113.
34. Rohrer F. *Pflüg. Arch. Ges. Physiol.* 1915, **162**, 225.
35. Bain J. A. and Spoerel W. E. *Can. Anaesth. Soc. J.* 1972, **19**, 426; Henville J. D. and Adams A. P. *Br. J. Anaesth.* 1975, **47**, 1024; Henville J. D. and Adams A. P. *Anaesthesia* 1976, **31**, 247; Gwilt D. J. et al. *Br. J. Anaesth.* 1978, **50**, 127; *see also* Adams A. P. and Henville J. D. in: *Recent Advances in Anaesthesia and Analgesia*—13 (Hewer C. L. and Atkinson R. S. ed.). Edinburgh: Churchill Livingstone, 1979, Ch. 2.
36. Macintosh R. R. and Mushin W. W. *Medical Times* 1945, **73**, 53; Macintosh R. R. and Pask E. A. *Br. J. Indust. Med.* 1957, **14**, 168. (The late E. A. Pask very staunchly allowed himself to be anaesthetized with ether on many occasions, during these experiments.)
37. Hannallah R. and Rosales J. K. *Can. Anaesth. Soc. J.* 1974, **21**, 511; Mansell W. H. *Anaesth. Soc. J.* 1976, **23**, 227.
38. Henville J. D. and Adams A. P. *Anesthesiology* 1976, **31**, 247; Baraka A. *Br. J. Anaesth.* 1969, **41**, 527; Bain J. A. and Spoerel W. E. *Can. Anaesth. Soc. J.* 1973, **20**, 629; Bain J. A. and Spoerel W. E. *Can. Anaesth. Soc. J.* 1975, **22**, 34; Bain J. A. and Spoerel W. E. *Can. Anaesth. Soc. J.* 1977, **24**, 559; Solimen M. G. and Laberge R. *Can. Anaesth. Soc. J.* 1978, **25**, 276.
39. Conway C. M. et al. *Br. J. Anaesth.* 1977, **49**, 1245; Rose D. K. et al. *Can. Anaesth. Soc. J.* 1978, **25**, 353.
40. Alexander J. P. *Br. J. Anaesth.* 1982, **54**, 1034.
41. Adams A. P. and Henville J. D. in: *Recent Advances in Anaesthesia and Analgesia*—13 (Hewer C. L. and Atkinson R. S. ed.). Edinburgh: Churchill Livingstone, 1979, Ch. 2.
42. Nott M. D. and Norman J. *Anaesthesia* 1983, **53**, 392.
43. Adams A. P. *Br. J. Clin. Equip.* 1976, **1**, 133.
44. Lack J. A. *Anaesthesia* 1976, **31**, 259; Lack J. A. *Anaesthesia* 1976, **31**, 576; Lack J. A. and Davies R. J. *Anaesthesia* 1976, **31**, 951, and addendum, 1253.
45. Humphrey D. *J. R. Soc. Med.* 1982, **75**, 513.
46. Radford E. P. *J. Appl. Physiol.* 1955, **7**, 451.
47. Christensen K. N. et al. *Acta Anaesthesiol. Scand.* 1978, **22**, 27; Jorgensen S. *Acta Anaesthesiol. Scand.* 1974, **18**, 29; Jorgensen S. and Thomsen A. *Acta Anaesthesiol. Scand.* 1976, **20**, 409; Thomsen A. and Jorgensen S. *Acta Anaesthesiol. Scand.* 1976, **20**, 395.
48. Miller D. M. *S. Afr. Med. J.* 1979, **55**, 721; Miller D. M. and Couper J. L. *Br. Med. J.* 1983, **55**, 569.
49. Burchett K. R. and Bennett J. A. *Anaesthesia* 1985, **40**, 181.
50. Humphrey D. *Anaesthesia* 1983, **38**, 361.
51. *See also* Farman J. V. *Anaesthesia and the E.M.O. System.* London: English Universities Press, 1973.
52. Ruben H. *Anesthesiology* 1955, **16**, 643; Ruben H. and Ruben A. *Lancet* 1957, **2**, 373.
53. Ayre T. P. *Lancet* 1937, **1**, 561; *Curr. Res. Anesth. Analg.* 1937, **16**, 330; *Br. J. Surg.* 1937, **35**, 131 (reprinted in 'Classical File', *Surv. Anesthesiol.* 1967, **11**, 400); *Br. J. Anaesth.* 1956, **28**, 520; *Anaesthesia* 1967, **22**, 359.
54. Flowerdew R. M. M. *Can. Anaesth. Soc. J.* 1979, **26**, 367.
55. Rees G. J. *Br. J. Anaesth.* 1960, **32**, 132.
56. Hewer C. Langton *Br. J. Anaesth.* 1923–1924, **1**, 113.
57. Boulton T. B. *Anesthesia* 1965, **20**, 442.
58. Boulton T. B. Presidential Address, Section on Anaesthetics, Royal Society of Medicine, London, 4 Nov. 1983.
59. Marrett R. *Br. Med. J.* 1942, **1**, 643.
60. Snow J. *Lond. Med. Gaz.* 1851, **12**, 622.

61. Kuhn F. *Dtsch. Zeit. Chir.* 1906, **81**, 63.
62. Reinhold H. in: *Anaesthesia; Essays on its History* (Rupreht J. and van Lieburg M. J., ed.). Berlin: Springer-Verlag, 1985.
63. Jackson D. E. *J. Lab. Clin. Med.* 1915, **1**, 1 (reprinted in 'Classical File', *Surv. Anesthesiol.* 1965, **9**, 98).
64. Waters R. M. *Curr. Res. Anesth. Analg.* 1924, **3**, 20.
65. Sword B. C. *Curr. Res. Anesth. Analg.* 1930, **9**, 198 (reprinted in 'Classical File', *Surv. Anesthesiol.* 1981, **25**, 65).
66. Primrose W. B. *Br. Med. J.* 1934, **1**, 478; **2**, 339.
67. Mapleson W. W. *Br. J. Anaesth.* 1960, **32**, 298.
68. Wilson R. C. *J. Ind. Eng. Chem.* 1920, **12**, 1000.
69. Waters R. M. *Curr. Res. Anesth. Analg.* 1926, **5**, 160; *Ann. Surg.* 1936, **38**, 103; *Proc. R. Soc. Med.* 1936, **30**, 11.
70. Sword B. C. *Curr. Res. Anesth. Analg.* 1930, **9**, 198.
71. Eger E. I. *Anesthetic Uptake and Action.* Baltimore: Williams and Wilkins, 1974.
72. *See also* Adams A. P. and Henville J. D. *Recent Advances in Anaesthesia and Analgesia—13* (Hewer C. L. and Atkinson R. S. ed.). Edinburgh: Churchill Livingstone, 1979; Haper M. and Eger E. I. *Anesth. Analg.* 1976, **55**, 724; Nunn J. F. *Br. J. Anaesth.* 1978, **50**, 733; Aldrete J. A. and Virtue R. W. *Low Flow and Closed System Anesthesia.* New York: Grune and Stratton, 1979.
73. Holmes C. McK. and Spears G. F. S. *Anaesthesia* 1977, **32**, 846.
74. Barton F. and Nunn J. F. *Br. J. Anaesth.* 1975, **47**, 350.
75. Bushman J. A. et al. *Br. J. Anaesth.* 1977, **49**, 575.
76. Smith W. D. A. *Br. J. Clin. Equip.* 1978, **3**, 49; DHSS Health Circular, No. HC (76) 38, London: HMSO, 1976.
77. Davenport H. T. et al. *Br. Med. J.* 1976, **2**, 1219.
78. Vaughan R. S. et al. *Anaesthesia* 1977, **32**, 339.
79. Bethune D. W. et al. *Anaesthesia* 1976, **31**, 1254.
80. Vaughan R. S. et al. *Br. Med. J.* 1973, **1**, 727.
81. Schimmelbusch C. *Anleitung Z. aseptischen Wundbehandling.* Berlin: Hirschwald, 1894.
82. Skinner T. *Retrosp. Pract. Med.* 1862, **46**, 185.
83. Curt Schimmelbusch, assistant to the Berlin surgeon, von Bergmann, a pioneer in the aseptic system of surgery. *Polytechnik (Bern)*, 1890, **12**, 203.
84. Bellamy Gardner G. H. *Br. Med. J.* 1907 **2**, 1516; *Br. Med. J.* 1910, **2**, 766.
85. Epstein H. G. and Macintosh R. R. *Anaesthesia* 1956, **11**, 83; Leatherdale R. A. L. *Anaesthesia* 1966, **21**, 504; *see also* Hill D. W. *Br. J. Anaesth.* 1968, **40**, 648.
86. Epstein H. G. et al. *Lancet* 1941, **2**, 62.
87. Marsh D. R. G. and Herbert P. *Anaesthesia* 1983, **38**, 575.
88. Schaefer H-G. and Farman J. V. *Anaesthesia* 1984, **39**, 171.
89. Macintosh R. R. *Br. Med. J.* 1953, **2**, 202.
90. Parkhouse J. *Anaesthesia* 1966, **21**, 498; Schaefer H-G and Farman J. V., *Anaesthesia* 1984, **39**, 171.
91. Green R. A. *Anaesthesia* 1986, **41**, 129.
92. Wilson M. E. and Burleton A. S. *Br. J. Anaesth.* 1982, **54**, 572.
93. Boidin M. P. *Br. J. Anaesth.* 1985, **57**, 306.
94. Guedel A. E. *JAMA* 1933, **100**, 1862 (reprinted in 'Classical File', *Surv. Anesthesiol.* 1966, **10**, 515).

Chapter 10   # INHALATION ANAESTHESIA

Clinical Signs of Anaesthesia

Since the early days of anaesthesia, it has been apparent that the anaesthetist must rely on a series of physical signs to indicate the onset of anaesthesia and to determine its depth. This was appreciated by the early anaesthetists, including

John Snow (who described 'five stages of narcotism')[1] and Francis Plomley,[2] but it was not until Arthur Eames Guedel,[3] then of Indianapolis, developed his classic table of the signs of anaesthesia with division, into stages and planes, using open ether, that a really detailed system became generally accepted.

The Stages of Anaesthesia

The clinical signs of anaesthesia are the signs of: (1) a progressive increase of muscular paralysis (eyeball muscles, intercostals, diaphragm); (2) a progressive abolition of reflex response. (*Fig. 10.1*).

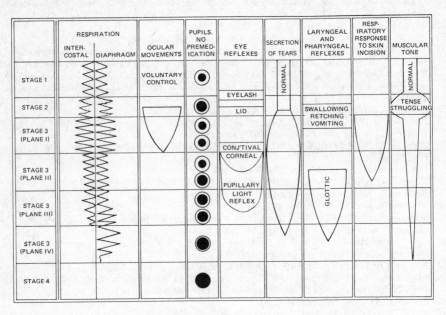

Fig. 10.1. The levels of disappearance of reflexes (*after Guedel*).

First Stage—Analgesia

From beginning of induction to loss of consciousness.

Second Stage—Excitement or Uninhibited Response

From loss of consciousness to onset of automatic breathing. There may be struggling, breath-holding, vomiting, coughing, swallowing, etc.

Third Stage—Surgical Anaesthesia

From onset of automatic respiration to respiratory paralysis. Guedel divided it into four planes:

Plane 1. From onset of automatic respiration to cessation of eyeball movement.

Plane 2. From cessation of eyeball movement to commencement of intercostal paralysis. Breathing remains regular and deep, not very different from Plane 1.

Plane 3. The plane of progressive intercostal paralysis, first described by John Snow;[4] later by Paul Bert (1833–1886) of Paris, and again in 1899 by J. Hughlings Jackson (1835–1911) and James Collier, both London physicians. Recognized as a sign of anaesthesia in 1924 by Albert Miller (1872–1959)[5] of Rhode Island (who

named it 'ascending respiratory paralysis') and placed in its correct position in Guedel's table by Ralph Waters. From commencement to completion of intercostal paralysis. The force of expiration is reduced with increasing depth of anaesthesia with volatile agents.[6] Rapid breathing may persist well into Plane 3. Slow breathing is usually associated with administration of narcotic analgesics.
Plane 4. From complete intercostal paralysis to diaphragmatic paralysis.

More recently there has been a tendency to divide the stage of surgical anaesthesia into only three planes:
Light anaesthesia. Until the eyeballs become fixed.
Medium anaesthesia. Increasing intercostal paralysis.
Deep anaesthesia. Diaphragmatic respiration.

Fourth Stage—Overdosage
From onset of diaphragmatic paralysis to apnoea and death. All reflex activity lost and pupils widely dilated.

Eye Signs

Extrinsic Muscles
Activity of the muscles of the eyeball is progressively reduced until it is abolished at the bottom of Plane 1.

Pupils
Opiates as premedication tend to produce miosis; atropine and hyoscine in large doses, mydriasis. If both are given the opiate effect usually predominates. In the 2nd stage the pupils may be dilated, reflexly, due to emotion and psychosensory impulses. In Stage 3, Plane 1, the pupils return to normal and then progressively dilate until the maximum is reached in Plane 4. Dilatation of the pupil occurs also after the administration of ganglion-blocking drugs (e.g. hexamethonium, trimetaphan).

Other Eye Reflexes
1. *Eyelash.* Gently touching eyelashes causes contraction of the lids. Reflex disappears on entering second stage.
2. *Eyelid.* Gently raising the upper lid causes contraction of the lids. Reflex disappears on entering third stage.
3. *Conjunctival.* Gently touching palpebral conjunctiva causes blinking, a reflex which disappears at bottom of Stage 3, Plane 1.
4. *Corneal.* Gently touching cornea produces contraction of lids. Reflex disappears in middle of Plane 2. Should seldom be used.
5. *Light.* Exposure to strong light causes the pupil to contract. Light reflex abolished in upper Plane 3.
6. *Lacrimation.* This is greater than normal in Planes 1 and 2, and is a useful sign of light anaesthesia. Some anaesthetists cover the eyes with adhesive tape to prevent drying of the eyes in deeper planes.

Other Reflexes

1. Swallowing
Occurs at upper border of Stage 3, Plane 1. Rapid deepening of anaesthesia at this point may avoid vomiting.

2. Vomiting

Occurs at lower border of Stage 2. These signs are also of importance in ascent from deeper anaesthesia, when swallowing may be a warning of impending vomiting. Vomiting may be associated with hypoxia or hypotension in the conscious subject.

3. Skin

Movement of limbs and deep breathing are the reflex responses to skin stimulation. Response to skin incision progressively depressed: (*a*) Gross limb flexion which interrupts the surgical operation; (*b*) Minor limb movements which do not interfere with surgery; (*c*) Subtle movements of facial muscles or digits, usually only noticed by the anaesthetist; (*d*) No movement, but an increase in the depth of respiration; (*e*) No response.

4. Cough

Progressively depressed in deeper planes. (*a*) Muscles of trunk, neck and limbs participate in the response; (*b*) Confined to the respiratory muscles; (*c*) Cough is present but ineffective; (*d*) No cough, but expiration is forceful; (*e*) No response.

5. Laryngeal

Coughing and adduction of the cords are produced by stimulation of the nerve endings in the larynx and epiglottis. Reflex abolished in upper Plane 2. Laryngeal spasm due to stimuli arising in the abdomen, anus or cervix uteri, etc. (Brewer–Luckhardt reflex)[7] may not be abolished until Plane 4. Inflammation of upper respiratory tract increases its reflex irritability, so that coughing may persist well into Plane 2 or even Plane 3. Smoking has the same effect.

6. Sweating

May be seen in light planes of anaesthesia and can occur even when the patient is completely paralysed by muscle relaxants. Sometimes abolished by atropine (*see also* p. 136).

7. Tracheal Tug

This jerky depression of the thyroid cartilage, synchronous with inspiration, is often seen when the intercostal muscles are paralysed, either by deep anaesthesia or by a relaxant (*see also* Chapter 14). It is more commonly seen in unfit patients.

8. Carinal

Stimulation of the carina as by tracheal suction, a long tracheal tube or bronchoscope may cause coughing anywhere above Stage 4.

The Signs with Different Anaesthetic Agents

With di-ethyl ether the stimulus of the strong vapour is intense and once the patient has accepted it without coughing or laryngospasm, the patient is unlikely to react to the skin incision. With the modern potent inhalation agents, halothane, enflurane and isoflurane, this is not so and a patient may be breathing quietly but still react to the skin incision. The use of muscle-relaxant drugs modifies all the signs of anaesthesia, as muscle tone and reflex activity may be abolished in light planes of anaesthesia; only autonomic responses (e.g. sweating, changes in the heart rate, dilatation of the pupil, etc.) then remain for the guidance of the anaesthetist. If the angle of the jaw is pushed firmly forward, the patient will often dorsiflex both feet; when this reflex is abolished a pharyngeal airway can be inserted without untoward response.[8]

Recovery

As anaesthesia lightens there is return of muscle tone and of reflex responses, though sometimes the latter remain sluggish until consciousness has almost returned.

Emergence delirium may occur as the patient ascends through the second stage.

Balanced Anaesthesia

The concept of balanced anaesthesia started in 1911 when George Washington Crile (1864–1943) of Cleveland, Ohio, taught that psychic stimuli must be obliterated by light general anaesthesia, while the noxious impulses due to surgery must be blocked by local analgesia—the so-called theory of anoci-association.[9] In 1926 John S. Lundy (1894–1972) of the Mayo Clinic introduced the term 'balanced anaesthesia' for a combination of agents such as premedication, regional analgesia and general anaesthesia with one or more agents, so that pain relief was obtained by a nice balance of agents and techniques.[10]

The Triad of Anaesthesia

Rees and Gray[11] of Liverpool divided anaesthesia into three basic components: (1) Narcosis; (2) Analgesia; (3) Relaxation. Gray[12] renamed the triad: (1) Narcosis; (2) Reflex suppression; (3) Relaxation. With selective drugs, it is possible to vary one component of the triad without affecting the others. In this context it is possible to avoid deep levels of central brain depression. The patient need not be 'deeper' than just unconscious, providing there is no awareness.

Anaesthesia (or analgesia) is a process of modification of the normal physiological reflex response to the stimuli provided by surgery (and anaesthesia). The triad of anaesthesia may be considered as: (1) Inhibition of the afferent part of the reflex system; (2) Depression of the central synaptic mechanisms of co-ordination; (3) Block of the efferent part of the reflex arc.

Inhalation Anaesthetic Agents

Nitrous Oxide

History

Gas[13] first prepared by Priestley (1733–1804) in 1772. Anaesthetic properties suggested by Sir Humphry Davy (1778–1829) in 1799. In 1808, P. C. Barton (1786–1808), of Philadelphia, again described the exhilarating effects of nitrous oxide. Both he and the distinguished surgeon Willard Parker (1800–1884) of New York may have influenced Colton who demonstrated its effects to Horace Wells (1815–1848), dentist of Hartford, in 1844, who in turn used it in dentistry and had one of his own teeth painlessly extracted by John M. Riggs on 11 December. After an unsuccessful demonstration before John Collins Warren (1778–1856) the surgeon and the students at the Massachusetts General Hospital, Wells continued to use it in his practice, but its use was temporarily forgotten and it was overshadowed by ether. Gardner Quincy Colton (1814–1898, a pupil of Parker) revived its use in 1867–1868 and this time the American dental profession showed considerable interest. In 1863 he established himself in practice in New York City and there founded the Colton Dental Association. T. W. Evans (1823–1897), US dentist working in Paris, introduced it to his colleagues in London in 1868,[14] having learnt its use the previous year from Colton at the International Congress of Medicine in Paris. Later in the same year, the gas was supplied compressed into cylinders and became available two years later as liquefied N_2O. Edmund Andrews (1824–1904)[15] of Chicago, combined it with oxygen, to give longer anaesthesia, in 1868. In 1878 Paul Bert (1830–1886), of France, administered it in a hyperbaric chamber.[16] In 1868 J. T. Clover (1825–1882), London anaesthetist, successfully demonstrated its use at the Radcliffe Infirmary, Oxford,[17] and proved it to be a true anaesthetic, not a means of causing asphyxia. Bert was an early user of Edmund Andrew's nitrous-oxide–oxygen mixture to prolong anaesthesia and to avoid asphyxia.[18] First apparatus for the sequential use of nitrous oxide and ether described by Clover.[19] Early users of the nitrous oxide, oxygen, chloroform ether sequence were F. J. Cotton (1869–1938); W. M. Boothby (1880–1953) of Boston; J. T. Gwathmey (1863–1944) of New York City; Geoffrey Marshall (1887–1982) and H. E. G. Boyle (1875–1941) of London (*see also* Boulton T. B. 'Classical File', *Surv. Anesthesiol.* 1985, **29**, 201). A reducing valve was described in 1873.[20] Sir F. Hewitt (1857–1916)[21] and E. I. McKesson (1881–1935), an early pioneer of careful notekeeping in anaesthesia,[22] have been pioneers in its use, and today it is widely used in anaesthesia along with a relaxant and an intravenous barbiturate. The book *Nitrous-oxide–Oxygen Anesthesia* by F. W. Clement (1892–1970) appeared in 1939. The book *Untoward Effects of Nitrous Oxide Anaesthesia* by C. B. Courville, Los Angeles neuropathologist, appeared in 1939. It dealt with acute asphyxia caused by McKesson's technique of secondary saturation.[23,24] In 1956 H. C. A. Lassen, Copenhagen physician, reported that very prolonged nitrous-oxide–oxygen anaesthesia could cause bone-marrow aplasia.[25] May cause macrocytic anaemia by inhibiting vitamin B_{12}. (*See also Under the Influence*, Smith W. D. A. London: Macmillan, 1982 and Frost F. A. M. in: *Nitrous Oxide* (Eger E. L. ed.) London: Arnold, 1985, Ch. 1.)

Manufacture

By heating ammonium nitrate in an iron retort to 240 °C. The issuing gas is collected, purified and compressed into metal cylinders at $50 \, kPa \times 100$ (750 lb/in^2). The cylinders are painted French blue (in Britain) and common sizes are 200 gal (907 litres) and 400 gal (1814 litres).

$$NH_4NO_3 \rightarrow 2H_2O + N_2O$$

Nitric oxide (NO) and nitrogen dioxide (NO_2) are produced as impurities so that the gases evolved must be washed with water and caustic soda, in turn, before being passed through activated alumina to remove water vapour. At various stages, monitors are used to detect the presence of higher oxides of nitrogen. As a further check, regular random sampling of cylinders is carried out.

The amount present in the cylinder can only be ascertained by weighing, as the gas is in liquid form and the gas pressure above the liquid level remains reasonably constant as long as any liquid remains. In fact some fall in pressure occurs due to fall in temperature as the liquid nitrous oxide evaporates using latent heat.[26] Up to four-fifths of the contents of a full cylinder is in the liquid state, so, in use, cylinders must have their valves elevated above the horizontal. Just before exhaustion of the cylinder, when all the liquid is vaporized, the pressure very quickly drops to zero. Cylinders are filled to a filling ratio (ratio of weight of nitrous oxide to weight of water the cylinder could hold) of 0·75 in temperate and 0·67 in tropical climates. The cylinder weights, full and empty, are stamped on it; 100 gallons of nitrous oxide weigh 850 g or 30 oz (1 US gallon = ⅝ Imperial gallon; 1 cubic foot = 6¼ Imperial gallons; 1 Imperial gallon = 4½ litres).

Physical Properties
Sweet smelling, non-irritating, colourless gas; the only inorganic gas in common use possessing anaesthetic properties. Boiling point −89 °C. Molecular weight 44. Critical pressure 71·7 atmospheres. Critical temperature 36·5 °C. Specific gravity 1·5—that is, 1½ times heavier than air. Density at 15 °C and 1 atmosphere is 1·875 g/litre. Velocity of sound in nitrous oxide is 262 m/sec (compared with 317 for oxygen) and a suitable whistle can be used to differentiate the two gases. Change from oxygen to nitrous oxide causes the pitch to fall one and a half tones.[27] Neither flammable nor explosive, but supports the combustion of other agents, even in the absence of oxygen, if a high temperature (above 450 °C) is supplied to initiate decomposition into nitrogen and oxygen. The oil/water solubility ratio is 3·2. Water will take up 100 vol %, while blood plasma dissolves 45 vol %. Nitrous oxide is fifteen times more soluble than oxygen. The partition coefficient is 0·47 between blood and gas, 1·0 between brain and blood, and 3·0 between fat and blood.

It is eliminated unchanged from the body, mostly via the lungs. It is stable and is unaffected by soda-lime.

For estimation of blood nitrous oxide levels *see* Saloojee Y. and Cole P. *Anaesthesia* 1978, **33**, 779; *see also* Grant W. J. *Medical Gases; Their Properties and Uses.* Aylesbury: H. M. and M. Publishers, 1978, p. 104.

(*See also* Robinson J. S. *Br. J. Anaesth.* 1983, **55**, 807.)

Impurities in Nitrous Oxide
Two cases of poisoning in the UK were reported in detail by Clutton-Brock.[28] Investigation showed that a batch of nitrous oxide had become contaminated with nitric oxide (NO) and nitrogen dioxide (NO_2). Both these substances are toxic. One patient died.

The clinical features are: (1) Cyanosis (methaemoglobinaemia). (2) Respiratory difficulty. (3) Circulatory failure.

A crude test for contamination[29] is to put a piece of moistened starch-iodide paper into a large syringe and then fill this with the suspected nitrous oxide mixed with 25% oxygen and wait for 10 min. If the gas is contaminated by over 300 parts per million, the starch iodide will turn blue.

See also a series of papers on the subject, *Br. J. Anaesth.* 1967, **39**, 343 et seq. and Editorial, *Lancet* 1967, **2**, 930.

Mode of Action
Nitrous oxide is a potent analgesic but a weak anaesthetic (MAC = 105 vol %). Anaesthesia is induced relatively rapidly due to the low blood/gas partition coefficient. In practice, at least 70% is required to guarantee

Table 10.1. Physical properties of some inhalation anaesthetics

Anaesthetic	Molecular weight	Boiling point (°C)	Vapour pressure @ 20°C (mmHg)	Liquid density	Oil/water solubility	Limits of flammability a = in air b = in oxygen (percent)	Vapour concentration for anaesthesia (vol%)	Minimal Alveolar Concentration for anaesthesia (vol%)	Blood/gas partition coefficient
Diethyl ether $C_2H_5\text{-}O\text{-}C_2H_5$	74	36·5	425	0·7	3·2	a. 1·85–48 b. 2–82	3–20	1·92	12
Cyclopropane C_3H_6	42	−34	—	—	34·4	a. 3·0–10·0 b. 2·5–50	7–23	9·2	0·46
Trichloroethylene C_2HCl_3	131	87·5	60	1·47	400	a. nonflammable b. 10–64	0·2–2	0·17	9
Nitrous oxide N_2O	44	−89	5200	1·2	2·2	nonflammable	50–80	105	0·47
Halothane $CF_3CHClBr$	197	50	243	1·87	220	nonflammable*	0·5–2	0·75	2·3
Enflurane $CHF_2\text{-}O\text{-}CF_2CHFCl$	184	56·5	174·5	1·52	120·1	nonflammable*	1·5–3	1·68 in oxygen 1·28 in 70% N_2O	1·9
Isoflurane $CHF_2O\text{-}CHCl\text{-}CF_3$	184	48·5	238	1·50	120·1	nonflammable	1–2·5	1·15 in oxygen 0·66 in 70% N_2O	1·4

*But see Leonard P. F. Anesth. Analg. (Cleve.) 1975, **54**, 238.

unconsciousness. It may cause the release of encephalin in the central nervous system. Endorphins may be involved in nitrous oxide analgesia and depletion of endorphin stores may lessen this effect.[30]

Side-effects of Nitrous Oxide

Nitrous oxide is usually regarded as a non-toxic anaesthetic agent, provided that it is administered with a sufficient concentration of oxygen. Undesirable effects may, however, sometimes occur:

1. Nitrous oxide in the alveolar gases will equilibrate with blood, tissue and gas-containing spaces within the body more rapidly than nitrogen diffuses out into alveolar gas. There is a thirty-five-fold difference in the blood/gas partition coefficients of the two gases (nitrous oxide 0·47, nitrogen 0·013) and for every molecule of nitrogen removed from air spaces, 35 molecules of nitrous oxide will pass in. There is thus an increase in the volume of the gas space when that space is compliant (gut, air embolus) and an increase in pressure when the space cannot expand (sinuses, the middle ear, in pneumo-encephalography). Postoperative hearing loss has been attributed to changes in middle-ear mechanics and rupture of the ear drums.[31] The increased middle ear pressure may cause problems in otological surgery (e.g. myringoplasty) and should nitrous oxide be undesirable, oxygen or oxygen-enriched air may be used as the carrier gas.[32] The pressure in a pneumothorax cavity may increase. The bowel may become distended with the gas, while in the gut it may become metabolized by anaerobic organisms through a reduction pathway.

2. Nitrous oxide inactivates the vitamin B_{12} component (i.e. cobalamin) of the enzyme methionine synthetase. The onset of inhibition has been studied in the rodent,[33] but is thought to be much slower in man.[34] Significant falls in plasma methionine concentrations during routine minor and intermediate surgery have not been demonstrated,[35] a period of at least 8 hours of nitrous oxide anaesthesia probably being needed to demonstrate a fall.[36] Recovery of the enzyme system is slow so that changes may be observed in the postoperative period.

Nitrous oxide interferes with folate metabolism and impairs DNA synthesis following prolonged inhalation.[37] Bone-marrow aplasia and fatal agranulocytosis[25,38] have followed prolonged administration of nitrous oxide in the treatment of poliomyelitis and tetanus. Exposure of patients to nitrous oxide for periods up to 6 hours or longer may result in megaloblastic anaemia.[39] Occupational exposure to nitrous oxide may result in myeloneuropathy, resembling subacute combined degeneration of the cord, the result of axonal degeneration. This emphasizes the need for the avoidance of pollution of the atmosphere of the operating room[40] and dental surgery.[41] Estimation of the urinary nitrous oxide is a simple and accurate method of biological monitoring of exposure to the gas in the atmosphere.[42] (*See also* Sharer N. M. and Nunn J. F. *Br. J. Anaesth.* 1983, **55**, 693; Amos R. J. and Amess J. A. et al. *Br. J. Anaesth.* 1984, **56**, 103; Sweeney B. and Bingham R. M. et al. *Br. Med. J.* 1985, **291**, 567.)

3. Teratogenic changes have been observed in pregnant rats exposed to nitrous oxide for prolonged periods. Nitrous oxide may affect the chromosomes in rat spermatozoa.[43] The critical time is when the embryo is 8 days old, corresponding to the human fetus of 6 weeks.

4. Nitrous oxide augments the respiratory depressant action of thiopentone, especially after opiate premedication.

5. Tolerance can be demonstrated in rats exposed to nitrous oxide for 72 h.[44]

Diffusion Hypoxia[45]

Immediately the mask is removed from a patient who has been breathing nitrous oxide mixture, hypoxia may occur, as both nitrogen and nitrous oxide occupy space in the alveolar gas at the expense of oxygen. As diffusion hypoxia (alveolar diffusion effect) it may be harmful in ill or handicapped patients. The remedy is to add high concentrations of oxygen to the inspired air during the quarter of an hour following cessation of nitrous oxide anaesthesia.

Nitrous Oxide in Anaesthesia

When the patient breathes nitrous oxide the tidal volume is decreased, respiratory rate is increased, the Pa_{CO_2} remains normal. It increases muscle tone. Nitrous oxide is a weak anaesthetic agent, and smooth anaesthesia with the sole agent is difficult to obtain consistently, even for short operations; it is used as an adjuvant and as a gaseous vehicle for the administration of more potent volatile agents. Nitrous-oxide–oxygen mixtures are usually administered after premedication, intravenous induction and with a volatile or intravenous supplement. Muscle relaxants may be used not only to provide full muscular relaxation, but also to obtund reflex activity. Under these circumstances it is possible to have very light planes of anaesthesia in a totally paralysed patient. Factors which may be considered are:

1. Reports of awareness[46] (*see also* Chapter 18). These would seem to be more common where sedative premedication has been omitted and other adjuvants used in minimal dosage (e.g. in Caesarean section).

2. Recollection of incidents occurring during operation when the patient is later subjected to hypnosis, though this does not necessarily indicate awareness at the time.

3. The cerebral function monitor[47] may have a place in determining the level of consciousness when intravenous agents are administered, but further work is required to assess its usefulness in inhalation anaesthesia.

4. The aware, paralysed, terrified patient may show sympathetic activity, e.g. dilatation of pupil, rapid bounding pulse.

It is now common practice to ensure against awareness by adding small amounts of a volatile agent to the nitrous-oxide–oxygen mixture. Heavy premedication, the use of intravenous narcotic analgesics and hypocapnia due to hyperventilation may achieve the same result.

Factors causing awareness during operation.[48] These include: (1) Induction. The risk is increased when ultra-short-acting intravenous agents are used for induction prior to intubation under full paralysis; (2) Ventilators may mix air or oxygen with the anaesthetic gases due to faulty adjustment or leaks; (3) Faults in the anaesthetic machine, e.g. oxygen bypass left on or failure of N_2O supply; (4) With closed systems it takes time to build up adequate alveolar tension of an agent. High flow-rates of N_2O during induction help to prevent awareness as also does the administration of premedication, e.g. lorazepam, 4 mg/70 kg.[49]

Premixed Nitrous Oxide/Oxygen

Premixed nitrous oxide/oxygen (80:20) at a maximum cylinder pressure of 47 kPa $\times$ 100 (700 lb/in²) was used in the US in 1945.[50] Certain mixtures of nitrous oxide and oxygen will remain in the gaseous phase at pressures and temperatures at which nitrous oxide by itself would normally be a liquid (Poynting effect). *Entonox* (50:50 mixture) is sold commercially.[51] The top is painted white and the body French blue. If such cylinders are exposed to cold (−7°C), some of the nitrous oxides separates as a liquid and may lead to delivery of uneven mixtures, too much oxygen at the beginning and too much nitrous oxide at the end of the cylinder life. Cooling due to expansion of gases while in use is not likely to cause this. Danger of separation can be avoided by immersing the cylinder in water at 52°C and inverting it three times, or by keeping it in a room at or above a temperature of 10°C for 2 h before use. Uses of *Entonox* include the relief of pain from dressing surgical wounds, chest physiotherapy, removal or changing of thoracotomy drains, coronary infarction. The apparatus can be used in ambulances, for IPPV in the intensive therapy unit, where it provides good analgesia without marked cardiovascular depression, and in dental anaesthesia and obstetric analgesia. The English National Board for Midwifery permit its use by midwives on their own responsibility. (*See also* Tunstall M. E. *Br. J. Anaesth.* 1968, **40**, 675; Baskett P. *Proc. R. Soc. Med.* 1971, **64**, 42; Parbrook, G. D. *Proc. R. Soc. Med.* 1971, **64**, 47.)

Premixed 50% nitrous oxide and 50% oxygen can also be supplied by pipeline and this has been shown to be safe and practical.[52]

Nitrous Oxide and Analgesia

Nitrous oxide is a good analgesic agent, a 25% concentration in oxygen being compared favourably with morphine for relief of postoperative pain while having little general effect on consciousness. Psychomotor performance is not affected at concentrations of nitrous oxide below 8–12%.[53] There is evidence that opiate receptors and endorphine may be involved in analgesia caused by nitrous oxide (and other inhalation agents), and that this may be reversed by naloxone.[54] The use of nitrous oxide in obstetrics is discussed in Chapter 27. For effects on vitamin B_{12} *see above*.

This very useful agent which has been in use for over 140 years is now being criticized as some workers think that its undesirable properties outweigh its benefits. The case is well argued, both pro and con in *Nitrous Oxide* (Eger E. I. ed.) London: Arnold, 1985.

Cyclopropane, BP

History

Cyclopropane or trimethylene was first synthesized by August von Freund (1835–1892) of Poland[55] who reduced trimethylene dibromide with sodium in an alkaline solution in 1882; its anaesthetic properties were shown by G. W. H. Lucas and V. E. Henderson (1877–1945), of Toronto, in 1929,[56] while investigating the narcotic properties of propylene in an effort to find a more satisfactory agent than ethylene. First used on a human volunteer by W. Easson Brown, the patient being Professor Henderson, soon followed by Lucas and Banting (of insulin fame) (1891–1941). As its use was not encouraged by the anaesthetic staff of the Toronto General Hospital it was developed by workers in the Anesthetics Department of the State of Wisconsin Hospital at Madison: clinical reports by Waters and his colleagues followed in the years after 1930, when he started its use.[57] Harold Griffith (1894–1985) began using the agent in Montreal about the same time. First used in the UK by Stanley Rowbotham (1890–1979).[58]

(*See also* The discovery of cyclopropane. Lucas G. W. H. *Anesth. Analg. Curr. Res.* 1961, **40**, 15; Bamforth, Betty, in: *Anaesthesia; Essays on its History.* (Rupreht J. et al. ed.). Berlin: Springer-Verlag, 1985, p. 269.)

Physical Properties[59]

Colourless gas with sweet smell. Molecular weight 42. Boiling point $-34\,°C$. One and a half times heavier than air. Critical temperature $175\,°C$. Critical pressure 54 atmospheres. Liquefies at ordinary temperatures if pressure of 5 atmospheres is applied: hence is stored in light-alloy cylinders (painted orange) as a liquid at a pressure of $5\text{ kPa} \times 100$ (75 lb/in^2) no reducing valves being required. Partition coefficients, blood/gas 0·46 (low), so induction and recovery are both rapid, fat/blood 20, oil/water 34·4, MAC 9·2. Very explosive with oxygen (between 2·5 and 50%) and nitrous oxide throughout the anaesthetic range; explosive in air between 3% and 10%. It is not decomposed by soda-lime, but slowly diffuses through rubber. There are no toxic products of its metabolism.

Pharmacology

Taken up and excreted via the lungs with little metabolism. Both induction of anaesthesia and recovery are relatively fast. There is progressive depression of the central nervous system as the inhaled concentration is increased. Cyclopropane is a powerful respiratory depressant. Hypercapnia is likely to occur in the absence of assisted or controlled respiration. Muscle-relaxant drugs can be used with light cyclopropane anaesthesia and IPPV. Cardiac output is usually increased with arterial pressure well maintained. At high concentrations and after morphine premedication cardiac output may fall.

Vagotonic Dysrhythmias. Bradycardia (below 50/min). Nodal rhythm.

Ventricular Ectopic Beats. These may occur singly, as coupled beats or as runs of ventricular tachycardia. Ventricular fibrillation, with sudden death, can occur. Factors which predispose to ventricular dysrhythmias: (1) Overdosage with cyclopropane; (2) Carbon dioxide retention; (3) Catecholamines; (4) Hypoxia; (5) Atropine. *See* Price H. L. et al. *Anesthesiology* 1958, **19**, 457; 1958, **19**, 619; 1959, **20**, 563; 1960, **21**, 380; 1963, **24**, 1.

Techniques of Administration

Induction with cyclopropane and oxygen.[60] It is always used in a closed system. Cyclopropane is a potent agent and rapid induction can be achieved, a few breaths of 50% cyclopropane in oxygen being enough to render a patient unconscious.

When administering cyclopropane these facts should be borne in mind: (1) The gas is explosive; (2) The agent is puissant and deaths have been reported from ventricular fibrillation; (3) The agent is a potent respiratory depressant and hypercapnia is a factor in the development of dysrhythmias.

Cyclopropane and intermittent positive pressure ventilation. If respiration is controlled and a state of hypocapnia is maintained by hyperventilation, then many of the serious complications of cyclopropane anaesthesia are considerably minimized.

Uses of Cyclopropane

Cyclopropane is a reasonably safe drug which can be used for a wide range of operations provided precautions against the explosive risk are taken. As the drug is excreted largely unchanged and recovery is rapid, some anaesthetists find it a useful agent in old, ill and shocked patients. It is also popular for induction in children.

Sequelae
Nausea and vomiting, cardiac dysrhythmias and emergence delirium are more common than with the popular nitrous-oxide–oxygen-relaxant techniques.

Contraindications
1. During operations involving use of diathermy or cautery.
2. When adrenaline is to be used. The danger is much greater than when adrenaline is injected during trichloroethylene or halothane administrations.

Other Gases

Ethylene [C_2H_4]
Discovered by Johannes Ingenhousz (1730–1799) in 1779 or by Johan Joachim Becher (1638–1682) of Mainz. May have been given as early in 1849 by Thomas Nunnelly (1809–1870) of Leeds.

Anaesthetic properties first noticed by Hermann in 1864. Crocker and Knight (1908), the botanists, proved that ethylene contained in illuminating gas would prevent carnation buds from opening. Has since been used to ripen fruit. Investigated by A. B. Luckhardt (1885–1957) and Jay Bailey Carter of Chicago in 1923, and by W. Easson Brown (1891–1957) of Toronto in 1923, and they introduced it into clinical medicine, along with Isabella Herb (1869–1943), who independently employed it in the Presbyterian Hospital, Chicago, in March 1923.[60]

Ethylene is similar to nitrous oxide in its anaesthetic properties, though rather more powerful, and hence a greater concentration of oxygen can be used. It never gained much popularity due to its explosive properties and its unpleasant smell. Cylinder colour is violet.

Xenon[61]
Isolated in 1898 by William Ramsey (1852–1916), Nobel prizeman in chemistry 1904. First used in 1951. Radioactive xenon used in cerebral blood-flow studies.

Volatile Agents

Ether [$CH_3.CH_2—O—CH_2.CH_3$]

History
Prepared originally in 1540 by Valerius Cordus (1515–1544), who called it sweet oil of vitriol. Sigmund August Frobensius, the German chemist, physician and botanist from Wittenberg, named it ether.[62] Used clinically for anaesthesia by W. E. Clarke (1818–1878) of Rochester, NY, in January 1842, when Dr Elijah

Pope extracted a tooth from a Miss Hobbs,[63] and by Crawford Long* (1815–1893) of Jefferson, Georgia, on 3 March 1842,[64] but they did not publish their results until later.[65] Introduced to the profession by W. T. G. Morton of Boston (1819–1868) on 16 October 1846[66] who was continuously supported by the influential John Collins Warren (1778–1856) and Henry (1818–1890), his father, and Jacob Bigelow (1786–1879), the first two surgeons, the third a professor of materia medica and a famous botanist at Harvard. The operation was for the removal of a vascular tumour from just below the mandible; the patient (who gave 'informed consent') was Gilbert Abbott. After the operation he remained in hospital for 7 weeks. The first account of its pharmacological and clinical properties appeared in John Snow's book *On the Inhalation of Ether*, published in 1847. François Malgaigné of Paris was the first to use ether in France. It did not attain much popularity in Britain until B. Joy Jeffries came from the US, advocating the safer ether instead of chloroform, with the American towel cone method of forcible induction, in 1872. Two years later Clover introduced his gas–ether sequence.[67] Before this time, chloroform had been used almost as a routine. 'Open ether' was reintroduced by Prince in America in 1895,[68] and popularized in the UK by Robert Lawson Tait (1845–1899), the well-known Birmingham surgeon and gynaecologist, former assistant to J. Y. Simpson.[69] It is still the safest all-purpose anaesthetic. 'I hold it therefore to be almost impossible that a death from this agent [ether] can occur in the hands of a medical man who is applying it with ordinary intelligence and attention' (John Snow, *On Chloroform and Other Anaesthetics*, 1858). In 1847, at least 25 books were published on the use of ether (Ole Secher).

Physical Properties
Colourless volatile liquid of molecular weight 74, and specific gravity of 0·719. Boiling point 35 °C; saturated vapour pressure at 20 °C is 425 mmHg; specific gravity of vapour 2·6. Oil/water solubility ratio 3·2. Oil/gas partition coefficient is low—65. Blood/gas partition coefficient 12·0. This is high, giving slow induction and recovery. Minimal alveolar concentration for anaesthesia 1·92. Ether vapour is flammable in air between 1·83% and 48%. Explosive in oxygen between 2% and 82%.

Chemical Properties
Relatively inert. Should be stored in a dark cool place.

It is largely unaltered in the body, 85–90% being eliminated by the lungs, a small amount metabolized to relatively non-toxic substances, alcohol, acetaldehyde and acetic acid.

Pharmacodynamics
Circulatory system. Heart rate is increased at first due to: (1) Catecholamines liberated; (2) Sympathetic stimulation; and (3) Vagal depression. Later, the heart rate is relatively unchanged. Blood pressure is well maintained if the autonomic system is intact.

---

*Born in Danielsville, Georgia, 1 Feb. 1815, the son of a state senator. Educated at the precursor of the University of Georgia and apprenticed to Dr Grant of Jefferson Ga. Further education at the University of Pennsylvania. Graduated 1839 and after working in New York settled with his former tutor in Jefferson. Removed a cyst from the neck of James Venables under ether anaesthesia 3 March 1842. A museum built on the site of Long's original office was dedicated in 1957, in Jefferson Ga.

Myocardium is depressed, but liberation of catecholamines offsets this. In deep ether anaesthesia β-blockade may be dangerous.

Dysrhythmias are rare. Adrenaline is relatively safe with ether.

Respiratory system. Respiratory movements first increase. This effect may be masked when a barbiturate or opioid has been given. They later decrease as anaesthesia deepens. In deep anaesthesia, as progressive respiratory depression develops, the respiratory centre is paralysed before the vasomotor centre. Respiratory rate increases, while amplitude decreases, as anaesthesia deepens. Salivary, but not bronchial, secretions are increased, while bronchial muscles are relaxed. Vapour is irritating, producing cough and laryngeal spasm, if introduced too rapidly. Hence induction of anaesthesia should be gradual, starting with a low ether tension.

Central nervous system. First analgesia, followed by excitement and then anaesthesia. Medullary depression is late and precedes serious cardiac depression. Cerebral blood flow is increased. Pressure of CSF rises. Ether clonus, an exaggerated response to stretch reflexes, is sometimes seen during light anaesthesia.

The sympathetic nervous system. Central stimulation, resulting in increase of plasma catecholamines with which is associated: (1) Increase of heart rate; (2) Increased production of glycogen and a raised blood-sugar level; (3) Contraction of spleen; (4) Dilatation of the gut and inhibition of its movements; (5) Bronchial dilatation; (6) Dilatation of coronary arteries; (7) Progressive dilatation of pupils; (8) Decreased limb blood flow with increased vascular resistance; (9) Increase in respiratory rate.

The parasympathetic system. Central depression.

Alimentary system. Nausea and vomiting occur in more than 50% of patients after ether anaesthesia. However, after use in minimal concentrations (2–3%) in air with muscle relaxants for major surgery, it is no worse than with other methods. Salivary and lacrimal glands are stimulated during induction and depressed later. Thus the tear in the corner of the eye is a useful sign of light, and the dry cornea of deep anaesthesia.

The urinary system. Urinary flow is diminished temporarily because of renal vascular constriction.

Skeletal muscle. Relaxation, which is good.

The pregnant uterus. Muscle tone inhibited, so that in deep anaesthesia relaxation is good. Ether passes the placental barrier and soon reaches the fetal blood.

Methods of Administration *(see* Chapters 9 and 30).

Advantages of Ether

1. It is relatively non-toxic especially in light planes of anaesthesia.

2. It will produce excellent relaxation without severe respiratory depression.

3. Respiratory depression with over-dosage is not accompanied by cardiac depression in the absence of hypoxia. IPPV will usually overcome this effect.

4. The products of its metabolism, alcohol, acetaldehyde and acetic acid are relatively non-toxic.

5. It has little tendency to cause dysrhythmias.

6. Thus ether is a very safe anaesthetic in the absence of severe hypoxia. For the unskilled anaesthetist dealing with the unfit patient it has a lot to commend it. It might be used more frequently today were it less flammable.

For more than a hundred years ether provided safe and efficient anaesthesia world-wide, and during most of that time it was given by the open-drop method on to a gauze mask.

Ether vapour 3% in air as from an EMO inhaler, with a muscle relaxant, produces a very safe, economical and acceptable anaesthetic.[70].

Disadvantages of Ether

1. Mucus secretion from the salivary glands and upper airway.
2. Nausea and vomiting, postoperatively.
3. The explosive risk, when used with oxygen or nitrous oxide.
4. Slow induction and recovery from anaesthesia (high blood/gas partition coefficient (12·0)). Irritative properties prevent rapid increase in vapour strength.

Light anaesthesia is obtained with an inspired concentration of 3–6%. Muscle relaxation requires up to 13%.

Ether Convulsions

The first use of barbiturates[71] (pentobarbitone) in the treatment of this condition was in 1933 and of curare in 1946.[72] The classic case is the feverish child with a perforated appendix, on a hot day, who receives atropine premedication and ether anaesthesia, with the surgeon continually requesting more relaxation. They are not due exclusively to ether and may occur during any inhalation anaesthetic. Convulsions occur most often in children and young adults and, as relaxation is now usually produced by the use of muscle relaxants, are seldom seen today.

Treatment. (1) Ventilate with oxygen. Stop administration of ether; (2) Abolish convulsive movement: (*a*) By use of a muscle relaxant; (*b*) By intravenous injection of thiopentone, 50–100 mg, or diazepam; (3) Prevent or treat hyperpyrexia.

Prevention. The possibility of convulsions must be borne in mind when deep ether is being given to produce muscular relaxation to patients who are hot (when it is better avoided).

Divinyl Ether [(C$_2$H$_3$)$_2$O]

History

Known also as divinyl oxide. Proprietary names, Vinesthene in Britain, Vinethene in the USA, Vinydan in Scandinavia. Originally prepared by F. W. Semmler (1865–1931) of Germany in 1887; anaesthetic properties discovered by Chauncey Depew Leake (1896–1978), American pharmacologist, and Mei-Yu Chen, Chinese pharmacologist, in the USA in 1930,[73] in an effort to combine the advantages of diethyl ether and ethylene. Used clinically by S. Gelfen, physiologist, and I. R. Bell (1882–1953), physician, of the University of Alberta in 1932.[74] (*See also* McConnell W. S. *Anaesthesia* 1975, **30**, 630.) No longer available in the UK. (For further information *see* earlier editions of this *Synopsis*; an obsolete drug.)

Ethyl Chloride [C$_2$H$_5$Cl]

History

Prepared by Guillaume Francis Rouelle (1703–1770), pharmacist of Paris, in 1759, and again by Marie-Jean Pierre Flourens (1794–1867) in 1847,[75] who described its anaesthetic properties. First used clinically by the surgeon, Ferdinand Martin

Heyfelder (1798–1869),[76] of Erlangen, Germany, in 1848, but was used thereafter for many years only as a local analgesic. Claes Hjalmat Carlson (1858–1937), Stockholm dental surgeon, in 1894, used it as a local spray to ease the pain of dental extraction and succeeded unexpectedly in producing general anaesthesia as the vapour was inhaled. Popularized by McCardie of Birmingham in 1901, by Lotheissen of Innsbruck in 1896, and in the USA by Ware in 1902. J. B. Bengué, a French anaesthetist, designed a suitable container fitted with an ingenious stopper which provided easy control of the flow of this very volatile liquid. Used in the first 4 decades of the 20th century for induction of anaesthesia on 'the open mask', prior to 'open-drop' ether, or as a sole agent for short operations. Now discarded. (For further information, *see* earlier editions of this *Synopsis*.)

Chloroform [CHCl₃]

History
As chloroform played a very important part in the introduction and development of surgical anaesthesia, its history is given here in some detail. Prepared in 1831 by Justus von Leibig (1803–1873) of Darmstadt, by Samuel Guthrie (1782–1848), of Sacketts Harbor, NY, in 1832 (*see* Pawling J. R. *Dr Samuel Guthrie: Discoverer of Chloroform*. Watertown, NY: The Brewster Press, 1947), and by Eugène Soubeiran (1793–1858), Paris pharmacist, in 1831. It was known as 'chloric ether', 'Dutch liquid', 'bichloric ether', 'chloride of carbon' and 'perchloride of formyle'. Jean-Baptiste André Dumas (1800–1884), Paris chemist, described its physical and chemical properties in 1834 and gave it the name 'chloroform' because of its relationships to chlorine and formic acid.[77] Anaesthetic properties discovered by Jean Pierre Marie Flourens (1794–1867),[78] Paris physiologist, in 1847 in animals before Simpson used it in humans. Used (in the form of chloric ether) at St Bartholomew's Hospital by Holmes Coote (at the suggestion of Furnell) in the spring of 1847,[79] 6 months before Simpson. Introduced to clinical practice and popularized by James Young Simpson and his assistants, James Mathews Duncan (1826–1890) and George Keith, after experimenting on themselves, in Edinburgh in November 1847, at the suggestion of David Waldie (1813–1889), a Liverpool chemist.[80] Within a few months chloroform superseded ether as the most popular anaesthetic agent. The first reported death due to chloroform was that of Hannah Greener of Winlayton, near Newcastle-upon-Tyne, little more than two months after its introduction (28 Jan. 1848). The anaesthetic was given for a minor operation by Dr Meggison. John Snow gave over 4000 chloroform anaesthetics without a death and, early on, recommended that for safety a concentration of not more than 4% in air should be used. To increase its safety, its administration with oxygen was recommended in 1850.[81] It was the favourite anaesthetic agent used by surgeons in the South (but not in the North) during the American Civil War, and in the Franco–Prussian War. Following 1890, reports of liver damage appeared in the literature (Guthrie, 1894).[82] The dangers of the drug were early recognized and in 1864 the first of many investigations into the causes of these was set up by the Royal Medico-Chirurgical Chloroform Committee. Their report recommended a mixture of chloroform with ether, e.g. ACE mixture (Alcohol 1 part, Chloroform 2 parts and Ether 3 parts) of Harley (1829–1896) described in 1860. It led to the first disenchantment with chloroform.[83] In 1888–1889, the First and Second Hyderabad Commission

suggested that chloroform depressed the respiration before the heart, a fact now known to be incorrect. In 1911, Goodman Levy (1856–1954) showed that death due to ventricular fibrillation might occur in light anaesthesia, never in deep anaesthesia, irrespective of concentration of vapour or over-dosage.[84]

Light chloroform analgesia given to Queen Victoria by John Snow for birth of her last two children, Prince Leopold (7 May 1853) and Princess Beatrice (14 May 1857). This removed the social stigma formerly associated with obstetric analgesia.

See also Sibson S. F. (1814–1876) 'On death from chloroform' *Lond. Med. Gaz.* 1848, **42**, 108; Featherstone H. *Anesthesiology* 1947, **8**, 362; Kindschi D. R. *Anesthesiology* 1948, **9**, 1; Sykes W. S. *Essays on the First Hundred Years of Anaesthesia*, Vols I and II. Edinburgh: Livingstone, 1960, 1961; *Chloroform, A Study after One Hundred Years* (Waters R. ed.). Madison: University of Wisconsin Press, 1951; Little D. A. *Surv. Anesthesiol.* 1965, **9**, 508; Atkinson R. S. *Simpson and Chloroform*. London: Priory Press, 1973; Thomas K. Bryn *Proc. R. Soc. Med.* 1974, **67**, 723; Poobalasingham N. and Payne J. P. *Br. J. Anaesth.* 1978, **50**, 305; Payne J. P. *Br. J. Anaesth.* 1981, **53**, 115; Jones I. W. 'Chloroform anaesthesia in Liverpool' *Anaesthesia* 1983, **38**, 578.

Pharmacodynamics
Prolonged inhalation of 2% vapour may produce respiratory arrest, but induction will require about 4%. Its use is largely given up because of tissue toxicity and action on heart.

Cardiovascular system. Blood pressure: Gradually falls as with halothane.

Sudden cardiac standstill, occurring during light anaesthesia,[85] may be due to:

1. *Ventricular fibrillation* (first described by McWilliam in 1890).[86] Over half the deaths from chloroform occur in the first few minutes of induction and are due to this cause.[87] Adrenaline, endogenous or exogenous, acts on the chloroform-sensitized myocardium to produce dysrhythmia which may end as ventricular fibrillation. *Thus, adrenaline is contraindicated during chloroform anaesthesia.* An increase in the P_{CO_2} predisposes to ventricular fibrillation.

2. *Vagal inhibition.*[88] E. Weber and W. D. Weber in 1845 discovered that peripheral stimulation of the vagus would inhibit cardiac action. A sudden inhalation or insufflation of a strong chloroform vapour may stimulate the vagus and so cause syncope. Atropine may be protective.

3. *Depression of the myocardium.* Depression increases with depth of anaesthesia.

Delayed chloroform poisoning.[89] A toxic hepatitis. First described by Caspar[90] (1796–1864) in 1850. May occur from the first to the third day after anaesthesia. More likely to follow repeated administrations. The symptoms are increasing nausea and vomiting, with jaundice, prostration and coma, and perhaps death.

Disadvantages
Occasional sudden death, even in experienced hands.

(For a fuller account of chloroform, *see* earlier editions of this *Synopsis*.)

Trichloroethylene, BP [CCl₂CHCl]
(Trichlorethylene, Trilene, Trimar)

History
First described in 1864 by E. Fischer (1852–1919), chemist, of Jena,[91] since when

it has been used in industry both as a fat solvent and in the dry-cleaning trade. Its poisonous properties have been long recognized (Plessner, 1916),[92] especially its power to produce analgesia in distribution of fifth cranial nerve (Oppenheim, of Berlin, 1915). On this account it has been used to relieve the pain of trigeminal neuralgia. Relief afforded is probably not a local action but part of a general analgesia. General anaesthetic effects described by Karl B. Lehmann (1858–1940) of Würzburg in 1911[93] and by Dennis Jackson[94] of Cincinnati in 1933.

Cecil Striker[95] (1897–) used it to anaesthetize 300 patients in 1935, but its introduction to clinical anaesthesia was due to Christopher Langton Hewer (1896–1986) of St Bartholomew's Hospital, London, who published case reports in 1941.[96]

Physical Properties
Colourless liquid. Molecular weight 131·4. Specific gravity 1·47. Boiling point high 87 °C, and saturated vapour pressure at 20 °C is 60 mmHg, so volatility is low. Partition coefficients: oil/water 400, blood/gas 9·0 (hence induction and recovery are slow), fat/blood 106·7. MAC 0·17 vol %. Will not burn or explode under clinical conditions. May be decomposed into phosgene ($COCl_2$) and hydrochloric acid at temperatures above 125 °C as by the cautery, especially in the presence of oxygen. Vapour density 4·35 (air = 1). Stored in amber glass or aluminium containers, as it is decomposed by sunlight. For anaesthesia the proprietary form of the drug known as 'Trilene' is used. It is coloured blue for identification purposes (1:200 000 waxoline blue) and contains 0·01% of thymol, to retard decomposition.

Pharmacology
Central nervous system. Trichloroethylene should not be used to produce deep anaesthesia, since untoward side-effects (*see below*) are likely to develop. It is useful for the production of analgesia without loss of consciousness.
Trichloroethylene and soda-lime. If used in a closed circuit with soda-lime, toxic products may be formed,[97] the most important being dichloracetylene:

$$C_2HCl_3 + NaOH \rightarrow C_2Cl_2 \text{ (dichloracetylene)} + NaCl + H_2O$$

This is a potent nerve poison and may produce paralysis of cranial nerves or even death. The fifth and seventh nerves are most commonly involved, but interferences with the third, fourth, sixth, tenth and twelfth nerves have been reported. These lesions may be temporary or permanent. This danger is much less with modern brands of soda-lime which do not get so hot. The reaction to form dichloracetylene is much accelerated about 60 °C whereas present-day soda-lime does not get much above 40 °C.
Cardiovascular system. Cardiovascular stability is seen with this agent and constitutes one of its main advantages. The main effect is the production of dysrhythmias. These may be vagal (nodal rhythm) or sympathetic (ventricular ectopic beats).

Trichloroethylene sensitizes the heart to the effects of adrenaline and other beta-adrenergic stimulants and many anaesthetists believe that the two drugs should not be used in the same patient. Others permit their careful use.
Respiratory system. Tachypnoea is probably due to a peripheral action in the lung,[98] which is less efficient in terms of gaseous exchange than slow deeper

breathing, for the same minute volume. Thus a fall in Po_2 has been found with severe tachypnoea, and there is a rise in Pco_2, which in turn may predispose to dysrhythmias. Narcotic analgesics are useful in controlling tachypnoea and in providing an alternative analgesic supplement if dysrhythmias occur.

Alimentary system. Postoperative nausea and vomiting more common than after halothane. Not hepatotoxic.

Muscular system. Relaxation is poor.

Pharmacokinetics. Induction is relatively slow and it takes a long time for the patient to become saturated. The longer the exposure to trichloroethylene, the longer the recovery time, and the sooner the agent should be discontinued before the end of operation.

A small amount undergoes change in the body with the formation of trichloracetic acid, which is pharmacologically inert, and which is excreted by the kidneys over a period of several days.

Toxicity. Biotransformation is greater than with any other volatile agent. After chronic exposure to trichloroethylene vapour (in industry) a diagnosis of trichloroethylene intoxication can be made if more than 7·5 mg of trichloracetic acid/100 ml of urine are present. There have also been identified two other metabolites, monochloracetic acid, a toxic agent found in small amounts, and trichloroethanol (similar to tribromethanol in its action) in larger amounts.

Methods of Adminstration
Trichloroethylene is used either as a supplement to nitrous-oxide–oxygen in the production of full surgical anaesthesia at a light plane, or as an agent in its own right for the production of a state of analgesia.

1. Trichloroethylene and surgical anaesthesia. An opioid is desirable to prevent tachypnoea, either with the premedication or during the administration. It is wise to give something more than a sleep dose of thiopentone for induction, so that a reasonable level of 'basal narcosis' will exist and trichloroethylene will not have to be 'pushed'. Following thiopentone, trichloroethylene should be added gradually to nitrous oxide and oxygen. It may be necessary to give a relatively high concentration for a few minutes to settle the patient, but this can later be reduced.

The maintenance concentration of vapour should be of the order of 0·5%, that is, slightly more than can just be appreciated by smell.

This method of administration is useful in a wide range of surgical operations where muscular relaxation is not necessary, but tolerance of a tracheal tube is required. It is also useful as a supplement to nitrous oxide oxygen, to prevent awareness during IPPV with full doses of muscle relaxant drugs.

Trichloroethylene in air has been used with muscle relaxants for major surgery with good results.[99] The slow induction time and cumulative effect (due to the high blood/gas partition coefficient) can be easily overcome by starting off with a loading dose (0·5%) then gradually reducing to 0·2%.[100]

2. Trichloroethylene and analgesia. This agent produces excellent analgesia in labour, 0·5% w/v in air being a suitable concentration for intermittent inhalation lasting several hours.

Advantages of Trichloroethylene
(1) A good analgesic; useful supplement of nitrous-oxide–oxygen; (2) Relative lack of irritation of upper respiratory tract; (3) Non-flammable; (4) Does not depress cardiovascular system; (5) Does not depress respiration; (6) Vastly less

expensive than halothane, enflurane or isoflurane. Can be used as the analgesic component of balanced anaesthesia, using 0·2% with IPPV.[101]

Disadvantages
(1) Tachypnoea may occur; (2) Dysrhythmias may occur; (3) Does not provide muscular relaxation; (4) May cause postoperative nausea and vomiting; (5) Cannot be used with soda-lime; (6) Addiction has been reported; (7) The slight possibility of mutagenic effects in pregnancy.

Uses of Trichloroethylene
   1. To maintain light anaesthesia.
   2. As a non-depressant inhalation supplement during induction of anaesthesia for transplant surgery, cardiac and liver.
   3. To produce analgesia in obstetrics and in various painful surgical procedures.
   4. To avoid 'awareness' and diminish sensory input during maintenance, when muscle relaxants and IPPV are used.
   In the authors' opinion this drug has a useful place in modern anaesthetic practice.
   See also Ostlere G. *Trichloroethylene Anaesthesia.* Edinburgh and London: Livingstone, 1953; review article, Atkinson R. S. *Anesthesiology* 1960, **21**, 67; Dobkin A. B. and Byles P. H. in: *Clinical Anaesthesia—Halogenated Anaesthetics* (Artusio J. F. ed.). Oxford: Blackwell, 1963, Ch. 3; Hewer C. L. *Anaesthesia* 1975, **30**, 476.

Halothane *(Fluothane)*
This is 2,bromo-2-chloro-1,1,1,trifluoroethane.

History
Synthesized in the laboratories of Imperial Chemical Industries near Manchester by C. W. Suckling in 1951[102] and studied pharmacologically by James Raventós (1905–1983)[103] in succeeding years. Used clinically in 1956 by M. Johnstone[104] of Manchester followed by Bryce-Smith and O'Brien[105] of Oxford.

Physical Properties
A colourless liquid volatile anaesthetic with molecular weight 197, specific gravity 1·87, boiling point 50°C, saturated vapour pressure at 20°C 243 mmHg. Minimal alveolar concentration for anaesthesia 0·75 vol %. Has a characteristic odour. Oil/water solubility coefficient 220. Blood/gas partition coefficient 2·5 (which is low); fat/blood 60·0; brain/blood 2·6. Decomposed by light (stabilized by 0·01% thymol), but is stable when stored in amber-coloured bottles. It can be used safely with soda-lime. The vapour is absorbed by rubber (rubber/gas partition coefficient at 20°C is 120). In the presence of moisture it attacks tin, brass and aluminium in vaporizers and circuits. Non-flammable and non-explosive when its vapour is mixed with oxygen in any concentration (or under hyperbaric conditions) used clinically. May be decomposed by an open flame liberating bromine.

Pharmacodynamics
A potent anaesthetic agent. Vapour is pleasant to smell and is non-irritant. For

induction of anaesthesia, 2–4% vapour is necessary; for maintenance, 0·5–2%. It is a very potent agent and has caused deaths from cardiovascular depression, often because of relative over-dosage.

Cardiovascular system

Arterial pressure falls, though not invariably. Cardiac output falls as a result of depression of the myocardium.[106] Dilatation of the smooth muscles of blood vessels (including the coronary arteries), sympathetic ganglionic blockade and central vasomotor depression contribute to a fall in arterial pressure. Cardiac output may fall as a result of bradycardia due to halothane, an effect reversed by atropine. Treatment with beta-blocking drugs does not contra-indicate careful halothane anaesthesia.[107]

During halothane anaesthesia, care must be taken when the patient is moved or when ganglionic blocking drugs are given in case hypotension is exacerbated. Blood volume should be maintained by infusion or transfusion.

Dysrhythmias. (1) Increased myocardial excitability; ventricular extrasystoles, ventricular tachycardia and even ventricular fibrillation. Factors which increase the likelihood of ventricular dysrhythmias include carbon dioxide retention, sensory stimulation in light anaesthesia, and the injection of drugs with a beta-stimulant effect. Cardiac arrest has been reported following adrenaline infiltration during halothane anaesthesia. Other workers have used the combination without incident. Intravenous infusions of adrenaline or noradrenaline during halothane anaesthesia at rates of more than 10 µg/min have been found to provoke dysrhythmias.[108] It has been recommended[109] that adrenaline infiltration may be safely used in a dosage of 10 ml of 1 in 100 000 concentration in a 10-min period or 30 ml/h, provided ventilation is adequate. (2) Bradycardia, which may be associated with hypotension. Atropine given intravenously may speed the pulse rate and produce a rise in blood pressure,[110] but it should be given slowly as it may itself produce ventricular dysrhythmias. Nodal rhythm; rarely of serious import. Dysrhythmias may be treated by the withdrawal of halothane, substituting another drug; by ensuring that arterial tensions of oxygen and carbon dioxide are within normal limits; and rarely by administration of a beta-blocking agent.

Alimentary system. The secretion of saliva, mucus and gastric juice is not stimulated, while postoperative nausea and vomiting are seldom severe. Motility of gastrointestinal tract inhibited.

Central nervous system. It is a potent anaesthetic, but not a good analgesic at low concentrations. It increases cerebral circulation and raises the CSF pressure.

Respiratory system. A respiratory depressant. Respiratory rate increased and depth decreased. Bronchial relaxation may be due to blockage of reflex pathways causing bronchoconstriction, rather than to depression of bronchial muscular tone. Not a bronchial irritant; pharyngeal and laryngeal reflexes depressed early, and secretions not stimulated. Control of respiration is facilitated by halothane but care is necessary to prevent rapid uptake as a result of increased alveolar ventilation with consequent hypotension due to myocardial depression.

Muscular system. Moderate relaxation is produced by anaesthetic concentrations and the masseters are relaxed early, making laryngoscopy relatively easy. Abdominal relaxation can be produced by deep planes of anaesthesia.

The uterus. Halothane may cause uterine atony and post-partum haemorrhage if used in obstetrics. This makes it potentially dangerous as an anaesthetic agent for operative delivery, though it is an excellent anaesthetic for external version. Many anaesthetists find it useful in operative delivery if used in low concentration (0·5%) so as to preserve uterine tone, while maintaining or even increasing placental blood flow, but this practice is not recommended for the tiro.

Halothane, even in concentrations as low as 0·5% may produce increase in blood loss during therapeutic abortion,[111] even when oxytocin is administered. It may be that the uterine muscle behaves differently in late pregnancy as compared with the earlier trimesters.

The liver. We believe that halothane hepatitis is a real clinical entity.[112] Massive hepatic necrosis following halothane anaesthesia was reported in 1958,[113] though widespread attention was not drawn to the problem until 1963. Subclinical 'halothane-hepatitis' may also occur.[114] Since 1964 there have been large retrospective surveys,[115] including the National Halothane Study carried out by the American National Academy of Sciences.[116] The general conclusion was that the incidence of liver failure is no higher after halothane than after other anaesthetics, and there was no evidence that patients with biliary tract disease were unduly susceptible. It is now accepted that on rare occasions halothane may be toxic to the liver. Theories include:

1. *Toxic reaction to a metabolite.* Up to 20% of halothane in body tissue may be degraded. Biotransformation is complex, many compounds being formed, but it is considered by many workers that the products of the reductive metabolic pathways are more dangerous than those arising from oxidative metabolism. Patients who suffer from hypoxaemia during or after operation may be at risk and this includes those of middle age, especially females, and the obese. Nitrous oxide has been shown to potentiate the hepatotoxicity of hypoxic, enzyme-induced rats. Nitrous oxide has complex effects on both folate and methionine metabolism and may thereby increase the likelihood of liver damage from toxic agents.[117]

2. *Hypersensitivity reactions.* The anaesthetist should be wary of repeated administration within 100 days. There may be hypersensitivity reactions to halothane.[118] or a halothane metabolite which may be present in higher concentrations during states of enzyme induction which may be associated with the administration of other drugs or with stress associated with the surgical condition. Patients at particular risk may include those with a tendency to develop organ-specific autoimmune disease. There is evidence that covalent binding to plasma proteins may be important.

3. *Genetic factors.* These may be of importance.

The jaundice, which may be associated with halothane anaesthesia, is hepatocellular. Biochemical changes include elevation of aminotransferases.

Histology may be able to exclude other causes of jaundice following liver biopsy, but it is difficult to differentiate between virus A and drug hepatitis.

Animal experiments show a correlation between cytochrome P450 enzymes and liver damage. Lipid peroxidation occurs in man after administration of clinical concentrations of halothane for 2 h. The importance of these investigations is not fully understood and more work remains to be done.

In a full and comprehensive survey of the present position,[119] the conclusions reached are that

1. Halothane can be given to children repeatedly as there is a very small risk factor.

2. Pre-existing liver disease, provided that it is not due to a previous halothane administration, is no contraindication, although acute liver dysfunction from any cause may well contraindicate any form of surgery and anaesthesia.

3. Severe liver damage is unlikely to follow a single administration of halothane.

4. Repeated administration to adults, particularly obese, middle-aged women, at intervals less than say 12 weeks, may cause acute liver damage. There is no means of predicting this, and the exact 'safe interval' is not known.

5. If a repeated halothane administration is contemplated, the reasons for the anaesthestist's choice should, for medicolegal reasons be charted, while the records of the earlier administration should if possible be scrutinized for any problems that may have arisen. Should these have been present, then no second administration should be undertaken.

The cause of the condition is unclear and there is no test that is specific for halothane induced liver damage, so that the diagnosis must be made by a process of elimination of all other possible causes. Metabolic problems alone are an unlikely cause.

Other causes of postoperative jaundice include the effect of drugs (such as phenothiazines, monoamine oxidase inhibitors, intravenous tetracycline), blood transfusion, shock, benign postoperative cholestasis, septic cholangitis, coincidental virus hepatitis.[120] Hepatitis B antigen[121] should be excluded. Stress and starvation may produce overt jaundice in subjects with Gilbert's syndrome[122] (familial unconjugated hyperbilirubinaemia) but the serum transaminases remain normal.

Metabolism of halothane.[123] Evidence in humans that enzymatic metabolism occurs include the appearance of bromide, chloride, trifluoracetylethanolamide chlorobromodifluoroethylene, and trifluoroacetic acid in the urine. This last is relatively non-toxic and is the main oxidative metabolite. Metabolites are slowly cleared from the body for as long as 3 weeks.

Renal function. Progressive reduction in renal blood flow and glomerular filtration rate as anaesthesia deepens. Urinary flow decreased. Antidiuretic hormone released. Hypotension may be responsible for some of these changes.

Hormonal effects. There is an increase in plasma growth hormone during operation under halothane anaesthesia. Adrenocortical responses are evoked via the anterior pituitary. Serum thyroxine levels are increased, but not pituitary thyroid-stimulating hormone. Plasma insulin levels do not change appreciably.

Blood sugar is not affected, but sensitivity to insulin is increased. Care should be taken when halothane is administered to a diabetic patient receiving insulin lest hypoglycaemia should occur.

Use with muscle relaxants. Non-depolarizing relaxants are potentiated. The ganglionic-blocking effect of tubocurarine is potentiated and hypotension may result. Halothane somewhat antagonizes the effects of suxamethonium, but this is not important clinically.

Temperature. Induction of anaesthesia with halothane is soon followed by a drop of up to 1 °C in oesophageal temperature, together with a rise of up to 4 °C in skin temperature. This is thought to be due to a redistribution between core and peripheral tissues. Later, skin temperature may fall as peripheral vasodilatation aids heat loss. Hence sometimes used during surface cooling to obtain hypothermia.

Shivering. Shivering and tremor have frequently been reported during the immediate postoperative period following halothane anaesthesia. It may be associated with a generalized increase in muscle tone, clonic or tonic. There may sometimes be an association between shivering and temperature falls during anaesthesia, and it has been suggested that the former can be prevented by delivering warmed humidified gases to patients during surgery.[124] Methyl phenidate (Ritalin) up to 20 mg i.v. or opioids have been recommended for treatment.

Immune system. It has been known for 80 years that volatile anaesthetic agents impair the ability of human neutrophil leucocytes to kill bacteria. Recent work[125] suggests that decreased mobilization of intracellular calcium appears to be one of the mechanisms by which the volatile agents halothane, and to a lesser extent enflurane and isoflurane inhibit the generation of superoxide ions (O_2^{-1}) in human neutrophils. This is related to their ability to kill bacteria and to destroy metastatic cancer cells. It is also suggested that prolonged anaesthesia with these agents may call for extra prophylaxis against infection and metastatic tumour cell survival.

Clinical Use

Premedication. Because halothane is a respiratory depressant, premedication with an opioid may be avoided unless it is intended to assist or control respiration. Atropine may prevent the development of bradycardia and reverse the decrease in cardiac output.[126]

Halothane in a high gas flow system. Halothane is often used as a supplement to thiopentone–nitrous-oxide–oxygen. The analgesic properties are poor so that reflex activity (e.g. movement with skin incision) may occur in light planes. The potency of halothane, however, allows rapid increase of depth of anaesthesia so that the patient will tolerate surgical stimulation or a tracheal tube and exhibit moderate degrees of muscular relaxation.

Halothane in a low gas flow system with rebreathing. Halothane can be administered in conjunction with either a to-and-fro or a circle absorption system. The authors find that a fresh gas flow of 1 litre/min of oxygen, together with 2–3% halothane is satisfactory for maintenance of anaesthesia. This is economical and causes little pollution of the atmosphere. The theory of administration differs according to whether the vaporizer is within the rebreathing system, or in the flow of fresh gases to that system.[127]

Vaporizer outside circuit (VOC)[127]: Halothane is vaporized by the flow of fresh gases to the circuit. The carrier gas may be nitrous oxide with 50% of oxygen or pure oxygen. If this flow is small, it follows that the vaporizer must be very efficient, and calibrated for low flows. Higher flows can be used if the expiratory valve is opened.

Vaporizer in circuit (VIC)[127] (e.g. the Goldman inhaler in a circle system). Halothane is vaporized by the patient's own respiratory effort. The deeper the breathing, the more halothane is vaporized. As anaesthesia deepens, respirations become depressed and less halothane is vaporized. The vaporizer must be relatively inefficient (cf. VOC) to prevent over-dosage, and must offer little resistance to respiration. Controlled or assisted respiration must be used with the greatest care, since they result in the addition of a large amount of halothane vapour into the system. Now seldom used.

The safety of closed system administration depends on the fact that saturation of the body tissues with halothane is not achieved for many hours.[128] This is because of the very high oil/water partition coefficient which is 220. Halothane is continually being removed from the blood as it passes to fat, and this is balanced by uptake of halothane from the alveoli. Hence the halothane concentration added to the system becomes diluted (VOC). The inspired concentration is, therefore, always less than the concentration delivered from the vaporizer (VOC), and if the vaporizers are switched off (VOC or VIC) the plane of anaesthesia lightens, even if there is apnoea.

Vaporizers. Because of the potency of halothane, accurate and fine control of vapour strength is required, and calibrated vaporizers have been designed:

1. *Fluotec vaporizer* (Cyprane Ltd).[129] Remains accurate despite changes in temperature, passage of time, amount of liquid in the container and gas flow (within limits). It utilizes the principle of a bimetallic strip as a temperature compensator. The entering gas is split into two streams, one bypassing the vaporizer, the other entering the vaporizing chamber where it becomes saturated with the volatile agent being used. When the two streams rejoin, the concentration of the issuing vapour can be calculated if the saturated vapour pressure of the volatile agent and the splitting ratios of the two flows are known. Mark 3[130] is superior to the Mark 2 vaporizer in that it does not give a relatively higher output at low flows and the back-pressure effect during IPPV is negligible. New modifications include the Selectatec for easy change of vaporizer. They should always remain upright so that liquid cannot reach the upper chamber.

There is a small difference in halothane output according to whether oxygen or nitrous oxide is used as the carrier gas.[131] At 0·5% and 1% settings the output is higher with oxygen (related to carrier gas density). At 2, 3 and 4% settings the output is higher with nitrous oxide (related to gas viscosity).

2. *The Goldman vaporizer.*[132] A simple apparatus without temperature control, commonly used with an intermittent nitrous-oxide–oxygen machine (Walton or McKesson) or a Boyle machine. *Table 10.2* indicates the halothane percentage delivered (v/v) with 20 ml in bowl at 20 °C after 1 min for the Mark 2 vaporizer.

Table 10.2. Halothane percentage delivered

Position	Gas flow Litres/min		
	2	8	30
1	0·1	0·1	0·1
2	0·5	1·0	1·0
3	1·5	2·5	1·5
ON	1·5	3·0	1·5

From Goldman V. *Anaesthesia* 1962, **17**, 537.

The incorporation of a wick made from blotting paper increases the maximal concentration by about 1%, and enhances clinical efficiency.[133] The McKesson vaporizer acts similarly.

3. *The Copper Kettle.*[134] This is a very efficient vaporizer described in 1952. It employs the principle of metering the variable flow of oxygen as a carrier gas through liquid anaesthetic, and subsequently mixing the saturated vapour with known volumes of diluent gases to provide delicate control over the resultant vapour concentration as though the vapour itself were being metered.

4. *The Halox vaporizer.*[135] This works on a similar principle to the Copper Kettle, but is made of glass. A thermometer is built in so that the temperature of the liquid halothane is known.

5. *The Dräger vaporizer.* A temperature-compensated vaporizer which delivers constant and accurate concentrations of vapour over a range of gas flows between 0·3 and 12 litres/min. It is unaffected by pressure fluctuations produced by the action of a ventilator but offers a high resistance so cannot be used in the breathing system. Very accurate.

6. *The Oxford miniature vaporizer,*[136] with a range of up to 3·5%, originally designed to pave the way for an ether maintenance, but can be used as a vaporizer in its own right.

7. *The Penlon drawover vaporizer, Mark 2.* This is thermocompensated, is efficient at flows from 4 to 14 litres/min and provides a concentration of up to 6%.

8. *The Blease universal vaporizer.* This is a development of the Gardner vaporizer which can be used for vaporizing all volatile anaesthetic agents.

9. *The Fluoxair* (*see* Chapter 30).

10. *The EMO draw-over apparatus* with air as the carrier gas.

Vaporizers should be drained regularly to prevent accumulation of thymol[137] which can reach a concentration 19 times that usually present.

Indications

The introduction of halothane revolutionized anaesthetic practice 30 years ago and with enflurane and isoflurane, has wide applications in nearly all types of surgery. Particularly useful in patients with chronic respiratory disease and for cystoscopy in day-stay patients. Useful for external version in obstetrics. Reduces bleeding by producing mild hypotension in suitable patients. Widely used in dental outpatient anaesthesia.

Disadvantages

1. Potency. The drug is very potent and an overdose is easily given.

2. Poor analgesic properties. Full surgical anaesthesia must be achieved to prevent reaction to painful stimuli. There is also little or no postoperative analgesia.

3. May cause uterine relaxation with consequent haemorrhage in obstetric practice.

4. Hypotension, which may or may not be undesirable.

5. Dysrhythmias may occur, though they are seldom serious.

6. It may cause shivering or tremor, sometimes of a severe nature, in the immediate postoperative period.

7. Remote possibility of liver toxicity, especially with repeated administrations.

Advantages

1. Rapid smooth induction.

2. Non-irritant to respiratory tract.

3. May produce bronchodilatation.

4. Produces vasodilatation.

5. Relatively rapid recovery.

Halothane may be used in clinical anaesthesia: (1) In minimal concentrations as a supplement to thiopentone–nitrous-oxide–oxygen, as part of a balanced technique; (2) In greater concentration as the main anaesthetic agent. In the latter case addition of nitrous oxide to the anaesthetic mixture has little advantage,[138] although it slightly reduces the amount of halothane needed.

The authors find halothane an excellent anaesthetic, though it can cause grave circulatory depression. Should this occur, the reservoir bag should be emptied, the halothane vaporizer turned off, the patient ventilated with pure oxygen and the table tilted head-down. This will usually reverse the depression. Anaesthesia can then be continued using an alternative agent. Occupational exposure to halothane may result in enzyme induction in anaesthetists; this may be either beneficial or harmful.[139]

Its introduction by Suckling, Raventos and Johnstone in 1956 had an enormous influence on clinical anaesthesia.

It is our current opinion (like that of many professors of anaesthesia in the UK)[168] that we favour its use if we think that it is clinically indicated. We advise that reasons for repeated use should be documented.

Enflurane *(Ethrane, Alyrane)*

History
The first clinical account on enflurane appeared in 1966.[140] Developed by Ross Terrell in the USA in 1963.

Physical Properties
This is 1,1,2-trifluoro-2-chloroethyl difluoromethyl ether (CHF_2-O-CF_2CHFCl) with molecular weight 184, boiling point 56·5; vapour density 180; MAC 1·68 in oxygen, 1·28 in 70% nitrous oxide; partition coefficients at 37 °C blood/gas 1·91; oil/gas 98·5; water/gas 0·78. Concentrations above 4·25% are flammable in 20% oxygen in nitrous oxide. Stable with soda-lime and metals. Contains no preservative.

Pharmacodynamics
The central nervous system. A potent anaesthetic. EEG changes of an epileptiform nature may occur which are more common during hypocapnia and may persist for several weeks.[141] Cerebral blood flow increased.
The cardiovascular system. As depth of anaesthesia is increased, there is a reversible fall in arterial pressure due to myocardial depression. Serious dysrhythmias uncommon. Relatively safe when adrenaline infiltration used; up to three times the dose permitted with halothane is reported to be safe.[142]
The respiratory system. Pulmonary ventilation depressed; tidal volume decreased, perhaps with a rise in respiratory rate. Salivary and bronchial secretions not increased. May cause occasional sighing respiration.
Muscular relaxation. Produces moderate relaxation. The activity of non-depolarizing relaxants is enhanced;[143] activity of suxamethonium not altered.
The liver.[144] Cross-sensitization between halothane and enflurane has been postulated.[145]
Pharmacokinetics. Mostly by lungs. About 3% is metabolized in the body and the fluoride ion excreted by the kidney.
Use in obstetrics. Has been used successfully in low concentrations (0·5–0·8%) in anaesthesia for Caesarean section without causing depression of the fetus.[146]

Clinical uses. Less potent than halothane and therefore a higher concentration is required for equivalent effect. Levels of anaesthesia can be changed quickly, while emergence is smooth and reasonably rapid, with shivering, nausea and vomiting infrequent. For induction up to 5%, for maintenance 1·5–3%.

Contraindications. Renal failure.

See also 'Symposium on Enflurane', *Acta Anaesth. Belge* 1974, **25**, No. 2; Savege T. M. in: *Recent Advances in Anaesthesia*—13 (Hewer C. L. and Atkinson R. S. ed.). Edinburgh: Churchill Livingstone, 1979; Black G. W. *Br. J. Anaesth.* 1979, **51**, 277; Editorial, *Anaesthesia* 1979, **34**, 755.

Isoflurane *(Forane; Aerrane; Nederane)*. [$CH_2.OCHCl.CF_3$] An isomer of enflurane

History

Isoflurane is a fluorinated methyl ethyl ether synthesized by Ross Terrell in 1965. The same worker had synthesized enflurane in 1963.[147] Used in clinical anaesthesia by Dobkin et al., 1971[148] and Stevens et al.[149]

Physical Properties

A colourless volatile liquid with properties outlined in *Table 10.1*. The saturated vapour pressure is similar to that of halothane. Theoretically it could be used in the same vaporizer as halothane though this is not recommended on safety grounds. Induction and recovery are rapid, partly because the blood/gas partition coefficient is lower (1·4) than that of halothane or enflurane, but also because the fat solubility is only about half that of halothane. MAC is 1·15 in oxygen and 0·66 in 70% nitrous oxide. Isoflurane is stable and no preservatives are necessary to prevent its decomposition. It does not react with metal in breathing systems. BP 48·5 °C.

Pharmacodynamics

Cardiovascular system. Isoflurane is a myocardial depressant[150] but it has less effect on the heart muscle than either halothane or enflurane. Systemic arterial blood pressure falls during isoflurane anaesthesia,[151] principally as a result of a fall in systemic vascular resistance.[152] It is, therefore, in theory, a better agent to produce deliberate hypotension than halothane (which causes a fall in cardiac output). Isoflurane anaesthesia is associated with a stable cardiac rhythm and the myocardium is not sensitized to catecholamines.[153] Heart rate may increase, especially in young patients.

Respiration. Like halothane and enflurane, isoflurane causes a decrease in tidal volume and increase in respiratory rate.[154] In terms of respiratory depression, it occupies a position intermediate between halothane and enflurane. Isoflurane depresses the respiratory response to hypoxaemia and hypercapnia. The incidence of coughing and laryngospasm during induction is greater than with halothane[155] as the vapour is mildly irritant.

Central nervous system. Low concentrations do not cause any increase in cerebral blood flow, provided that the $Paco_2$ is normal.[156] Therefore it has some superiority over halothane and enflurane in neurosurgical anaesthesia. However, larger concentrations do increase cerebral blood flow. It has no protective effect on the development of post-traumatic cerebral oedema[157] and does not produce changes in the EEG. It may, however, offer some protection against the cerebral effect of hypoxia.[158]

Muscle tone. Like halothane and enflurane, isoflurane relaxes muscles, often satisfactory for abdominal surgery, but at the expense of cardiorespiratory depression.

The reproductive system. The effect on the pregnant uterus is similar to that of halothane and enflurane and is dose related. In a concentration of 0·74% it has been used successfully in Caesarean section.[159]

Pharmacokinetics

Only about 0·2% of inhaled isoflurane can be recovered as urinary metabolites.[160] Serum fluoride after 3 MAC hours' exposure amounts to only about 5% of the levels associated with renal toxicity.[161] The likelihood of renal or hepatic toxicity following isoflurane anaesthesia is thought to be very low. Its ability to provoke malignant hyperpyrexia in susceptible subjects has not yet been evaluated.

Indications

Of the various inhalation agents available, isoflurane has the advantage of providing stability of cardiac rhythm and lack of sensitization of the heart to exogenous and endogenous adrenaline. Rapid awakening may be an advantage in the day-stay patient. The drug has a stable molecule and is unlikely to be toxic to the vital organs. It produces hypotension with less cardiac depressant action than halothane. It has been estimated that in the USA where the drug has been available for some years, about one-half of the anaesthetics administered with volatile agents incorporate isoflurane. For maintenance 1–2·5%.

The high cost of isoflurane limits its use in the UK at present, when no clear indication for its choice exists. The use of rebreathing systems[162] are likely to make the administration of the agent more economical. (*See also* Eger E. I. *Anesthesiology* 1981, **55**, 559 and Jones R. M. in: *Recent Advances in Anaesthesia and Analgesia—15* (Atkinson R. S. and Adams A. P. ed.) Edinburgh: Churchill Livingstone, 1985, p. 1.)

Fluroxene (*Fluoromar*)

This volatile agent, the first fluorine-containing anaesthetic, is trifluoroethyl vinyl ether. It was synthesized in the USA by Shukys, described by Lu and Krantz, and investigated by Krantz in 1953[163] (the first human to be anaesthetized by a fluorine-containing volatile anaesthetic was Dr Max Sadove (1914–) of Chicago—the anaesthetist being J. C. Krantz (1899–)) and by William Dornette (1922–) in 1956.[164]

Methoxyflurane (*Penthrane*) [$CHCl_2.CF_2OCH_3$]

Methoxyflurane is a halogen-substituted methyl ethyl ether. First used in clinical anaesthesia by Artusio and Van Poznak in 1960.[165] For induction, 2–3%, and for maintenance, 0·5–1% have been used.

Physical Properties

Volatile liquid, boiling point 104·6 °C. Blood/gas partition coefficient 13 and so induction time and recovery are slow. MAC 0·16 vol %. Non-flammable, non-explosive. No reaction with soda-lime.

Pharmacodynamics

Induction is slow due to its low volatility, though the minimal alveolar concentration of 0·16 (0·07% if given with 60% nitrous oxide)[166] indicates that it is potent. A good analgesic. Like other volatile agents it increases the brain bulk.

Metabolism

Most of the drug administered is excreted unchanged via the lungs, but a significant amount is metabolized. Metabolites are excreted in the urine over a period of up to 12 days, and fluoride is toxic to the kidney.

Toxicity

High output renal failure may follow methoxyflurane anaesthesia.[167] Not now in clinical use. Like fluroxene its interest is largely historical. For a fuller account *see* the 9th edition of this *Synopsis*.

References

1. Snow J. *On the Inhalation of Ether in Surgical Operations*, London, 1847.
2. Plomley F. *Lancet* 1847, p. 134 (30 January) (reprinted in 'Classical File', *Surv. Anesthesiol.* 1970, **14**, 88).
3. Guedel A. E. *Inhalation Anesthesia* 1937 and 2nd ed. London: Macmillan, 1951.
4. Snow J. *Chloroform and Other Anaesthetic Agents*. London: Churchill, 1858.
5. Miller A. H. *JAMA* 1925, **84**, 201 (reprinted in 'Classical File', *Surv. Anesthesiol.* 1979, **23**, 400).
6. Morton H. J. V. *Proc. R. Soc. Med.* 1945, **38**, 441.
7. Brewer N. et al. *Curr. Res. Anesth. Analg.* 1934, **13**, 257.
8. Ballantine R. I. W. *Anaesthesia* 1982, **37**, 214.
9. Crile G. W. *Lancet* 1913, **2**, 7; *Surg. Gynecol. Obstet.* 1911, **13**, 170; *Ann. Surg.* 1908, **47**, 866; *Boston Med. Surg. J.* 1910, **163**, 893 (reprinted in 'Classical File', *Surv. Anesthesiol.* 1966, **10**, 291).
10. Lundy J. S. *Minnesota Med.* 1926, **9**, 399. (Reprinted in 'Classical File', *Surv. Anesthesiol.* 1981, **25**, 272.)
11. Rees G. J. and Gray T. C. *Br. J. Anaesth.* 1950, **22**, 83.
12. Gray T. C. *Ir. J. Med. Sci.* 1960, **419**, 499.
13. *Gas*, a word invented by the Flemish chemist Johannes Baptiste van Helmont (1577–1644) from the Greek work *Khos* = chaos.
14. Evans T. W. *Br. J. Dent. Sci.* 1868, **2**, 196.
15. Andrews E. A. *Chicago Med. Examiner* 1868, **19**, 656 (reprinted in 'Classical File', *Surv. Anesthesiol.* 1963, **7**, 74).
16. Bert P. *C. r. Soc. Biol. Paris* 1878, **87**, 728; 1879, **89**, 132.
17. Clover J. T. *Br. Med. J.* 1868, **2**, 201.
18. Bert P. *C. r. Acad. Sci. Paris* 1883, **96**, 1271.
19. Clover J. T. *Br. Med. J.* 1876, **2**, 74.
20. Hele W. *Trans. Odont. Soc.* 1873, **5**, 95.
21. Hewitt F. *Lancet* 1885, **1**, 840.
22. McKesson E. I. *Am. J. Surg. (Anesth. Suppl.)* 1916, **7**, February.
23. Courville C. B. *Medicine* 1936, **15**, 129 (reprinted in 'Classical File', *Surv. Anesthesiol.* 1958, **2**, 523, 660).
24. McKesson E. I. *Can. Med. Assoc. J.* 1921, **11**, 130.
25. Lassen H. C. A. *Lancet* 1956, **1**, 525.
26. Jones P. I. *Br. J. Anaesth.* 1974, **46**, 534.
27. Wright B. M. *Lancet* 1977, **2**, 1008.
28. Clutton-Brock J. *Br. J. Anaesth.* 1967, **39**, 388.
29. Kain M. L. et al. *Br. J. Anaesth.* 1967, **39**, 425.

30. Rupreht J. et al. 8th World Congress WSFA, Manila, 1984, **2**, A386.
31. Owen W. D. et al. *Anesth. Anal.* 1978, **57**, 283.
32. Mann M. S. et al. *Anaesthesia* 1985, **40**, 8.
33. Deacon R. et al. *Eur. J. Biochem.* 1980, **104**, 419; Koblin D. D. et al. *Anesthesiology* 1981, **54**, 318.
34. Koblin D. D. et al. *Anesth. Analg.* 1982, **61**, 75.
35. Nunn J. F. et al. *Br. J. Anaesth.* 1986, **58**, 1.
36. Amess J. A. L. et al. *Lancet* 1978, **2**, 339; Amos R. J. et al. *Lancet* 1982, **2**, 835.
37. Bank R. G. S. and Henderson R. J. *J. Chem. Soc. (A)* 1968, 2886.
38. Annotation, *Lancet* 1978; **2**, 613.
39. Nunn J. F. and Chanarin J. *Br. J. Anaesth.* 1978, **50**, 1089.
40. Layzer R. B. *Lancet* 1978, **2**, 1227.
41. Sweeney B. *SAAD Digest* 1985, **6**, 82.
42. Sonander H. et al. *Br. J. Anaesth.* 1983, **55**, 1225.
43. Vieira E. et al. *Anaesthesia* 1983, **38**, 319.
44. Rupreht J. et al. 8th World Congress WSFA, Manila, 1984, **2**, A439.
45. Fink B. R. *Anesthesiology* 1955, **16**, 511; Fink B. R. et al. *Fed. Proc.* 1954, **13**, 354.
46. Hutchinson R. *Br. J. Anaesth.* 1961, **33**, 463; Utting J. F. *Anaesth. Intensive Care* 1975, **3**, 334; Editorial, *Br. Med. J.* 1980, **1**, 811.
47. Maynard M. et al. *Br. Med. J.* 1969, **4**, 545; Dubois M. et al. *Anaesthesia* 1978, **33**, 157.
48. Waters D. J. *Br. J. Anaesth.* 1968, **40**, 259.
49. Cormack R. S. *Br. J. Anaesth.* 1979, **51**, 1051.
50. Barach A. L. and Rovenstine E. A. *Anesthesiology* 1945, **6**, 449.
51. Hill D. W. *Physics Applied to Anaesthesia*, 3rd ed. London: Butterworths, 1976, p. 44.
52. MacGregor, W. G. et al. *Anaesthesia* 1972, **27**, 14.
53. Allison R. H. *Br. J. Anaesth.* 1979, **51**, 177.
54. Yank J. C. et al. *Anesthesiology* 1980, **52**, 414.
55. von Freund A. *Monats. f. Chemie* 1882, **3**, 625.
56. Lucas G. H. W. and Henderson V. E. *Can. Med. Assoc. J.* 1929, **21**, 173.
57. Stiles J. A. et al. *Curr. Res. Anesth. Analg.* 1934, **13**, 56 (reprinted in 'Classical File', *Surv. Anesthesiol.* 1959, **3**, 250); Waters R. M. and Schmidt E. R. *JAMA* 1934, **103**, 975.
58. Rowbotham E. S. *Lancet* 1935, **2**, 1110; Magill I. W. *Br. Med. J.* 1979, **1**, 1348.
59. Grant W. J. *Medical Gases; Their Properties and Uses.* Aylesbury: HM & M Publishers, 1978, p. 177.
60. Nosworthy M. D. *Proc. R. Soc. Med.* 1941, **34**, 479.
61. Cullen S. C. and Gross E. G. *Science* 1951, **113**, 580; Pittinger C. B. et al. *Anesthesiology* 1953, **14**, 10; Grant J. W. *Medical Gases; Their Use and Properties.* Aylesbury: HM & M Publishers, 1978, p. 158.
62. Frobensius J. A. S. *Phil. Trans. R. Soc. Lond.* 1739, **36**, 283.
63. Bigelow H. J. *Am. J. Med. Sci.* 1876, **141**, 164.
64. Jeffereys J. *Lancet* 1872, **2**, 241; *Br. Med. J.* 1872, **2**, 499.
65. Long C. W. *Sth Med. J.* 1849, n.s. **5**, 705 (reprinted in 'Classical File', *Surv. Anesthesiol.* 1960, **4**, 120); *JAMA* 1965, **194**, 1008; Cole W. H. J. *Anaesth. Intensive Care* 1974, **2**, 92; Taylor F. C. W. *Long and the Discovery of Ether.* New York: Hoebner, 1928.
66. Bigelow H. J. *Boston Med. Surg. J.* 1846, **35**, 309 (reprinted in 'Classical File', *Surv. Anesthesiol.* 1957, **1**, February); Morton W. T. G. *Remarks on the Proper Mode of Administration of Sulphuric Ether by Inhalation.* Boston: Dutton & Wentworth, 1847.
67. Clover J. T. *Med. Times, Lond.* 1874, **2**, 603; Vandam L. *Anesthesiology* 1980, **52**, 62.
68. Prince L. H. *Chicago Med. Rec.* 1897, **17**, 232.
69. Shepherd J. A. *Lawson Tait, the Rebellious Surgeon.* Liverpool Medical Institution, Coronado Press, 1980.
70. Farman J. V. *Anaesthesia and the EMO System.* London: English Universities Press, 1973.
71. Wright A. D. *Br. Med. J.* 1933, **2**, 1210.
72. Greenfield I. *Anesthesiology* 1946, **7**, 299.
73. Leake C. D. and Chen M. Y. *Curr. Res. Anesth. Analg.* 1931, **10**, 1; Leake C. D. et al. *J. Pharmac. Exp. Ther.* 1933, **47**, 5 (reprinted in 'Classical File', *Surv. Anesthesiol.* 1965, **9**, 199).
74. Gelfen S. and Bell I. R. *J. Pharmac. Exp. Ther.* 1933, **47**, 1; Everitt E. F. *Br. J. Anaesth.* 1952, **24**, 201.
75. Flourens M.-J. P. *C R Seances Acad. Sci. [III]* 1847, **24**, 340, 482.
76. Heyfelder J. F. M. Erlangen: Heyder, 1848.
77. Dumas, J.-B. *Ann. Chim. (Phys.)* 1834, **56**, 115.

78. Flourens M.-J. P. *C R Seances Acad. Sci. [III]* 1847, **24**, 340.
79. Furnell M. C. *Lancet* 1871, **1**, 433; 1877, **1**, 934.
80. Simpson J. Y. *Lond. Med. Gaz.* 1847, n.s. **5**, 934; Simpson J. Y. *Lancet* 1847, **2**, 549; reprinted in *Foundations of Anesthesiology* (Faulconer A. and Keys T. E. ed.). Springfield, Ill.: Thomas, Vol. 1, p. 463; and also in 'Classical File', *Surv. Anesthesiol.* 1961, **5**, 93, *See also* Herdman N. *The Scotsman* 31 December 1959. (When Simpson, on being awarded a baronetcy, was looking for a suitable crest, it was suggested that there should be a picture of a 'wee naked bairn' with the motto 'Does your mother know you're oot?').
81. Duroy J. L. P. *J. Pharm. Chim., Paris* 1850, **18**, 64.
82. Guthrie L. *Lancet* 1894, **1**, 193, 257; 1903, **2**, 10 (reprinted in 'Classical File', *Surv. Anesthesiol.* 1967, **6**, August).
83. *Med. Chir. Trans.* 1864, **47**, 323.
84. Levy A. G. *Chloroform Anaesthesia.* London: Bale Son & Daniellson, 1922; *Proc. R. Soc. Med.* 1914, **7**, 57 (reprinted in 'Classical File' *Surv. Anesthesiol.* 1973, **17**, 477).
85. *See Proc. R. Soc. Med.* 1914, **7**, 57 (reprinted in 'Classical File', *Surv. Anesthesiol.* 1973, **17**, 383).
86. McWilliam J. A. *Br. Med. J.* 1890, **2**, 831.
87. Levy A. G. *Heart* 1913, **4**, 319; *J. Physiol.* 1911, **3**, 42; *Proc. R. Soc. Med.* 1914, **7**, 57 (reprinted in 'Classical File', *Surv. Anesthesiol.* 1973, **17**, 384).
88. Embley E. H. *Br. Med. J.* 1902, **1**, 817, 885, 951 (reprinted in 'Classical File', *Surv. Anesthesiol.* 1965, **9**, 511, 634); Cass N. *Anaesth. Intensive Care* 1979, **7**, 114.
89. *Chloroform: A Study after One Hundred Years* (Waters R. ed.). Madison: University of Wisconsin Press, 1951.
90. Caspar J. L. *Wochenschr. Ges Heilk.* 1850, **16**, 273.
91. Fischer E. *Jena Z. Med. Naturw.* 1864, **1**, 123.
92. Plessner W. *Berl. Klin. Wochenschr.* 1916, **53**, 25.
93. Lehmann K. B. *Arch. Hyg. Berl.* 1911, **74**, 1.
94. Jackson D. E. *Curr. Res. Anesth. Analg.* 1934, **13**, 198.
95. Striker C. et al. *Curr. Res. Anesth. Analg.* 1935, **14**, 68.
96. Hewer C. L. and Hadfield C. F. *Br. Med. J.* 1941, **1**, 924 (reprinted in 'Classical File', *Surv. Anesthesiol.* 1963, **7**, April); Hewer, C. L. *Proc. R. Soc. Med.* 1942, **35**, 463.
97. Morton H. J. V. *Br. Med. J.* 1943, **2**, 838; McAuley J. *Br. Med. J.* 1943, **2**, 713.
98. Whitteridge D. and Bulbing E. *Br. Med. Bull.* 1946, **4**, 85.
99. Prior F. N. *Anaesthesia* 1972, **27**, 66; Farman J. V. *Anaesthesia and the EMO System*, 1973 London: English Universities Press.
100. Reynolds F. *Anaesthesia* 1984, **39**, 932.
101. Davidson J. T. *Anaesthesia* 1984, **39**, 501.
102. Suckling C. W. *Br. J. Anaesth.* 1957, **29**, 466.
103. Raventós J. *Br. J. Pharmacol.* 1956, **11**, 394 (reprinted in 'Classical File', *Surv. Anesthesiol.* 1966, **10**, 183).
104. Johnstone M. *Br. J. Anaesth.* 1956, **28**, 392.
105. Bryce-Smith R. and O'Brien H. D. *Br. Med. J.* 1956, **2**, 969; *Proc. R. Soc. Med.* 1957, **30**, 193.
106. Prys-Roberts C. et al. *Br. J. Anaesth.* 1972, **44**, 634; Prys-Roberts C. et al. *Br. J. Anaesth.* 1974, **16**, 105.
107. Roberts J. G. *Br. J. Anaesth.* 1976, **48**, 315.
108. Andersen N. and Johansen S. H. *Anesthesiology* 1963, **24**, 51.
109. Katz R. L. *Anesthesiology* 1962, **23**, 597.
110. Barash P. G. et al. *Anesthesiology* 1978, **49**, 79.
111. Grant I. S. *Br. J. Anaesth.* 1980, **52**, 711.
112. Neuberger J. and Williams R. *Br. Med. J.* 1984, **289**, 1136.
113. Virtue R. W. and Payne K. W. *Anesthesiology* 1958, **19**, 562.
114. Lecky J. N. and Cohen P. S. *Anesthesiology* 1970, **33**, 371.
115. Mushin W. W. et al. *Br. Med. J.* 1964, **2**, 329; Green K. G. and Mungarim J. M. *Proc. R. Soc. Med.* 1964, **57**, 311; Pearce C. et al. *Med. Tijdschr. Geneesk.* 1966, **110**, 80.
116. Bunker J. P. *JAMA* 1966, **197**, 775; Gall E. A. *Anesthesiology* 1968, **29**, 233; McCaughey W. *Br. J. Anaesth.* 1972, **44**, 918.
117. Ross J. A. S. et al. *Br. J. Anaesth.* 1984, **56**, 527.
118. Neuberger J. et al. *Br. J. Anaesth.* 1983, **55**, 15.
119. Stock J. C. L. and Strunin L. *Anesthesiology* 1985, **63**, 424.
120. Johnstone M. *Br. J. Anaesth.* 1964, **36**, 718; Hart S. M. and Fitzgerald P. G. *Br. J. Anaesth.* 1975, **47**, 1321.
121. Blumberg B. S. et al. *Ann. Intern. Med.* 1967, **66**, 924.

122. Gilbert A. and Lereboullet P. *Semaine médicale, Paris* 1901, **71**, 241; Quinn N. W. and Gollan J. L. *Br. J. Oral Surg.* 1975, **12**, 285.
123. Geddes I. C. *Br. J. Anaesth.* 1972, **44**, 953.
124. Pflug A. E. et al. *Can. Anaesth. Soc. J.* 1978, **25**, 43.
125. Nakagawara M. et al. *Anesthesiology* 1986, **64**, 4; Welch W. W. Editorial, *Anesthesiology* 1986, **64**, 1.
126. Barash P. G. et al. *Anesthesiology* 1978, **49**, 79.
127. Mapleson W. W. *Br. J. Anaesth.* 1960, **32**, 294; Galloon S. *Br. J. Anaesth.* 1960, **32**, 310; Mushin W. W. and Galloon S. *Br. J. Anaesth.* 1960, **32**, 328.
128. Duncan W. A. M. and Raventós J. *Br. J. Anaesth.* 1959, **31**, 302.
129. Brennan H. J. A. *Br. J. Anaesth.* 1957, **29**, 332; Mackay I. M. *Can. Anaesth. Soc. J.* 1967, **4**, 235.
130. Paterson G. H. et al. *Br. J. Anaesth.* 1969, **41**, 109.
131. Diaz P. M. *Br. J. Anaesth.* 1976, **48**, 387.
132. Goldman V. *Anesth. Analg. Curr. Res.* 1959, **38**, 192.
133. Young T. M. *Br. J. Anaesth.* 1969, **41**, 120.
134. Morris L. E. *Anesthesiology* 1952, **13**, 587 (reprinted in 'Classical File', *Surv. Anesthesiol.* 1975, **19**, 577); Young T. M. *Anaesthesia* 1962, **17**, 328; Abajian J. et al. *JAMA* 1959, **171**, 535; Feldman S. A. and Morris L. *Anesthesiology* 1958, **19**, 650.
135. Young J. V. I. *Anaesthesia* 1966, **21**, 551; Collis J. M. *Anaesthesia* 1966, **21**, 558.
136. Parkhouse J. *Anaesthesia* 1966, **21**, 498.
137. Rosenberg P. H. and Alila A. *Anaesthesia* 1984, **38**, 581.
138. Wolfson B. et al. *Anesthesiology* 1978, **48**, 187.
139. Duvaldestin P. et al. *Anesthesiology* 1981, **54**, 57.
140. Virtue R. W. et al. *Can. Anaesth. Soc. J.* 1966, **12**, 233 (reprinted in 'Classical File', *Surv. Anesthesiol.* 1977, **21**, 210).
141. Julien R. M. and Kavan E. M. *J. Pharmacol. Exp. Ther.* 1972, **123**, 393; Grant I. S. *Anaesthesia* 1986, **41**, 1024; Nicoll J. M. V. *Anaesthesia* 1986, **41**, 927.
142. Reisner L. S. and Lippmann M. *Anesth. Analg.* 1975, **64**, 468; Johnston R. R. et al. *Anesth. Analg.* 1976, **55**, 709.
143. Lebowitz M. H. et al. *Anesthesiology* 1970, **19**, 355.
144. Denlinger J. K. et al. *Anesthesiology* 1974, **41**, 86; Reis L. V. D. et al. *JAMA* 1974, **227**, 76; Douglas H. J. *N. Engl. J. Med.* 1977, **269**, 553; Danilewitz M. D. et al. *Br. J. Anaesth.* 1980, **52**, 1151.
145. Sadove M. S. and Kim S. I. *Anesthesiology* 1974, **53**, 336.
146. Coleman A. J. and Downing J. W. *Anesthesiology* 1975, **43**, 354.
147. Vircha J. F. *Anesthesiology* 1971, **21**, 4.
148. Dobkin A. B. et al. *Can. Anaesth. Soc. J.* 1971, **18**, 264.
149. Stevens D. J. et al. *Can. Anaesth. Soc. J.* 1971, **18**, 500.
150. Beaupre P. N. et al. *Anesthesiology* 1983, **59**, A59.
151. Wade J. G. and Stevens W. C. *Anesth. Analg. (Cleve.)* 1981, **60**, 666.
152. Eger E. I. *Anesthesiology* 1981, **55**, 559.
153. Johnson R. R. et al. *Anesth. Analg. (Cleve.)* 1976, **55**, 707.
154. Calverley R. K. et al. *Anesth. Analg. (Cleve.)* 1978, **57**, 610; Fourcode H. E. et al. *Anesthesiology* 1971, **35**, 26.
155. Friesen R. H. and Lichter J. L. *Anesth. Analg. (Cleve.)* 1983, **62**, 411; Pandit V. A. et al. *Anesthesiology* 1971, **35**, A445.
156. Wade J. G. and Stevens W. C. *Anesth. Analg. (Cleve.)* 1981, **60**, 666; Eger E. I. *Anesthesiology* 1981, 55, 559.
157. Smith A. L. and Marque J. J. *Anesthesiology* 1976, **45**, 64.
158. Newberg L. A. and Michenfelder J. D. *Anesthesiology* 1983, **59**, 29.
159. Warren T. M. et al. *Anesth. Analg. (Cleve.)* 1983, **62**, 516.
160. Holaday D. A. et al. *Anesthesiology* 1975, **43**, 325.
161. Mazze R. I. et al. *Anesthesiology* 1974, **40**, 536.
162. O'Callaghan A. C. et al. *Br. J. Anaesth.* 1983, **55**, 1061; Yin C. Y. et al. *Anesthesiology* 1983, **59**, A478.
163. Go Lu et al. *Anesthesiology* 1953, **14**, 466. Krantz J. C. *Anesth. Analg. Curr. Res.* 1970, **49**, 511.
164. Dornette W. H. L. *Cal. Med.* 1956, **85**, 311.
165. Artusio J. F. et al. *Anesthesiology* 1960, **21**, 512 (reprinted in 'Classical File', *Surv. Anesthesiol.* 1968, **12**, 196).
166. Stoelting R. K. *Anesthesiology* 1971, **34**, 353.

167. Paddock R. B. et al. *Anesthesiology* 1964, **25**, 707; Crandell W. B. et al. *Anesthesiology*, 1966, **27**, 591; Richey J. E. and Smith R. B. *Anaesthesia* 1972, **27**, 9.
168. Adams A. P. et al. *Br. Med. J.* 1986, **293**, 1023.

Chapter 11   # GASES USED IN ASSOCIATION WITH ANAESTHESIA[1]

Oxygen [O₂]

Historical
John Mayow[2] (1643–1679) of Oxford showed that a component of air was used up by a burning candle or a live mouse. Priestley[3] (1772) discovered 'dephlogisticated air' and so did Carl Wilhelm Scheele (1742–1786) in 1771. Antoine-Laurant Lavoisier (1743–1794) and Pierre Simon Laplace[4] (1749–1827), who coined the term 'oxygène' (oxy=acid; gene=former) in 1779, were the first to show a quantitative relation between the heat production of animals and that resulting from combustion of carbon. They demonstrated a relationship between oxygen used and carbon dioxide produced. Justus von Liebig[5] (1803–1873), Darmstadt chemist, in 1851 showed that carbohydrates and fats were important substrates and not carbon itself. Thomas Beddoes (1760–1808) used oxygen in medical treatment in 1794 at Bristol. Barth compressed the gas into cylinders in 1868. Cylinders are painted black with white shoulders in the UK (International Standards Organization), blue in some European countries and green in the USA.

Modern use of oxygen was popularized in 1917 by J. S. Haldane (1860–1936) during the First World War,[6] and by Yandell Henderson, the New Haven physiologist (1873–1944).

Preparation
In the 1850s a French chemist, Boussingault, discovered that at a temperature of about 1000 °C barium monoxide would absorb oxygen from the atmosphere forming barium dioxide and at a higher temperature would give it off again. This process was patented by his pupils the Brin brothers in the 1880s.

Medical and industrial oxygen is now manufactured by the fractional distillation of liquid air (nitrogen comes off first), patented by Carl Linde of Germany. Boiling point of oxygen −182·5 °C; of nitrogen −195 °C. Oxygen is supplied in cylinders as the compressed gas at a pressure of 136 kPa × 100 (135 atmospheres) and in liquid form in insulated tanks at relatively low pressure. One volume of liquid oxygen is equivalent to 840 vol. of gas. Pipeline pressure is 410 kPa.

The oxygen concentrator produces oxygen from ambient air by preferential absorption of nitrogen on certain aluminosilicates. It is suitable for use in both hospitals and domestically. It is useful in remote areas, in developing countries and in military surgery. The resultant gas contains 6% of impurities, mostly argon. These are harmless. (*See also* Carter J. A. et al. *Anaesthesia* 1985, **40**, 560.) The Mini O₂ and the Healthdyne oxygen concentrators. Both work on the 'molecular sieve' principle.[7]

Properties
Molecular weight 32. Solubility in water at 37 °C, 2·4 vol. %; in water at 0 °C,

4·9 vol. %. Specific gravity 1105 (air is 1000). Critical temperature −118·4 °C. Critical pressure 50·8 atmospheres. Electric sparks convert it into ozone (O_3).

With oil or grease, oxygen under high pressure will cause an ignition. It encourages fires, although not itself flammable. Oxygen (and nitrous oxide) cylinders should be turned on outside the operating theatre, brought in faintly hissing, so that when the reducing value is connected, pressure is not built up in it suddenly, but gradually. At other times when the cylinders are turned on, the flow-metres should themselves be on.

Air

Air for medical purposes is supplied in cylinders painted grey with black and white shoulder quadrants in the UK. It is compressed to 137 atmospheres. In many hospitals it is also supplied by pipeline. It is used to drive ventilators, drills, etc. Respirable air as used by divers or airline pilots is supplied in special cylinders at a higher pressure than medical air.

Carbon Dioxide [CO_2]

Discovered by Jean Baptiste von Helmont (1597–1644) and isolated by Joseph Black (1728–1799) in 1757. Became popular with anaesthetists soon after the work of Haggard and Yandell Henderson (1873–1944)[8] in the USA (1921) who recommended 5 per cent of the gas in oxygen ('to overcome collapse due to anaesthesia') and John Scott Haldane (1860–1936) in Britain.[9] The gas should always be provided on anaesthetic machines. The stimulating effect on respiration was shown by Herman and Escher in 1870.[10]

In the eighteenth and nineteenth centuries the ill effects of inadequate ventilation were established as being due to oxygen lack. Anaesthetists only became aware of the possibility of CO_2 excess in their patients when Ralph Waters, then in private practice in Sioux City, Iowa, pointed it out.[11] He realized that the percentage of CO_2 could be controlled, at least in animals undergoing anaesthesia, following the publication of the work of D. E. Jackson, a Cincinnati pharmacologist.[12] John Snow was, of course, an even earlier pioneer of CO_2 absorption.[13] Water's first reason for the use of CO_2 absorption was economy and convenience; when he started to use cyclopropane economy became even more important. Only later did he stress the possible harm produced by excessive percentages of CO_2.[14] With the later introduction of the relaxants and the common practice of IPPV many anaesthetists tended to produce hypocapnia in their patients and several apparently good reasons were offered why this was not only harmless but positively beneficial.[17] It is perhaps not surprising that the pendulum is now swinging in the reverse direction and normocapnia is becoming respectable once again.

Properties
Colourless gas with a pungent odour in high concentration. Molecular weight 44. Dissolves in water 87·8 vol. % at room temperature. Critical temperature −31 °C. Critical pressure 73·8 atmospheres. Density 1·98 at 0 °C.

Preparation and Storage
In Britain obtained from four sources: (1) By-product of manufacture of

hydrogen. (2) By-product of fermentation in brewing of beer. (3) As a combustion gas from burning fuel. Only a small fraction of the CO_2 manufactured is used for medicinal purposes. (4) Manufactured by heating magnesium and calcium carbonate in the presence of their oxides. It is stored in cylinders at 50 atmospheres pressure (and for industrial purposes in refrigerated tanks). Solid CO_2 is stored and transported in insulated containers.

Cylinders of CO_2 are painted grey. The filling ratio is 0·75 in temperate and 0·67 in tropical climates. The liquid phase occupies about 90–95% of the cylinder capacity and the liquid phase disappears when about 83% of the gas has been discharged.

Carbon dioxide–oxygen premixed cylinders are available in various combinations. The cylinder colour is black with grey/white shoulder quadrants. Cylinders are filled to a pressure of 137 atmospheres.

Carbon dioxide–air cylinders are painted with grey (body) and black/grey/white/grey shoulder quadrants, and are filled to a pressure of 137 atmospheres.

Effects on Respiratory System. *See* Chapter 2
Five per cent carbon dioxide in air or oxygen is tolerated by the patient, but higher percentages cause distress, dyspnoea, headaches, etc. Above 10% the narcotic effect becomes more marked, while at 30% there is coma. At 40% breathing is depressed. This so-called carbon dioxide reversal may occur at concentrations of even 5%, if respiratory centre is deeply depressed by narcotics or hypoxia. Thus carbon dioxide should not be used for resuscitation in such cases.

Carbon dioxide narcosis was described in 1954[15] and is closely related to the fall in pH of the cerebrospinal fluid, and this may be independent of arterial pH. Pco_2 and the Pco_2 of cerebrospinal fluids. Narcosis begins when the Pco_2 is greater than 12 kPa and when the cerebrospinal fluid pH falls below 7·1 and reaches a maximum at pH 6·8. The narcosis resulting from carbon dioxide inhalation is thus likely to be due solely to the pH effect. Sudden reduction of hypercapnia as by hyperventilation may result in ventricular fibrillation.[16]

Carbon Dioxide in Anaesthesia
Inspired air contains 0·03%. Expired air contains 4%. Alveolar air contains 5·6%.

Clinical Use
1. To increase depth of anaesthesia rapidly when volatile agents are in use. The addition of a little carbon dioxide for no longer than 5 min stimulates depth of respiration, helps to overcome breath-holding and laryngeal spasm, and increases the speed of induction when volatile agents with a high blood/gas partition coefficient are administered (*see* Chapter 6).

2. To widen the glottis and facilitate blind intubation.

3. During induction of hypothermia, carbon dioxide has been used to increase peripheral vasodilatation and so lessen the degree of metabolic acidosis.

4. Has been given during anaesthesia to increase cerebral blood flow in arteriosclerotic patients undergoing surgery, and to increase the tolerance to cerebral ischaemia during carotid endarterectomy.

5. To stimulate the onset of respiration at the end of a period of controlled apnoea, following complete reversal of relaxant drugs.

6. In chronic respiratory obstruction, the retention of carbon dioxide accustoms the respiratory centre to a high tension of the gas. When obstruction is relieved, apnoea may follow unless carbon dioxide is added to the inspired gases, to be gradually reduced.

7. Added to inspired gases to prevent hypocapnia during hyperventilation in clinical anaesthesia.

Contraindications

1. Many anaesthetists find no use for carbon dioxide, but believe it to be a potential source of danger. In some areas, particularly outside the UK, carbon-dioxide rotameters are not fitted to anaesthetic machines.

2. In resuscitation, carbon dioxide is rarely of use. It is not rational to try to stimulate a respiratory centre depressed by overdose of drugs with carbon dioxide. It is more likely to be harmful.

3. In respiratory obstruction, carbon dioxide may be dangerous. Further increase in respiratory effort increases negative intrathoracic pressure and is exhausting.

Water Vapour

Water has a high specific heat. Inspired air is warmed to body temperature and humidified to saturation point by the time it reaches the trachea. With the trachea intubated these changes, though to a lesser extent, take place in the tracheobronchial tree; 50 mg of water may be required to bring each litre of inspired gas to body temperature and saturation. At a temperature of 20 °C air saturated with water vapour contains 20 mg of water per litre at partial pressure of 17·5 torr. At body temperature, 100% relative humidity is equivalent to a water content of 53 mg/litre at a pressure of 47 torr.

Helium [He]

Isolated by Sir W. Ramsey (1852–1916) (British chemist and Nobel prizewinner 1904 for his work on the inert gases) in 1895.

Preparation

From natural gas, the concentration being about 1% in some gas wells in North America. Natural gas from the North sea contains only 0·01–0·03%. Air contains 1 part in 200 000. Helium cylinders are painted brown, helium–oxygen cylinders are brown with brown/white shoulder quadrants. The pressure in a full cylinder is 137 atmospheres (1987 lb/in^2).

Properties

Inert, colourless, odourless gas. Molecular and atomic weights 4. Specific gravity 178 (air is 1000).

When helium replaces the nitrogen of air the resulting mixture of helium and oxygen has a specific gravity of 341 (air is 1000). Because of its low density the gas will flow through an orifice three times as fast as air, so in patients with partial respiratory obstruction, 20% of oxygen with 80% of helium will enable more oxygen to get to the alveoli with the same effort, or the same ventilation will take place with less effort than when air is inhaled. (There is a difference between viscosity and density when considering laminar and turbulent flow.) Absorption rate from alveoli very slow and it has been employed to prevent atelectasis. Helium has a low coefficient of solubility and high rate of diffusion, compared with nitrogen.

If fed through a nitrous-oxide flow-meter the reading must be multiplied by 3·3 to get the approximate rate of flow in litres per minute. It diffuses through rubber.

References

1. *See also* Grant W. J. *Medical Gases; Their Properties and Uses.* Aylesbury: HM & M Publishers, 1978; *Physiological Aspects of Anaesthetics and Inert Gases.* London: Academic Press, 1978.
2. Mayow J. *Tractactus Quinque Medico-physici*, No. 2. Oxford:1674.
3. Priestley J. *Phil. Trans.* 1772, **52**, 147; *Experiments and Observations on Different Kinds of Air*, Vol. 2, sect. III–V, pp. 29–103 (reprinted in 'Classical File', *Surv. Anesthesiol.* 1976, **20**, 81).
4. Lavoisier A.-L. and Laplace P. S. *Mém. Prés. Acad. Sci. Paris* 1780, **103**, 566.
5. von Liebig J. *Letters on Chemistry*, 3rd ed. 1851.
6. Haldane J. S. *Br. Med. J.* 1917, **1**, 181.
7. Harris C. E. and Simpson P. J. *Anaesthesia* 1985, **40**, 1206.
8. Henderson Y. *Br. Med. J.* 1925, **2**, 1170.
9. Haldane J. S. and Smith J. L. *J. Path. Bact.* 1893, **1**, 168.
10. Herman L. and Escher T. *Pflüger Arch. Ges. Physiolog.* 1870, **3**, 3.
11. Waters R. M. *Curr. Res. Anesth. Analg.* 1924, **3**, 20; Waters R. M. et al. *Curr. Res. Anesth. Analg.* 1931, **10**, 10.
12. Jackson D. E. *J. Lab. Clin. Med.* 1915, **1**, 1.
13. Foregger R. *Anesthesiology* 1960, **21**, 20.
14. Waters R. M. *Can. Med. Assoc. J.* 1927, **17**, 1500; Waters R. M. et al. *Curr. Res. Anesth. Analg.* 1931, **10**, 10.
15. Scurr C. F. *Br. Med. J.* 1954, **1**, 565; Westlake E. K. et al. *Q. J. Med.* 1955, **24**, 155.
16. Brown E. B. and Miller F. A. *Am. J. Physiol.* 1952, **169**, 56.
17. Geddes I. C. and Gray T. C. *Lancet* 1959, **24**.

Chapter 12   # TRACHEAL INTUBATION

History

Tracheal insufflation in animals was described by Andreas Vesalius (1514–1564) of Padua in 1555,[1] and by Robert Hooke (1635–1703) in 1667.[2] C. Kite of Gravesend described oral and nasal intubation for resuscitation of the apparently drowned in 1788.[3] Pierre Joseph Desault (1744–1795) and his pupil Marie F-X Bichat (1771–1802) were early intubators for laryngeal obstruction. Intubation from the neck, through a tracheotomy wound, was performed in 1858 by John Snow, in anaesthetizing animals. Friederich Trendelenburg (1844–1924) of Rostock used the method in man in 1871, occluding the trachea by an inflatable cuff.[4]

William MacEwen (1848–1924) of Glasgow in 1878 passed a tube from the mouth into the trachea, using his fingers as a guide in the conscious patient;[5] through it he gave chloroform and air for removal of a carcinoma of the mouth after first using it for the relief of obstruction in laryngeal diphtheria. Historically, tracheostomy was preferred to intubation as it was supposed that a laryngeal tube would not be tolerated. These early attempts were all made to prevent aspiration pneumonia in surgery of the upper air passages. Karl Maydl (1853–1903) of Prague employed the tube of J. P. O'Dwyer (1841–1898) of Cleveland,[6] designed for the treatment of laryngeal diphtheria, in anaesthesia.[7]

Franz Kuhn of Cassel (1866–1929) in 1901 extended the technique by using a flexible metal tube introduced on a curved guide through the mouth. A year later he described nasotracheal intubation.[8] His preference was for inhalation anaesthesia, the patient breathing to and fro along the tube.[9] (*See also* Zingharnell H. *Anaesthesist*, 1974, **23**, 308 and Sweeney B. *Anaesthesia* 1985, **40**, 1000).

In 1907, Barthélemy and Dufour of Nancy, France, blew chloroform vapour and air from a Vernon Harcourt (1834–1919) inhaler[10] and a rubber catheter, guided into the trachea by touch—the first use of the insufflation endotracheal technique.[11]

Samuel James Meltzer (1851–1920) and his son-in-law, John Auer (1875–1948), physiologists working in the USA at the Rockefeller Institute, New York City, pioneered insufflation endotracheal anaesthesia in animals in 1909.[12] This entailed blowing an anaesthetic vapour at a positive pressure through a narrow tube into the trachea near the carina, the gases returning either through a second tube or alongside the insufflation tube. It proved that life could be maintained without respiratory movements—apnoeic ventilation. Charles Albert Elsberg neurosurgeon (1871–1948) of New York and others,[13] in the same year, applied the technique to man, while in 1912 Robert Kelly (1879–1944) of Liverpool brought the method to Britain.[14]

Alfred Kirstein (1863–1922) of Berlin[15] and Gustav Killian (1860–1921) of Freiburg—the original bronchoscopist[16]—pioneered direct laryngoscopy in 1895 and 1912, respectively, and Chevalier Jackson (1865–1958) of Philadelphia published a book on the subject in 1907; this popularized direct laryngoscopy. Jackson did his first bronchoscopy in 1899.[17]

As a result of their experiences after the First World War, especially in plastic surgery, as anaesthetists to Sir Harold Gillies at the Queen's Hospital for Facial and Jaw Injuries at Sidcup (1919), Edgar Stanley Rowbotham (1890–1979) and Ivan Whiteside Magill[18] (1888–1986) used first insufflation through one, later two narrow gum-elastic tubes passed via a laryngoscope—one for insufflating gases in from a Shipway apparatus[19] (warm ether vapour) by the aid of an electric motor, the other for carrying them away—and later inhalation endotracheal methods, the patient breathing in and out through a single wide-bore tube.[20] Magill published his results of blind nasal intubation with a single wide-bore rubber tube during the years following 1928.[21] The first blind nasal intubation was performed by Stanley Rowbotham of London.[22]

Inflatable cuffs have been used for many years (e.g. by Dorrance[23]) but were reintroduced by Ralph Milton Waters and Arthur E. Guedel in 1928.[24]

A pilot balloon was described in 1893 by Victor Eisenmenger (1864–1932)[25] by Green in 1906[26] and was reintroduced by Langton Hewer in 1939.[27]

Before the days of muscle relaxants, blind nasal intubation was very popular as it was usually quicker than direct-vision oral intubation when inhalation agents were all that were available. The use of muscle relaxants to facilitate intubation (rather than deep anaesthesia) was pioneered by Bourne.[28]

Indirect laryngoscopy with a laryngeal mirror was pioneered by M. Garcia (1805–1906), a teacher of singing in London.[29]

(*See also* Gillespie N. A. in: *Endotracheal Anesthesia*, 2nd ed. (Bamforth B. J. and Siebeckar K. L. ed.) University of Wisconsin Press, 1943; Endotracheal anaesthesia; its historical development, Waters R. M. and Guedel A. E. *Anesth. Analg. Curr. Res.* 1933, **12**, 196 (Reprinted in 'Classical File', *Surv. Anesthesiol.* 1984, **28**, 76); Little D. M. 'Classical File', *Surv. Anesthesiol.* 1981, **25**, 195; Sir Ivan Magill's contributions to anaesthesia (Bowes J. B. and Zorab J. S. M. in: *Anaesthesia; Essays on its History* (Rupreht J. et al. ed.) Heidelberg: Springer-Verlag, 1985.)

Apparatus

Tubes
The traditional tubes are the wide-bore Magill tubes of mineralized rubber. They can be used for either nasal or oral intubation, the latter having thicker walls. The number of the tube corresponds to the internal diameter in millimetres.

Other tubes are made of semi-rigid material, the Portex plastic tubes (polyvinyl chloride) being useful. Portex tubes if boiled and left to cool on a curved wire stylet will permanently take the curve of the wire. Other plastic tubes are the PVC Cole tube with a narrower distal portion; for neonates,[30] a plastic tube provided with a communicating cross-piece which may be attached to the head of the baby, and through which it may be ventilated with minimal dead space. Variations on this theme are the Hale Enderby tube,[31] in which the nylon spiral is continued right to the proximal end of the tapered tube, and the Pollard tube[32] which has a narrower distal portion designed to facilitate microlaryngoscopy. The Oxford or inverted L-shaped tube[33] has two limbs which are shaped to conform to the passage from the mouth to the trachea and so cannot kink, even when the head is fully flexed. Its internal diameter is the same throughout but the thickness of the part which lies in the mouth and pharynx is twice that of the distal part. It has an anteroposterior bevel. The tube can be passed between the cords as it is or else on a curved stylet or a long gum-elastic introducer. An S-shaped tube with cuff has been described for use in faciomaxillary surgery.[34] Rae tubes are similar.
Cleaning. Tubes should be cleaned with soapy water outside and inside with a test-tube brush. Heating to 75 °C for 10 min (pasteurization) will kill vegetative organisms which are potentially harmful (although the relatively harmless spores will not be killed). Rubber tubes can be autoclaved up to six times without much deterioration. Disposable tubes are used in many hospitals and ITUs. Most tubes are now supplied already sterilized by gamma-rays.

(For physical aspects of tracheal tubes, see Williams A. *Anaesth. Intensive Care* 1979, **7**, 399.)

Laryngoscopes
The prototype is that of Chevalier Jackson (1865–1958),[35] later modified by Magill,[36] Paluel J. Flagg (1886–1970) of New York;[37] Miller[38] and Robert Macintosh of Oxford (1897–).[39] Magill's laryngoscope was modelled on that of William Hill, laryngologist to St Mary's Hospital, London. It had a blade, U-shaped on cross-section.[40] The light which was eventually supplied from a battery in the handle was originally powered from the electric mains. It can be fitted with fibreoptic illumination.[41] The blade and handle may be either parallel or set at an angle one to the other, the handle containing the 3-volt battery. Various types and sizes of blade are in use. While the Magill laryngoscope blade is

designed to lift the epiglottis forward, the Macintosh blade is shorter, curved and Z-shaped on cross-section, and its tip enters the vallecula, lifts the base of the tongue and, with it, the attached epiglottis, so that the cords can be visualized. Both aspects of the epiglottis are supplied by the internal branch of the superior laryngeal nerve. An additional advantage of the Macintosh instrument is that during intubation the tube does not hide the cords from view. A plastic version is now available made of acetyl co-polymer which can be boiled but not autoclaved.

While the blade of each instrument is designed to be inserted into the right side of the patient's mouth, moving the tongue over to the left, there is a blade available for the left side.[42] Full-size blades can be used for quite small children, but neonates and babies require special straight blades, e.g. the Oxford infant blade.[43] The relationship of the floor of the mouth to that of the pharynx was pointed out by Bannister et al.[44]

Some of the many modifications which are available include: The Bowen–Jackson laryngoscope,[45] a modification of Macintosh's design. It has a rather long blade and the smallest possible 'step' consistent with adequate tongue deflexion. The Polio laryngoscope can be used on patients in iron-lung respirators; the Macintosh-type blade makes an angle of approximately 135° with the handle.

Other modifications have been described,[46] including an obstetric laryngo-scope.[47] A flexible fibreoptic laryngoscope can be threaded through a tracheal tube and inserted nasally or orally into the trachea, directing the tip by remote control. It is then withdrawn, leaving the tube in place; this may be useful when the teeth are fragile or in other cases of difficulty.

(*See also* The Macintosh laryngoscope, Boulton T. B. 'Classical File', *Surv. Anesthesiol.* 1983, **27**, 396; History of the commercial development of the Macintosh laryngoscope, Jephcott A. *Anaesthesia* 1984, **39**, 474.)

Intubating Forceps

Magill's instrument is commonly used and is made in two sizes[48] and a modification with an antero-posterior grip has been described.[49] First used for the introduction of narrow gum-elastic catheters for insufflation anaesthesia. *See also*[177].

Angle-pieces

These connect the tracheal tube to the breathing tube of the gas machine. Several designs are in use and some provide an adjustable cap for insertion of a sucker tube where suction is required, e.g. Magill, Cobb. Gas flow is more turbulent and less laminar in right-angled than in curved connectors.

Catheter Mounts

These connect the angle-piece to the anaesthetic machine and are made of plain or corrugated rubber tubing; 22-mm taper connections are very widely used for such connections.

Inflatable Cuffs

As cuffs prevent leakage between the wall of the trachea and the outer wall of the tube, they are useful in IPPV. They also prevent gastric contents, blood, mucus and vomitus from entering the lungs and so are essential in intestinal obstruction with regurgitant vomiting, and in operations on the upper air passages.

The traditional cuff is 2–3 cm long and of the low-volume high-pressure type.

Used to ensure airtight tracheal anaesthesia, instead of pharyngeal gauze packing.[50] The Hewer pilot balloon shows the state of the cuff when it is hidden in the trachea.[51] There is the danger, when using a cuff, of causing sloughing of the tracheal mucosa. Measurement of the pressure exerted by the inflated cuff on the mucosa of the tracheal wall is difficult,[52] but indirect methods have been described.[53] Cuffs should not be inflated to a pressure greater than that needed to prevent audible leakage of gas when the reservoir bag is compressed.[54] Low-pressure large-volume cuffs have many advantages over the standard variety, but they too may injure the tracheal epithelium. Various cuffs exert different pressures. Large volume cuffs can have a pressure gauge in line. If inflated with normal saline, nitrous oxide will not diffuse in and increase the pressure. A continuous lateral wall pressure should not exceed $30\,cmH_2O$ or $22\,mmHg$ to avoid damage to the tracheal mucosa.[55] The integrity of the inflatable cuff must always be tested before use. N_2O has the ability of diffusing into air-inflated latex cuffs and may thus cause over-expansion, and trauma to the mucosa. Filling the cuff with anaesthetic gas mixtures is a simple way to prevent tracheal damage from increased pressure during anaesthesia.[56]

(*See also* Lindholm C-E. and Grenvik A. *Recent Advances in Intensive Therapy*. London and Edinburgh: Churchill Livingstone, 1977; Thompson W. R. and Oh T. E. *Anaesth. Intensive Care* 1979, **9**, 152; Latto I. P. in: *Difficulties in Tracheal Intubation* (Latto I. P. and Rosen M. ed.) London: Baillière Saunders, 1985; Patel R. J. et al. *Anaesthesia*, 1983, **38**, 44; *Anaesthesia* 1984, **39**, 866; Mehta S. *Br. J. Anaesth.* 1981, **53**, 1227; Mehta S. *Ann. R. Coll. Surg.* 1984, **66**, 426.)

Lubricants

A greasy or water-soluble lubricant, with or without a local analgesic (e.g. 2–4% lignocaine), reduces trauma.

Topical Analgesia

The use of cocaine to suppress the laryngeal reflex in general anaesthesia was first used by Rosenberg in 1895[57] and by Magill, to aid intubation, in 1928.[58] The solution should be sprayed onto the superior laryngeal aperture, the cords and the mucosa of the larynx and trachea. To avoid overdosage, lignocaine 3 mg/kg or 5 ml of 4% solution for a 75-kg man should not be exceeded. Prilocaine, 10 ml of 4% solution, is probably safe. Two per cent lignocaine spray is said to have cardiac stabilizing effects, so preventing excess cortisol excretion during intubation.[59]

Sprays

A spray, e.g. Vale[60] or Forrester,[61] is useful. The dental aerosol local analgesic spray, with specially long nozzle and measured dose, has been used. Sprays may become a source of infection.

Lignocaine ointment, 2 ml of 5%, applied to a tube can result in significant systemic absorption.[62]

Indications for Tracheal Intubation

About this, experienced opinions vary. There are workers who intubate almost every patient and others who are much more conservative: (1) In operations in which a free airway cannot be otherwise maintained; (2) In patients who may not have an empty stomach: reduces the chance of aspiration; (3) In many abdominal operations; (4) In intrathoracic operations, so that the airway is always patent, suction can be easily carried out, and control of intrapulmonary pressure and ventilation made easy; (5) In cases operated on in positions making control of the airway difficult, e.g. operation in prone position; (6) With the use of relaxants and IPPV. Manual ventilation, employing a face-mask, is uncomfortable and may result in inflation of the stomach; (7) In a majority of operations on the head and neck; (8) In patients likely to develop laryngeal spasm, e.g. some cases of cystoscopy, haemorrhoidectomy, etc.; (9) In paediatric anaesthesia where enthusiasts use it almost invariably.

In the authors' opinion tracheal intubation should not be abused and should not be employed without a real indication. The duration of an operation is not of itself an indication for tracheal intubation.

Intubation in Non-surgical Conditions
(1) To preserve the airway in any patient who is unconscious as a result of head injury, drug overdose, cardiac arrest, etc.; (2) In grave asphyxia neonatorum; (3) To overcome airway obstruction due to tumour or inflammation; (4) To facilitate bronchial and tracheal suction in the presence of sputum retention; (5) In prolonged IPPV.

(For discussion of prolonged intubation *see* Gilston A. *Anaesthesia* 1982, **37**, 209.)

Contraindications

These are relative: (1) Aneurysm of aortic arch: trauma of tracheal walls may cause rupture; (2) Acute laryngitis: trauma may make condition worse or cause oedema. Intubation may, however, be life-saving.

Technique of Blind Nasal Intubation

Distance between naris and carina averages 32 cm in males and 27 cm in females. It is essential that extreme gentleness should characterize the whole procedure. It is a knack, only acquired by practice. The experienced worker employs tubes of the size, shape and consistency to suit his individual technique.

1. The nares should be examined for patency by listening to the patient's breathing with each naris alternatively occluded. Nasal polypi should be excluded.

2. The nares and upper respiratory tract can be sprayed with 4% cocaine solution, realizing that it is toxic, or 1% ephedrine in oil can be instilled to shrink the nasal mucosa. An alternative is 3% lignocaine with 0·25% phenylephrine.[63]

3. Then select the largest size of tube that experience suggests will pass atraumatically through the larger naris: for a big man size 10, for a small woman sizes 5–7. The lumen of the tube must be clean and patent. On the curve of the tube depends the position of the patient's head. The greater the curve, the more flexed should be the head during intubation. An average position of the head, advised by Magill, is that adopted 'when sniffing the morning air', on a single pillow, with slight extension of the atlanto-occipital joint. The optimal position of the atlanto-occipital joint and the tube curvature differs between workers.

4. Following induction of anaesthesia, the anaesthetist must decide whether to attempt intubation with the patient fully relaxed and apnoeic (as after suxamethonium), or to allow spontaneous respiration with an inhaled mixture supplemented with carbon dioxide to stimulate respiration with widening of the glottis during inspiration.

5. The tube is inserted into the naris so that its concavity is directed to the patient's feet. It is thrust directly backwards, not upwards. Movement of the bevel by rotation of the tube may be necessary to overcome resistance, either at this stage or when the tube enters the nasopharynx from the nose.

6. The lower jaw should be slightly elevated to lift the epiglottis away from the posterior pharyngeal wall and the opposite nostril occluded so that all breathing is taking place through the tube. If the right naris is used the head should be inclined slightly to the right, and vice versa.

7. If the patient is breathing spontaneously the anaesthetist should listen carefully to the respiration. The audible tubular breathing conducted through the tube becomes maximal when the tip is immediately above the glottis. If the tube does not enter the larynx because it is wrongly directed, an adjustment can be made by rotation of the tube, rotation of the neck or digital movement of the larynx to meet the advancing tube. Should the tube enter the oesophagus it can be partially withdrawn and its tip directed anteriorly by increased extension of the neck or by the selection of a tube with a larger curvature. Occasionally the tip of the tube impinges on the anterior commissure of the larynx. It will then often enter the larynx if the neck is flexed.[64] As the tube passes the cords a slight snap is often noticeable and there may be some coughing or breath-holding in the lightly anaesthetized patient, even when muscle relaxant drugs have been employed. In the patient who is not paralysed the tube may enter the trachea during the explosive cough which may follow spasm of the cords. Failure to enter the larynx requires partial withdrawal of the tip into the oropharynx and then reinsertion.

8. The character of the breath sounds issuing from the proximal end of the tube shows that it is in the trachea. With a tube of reasonable length, if breath sounds are free, the distal end of the tube must lie in the trachea. If the tube can be inserted to its full extent and no breath sounds can be heard, it is probably in the oesophagus. Free breathing through the tube, while the lower jaw is pushed backwards firmly, suggests successful intubation. Capnography confirms this.

9. Blind intubation may also be accomplished in the patient who is paralysed by suxamethonium or a non-depolarizing relaxant. Some workers find this to be easier, since reflex laryngospasm does not occur.

10. In the case of failure to intubate through one naris, success may be achieved through the other, or with a tube of different curvature.

Difficulties

If unsuccessful, blind intubation should not be persisted in or trauma may result. Tubes, which must be supple and rather soft, should always be handled daintily and not forcibly rammed down the patient's throat. Difficulty may be encountered if the tube is not sufficiently curved. A radius of curvature of 10 cm is suitable. Should the tube not lie in the trachea it may be situated: (1) In the oesophagus, i.e. posterior to its correct position, either because the tube is not sufficiently curved or because the head is too flexed; (2) On the anterior commissure of the larynx, i.e. anterior to its correct position, for reasons the opposite to those above; (3) In the vallecula, between the base of the tongue and the epiglottis. Rotation of the tube, so that it slips down the lateral wall of the pharynx, should overcome this obstruction; (4) In one or other pyriform fossa, lateral to its correct position. This is likely where the nose is asymmetric, and is overcome by rotating the tube, by moving the larynx laterally to meet the tube or by rotating the patient's head; (5) Curled up in the pharynx. This will only occur with soft, worn-out tubes. Patients with ankylosing spondylitis and with ankylosis of the jaw may present special difficulties. It is important to select a tube with a curvature appropriate for the patient, whose neck may be fixed.

When blind intubation fails. Following the passage of the tube through the naris, the distal end can be guided into the trachea by: (1) The Magill intubating forceps,[48] (2) The use of a wire hook in the oropharynx to guide the tube backwards or forwards; (3) Passage of a plastic catheter through the cricothyroid membrane via a Tuohy needle into the larynx and out through the nose; the catheter is then used as a guide for the nasal tube; (4) The use of a fibreoptic endoscope.[65]

A prominent arch of the atlas vertebra may cause obstruction with the possibility of laceration of its overlying mucosa. To overcome this a small suction catheter may be threaded through the endotracheal tube and tension made on it as it is delivered through the mouth, thus displacing the tip of the tube and overcoming obstruction. Bony spicules on the spinous processes of the cervical vertebrae can, by interfering with the extension of the neck, make intubation difficult.

Epistaxis. This looks messy, but seldom interferes with the anaesthesia or causes postoperative discomfort. Partial obstruction of a nasotracheal tube by an avulsed piece of turbinate may occur.[66] Blood clot in the lumen may cause obstruction.

Partial occlusion of tube by nasal spurs, deflected septa, etc., causing respiratory obstruction. The opposite naris or the orotracheal route may have to be substituted. A laryngocele, a pathological enlargement of the saccule of the larynx, may complicate intubation.[67]

A 'Difficult Intubation Box' has been described.[68]

Indications for Blind Nasal Intubation

(1) When an oral tube is in the surgeon's way, e.g. in tonsillectomy, dental extraction and operations on tongue. (2) When the use of a laryngoscope is difficult owing to the anatomy of the patient. (3) In unanaesthetized unconscious patients, for improvement of the airway. (4) In the presence of dental crowns.

Some workers of experience find no use for this technique, believing that the danger of epistaxis, avulsion of nasal polyps, etc. with the risk of foreign material entering the tracheobronchial tree contraindicates the method. Others point to the dangers of the use of the laryngoscope with risk of damage to teeth, dental bridges, etc. and the possibility of inhalation of tooth fragments. The main indication for blind intubation is in the patient in whom direct laryngoscopy is likely to be difficult, or has failed. The anaesthetist will not succeed with blind intubation in these cases unless he is practised in the technique. The authors of this book regard it as a most useful method when it is indicated.

Technique of Direct-vision Nasal Intubation

This is necessary if blind intubation fails and if a nasotracheal tube is desirable.

The laryngoscope is inserted after anaesthesia is induced, as for direct orotracheal intubation. The tube tip, having been inserted as far as the hypopharynx, is guided between the cords, either by slight movement of the tube or with the aid of intubation forceps. If the tube is too curved or the head too extended it may impinge against the anterior commissure of the larynx and this can often be remedied by keeping the tube pressed against the anterior commissure, withdrawing the laryngoscope, flexing the head and pushing the tube home 'blind'. Occasionally a tube cannot be guided successfully into the trachea from the nose; it must then be withdrawn and inserted via the mouth.

Nasal intubation has been followed by bacteraemia in 12% of children[69] and in 17% of adults.[70] The significance of these findings in patients at risk of developing endocarditis, is not known.

Technique of Direct-vision Orotracheal Intubation[71]

Before induction, the shape of the jaws and the condition of the teeth are carefully assessed. A small pillow should usually be placed under the occiput to flex the neck and extend the atlanto-occipital joint.[21] Loose, filled or capped teeth, especially upper incisors, and the lips may be damaged by the blade of the laryngoscope and so should be protected by lead sheet, rubber, adhesive strapping, etc. The usual method consists of the injection of a sleep dose of barbiturate (e.g. thiopentone 100–500 mg) preceded or followed by ventilation with pure oxygen: if this is maintained for 3 min there will be no hypoxia following 4 min of suxamethonium apnoea. A little more barbiturate may be needed before the injection of suxamethonium 30–100 mg. Anaesthesia must be well established (in the second plane or below, with complete suppression of reflexes, if a volatile agent is being used), and relaxation must be profound. Less harm is done by getting the patient a little too deep than by using force in a patient with active reflexes and rigid neck muscles. Absence of reflexes and adequate muscular relaxation are necessary for laryngoscopy in all but expert hands.

Using the Curved Laryngoscope (Macintosh)
To convert the angular line from the tip of the upper incisor teeth, through the mouth to the pharynx and larynx, to a straight line with a laryngoscope blade, the occiput should be raised 8–12 cm, the neck flexed and the head extended at the atlanto-occipital joint.[72] Good muscular relaxation is necessary so that the tongue and soft tissues can be lifted anteriorly. The blade of the instrument should be inserted towards the right side of the patient's mouth to prevent his tongue from blocking the view of the larynx. The blade is passed along the tongue to the vallecula and is tilted forwards so that the epiglottis is drawn away to reveal the cords. A tube with a curve or on a curved introducer is important as a straight one is difficult to insert. The curved blade is usually easier to use if the patient has a full set of teeth. It may also cause less stretching of the faucial pillars and hence bruising than the straight blade. Backward pressure on the thyroid cartilage by an assistant may aid visualization of the cords. Otherwise a 60-cm gum-elastic introducer can be passed into the larynx more easily than a tube. Its proximal end is then inserted into a tracheal tube and this is slid into the larynx over the gum-elastic introducer.[73] The use of a rigid bronchoscope with a cuffed tracheal tube outside it, may facilitate a difficult intubation.[74]

Using the Straight Laryngoscope (Magill)

With the patient adequately anaesthetized and in the proper position, with some extension of the atlanto-occipital joint, and a pillow under the neck[21] with a strip of adhesive protecting the upper incisor teeth, and after ventilation of the lungs with oxygen, the lubricated laryngoscope blade is gently inserted into the mouth and progressively advanced. When the epiglottis is seen it is elevated by the tip of the blade, care being taken not to scratch the posterior pharyngeal wall. The tongue and epiglottis are now lifted forwards, i.e. in the direction of the ceiling. The upper teeth must not be used as a fulcrum. As the curtain of the epiglottis is lifted forwards, the cords are exposed to view and are identified by their pallor.

Difficulties

An experienced worker may fail to spot a case which will be difficult while a case expected to be difficult may prove quite easy to intubate. Grading of difficulty has been proposed according to the view obtained at laryngoscopy.[75] Difficulty, which may be expected in about 2% of patients[76] may be anticipated in patients with: (1) A reduction in the radiological distance between the occiput and the spinous process of C1 or the C1–C2 intergap;[77] (2) A short muscular neck with a full set of teeth; (3) A receding lower jaw; (4) Increased distance between the mental symphysis and the lower alveolar margin which requires wide depression of the lower jaw during intubation; (5) A long high arched palate and a narrow deep mouth; (6) Protruding upper incisors—'rabbit teeth'; (7) Carious, capped or insecure upper teeth; (8) Difficulty in opening the jaw, as in multiple arthritis involving the temporomandibular joints, and spondylitis of the cervical spine causing rigidity of the neck so that the head cannot be positioned; (9) Fusion of the atlanto-occipital joint and calcification of interspinous ligaments;[76,77] (10) Calcified stylohyoid ligament;[78] this causes difficulty in lifting the epiglottis from the posterior pharyngeal wall and may be accompanied by a skin crease over the hyoid bone;[79] (11) Scleroderma, neoplasms of the oropharynx, epiglottic cyst;[80] (12) Cicatricial conditions of the mouth and neck causing contraction of tissues; (13) Achondroplasia; (14) Trismus; (15) Contracture of tissue at the front of the neck from burns, resulting in flexion of the neck; (16) Tumours of the mouth or larynx; (17) Hypertrophy of the posterior one-third of the tongue; (18) Subglottic stenosis, following previous prolonged intubation. (*See also* Latto I. P. and Rosen M. *Difficulties in Tracheal Intubation*. London: Baillière Saunders, 1985.) It may well be unwise to abolish spontaneous respiration in some of these patients before intubation. Absence of the upper incisors usually makes intubation relatively easy.

Intubation is often facilitated by the use of a malleable gum elastic introducer with a tip curved anteriorly and projecting for 5 cm beyond the opening of the tube.[81] Difficulties due to gross obesity may be overcome by the use of the polio laryngoscope.

Transtracheal ventilation may be life-saving; a 14-gauge plastic-over-metal intravenous cannula is thrust into the larynx through the cricothyroid membrane and connected to a modified bronchoscope injector with a pressure of oxygen of about 345 kPa.[82]

The anterior larynx.[103] The atlanto-occipital joint may not be extensible because the posterior tubercle of the atlas makes contact with the occipital bone. This prevents extension of the joint and persistent attempts cause anterior bowing of the cervical spine and anterior displacement of the larynx. Preoperative testing should give a warning of this. For intubation, the occiput must be raised on a pillow. Conversely, good extension is usually associated with easy visualization of the cords.[83] The position of the larynx can be observed radiologically.

Technique of Orotracheal Intubation without Laryngoscope

This is very occasionally necessary when abnormal anatomy precludes the use of a laryngoscope or when the nasal route is undesirable.

1. With the patient deeply anaesthetized and the anaesthetist standing to the left of the patient and facing him, and an assistant drawing the tongue forwards, the anaesthetist passes two fingers of his left hand over the dorsum of the tongue, so that the epiglottis is hooked forwards. The tube, which must be fully curved, is guided by the two fingers in the mouth into the glottis. Curved introducers have been used to aid this procedure, which was the one favoured by Franz Khun in 1901.[8,9]

2. The anaesthetist stands in his usual place at the head of the table and inserts his left thumb into the patient's mouth with his forearm pronated and his fingers on the patient's chin. The tip of the thumb makes contact with the base of the tongue as far back as possible. This gives good control of the lower jaw which with the tongue can be moved forward and backward, the patient being deeply anaesthetized. The tube is guided into the glottis with the right hand.

3. The tube, which must not be too fully curved, can be passed 'blind' through a London Hospital prop held in the mouth, with the head of the anaesthetized patient in full extension.

Checking that the Tip of the Tube in in the Trachea
The anaesthetist must convince himself that all parts of each lung are receiving and expelling gas during ventilation. He should auscultate: (1) The trachea; (2) Each upper zone; (3) Each axilla; (4) The epigastrium.

Causes of diminished air entry into one lung are: (1) Endobronchial placement of tube; (2) Pneumothorax; (3) Collapse of lung; (4) Blockage of bronchus from stomach contents, blood, etc.; (5) Bronchial adenoma.[84]

For Technique of Fibreoptic Laryngoscopy
See Rogers S. N. and Nenumof J. L. *Anesthesiology* 1983, **59**, 569; Fibreoptic endoscopy in anesthesia (Patil V. U. et al. ed.) Chicago: Year Book Publishers, 1983.

Failed Intubation (*see also* pp. 212 and 217)

Oxygenation without aspiration is the watchword! An oesophageal gastric tube airway may be passed into the gullet and its cuff inflated with 35 ml of air. This displaces the larynx forward and provides an airway.[85,86]

To minimize failed intubation, the following equipment should be readily available: laryngoscope with two Macintosh, one Magill and one polio blade, Magill forceps; long gum-elastic bougies as introducers; malleable stylets; oesophageal gastric tube airways; and emergency transcricoid ventilation set.[86] (For modification of Tunstall's failed intubation drill, *see* Hyde P. R. *Anaesth. Intensive Care* 1983, **11**, 56; Campbell W. I. *Br. J. Anaesth*. 1983, **55**, 1040.)

Transtracheal ventilation can be carried out using a drip set, the sharp end of the drip chamber being inserted into the trachea, the other end connected to a source of oxygen. Such equipment is available in an emergency.[87]

Extubation

The normal response to extubation is a rise in blood pressure and pulse rate. This can be minimized by instilling 60 mg of lignocaine down the tube a few minutes before it is withdrawn,[88] or by injecting lignocaine, 1 mg/kg 2 min before withdrawal, i.v.[89] This may be useful in patients with coronary disease. After the operation the tube can be removed in the theatre, the air passages sucked clear, and a pharyngeal airway inserted. Otherwise the patient returns to the ward with the tube still in position. In the latter case it is better that it should remain until the return of the cough reflex, when it can be removed by the postoperative observation ward sister.

Laryngeal spasm after extubation is sometimes seen, so it is important to fill the lungs with oxygen before extubation and to verify that breathing is free after the tube is removed. Extubation spasm can usually be prevented or treated by: (1) Suxamethonium followed by ventilation with oxygen; (2) More neostigmine, if a non-depolarizing relaxant has been used; (3) Doxapram 1·5 mg/kg;[90] (4) Incremental doses of diazepam;[91] (5) Topical analgesia; (6) Physostigmine.[92]

Laryngeal spasm may result in acute pulmonary oedema[93] and can often be ameliorated by giving oxygen by mask while the chest is rhythmically compressed.

It may be due to high negative pressure in the alveoli disturbing the normal ratio between capillary-alveolar pressure and intracapillary interstitial pressure with seepage of fluid into the alveoli and lung parenchyma.[94]

Difficult respiration following laryngospasm due to extubation may be due to pulmonary oedema.[95]

Extubation with the patient in the lateral head-down position has much to recommend it.

Acute onset facial oedema in a patient with liver disease has been reported, following extubation.[96]

Difficulty in extubation has been reported in patients in whom intubation was easy. Acute oedematous laryngitis has resulted from this complication. It may be due to a fold of the cuff.[97]

Suction

Great care must be taken, especially in ill or handicapped patients, to avoid hypoxia from suction, which should be graduated and controlled.

Catheters

These are expressed in FG (French Gauge). Division by 3 gives the approximate external diameter in millimetres. Lengths vary between 38 and 55 cm. A suction catheter, the external diameter of which is half the internal diameter of the tracheal tube, allows sufficient free gas flow to prevent significant subatmospheric pressure in the lungs. For example, catheter FG 12 is satisfactory for an 8-mm tracheal tube.[98] Pharyngeal trauma may follow suction.[99]

Some Difficulties After Direct-vision Intubation

(1) Kinking of the tube causing respiratory obstruction. Use as firm a tube for orotracheal intubation as possible. A reinforced latex or Oxford tube kinks less easily than a plain rubber one. Kinking is rare with a nasotracheal tube though it may be compressed in the naris if the airway is narrow; (2) Partial respiratory obstruction caused by use of too small a tube; (3) Separation of anaesthetic connections from tube; (4) Blockage of tube by blood, mucus, etc. Tube may need to be sucked out; (5) Obstruction has resulted from a tube being pulled up so that its distal end becomes blocked by the inflated cuff; (6) Slipping out of tube owing to weight of attached breathing tubes, etc.; (7) Obstruction by apposition of the bevel of the tube against the tracheal wall; (8) Damage to teeth.[100] If a tooth is knocked out it must be accounted for by carefully examining the mouth and pharynx and prevented from disappearing into the trachea. If a radiograph shows it to be in a bronchus, it should be looked for with a bronchoscope as soon as possible. Enamel can be protected by the use of metal foil, e.g. the top of a milk bottle; (9) Grave laryngeal spasm, before insertion or on removal of tube. This will usually yield to a relaxant; if not, cricothyroid puncture with a wide-bore needle and subsequent oxygen insufflation may be life-saving;[101] In cases of grave laryngeal spasm a 10-gauge plastic needle and cannula can be inserted into the front of the trachea and an intermittent jet of oxygen given. Translaryngeal insufflation of oxygen under pressure through a Tuohy 16g needle, provides useful oxygenation, the jet acting as a Venturi, provided that there is no upper airway obstruction;[102] (10) Intubation of the right bronchus. Due to use of too long a tube. Average distance between central incisors and carina is 27 cm in an adult male and 23 cm in a female. Distance from nares to carina is an additional 4 cm. In a newborn baby, 5 cm separates the gums from the cords, and a similar distance separates the cords from the carina. Diagnosed by hypoxic appearance of patient, absence of air entry into left lung, unsatisfactory anaesthesia with jerky breathing and bucking. Entry of gas into both the left and right upper zones should always be checked by auscultation, following intubation.

Intubation of the Oesophagus

A tube inadvertently placed in the oesophagus and then connected to a reservoir bag may result in a 'tidal volume' of 50 ml with a rhythmically moving bag simulating a correctly placed tube.[104] Unwitting intubation of the oesophagus and subsequent hypoxia is a common cause of anaesthetic catastrophe.[105]

Intubation of the oesophagus is not uncommon. It can be diagnosed by: (1) Using a stethoscope over the epigastrium while the reservoir bag is squeezed; a gurgling sound results; (2) By blowing down the tracheal tube when a bubbling sound results and on taking the mouth away, no air returns through the tube; (3) By passing a fibreoptic bronchoscope down the lumen of the tube;[106] (4) By allowing the gas issuing from the tube to bubble through an Einstein CO_2 detector, as tracheal gas contains 4% CO_2;[107] Use of the capnograph as an end-expiratory CO_2 monitor is a rapid and reliable indicator that useful ventilation is taking place and that the tube is in the trachea when doubt arises. The typical CO_2 trace disappears if the oesophagus is intubated and reappears only when the tube is correctly placed in the trachea: it can be used in patients breathing spontaneously or with ventilation controlled.[108] (*See also* Pollard B. J. and Junius F. *Anaesth. Intensive Care* 1980, **8**, 183; Cundy J. *Anaesth. Intensive*

Care 1981, **9**, 76; Howells T. H. and Riethmuller R. J. *Anaesthesia* 1980, **35**, 984; Warden J. C. *Anaesth. Intensive Care* 1980, **8**, 377.) Estimation of oxygen saturation is also valuable;[109] (5) Oesophageal misplacement of a tracheal tube can often be detected by slightly overdistending the pilot balloon and clamping it off. It is now rapidly and intermittently squeezed while the other hand firmly palpates the front of the neck above the sternum. Transmitted pulsation gives a positive indication that the tube is in the trachea.[110] (For drill for cases of failed intubation, *see* Chapter 27 and Tunstall M. E. *Anaesthesia* 1976, **31**, 850; Hyde P. R. *Anaesth. Intensive Care* 1983, **11**, 56; Campbell W. I. *Br. J. Anaesth.* 1983, **55**, 1040; Swartman S. et al. *Br. J. Anaesth.* 1983, **55**, 1040.) Cricoid pressure can also be used in elective cases to prevent oesophageal intubation.[111]

Anaesthetic Agents in Relation to Tracheal Intubation

1. Suxamethonium. This short-acting muscle relaxant is probably the most popular drug used for making intubation quick, easy and atraumatic when combined with an intravenous barbiturate. A suitable dose is 25–100 mg. This is given after the patient is anaesthetized, it works in less than 1 min, while its effect, including apnoea, seldom lasts more than a few minutes. For *blind nasal intubation*, during or shortly following apnoea, a combination of thiopentone and suxamethonium can be used by experienced workers. Dosage suggested is 0·25 g of the barbiturate, with suxamethonium chloride 25–40 mg. The relaxant removes the tone from the laryngeal and neck muscles. Suxamethonium can be given intramuscularly if veins are difficult, e.g. in infants.

2. Non-depolarizing relaxants. These drugs take up to 3 min to exert their full effect and during this time, following the injection of thiopentone and the relaxant, the lungs must be gently inflated with oxygen. Additional doses of either thiopentone or the relaxant may be given as necessary. In those patients at risk of inhaling stomach contents, the relaxant drug may be given before the thiopentone, providing that venous access is secure, to shorten the time to intubation. Vecuronium is probably then the non-depolarizing agent of choice. Non-depolarizing drugs should never be given unless the anaesthetist is confident of his ability to ventilate the lungs using a face-mask (*see also* Chapter 15).

3. Inhalation agents. Intubation may be carried out under inhalation anaesthesia, the patient breathing spontaneously throughout. Any agent may be used but deep anaesthesia with ether probably produces the best conditions, without undue respiratory depression. Halothane is popular in children, though care must be taken not to administer too high a concentration, with resultant cardiorespiratory depression.

4. Intravenous induction agents. Intubation when any of these is used alone is not recommended. Laryngeal reflexes are usually active with the probability of causing laryngeal spasm, and cough reflexes usually remain active. These agents should therefore usually be combined with a muscle relaxant, or followed by deep inhalation anaesthesia.

5. Local analgesia and awake intubation (*see also* Murrin K. R. in: *Difficulties in Tracheal Intubation* (Latto I. P. and Rosen M. ed.), London: Baillière Saunders, 1985). Possible indications are: (*a*) A full stomach; (*b*) Upper airway obstruction, e.g. from laryngeal neoplasm; (*c*) Possible technical difficulties in intubation; (*d*) Bronchopleural fistula; (*e*) When the use of muscle relaxants is undesirable. One or more of the following methods may be used: (*a*) Sucking an analgesic lozenge; (*b*) Spray of the mouth and pharynx and cords; (*c*) Bilateral superior laryngeal nerve block[112] (q.v.); (*d*) Transtracheal injection. For intubation after *transtracheal injection* the patient should be calm. Thiopentone 50–150 mg, diazepam 5–10 mg, midazolam 2–7·5 mg or fentanyl 50–150 µg is injected i.v. and in 60–90 sec 3 ml of 4% lignocaine solution is injected in the midline into the airway, above or below the cricoid, checked for correct position by the ability to aspirate air. After expiration, the solution is injected and will produce an explosive cough. A 1-in 22-g plastic-over-metal cannula can be used for the injection, after withdrawing the metal; this reduces the risk of bleeding.[113] The patient is then given oxygen for 2–3 min, thiopentone is slowly injected until the jaw relaxes to enable the laryngoscope to be inserted and the cords to be visualized. Intubation follows, when the cords will usually be found to be abducted.[114,115] Voluntary hyperventilation, breathing pure oxygen,[116] for a few minutes before intubation, minimizes blood-gas alteration associated with this manoeuvre.

Failed Intubation[175]

Should the anaesthetist fail to intubate the trachea, the lungs must be inflated with an oxygen-rich mixture until spontaneous respiration returns. If vomiting, or regurgitation of stomach contents is considered possible, the patient's head should be lowered and the lateral position adopted, with the idea of keeping the respiratory tract free from contamination. Sometimes the wise course is to allow full return of consciousness. Anaesthesia may then be continued by: (1) Use of a face-mask and pharyngeal airway (all operations were conducted in this way before the 1930s); (2) Use of nasopharyngeal airways which may be bilateral;[117] (3) The laryngeal mask;[118] (4) The oesophageal obturator airway;[119] (5) The substitution of regional for general anaesthesia.[120]

Advantages and Disadvantages of Intubation

Advantages
(1) Avoidance of respiratory obstruction, and consequent absence of laboured respiration and capillary oozing. (2) Absence of straining due to laryngeal spasm. (3) Artificial ventilation and control of intrapulmonary pressure made easy. (4) Enables anaesthetist to keep away from the operative field. (5) In the presence of a full stomach lessens the chance of inspiration of foreign matter during the operation (with an inflated cuff). (6) Dead space reduced to a minimum.

Disadvantages
(1) Trauma to lip, teeth, nose, throat and larynx, resulting in hoarseness, dysphagia, pain, etc. Abrasion of the mucosa of the pharynx may result in extensive surgical emphysema; (2) Safe use of laryngoscope may require a deeper plane of anaesthesia than the surgical operation or the use of a muscle relaxant which would otherwise not be employed; (3) Lack of contact of inspired gases with the mucosa covering the turbinates leads to cold dry gases reaching the alveoli; the use of a closed system or humidifier prevents this; (4) Postoperative voice problems.[121]

Difficulty with tracheal intubation is one of the most important factors leading to maternal deaths attributed to anaesthesia.[120]

Lignocaine 2 mg/kg i.v. 1–5 min before intubation significantly reduces the incidence of coughing following the insertion of the tube in anaesthetized patients not receiving a muscle relaxant.[122] Such a dose given 2 min before intubation also attenuates the increase in intraocular tension, and so may be useful in dealing with patients with perforating eye injuries.[123]

Endotracheal Absorption of Drugs[124]

The following drugs can be given through a tracheal tube and are quickly absorbed; lignocaine, atropine,[125] adrenaline,[126] isoprenaline, naloxone.[127]

Reflex Circulatory Responses to Laryngoscopy and Intubation[176]

During light general anaesthesia, direct laryngoscopy and intubation, uncomplicated by hypoxia, hypercapnia or cough, cause an increase in heart rate, arterial pressure and dysrhythmia in up to 90% of patients because of stimulation of the nerve endings of the vagus and trigeminal nerves.[128] These changes are not of great clinical significance in healthy patients, but are made much worse by changes in the blood gases, while hypertensive subjects are likely to show an exaggerated response. Deep anaesthesia is however, protective. For this reason pre-oxygenation by inhalation of pure oxygen for a few minutes or inflation with oxygen should be carried out following the injection of a relaxant and before intubation. Adequate depression of reflexes as by topical analgesia reduces the incidence of this, and may be used in certain cases of myocardial disease for this reason. Sudden death, presumably from ventricular fibrillation, has been reported to result reflexly from intubation and from tracheal suction. To reduce the dangers of hypertension during intubation, e.g. in patients with intracranial aneurysm, coronary disease, leaking aortic aneurysm etc., hydralazine 0·4 mg/kg in 10 ml of saline injected i.v. 10 min before induction, has been recommended. It has no effect on possible tachycardia while the effects last 3–4 h.[130]

Tubocurarine may be associated with a lower incidence of reflex cardiac disturbance than suxamethonium, alcuronium than pancuronium.[131] These reflexes are not influenced by the type of laryngoscope blade used.[133] Pre-treatment with fentanyl, 5 μg/kg or alfentanil, 15 μg/kg may also be employed.[129] Intranasal instillation of nitroglycerine 60 mg in 2 ml of water may be used for the same purpose.[133] There is evidence that suppression of pressor responses to laryngoscopy and intubation require both alpha- and beta-adrenergic blockade.[134] Midazolam 0·3 mg/kg may be associated with fewer cardiovascular reflexes than thiopentone, when used as an induction agent.[135] Pre-treatment with 6–8 ml of 3·3% nebulized lignocaine by inhalation 3 min before laryngoscopy, reduces potentially harmful cardiovascular effects of intubation. Intravenous droperidol 150 μg/kg 5 min before induction has also been recommended. *See also* Chapter 14.

There may be a rise in intracranial pressure associated with tracheal intubation, especially when suxamethonium is employed.[136] This may also occur when non-depolarizing relaxants are used.[137]

Complications after Intubation

1. Non-specific Granuloma of the Larynx (Granuloma Pyogenicum)

This is usually superimposed on a contact ulcer and takes some time to develop. The usual site is the tip of the vocal process of one or both arytenoids in the posterior one-third of the rima glottidis. The tips of the vocal processes are prominent and are covered with mucoperichondrium. Contact ulcer is not necessarily due to trauma from the intubation but may be due to actual movements of the cords against the tube as it lies in the larynx. These movements are not necessarily abolished by anaesthesia. Granuloma of the carina has been reported[138] as have also uvulitis and oedema of the pharynx.[139]

The prognosis of a contact ulcer is good. Healing is usual but is hindered by phonation. If it is followed by granuloma formation, local removal will be necessary.

2. Acute Oedematous Stenosis

This is very rare, but may follow intubation prolonged for more than 2 or 3 days. More usual in children because of: (*a*) The amount of loose areolar tissue in the subglottic region; (*b*) The small lumen which is easily occluded. Obstructive laryngeal oedema, from whatever cause, has the following signs: (i) Indrawing, during inspiration, at any of the following sites: (*a*) The suprasternal notch; (*b*) Around the clavicles; (*c*) The epigastrium; (*d*) The intercostal spaces; (ii) Ashy grey pallor; (iii) Choking and waking in terror every time the child falls asleep; (iv) Restlessness.

Treatment. No sedatives. Further intubation contraindicated. Active humidification of inspired air. Low tracheostomy without delay.

3. Bruising of Larynx

This may result in dysphonia and dysphagia but usually clears up in a few days. It bears no constant relationship to the difficulty of intubation. The arytenoids may be dislocated.[145] Tracheal laceration may result in surgical emphysema.

4. Stretch Injury of Recurrent Nerves

This has been reported following intubation and results in a paralysed cord. Suggested causes: (*a*) Stretching of nerve during acute extension during intubation; (*b*) Stretching during difficult extubation; (*c*) Rough handling of patient after operation; (*d*) Neuropraxis due to inflation of the cuff within the larynx rather than in the trachea. A low-pressure large-volume cuff might avoid this.

Idiopathic palsy of the recurrent nerve, a transient cranial mononeuropathy can occur with a reasonable chance of a good recovery.[140] The law of F. Semon (1849–1921) states that in a disorder of the laryngeal motor nerves, the abductors of the cords are the first and occasionally the only muscles affected.[141]

5. Unilateral Vocal Cord Paralysis

Paralysis presumably due to asymmetrical inflation of a cuff, has been described.[142] Bilateral cord paralysis, perhaps due to pressure of the inflated cuff on the laminae of the thyroid cartilage and injury to the recurrent nerve.[143] (*See also* Annotation, *Lancet* 1986, **1**, 636.) Precise assessment of vocal fold impairment can be determined by laryngography following intubation.[144]

6. *Neuropraxis*

Neuropraxis of the lingual nerve due to acute compression or stretching in its course from the medial surface of the mandible to the underside of the tongue has been described. Although axonal function is impaired for a few days, anatomical continuity is preserved and the outlook is good.[146]

7. *Dislodgement of Nasal Polypi*

Each patient must demonstrate free nasal breathing before nasal intubation. Damage to turbinate bones;[147] ulceration of turbinates due to prolonged nasal intubation.[148]

8. *Sublingual Haematoma*[149]

Swelling in the neck due to haematoma may cause post-extubation obstruction.[150] (Bukht D. and Langford R. M. *Anaesthesia* 1983, **38**, 390.)

9. *Postoperative Sore Throat*[151]

The cause may be post-suxamethonium muscle pain and not local trauma.[152] Retropharyngeal abscess after traumatic intubation.[153]

Other Complications

10. *Permanent alteration of the voice* has been reported in 3% of patients after intubation.[121]

11. *Damage to the teeth* (*see* Wright R. B. and Mansfield F. F. V. Medical Protection Society Publication, London).

12. *Tracheal rupture* during anaesthesia.[154]

13. *Pharyngeal and oesophageal perforation.*[155]

14. *Swallowed tube in adults*,[156] and in children.

15. *Fracture-luxation of the cervical spine.* Careless movement of the head can result in serious injury, particularly in the presence of pathology involving the cervical spine, especially when muscle tone has been abolished by relaxant agents.[157] In the presence of recent trauma it may be wise to ask the surgeon to hold the head in a safe position during intubation.

16. *Trauma to the eye.*

17. *Ignition of the tube during laser surgery* (*see* Chapter 24).

   In longstanding cases it has been suggested that the tube may safely remain in situ for 7 days and should then be withdrawn and the larynx examined; in the absence of pathology it may be reinserted for a further 5 days.[158] Morbidity from long-term intubation in infants and children is small.[159]

The Laryngeal Mask Airway

A new form of airway has recently been described which is introduced blindly into the hypopharynx to form a seal around the larynx, so allowing either spontaneous or positive-pressure ventilation without penetration of the trachea or oesophagus. It can be used instead of the face-mask in routine anaesthesia and is valuable in ophthalmic, dental, throat, nose and ear operations and where difficulties with the airway are expected.[160]

Tracheal Intubation in Infants and Children

Anaesthesia may be induced by any of the volatile agents, or by cyclopropane or nitrous oxide. Halothane, up to 4% with oxygen is satisfactory. Other workers prefer to use an intravenous agent. Relaxants are satisfactory and if venepuncture proves difficult, suxamethonium 3 mg/kg can be injected intramuscularly. In neonates, awake intubation is sometimes preferred. The head and shoulders of the child must be held firmly by someone experienced in the technique and the larynx is pushed backwards. The tip of the laryngoscope blade is placed either deep (posterior) to the epiglottis or in the glosso-epiglottic fold; the blade is inserted at the side of the mouth and pushes the tongue to the left. The child's larynx differs from the adult larynx in being: (1) Higher up: the rima glottidis is opposite the 3rd–4th cervical interspace in the infant, in adults one interspace lower. (2) The epiglottis is relatively longer, being V-shaped, instead of flat as in the adult. It makes an angle of 45° with the anterior pharyngeal wall while in adults it lies closer to the base of the tongue. (3) The narrowest part of the larynx may be at the level of the cricoid cartilage, which is not distensible, as are the cords, the narrowest part in adults: thus a tracheal tube may be squeezed through the glottis, but be held up at the cricoid causing trauma and oedema. If this occurs, a smaller tube should be substituted. Laryngeal trauma may be dangerous in infants and oedema may result either from clumsy intubation or from irritation due to too large a tube being left too long in the larynx. In children under 3, both main bronchi come off the trachea at an equal angle, unlike the arrangement in adults. At birth, the trachea is 4 cm long and 6 mm wide. Calculation for length of tracheal tube:[161] distance from teeth to carina is age divided by 2 plus 12 cm.

For use in infants the Seward[162] or Robertshaw laryngoscope blade is popular and the Shrivastava[163] has been recommended.[164] The neck should not be extended during laryngoscopy. A well developed occiput may make intubation more difficult. When using a mask (e.g. Rendell Baker) for IPPV, care must be taken not to inflate the stomach.

In neonates it is sometimes safer to pass the tube while the child is still conscious, since this is often easy and it avoids the possibility of hypoxia due to spasm or obstruction. The anatomy of the infant is such that the straight-bladed laryngoscope is preferable while its tip should be inserted into the vallecula, anteriorly to the epiglottis, and gently raised.

Size of Tubes[161]

In the neonate the correct length of a tracheal tube is 12 cm, with proximal end at the lips. Length of tube in older children in centimetres is age divided by 2 plus 12 cm. Diameter of tube is 2·5 mm for infant under 1 kg; 3 mm if weight is 1–2 kg; 3·5 mm for the neonate; 4 mm up to 2 years; 4·5 mm up to 3 years; 5 mm up to 4 years; 5·5 mm up to 6 years; another method of determining diameter required is: up to 6 years, age divided by 3 plus 3·5; over 6 years, age divided by 4 plus 4·5. Occasional subglottic stenosis will require a smaller tube than expected. This is especially likely in the presence of imperforate anus.[165] A tube has been designed which is of much larger diameter in the pharynx than below the glottis. This minimizes obstruction to air flow and avoids inadvertent endobronchial intubation. It is modelled on an early version designed by Magill for the operation of repair of cleft palate. Topical analgesic or lubricant is not necessary.[166] In small children and infants it is important to confirm that the tracheal tube has not entered either main bronchus. Inspection and auscultation of the chest should be carried out. For resistance to breathing in tracheal tubes in infants, *see* Hatch D. J. *Anaesthesia* 1978, **50**, 959.

Endobronchial Intubation in Infancy

The following technique has been recommended.[167] A plain Portex tube is taken, 1 cm longer than the distance from mouth to carina as measured on a lateral chest X-ray. When this is passed it enters the bronchus on the opposite side to the bevel. It is then rotated through 180° so that the upper lobe bronchus is not obstructed. The bevel must be cut for the appropriate side with an extension to avoid the orifice of the upper lobe orifice on the right side. For transtracheal ventilation in paediatric patients, *see* Smith R. B. et al. *Br. J. Anaesth.* 1974, **46**, 313.

Ayre's T-Piece[168]

Philip Ayre (1902–1979) Newcastle anaesthetist. Originally used in neuro-surgery. Ayre's method (Mapleson E system) does away with valves and rubber bags and allows the circuit to be open to the outside air thus there is no obstruction to expiration. One end of the cross-piece of a metal T-tube 1 cm in diameter is connected to an angle-piece of an endotracheal tube by about 2·5 cm of tubing. The upright of the T-piece is connected to a continuous-flow gas machine. Nitrous oxide, oxygen and, if necessary, a volatile supplement are delivered by a small inlet tube at right-angles to the main limb (the upright of the T). The other cross-piece has fixed to it rubber tubing—open to the air—which constitutes a small reservoir for the anaesthetic gases, most of which would otherwise escape into the outside air. The internal diameter of the reservoir tube should be 1 cm so that each 2·5 cm in length will have a capacity of about 2 ml. (For adults a slightly larger tube with an internal diameter of 1·25 cm and a capacity of 1 ml/cm in length may be used.) These measurements should not be exceeded, otherwise increased dead space will result. The fresh gas inflow should average twice the minute volume of the patient. *Table 12.1* is a guide to the gas inflow and tube (reservoir) capacity required for children of different ages. Breathing is of course spontaneous.[169] As originally suggested by Philip Ayre[168] a reservoir volume in the open ended tube of one-third of that of the tidal volume will prevent dilution with air.[170]

The T-piece principle can be modified by the addition of a small reservoir bag open at one end fitted on to the end of the reservoir tube. This enables IPPV with

Table 12.1 Gas inflow and tube capacity for children[168] (Ayre's T-piece)

Age	Gas inflow in litres/min	Reservoir tube capacity in ml
0–3 months	3–4	6–12
3–6 months	4–5	12–18
6–12 months	5–6	18–24
1–2 years	6–7	24–42
2–4 years	7–8	42–60
4–8 years	8–9	60–72

gas and oxygen to be employed, following the use of an intravenous barbiturate with a relaxant.[171] A scavenging system has been described to prevent atmospheric pollution.[172] Modifications of the T-piece have been described.[173]

In children the laryngeal reflexes are very active, while the glottis is smaller relative to body size. A tube may pass readily into a naris, but be too big for the larynx, the narrowest part of which is at the level of the cricoid cartilage. The largest tube in a child's larynx, because of its rubber walls, reduces the capacity of the larynx very considerably. The morbidity from long-term intubation, even up to several weeks, is small.[174]

The larynx is well anterior in infants and children.

References

1. Wedley J. R. *Br. J. Clin. Equip.* 1979, **4**, 49.
2. Hooke R. *Phil. Trans. R. Soc.* 1667, **2**, 539.
3. Davison M. H. A. *Br. J. Anaesth.* 1951, **23**, 238.
4. Trendelenburg F. *Arch. Klin. Chir.* 1871, **12**, 121.
5. MacEwen W. *Br. Med. J.* 1880, **2**, 122 (reprinted in 'Classical File', *Surv. Anesthesiol.* 1969, **13**, 105).
6. O'Dwyer J. *Med. Rec.* 1887, **32**, 557.
7. Maydl K. *Wien. Med. Wochenschr.* 1893, **43**, 102.
8. Kuhn F. *Münch. Med. Wochenschr.* 1902, **49**, 1456.
9. Kuhn F. *Zbl. Chir.* 1901, **28**, 1281.
10. Harcourt V. *Br. Med. J.* 18 July 1903.
11. Barthélemy and Dufour, *Presse Méd.* 1907, **15**, 475.
12. Meltzer S. J. and Auer J. *J. Exp. Med.* 1909, **2**, 622.
13. Elsberg C. A. *N.Y. Med. Rec.* 1910, **77**, 493; *Ann. Surg.* 1910, **52**, 723.
14. Kelly R. E. *Br. Med. J.* 1912, **2**, 617, 1121.
15. Kirstein A. *Allg. Med. ZentZtg* 1895, **34**, 110; Kirstein A. *Lancet* 1895, **1**, 1132; Hirsch N. P. et al. *Anaesthesia* 1986, **41**, 42.
16. Zollner F. *Arch. Otolaryngol.* 1965, **82**, 656.
17. Jackson C. *Tracheobronchoscopy, Esophagoscopy and Gastroscopy.* St Louis: Mosby, 1907.
18. Rowbotham E. S. and Magill I. W. *Proc. R. Soc. Med.* 1921, **14**, 17; Magill I. W. *Lancet* 1923, **2**, 228; Rowbotham E. S. *Br. Med. J.* 1920, **2**, 590; Magill I. W. *Anaesthesia* 1975, **30**, 476.
19. Shipway F. *Lancet* **1**, 70, 1916.
20. Rowbotham E. S. and Magill I. W. *Proc. R. Soc. Med.* 1921, **14**, 17; Magill I. W. *Proc. R. Soc. Med.* 1929, **22**, 83 (reprinted in 'Classical File', *Surv. Anesthesiol.* 1978, **33**, 580).
21. Magill I. W. *Br. Med. J.* 1930, **2**, 817.
22. Rowbotham E. S. *Br. Med. J.* 1920, **2**, 590.
23. Dorrance G. M. *Surg. Gynecol. Obstet.* 1910, **11**, 160.
24. Guedel A. E. and Waters R. M. *Curr. Res. Anesth. Analg.* 1928, **7**, 238 (reprinted in 'Classical File', *Surv. Anesthesiol.* 1984, **28**, 71).
25. Eisenmenger C. *Wien. Med. Wochenschr.* 1893, **43**, 199.
26. Green N. W. *Surg. Gynecol. Obstet.* 1906, **2**, 512.
27. Hewer C. L. *Recent Advances in Anaesthesia and Analgesia* 3rd ed. London: Churchill, 1939, p. 115.
28. Bourne J. G. *Br. Med. J.* 1947, **2**, 654.
29. Garcia M. *Proc. R. Soc. Lond.* 1855, **7**, 399.
30. Cole F. *Anesthesiology* 1945, **6**, 627.
31. Enderby G. E. H. *Lancet* 1961, **2**, 693.
32. Pollard B. J. *Anaesthesia* 1968, **23**, 534.
33. Alsop A. F. *Anaesthesia* 1955, **10**, 401.
34. Read D. H. and Du Boulay M. *Anaesthesia* 1982, **37**, 940.
35. Jackson C. *Surg. Gynecol. Obstet.* 1913, **17**, 507.
36. Magill I. W. *Lancet* 1926, **1**, 500.

37. Flagg P. J. *Arch. Otolaryngol.* 1928, **8**, 716.
38. Miller R. A. *Anesthesiology* 1941, **2**, 317.
39. Macintosh R. R. *Lancet* 1943, **1**, 205.
40. Hill W. *Br. Med. J.* 1909, 16 October.
41. Scott D. L. *Anaesthesia* 1983, **38**, 695.
42. Pope E. S. *Anaesthesia* 1960, **15**, 326.
43. Bryce-Smith R. *Br. Med. J.* 1952, **1**, 217.
44. Bannister F. B. and Macbeth R. G. *Lancet* 1944, **2**, 651.
45. Bowen R. A. and Jackson I. *Anaesthesia* 1952, **7**, 254.
46. Grant G. C. *Anaesth. Intensive Care* 1977, **5**, 263; Seward E. H. *Lancet* 1957, **2**, 104; Robertshaw F. L. *Lancet* 1962, **2**, 1034.
47. Kessel J. *Anaesth. Intensive Care* 1977, **5**, 265.
48. Magill I. W. *Br. Med. J.* 1920, **2**, 670.
49. Libermann H. *Anaesth. Intensive Care* 1978, **6**, 162.
50. Guedel A. E. and Waters R. M. *Curr. Res. Anesth. Analg.* 1928, **7**, 238.
51. Hewer C. L. *Recent Advances in Anaesthesia and Analgesia* 3rd ed. London: Churchill, 1939, p. 115.
52. Wu W-H. et al. *Crit. Care Med.* 1973, **1**, 197; Black A. M. S. and Seegobin R. D. *Anaesthesia* 1981, **36**, 498.
53. Dobrin P. B. et al. *Anesth. Analg. (Cleve.)* 1974, **53**, 456.
54. Guedel A. E. and Waters R. M. *Ann. Otol. Rhinol. Lar.* 1931, **40**, 1139.
55. Seegobin R. D. and Van Hassalt G. L. *Br. Med. J.* 1984, **288**, 965.
56. Revenas B. and Lindholm C.-E. *Acta Anaesthesiol. Scand.* 1976, **20**, 321; Reader J. C. et al. *Anaesthesia* 1985, **40**, 444.
57. Rosenberg P. *Berl. Klin. Wochenschr.* 1895, **32**, 14.
58. Magill I. W. *Proc. R. Soc. Med.* 1929, **22**, 83.
59. Lehtinen A-M. et al. *Br. J. Anaesth.* 1984, **56**, 239.
60. Vale R. *Anaesthesia* 1967, **22**, 314.
61. Forrester A. C. *Br. J. Anaesth.* 1974, **46**, 413.
62. Sellers W. F. S. and Dye A. *Anaesthesia* 1985, **40**, 483.
63. Gross J. B. et al. *Anesth. Analg. (Cleve.)* 1984, **63**, 915.
64. Walker W. E. and Bender H. W. *Surg. Gynecol. Obstet.* 1981, **152**, 87.
65. Messiter K. H. and Patterson K. I. *Anaesthesia* 1980, **35**, 294.
66. Boysen K. *Anaesthesia* 1985, **40**, 1024.
67. Divekar V. M. et al. *Can. Anaesth. Soc. J.* 1979, **26**, 141.
68. Rendell-Baker L. *Br. J. Anaesth.* 1978, **50**, 407; Allen C. T. B. *Anaesthesia* 1976, **31**, 263.
69. Berry F. A. et al. *Pediatrics* 1973, **51**, 476.
70. McShane A. J. and Hone R. *Br. Med. J.* 1986, **292**, 26 and 410.
71. Dunkin L. J. *Br. J. Hosp. Med.* 1980, **23**, 77.
72. Jackson Chevalier, and Jackson C. L. *Bronchoscopy, Esophagoscopy and Gastroscopy* 3rd ed. Philadelphia: Saunders, 1934, p. 85.
73. Tomlinson A. A. *Anaesthesia* 1985, **40**, 496.
74. Rigg D. and Dwyer B. *Anaesth. Intensive Care* 1985, **13**, 431.
75. Cormack R. S. and Lehane J. *Anaesthesia* 1984, **39**, 1105.
76. White A. and Kander P. L. *Br. J. Anaesth.* 1975, **47**, 468.
77. Zuck D. *Br. J. Anaesth.* 1976, **48**, 395; Payne K. A. *Anaesth. Intensive Care* 1980, **8**, 84.
78. Kinyemi O. O. and Elegbe E. O. *Can. Anaesth. Soc. J.* 1981, **28**, 80.
79. Sharwood-Smith G. H. *Anaesthesia* 1976, **31**, 508.
80. Kloss J. and Petty C. *Anesthesiology* 1975, **43**, 380.
81. Macintosh R. R. *Br. Med. J.* 1949, **1**, 28.
82. Spoerel W. E. et al. *Br. J. Anaesth.* 1971, **43**, 932; Layman P. R. *Anaesthesia* 1983, **38**, 478; Brian-Smith R. et al. *Can. Anaesth. Soc. J.* 1975, **22**, 607.
83. Nichol H. C. and Zuck D. *Br. J. Anaesth.* 1983, **55**, 141.
84. Him D. Y. K. *Anaesth. Intensive Care* 1982, **10**, 158.
85. Boys J. E. *Br. J. Anaesth.* 1983, **55**, 187.
86. Tunstall M. E. *Clin. Obstet. Gynecol.* 1980, **7**, 665; *Br. J. Anaesth.* 1984, **56**, 659.
87. Debenham T. R. *Anaesthesia* 1985, **40**, 599.
88. Bidwai A. V. et al. *Can. Anaesth. Soc. J.* 1978, **25**, 416.
89. Bidwai A. V. et al. *Anesthesiology* 1979, **51**, 171.
90. Owen H. *Anaesthesia* 1982, **37**, 1112.
91. Thind G. S. *Anaesthesia* 1983, **38**, 393.

92. Ruphreht J. and Dworacek B. *Anaesthesia* 1983, **38**, 394.
93. Kamal R. S. and Agha S. *Anaesthesia* 1984, **39**, 464; Jenkins J. C. *Anesthesiology* 1984, **60**, 611.
94. Cozanitis D. A. et al. *Anaesthesia* 1982, **37**, 1198.
95. Melnick B. M. *Anesthesiology* 1984, **60**, 517.
96. Conacher I. D. *Anaesthesia* 1981, **36**, 45.
97. Lal N. G. *Anaesthesia* 1980, **35**, 500.
98. Rosen M. et al. *Br. J. Anaesth.* 1963, **35**, 125; Henville J. D. *Br. J. Clin. Equip.* 1977, **2**, 125.
99. Das P. K. and Thomas W. J. W. *Anaesth. Intensive Care* 1980, **8**, 375.
100. Wright R. B. and Manfield F. F. V. *Anesth. Analg. Curr. Res.* 1974, **53**, 4.
101. Dobbinson T. L. *Anaesth. Intensive Care* 1980, **8**, 72.
102. Pottecher T. et al. *Ann. Fr. d'Anaes. Réanim.* 1984, **3**, 54.
103. Zuck D. *Anaesthesia* 1985, **40**, 1016.
104. Robinson J. S. *Br. Med. J.* 1974, **3**, 275.
105. Utting J. E. et al. *Can. Anaesth. Soc. J.* 1979, **26**, 472; Pollard J. and Junius F. *Anaesth. Intensive Care* 1980, **8**, 183; Stirt J. A. *Anaesth. Intensive Care* 1982, **10**, 274.
106. O'Brien D. O. and Curran J. *Anaesthesia* 1985, **40**, 73.
107. Burman J. A. and Furgiuele J. J. *Anesthesiology* 1984, **60**, 613.
108. Ionescu T. *Anaesthesia* 1981, **36**, 422; Murray I. P. and Modell J. H. *Anesthesiology* 1983, **59**, 344.
109. Hanning C. D. *Br. J. Anaesth.* 1985, **57**, 359.
110. Munro T. N. *Anaesthesia* 1985, **40**, 919; Triner L. *Anesthesiology* 1982, **57**, 548.
111. Woodhall N. M. *Anaesthesia* 1985, **40**, 1244.
112. Gotta A. W. and Sullivan C. A. *Br. J. Anaesth.* 1981, **53**, 1055.
113. Stiffel P. and Hameroff S. R. *Anesthesiology* 1979, **51**, 274.
114. Bromage P. R. *Epidural Analgesia.* Philadelphia: Saunders, 1978, p. 476.
115. Golla A. W. and Sullivan C. A. *Br. J. Anaesth.* 1981, **53**, 1055.
116. Meyer R. J. *Anaesth. Intensive Care* 1982, **10**, 64.
117. Elam J. O. et al. *Anesth. Analg. Curr. Res.* 1969, **48**, 307.
118. Brain I. A. J. *Br. J. Anaesth.* 1983, **55**, 801.
119. Donen M. et al. *Can. Anaesth. Soc. J.* 1983, **30**, 194.
120. Lyons G. *Anaesthesia* 1985, **40**, 759.
121. Kark A. E. et al. *Br. Med. J.* 1984, **289**, 1412.
122. Yukioka H. et al. *Anesth. Analg. (Cleve.)* 1985,. **64**, 1189.
123. Drenger B. et al. *Anesth. Analg. (Cleve.)* 1985, **64**, 1211.
124. Donegan J. H. *Anesth. Analg. (Cleve.)* 1981, **60**, 100.
125. Greenberg M. I. et al. *Ann. Emerg. Med.* 1982, **11**, 546.
126. Chernow et al. *Anesth. Analg. (Cleve.)* 1984, **63**, 829.
127. Berlot G. et al. *Anaesthesia* 1985, **40**, 819.
128. Reid L. C. and Brace D. E. *Surg. Gynecol. Obstet.* 1940, **70**, 157.
129. Black T. E. et al. *Anaesthesia* 1984, **39**, 883.
130. Davies M. J. et al. *Anaesthesia* 1981, **36**, 147.
131. Cummings M. F. et al. *Br. J. Anaesth.* 1983, **55**, 619.
132. Cozanitis D. A. et al. *Can. Anaesth. Soc. J.* 1984, **31**, 155.
133. Fassoulski A. and Kaniaris A. *Br. J. Anaesth.* 1983, **55**, 49.
134. Derbyshire D. R. et al. *Br. J. Anaesth.* 1983, **55**, 855.
135. Boralassa H. et al. *Anaesthesia* 1983, **38**, 623.
136. Shapiro H. M. et al. *Anesthesiology* 1972, **37**, 399; Burney R. G. and Winis R. *Anesth. Analg. (Cleve.)* 1975, **54**, 687.
137. Moss E. et al. *Br. J. Anaesth.* 1978, **50**, 353.
138. Abeyewickreme N. et al. *Br. Med. J.* 1977, **2**, 868.
139. Ravindran R. et al. *Anesthesiology* 1978, **48**, 374.
140. Blau J. N. and Kepadia R. *Br. Med. J.* 1972, **4**, 259.
141. Semon F. *Arch. Laryngol.* 1881, **2**, 197.
142. Hahn F. W. et al. *Arch. Otolaryngol.* 1970, **92**, 226; Ellis P. D. M. *Anesthesiology* 1977, **46**, 374.
143. Gibbin K. P. and Egginton M. J. *Br. J. Anaesth.* 1981, **53**, 1091.
144. Gleeson M. J. and Fourcin A. J. *J. R. Soc. Med.* 1983, **76**, 928.
145. Chatterji S. et al. *Anaesthesia* 1984, **39**, 246; Nicholls B. J. and Packham R. N. *Anaesth. Intensive Care* 1986, **14**, 196.
146. Teichner R. I. *Br. J. Anaesth.* 1971, **43**, 413; Jones B. C. *Br. J. Anaesth.* 1971, **43**, 730; Loughman E. *Anaesth. Intensive Care* 1983, **11**, 171.
147. Scammon F. L. and Babin R. W. *Anesthesiology* 1983, **59**, 352.

148. Sherry K. M. *Anesthesiology* 1983, **59**, 148.
149. McGoldrick K. E. and Donlon J. V. *Anesth. Analg. (Cleve.)* 1979, **58**, 343.
150. Bukht D. and Langford R. M. *Anaesthesia* 1983, **38**, 390.
151. Loeser F. A. et al. *Can Anaesth. Soc. J.* 1980, **27**, 56.
152. Caplan I. M. et al. *Anesthesiology* 1984, **59**, 202.
153. Majumdar B. et al. *Anaesthesia* 1982, **37**, 67.
154. Smith B. A. C. and Hopkinson R. B. *Anaesthesia* 1984, **39**, 894; Correspondence, *Anaesthesia* 1985, **40**, 211 and 212; Gaukroger P. B. and Anderson G. *Anaesth. Intensive Care* 1986, **14**, 199.
155. O'Neill J. et al. *Anesthesiology* 1984, **60**, 482.
156. Hoffman S. et al. *Anesth. Analg. (Cleve.)* 1984, **63**, 487.
157. Stauffer J. L. et al. *Am. J. Med.* 1981, **70**, 65.
158. Sellery G. R. et al. *Can Anaesth. Soc. J.* 1978, **25**, 140.
159. Battersby E. F. et al. *Anaesthesia* 1977, **32**, 154.
160. Brain A. I. J. *Br. J. Anaesth.* 1983, **55**, 801; Brain A. I. J. and McGhee T. D. *Anaesthesia* 1985, **40**, 356.
161. Keep P. J. and Manford M. L. M. *Anaesthesia* 1974, **29**, 181.
162. Seward E. H. *Anaesthesia* 1951, **6**, 54.
163. Srivastava R. K. *Anaesthesia* 1963, **18**, 532.
164. Inkster J. S. in *Recent Advances in Anaesthesia and Analgesia*—12 (Hewer C. L. and Atkinson R. S. ed.). Edinburgh and London: Churchill Livingstone, 1976, p. 60.
165. Inkster J. S. in *Recent Advances in Anaesthesia and Analgesia*—12 (Hewer C. L. and Atkinson R. S. ed.). Edinburgh and London: Churchill Livingstone, 1976, p. 61.
166. Bush G. H. in *General Anaesthesia* (Gray T. C. and Nunn J. F. ed.), 3rd ed., London: Butterworths, 1971, Vol. 2, Ch. 31.
167. Cullum A. R. and others. *Anaesthesia* 1973, **28**, 66.
168. Ayre T. P. *Lancet* 1937, **1**, 561; *Br. J. Surg.* 1937, **25**, 131; *Br. J. Anaesth.* 1956, **28**, 520; *Anaesthesia* 1967, **22**, 359.
169. Rose D. K. and Froese A. B. *Can. Anaesth. Soc. J.* 1979, **26**, 104.
170. Naunton A. *Br. J. Anaesth.* 1985, **57**, 803.
171. Rees G. J. *Br. Med. J.* 1950, **2**, 1419; *Br. J. Anaesth.* 1960, **32**, 132.
172. Steward D. J. *Can. Anaesth. Soc. J.* 1972, **19**, 670.
173. Harrison G. A. *Br. J. Anaesth.* 1964, **36**, 115.
174. Battersby E. F. and Hatch D. J. *Anaesthesia* 1977, **32**, 154.
175. Tunstall M. E. *Anaesthesia* 1976, **31**, 850.
176. Ng W. S. in *Difficulties in Trachael Intubation* (Latto I. P. and Rosen M. ed.) London: Baillière Saunders, 1985.
177. Pelimon A. and Simunovic Z. *Anaesthesia* 1987, **42**, 83.

Chapter 13   # INTRAVENOUS ANAESTHETIC AGENTS

Intravenous anaesthetic agents may be used for: (1) The induction of anaesthesia; (2) As the sole agent for short operations; (3) To supplement general anaesthesia or regional analgesia; (4) For sedation. The injection of a potent drug into the bloodstream cannot be readily withdrawn, whereas inhalation agents can be more easily eliminated.

History

Johann Sigmund (1623–1688), a German physician, injected opium intravenously, to produce unconsciousness in 1665. Pierre-Cyprien Oré (1828–1891),[1] Professor of Physiology at Bordeaux, used chloral hydrate intravenously in 1872 in a patient suffering from tetanus. The hypodermic syringe and needle were not, as popularly supposed, invented by the Frenchman, Charles Gabriel Pravaz (1791–1853) of Lyon.[2] Francis Rynd (1801–1861) of Dublin in 1845[3] used a trocar and cannula with morphine for the treatment of trigeminal neuralgia; he did not use a syringe. Alexander Wood (1817–1884)[4] of Edinburgh was the true founder of hypodermic medication. He used a Ferguson syringe. The Record syringe of metal and glass was introduced about 1906 in Berlin, and the French Luer followed it.[5] The first needle to remain patent, for multiple injections was described by Torsten Gordh in 1945. (Syringe from Gr *Syrinx* = a tube or pipe.)

Intravenous hedonal was used in 1905 by Krawkow of St Petersburg, Russia,[6] and in 1912 by Max Page in London; in 1909 Burckhardt gave chloroform and ether by the intravenous route.[7]

Barbituric acid synthesized by Adolf v. Baeyer (1835–1917) of Munich in 1864 but its narcotic effects not discovered. Later, also in Munich, barbiturate was synthesized by Emil Fischer (1852–1918) and Joseph Friederich von Mering (1849–1908) in 1903:[8] this was diethyl barbituric acid or Veronal. Phenobarbitone was discovered in 1912. Somnifaine was the first barbiturate to be given intravenously; it is a combination of diethyl and diallyl barbituric acids, and was used in France by Bardet- in 1924.[9] Noel and Souttar used intravenous paraldehyde in 1913.[10] Intravenous morphine and hyoscine were employed for 'twilight sleep' in 1916.[11]

In 1927 Bumm introduced Pernocton[12] while Zerfas, in the USA, used sodium amytal intravenously two years[13] later. This was soon followed by Nembutal (pentobarbitone).[14] Magill was the first to demonstrate this clinically in Britain[15] and John Silas Lundy[16] (1890–1974) of the Mayo Clinic in the USA in 1931.

Martin Kirschner (1879–1942) of Heidelberg gave Avertin (bromethol) intravenously in 1929.[17]

Hexobarbitone was the first drug to make intravenous anaesthesia popular and was used by Helmut Weese (1897–1954), professor of pharmacology at Dusseldorf and later director of pharmacology at Bayer (Wuppertal-Elberfeld), and the true father of intravenous anaesthesia, and Walter Scharpff in 1932,[18] having been synthesized by Kropp and Taub in Elberfeld. It was first given in Great Britain in 1933 by Ronald Jarman (1898–1973) and L. Abel in London.[19]

Pentothal sodium (thiopentone) was synthesized in 1932 by Ernest Henry Volwiler and Donalee Tabern[20] and introduced into clinical practice by Lundy of the Mayo Clinic on 18 June 1934,[21] and by Waters of Madison on 3 March 1934,[22] the former being the more influential. First used in Great Britain by Jarman and Abel in 1935.[23] Its fate in the body and distribution described by Brodie in 1950.[24] Methohexitone, a methyl barbiturate, first used by Stoelting in 1957.[25] Thiopentone was originally employed as the sole anaesthetic and this led to many deaths, e.g. at Pearl Harbour on 9 December 1941.[26] Intermittent doses along with nitrous oxide and oxygen, first described by Geoffrey Stephen William Organe (1908–) and Broad in 1938.[27] Thiopentone and methohexitone are the most useful barbiturates for intravenous anaesthesia. (*See also* The 50th Anniversary of the Use of Thiopentone, Editorial, Papper E. M. *Anaesthesia* 1984, **39**, 517; Editorial, Dundee J. W. *Br. J. Anaesth.* 1984, **56**, 211.)

Intravenous ether was used in animals by Nikolai Ivanovitch Pirogoff (1810–1881) in Russia in 1847, a year after Morton's use of ether by inhalation. Used in surgery by Ludwig Burckhardt (1872–1922), Nuremberg surgeon, in 1909. A 2·5–5% solution in normal saline or glucose 5% was used.

Many intravenous anaesthetic agents have been tried but have not survived. Examples include hydroxydione in 1955; propanidid in 1956;[28] gamma-hydroxy-butyric acid in 1960 and alphaxadone/alphadolone (Althesin) in 1971.[29,30] (*See also* Dundee J. W. and McIlroy P. D. A. *Anaesthesia* 1982, **37**, 726 and Dundee J. W. in: *Anaesthesia; Essays on its History* (Rupreht J. et al. ed.) Berlin: Springer-Verlag, 1985, p. 88.)

Technique of Intravenous Injection

Good illumination and a sharp needle are essential for successful intravenous injection. The Butterfly needle is most convenient and comes in several sizes, e.g. 21 or 23. The easiest and most accessible vein should be chosen.

Suitable sites are: (1) The forearm; (2) The back of the hand; (3) Anterior to the elbow-joint; (4) Anterior to the wrist joint; (5) The internal saphenous vein, anterior to the medial malleolus—the skin overlying this is tough; (6) The external jugular vein; (7) Subclavian vein—by supraclavicular puncture; (8) A scalp vein in infants; (9) The femoral vein, medial to the artery.

When the arm is chosen, the veins are made as prominent as possible by the use of a venous tourniquet, such as a length of rubber tubing around the arm secured and released by means of an artery forceps. Applied near the site of injection, the tourniquet steadies the vein proximally, while the anaesthetist's finger, by stretching the skin, steadies it distally. This is very important in thin old people whose veins, although prominent, very readily slip about beneath the skin and may run away from the point of the needle.

The artery must not be occluded in addition to the vein; the presence of arterial pulsation is a most useful guide to the position of an artery and hence to avoidance of injection into it.

Soaking the whole arm in hot water to produce hyperaemia or light general anaesthesia by causing venodilatation, makes injection easier (and pleasanter). If a cream containing 5% lignocaine and 5% prilocaine is rubbed into the skin and left on as a dressing for 1 hour, the subsequent puncture of the skin is rendered painless.[31]

When the skin has been well cleaned with an antiseptic (thought by many workers to be a waste of time and effort), the needle is inserted so that it comes to lie between the skin and the vein wall. The point is now advanced and the vein wall is pierced at a different level from the skin puncture. This tends to prevent transfixion of the vein and lessens haematoma formation when the needle is withdrawn. With the needle point within the lumen of the vein it should, if possible, be advanced for a short distance to prevent slipping out.

A few drops of procaine can be injected into the dermis with an intradermal needle before the larger needle is inserted, if necessary, to reduce pain caused by the larger needle. Otherwise the tip of the needle is pressed on to the skin to blanch it, for 10 sec, before the needle is advanced through the skin.

With the needle in the vein, the aspiration test is performed and injection can commence. After withdrawal of the needle oozing should be checked by firm pressure for several minutes and elevation of the limb, if necessary. For technique of setting up an intravenous drip *see* Chapter 42. Nitroglycerin ointment may aid venepuncture by increasing skin vasodilatation.[32]

Barbiturates

Thiopentone Sodium BP Thiopental USP (*Pentothal; Trapanal; Penthiobarbital; Intraval; Nesdonal; Farmotal*).

This is sodium ethyl (1-methyl butyl) thiobarbiturate. It is the sulphur analogue of pentobarbitone. Introduced commercially as Pentothal sodium in 1935.

It is a yellow amorphous powder with odour resembling H_2S. It is soluble in water and alcohol and forms a 2·5 or 5% solution in distilled water of pH 10·5, which is highly alkaline (pH of blood 7·4). To prevent formation of free acid by carbon dioxide from the atmosphere, 6% anhydrous sodium carbonate is added to the powder, which is prepared in an atmosphere of nitrogen. In solution it is not very stable, but can be left for 24–48 h or longer without harm resulting on subsequent injection, provided solution remains clear. A solution which is cloudy should be discarded. The oil/water coefficient is 4·7.

It is supplied in ampoules, with sterile distilled water sufficient to make a 2·5% solution, which, in the writers' opinion, is the preferred strength. Anaesthesia with thiopentone should never be undertaken lightly. Average dose 4–7 mg/kg i.v.

Pharmacodynamics

The central nervous system. Like other barbiturates, it causes sedation, hypnosis, anaesthesia and respiratory depression, depending on the dose injected and the rate of injection. There is an anticonvulsant action. The cerebral cortex and the ascending reticular-activating system are depressed before the medullary centres. Cerebral blood flow and CSF pressure are reduced, and intracranial pressure falls. Cerebral oxygen consumption is reduced. Thiopentone in doses insufficient to cause unconsciousness is antanalgesic,[33] and this sensitivity to pain lasts into the postoperative period.

There is a reasonably consistent correlation between depth of anaesthesia and EEG pattern, though not with plasma barbiturate levels.

In monkeys, thiopentone in doses greater than would be required for anaesthesia will, if given soon after acute global brain ischaemia (e.g. after cardiac standstill), reduce the degree of cerebral damage. Other work,[34] however, has failed to reproduce these results, while application to human patients remains to be evaluated.[35]

Acute Tolerance.[36] There is a relationship between the induction dose of thiopentone and the blood thiopentone level at which patients awake from anaesthesia. With larger induction doses the patient wakes at a higher blood level. A high initial concentration of thiopentone in the brain may result in an increased acute tolerance to supplementary doses. The greater the initial dose, the greater will be the increments of drug required to maintain surgical anaesthesia. For these reasons it is impossible to correlate blood levels with depth of anaesthesia.

pH effect. Thiopentone has a pK value of 7·6. Acidosis reduces the thiopentone concentration in the plasma of experimental animals by up to 40%, with return to control levels on return of pH to normal.

Protein Binding. About 70% of the thiopentone in peripheral blood is bound to plasma proteins, chiefly albumin, and so is inactivated. The tissues are in equilibrium only with the unbound fraction. pH changes may affect the ratio of bound to unbound thiopentone,[37] maximum binding occurring at pH 8. The degree of binding also varies according to the concentration of thiopentone, being greatest when the concentration is low. Thiopentone enters red blood cells in a concentration about 40% of that found in plasma.

Respiratory system. The chief effect is depression of the respiratory centre, depending on the dose and rate of injection. The sensitivity of the respiratory centre to CO_2 is reduced. A deep breath or two, or a yawn, may precede the depression, which is a reduced depth rather than a reduced rate of respiration. It is because of the hypoxia produced by this depressant action that thiopentone may be dangerous from the respiratory viewpoint. The depth of breathing is related to the surgical stimuli, which increases it and to the respiratory depressant activity of drugs given for premedication, which decreases it. If, after respiratory arrest, oxygen is supplied to the lungs, the rapid distribution of the drug in the tissues will usually soon occur, and spontaneous breathing will recommence. Depression of respiration is usually only temporary.

Cardiovascular system. Cardiac output is reduced, but this is of no importance in normal hearts in fit patients receiving moderate doses of the drug; effects are less when injection is slow. *The tone of systemic capacitance vessels is reduced*, leading to pooling of the blood, in the periphery. This shift causes reduction in the left ventricular diastolic filling and stroke volume. The drug is especially dangerous when the pathological condition of the heart does not allow for changes in rate or cardiac output to compensate for changes in vascular haemodynamics, e.g. constrictive pericarditis, tight valvular stenosis, complete heart block. *The blood pressure is depressed*, depending on rate and amount of drug injected: it is probably due to dilatation of the vascular bed especially in skin and muscle, perhaps due to depression of the vasomotor centre, and the effect usually passes off within minutes. Blood pressure falls are likely to be greater in hypertensive or hypovolaemic patients and in those with cardiac or adrenocortical insufficiency. *Rapid injection of too much thiopentone may have a most grave effect on the circulatory system.*

Larynx. The respiratory tract is hypersensitive to stimuli arising during light thiopentone anaesthesia. Laryngeal spasm may occur.

Eyes. Pupils first dilate, then contract. Sensitivity to light remains until the patient is deep enough to permit incision of the skin, and at this stage the eyeballs are usually centrally placed. It reduces intraocular tension.

Pregnant uterus. Thiopentone has no effect on its tone, and so is a poor agent used alone for external version. It readily passes the placental barrier, achieving its maximal concentration in fetal blood very soon after its injection into the mother.

Kidney. Specific effects are unimportant. A powerful stimulator of ADH.

Pharmacokinetics

After a single small dose of thiopentone, its level in the plasma falls rapidly and the patient regains consciousness due to the redistribution of the drug to viscera, lean body mass (muscles, etc.) and fat during the first 30 min after intravenous injection. After a single large dose, or repeated small ones, however, the resulting equilibrium plasma level may be high enough to cause anaesthesia and because of the slow metabolism of thiopentone anaesthesia is prolonged. Anaesthesia depends not only on the concentration of the drug, but also on the length of time of exposure of tissues to the drug. It rapidly crosses the blood–brain barrier due to its low degree of ionization and its high lipid solubility. It is the un-ionized part which crosses the barrier and its concentration in the cerebrospinal fluid approaches that in the plasma in 15 min. Equilibrium between plasma and brain is established 1 min after intravenous injection. The initial high uptake of thiopentone by the brain due to its high lipid solubility and non-ionization accounts for the rapidity of the onset of anaesthesia. There is a small decrease in plasma potassium following injection.

It is almost completely metabolized in the body. The liver is the principal site of breakdown and this may be a more important factor than generally supposed in the early recovery from its effects. Between 10 and 15% of the drug in the body is metabolized each hour; muscular tissue may help in its detoxication as may the kidneys. The degree of liver dysfunction must be considerable before a patient shows diminished tolerance to thiopentone, and tolerance is decreased only to intermittent doses given over a long period. The products of its breakdown are removed via the kidneys, but renal disease is not a contraindication to its use, although a uraemic patient will require smaller amounts than a normal patient. A high blood urea prolongs thiopentone narcosis. Eliminated more rapidly in the young than in the old so the old require smaller doses. For estimation of plasma thiopentone *see* Toner W. et al. *Anaesthesia* 1979, **34**, 657.

Miscellaneous effects. It passes into the breast milk shortly after injection. There is a positive relationship between the induction dose and the plasma urea and the plasma haemoglobin levels, both due to plasma binding of the drug.[38] Barbiturates induce the secretion of enzymes from the liver which metabolize warfarin and related anticoagulants. In some patients a localized muscular spasm is seen following injection. It usually takes the form of pronation of the forearm receiving the injection which can be lessened by narcotic analgesics.

Skin rashes have been very occasionally reported following its use. Anaphylactic response has been described.[39] This is the classic anaphylactic reaction type 1 sensitivity mediated by immunoglobulin E (*see below*).

Causes muscular necrosis if injected into muscular tissue.

It is a poor relaxer of the muscles but following a rapid induction dose, examinations under anaesthesia are usually possible (e.g. gynaecology) while manipulations of the spine or joints can be carried out if dosage is sufficient.

Course of Anaesthesia

At the time of operation, the stomach and bladder should be empty. When an intravenous anaesthetic is given the following should be at hand in case of need: (1) A laryngoscope; (2) Tracheal tubes; (3) Oxygen; (4) A mask and reservoir bag; (5) A tilting table; (6) Suction apparatus; (7) Suitable syringes and needles, e.g. the Butterfly needle. Guedel's classification of stages of anaesthesia does not apply. The patient is either too light (he reacts to surgical stimuli); he is properly anaesthetized; or he is too deep (his respirations are very shallow, his blood pressure depressed). The first injection should be 4–8 ml of 2·5% solution and it can be made quite rapidly in fit subjects; more slowly in others. The concentration of the drug reaching the brain in arterial blood immediately after injection is determined by the rate of injection. If the patient counts at a uniform rate, an indication of his reaction to the drug is obtained. Just after the onset of unconsciousness, there is often a deep breath, followed by a period of respiratory depression. During this period no further injection should be made. Consciousness is lost in one arm–brain circulation time, but maximum depth of anaesthesia occurs some 30–60 sec later. With normal breathing re-established, further thiopentone is given according to the needs of the patient. If a little is injected at frequent intervals, observing its effects, no danger is likely to be encountered, though the drug is cumulative. *Thiopentone anaesthesia, except in the shortest and most minor operations, should always be accompanied by nitrous oxide and oxygen. This enables the depth of respiration to be accurately assessed, reduces the amount of thiopentone needed by about 50%, produces smoother anaesthesia, and guards against hypoxia.*

The criteria of depth are: (1) The activity of respiration in relation to surgical stimuli. (2) Reflex movements of the patient in relation to such stimuli. When stimuli are severe, depth may have to be increased, e.g. when skin is incised or sutured.

Doses of thiopentone required vary from 0·1 to 1·0 g. Seldom should a larger dose be injected. A small dose in a fit patient results in a short period of narcosis, but larger doses may be followed by prolonged sleep. Additional doses within 36 h cause cumulation. A patient may respond to gentle face slapping in the theatre, only to return to the quiet and warmth of his bed and there meet death from an unobserved respiratory obstruction.

Control of the airway is of primary importance in intravenous anaesthesia. Occasionally a pharyngeal airway or a nasopharyngeal tube is necessary, but these should only be used if the airway becomes obstructed without them, as they may stimulate pharyngeal reflexes which upset the smooth course of the anaesthesia. They may also cause laryngospasm.

A trace of volatile agent, given before the pharyngeal airway is inserted, will frequently depress coughing and gagging reflexes, but should not, in the authors' opinion, be used routinely.

Respiratory obstruction or relative over-dosage resulting in apnoea causes hypoxia, which, added to the depressing effect of the barbiturate, may soon inactivate the respiratory centre. The remedy for this respiratory depression or arrest is to secure a free airway and to ventilate the lungs with oxygen or air. The surgeon should, if necessary, be asked to wait until control of the airway is regained. The intravenous injection of a short-acting relaxant, e.g. suxamethonium, will also abolish spasm of the larynx due to this cause. Patients vary greatly in the amounts of drug they require to abolish reflex response to stimuli. Males need more than females; the fat need more than the thin; the young need more than the old.

Recovery from Anaesthesia
Rate of recovery is influenced by the amount of premedication and the amount of thiopentone injected. Postoperative restlessness is rare and vomiting is infrequent. During the immediate postoperative period the airway and the tidal exchange must be carefully watched. The return of normal mental faculties does not accompany apparent return of full consciousness. Outpatients should always be accompanied after thiopentone anaesthesia and must not drive a car to their home or engage in responsible activity. For studies in the recovery of intravenous agents *see* Korttila K. et al. *Anesthesiology* 1975, **43**, 291; Epstein B. S. *Anesthesiology* 1975, **43**, 285; Bahar M., Dundee J. W. et al. *Anaesthesia* 1982, **37**, 1171.

Agents used to Supplement Thiopentone
Thiopentone is seldom used as the sole agent in modern anaesthetic practice, nitrous oxide and oxygen are usually administered, with or without an intravenous narcotic analgesic, or inhalation supplements. Small doses of muscle relaxants

(e.g. tubocurarine 3–5 mg) will often reduce muscular movement (e.g. raising of the legs), without markedly depressing respiration.

Complications of Thiopentone Anaesthesia
Local complications
1. *Perivenous injection*. This may cause pain, redness and swelling; haematoma formation; bruising; rarely ulceration (due to alkalinity of the solution). It may lead to median nerve injury if injection is made into the medial side of the antecubital fossa. Should solution be deposited outside the vein, 10 ml of 1% procaine can be injected into the area. This dilutes the thiopentone solution and, by promoting vasodilatation, aids absorption.

2. *Intra-arterial injection*. This may follow misplacement of the needle or accidental injection into an arterial cannula. Warning of the possiiblity of this was first pointed out in 1943.[40] When it occurs the patient usually, but not always, feels severe burning pain down the arm and hand. It can be avoided by seeing that the artery is not occluded by the tourniquet before injection and by injecting 2 ml of solution, and inquiring as to any pain experienced by the patient. Only if this is absent should the main injection proceed. This mishap may be dangerous and has led to necrosis and amputation of the hand. Sudden death from this cause has been reported. Accidental intra-arterial injection into arteries around the ankle and back of hand may occur. *Immediate signs* may include: (i) A white hand with cyanosed fingers due to arterial spasm, which may be accompanied or followed by arterial thrombosis. (ii) Patches of skin discoloration. (iii) Onset of unconsciousness may be delayed. *Late signs* may include: (i) Ulcers or blisters. (ii) Oedema of forearm and hand. Oedematous areas may recover, the cause of such cases being spasm rather than thrombosis. Gangrene following the intra-arterial injection of 2·5% solution is extremely rare.[41]

Anatomy: Division of the brachial artery above the elbow joint occurs in 10% of patients. When division is high, the ulnar artery reaches the forearm by running superficial to the flexor muscles and may run: (i) below the deep fascia all the way down; (ii) below the deep fascia proximally, later becoming subcutaneous; (iii) subcutaneous near the elbow, later becoming deep to the deep fascia. It is this abnormal ulnar artery in its superficial position immediately deep to the median cubital vein, and without the protection of the aponeurotic tendon of the biceps, which may be accidentally punctured and used for injection.

When the brachial artery divides above the elbow, the common interosseous branch of the ulnar artery is usually given off from the radial artery, so if ulnar artery is punctured its deep common interosseous branch is usually not involved.

Some of the bad effects of the intra-arterial injection of drugs are due to the thrombosis of the small arteries supplying nerves, and so interfering with their conduction of motor impulses.

The pH of 2·5% solution of thiopentone in water is 10·8 (pH of blood is 7·4). It is thus a strong alkaline irritant.

Pathology: (i) The changes in pH of thiopentone which occur when it is mixed with blood in an artery result in precipitation of solid crystals of thiopentone which are swept along and eventually block small vascular channels at arteriolar and capillary levels. The crystals remain in the small vessels and their irritant properties cause a local release of noradrenaline with subsequent vascular spasm. Thus the greater the weight of the drug injected, the greater will be the effect—an additional argument in favour of the use of 2·5% solution; (ii) The essential lesion is arterial thrombosis, and it may not become complete for 15 days; (iii) Endothelial damage may be a factor.

Treatment: When thiopentone has been injected into the lumen of an artery during induction of anaesthesia the suggested lines of treatment are as follows: (i) Leave needle in the lumen of the artery; (ii) Dilution of injected thiopentone with saline; (iii) Relief of arterial spasm and the pain it causes; (iv) Prevention of thrombosis; (v) Later treatment of such symptoms as may arise.

If possible abandon the proposed operation and institute intensive anticoagulant therapy with heparin.[42] It can be given into the artery. The oral, longer-acting anticoagulants may be necessary for the 2 weeks following. If postponement of operation is impossible, neurectomy of the sympathetic supply to the affected limb may be performed surgically. The increase in blood flow resulting will probably discourage thrombosis in the vessel damaged by thiopentone.

Additional management: (i) Through needle in the artery inject: (*a*) Procaine hydrochloride 10–20 ml of 0·5% solution; (*b*) Papaverine 40–80 mg in 10–20 ml of saline; (*c*) Tolazoline (Priscol) 5 ml of 1% solution, or as a continuous drip; this is a noradrenaline antagonist; (*d*) Phenoxybenzamine, either 0·5 mg which does not appreciably affect the general circulation or as a drip diluted with saline 50–200 µg/min. (*e*) Urokinase.[43] These solutions can also be injected into the subclavian artery following a brachial plexus or stellate ganglion block. (ii) Continue anaesthesia as an effective method of securing vasodilatation, using halothane. Perform a brachial plexus or stellate ganglion block to remove all vasoconstrictor impulses. (iii) Elevate limb, wrap in sterile towels and keep it warm.

3. *Thrombophlebitis*.[44] This may occur in spite of a clean, aseptic venepuncture and is due to chemical irritation of the vein wall. It may follow the injection or be postponed for 7–10 days. It should be treated by heat and rest.

4. *Injury to Nerves*, especially the median, following injection into the medial side of the antecubital fossa. Accidental injection into the median nerve is likely to produce an intense shooting pain in the distribution of the nerve, together with sudden flexion of the wrist and thumb. The area should be generously infiltrated with a local analgesic solution and in severe cases, a neurological opinion sought.

5. *Broken Needle*. As the fracture usually occurs between the hub and the shaft, at least 0·5 cm of shaft should always be outside tissues.

6. *Auto-erythrocyte sensitization syndrome; the painful bruising syndrome.*[45]

7. *Contamination of the solution with glass spicules* (not confined to thiopentone); suggested use of a filter.[46]

General complications

1. *Respiratory depression*. For treatment, *see above*. Apnoea during intravenous anaesthesia may be due to: (i) Relative over-dose of drug; (ii) Respiratory obstruction above the glottis, e.g. the tongue falling back; (iii) Laryngeal spasm.

2. *Circulatory collapse*. This is usually due to a relative over-dose causing vasodilatation and myocardial depression. *Treatment*: Raise the legs; give oxygen by IPPV; infuse fluids intravenously.

3. *Laryngeal spasm*. This may result from: (i) Direct local stimulation by an airway, saliva, blood, etc.; (ii) Stimulation of some remote area, e.g. anal sphincter, cervix uteri, etc. (Brewer–Luckhardt reflexes); (iii) Part of a general anoxic spasm. Thiopentone predisposes to laryngeal spasm. Oxygen should be administered under pressure. Intravenous injection of 20–30 mg of suxamethonium may be required to relax the spasm.

4. *Coughing*. Depth should be gradually increased. Nitrous-oxide–oxygen, volatile or analgesic agents may be required in resistant cases. Hiccup occasionally seen.

5. *Postoperative vertigo, euphoria and disorientation*. Because of the possibility of this condition, outpatients should be accompanied home and not allowed to drive a car or to cook.

6. *True cutaneous allergy* can occur either in the form of a scarlatiniform rash or as true angioneurotic oedema. Photosensitivity to thiopentone in patients recently exposed to sunlight has been reported.

7. *Severe anaphylactic reactions. See below*. These reactions, although rare, are of serious import. They may take the form of cutaneous manifestations (rashes, weals, flushes, oedema), cardiovascular collapse (hypotension, tachycardia), bronchospasm, laryngospasm and muscle rigidity or abdominal pain. There is a positive association between a patient's allergic diathesis and hypersensitivity reactions to intravenous anaesthetics.[36]

For mechanism of histamine release, anaphylactic and anaphylactoid reaction, *see* Baxter A. D. *Anaesthesia* 1978, **33**, 349; Whitwam J. G. *Br. J. Anaesth.* 1978, **50**, 677. For intradermal testing, *see* Fisher M. M. *Anaesth. Intensive Care* 1979, **7**, 58.

Advantages and Disadvantages of Thiopentone Anaesthesia

The advantages are: (1) Ease and rapidity of induction; (2) Absence of stage of delirium; (3) Rapid recovery (with correct dosage) and relative freedom from vomiting and postoperative discomfort, etc.; (4) Ability to increase depth rapidly.

The disadvantages are: (1) Respiratory depression; (2) Tendency to laryngeal spasm; (3) Poor abdominal relaxation with safe dosage; (4) Circulatory depression in poor-risk patients.

Indications

These are legion, almost every operation in surgery having been performed under intravenous barbiturate anaesthesia. It is specially useful: (1) For induction of general anaesthesia; (2) For short operations, orthopaedic manipulations, minor gynaecology, examinations under anaesthesia, etc.; (3) Under Service conditions where portability and relative ease of administration are advantages; (4) For supplementing regional analgesia; (5) For controlling convulsions during general or local anaesthesia, eclampsia, epilepsy, tetanus, etc.; (6) For narco-analysis in psychiatry, and for electroconvulsive therapy.

Conditions Requiring Special Consideration

In the following procedures and types of case, special care is needed, and oxygen or nitrous-oxide–oxygen should be given in addition:

1. Porphyria,[47] which may be congenital or appear as acute attacks of abdominal pain somewhat resembling lead poisoning, with the passage of urine, which assumes a dark reddish colour after being left exposed to daylight for some hours. Barbiturates may precipitate lower motor neuron paralysis and perhaps death, and are absolutely contraindicated. If suspected, the urine should be tested for porphyrins. It has been suggested that not all patients with porphyria are sensitive to barbiturates. *See also* Chapter 22.

2. A history of thiopentone anaphylaxis, which has a high mortality.

3. Shocked, debilitated, severely anaemic and uraemic cases: small doses are required. The drug causes vasodilatation and reduces cardiac output. The administration of pure oxygen is useful in handicapped patients before anaesthesia is induced. It also aids the removal of nitrogen from the lungs and allows nitrous oxide to exert its analgesic effects more quickly, so reducing the need for thiopentone.

There may be a dose of the drug small enough for induction of anaesthesia with safety in even the most decrepit patient, but in the gravely ill inhalation methods have some advantages.

4. Children under 4: because while their respiratory centres are easily depressed, their upper respiratory passages are relatively small, these factors predisposing to hypoxia. Many workers disagree. Children do not like needles;

5. Patients with gross dyspnoea due to cardiac or respiratory disease. It should be used with extreme caution—if at all—in cases of constriction pericarditis, tight valvular stenosis and complete heart block. There is sudden perfusion of the drug into coronary vessels in right-to-left shunt.

6. Patients with respiratory obstruction or status asthmaticus.

7. Operations in which the return of reflexes immediately after operation is desirable. It is difficult to have a patient adequately anaesthestized one minute and coughing the next, e.g. in tonsillectomy.

8. Cases of acute intestinal obstruction. Regurgitation may follow loss of consciousness, while aspiration of stomach contents may cause dangerous laryngeal spasm unless proper care is taken to prevent it.

9. Patients with acute inflammation about the mouth, jaw and neck. Several deaths have occurred under thiopentone anaesthesia in such patients. A likely cause of death is interference with the airway associated with spasticity of the jaw due to inflammatory oedema.

10. Obstetrics: for external version, thiopentone is a poor relaxant; for delivery, no more than an induction dose should be used (250 mg).

11. In any severely ill patient, the drug should be used cautiously in minimal dosage.

12. Cases of dystrophia myotonica. *See* Chapter 22. The patients react normally to curare, but abnormally to thiopentone[48] as to most respiratory depressants and prolonged apnoea may follow injection of more than 100 mg.

13. Alcoholics taking disulfiram (Antabuse) and patients suffering from poisoning with dinitro-orthocresol, a weed killer (barbiturates and DNC have a synergistic depressant effect on cellular respiration).

14. Hyperkalaemic familial periodic paralysis.

15. Huntington's chorea. *See* Chapter 22.

16. Patients with difficult veins. There is no excuse for subjecting a patient to the painful experience of multiple needle punctures in an effort to provide a pleasant induction of anaesthesia.

17. Thermally injured children between the ages of 6 and 16 who have recovered from their injuries require about 60% more thiopentone than similar normal children and an induction dose of 7–8 mg/kg may be required.[49]

Methohexitone (*Brietal; Brevital; Methohexital USP; Sombulex*)
First described by Chernish S. M. et al. in 1956[50] and used clinically by Stoelting in 1957[25] in the US and by Dundee and Moore in 1961 in the UK.[51]
This is a methylated oxybarbiturate with the chemical name sodium α-*dl*-1-

methyl-5-allyl-5-(1-methyl-2-pentynyl) barbiturate. To each 500 mg of powdered drug is added 30 mg of sodium carbonate. When used in 1% solution the pH is 11·1; 2% solution is also satisfactory. While it is two and a half to three times as potent as thiopentone complete recovery is quicker. Less irritating than thiopentone solution when injected into tissues, but intra-arterial methohexitone is as irritant and dangerous as thiopentone in the same concentration, but the 1% solution as commonly used is less dangerous than 2·5% thiopentone. Sometimes causes pain on intravenous injection. This can often be abolished by injecting 1·5 ml of 1% solution of plain lignocaine, and keeping the tourniquet in position for 15 s, followed by the injection of the drug.[52] Causes less cardiovascular depression than thiopentone, although it results in vasodilatation by an action on the sympathetic nervous system, but more abnormal muscular movements with tremor, coughing and hiccups; these are reduced after premedication with narcotic analgesics, e.g. fentanyl, 0·1 mg i.v.[53] Methohexitone has been found to cause abnormal spike discharges in epileptic subjects. It does not suppress epileptic manifestations, and may be implicated in the aetiology of fits during anaesthesia. Can cause anaphylactic, histaminoid reactions. The drug is redistributed and then detoxicated in the liver.

Induction of anaesthesia results in a slight fall in the plasma potassium level. Dosage of the 1% solution is about 1 mg/kg for induction (50–120 mg) (similar in volume to 2·5% thiopentone) and this is usually followed by nitrous oxide and oxygen. The aqueous solution is stable for at least 6 weeks at room temperature. Useful for induction of anaesthesia in the dental chair[54] and for operations on outpatients, for electroplexy, minor gynaecological, minor surgical, orthopaedic operations and for induction of anaesthesia in general surgery (5–12 ml of 1% solution). The only barbiturate which competes clinically with thiopentone, especially when rapid recovery is required. Useful as an aid to diagnosis in electro-encephalography.

Pharmokinetics of methohexitone; it has a terminal half-life of 97 min. Total body plasma clearance four times greater than that of thiopentone. Thus it may be preferable to thiopentone when a rapid recovery is required, especially after large or repeated doses.[55]

Intramuscular Methohexitone

This is reported to give satisfactory pre-anaesthetic sedation in about 85% of paediatric cases. The dose recommended is 6·6 mg/kg in 2% solution given into the upper and outer quadrant of the buttock. Sleep usually comes on in under 10 min. Abscesses and sloughs are rare.

Has also been given per rectum, 15–20 mg/kg.

Etomidate (Hypnomidate)

This is a carboxylated imidazole (ethyl-1-(α-methyl-benzyl) medazole-5-carboxylate) ($C_{14}H_{16}N_2O_2$). It was synthesized and studied by Janssen and co-workers in 1971[29] and used in man by Alfred Doenicke of Munich and colleagues in 1973.[30] It is a white crystalline powder, soluble in a wide range of solvents including water, ethanol and propylene glycol. The commercial preparation is presented in 10-ml ampoules containing 2 mg/ml of the drug dissolved in water with 35% propylene glycol. The pH is 8·1.

Pharmacodynamics

Etomidate is used as an intravenous induction agent. In the blood it distributes equally between red blood cells and plasma and the protein binding is 76·5%. Only 2·5% of the injected dose remains in the circulation 2 min after administration, at which time peak concentrations are found in the brain and major organs. The drug is thought to be metabolized rapidly in the liver and the decomposition products excreted in urine and bile. Recovery is rapid. Most patients wake following a single induction dose in 6–8 min and the quality of recovery is good. Repeated doses are not cumulative.[56]

The incidence of pain at the site of injection is high, occurring in a quarter to a half of patients. It can be reduced by fast injection, by use of a large vein in the antecubital fossa and by the addition of 0·1% lignocaine.[57] Or the patient may be made unconscious by the injection of a small amount of thiopentone.[58]

Muscle movements associated with induction are commoner than after thiopentone, Althesin or propanidid. The incidence is decreased when narcotic analgesics are used in premedication and increased by even mild reflex stimulation. It potentiates both types of muscle relaxants.[59]

Histamine release has not been reported.[30] No interaction with suxamethonium.

Central nervous system. The EEG changes are similar to those seen in association with thiopentone and Althesin. The muscle movements frequently seen during induction with etomidate are not associated with epileptiform discharges. The origin of these movements therefore probably lies in deep cerebral structures or the brain stem.

Etomidate is a good hypnotic but it does not prevent movement as a result of surgical stimulation. Autonomic responses are not blocked.

Cerebral blood flow is reduced. Intraocular pressure is reduced in premedicated patients.

Cardiovascular system. There is no overt depression of the cardiovascular system[60] as a rule although both myocardial ischaemia and asystole have been reported. This could have been due to the polyethylene glycol in the ampoule.[61]

Respiratory system. Respiratory rate slows and tidal volume rises for a brief period following induction. Respiration may then be shallow, but apnoea is likely to be brief and is less common than after thiopentone. Coughing and hiccup are uncommon.

Alimentary system. Nausea and vomiting occur more commonly than following other intravenous induction agents.[62]

Metabolism. No significant effects have been described in terms of liver function or plasma electrolytes. It is broken down by plasma and liver esterases.

Clinical Use

Cardiovascular stability and rapid recovery are features which commend its use as an induction agent in sick and shocked patients. Anaesthesia is then continued using other agents. A single shot dose by itself is unsatisfactory owing to the pronounced muscle movements often seen; use of adjuvant agents then may hinder recovery. Dose 0·3 mg/kg. Etomidate may, very rarely cause an anaphylactoid reaction.[63]

Etomidate infusion suppresses the secretion of cortisol and aldosterone for up to 22 h following its termination and is not now recommended. An increased mortality was associated with etomidate infusion in the ITU.[64] The drug also causes a depression of the normal increase in plasma cortisol concentration which occurs during surgery.[65] A single injection of etomidate is reported to cause a significant reduction in secretion of cortisol[66] but there is controversy whether this has clinical importance.[67]

(*See also* Savege T. M. in: *Recent Advances in Anaesthesia and Analgesia—13* (Hewer C. L. and Atkinson R. S. ed.) Edinburgh: Churchill Livingstone, 1979.)

Di-Isopropyl Phenol (Disoprofol; Diprivan; propofol)

First reported use in 1977.[68] The original product was dissolved in Cremophor EL and showed promise as a new induction agent.[69] Because of doubt about possible anaphylactoid reactions due to the solvent, there is now a new formulation, propofol.

Propofol is a 1% formulation in an oil and water emulsion containing 10% soya bean oil, 1·2% egg phosphatide and 2·25% glycerol. The recommended dose is 2·5 mg/kg for induction of anaesthesia in non-premedicated patients.[70] Some depression of arterial pressure and of respiration has been reported, and the incidence of pain on injection is significant. The drug appears to be a promising agent for the smooth induction of anaesthesia though it must be viewed with reserve in the hypovolaemic patient and in those anaesthetized in postures other than the supine horizontal.[71] Infusion has been used as a sedative.

Althesin[72] (Alphathesin; Alphadione)

This is no longer manufactured. It was a mixture of two steroids, alphaxalone 9 mg/ml and alphadolone 3 mg/ml. The latter has about half the potency of the former and is made up as follows: 3α-hydroxy-5α-pregnane-11,20-dione 0·9%, 21-acetoxy-3α-hydroxy-5α-pregnane-11,20-dione 0·3%, Cremophor EL (to aid solubility) 20% (is polyoxyethylated castor oil), sodium chloride 0·25%, with water to 100%. Total steroids per ml of Althesin is 12 mg. The solution was isotonic. It may be further diluted with normal saline if desired.

Before the preparation was withdrawn the makers received reports of an unacceptable number of adverse effects, following either first exposure to the drug, mediated either by the alternative complement pathway or as direct pharmacological effect, or after repeated exposure when the effect was probably mediated by the classical complement pathways. It seems probable that the Cremophor, the solubilizing agent, a polyoxyethylated castor oil, was the cause of these adverse reactions, most of them being relatively benign.

The Benzodiazepines

History
In the mid-1950s work on the existing tranquillizers was extended—these included chlorpromazine, reserpine and meprobamate. The benzheptodiazepines had been studied in Cracow, Poland in the 1930s[74] and elsewhere. Chlordiazepoxide was prepared in 1960[75] and named Librium, the pharmacology having been worked out by Randall.[76] First used clinically in 1961.[77] First reported as an intravenous anaesthetic in the UK in 1966 (diazepam).[78] Includes chlordiazepoxide (Librium) 1960, the first of the series to be used clinically diazepam, 1963 (Valium, Diazemuls), nitrazepam (Mogadon), temazepam (Normison), midazolam (Hypnovel), oxazepam, 1965 (Serenid D), medazepam (Nobrium), chloraze-

pate (Transcene), lorazepam, 1977 (Ativan), flunitrazepam[79] (Rohypnol) and flurazepam, 1970 (Dalmane).

The benzodiazepines differ from the barbiturates in four respects: (1) Habituation unusual; (2) Withdrawal effects may occur; (3) No significant enzyme induction; (4) REM sleep not greatly inhibited.

The benzodiazepines are depressors of the limbic system and are classed as minor tranquillizers. They depress emotional response and alertness, are anticonvulsant from their centrally acting muscle relaxant effects. GABA (the neurotransmitter) release is facilitated and they may depress noradrenaline secretion. Biotransformation to active metabolites may occur.

Diazepam

A base, insoluble in water but prepared commercially in an organic solvent containing propylene glycol. When dissolved in Cremophor EL pain on injection is less if mixed in a syringe with aspirated blood[80] or Intralipid. Suspected anaphylactic reaction to Cremophor EL has been reported.[81] Now available as a soya bean oil/water emulsion (Diazemuls)[82] which is less painful[83] and also as Valium Roche Mixed Micelles, using lecithin-bile acid-water solvent.[84]

Pharmacodynamics

Central nervous system. The actions of benzodiazepines on the central nervous system are mediated by facilitation of the inhibition of synaptic transmission by gamma-aminobutyric acid (GABA). Relieves tension and anxiety. Causes drowsiness and controls convulsions. Not analgesic. Its effects summate with those of other sedatives including alcohol. Can be safely given to patients receiving mono-amine oxidase inhibitors. Thought to depress the limbic system and the amygdala where fear, anxiety and aggression are generated. Cortex not depressed. Causes anterograde amnesia of about 10 min duration after intravenous injection. Used to control drug-induced dyskinesias. Does not cause nausea or vomiting. Does not increase cerebral blood flow and can be used in patients with head injury.

Respiratory system. Causes a slight depression of breathing,[85] usually not serious.

Cardiovascular system. Myocardial depression and hypotension not common but can cause collapse.

Muscular system. Potentiates non-depolarizing relaxants and reduces the amount of relaxation due to suxamethonium. Relieves muscle spasm and spasticity.

Metabolism. The major active metabolite is desmethyldiazepam with an elimination half-life of 24 hours.[86] Allergy to diazepam has been reported. Benzodiazepine blood levels are increased, owing to inhibition of their metabolism, by cimetidine.

For estimation of plasma diazepam level *see* Gamble J. A. S. et al. *Anaesthesia* 1975, **30**, 159.

Excretion. Mostly in the urine.

For current theories of the actions of the benzodiazepines, *see* Richter J. J. *Anesthesiology* 1981, **56**, 66.

Benzodiazepine receptors have been demonstrated in man and may be found in the brain cortex, spinal cord and other tissues.[87]

Clinical Uses

Diazepam has been recommended for many purposes. Among them are the following: (1) For premedication to relieve anxiety. Dose 10 mg intravenously; 10–12 mg intramuscularly or 20–30 mg by mouth. Is a more effective sedative when given by mouth than after intramuscular injection into the outer side of the thigh.[88] Acts more rapidly after injection into the deltoid. In children has been given per rectum 0·75 mg/kg, maximum dose 20 mg;[89] (2) For induction of anaesthesia (0·2–0·6 mg/kg intravenously), especially in poor-risk cases; (3) As an adjunct to light intravenous anaesthesia, e.g. in conservative dentistry; (4) To provide basal sedation during regional analgesia; (5) As the sole anaesthetic in cardioversion; (6) Before bronchoscopy under local analgesia; (7) Before local analgesia in dental surgery; (8) To control postoperative restlessness; (9) As an anticonvulsant in status epilepticus; (10) To control drug-induced dyskinesia; (11) In the treatment of tetanus; (12) In obstetrics to allay anxiety and promote relaxation. In the treatment of eclampsia diazepam crosses the placental barrier; (13) For cardiac catheterization; (14) To reduce hallucinations after ketamine; (15) For fibre-endoscopy of stomach, etc. It suppresses the laryngeal closure reflex. To control secretions, atropine must be given first. Rapid injection can cause apnoea; (16) For the relief of angina pectoris (by dilating coronary vessels).

Diazepam should not be mixed with other drugs and should be injected into large veins to reduce the incidence of thrombophlebitis.

It is available in the form of tablets, syrup and ampoules for injection (5 mg/ml in polyethylene glycol). Also as rectal suppository, 5 and 10 mg.

Following intravenous injection there is a small fall in plasma potassium. Car driving should be prohibited for 10–12 h after an active dose of diazepam.

Lorazepam (*Ativan*)

May be given orally or by injection. Long duration of action. Has an elimination half-life of 12 h and has no pharmacologically active metabolites. Produces sedation, drowsiness and amnesia. Useful for premedication[90]—oral dose 1–5 mg or may be given intramuscularly, dose 4 mg. Used also for sedation of patients in the intensive therapy unit. For comparison between lorazepam and diazepam, *see* Dundee J. W. et al. *Br. J. Anaesth.* 1979, **51**, 439.

Midazolam[91] (*Hypnovel*)

This is a water-soluble benzodiazepine which can be used for induction of anaesthesia. The duration of action is short and it does not irritate veins.[92] Apnoea has been observed with a dosage of 0·15 mg/kg which is not sufficient to induce anaesthesia reliably in unpremedicated subjects. Anterograde amnesia and drowsiness are common. Cardiovascular stability is seen. Midazolam has a slower induction time than thiopentone with more variation of dose response.[93] Has been used for induction of anaesthesia in patients undergoing cardiovascular surgery because of its minimal effect on the cardiovascular system in a dose of 0·3 mg/kg.[94] Midazolam is suitable for a slow induction in elderly patients.[95]

(*See also* Dundee J. W. and Wyant G. M. *Intravenous Anaesthesia*. Edinburgh: Churchill Livingstone, 1974; Committee on the Review of Medicine, *Br. Med. J.* 1980, **1**, 910; Dundee J. W. *Intravenous Anaesthetic Agents*. London: Arnold, 1979; Pharmacodynamics of intravenous agents, *see* Sear J. W. *Anaesthesia* 1983, **38**, Suppl. 10; Gamble J. A. S. et al. *Anaesthesia* 1981, **36**, 868.)

Antagonists
Aminophylline 3 ml of 2% solution, i.v. cautiously.[96] Physostigmine is not a reliable antagonist.[97] True antagonists have been formulated (Ro. 15–1788 and Ro. 15–3505).[98]

Neurolept Analgesia

This is a neologism which has been used to describe the state of a patient following the administration of one of the newer, very potent analgesic agents, such as phenoperidine, pentazocine 1–2 mg/kg or fentanyl, together with a sedative drug of the butyrophenone series such as haloperidol and droperidol. Thalamonal (Innovar) is a premix of 50:1 droperidol and fentanyl, each millilitre comprising droperidol 2·5 mg with 0·05 mg of fentanyl.

The term 'neurolepsis' was coined by Delay in 1959[99] and 'neurolept analgesia' was introduced by J. A. De Castro and Mundeleer of Brussels in the same year.[100] A development of the artificial hibernation, neurovegetative block, ataralgesia concepts. All neuroleptic agents and phenothiazines used in anaesthesia are chemically based on methyl ethylamine and are related to gamma-hydroxybutyric acid (GABA).

Short-acting Narcotic Analgesics

Phenoperidine Hydrochloride (*Operidine*) and **Fentanyl Citrate** (*Phentanyl; Sublimaze*)
These are chemically related to pethidine but are much more potent.[101] Like it they possess all the properties of narcotic analgesics such as psychological dependence, intense analgesia, respiratory depression which outlasts the analgesia, small pupil, nausea and vomiting, depending on the dose used. Phenoperidine 2 mg has the analgesic potency of morphine 10 mg. Fentanyl 0·1 mg has the analgesic potency of morphine 10 mg or pethidine 75–100 mg. Their effects on the cardiovascular system are minimal, although the heart rate may be slowed, a vagal effect. Nitrous oxide may also cause cardiovascular instability when used with doses of fentanyl,[102] while respiratory depression can be antagonized by naloxone and its congeners. The analgesic effects of phenoperidine last from 40 to 60 min, those of fentanyl up to 30–60 min when given i.v. Fentanyl is partly excreted into the stomach and reabsorbed from the alkaline juices of the small bowel.[114] Phenoperidine is metabolized and excreted in the urine in equal amounts; fentanyl is mostly destroyed in the liver and about 10% excreted in the urine. Should be used carefully in patients who have been taking mono-amine oxidase inhibitors within 14 days. Effects during early pregnancy not known. There is no evidence that fentanyl and droperidol are toxic to bone-marrow cells.

Alfentanil (*Rapifen*)
First used in 1981.[103] A narcotic analgesic with potency about one-quarter that of fentanyl. Onset of action is four times faster than that of fentanyl and duration about one-third as long. It may be used as a supplement to anaesthesia in the same way as fentanyl, but because of its rapid action is particularly suitable in short precedures and in day case surgery. May also be used in repeated dosage or continuous infusion in major surgery. To prevent metabolic and endocrine responses to surgery, high doses are necessary before the start of the operation,

not after it has begun.[104] Dosage up to 500 µg with spontaneous respiration, 30–50 µg/kg with IPPV; supplementary doses should be one-half the initial dose. (*See also* Kay B. *Br. J. Anaesth.* 1982, **54**, 1011; Hull C. J. *Br. J. Anaesth.* 1983, **55**, 1578; Symposium on Alfentanil, *Br. J. Anaesth.* 1983, **55**, Suppl 2.; Sinclair M. E. and Cooper G. M. *Anaesthesia* 1983, **38**, 435.)

Sufentanyl
For pharmacodynamics, *see* Bovill.[105]

Clinical Uses
1. Together with droperidol to produce neurolept anaesthesia. Doses: either phenoperidine 2–5 mg or fentanyl 0·1–0·6 mg with droperidol 5 mg. Or as Thalamonal (Innovar), each millilitre of which contains fentanyl 0·05 mg and droperidol 2·5 mg (1:50). Incremental doses of 0·5 ml of Thalamonal. Fentanyl and phenoperidine produce short-lived rise in intrabiliary pressure.[106] A dose within 30 min of the end of the operation may result in respiratory depression[106] which may recur after an interval.[107]
2. To produce apnoea when it is desired to institute or maintain mechanical ventilation in the intensive therapy unit, e.g. chest injuries. Doses: phenoperidine up to 5 mg or fentanyl up to 0·6 mg intravenously.
3. As analgesics: phenoperidine 1 mg intravenously (fentanyl 0·05 mg). Effects come in 2–3 min, reach peak in 5 min and wear off in 20 min. A dose of fentanyl 0·05 mg causes intense analgesia with bradycardia and perhaps some depression of breathing requiring assisted respiration. Light general anaesthesia with or without a relaxant may be used additionally. Has been employed in day-stay surgery, together with methohexitone and nitrous oxide and oxygen; dose 0·075–0·15 mg fentanyl. Large doses may result in muscular rigidity, making IPPV difficult, but a relaxant will overcome this effect. Delayed respiratory depression following apparent recovery of respiratory activity after fentanyl has been reported.[108]
4. Fentanyl has been used in high dosage, up to 25 µg/kg to attenuate stress responses during surgery. Doses of 50 µg/kg have been used with oxygen, with or without diazepam for cardiac surgery.

Butyrophenones

Droperidol[109] (*Dehydrobenzperidol; Droleptan; Inapsine*)
One of the butyrophenone series of drugs which causes mental detachment, absence of voluntary movements (catatonia), a specific inhibitory effect on the chemoreceptor trigger zone controlling nausea and vomiting (apomorphine antagonism), a weak α-adrenergic receptor blocking action (sometimes causing hypotension, a mechanism doubted by others)[110] and amphetamine antagonism. The butyrophenones compete with GABA at postsynaptic receptor sites. They have similar actions to the phenothiazines and are dopaminergic antagonists. Onset of effect 3–20 min after i.v. injection. Duration of effect up to 12 h. It acts quickly and is much more potent than haloperidol. Large doses may cause extrapyramidal dyskinesia which can be overcome by anti-Parkinson agents (other than laevo-dopa) atropine or promethazine. Reticular activating system not unduly depressed. Gives some protection against catecholamine-induced dysrhythmias during anaesthesia. Reduces body oxygen consumption. Following

the injection of **Haloperidol** (*Serenace*), an allied drug, its effect is noticed in 10 min and lasts 24–48 h. Has little effect on liver, heart or respiratory function. Mostly broken down in liver, but 10% excreted in urine. Liver disease calls for smaller dosage than usual. Has very little effect on metabolism (For current theories of the actions of butyrophenones, *see* Richter J. J. *Anesthesiology* 1981, **56**, 66.) Haloperidol crosses the placenta.[111]

Uses of Neurolept Analgesia

1. As premedication, 0·5–2 ml of Thalamonal. Occasionally unpleasant subjective sensations and muscular dyskinesia are experienced. Analgesia varies with the amount of the analgesic component but if dosage is adequate, burns dressings, needle punctures, sutures and other minor traumata are tolerated.

2. In certain neurosurgical operations when the patient's conscious co-operation is required during surgery, e.g. in stereotactic surgery and antero-lateral tractotomy. It reduces the cerebrospinal fluid pressure in normal patients and those with space-occupying lesions. No significant effect on cerebral blood flow or oxygen consumption. May raise intracranial pressure in head injury or cerebral tumour.

3. In diagnostic procedures, e.g. aortography, angiocardiography, bronchos-copy and oesophagoscopy, fibreoptic gastroscopy.

4. As a supplement to thiopentone, relaxant and gas–oxygen anaesthesia. Rigidity of the chest wall may arise and may cause impaired breathing if this is spontaneous. IPPV is more commonly employed. Droperidol, 5–20 mg, is followed by incremental doses of fentanyl until apnoea occurs. Nitrous oxide, oxygen and relaxants are then administered and the trachea intubated. It prevents awareness during these operations. Naloxone may be needed at the end of the operation. Additional injections of analgesic may be required if there is movement, sweating, a rise in blood pressure or pulse rate.

5. As an alternative to conventional anaesthesia, given in large doses to provide suitable conditions for surgery. A typical regime might be: premedica-tion, droperidol 10 mg; induction, phenoperidine 2 mg i.v. followed by infusion of phenoperidine 20 mg and droperidol 50 mg in 500 ml of 5% dextrose. Tracheal intubation is employed with IPPV using air. Muscle relaxants, as required, and naloxone given at the end of surgery. This technique has advocates in European countries, but is not popular in the UK.

6. To provide sedation during operations under regional analgesia.

7. During bypass in cardiovascular surgery in order to avoid the cardiodepres-sant and dysrhythmic effects of volatile agents.

8. In ophthalmology to provide sedation in patients undergoing intraocular operations under local analgesia.

9. For dressing of burns.

10. Should not be used in the first trimester of pregnancy, and only with great care in patients receiving mono-amine oxidase inhibitors.

11. In the intensive therapy unit to facilitate intubation and IPPV.

12. To increase afferent block during halothane anaesthesia.

Car driving should be discouraged during the 24 h following 10 mg droperidol. Other narcotic analgesics (e.g. pentazocine) can be used with droperidol.[112]

(*See also* Dundee J. W. and Wyant G. M. *Intravenous Anaesthesia*. Edinburgh: Churchill Livingstone, 1974.)

The Phenothiazine Derivatives

This group of drugs includes, among hundreds of others:

Promethazine Hydrochloride, BP (*Phenergan, Atosil*)
(N-(2-dimethylamino-*n*-propyl)-phenothiazine hydrochloride). It is thought to stabilize cell membranes and the coverings of the endoplasmic reticulum. First used in anaesthesia in the 'lytic cocktail'.[113] Its effects are similar to those of chlorpromazine but it has, among others, the following differences: (*a*) It has less antagonism to adrenaline; (*b*) It has 100 times more antagonism to histamine by its effect on H_1 receptors; (*c*) It is a more potent depressant of upper respiratory tract reflexes and is a bronchodilator; (*d*) It has slight atropine-like activity; (*e*) It is a powerful hypnotic in its own right and potentiates barbiturates and narcotic analgesics, possibly by an influence on liver cells;[114] (*f*) It is said to increase sensitivity to pain.[114] (*g*) It opposes 5-hydroxytryptamine. It is supplied as 2·5% solution and as tablets, 25 mg, and elixir, 5 mg/5 ml. Dose for premedication 25–50 mg i.m. *See* Chapter 8.

Trimeprazine Tartrate BPC (*Vallergan*)
This is the neutral tartrate of trimeprazine, 10-(3-dimethylamino-2-methyl-propyl)-phenothiazine. It is a powerful antihistaminic, serotonin antagonist, anti-emetic and spasmolytic agent and is also a good antipruritic. It does not possess the anti-adrenaline properties of chlorpromazine and it is shorter-acting. Almost no effect on either heart or blood pressure. Some anti-cholinergic activity. It is a satisfactory drug for preoperative sedative medication in children given by mouth as a syrup (6 mg/ml), dose (3–4 mg/kg) 1–2 h before anaesthesia.

Perphenazine, BP (*Fentazin, Trilafon*)
A phenothiazine derivative, five times as potent as chlorpromazine and less toxic and with fewer side-effects. Useful in treatment of nausea and vomiting associated with anaesthesia (2–4 mg thrice daily). Perhaps should not be given during the first trimester of pregnancy. No evidence that it is toxic to the liver or bone marrow. Is a powerful central nervous system depressant. May cause dyskinesia (treatment: diazepam). Intramuscular dose 2·5–5 mg.

Promazine Hydrochloride, BP USP (*Sparine*)
Differs chemically from chlorpromazine by the absence of a chlorine atom in the molecule, and is one-third as potent. Similar effects to the parent drug but causes less hypotension and less liver damage. It does not cause much pain when injected intramuscularly. Average dose 25–50 mg.

Prochlorperazine Maleate, BP USP (*Stemetil, Compazine*)
Has been used to control vertigo after inner and middle-ear operations. Dose 12·5 mg i.m.; 15–30 mg *per oram*.

Fluperazine Hydrochloride, BP USP (*Modicate, Moditen, Permitil, Prolixin*)
Used to prevent (1 mg by mouth twice daily) and to treat (5 mg i.m.) postoperative vomiting.

Chlorpromazine Hydrochloride, BP (*Largactil, Thorazine, Megaphen, Hibernal*)
(2-chloro-10(3'-dimethylamino-*n*-propyl)-phenothiazine hydrochloride).

The description which follows applies primarily to *chlorpromazine*.

History

Chlorpromazine was synthesized in France by Charpentier in 1950. Pharmacology worked out by Courvoisier and others.[115] With promethazine (synthesized in 1945) it was used in psychiatry in 1952 and in anaesthesia by Laborit and Huguenard in 1951,[116] (who coined the names 'potentiated anaesthesia', 'lytic cocktail', 'anaesthesia without anaesthetics'), and in Britain in 1953.[117] In the same year it was used together with surface cooling to facilitate hypothermia.[118]

Physical Characteristics

pH of 5% solution is 4·5—so it should be well diluted to avoid irritation. It is prepared in 1% and 2·5% solutions, which should not be exposed to light; in tablets, each containing 10 or 25 mg; and as 100-mg suppositories. It may cause cloudiness when mixed with certain solutions of dextrose and saline.

Pharmacodynamics of Chlorpromazine

It is very variable in its effect especially when taken by mouth. A dopamine antagonist.

The central nervous system. It depresses the reticular formation of the brain and has an inhibitory effect on all cellular activity, the so-called narcobiotic effect (Decourt). It produces drowsiness and relieves anxiety but does not inhibit the higher psychic centres. With sufficient dosage it will cause unconsciousness. It potentiates all anaesthetics and sedatives. It antagonizes drugs, other than strychnine, having a stimulating action on the brain stem, e.g. nikethemide, nicotine and caffeine. The EEG changes are those of normal sleep and differ from the changes resulting from barbiturates.

Autonomic nervous system. It inhibits sympathetic activity centrally by depressing the centres in the diencephalon and thus prevents responses to stimuli mediated through sympathetic nerves, e.g. vasoconstriction following haemorrhage, trauma and shock. This central inhibition of vasomotor reflexes is one of the chief characteristics of the drug. It may also depress the heat-regulating centre in the diencephalon. It greatly reduces the effects of adrenaline on the α-receptor sites. Produces pallor.

Respiratory system. Pulmonary ventilation may be reduced; bronchial and laryngeal reflexes and secretions are depressed. It may cause Cheyne–Stokes respiration.[119] Has been used with success in the treatment of asthma. Increases respiratory rate depressed by pethidine.

Cardiovascular system. Chlorpromazine reduces blood pressure by causing peripheral vasodilatation, the result of central vasomotor depression. If given before the onset of shock—but not after its development—the drug prevents the intense and prolonged vasoconstriction with its accompanying visceral ischaemia. Chlorpromazine is a mild α- and β-blocker.

Vomiting. It is a mild anti-emetic.

Temperature regulation. (*a*) Depresses the tone of muscle; (*b*) May depress the heat-regulating centre; (*c*) Causes peripheral vasodilatation so that the patient becomes strongly influenced by the surrounding temperature; (*d*) Inhibits shivering by a central effect. Oxygen consumption is reduced only if the patient's temperature is made to fall.

Other actions. Chlorpromazine is a local analgesic. It potentiates the effects of anaesthetics, analgesics, hypnotics and muscle relaxants. The secretions of the mouth, pharynx and upper respiratory tract are inhibited. It is an antipruritic. Has a membrane-stabilizing effect, and depresses muscarinic receptors.

Side-effects and toxic actions. (*a*) Faintness and dizziness due to postural hypotension; (*b*) Liver damage following prolonged administration, but a case following a single dose of 50 mg has been reported; shown by an enlarged, tender liver and jaundice of cholestatic type; patients having alcoholic liver disease are very sensitive to phenothiazines. The kidneys are not harmed by the drug; (*c*) Contact dermatitis and photosensitivity; (*d*) Agranulocytosis, following prolonged administration.

Pharmacokinetics
Broken down in body into chlorpromazine sulphoxide, perhaps partly by the liver. Small amounts excreted in the urine, which may be coloured pink or purple.

Clinical Uses of Chlorpromazine (and Promethazine)
In anaesthesia

1. *As premedication*. Various techniques have been described; 12·5–50 mg of each drug and 50–100 mg of pethidine, i.m., 1½ hours preoperatively.

2. *As part of the anaesthetic technique*. Again, various methods of administration have been advocated, including: (i) The slow intravenous drip of 500 ml of dextrose containing, for example, chlorpromazine 50–100 mg, promethazine 50–100 mg and pethidine 50–100 mg, the so-called 'lytic cocktail' which produces the state unfortunately named 'artificial hibernation'. The drip can be slowed down when the desired result has been obtained. (ii) The same amount of the three drugs can be dissolved in 20 ml of dextrose solution and given slowly i.v. or i.m. before anaesthesia commences. The patient is likely to be sleepy for 5–10 h after the administration of these amounts, and of course general anaesthetic agents will be used in smaller doses than normal.

3. To reduce or cure postoperative vomiting.

4. To aid induced hypothermia by surface cooling.

5. To promote sleep during operations performed under regional analgesia.

In general therapeutics chlorpromazine has been used for: (*a*) The potentiation of analgesics in inoperable carcinoma; (*b*) To cure vomiting, due to digitalis, radiation, carcinomatosis, labyrinthitis, acute alcoholism, anaemia, etc. (*c*) In organic psychoses, e.g. schizophrenia, and delirium tremens to control excitement and relieve mental tension; (*d*) To control intractable hiccups.

For current theories of the actions of the phenothiazines, *see* Richter J. J. *Anesthesiology* 1981, **56**, 66.

Dissociative Anaesthesia

Ketamine (*Ketalar; Ketaject*)
Ketamine is 2-*o*-chlorophenyl-2-methylaminocyclohexanone hydrochloride. It is a white crystalline substance with a characteristic smell. Readily soluble in water, pH 3·5–4·1 in 10% solution. Supplied in 1, 5 and 10% solutions. Forms a precipitate with barbiturates.

History
A related compound, phencyclidine (Sernyl) was synthesized by Victor Maddox

of Detroit, investigated by Chen of Ann Arbor[120] and was used in anaesthesia,[121] but was withdrawn because of the high incidence of hallucinations, though it is still used in animals. Ketamine was synthesized by Stevens of Detroit and tested on volunteers from a state prison in Michigan in 1964. It was used in anaesthesia in 1965 by Domino and Corssen.[122] It proved a promising new agent, particularly for use in underdeveloped countries or in the field situation. Since then considerable interest has developed in this compound which has certain properties not shared by other agents. (*See* Corssen G. in: *Anaesthesia; Essays on its History* (Rupreht J. et al., ed.) Berlin: Springer-Verlag, 1985, p. 92.)

Pharmacodynamics
Ketamine is rapidly absorbed after oral, intramuscular or intravenous administration. The injection of a therapeutic dose of ketamine produces a state of *dissociative anaesthesia*. The sleep produced is somewhat different from that of conventional anaesthesia. It occurs within minutes of intramuscular or intravenous injection and lasts for up to 15 min. Analgesia is a marked feature.

Cardiovascular system. Systolic and diastolic blood pressures are raised and pulse rate increases. It has been suggested that the changes are due to central sympathetic stimulation[123] and depression of baroreceptors. There is evidence that ketamine is a direct myocardial stimulant since the rise in blood pressure can be prevented by administration of verapamil, a calcium ion antagonist. It causes pulmonary vasoconstriction and undesirable strain on the right heart in some cases of valvular heart disease. Ketamine may act by increasing the availability of calcium ions across cell membranes. The chronotropic effect is not blocked by verapamil. There is a rise in plasma noradrenaline which can be reduced by prior administration of droperidol. Premedication with propranolol or atropine does not prevent rise of blood pressure and increase of pulse rate when ketamine is used.[124] There is an antidysrhythmia effect. Ketamine prevents reflex adrenergic responses of peripheral blood vessels to surgical stimuli.

Respiratory system. Respiration is not depressed, except by large doses, and is usually mildly stimulated. The prevention of aspiration under ketamine cannot be guaranteed. Salivation may be produced.

Alimentary system. Has analgesic effects when taken by mouth.[125]

Ocular. Some rise of intraocular pressure may occur, but this is transient and ketamine has been recommended for tonometry in children.[126] Eye movements and nystagmus may occur.

Skin. Transient erythema has been reported in 15% of patients and is of little consequence.[126]

Cerebral. Increases cerebral blood flow and intracranial pressure with marked regional variations.[127] When used for a prolonged period, it has increased the frequency of attacks in epileptic patients.[128]

Onset and duration of effect. An intravenous dose of 2 mg/kg will result in anaesthesia in 30 sec, lasting for 5–10 min. An i.m. dose of 10 mg/kg gives anaesthesia in 3–4 min, lasting 10–20 min.

Pharmacokinetics
It is converted into water-soluble metabolites by N-demethylation and hydroxylation of the cyclohexanone ring. These are excreted in the urine.

Clinical Uses
Ketamine is a rapidly acting parenteral anaesthetic causing sedation, profound

analgesia, catalepsy, some increase in striated muscle tone, mild cardiovascular stimulation, but only slight diminution of pharyngolaryngeal reflexes. Not very efficient as an obtundor of visceral pain. It increases salivation so that atropine should always be used. Intravenous injection should take 60–120 s. Has been employed: (1) As the sole agent for minor operations; (2) As an induction agent before general anaesthesia; (3) When airway control is difficult; (4) For certain neurological radiodiagnostic and therapeutic procedures in children to abolish movement; (5) When maintenance of blood pressure is important, e.g. in states of shock and in some poor-risk patients and in the elderly; (6) In open heart surgery, (7) For manipulations; (8) For dressing of burns, skin débridement, skin grafts, etc.; (9) For dealing with mass casualties; (10) In developing countries or when anaesthetists are unavailable. (11) When intramuscular injection is more convenient than intravenous. (12) Subanaesthetic doses have been used to produce analgesia.[129] (13) For induction of anaesthesia in small children. A 0·1% solution in 5% dextrose[130] has been given as a slow i.v. drip for postoperative pain relief and for analgesia in patients in the intensive care unit. (For pharmacokinetic effects of ketamine infusions, *see* Idvall J. et al. *Br. J. Anaesth.* 1979, **51**, 1167.)

Dosage

For i.v. use, 1–2 mg/kg, and supplementary doses of 0·5 mg/kg as required, of 1% solution. For i.m. use, 10 mg/kg of 5% solution. The solution is not irritant to tissues or veins. Slow i.v. infusions of ketamine have been used (0·1%), the maintenance dose during surgery being about 0·5–0·75 mg/min.[131]

Adverse reactions. These include rise of blood pressure and pulse rate which may be disadvantageous in the hypertensive. Transient erythematous rashes have been reported.

Dreams. Vivid unpleasant dreams have been reported.[132] and occasionally true hallucinations. These are a problem in adults, but not in children. It has been suggested that the phenomena are related to those found in acute sensory deprivation.[133] The incidence of these emergence phenomena can be reduced by: (1) Leaving the patient without stimulation in the recovery period; (2) Use of opiate–hyoscine premedication; (3) Injection of droperidol (2·5–7·5 mg, i.m. or i.v.) towards the end of surgery; (4) Small amounts of diazepam, lorazepam or thiopentone. (5) Preoperative psychotherapy.[134] These dreams occur during surgery as well as after it. 4-aminopyridine, 0·3 mg/kg, aids recovery from ketamine (and diazepam) unconsciousness.[135]

Used in Bier's technique for intravenous regional analgesia, it produces analgesia in the arm, unfortunately followed by unconsciousness a few minutes after release of the tourniquet[136] and extradurally, 4 mg in 10 ml of 5 % dextrose in water when it is reported to give good pain relief after operation without side-effects.[137]

Contraindications

1. *Age*. Many anaesthetists believe that ketamine is more suitable for use in children than adults owing to the incidence of emergence phenomena.

2. *Hypertension*. It has been suggested that it should not be used in patients with systolic blood pressure higher than 160 mmHg,[138] at least until more information is available, or in cases of eclampsia or pre-eclampsia. It may raise the cerebrospinal fluid pressure and increase cerebral blood flow. Not very suitable in chronic alcoholics or patients who are drunk.

Ketamine produces only transient hormonal changes which are minor in comparison with those superimposed by surgery.[139] Ketamine analgesia is partially reversed by naloxone.[140] Ketamine has been used for intradural analgesia in war surgery.[141] It can also be given orally.[142]

(*See also* Ketamine; its pharmacology and therapeutic uses. White P. F. et al. *Anesthesiology* 1982, **56**, 119.)

Narcotic Analgesics

Neurolept drugs, morphine, pethidine, etc. can be used to supplement light anaesthesia produced by barbiturates, etc. and nitrous oxide, oxygen. *Intravenous pethidine* during anaesthesia was first used in 1947 by Neff and his colleagues in the USA[143] and by Mushin and Rendell-Baker in 1949[144] in Britain. It reduces the rapid ventilation rate sometimes seen after even small amounts of trichloroethylene and postpones and reduces the need for postoperative sedation. It causes respiratory depression and slow breathing. It contracts the sphincter of Oddi and so may interfere with successful exploration of the common bile duct. For pharmacology *see* Chapter 8.

Total Intravenous Anaesthesia

Given a satisfactory total intravenous technique the problem of pollution of the operating theatre atmosphere would disappear. This can be achieved relatively easily when regional analgesia is employed, but such methods are applicable to only a limited range of surgical operations. Intravenous agents can be used in association with muscle-relaxant drugs provided ventilatory exchange is maintained by IPPV with air, enriched with oxygen if necessary, but it is then difficult to ensure that the patient remains asleep and awareness may be a problem.

Recently techniques have been explored using a combination of hypnotic agent, analgesic drugs and muscle relaxants.[145] The use of short-acting agents allows recovery to be reasonably rapid. The following agents have been used: barbiturates, etomidate, propofol, ketamine, GABA, and narcotic analgesics.

The *cerebral function monitor*[146] has been used to assess depth of anaesthesia when muscle relaxants might mask the signs of either deep cortical depression or awareness. The signal is derived from the EEG and uses two biparietal electrodes. The voltage measured varies with amplitude and frequency of cerebral waves and the variation in voltage is plotted against time on a semi-logarithmic scale. When intravenous induction agents are administered a characteristic pattern emerges and with experience the anaesthetist gains valuable information.[147]

Ketamine has also been given in a continuous infusion (1 mg/ml). A suggested technique is premedication with diazepam and induction with diazepam, 0·3 mg/kg, supplemented by ketamine 1–1·5 mg/kg. Muscle relaxants are given and IPPV instituted with nitrous oxide and oxygen. The ketamine infusion is maintained at a rate of 0·5–0·75 mg/min. This is not strictly a total intravenous technique, but it seems likely that such a method could be modified by the substitution of intravenous analgesic drugs for nitrous oxide. (*See also* Knell P. J. W. *Anaesthesia* 1983, **38**, 586; Symposium Total Intravenous Anaesthesia (Morgan M. ed.); *Anaesthesia* 1983, **38**, Suppl. July; Dundee J. W. and McMurray, T. J. *J. R. Soc. Med.* 1984, **77**, 669.)

A knowledge of the fate of intravenous drugs used in the body, is necessary for the rational use of continuous i.v. anaesthesia.

(*See also* Sear J. W. *Anaesthesia* 1983, **38**, Suppl. July, 10.)

Untoward Reactions to Intravenous Anaesthetic Drugs[148]

Possible Mechanisms

(1) A direct release of histamine from circulating basophils. This is dose related and no previous administration of the drug is necessary. May result in erythema and/or hypotension; (2) Complement activation (the alternative pathway) by the drug, causing histamine release; (3) A true type 1 hypersensitivity response, depending on previous exposure to the drug.[149]

Prevention

(1) Slow rate of injection of all intravenous agents; (2) Special care with those patients with a history of allergy or atopy, especially those with high levels of IgE; (3) Pre-treatment with an H_1 receptor antagonist may be helpful.

Causes

1. *Over-dose.* (*a*) Direct effects of the drug; (*b*) Side-effects of the drug; (*c*) Depression of an abnormal organ by a normal dose.
2. *Abnormal sensitivity to the drug or its solvent.* (*a*) Idiosyncrasy, which may be congenital; (*b*) Allergic, hypersensitivity, anaphylactic or histamine response on the first or subsequent exposure to the same (or even another) drug. An anaphylactoid phenomenon is a hypersensitivity response which is clinically indistinguishable from anaphylaxis but without proven antibody involvement. Intradermal testing, using 1:1000 solutions of the suspected drug, is a useful diagnostic test; a red weal or flare indicates sensitivity. (For intradermal skin testing *see* Sage D. *Anaesth. Intensive Care* 1981, **9**, 381; Laxenaire M-C. et al. *Anaesthesia* 1983, **38**, 147; Moss J. and Rosow C. E. *Anesthesiology* 1983, **59**, 330; Fisher McD. and Roffe D. J. *Anaesthesia* 1984, **39**, 213.) Commoner in females, in those with atopic conditions, e.g. hay fever, asthma, eczema, other drug allergies,[150] and in those with a high level of immunoglobulin G. All degrees of sensitivity exist from cutaneous flushing to rapidly fatal collapse. The commonest signs are: (i) Cutaneous: flushing, urticaria, oedema (e.g. of eyelids); (ii) Cardiovascular: collapse, tachycardia, hypotension; (iii) Respiratory: broncho-spasm, laryngospasm, cyanosis; (iv) Abdominal: pain, colic, pyrexia; (v) Various other target organs may be damaged, e.g. the liver.

The complement activation sequence is triggered and may be detected by CIq, C3 and C4 immunoassay. Lymphocyte cultures and gas–liquid chromotography are used to measure immune complexes.

3. *Reactions with other drugs*, e.g. pethidine and mono-amine oxidase inhibitors.
4. *Toxic reactions to metabolites of the drug*, e.g. ethanol.
5. *Others*, e.g. malignant hyperpyrexia.

Several factors, including pregnancy and re-exposure, may predispose to hypersensitivity reactions following the injection of solutions containing Cremophor EL.[151] Intradermal testing must be used and interpreted with caution.[152]

Treatment

Over-dose: supportive therapy and, occasionally, dialysis. Allergic reactions:[153] head-down tilt; rapid infusion of 1–2 litres of a plasma expander, colloid or crystalloid; for bronchospasm, aminophylline 250–300 mg or salbutamol 0·25–0·5 mg, hydrocortisone hemisuccinate 100–200, but this will take some time to act; tracheal intubation and IPPV; possible use of an antihistamine in the treatment of glottic oedema and urticaria, e.g. chlorpheniramine (Piriton) 10–20 mg. i.v.

(*See also* Dundee J. W. *Intravenous Anaesthetic Agents*. London: Arnold, 1979; Fisher McD. and Morr D. G. *Anaesth. Intensive Care* 1981, **9**, 226; Fisher McD. *Anaesth. Intensive Care* 1981, **9**, 235; Fisher McD. *Anaesth. Intensive Care* 1981, **9**, 242.)

References

1. Oré P.-C. *Bull. Soc. Chirurg.* 1872, **1**, 400; *see also* Sabathié M. and Delperier A. *Progress in Anaesthesiology*. Amsterdam: Excerpta Medica, 1970, p. 841.
2. Pravaz C. G. *C. R. Seances Acad. Sci.* 1853, **36**, 88.
3. Rynd F. *Dublin Med. Press*, 1845, **13**, 167.
4. Wood A. *Edin. Med. Surg. J.* 1855, **82**, 265.
5. Howard-Jones N. J. *J. Hist. Med.* 1947, **2**, 201.
6. Krawkow N. F. *Arch. Exp. Path. Pharmak*. 1908, Suppl. 317.
7. Burckhardt L. *Münch. Med. Wochenschr.* 1909, **2**, 2365.
8. Fischer E. and von Mering J. *Ther. d. Gegenw.* 1903, **5**, 97.
9. Bardet D. *Bull. Gen. Therap.* 1921, **1**, 27; Fredet P. and Perlis R. *Bull. et Mém. Soc. Nat. de Chir.* 1924, **50**, 789.
10. Noel H. and Souttar H. S. *Ann. Surg.* 1913, **57**, 64.
11. Bredenfeld E. *Z. Exp. Path. Ther.* 1916, **18**, 80.
12. Bumm R. *Klin. Wochenschr.* 1927, **6**, 725.
13. Zerfas L. G. and McCallum J. T. C. *J. Ind. Med. Assoc.* 1929, **22**, 47.
14. Fitch R. H. et al. *Am. J. Surg.* 1930, n.s. **9**, 110.
15. Magill I. W. *Lancet*, 1931, **1**, 74.
16. Lundy J. S. *Surg. Clin. North Am.* 1931, **11**, 909.
17. Kirschner M. *Chirurg.* 1929, **1**, 673; Macintosh R. R. et al. *Lancet*, 1941, **2**, 10; Thornton H. L. et al. *Anesthesiology* 1945, **6**, 583.
18. Weese H. and Scharpff W. *Dtsch. Med. Wochenschr.* 1932, **58**, 1205.
19. Jarman R. and Abel L. *Lancet*, 1933, **2**, 18.
20. Tabern D. L. and Volwiler E. H. *J. Am. Chem. Soc.* 1935, **57**, 1961.
21. Lundy J. S. and Tovell R. M. *North West Med.* 1935, **33**, 308; Lundy J. S. *Proc. Staff Meet. Mayo Clin.* 1935, **10**, 536 (reprinted in 'Classical File', *Surv. Anesthesiol.* 1958, **2**, 231); Corssen G. in: *Anaesthesia; Essays on its History* (Rupreht J. et al. ed.) Berlin: Springer-Verlag, 1985, p. 88.
22. Pratt T. W. et al. *Am. J. Surg.* 1936, **31**, 464.
23. Jarman R. and Abel L. *Lancet*, 1936, **1**, 422.
24. Brodie B. B. et al. *J. Pharmacol. Exp. Ther.* 1950, **98**, 85 (reprinted in 'Classical File', *Surv. Anesthesiol.* 1965, **9**, 391).
25. Stoelting V. K. *Anesth. Analg. Curr. Res.* 1957, **36**, 49.
26. Halford F. J. *Anesthesiology* 1943, **4**, 67.
27. Organe G. S. W. et al. *Lancet*, 1938, **2**, 1170.
28. Dundee J. W. and Clarke R. S. J. *Br. J. Anaesth.* 1964, **36**, 100.
29. Janssen P. A. J. et al. *Arzneimittel-Forschung*, 1971, **21**, 1234.
30. Doenicke A. et al. *Anaesthesist* 1973, **22**, 357; Krumholz W. et al. *Anaesthesist* 1984, **33**, 161.
31. Hallén B. et al. *Anaesthesia* 1984, **39**, 969; Hallén B. et al. *Br. J. Anaesth.* 1985, **57**, 326.
32. Hecker J. F. *Lancet* 1983, **1**, 332.
33. Dundee J. W. *Br. J. Anaesth.* 1960, **32**, 407; Clutton-Brock J. *Anaesthesia* 1962, **16**, 80; Clutton-Brock J. *Br. J. Anaesth.* 1966, **38**, 413.
34. Grisvold S. E. et al. *Crit. Care Med.* 1982, **10**, 466.

35. Aitkenhead A. R. *Br. J. Anaesth.* 1981, **53**, 1011.
36. Dundee J. W. et al. *Br. J. Anaesth.* 1956, **28**, 344; Mark, L. C. Papper, E. M. et al. *New York Med.* 1949, **49**, 1546.
37. Brodie B. B. et al. *J. Pharmac. Exp. Ther.* 1950, **98**, 85 (reprinted in 'Classical File', *Surv. Anesthesiol.* 1965, **9**, 391).
38. Dundee J. W. and Hassard T. H. *Anaesthesia* 1983, **38**, 26.
39. Clark M. M. and Cockburn H. A. *Br. J. Anaesth.* 1971, **43**, 185; Anderton J. M. and Baldwin A. C. *Anaesthesia* 1979, **34**, 333.
40. Macintosh R. R. and Heyworth P. S. A. *Lancet*, 1943, **2**, 571.
41. Davies D. D. *Br. J. Anaesth.* 1966, **38**, 530; Dundee J. W. *Anesthesiology* 1983, **59**, 154.
42. Lazarus H. M. et al. *J. Surg. Res.* 1977, **22**, 46.
43. Corser G. et al. *Anaesthesia* 1985, **40**, 51.
44. Jamieson D. et al. *Can. Anaesth. Soc. J.* 1972, **19**, 659; Baxter A. D. *Anaesthesia* 1978, **33**, 349.
45. Hales P. *Anaesth. Intensive Care* 1981, **9**, 390.
46. Purdie H. R. M and Punchihewa V. G. *Anaesthesia* 1982, **37**, 101.
47. Dundee J. W. and Riding J. E. *Anaesthesia* 1955, **10**, 55; Dundee J. W. et al. *Anesth. Analg. Curr. Res.* 1962, **41**, 567; Bush G. H. *Proc. R. Soc. Med.* 1968, **61**, 171.
48. Dundee J. W. *Curr. Res. Anesth. Analg.* 1952, **31**, 257; Lodge A. B. *Br. Med. J.* 1958, **1**, 1043; McClelland R. M. A. *Br. J. Anaesth.* 1960, **32**, 81.
49. Coté C. J. and Petitau A. J. *Anesth. Analg. (Cleve.)* 1985, **64**, 1156.
50. Chernish S. M. et al. *Fed. Proc.* 1956, **15**, 409.
51. Dundee J. W. and Moore J. *Anaesthesia* 1961, **16**, 50.
52. Burnell J. C. *Anaesthesia* 1984, **39**, 286.
53. Whitwam J. G. *Br. J. Anaesth.* 1982, **54**, 900.
54. Drummond-Jackson S. L. *Br. Dent. J.* 1962, **113**, 404.
55. Hudson R. J. et al. *Anesthesiology* 1983, **59**, 215.
56. Spanos A. et al. *Anaesth. Intensive Care*, 1978, **6**, 337.
57. Brown P. M. *Anaesthesia* 1981, **36**, 814.
58. Cundy J. M. *Br. Med. J.* 1982, **285**, 378.
59. Fragen R. J. et al. *Br. J. Anaesth.* 1983, **55**, 433.
60. Rifat K. et al. *Can. Anaesth. Soc. J.* 1976, **23**, 492.
61. Van den Hurk A. W. and Teijen H. J. *Anaesthesia* 1983, **38**, 1183.
62. Holdcroft A. et al. *Br. J. Anaesth.* 1976, **48**, 199.
63. Sold M. J. *Anaesthesia* 1985, **40**, 1014.
64. Ledingham I. McA. and Watt I. *Lancet* 1983, **1** 1270.
65. Moore R. A. and Allen M. C. *Anaesthesia* 1985, **40**, 124.
66. Yeoman P. M. et al. *Br. J. Anaesth.* 1984, **56**, 1291P.
67. Duthrie D. J. R. et al. *Br. J. Anaesth.* 1985, **57**, 156; Byrne A. J. and Yeoman P. M. *Br. J. Anaesth.* 1985, **57**, 1264.
68. Kay B. and Rolly G. *Acta Anaesthiol. Belg.* 1977, **28**, 303.
69. Rogers K. M. et al. *Br. J. Anaesth.* 1980, **52**, 407; Kay B. and Stephenson D. K. *Anaesthesia* 1980, **35**, 1182; Rutter D. V. et al. *Anaesthesia* 1980, **35**, 1188; Kay B. *Anaesthesia* 1981, **36**, 863; Major E. et al. *Br. J. Anaesth.* 1981, **53**, 267.
70. Cummings G. C. et al. *Anaesthesia* 1984, **39**, 1168.
71. Fahey L. T. et al. *Anaesthesia* 1985, **40**, 939.
72. Child K. J. et al. *Br. J. Anaesth.* 1971, **43**, 2; Campbell D. et al. *Br. J. Anaesth.* 1971, **43**, 14; Savege T. M. et al. *Anaesthesia* 1971, **26**, 401; Clarke R. S. J. et al. *Anaesthesia* 1971, **26**, 512; Bradford E. M. W. et al. *Br. J. Anaesth.* 1971, **43**, 940; Swerdlow, M. et al. *Br. J. Anaesth.* 1971, **43**, 1075; Aronski A. et al. *Anaesthesia* 1976, **31**, 195; Coleman A. J. *Anaesthesia* 1972, **27**, 373; Tammisto T. et al. *Br. J. Anaesth.* 1973, **45**, 100.
73. Sternbach L. H. *J. Med. Chem.* 1979, **22**, No. 1.
74. Dziewonski K. and Sternbach L. H. *Chem. Abst.* 1936, **30**, 2971.
75. Sterbach L. H. et al. *J. Am. Chem. Soc.* 1960, **82**, 475.
76. Randall L. O. *J. Pharmacol. Exp. Ther.* 1960, **129**, 163.
77. Randall L. O. et al. *Anesth. Analg. Curr. Res.* 1961, **3**, 405.
78. Cushman R. P. A. *Lancet*, 1966, **1**, 1042.
79. Male C. G. et al. *Br. J. Anaesth.* 1980, **52**, 429; Clarke R. S. J. et al. *Br. J. Anaesth.* 1980, **52**, 437.
80. Thakuria S. P. *Anaesthesia* 1980, **35**, 392.
81. Dye D. and Watkins J. *Br. Med. J.* 1980, **2**, 1353.
82. Jeppsson R. and Ljungberg S. *Acta Pharmacol. Toxicol* 1975, **36**, 312.

83. Scholl Olesen A. and Hüttel M. S. *Br. J. Anaesth.* 1980, **52**, 609.; Von Dardel O. et al. *Br. J. Anaesth.* 1983, **55**, 41.
84. Mattila M. A. K. and Suistomaa M. *Anaesthesia* 1984, **39**, 879.
85. Clergue F. et al. *Br. J. Anaesth.* 1981, **53**, 1059.
86. Garrattini S. et al. *The Benzodiazepines.* New York: The Raven Press, 1973.
87. Whitwam J. G. *Anaesthesia* 1983, **38**, 93; Mohler H. and Okada T. *Br. J. Psychiatry* 1978, **133**, 261.
88. Dundee J. W. et al. *Br. J. Anaesth.* 1970, **42**, 54; Assaf R. A. E. et al. *Anaesthesia* 1975, **30**, 152, 164; Gamble J. A. S. et al. *Br. J. Anaesth.* 1973, **45**, 1085.
89. Haagensen R. E. *Anaesthesia* 1985, **40**, 956.
90. Kanto J. *Br. J. Anaesth.* 1981, **53**, 1179.
91. Conner J. T. et al. *Anesth. Analg. (Cleve.)* 1978, **57**, 1; Fragen R. J. et al. *Anesthesiology* 1978, **49**, 41; Reeves J. G. et al. *Can. Anaesth. Soc. J.* 1979, **26**, 42; Forster A. et al. *Br. J. Anaesth.* 1980, **52**, 907.
92. Jensen S. et al. *Br. J. Anaesth.* 1981, **53**, 1083.
93. Hughes T. J. and Thornton J. A. *Anaesthesia* 1981, **36**, 868; Gamble J. A. S. et al. *Anaesthesia* 1981, **36**, 868.
94. Al Khudhairi D. et al. *Br. J. Anaesth.* 1982, **54**, 831.
95. Kanto J. et al. *Anesth. Analg. (Cleve.)* 1986, **65**, 15.
96. Arvidsson S. B. et al. *Lancet* 1982, **2**, 1467.
97. Spaulding B. C. et al. *Anesthesiology* 1984, **61**, 551.
98. Darragh A. et al. *Lancet* 1981, **2**, 8; O'Boyle C. et al. *Br. J. Anaesth.* 1983, **55**, 349; Wolff J. et al. *Anaesthesia* 1986, **41**, 1001; Kirkegaard L. et al. *Anaesthesia* 1986, **41**, 1184.
99. Delay J. *Psychopharmacological Frontiers.* Boston: Little, Brown & Co., 1959.
100. De Castro J. and Mundeleer P. *Anesth. Anal. Paris*, 1959, **16**, 1022.
101. Janssen P. A. J. *Br. J. Anaesth.* 1962, **34**, 260.
102. Eisle J. H. et al. *Anesthesiology* 1976, **44**, 16.
103. Niemeggers C. J. E. and Janssen P. A. J. *Drug Dev. Res.* 1981, **1**, 83.
104. Bent J. M. and Paterson J. L. *Anaesthesia* 1984, **39**, 19.
105. Bovill J. G. et al. *Anesthesiology* 1984, **61**, 502.
106. Holderness M. C. et al. *Anesthesiology* 1963, **24**, 336 (reprinted in 'Classical File', *Surv. Anesthesiol.* 1975, **19**, 310).
107. Stoeckel H. et al. *Br. J. Anaesth.* 1979, **51**, 741.
108. Adams A. P. and Pybus D. A. *Br. Med. J.* 1978, **1**, 278.
109. Janssen P. A. J. et al. *Arzneimittel-Forsch.* 1963, **13**, 205.
110. Johnstone M. *Lancet.* 1979, **1**, 378.
111. Whalley L. J. et al. *Br. Med. J.* 1981, **1**, 1746.
112. Morgan M. et al. *Br. J. Anaesth.* 1974, **46**, 288.
113. Laborit H. and Huguenard P. *Pratique de l'Hibernothérapie.* Paris: Masson, 1954.
114. Dundee J. W. *Anaesthesia* 1961, **16**, 61.
115. Courvoisier S. et al. *Arch. Int. Pharmacodyn. Thér.* 1953, **92**, 305.
116. Laborit H. and Huguenard P. *Presse Méd.* 1951, **59**, 1329.
117. Smith A. and Fairer J. G. *Br. Med. J.* 1953, **2**, 1247.
118. Dundee J. W. et al. *Br. Med. J.* 1953, **2**, 1237.
119. Stokes W. (1804–1878), *The Diseases of the Heart and Aorta.* Dublin, 1854; Cheyne J. (1777–1836), *Dublin Hosp. Rep.* 1818, **2**, 216.
120. Chen G. et al. *J. Pharmacol. Exp. Ther.* 1966, **152**, 332.
121. Johnstone M. et al. *Br. J. Anaesth.* 1959, **31**, 433; Muir B. J. et al. *Br. J. Anaesth.* 1961, **33**, 51; Camilleri J. G. *Anaesthesia* 1962, **17**, 422; Mallick N. P. *Lancet*, 1963, **1**, 392.
122. Domino E. F. et al. *Clin. Pharmacol. Ther.* 1965, **6**, 279; Corssen G. and Domino E. F. *Anesth. Analg. Curr. Res.* 1966, **45**, 29.
123. Chadoff P. *Anesth. Analg. Curr. Res.* 1972, **51**, 247.
124. Bovill J. G. and Dundee J. W. *Anaesthesia* 1972, **27**, 309.
125. Morgan A. J. and Dutkiewicz T. W. S. *Anaesthesia* 1983, **38**, 293.
126. Dillon J. B. *Proc. R. Soc. Med.* 1971, **64**, 1153.
127. Hougaard K. et al. *Anesthesiology* 1974, **41**, 562.
128. Bennett D. R. et al. *Neurology* 1973, **23**, 449.
129. Sher M. H. *Anaesth. Intensive Care.* 1980, **8**, 359; Currie M. A. and Currie A. L. *Ann. R. Coll. Surg.* 1984, **66**, 424.
130. Ito Y. and Ichiyanagi K. *Anaesthesia* 1974, **29**, 222.

131. Hatano S. et al. *Can. Anaesth. Soc. J.* 1976, **23**, 648; El Naggar M. et al. *Anesth. Analg. (Cleve.)* 1977, **56**, 279; Lilburn J. K. et al. *Anaesthesia* 1978, **33**, 315.
132. Bovill J. G. et al. *Br. J. Anaesth.* 1971, **43**, 600; Pandit S. K. et al. *Br. J. Anaesth.* 1971, **43**, 362.
133. Collier B. B. *Anaesthesia* 1972, **27**, 120.
134. Sklar G. S. et al. *Anaesthesia* 1981, **36**, 183.
135. Agoston S. et al. *Br. J. Anaesth.* 1980, **52**, 312.
136. Amiot J. F. et al. *Anaesthesia* 1985, **40**, 899.
137. Islas J. A. et al. *Anesth. Analg. (Cleve.)* 1985, **64**, 1161.
138. Dillon J. B. *Proc. R. Soc. Med.* 1971, **64**, 1153.
139. Lacoumenta S. and Walsh E. S. *Br. J. Anaesth.* 1984, **56**, 493.
140. Finck A. D. and Ngai S. H. *Anesthesiology* 1982, **56**, 291.
141. Bion J. F. *Anaesthesia* 1984, 39, 1023.
142. Hain W. R. *Anaesthesia* 1983, **38**, 810.
143. Neff W. B. et al. *Calif. Med.* 1947, **66**, 67.
144. Mushin W. W. and Rendell-Baker L. *Br. Med. J.* 1949, **2**, 472.
145. Dallas S. N. *Anaesthesia* 1981, **36**, 427.
146. Maynard M. et al. *Br. Med. J.* 1969, **4**, 545; Dubois M. *Anaesthesia* 1978, **33**, 157.
147. Savege T. M. in: *Recent Advantages in Anaesthesia and Analgesia*—13 (Hewer C. L. and Atkinson R. S. ed.). Edinburgh: Churchill Livingstone, 1979.
148. *See also* Clarke R. S. J. in *Recent Advances in Anaesthesia and Analgesia*—14 (Hewer C. L. and Atkinson R. S. ed.) Edinburgh, Churchill Livingstone, 1982.
149. Thornton J. A. *Br. J. Anaesth.* 1982, **54**, 1.
150. Dundee J. W. et al. *Br. J. Anaesth.* 1978, **50**, 793.
151. Simpson P. J. et al. *Anaesthesia* 1985, **40**, 420.
152. Macdonald A. R. and Emery F. M. *Anaesthesia* 1985, **40**, 549.
153. Annotation, *Br. Med. J.* 1981, **1**, 1011.

Chapter 14   **THE MUSCLE RELAXANTS**

It is usual to classify muscle relaxants used in anaesthesia as: (1) Non-depolarizing agents, e.g. tubocurarine, atracurium, vecuronium, pancuronium, alcuronium (tachycurares), and (2) Depolarizing agents, e.g. decamethonium, suxamethonium (leptocurares). Under certain circumstances the depolarizing drugs can exert a non-depolarizing effect, the so-called dual or biphasic block. Muscular relaxation can also be produced centrally by deep general anaesthesia or peripherally by local nerve block. Most relaxants in clinical use are highly ionized and therefore are confined to the extracellular fluid.

History

1596 Sir Walter Raleigh (1552–1618) mentioned the arrow poison in his book *Discovery of the Large, Rich, and Beautiful Empire of Guiana*. It is possible that the poison he described was not curare at all.[1]

1811–1812 Sir Benjamin Collins Brody (1783–1862)[241] experimented with curare (*Phil. Trans.* 1811, **101**, 194; 1812, **102**, 205). He was the first to show that artificial respiration could maintain life in curarized animals.

1825 Curare brought to Europe by Charles Waterton (1782–1865)—*Wanderings in South America*. He described a classic experiment in which he kept a curarized she-ass alive by artificial ventilation with a bellows through a tracheostomy.[2]

1850 Claude Bernard (1813–1878),[3] The great French physiologist, stimulated by Francois Magendie (1783–1855), showed that curare acts by paralysing the myoneural junction. This led to his discovery of the concept of the motor end-plate. George Harley (1829–1896), of ACE anaesthetic mixture fame, showed that curare (wourali) was an efficient antidote to strychnine poisoning and also to tetanus.[4]

1858 Lewis Albert Sayer (1820–1900) used curare to treat tetanus in New York.[5]

1862 Curare used by Chisholm, in the American Civil War.

1872 Curare used by Demme in the treatment of tetanus.

1894 R. Boehm (1844–1926), the German pharmacologist, separated curare into 'pot', 'gourd' and 'tube' curare according to the method used for storing it by the South American Indians. In 1897 he isolated highly active extracts from calabash curare.[6]

1912 Curare used by Arthur Läwen (1876–1958) of Konigsberg[7] in an effort to reduce the amount of ether employed in abdominal surgery with IPPV.

1914 Physiological actions of acetylcholine described by Dale (1875–1968).[8] Twenty-five years later he showed that acetylcholine is responsible for neuromuscular transmission, an effect blocked by curare.[9]

1934 First therapeutic use of curare in the UK (the treatment of tetanus) at Cambridge by Cole.[10]

1935 King (1887–1956)[11] of London, working in Sir Henry Dale's laboratory, isolated d-tubocurarine chloride from the crude drug and established its chemical structure and Ranyard West used it in the treatment of tetanus.[12]

1938 Richard C. Gill (1902–1958), American explorer, drew attention to it in his book *White Water and Blue Magic*, 1940, New York.

1939 Abram Elting Bennett[13] of Omaha (Neb) employed curare to modify metrazol-induced convulsive therapy. Later used by H. Palmer,[13] of Hill End Hospital, Hertfordshire. Curare came to anaesthesia via psychiatry (electroplexy). Bennett arranged for crude curare to be given by Gill to McIntyre of the University of Nebraska who first standardized the drug.

1942 Harold R. Griffith (1894–1985) and Enid Johnson (now of Nova Scotia) used curare (the commercial preparation Intocostrin, prepared by Horace Holaday) at the suggestion of Dr Lewis Wright of E. M. Squibb Co.,[14] deliberately to give relaxation during surgery on 23 January in Montreal, Canada. A famous day in the history of anaesthesia.[15] Messrs Squibb obtained their supply of curare from R. C. Gill who brought it back from an expedition to Ecuador.

1943 Extraction of tubocurarine from *Chondrodendron tomentosum* by Winter-steiner[16]—the source of the drug as used today. First publication of Stuart Chester Cullen (1909–1979), a US pioneer of its use.[17] When given a sample of the preparation 'Intocostrin', Cullen first tried it on animals, and producing apnoea, was not able easily to ventilate them artificially, and so did not proceed to use it on humans. Griffith was also given a sample, but as he was familiar with the management of apnoea due to cyclopropane with IPPV the apnoea caused by curare was not a problem. Thus he rightly claimed priority for the introduction of relaxants into anaesthetic practice.

1944 Earliest mention of the use of curare with unsupplemented nitrous oxide and oxygen by Waters in abdominal surgery;[18] also by Harroun in thoracic surgery.[19]

1945 First reported use in Britain of curare (Intocostrin) by Barnett Mallinson.[20]

1946 T. C. Gray (1913–) and John Halton (1904–1969) of Liverpool established the position of curare in Britain.[21]

1947 Bovet described gallamine triethiodide.[22] This was used clinically in France by Huguenard and Boué in 1948[23] and by Mushin in 1949 in Britain.[24] Influential article describing use of gas, oxygen, pethidine and curare by Neff.[25]

1948 Decamethonium described by Barlow and Ing[26] and by William Drummond Macdonald Paton (1917–) and Eleanor Zaimis (1915–1982).[27] Used clinically by Organe in 1949.[28]

1949 Daniel Bovet of Paris and Rome, and others introduced suxamethonium.

1951 Suxamethonium first used in anaesthesia by von Dardel, in Stockholm[29] and by Otto Mayerhofer in Vienna.[30] Cyril Fredrick Scurr introduced it into Britain.[31]

1954 Sensational article by Henry Knowel Beecher (1907–1976) and D. P. Todd suggesting that the use of relaxants increased deaths due to anaesthesia nearly sixfold.[32] This has, of course, been completely disproved.

1956 W. D. M. Paton made the distinction between depolarizing and non-depolarizing relaxants.[33]

1958 A new relaxant from strychnos toxifera later named alcuronium, described.[34]

1961 Alcuronium first used.[35]

1967 Pancuronium (Pavulon) described clinically,[36] following pharmacological investigations in 1966.[37]

1968 Pancuronium introduced by Burkett W. R. et al.[38]

1970 Correct structure of tubocurarine molecule worked out.[39]

1979 Org.NC.45 (Vecuronium) introduced by Durant et al.[40]

1980 First clinical use of vecuronium (Norcuron).[41]
Atracurium used in man by Hunt and Payne.[42]

1981 Atracurium described by Hughes and Payne.[43]

(*See* Cullen S. C. *Anesthesiology* 1947, **8**, 479; Robbins B. H. and Lundy J. S. *Anesthesiology* 1947, **8**, 252; McIntyre A. R. *Curare; Its History, Nature and Clinical Use.* Chicago: Univ. of Chicago Press, 1947; Thomas K. B. *Curare. Its History and Usage.* London: Pitman, 1964; Stovner J. in: *Muscle Relaxants* (Katz L. ed.). Amsterdam: Excerpta Medica, 1975, Chap. 10; Betcher A. M. *Anesth. Anal.* 1977, **56**, 305; Crul J. F. *Acta Anaesthesiol. Scand.* 1982, **26**, 409; Humble R. M. The Gill Merritt Expedition. *Anesthesiology* 1982, **57**, 519; Suxamethonium, the development of a modern drug from 1906 to the present day. Dorkin H. R. *Med. Hist.* 1982, **26**, 145.)

The Physiology of the Neuromuscular Junction

It was shown by Sir Henry Dale (1875–1968), in 1934, that acetylcholine is responsible for neuromuscular transmission, an effect blocked by curare,[44] and, in 1936, that a motor nerve liberates acetylcholine from the dense projections in the nerve terminal at the myoneural junction on the arrival of a nerve impulse.[45] Acetylcholine crosses the junctional cleft and becomes fixed at lipoprotein receptors on the junctional folds of the end-plate membrane and permits entry of sodium which causes a sudden depolarization with exit of potassium from the muscle fibre. The depolarization passes along the membrane of the muscle fibre and is the final stimulus for causing the contraction of the contractile part of the muscle fibre. The released acetylcholine is meanwhile hydrolysed by acetylcholinesterase in the region of the motor end-plate, so that when the excited muscle fibre has come out of its refractory state it will not become excited again by a depolarized end-plate unless a new nerve impulse has arrived and released a new supply of acetylcholine.

Depolarization causes Ca^{++} to enter the nerve terminal. Increased permeability of the special sodium (Na^+) channels in the neuromuscular junction to Na^+ is the trigger which leads to the propagating action potential. Na^+ enters the fibre, then K^+ leaves, as the action potential proceeds. A change of resting potential of 20 mV is adequate to initiate this process. Fresh acetylcholine (ACh) is synthesized in the axoplasm of the nerve terminal from choline obtained from the ECF and is transferred to vesicles ready for use. This process may be defective in the shocked, acidotic or toxaemic patient, making reversal of relaxants impossible. ACh exists in the nerve terminals in two forms—storage and releasable. ACh release is a self-potentiating process, leading to greater release and giving access to the storage granules for further and subsequent release. Relaxant drugs act on the postjunctional receptors of the neuromuscular junction, and also the prejunctional receptors on the last part of the nerve fibre, where they prevent this self-potentiating release of ACh, causing the characteristic 'fade' seen on neuromuscular monitoring during partial relaxation.

ACh release and receptor stimulation in response to a nerve action potential is far greater than that required to elicit a single muscle fibre contraction. This large 'safety factor' means that up to 70–80% of the receptors can be occupied before surgical relaxation develops, and, conversely, reversal can be clinically adequate, even though many receptors are still blocked. Postoperative introduction of drugs which interact with relaxants may cause paralysis to re-develop.[46]

There are three receptors at the neuromuscular junction (two in the muscle and one in the nerve ending), which respond to ACh, by opening an ion channel: prejunctional, postjunctional and extrajunctional.

1. The Postjunctional Receptors

These are 8–9 nM in diameter with a central pit. The mouth of these special sodium channels is surrounded by five protein moieties, two of which (α) are cholinoceptors which respond to ACh or depolarizing relaxants, causing the other three subunits to rotate to a new conformation with opening of the channel. Na^+ and Ca^{++} move into the muscle and K^+ moves out.[47] Non-depolarizing blockers bind to α units, preventing access of ACh, blocking the channel closed. (Depolarizing relaxants block the channel open, with initial stimulation, e.g. muscle fasiculations.) There are several hundred thousand receptors in each neuromuscular junction. Other drugs blocking these receptors are: local analgesics, aminoglycoside, lincosamine and polymyxin antibiotics, barbiturates, procainamide, quinidine, disopyramide. Other reactions in postjunctional receptor channels: (i) Desensitization, occurring within the receptor molecule, agonist binding failing to cause an opening reaction. Caused by agonists (carbachol, suxamethonium, decamethonium), barbiturates, ACh inhibitors (neostigmine, edrophonium, pyridostigmine, DFP), Ca^{++} channel blockers, (verapamil) local analgesics, phenothiazines, phencyclidine, volatile anaesthetics, aminoglycoside antibiotics, substance P, alcohol. (ii) Physical channel blockade. This prevents normal flow of ions through the tube and thus depolarization. May be caused by local analgesics (on the Na^+ channel of nerve), and Ca^{++} antagonists (on the Ca^{++} channels of heart and blood vessels). This blockade can occur in two modes, blocked when open and blocked when closed. Physical blockage by a molecule of an open channel (by cationic drugs only) relies on the channel being open in the first place, and the development of this is proportional to the frequency of channel opening. Physical blockade of a closed channel may be caused by hexamethonium, tricyclic drugs, and naloxone. Muscle relaxants e.g. decamethonium and suxamethonium, have been known to cause physical channel blockade. (iii) Blockade of the intracellular mechanism, e.g. by entry of decamethonium, dantrolene (Dantrium).

Phase II block involves the above mechanisms at different subphases (*see below*).

2. Prejunctional Receptors

These control an ion channel that is specific for Na^+ (which is essential for synthesis and mobilization of transmitter). They are blocked by curare, resulting in 'fade' and exhaustion. They are blocked by aminoglycoside, lincosamine and polymyxin antibiotics.[48] The action of polymyxin here is due to competition with Ca^{++},[49] does not produce 'fade', can be reversed by Ca^{++} administration, and is made worse by neostigmine. Corticosteroids, barbiturates, anticonvulsants, antidysrhythmics, β-blockers, and lithium may also cause this effect, potentiating muscle relaxants.

Prejunctional block due to relaxants is quite different from that due to Mg^{++} or aminoglycoside and polymyxin antibiotics.

3. Extrajunctional Receptors

These appear all over the surface of the muscle fibre, when the muscle is denervated or deprived of nerve stimulation, by injury, stroke or even disuse.[50] They are similar to, but more responsive than junctional receptors to depolarizing agents, and less responsive to non-depolarizing agents.[51] When these receptors are present in large numbers, suxamethonium causes substantial flow of ions across the membrane producing hyperkalaemia, which is difficult to suppress by prior non-depolarizing drugs (tubocurarine can act as an agonist on these receptors.[52]) They are present before birth and in infancy, without causing problems for the anaesthetist!

α-adrenergic receptors have also been found on the nerve terminals. They may be involved in the improved muscle performance seen when adrenaline is flowing!

Characteristics of Muscle

A skeletal muscle fibre is a very long cell, and may run the whole length of the muscle. There are many myofibrils in each cell, with neuromuscular junctions extending throughout the length of the muscle. The external ocular muscles are different, having multineuronal innervation of fibres and a tonic response to suxamethonium.

The features of a drug which determine its performance as a muscle relaxant include:

1. Its electrostatic characteristics (particularly the position and number of its quaternary nitrogen groups). An interonium distance of 11 Å, as in pancuronium, was thought to be an effective spatial arrangement, allowing the second nitrogen

to repel incoming ACh electrostatically. That a bond is formed between a non-depolarizing relaxant and a neuromuscular postjunctional cholinoceptor is shown by the fact that the effect of tubocurarine is not proportional to its plasma concentration, but continues after decline of this level. (However, depolarizing relaxants do show the 'washout phenomenon'.) The high level of ionization of relaxants means that they are confined to the extracellular space, and undergo no renal tubular reabsorption.

2. Its steric nature, i.e. the way it fits the neuromuscular receptors. Receptor occupancy varies between one relaxant and another, and the steeper the occupancy/concentration profile, the more rapid is a drug's onset and wear-off characteristic. Atracurium is faster than tubocurarine. For clinical relaxation, the human diaphragm requires 90% receptor occupancy, while the tibialis anterior needs only 20%. An average value is around 70%. Adductor pollicis may thus still be completely paralysed, even after the patient has resumed normal respiration. This is significant, since adductor pollicis is often used for monitoring.

3. The balance between its hydrophilic and hydrophobic characteristics.

4. Its optical isomerism (e.g. l-tubocurarine is ineffective).

Characteristics of Non-depolarizing Neuromuscular Blockers

1. Do not cause muscular fasciculation.

2. Mostly mono- or bis-quaternary salts with interonium distances of 7–14 Å, and high electrostatic characteristics, i.e. very hydrophilic.

3. Relatively slow onset (1–5 min). Dacuronium is faster.

4. Reversed by neostigmine and other anticholinesterases.

5. Effects reduced by adrenaline and acetylcholine. Also by suxamethonium (but not in myasthenics).

6. The relaxed muscle is still responsive to other (mechanical and electrical) stimuli.

7. In partial paralysis, neuromuscular monitoring shows: (i) 'fade', (ii) post-tetanic facilitation, followed by exhaustion, (iii) depression of muscle twitch.

8. Potentiated by volatile agents, and Mg^{++}.[243]

9. Slow dissociation constant at receptors.

10. Mild cooling antagonizes their effects.

11. Greater cooling below the critical temperature (about 33°C) potentiates them.

12. Repeated tetanic bursts cause their effect to wear off.

13. Acidosis increases duration and degree of non-depolarizing block.[53]

Characteristics of Depolarizing (Phase 1) Blocking Drugs

1. Cause muscular fasciculation (but not in myasthenic man and in some other species).

2. The depolarized muscle fibres are unresponsive to other stimuli. The Na^+ channels are blocked open.

3. Repolarization is interfered with. The resting membrane potential is held up until phase II block develops, when it returns to $-70\,mV$.

4. Not reversed by neostigmine and other anticholinesterases (rather the opposite in the case of suxamethonium).

5. In partial paralysis, the neuromuscular monitoring shows: (i) depression of muscle twitch, (ii) no 'fade', but a well sustained response, (iii) no post-tetanic facilitation (*see below*).

6. Potentiated by isoflurane, enflurane, acetylcholine, respiratory alkalosis, hypothermia and Mg^{++}.[243]

7. Antagonized by ether, halothane, acidosis, and non-depolarizing relaxants.

8. Fast dissociation constant at receptors. There is little or no bond between drug and receptor.

9. Repeated or continuous use leads to 'phase II block' (*see below*).

Neuromuscular Monitoring with or without the Electromyogram (EMG)[54]

The electric stimulus is a rectangular pulse of $0\cdot2\,ms$ of supramaximal intensity ($100–200\,V$, transcutaneous). The ulnar nerve at elbow or wrist is a convenient site, while avoiding the twin dangers of: (1) having the stimulating electrodes too close to the recording electrodes, and (2) directly stimulating the long flexors of the forearm. If an EMG is not available, a useful measure can be made by watching or feeling the fingers and thumb or by using an ECG, with electrodes on the thenar and hypothenar eminences and the back of the hand. For a tetanic burst, $50\,Hz$ is adequate. A negative response to stimulation may mean that (1) the neuromuscular junction is blocked, (2) the stimulator is not working! (3) the ulnar nerve is not in its usual position.

The neuromuscular transmission monitor compares well with the old force transducers.[55] Paraesthesia after neuromuscular twitch monitoring has been described postoperatively.[56]

Response to Electrical Stimulation
First use of nerve stimulator to assess neuromuscular transmission in man in 1949.[57] Electrical responses to nerve stimulation recorded on EMG in 1952.[58] Mechanical responses first recorded in the same year.[59]

In the absence of complete paralysis due to *non-depolarizing* block the single twitch and tetanic stimulation lead to a successive fade in the response. Following a tetanic stimulus, a single-twitch stimulus causes an increased response, i.e. post-tetanic facilitation (thought to be due to release of increased quanta of acetylcholine for a few seconds). Post-tetanic facilitation is followed by a period of post-tetanic exhaustion due to depletion of readily available acetylcholine.

In contrast, with *depolarizing agents* there is a well-sustained response to successive stimuli following both a single-twitch stimulus and fast tetanic stimuli. The response to a single-twitch stimulus after a series of tetanic stimuli is not increased, i.e. there is no post-tetanic facilitation.

'Train-of-Four' Stimulation[60]
Four stimuli are given in succession, the resulting contractions give as much information as a tetanic burst, and may be repeated more frequently. It is less painful than tetanic stimulation. The ratio of the amplitude of the fourth evoked

response to that of the first is used as a measure of neuromuscular transmission and compares well with clinical tests of recovery.[61] The fourth is eliminated at about 75% depression of the control, the third at 80% and the second at 90%. Absence of all four indicates complete block.

A T_4/T_1 ratio > 60% is equivalent to being able to raise the head from the bed and having normal respiratory function tests.[62]

A T_4/T_1 ratio > 75% is equal to being able to cough properly, open the eyes and protrude the tongue on command.

Post-tetanic count (PTC) is a new method of evaluating an intense non-depolarizing neuromuscular block. The number of single twitch responses to nerve stimuli at 1 Hz following a 5-sec tetanus at 50 Hz is an indication of recovery from a relaxant, when the 'train-of-four' stimulation shows nothing.[63] Commonly, 1–5 twitch responses occur.

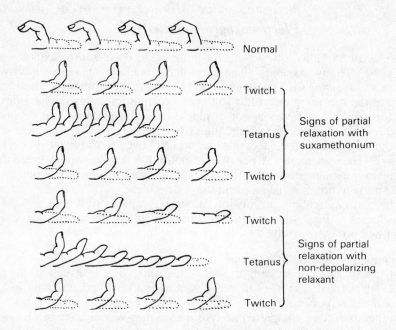

Fig. 14.1. Finger twitch response to ulnar nerve stimulation.

Electromyography has been made easy and practical for the anaesthetist.[64]

Dantrolene, an agent used for the treatment of malignant hyperpyrexia, is a muscle relaxant, acting on the sarcoplasmic reticulum, reducing calcium flux.

NON-DEPOLARIZING RELAXANTS

Pharmacokinetics[65]

Mainly on a two-compartment model. Clearance from the central compartment (plasma) = $V_1 \times K_{10}$.

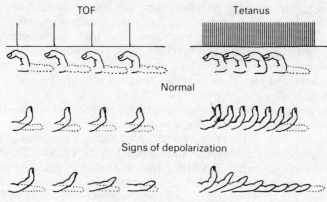

Fig. 14.2. Finger twitch response to 'train-of-four' and tetanic stimulation of ulnar nerve.

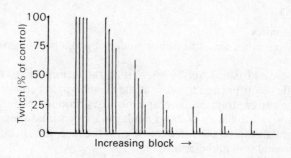

Fig. 14.3. Measured responses to 'train-of-four' stimuli during progressive non-depolarizing relaxation. At 80% block (reasonable abdominal relaxation), T_4 disappears. At 90% block (excellent abdominal relaxation) T_2 has disappeared.

Volumes of Distribution (l/kg)

Alcuronium	0·37	atracurium	0·16	gallamine	0·23
metocurine	0·45	pancuronium	0·28	tubocurarine	0·45
vecuronium	0·35	pipecuronium	1·2		

Clearance (ml/kg/min)

Alcuronium	1·3	atracurium	5·0	gallamine	1·2
metocurine	1·2	pancuronium	1·8	tubocurarine	3·0
vecuronium	5·0	pipecuronium	14·0		

Effective Blood Concentration (mg/l)

Alcuronium	0·8	atracurium	1·3	gallamine	10·0
metocurine	0·6	pancuronium	0·3	vecuronium	0·2
tubocurarine	1·0				

Poorly bound to plasma proteins, and excepting atracurium, eliminated unchanged by the kidneys, and to a smaller extent in the bile (except gallamine). Biliary excretion increases in renal failure. The drugs are concentrated in the kidneys, liver and cartilage. Early hepatic uptake lowers the plasma concentration of these drugs (except gallamine and atracurium). These pharmacokinetics are altered in liver disease, increasing the terminal elimination half-life ($T_{\frac{1}{2}\beta}$) by about 50%.[66]

Absorption and excretion. Absorbed when administered intravenously, intramuscularly, subcutaneously, intraperitoneally, sublingually and per rectum. In practice, nearly always given intravenously, occasionally intramuscularly. Most of them are metabolized in the liver, and excreted by the kidneys. Plasma proteins, especially gamma-globulins, have the power of binding competitive relaxants and this influences their fate in the body, and there seems to be a positive correlation between the relaxant requirements and the serum level of gamma-globulin, e.g. in cirrhosis of the liver and other hepatic disorders. Atracurium undergoes Hofmann elimination and hydrolysis in the plasma and elsewhere in the body. It has been recommended as the non-depolarizing agent of choice in patients with renal impairment.[70]

Pharmacodynamics

The drugs have neither anaesthetic nor analgesic properties when given in clinical doses.

Effect on motor end-plate. Act by preventing the adsorption of acetylcholine to the cholinergic receptors and so prevent the changes in the end-plate which cause muscular tone and contraction. Therapeutic doses produce the following effects in sequence: ptosis, imbalance of extra-ocular muscles with diplopia (which rarely may last several days), relaxation of muscles of the face, jaw, neck and limbs, and, finally, abdominal wall and diaphragm.

Effects on respiration. Paralysis of the muscles of respiration causing 'square-wave' respiration; the diaphragm, being less sensitive than other muscles, is usually the last one to be paralysed.

Effects on circulation. There may be hypotension[67] with tubocurarine, hypertension with pancuronium, tachycardia with gallamine and skin flushing with atracurium.

Synergy of relaxants. This is potentiation of one by another, when used together.[54,68] For example, ⅕ of the usual dose of tubocurarine or pancuronium will double the effect of atracurium.

Allergic effects.[54] Any of these drugs may cause histamine release at the first injection. Tubocurarine is the most likely to do so, and vecuronium probably the least likely. A second injection on the same day will not do so (owing to the great rapidity with which the histamine release develops tachyphylaxis). Development of true allergy with antibody formation, may of course occur in days or weeks following exposure to any drug.

Gastrointestinal system. The cardiac sphincter is probably not relaxed completely and still has an opening pressure of 25 cm of water.

Technique of Clinical Use

Following induction of anaesthesia the relaxant is injected intravenously. The patient's lungs are gently inflated with nitrous oxide, oxygen and volatile agent. Care must be taken not in inflate the stomach. After 1–3 min, when the effect of the muscle-relaxant drug is maximal, intubation of the trachea is carried out. IPPV is maintained, and additional doses of muscle relaxant are given as required.

Assisted or controlled respiration should be used as the tidal exchange is reduced or abolished.

During thiopentone–gas–oxygen–relaxant anaesthesia, the following signs often indicate the need for more relaxant: (1) Hiccup, due to contraction of the periphery of the diaphragm; (2) Rigidity of the abdominal wall; (3) Increased resistance to inflation of the lung (in the absence of respiratory obstruction), i.e. decreased compliance; (4) Bucking or coughing on the tracheal tube; (5) As indicated by neuromuscular monitoring; (6) Measurement of the ocular inter-limbic distance with a vernier caliper can be used to monitor incremental doses.[71]

Analgesic supplements may be required if: (1) The patient moves his skeletal muscles in response to the surgical stimulus, e.g. face, limb or neck muscles, especially swallowing or frowning; (2) Rise of blood pressure and pulse; (3) Sweating, unexplained by other causes, occurs; (4) There is reflex response to surgical stimuli, e.g. hiccups. Many anaesthetists routinely administer an intravenous or inhalation supplement to prevent possible awareness.

Reversal of relaxant by neostigmine (2·5–5 mg in adults) or edrophonium 1 mg/kg with atropine or glycopyrronium to prevent side-effects.

Whenever muscle relaxants are used, it is of paramount importance to see that the patient is breathing reasonably deeply before he leaves the operating table. In a recent investigation[72] it was found that a relatively large number of patients have a defect in neuromuscular transmission on their arrival in the postoperative room. Respiratory depression at the end of the operation should be treated either by IPPV until the tidal volume becomes normal or, more usually, by the injection of neostigmine with atropine. The use of a nerve stimulator to monitor the proper recovery of the neuromuscular junction can be employed.

Signs of Incomplete Reversal

(1) Shallow respiration. (2) Jerky respiration. (3) 'Tracheal tug', and 'see-saw' respiration, where, as the abdomen moves out, the chest moves in. (4) Cyanosis. (5) A restless, frightened, struggling patient, who says that he cannot breathe. (6) Diplopia. (7) Inability to raise head or extrude tongue.

Management of Incomplete Reversal ('The Incomplete Reversal Drill')

1. IPPV is given with a mask and oxygen, while the degree of incomplete reversal is assessed.

2. If mild (T_4/T_1 ratio > 50%, respiration is almost adequate) more neostigmine or other anticholinesterase is given.

3. If severe (T_4/T_1 ratio < 50%, respiration is obviously inadequate) the patient is sedated (e.g. with diazepam) intubated and IPPV continued with a ventilator for at least an hour, acid–base status is determined, and corrected. The serum electrolytes are estimated and normalized. Re-assessment is performed using a nerve stimulator and neuromuscular monitoring performed.

4. A diuresis is promoted to reduce the plasma concentration of the drug, e.g. using frusemide.

5. Alternative diagnoses are considered—overdose of inhalation agents, opioids, antibiotics; barbiturates, renal failure, botulism, myasthenia gravis,

myasthenic syndrome, adrenal failure, hypothermia, renal failure, overdose of relaxant.

Infants and children tolerate muscle relaxants well if the dosage is suitably adjusted to their general condition and body weight (*see* Chapter 28).

Choice of Non-depolarizing Relaxant

Every anaesthetist has his favourite relaxants, which work best for him. However, the following suggestion for preferred relaxants may help the tyro:

In renal failure—vecuronium or atracurium; in myasthenia gravis—if relaxants are essential, one-tenth of the normal dose of atracurium; in hepatic failure—atracurium; in arterial surgery, to maintain arterial pressure—pancuronium; to deliberately reduce blood pressure—tubocurarine; in obstetrics—any relaxant except gallamine; in short cases—atracurium; for 'crash induction' without using suxamethonium—alcuronium or vecuronium.

Emphasis must be placed on the danger of the patient returning to bed with a poor tidal exchange which will not only cause oxygen lack and carbon dioxide excess, but will also predispose to the formation of patches of collapse of the lungs. Inspiratory stridor, due to atony and indrawing of the vocal cords, has been described following the use of relaxants.

Occasionally some residual paresis of the muscles of accommodation persists for 24 hours after operation, making reading difficult.

The drugs must be used with special care if given to the same patient on two occasions within 24 hours, as a cumulative effect may occur.

Atracurium Besylate (Tracrium)[54]

First used in 1980.[73]

Pharmacy
Mol Wt 1243. pH of solution 3·5, stored at 4 °C in refrigerator.

Pharmacokinetics
1. Absorption—From i.m. and i.v. routes.
2. Distribution—Throughout ECF. No effective crossing of the placenta.[74]
3. Metabolism—Hofmann degradation and alkaline ester hydrolysis in the plasma and elsewhere in the body (producing a monoquarternary alcohol at first). (A. W. von Hofmann (1818–1892) German chemist who made his discovery in 1848.)[75] Elimination half-life for atracurium is 20 min. The resulting tertiary amine, laudanosine,[242] has slow renal elimination and crosses the blood–brain barrier. This increases the MAC of halothane by 30% in high concentrations (unlikely to be found in clinical situations). Mean half-life for the monoquarternary alcohol is 39 min, that for laudanosine is 234 min.

Pharmacodynamics
1. Bolus dose—average 0·5 mg/kg. Infusion—average 0·5 mg/kg/h. Potentiated by enflurane and isoflurane, less so by halothane.[76]

Infants are slightly more resistant than adults.[77] Dose for premature neonates is 0·3 mg/kg.

2. Speed of onset 1–2 min. This can be halved by the 'Priming technique', where 0·1 mg/kg is injected 3–5 min before the main dose (unpleasant for patient).

3. Duration 20–40 min, even in anephric patients,[78] the elderly and severely ill.[79] Duration doubled at 25 °C.[80]

4. Quality of reversal with neostigmine or edrophonium is extremely good.[81]

5. Side-effects (no vagolytic effects on the heart. This may allow bradycardia to occur). Angioneurotic oedema has occurred.[82] Histamine release[54] does not occur when the drug is injected slowly over 75 s,[83] or when less than 0·6 mg/kg is injected.

The clinical signs sometimes following atracurium (e.g. flushing of the skin, maculopapular, pruritic rash, suggestive of mediator release from mast cells in the presence of IgE) do not correlate with plasma histamine levels,[84] nor with complement C_3 conversion.[85] These effects are however abolished by pretreatment with i.v. cimetidine 4 mg/kg and chlorpheniramine 0·1 mg/kg or phenylhydramine 0·3 mg/kg.[86] Intraocular pressure—no change, or a fall.[87] Intracranial pressure—unaltered.

Suitable in anephric patients—the relaxant of choice.[88] Suitable in patients with atypical cholinesterase.[89] Suitable in short cases—a relaxant of choice.[90] Long cases—suitable with intermittent injection or continuous infusion.[91] Infusion rate 0·5 mg/kg/hr with cessation at 15 min before the estimated end of the operation (e.g. at closure of the peritoneum in an abdominal case). Simple neuromuscular monitoring is desirable but not essential. Caesarean section—suitable.[92] Cardiopulmonary bypass with hypothermia—suitable.[80] With tourniquets—suitable.[93] Organophosphorus poisoning—suitable.[94] Myasthenia gravis—suitable.[95]

Vecuronium Bromide (Norcuron)[54]

First used in 1979 in France.[40,41]

Chemical Basis
It has rings A and D. The D ring is similar to pancuronium. The A ring is modified by a tertiary nitrogen at 2B, giving less stability in solution, a shorter time-course and lack of cumulation *in vivo*.[96] The solution (pH 4) is stable for 24 hrs at 25 °C. Mol Wt 638.

Pharmacokinetics
Absorption—from i.m. or i.v. route; distribution—throughout the ECF. The lipophilic effect of the single quarternary nitrogen enhances rapid uptake into hepatocytes. No effective crossing of the placenta. Metabolism—theoretically in the liver with excretion in the urine.

Pharmacodynamics
Bolus dose average 0·1 mg/kg (adults, infants and elderly). Infusion 0·2 mg/kg/hr. Potentiated (but not much extended) most by enflurane, >isoflurane>halothane. Potentiated and prolonged by previous suxamethonium. Time of onset 1–2 min (can be shortened by preloading with a small dose, 6 min before the main dose).[97] Duration 10–20 min (much longer with higher doses), not influenced by renal failure. Side-effects—no effect on vascular system in clinical doses. (*See also Clinics in Anesthesiology*. 1985, **3**, 347.)

Tubocurarine Chloride BP (Tubarine)

Source from bark, leaves and vines of *Chondrodendron Tomentosum* growing near upper reaches of the Amazon. Has long been used by Amazonian Indians to poison the heads of their arrows. They transport it in bamboo tubes, hence the name tubocurarine. It is a monoquarternary alkaloid, an isoquinoline derivative.

Pharmacokinetics
Dose—0·5 mg/kg onset 3 min after i.v. injection; 10 min after i.m. injection. Duration about 40 min, prolonged by volatile anaesthetics, shortened by alkalosis. Cumulation occurs. Distribution—to extracellular fluid, muscles, liver, kidney, and cartilage. It is retained in spleen, heart and lungs in an inactive state. It is bound to serum albumin.

Pharmacodynamics
Non-depolarizing block with pre- and post-junctional components. Reversal by anticholinesterases is satisfactory, except in acidosis, hypokalaemia or overdose.

Side-effects
Respiration: Paralysis of muscles of respiration, occasionally bronchospasm, notably in asthmatic patients.
Histamine release: Circulatory collapse due to this has been reported, but is rare, while anaphylactoid response has occurred.
Circulation: Hypotension[67] due to ganglion blockade, potentiated by halothane and reversed by calcium. Decreased blood coagulation has been observed, possibly due to release of heparin from mast cells. Allergic circulatory collapse due to histamine release has been reported, but is rare, while anaphylactoid response has occurred.[69] There is an antifibrillatory action on the ventricles and a decreased likelihood of dysrhythmia. The drug is strongly concentrated in heart muscle. In enormous doses it may have a negative inotropic effect. When hypotension is thought to be due to tubocurarine, it may be reversed by intravenous calcium. Should be used carefully in patients with myocardial ischaemia or with hypokalaemia.
Gastrointestinal system: The cardiac sphincter is probably not relaxed and still has an opening pressure of 25 cmH$_2$O.

Other Features
Small amounts cross the placenta, not affecting the baby in clinical dose. Patients with liver disease may require more tubocurarine than usual. (The real reason for this is still obscure.)

Potency enhanced by inhalation agents, 1·5–2 times (enflurane > isoflurane > halothane), and by previous injection of suxamethonium.[98]

Gallamine Triethiodide BP (Flaxedil)

A synthetic curarizing agent producing non-depolarizing neuromuscular block. The least expensive non-depolarizing relaxant.

Pharmacodynamics and Pharmacokinetics

Shows an atropine-like vagal blocking effect on the post-ganglionic nerve endings of the heart which results in tachycardia, even with small doses, e.g. 20 mg. Additional reasons for the rapid heart action may be its blockage of the muscarinic effect of acetylcholine liberated from the post-ganglionic vagal nerve endings, and a direct stimulating effect on intracardiac β-receptors.[99] This outlasts the relaxant effect. It often causes a slight rise in blood pressure, and this with the tachycardia may result in more bleeding than in comparable anaesthesia utilizing tubocurarine.[100] Allergic reactions have been reported following its use.[101] It passes the placental barrier and perhaps should not be used in obstetrics routinely, although many workers have found it satisfactory in clinical obstetric practice. Between 15 and 40% of the drug is degraded, and the 3-hydroxy metabolite has about half the neuromuscular blocking activity of the parent drug. About 80% is excreted by the kidneys, and it should not be used in patients with renal disease, in case prolonged curarization results. Hypocapnia, following hyperventilation, potentiates its effects.

Clinical Uses

Given intravenously the first dose usually loses its effect in half an hour. To relax the abdominal wall or pass a tracheal tube in an average patient, a dose of from 60 mg to 160 mg is needed. Indications for its use include the presence of heart block and in short operations.

It is possibly better avoided: (1) When there is pre-existing tachycardia; (2) When there is renal impairment: there is a relationship between the duration of action of the drug and renal excretion. Prolonged apnoea due to the defective renal excretion of the drug may be treated by diuresis and if necessary by dialysis.[102] If there is inadequate renal excretion due either to pre-existing renal disease or the renal inadequacy consequent on the operation (e.g. left heart failure or shock), recurarization may result after reversal with neostigmine. This may require additional doses of the anticholinesterase drug during the first 24 h after operation; (3) In obstetrics.

Dosage

40 mg will usually paralyse muscles of limbs, without greatly affecting respiration; 80–100 mg will usually cause apnoea; 120–160 mg is required for smooth intubation. For children, 1·5 mg/kg.

Duration of Effect

About 20 min. Muscular paralysis prolonged by hyperventilation, volatile anaesthetic agents, but not by neurolept or opioid drugs.

Alcuronium Chloride, Diallyl Nortoxiferine
(Alloferin)

This is derived synthetically from toxiferin,[103] an alkaloid of calabash curare. It was used clinically in 1961.[35] It is a medium-acting non-depolarizing relaxant. Deteriorates on exposure to air and sunlight and so is sold in coloured ampoules. Is miscible in the same syringe with methohexitone but not with thiopentone. Little effect on pulse rate, but it may result in a small fall in blood pressure.[104]

Does not release histamine from the tissues. Said to be twice as potent as tubocurarine. Does not cross the placenta in significant amounts.[105]

There is a positive co-relationship between serum-albumin and alcuronium requirements. It is bound to serum albumin.

Suggested dosage: 0·16 mg/kg and double this for intubation (10–20 mg). In children, 0·125–0·2 mg/kg. Duration of activity, 20–40 min.

Its effects are reversed by anticholinesterases. pH changes have little effect on the action of alcuronium.[106]

A reliable, easily reversible relaxant of good repute, which should be avoided in renal failure.[107] Anaphylactoid reactions have been reported.[108]

Very rapidly produces extremely good intubating conditions.

After the distribution phase (20 min) it is metabolized very slowly.

Reversal can be difficult after large doses.

Pancuronium Bromide *(Pavulon)*

First described in 1967.[109]

Pharmacodynamics

A bis-quaternary amino-steroid, devoid of hormonal activity, first synthesized by Savage and Hewett in 1964 and used clinically in 1967.[36,37] Relatively inexpensive. Interonium distance 1·1 nm. Can release histamine[110] but is the least likely of the available relaxants to cause a major anaphylactic incident (Galletly D. C. and Treuren B. C. *Anaesthesia* 1985, **40**, 329). An insignificant proportion of it crosses the placental barrier. It causes noradrenaline release, and 30% is excreted by the kidney, 25% excreted in bile (one-third of this as hydroxylated drug). It should be avoided in renal failure.[111] Does not cross the blood–brain barrier. It becomes strongly bound to gamma-globulin and moderately bound to serum albumin, so less than 13% of a dose in the clinical range is unbound and active.[112] It is said to reduce the requirement for halothane,[113] while it lasts longer in patients under halothane.[114] A non-depolarizing relaxant with onset and duration similar to those of tubocurarine, and which is about five times as potent. It shows no evidence of cumulative effect and is well reversed by neostigmine and atropine. Its effect on the cardiovascular system is minimal,[115] although sometimes it stimulates the myocardium[116] and causes rise in pulse rate and blood pressure and blocks vagal muscarinic receptors.[117] It can release histamine from the tissues. Useful in obstetrics.[118] Partly metabolized by hepatic microsomal enzymes. In cirrhosis of the liver larger doses are required with the risk of prolonged apnoea postoperatively.[119] In total biliary obstruction the drug should be used with care.[120] In hypokalaemia small doses are required and relatively large doses of neostigmine may be necessary.[121] May be safe in patients susceptible to malignant hyperpyrexia.[122] Duration: 20–30 min.

Dosage[123]

0·06–0·1 mg/kg. For doses in neonates *see* Chapter 28. Each ampoule contains 4 mg in 2 ml of saline and also acetate buffer and 1% benzyl alcohol.

Fazadinium Bromide *(Fazadon)*[124]

A non-depolarizing muscle relaxant first used in 1972 with short onset of action. It is claimed that conditions for rapid intubation are comparable with those using suxamethonium, though this is not borne out in practice.[125] Seldom used today.

Dimethyl Tubocurarine Iodide *(Metubine, Meto-curarine)*, Bromide *(Diamethine)* and Chloride *(Mecostrin)*

Prepared by King and Dutcher (1935). Pharmacological properties described by Collier in 1948.[126] This non-depolarizing relaxant is two to two and a half times more potent than tubocurarine. It lasts for 1·5–2 h, and is easy and predictable for reversal. Seventy per cent of the injected dose is bound to plasma proteins, and it is devoid of autonomic ganglionic-blocking action. It neither speeds nor slows the heart rate and does not cause hypotension. Excreted in the urine. Recent work suggests that this drug should be more widely used, especially in patients with myocardial ischaemia.[127] Dose: 0·15–0·3 mg/kg.

Other Relaxants

Duador
Dose 0·5 mg/kg, duration 25 min.

BW444U
Dose 0·2 mg/kg, duration 1 h antagonized by plasma cholinesterase.

Pipecuronium *(Arduan)*
Dose 0·05 mg/kg.[130] Chemistry—analogue of pancuronium with quarternary nitrogen at the 2 and 16 positions and longer interonium distance.
Pharmacy—4 mg powder/ampoule, solution stable 24 h at 4 °C.
Pharmacokinetics—two-compartment model. Concentrated in kidney, liver and spleen; 40% is excreted by the kidneys. Does not cross the placenta. Cumulation occurs. Potentiated by enflurane.
Pharmacodynamics— reversibly inhibits serum cholinesterase. Duration 1–2 h.
Side-effects—very little on circulation.

Antagonists to Non-depolarizing Relaxants

Anticholinesterase Drugs

Neostigmine

History
Neostigmine methylsulphate (Prostigmine) was synthesized by Aeschlimann and Reinert in 1931.[128] It is twice as powerful as physostigmine (isolated in 1864 from the calabar bean by Sir T. R. Fraser (1841–1920), Scottish pharmacologist who also showed that atropine counteracts its effects, *Trans. R. Soc. Edinburgh* 1866/67, **24**, 715, and discovered the drug strophanthin), the anticurare action of which was discovered by Jacob Pal (1863–1936) in 1900,[129] and used in animal experimentation in 1909.[131]

It prevents the normal hydrolysis of acetylcholine and so allows it to accumulate.

Pharmacokinetics
It is partly broken down by serum cholinesterase and partly excreted unchanged by the kidneys. Renal failure reduces the clearance of this drugs by up to four times.[132] Binds to the esteratic subsite of cholinesterase with its carbonate group.

Neostigmine is also a depolarizer and can cause on its own a depolarizing type of block.[133] This is due to the build-up of acetylcholine, following the inhibition of cholinesterase. Phase 2 block can eventually result. The amount needed to cause paralysis by persistent depolarization is much greater, normally, than that required to antagonize an effective dose of tubocurarine or its congeners.

Non-depolarizing block due to the following is not always reversed by neostigmine: (1) That due to aminoglycoside antibiotics; (2) That due to phase 2 block following suxamethonium.

When injected into a conscious patient it may cause muscular fasciculations. In addition, it is a direct stimulant of cholinergic effector cells. It has nicotinic effects and has a direct stimulant action on muscle. In small doses it stimulates and in larger doses it depresses autonomic ganglia. It also has muscarinic properties (from *Amantia muscaria*) which are blocked by atropine, e.g. bradycardia, intestinal peristalsis and spasm, bronchial and salivary secretion and bronchospasm, stimulation of the sweat glands, contraction of the pupil and contraction of the bladder. Dysrhythmias and asystole can be prevented by avoiding hypercapnia and hypoxia, by titrating the exact dose of neostigmine and atropine (2·5:1) with the aid of a nerve stimulator, and by the slow administration of the drug, after or with atropine. Dose is 2·5 mg carefully repeated up to a total of 5 mg,[134] with atropine 1·5 mg or glycopyrronium. Some workers of experience use 5 mg as the average dose. For injection the methylsulphate is used; for oral administration, the bromide. The blood concentration decreases rapidly within 2–5 min after intravenous injection, but some can be detected after 60 min.[135] Renal excretion accounts for 50% of its clearance.[137] Its effects last for up to 2 hours.

Edrophonium *(Tensilon)*
It has, like neostigmine, anticholinesterase, depolarizing and direct stimulating actions on the motor end-plate. It may cause fasciculation; quicker in onset, but not as long lasting as neostigmine, consequently hypoventilation and recurarization may follow an initial stimulant effect on the respiration (although this is not seen following repeated injection of 20 mg at 3-min intervals).[138] Dose is 10–70 mg, although more recent work suggests that it reverses myoneural block following pancuronium as efficiently as does neostigmine if given in adequate doses; neostigmine is 16 times more potent than edrophonium.[139] Edrophonium binds electrostatically to the anionic subsite of cholinesterase and also by hydrogen bonding. This type of bonding is easily reversible. It is rapidly metabolized, in small doses (10 mg) but not in large doses (70 mg)[140] when its pharmacokinetics are similar to pyridostigmine and neostigmine.[141]

Pharmacodynamics
Faster onset against vecuronium[142] and atracurium,[81] than neostigmine, and greater anti-fade activity, suggesting more prejunctional effects.[143]

Pyridostigmine[136] *(Mestinon; Regonol)*
This is the dimethyl carbonic ester of *n*-methyl pyridium bromide. It has one-quarter the potency of neostigmine but a longer duration of action and a slower onset. Cardiac dysrhythmias less common.[144] It has nicotinic action on end-plates and muscarinic side-effects, e.g. salivation, colic and diarrhoea though these are less than with neostigmine. Its duration of action makes it especially suitable for reversal of relaxants in cases of renal failure where the excretion of the relaxant may be delayed.[145] Dose: 10 mg, the equivalent of 2·5 mg of neostigmine. Reports suggest that it is equal to neostigmine and superior to edrophonium, causing less oropharyngeal secretion than the former, with less bradycardia.[146] It is capable of penetrating the blood–brain barrier and increases the plasma cortisol level above normal limits.

The above three drugs are used also in the diagnosis and treatment of myasthenia gravis.

Physostigmine Salicylate *(Antilirium)*[147]
An alkaloid obtained from the West African calabar bean. An anticholinesterase with a tertiary amine structure which can cross the blood–brain barrier. Used to treat the anticholinergic syndrome (*see* p. 139) produced by hyoscine and other related alkaloids. It does not adequately antagonize neuromuscular block in doses up to 4 mg. It shortens the time taken to recover from ketamine[148] and sodium hydroxybutyrate.[149] It antagonizes the sedative and respiratory depressant effects of morphine without affecting the analgesic activity.[150] Glycopyrronium antagonizes the peripheral side-effects of the drug.[151]

4-Aminopyridine[152]
This drug potentiates both neostigmine and pyridostigmine[153] and antagonizes block due to non-depolarizing muscle relaxants and also that due to antibiotics. There is no muscarinic effect and atropine is not required. It releases acetylcholine from nerve terminals and blocks potassium channels. It has little effect on either smooth muscle or on the autonomic nervous system. It reverses morphine-induced respiratory depression.[154] Unfortunately it is a central nervous system stimulant and causes postoperative restlessness and confusion, but it may have a use in conjunction with pyridostigmine or neostigmine as smaller doses of each agent are then required. Duration of activity longer than neostigmine. It is not an anticholinesterase. It may have a use where routine measures have failed, e.g. the Eaton–Lambert syndrome, myasthenia gravis, and following certain antibiotics.[155] Dose: 20–70 mg/kg.

Clinical Uses of Neostigmine
1. The muscarinic effects, especially bradycardia, must be prevented by atropine (1·5 mg for each 2·5 mg) or glycopyrronium (0·6 mg) which can be given before, or with,[156] the neostigmine—good reasons are advanced for each of these times. Simultaneous injection of the two drugs appears to be safe. To minimize salivation, atropine should be given before neostigmine.

2. The maximal dose should probably seldom exceed 5 mg as neostigmine can itself cause myoneural block of a depolarizing type.

3. Neostigmine prolongs the action of suxamethonium by antagonizing serum cholinesterase.

Before it is injected, the patient should not be acidotic, and have a normal Pa_{O_2}.

In the average case, towards the end of the operation, Pa_{CO_2} should be normalized. Atropine and neostigmine are given in small and if necessary repeated doses. If 3 mg of neostigmine does not reverse the block, the following factors should be considered: (1) Has enough time been allowed? Twitch height using a nerve stimulator may take up to 15 min to recovery, or up to 30 min when height is less than 20% of control; (2) Has too much relaxant been given? (3) What is the acid–base and electrolyte status? (4) What is the temperature? (5) Is the patient receiving other drugs which might make antagonism difficult? (6) Has excretion of the relaxant been impeded? Breathing can be stimulated by moving the tube within the trachea and by application of a suction catheter to the carina. CO_2, 5%, can also be given for a short period at this time. IPPV must be carried out until the patient can ventilate himself adequately. Low blood pressure and poor tissue perfusion may retard reversal.

It has been shown that neostigmine causes increased peristalsis and this may account for leaks from intestinal anastomoses, especially those involving the ileum. Atropine delays this increase in intraluminar pressure but it can be completely prevented by halothane.[157]

Signs of adequate decurarization after injection of neostigmine:[158] (1) Return of normal tidal exchange measured either by an anemometer or by the flow-meters of the anaesthetic machine using a Ruben or other non-rebreathing valve; (2) Effective coughing on tracheal tube; (3) Ability to open eyes and keep them open; (4) Presence of tone in the masseters; (5) Ability to raise the head from the pillow or to lift arm;[159] (6) Return of full muscular activity shown after electrical nerve stimulation.

Signs of incomplete decurarization: *see* p. 265.

Reversal in children: This is quicker and easier than in adults.[160]

Deaths have occurred following the use of neostigmine and atropine. Possible causes are: (1) Cardiac inhibition; (2) Adrenergic effects of atropine causing ventricular fibrillation; (3) The atropine itself causing dysrhythmia, especially in the presence of hypercapnia. There is evidence that harm from neostigmine is only likely if it is given while the patient has hypercapnia or hypoxia. Respiratory alkalosis seems to protect the heart. It is of fundamental importance that the anaesthetist should not leave the patient until he is able to ventilate himself adequately and his muscular power has returned. If this is not so, IPPV should be continued.

For paediatric dosage *see* Chapter 28.

DEPOLARIZING RELAXANTS

Decamethonium Iodide
This is *bis*-methylammonium decane di-halide and was originally known as C.10.

Chemistry
Soluble in water, neutral in solution, stable and resistant to heat. The solution mixes well with thiopentone and alkaloids and is non-irritant to tissues.

Pharmacodynamics
Muscular system. It causes neuromuscular block by prolonged depolarization of the postjunctional membrane of the motor end-plate in skeletal muscles and its action extends to the muscle fibres themselves on each side of the end-plate and makes them unexcitable. It acts like acetylcholine, which cannot be hydrolysed. Muscular twitching may be seen. It does not liberate histamine. The subsequent muscle pains differ from those caused by suxamethonium. It is not antagonized by the anticholinesterases. Repeated use of this relaxant may lead to the depolarization at the end-plate giving place to a non-depolarization, the so-called phase 2 block and this, if present, can be reversed by edrophonium or neostigmine. Side-effects minimal. Does not cross the placental barrier. Excreted via the kidneys.

Patients with myasthenia gravis are said to be less affected by the drug than are normal people and a single injection results in dual block which is antagonized by edrophonium and neostigmine.

Dosage
3 mg are roughly equipotent to 15 mg of tubocurarine. Maximum dosage, 10 mg. Duration of effect, 15 min approx.

Clinical Uses
The drug causes a depolarizing block which is active but does not last long. It gives place to a non-depolarizing block, which, although incomplete, is longer lasting: with increasing amounts the non-depolarizing block becomes more complete. For intubation it can be mixed in the same syringe with suxamethonium.

If the operation is nearing its end, suxamethonium 10–20 mg may be given and repeated. A useful relaxant for short operations.

It has been shown that, as in the case of suxamethonium, second and subsequent doses of decamethonium may cause cardiac slowing. A useful and safe muscle relaxant which has stood the test of time.

Suxamethonium Chloride, Succinylcholine *(Scoline, Anectine, Curaryl)*

History
Prepared in 1906 by Reid Hunt (1870–1948) and Taveau of Boston.[161] In 1949 Bovet and his colleagues[162] and J. C. Castillo and Edwin de Beer[163] described the paralysing action of the *bis*-choline esters of succinic acid, showing that they produced muscular paralysis of short duration and rapid onset. Used in anaesthesia in 1951.[164] Prolonged apnoea found to be associated with an abnormal cholinesterase value by James G. Bourne of London and his colleagues in 1952.[165] The hereditary nature of this abnormality was shown in 1953[166] (*see also* Dorkin, Huw R. *Med. Hist.* 1982, **26**, 145).

Chemistry
The dicholine ester of succinic acid. The active part of the molecule is the cation, formed by the succinic radical with a quaternary ammonium group at each end of the molecular chain. If these end-groups contain three methyl groups (CH_3), the substance is a suxamethonium compound; if two methyl and one ethyl

(C_2H_5), then it is an ethonium compound—hence suxamethonium and suxethonium. Solutions deteriorate in hot environments.

Dose

1 mg/kg (more in neonates < 10 wks old) Infusion 16 µg/kg/min. Onset in 10–30 sec. Duration of bolus 1–5 min. Average dose for intubation 25–100 mg.

Pharmacy

Hydrolysis occurs at room temperature. The drug should be stored at 4 °C.

Pharmacokinetics[167]

Absorption. i.m., i.v., or s.c.

Distribution. Throughout the ECF, and slightly across the placenta.

Metabolism. Hydrolysis to succinyl monocholine, then to choline and succinic acid by plasma cholinesterase. (EC 3.1.1.8.) Dibucaine number (DN) 75–85. This is the percentage inhibition of cholinesterase by 10^{-5} molar solution of dibucaine. The 'Fluoride number' is the percentage inhibition of cholinesterase by 5×10^{-5} molar sodium fluoride. Urea inhibition has also been used. Plasma cholinesterase is found in plasma but not in red cells; also in the liver, brain, kidneys and pancreas. It also hydrolyses ester-linked local analgesics. Plasma cholinesterase is a lipoprotein synthesized in the liver. Failure of its action due to abnormality or deficiency prolongs the action of suxamethonium. Of the population 94% are normal $E_1^U E_1^U$ genotypes with normal enzyme activity and a DN of 75–85. Three abnormal genes exist: E_1^A (atypical) homozygotes comprise 0·03% of the population; E_1^F (fluoride-resistant) homozygotes comprise 0·0003% of the population; E_1^S (silent) homozygotes comprise 0·001% of the population. Normal serum cholinesterase level about 80 units/ml.

Abnormalities of suxamethonium metabolism:[168]

1. Abnormal plasma cholinesterase (inherited)[169]

> 1.1 Atypical cholinesterase—Mendelian recessive $E_1^A E_1^A$ Homozygotes (1/3000 of population) have 1–2 hr apnoea, during which phase II block develops (DN 16–25). Heterozygotes (1/25 of population) have little or no disturbance (DN 50–65), with apnoeas up to 10 min.
>
> 1.2 Fluoride-resistant cholinesterase. Homozygotes have 1 hr apnoea, during which phase II block develops (DN 16–25). Heterozygotes have 10 min apnoea (DN 50–65).

All the possible combinations of heterozygotes exist (1 in 25 of the population, with apnoeas around 10 min).[170]

2. Plasma cholinesterase deficiency.

> 2.1 *Acquired*—after X-ray therapy, after organophosphorus poisoning, in hyperpyrexia, in cardiac failure, in hepatic failure, uraemia, hypoproteinaemia due to malnutrition or plasmapheresis, e.g. in lupus erythematosus, myasthenia gravis, Goodpasture's syndrome, and Rh incompatibility,[171] in trophoblastic disease,[172] pregnancy, puerperium, myxoedema, obesity and following treatment with: cyclophosphamide, ecothiopate, procainamide, quinidine, phenothiazines, ketamine, trimetaphan, pancuronium, propanidid, and metrifonate (antibilharzial drug).[169]

2.2 *Congenital*—presents unexpected danger to the patient. Hydrolysis proceeds only at the rate of 5% per hour. Inherited absence due to the silent gene E_1^S.[173] Homozygotes have 1–2 h apnoea, and phase II block develops in the course of this. Heterozygotes have normal DN and FN[149] but only half the normal plasma cholinesterase activity.[169]

3. Plasma cholinesterase antagonism by anticholinesterases and tacrine.

4. Plasma cholinesterase excess. The result is shortening of the duration of activity of the drug.

4.1 *Acquired*—in obesity, toxic goitre, nephrosis, depression, psoriasis, and alcoholism.

4.2 *Congenital*—the C_5 variant.

Pharmacodynamics
Muscular system
Phase I block preceded by muscle fasciculation (*see above*), potentiated by isoflurane, anticholinesterases, magnesium and lithium.

Phase II block accompanies the prolonged action of suxamethonium, whether due to infusion or to abnormal cholinesterase activity. This development is slightly potentiated by enflurane and rather less so by halothane.[174] The development has 4 phases:[175]

Phase A—depolarizing block which may last 30–50 min.

Phase B—non-depolarizing block develops quite quickly.

Phase C—A plateau 30-min period of no change.

Phase D—A 'wearing-off phase' up to 2 hr long.

In infants, phase II block may not be associated with prolonged paralysis.[176]

Reversal—phase II block has been reversed by neostigmine and other anticholinesterases, but the results are not consistent, thus this approach is not in routine use. A test dose of edrophonium can be used as a pointer to the likely response.[177]

Side-effects
Prolonged apnoea. This was first reported in 1952.[178] After a single dose of suxamethonium the commonest causes are:

1. Atypical serum cholinesterase. Homozygotes for the atypical gene show this. A heparinized sample of blood and a full clinical history will be required. Over 25% of patients with suxamethonium apnoea have normal enzymes.[179,181]

2. Dehydration and electrolyte imbalance leading to the development of dual block at a very early stage.

3. An over-dose of the relaxant drug, i.e. more than 1 g in an infusion. In order to prevent over-dosage of suxamethonium, there are those who advise that apnoea should never be allowed to occur and assisted rather than controlled ventilation should be employed. Tachyphylaxis may occur and result in over-dosage.[180]

4. A low serum cholinesterase level in the blood. This seldom causes prolonged apnoea if 50 mg is not exceeded, a dose adequate for most patients requiring a single injection, e.g. for intubation or ECT. It is unlikely to be the cause of apnoea prolonged beyond 20–30 min, if the serum cholinesterase level is more than 25 units. Apnoea due to a low cholinesterase value may be reversed by a blood transfusion as even stored blood contains 30 units of cholinesterase to each

millilitre and retains 80% of its cholinesterase activity after storage for 25 days at 6 °C. 0·5 litre of fresh blood restores the serum cholinesterase level by 10 units/ml; 0·5 litre of stored blood restores it by 5 units/ml. Reconstituted plasma is also useful as it contains 36–40 units/ml. Over 25% of patients with apnoea following suxamethonium are said to have normal enzymes.[181] Cholinesterase activity should be measured in patients who have undergone plasmapheresis and in whom the use of suxamethonium is contemplated.[182]

5. An excessive formation of succinyl monocholine. In 1952 it was pointed out that the hydrolysis of succinylcholine takes place in two stages, succinyl monocholine being the intermediate product.[183] This has between 5% and 20% the relaxing effect of the parent compound,[184] but as it is hydrolysed rather slowly by both acetyl and serum cholinesterase, it may accumulate in the bloodstream, but only if relatively large amounts of suxamethonium (more than 0·5 g) have been used, e.g. as drip infusion.

6. Phase II block (dual block), a phenomenon described by Zaimis[185] in 1953.

Other causes of prolonged apnoea
1. Central depression of the respiratory centre by a narcotic analgesic, thiopentone, or volatile anaesthetics.

2. Hypocapnia: in this case respiration will recommence if the blood carbon dioxide level is allowed to rise.

3. Hypercapnia: deficient carbon dioxide elimination from the anaesthetic circuit can poison the respiratory centre and cause apnoea. Theoretically this could lead to ventricular fibrillation;[186] unlikely in practice.

4. Depression of the Hering–Breuer mechanisms during controlled respiration. This will usually yield to more gentle inflation together with the addition of a little carbon dioxide for short periods.

5. Reflex laryngeal apnoea. Due to the presence of a tracheal tube. Removal of the tube or deflation of the cuff leads to restoration of spontaneous respiration.

6. Head injury and acute rise of intracranial pressure.

7. Moribundity. There are some gravely ill patients who breathe again only with difficulty once they become apnoeic. In such patients it may be wise not to abolish voluntary respiration at all.

8. Metabolic acidosis can cause a clinical picture similar to that of myoneural block. The cause of prolonged apnoea is not always fully understood.[187]

Diagnosis of the cause of prolonged apnoea
1. Electrical stimulation of a peripheral nerve to differentiate central depression from neuromuscular block (*see above*).

2. Examination of an arterial blood specimen to assess Pco_2 and cholinesterase level.

3. Edrophonium, to exclude dual block once shallow respiration has commenced.

Differential diagnosis between hypopnoea due to central depression and that due to peripheral paralysis
1. *Central Depression.* Breathing slow, reasonably deep. No tracheal tug; no pause at end of inspiration.

2. *Peripheral Paralysis* (myoneural block). Breathing jerky, shallow and of

normal rate. Pause after inspiration and again after expiration (Morton's rectangular breathing).[188] Tracheal tug.

Electrical stimulation of a peripheral nerve, always supposing that myoneural block is not complete, should settle any doubt.

Management of unexpectedly prolonged apnoea after suxamethonium

1. IPPV and sedation are maintained until monitoring shows the block to have worn off.

2. A blood sample is taken for cholinesterase analysis.

3. Plasma or cholase is administered to correct the deficiency. Dried plasma contains one-third of the cholinesterase activity of blood.[189] It should be infused slowly because of its high K^+ content.

4. Near relatives are screened and issued with warning cards or bangles.

Management of known or suspected suxamethonium-sensitive patients

1. Suxamethonium is avoided if possible.

2. If suxamethonium is indicated for the anaesthetic sequence, (e.g. for ECT) it may be given to documented heterozygotes only, in very small test doses, e.g. 0·05–0·1 mg/kg, when it produces a normal response.[190] A normal dose of 1 mg/kg, when given to a heterozygote, produces apnoea for 10 min, and very rarely up to an hour.

3. In homozygotes, a rapid-onset, short-acting non-depolarizing drug may be used (e.g. atracurium).

Hyperkalaemia. Potassium is released from muscles following suxamethonium injection, causing a rise of serum potassium of 0·2–0·4 mmol/l. Much greater hyperkalaemia occurs after burns (3 wks–3 months), tetanus and spinal cord injuries. Also in patients with upper and lower motor neurone lesions congenital cerebral palsy, Duchenne's muscular dystrophy, wasting secondary to chronic arterial insufficiency, and severe intra-abdominal infection. This great release is the result of extrajunctional receptor stimulation (*see above*).

Raised intraocular pressure (this may be important in the presence of a perforating eye injury). Suxamethonium, 1 mg/kg, raises the pressure an average of 7 mmHg, partly due to tonic contraction of the extraocular muscles, with return to normal pressure in 10 minutes, due to absorption of aqueous humour (the extraocular muscles may remain contracted for 30 min, upsetting the calculations used in squint correction). The lens is left nearer the corneal endothelium, with greater risk of damage during lens extraction and implants. Some workers view its use in severe glaucoma with reserve.

Muscle pains. ('The body all aching and racked with pain' syndrome). These were first observed in 1950.[191] The pain is influenced by age, sex and physical fitness. It is suggested that uncoordinated muscle contractions that precede paralysis are the cause of the pain[192] but this is probably not so.[193] Pains more frequent in women and middle-aged patients than in those at the extremes of age and in men. The incidence is reduced during pregnancy.[194] The longer the interval between the injection of an intravenous barbiturate and the suxamethonium, the more intense the postoperative discomfort. Pains may be delayed until the third or fourth postoperative day. Post-suxamethonium sore throat may be a muscle-produced pain and not due to trauma.[195]

Pain is less frequent in patients who are muscularly 'fit' than in the 'unfit' and when the injection is given slowly.

Prevention

1. Pre-curarization,[196] the i.v. injection of a small dose of a non-depolarizing

relaxant (e.g. tubocurarine, 3–5 mg[197] or gallamine, 5–20 mg) 3 min before the suxamethonium. Larger doses (tubocurarine, 10 mg or gallamine, 60 mg) given 1 min before the suxamethonium are said to be equally efficient and to cause no problems with either intubation or prolonged apnoea. Muscle fasciculations may also be reduced by i.v. injection of suxamethonium, 10 mg, and injection of the rest of the dose after a 1-min interval,[198] or when it is given in a drip at a rate of less than 2 mg per sec.[199]

2. Intravenous injection of lignocaine 2–6 mg/kg following thiopentone and 3 min before the relaxant.[200] This also prolongs apnoea. Intravenous lignocaine may cause significant sinus bradycardia or even asystole.[238] It restricts increase in serum potassium and decrease in serum calcium.[239]

3. Tacrine (*see below*) and hexafluorenium (*see below*).

4. Diazepam, 10 mg, before suxamethonium reduces the incidence of muscle pains.[201]

5. Dantrolene; there is evidence that a single oral dose of 100–150 mg, at least 2 hours preoperatively reduces the incidence of muscle pains.[202]

It is suggested that the muscle-spindle injury—as shown by the creatinine phosphokinase level[200]—is produced by suxamethonium given intermittently, especially if the patient is receiving halothane. This may result in myoglobinuria which may, among other things, give a positive Haemostix reaction in urine. Visible fasciculations are not constantly related to the severity of any subsequent symptoms.[200,203] Some recent work suggests that routine efforts to reduce these muscle pains after major abdominal surgery are unjustified.[204] (*See also* Ferguson A. et al. *Anaesthesia* 1981, **36**, 661).

These muscle pains may not be prevented by fazadinium or atracurium.[205] A rise in myoglobin can be detected in some patients who receive suxamethonium; this can be prevented by the prior injection of a non-depolarizing relaxant.[206]

Effect in malignant hyperpyrexia. It is one of the drugs most commonly implicated in this condition. Incidence 1:100 000 adult anaesthetics. It then causes muscle rigidity, not relaxation. *See* Chapter 18.

Cardiovascular system. Bradycardia and cardiac arrest may occur on the second, or even the first injection. Prevented by prior atropine or gallamine. Cardiac arrest due to hyperkalaemia may occur when suxamethonium is given to patients with existing hyperkalaemia, 3-wk old burns, crush injuries, widespread denervation, or tetanus. The treatment is standard CPR with lignocaine to prevent dysrhythmias, and measures to reduce serum potassium.

Suxamethonium may cause a rise in blood pressure, perhaps due to ganglion stimulation, a nicotinic response.

Central nervous system. Muscarinic effects may occur.

Alimentary system. Muscarinic effects, salivation and gastric secretion. Increase in intragastric pressure to more than 20 mmHg, due to severe muscle fasciculation. The cricopharyngeal sphincter loses its tone.

Placental barrier. Small amounts of this highly polarized drug do in fact reach the fetus, but are without effect on the baby. Excellent for operative obstetrics and Caesarean section.

Histamine release. True anaphylaxis without previous exposure, has been reported, with bronchospasm, hypotension, acute circulatory collapse,[207] pharyngeal and facial oedema, and a positive transfer (Prausnitz–Kustner) reaction.

Prevention of Side-effects (Except perhaps rise of intraocular pressure)
1. Self-taming by 10 mg suxamethonium injected a minute before induction of anaesthesia (unpleasant for the patient).
2. Precurarization 3 min before induction of anaesthesia; gallamine 20 mg, tubocurarine 3 mg, vecuronium 0·5 mg,[208] dimethyltubocurarine[209] or other non-depolarizing drug. *See also* under 'muscle pains'.

The *continuous suxamethonium drip* is used as a controllable and rapid method of maintaining relaxation of different degrees during abdominal and other surgical procedures. Various strengths have been described, a popular one containing 10 ml (500 mg) of suxamethonium chloride in 500 ml of saline, giving a dilution of 0·1%.[210]

The amount used varies between 4 and 10 mg/min. When the peritoneum is sutured, the drip may be stopped. Average rate of drip, 30–60 drops a minute or 150–400 ml each hour.

Some workers prefer serial injections given at carefully judged intervals to the continuous drip. A colouring agent, e.g. methylene blue, may be added to the bottle to prevent confusion between this potentially lethal infusion and other infusions.

The Potentiation of Suxamethonium by the Use of Extenders

Duration of effect increased by a factor of 2 with neostigmine, by a factor of 3–4 with tacrine, and by a factor of 8–10 by hexafluorenium.
1. By *tacrine hydrochloride* BPC (Romotal, THA, tetrahydroaminacrine). Chemically this is 5-amino-1,2,3,4,-tetrahydroacridine, and it was introduced into clinical medicine in 1949.[211] Dose 10 mg. This will prolong the effect of the second and subsequent doses of the relaxant about three times.
2. By *hexafluorenium* (Mylaxen). This is a *bis-quaternary* ammonium compound which was synthesized by Cavallito in 1954[212] and was first used in clinical anaesthesia in the following year.[213] The dose suggested is 0·5 mg/kg.

Use of Different Relaxants in the Same Patient

The effects of non-depolarizing relaxants are additive and so are those of decamethonium and suxamethonium. In general, depolarizers should not be used after non-depolarizers. Only if the effects of the first drug have worn off should one of the other group be used.

Suxamethonium given to a patient recovering from non-depolarizing block causes a mixed block. Effects vary with the degree of recovery from the non-depolarizing block; early in recovery suxamethonium reverses non-depolarizing block without paralysis but, when given later, initial recovery from non-depolarizing block is followed by paralysis.[214]

Mephenesin (Myanesin)

For further information, *see* earlier editions of this Synopsis. A drug very little used today.

Some Factors Influencing Neuromuscular Block

In Disease

1. Myasthenia gravis (*see* Chapter 22). Patients are abnormally sensitive to non-depolarizers and resistant to depolarizers.

2. Myasthenic (Eaton–Lambert) syndrome (*see* Chapter 22).

3. Patients with hepatic failure may show resistance to curare, gallamine and pancuronium. This is not related to low cholinesterase or to increased protein binding. They may show abnormal sensitivity to suxamethonium. Obstructive jaundice, without liver damage, may, on the other hand, require smaller doses of non-depolarizers than normal. True cholinesterase is not formed in the liver nor does it hydrolyse suxamethonium.

4. Patients with renal failure when the filtration rate is reduced in hypotension, may excrete gallamine and decamethonium more slowly than normal. Saturation of depot sites by the relaxant may cause difficulty in reversal. Dehydrated patients require less drug, so fluids should be infused if apnoea persists. Frusemide may prevent circulatory overload.[215] Non-depolarizing relaxants are removed during haemodialysis, as also are the products of hydrolysis of suxamethonium.

5. Patients with electrolyte imbalance. Hypokalaemia and hyponatraemia produce increased sensitivity to non-depolarizing relaxants. Low calcium and high magnesium blood levels increase the effects of relaxants.[216]

The magnitude of the end-plate potential can be considered to bear a direct relationship to the ratio of intracellular to extracellular potassium concentration.

a. Relative fall in extracellular potassium. It is the ratio of intra- to extracellular potassium which is important, not the absolute value of either. Cell membrane is hyperpolarized with resistance to the action of acetylcholine. Non-depolarizers are potentiated, depolarizers antagonized. Response to neostigmine normal.

b. Relative rise in extracellular potassium. Resting membrane potential is lowered—less highly polarized. Increased sensitivity to depolarizers, resistance to non-depolarizers. Potassium liberation is absent after non-polarizing agents. It may be associated with malignant hyperpyrexia. In cases of peripheral nerve injury, a tourniquet may be able to isolate the denervated limb and so prevent the access of suxamethonium to denervated muscle cells and consequent hyperkalaemia.[217]

c. Fall in both intracellular and extracellular potassium. The commonest situation in clinical practice. Resting membrane potential relatively unaffected, and response to muscle relaxants normal. The danger lies in the lack of reserve, a relatively small shift of potassium into the cells may precipitate symptoms of hypokalaemia (e.g. metabolic and respiratory acidosis, administration of glucose). Cyclophosphamide, thiotepa, carbenoxolone, thiazide diuretics and corticosteroids may potentiate non-depolarizing agents, if they cause hypokalaemia.

(*See also* Vaughan R. S. and Lunn J. N. *Anaesthesia* 1973, **28**, 118.)

6. Patients with collagen diseases, for example, systemic lupus erythematosus, polymyositis, dermatomyositis,[240] etc., may show increased sensitivity to non-depolarizing relaxants, as in myasthenia.

7. Multiple neurofibromatosis (Von Recklinghausen's disease) may potentiate the effects of non-depolarizing block.[218]

8. Dose of relaxants required in relation to serum proteins. Tubocurarine becomes partly bound to plasma globulin. Tubocurarine requirements are directly correlated to plasma-globulin levels. Alcuronium requirements are correlated to plasma-albumin levels. Gallamine requirements are also related to plasma-albumin levels whereas plasma-protein levels do not appear to affect the activity of pancuronium.[219]

9. *Motor neuron disease.* There may be differences in response to electrical stimulation between muscles affected by this condition and normal muscles, making the peripheral nerve stimulator an unreliable guide to the state of relaxation.[220]

10. *Dystrophia myotonica.* Following the injection of suxamethonium, myotonic spasm without fasciculation may be seen. If this occurs its cause should be sought and it is unwise to give further suxamethonium or other triggering agents of malignant hyperpyrexia, as spasm may be a warning.[221]

11. *Hypothermia* potentiates the effects of depolarizing and diminishes the activity of non-depolarizing relaxants, especially in neonates and in old age as both hepatic and renal excretion are reduced.

12. *Repeated plasmapheresis* may lead to progressive depletion of serum cholinesterase.[222]

13. *Puerperal patients.* Smaller doses of suxamethonium than normal are required (e.g. during tubal ligation operations) due to reduced plasma cholinesterase activity.[223]

All non-depolarizing relaxants are fully ionized quarternary ammonium compounds and so will cross the placenta slowly; effect on the fetus is unlikely with reasonable dosage.

Effect of Drugs

1. *Aminoglycoside antibiotics.* Neomycin (first reported by Pridgen J. E. *Surgery* 1956, **40**, 571), streptomycin, kanamycin, gentamicin, tobramycin, bacitracin, colimycin, polymixin, clindamycin and colistimethate, if given parenterally or intraperitoneally, may cause a non-depolarizing block which will be potentiated by tubocurarine and gallamine, and by ether and cyclopropane even if given 24 h before. It is not always reversed by neostigmine. The membrane potential of the end-plate is dependent on the presence of calcium ions and this is reduced by the antibiotics. Intravenous calcium chloride (0·5–1 g) or gluconate may have both a prophylactic and a therapeutic use in these cases.[224] Neostigmine and perhaps 4-aminopyridine 0·5 mg/kg are also useful.[106] They do not interfere with the antibacterial effects of the antibiotics.[225] Tetracycline and penicillin show no neuromuscular blocking activity.

2. *Ganglionic blocking agents.* Hexamethonium, trimetaphan and phenactropinium all produce neuromuscular block.

3. *Oxytocin (Syntocinon).* Prolonged intravenous infusion of oxytocin modifies the action of suxamethonium. Fasciculations are minimal or absent and normal doses are ineffectual in causing apnoea. The occasional case of prolonged apnoea in labour following suxamethonium may be due to the low maternal level of cholinesterase in late pregnancy and the puerperium.

4. *Digitalis.* In the fully digitalized patient, although there is no alteration in the muscle relaxation produced by suxamethonium, this relaxant may result in ventricular dysrhythmias: these can be abolished by tubocurarine (as can the dysrhythmias of digitalis intoxication). Thus in fully digitalized patients, e.g. in

cardiac surgery, there is an argument against the use of suxamethonium. The transmembrane flux of potassium may be implicated in causation.

5. *Quinidine.*[226] The *d*-stereo isomer of quinine potentiates both depolarizing and non-depolarizing relaxants. Quinine acts similarly.[227]

6. *The anti-dysrhythmic agents.* Procainamide, lignocaine, β-blockers and diphenyl hydantoin increase the patient's sensitivity to tubocurarine.

7. *Diazepam (Valium).* This increases the duration of non-depolarizing block.

8. *Aprotinin (Trasylol).* Slightly reduces the serum cholinesterase activity of the blood, but unless its level is already very low from other causes, prolonged apnoea is very unlikely.

9. *Ecothiopate eye drops* which are an anticholinesterase and are used in the treatment of glaucoma. Apnoea from an intubating dose of suxamethonium may be prolonged. The effects of ecothiopate drops may last for 3 weeks.

10. *Metriphonate*, used in the treatment of urinary schistosomiasis, reduces serum cholinesterase.[228]

11. *Verapamil (Isotopin).* This may potentiate both types of relaxant. It causes blockade of the slow calcium ion influx into conductive and contractile myocardial cells which results in slowing of conduction, prolonged refractory period and depression of contractility.

12. *Lithium Salts.* Lithium was introduced for the control of mania in 1949.[229] Now used for the treatment of unipolar and bipolar manic-depressive states. A raised blood lithium level potentiates the effects of anaesthesia and relaxants and it is suggested that at least two doses should be omitted before anaesthesia.[230] Delayed onset and prolongation of suxamethonium block may result.[231] Potent diuretics may increase its toxicity.[232] Preoperative dehydration is to be avoided as this may cause lithium toxicity.[233] (*See also* Mogelinsky S. *Anesth. Analg. (Cleve.)* 1977, **56**, 562; Ominsky A. J. *Anesth. Analg. (Cleve).* 1977, **56**, 463; Freeman C. P. L. *Br. J. Hosp. Med.* 1979, **21**, 281; *Drug. Ther. Bull.* 1981, **19**, 21.)

Blood Flow
The greater the blood flow in a muscle, the sooner the onset and the quicker the recovery from myoneural block.

Body Temperature (Hypothermia)
With depolarizing agents, low temperature prolongs block. The intensity of pancuronium block is reduced by a low temperature down to a critical point around 30–34 °C when there is sudden potentiation of activity.[234] During hypothermia there is a delayed onset of activity of tubocurarine and larger doses than normal may be required; no change in the rate of recovery.[235] The action of atracurium may be prolonged, perhaps as a result of slowing of the Hofmann elimination process.[236]

Carbon Dioxide
Respiratory acidosis prolongs and alkalosis reduces the effects of myoneural block due to atracurium, vecuronium and tubocurarine in man. This may have some clinical importance. Respiratory acidosis decreases and alkalosis increases the myoneural blocking effect of gallamine and suxamethonium. Alcuronium block is not affected by changes in the Pa_{CO_2} in man. Pancuronium block is prolonged by hypercapnia and unaffected by hypocapnia.[237]

Changes in blood pH within the clinical range have little effect on the plasma distribution of tubocurarine.

Laboratory studies of acid–base changes do not always agree with clinical findings.

Children and Neonates (*See* Chapter 28)
Neonates are very sensitive to relaxants.

Exercise
Fatigue prolongs non-depolarizing block and makes suxamethonium pains worse.

Differential Effect on Various Muscle Groups
The higher the cholinesterase content of a muscle, the more sensitive is it to non-depolarizing relaxants. The external eye muscles, the diaphragm and the heart have cholinesterase in decreasing amounts.

The Placental Barrier
It is now known that most of the non-depolarizing relaxants can pass the placental barrier from mother to fetus in small doses. Normal clinical amounts of tubocurarine, pancuronium, atracurium, vecuronium and alcuronium are reasonably safe in this respect, gallamine is less so. Suxamethonium is now known to cross the barrier in doses larger than 50–100 mg.

Acidosis
Both respiratory and metabolic prolongs the action of tubocurarine and alkalosis has the opposite effect. With gallamine the effects are reversed. With pancuronium and alcuronium there is no alteration of effect.

References

1. Carman J. A. *Anaesthesia* 1968, **23**, 706.
2. Reprinted in 'Classical File', *Surv. Anesthesiol.* 1978, **22**, 98; McDowall G. *Anaesth. Intensive Care* 1982, **10**, 4; Symposium on Charles Waterton, *Br. J. Anaesth.* 1983, **55**, 221; Maltby J. R. in: *Anaesthesia; Essays on its History* (Rupreht J. van, Lieburg M. J. et al. ed.), Ch.2.4. Berlin: Springer-Verlag, 1985.
3. Bernard C. *C. R. Soc. Biol. Paris* 1851, **2**, 195; *Leçon sur les Effets des Substances Toxiques et Médicamenteuses.* Paris: Baillière, 1851.
4. Paton A. *Practitioner* 1979, **223**, 849.
5. Sayer L. A. *N.Y. J. Med.* 1858, **4**, 250.
6. Boehm R. *Arch. Pharm.* 1897, **235**, 660.
7. Läwen A. *Beitr, Klin. Chir.* 1912, **80**, 168.
8. Dale H. H. *J. Pharmacol. Exp. Ther.* 1914, **6**, 147.
9. Dale H. H. *Br. Med. J.* 1934, **1**, 835.
10. Cole L. *Lancet* 1934, **2**, 475.
11. King H. *J. Chem. Soc.* 1935, **57**, 1381; *Nature* 1935, **135**, 469.
12. West R. *Lancet* 1936, **1**, 12.
13. Bennett A. E. *JAMA* 1940, **114**, 322; Bennett A. E. et al. *JAMA* 1940, **114**, 1791; Bennett A. E. *Am. J. Psychiatry* 1941, **97**, 1014; Palmer H. *J. Ment. Sci.* 1946, **92**, 411.
14. Betcher A. M. *Anesth. Analg. (Cleve.)* 1977, **56**, 305.
15. Griffith H. R. and Johnson G. E. *Anesthesiology* 1942, **3**, 418 (reprinted in 'Classical File', *Surv. Anesthesiol.* 1957, **1**, 174).
16. Wintersteiner O. and Dutcher J. D. *Science* 1943, **97**, 467.
17. Cullen S. C. *Surgery* 1943, **14**, 261.

18. Waters R. *Anesthesiology* 1944, **5**, 618.
19. Harroun P. et al. *Anesthesiology* 1946, **7**, 24.
20. Mallinson F. B. *Lancet* 1945, **2**, 75.
21. Gray T. C. and Halton J. A. *Proc. R. Soc. Med.* 1946, **39**, 400 (reprinted in 'Classical File', *Surv. Anesthesiol.* 1974, **18**, 500); Gray T. C. *Br. J. Anaesth.* 1983, **55**, 227.
22. Bovet D. et al. *C. R. Séances Acad. Sci.* 1947, **225**, 74.
23. Huguenard P. and Boué A. *C. R. Acad. Sci.* **17**, 1948.
24. Mushin W. W. et al. *Lancet* 1949, **1**, 726.
25. Neff W. B. et al. *Calif. Med.* 1947, **66**, 67.
26. Barlow R. B. and Ing H. R. *Nature* 1948, **161**, 718; *Br. J. Pharmacol.* 1948, **3**, 298 (reprinted in 'Classical File', *Surv. Anesthesiol.* 1961, **5**, 213).
27. Paton W. D. M. and Zaimis E. J. *Nature* 1948, **162**, 810.
28. Organe G. S. W. et al. *Lancet* 1949, **1**, 21.
29. von Dardel O. and Thesleff S. *Nord. Med.* 1951, **46**, 1308; *Acta Chir. Scand.* 1952, **103**, 321 (translated in 'Classical File', *Surv. Anesthesiol.* 1967, **11**, 176).
30. Brücke H. et al. *Wien. Klin. Wochenschr.* 1951, **47**, 885; Mayerhofer O. *Br. Med. J.* 1952, **2**, 1332.
31. Scurr C. F. *Br. Med. J.* 1951, **2**, 831.
32. Beecher H. K. and Todd D. P. *Ann. Surg.* 1954, **140**, 2 (reprinted in 'Classical File', *Surv. Anesthesiol.* 1971, **15**, 394, 496).
33. Paton W. D. A. *Br. J. Anaesth.* 1956, **28**, 470.
34. Bernauer K. et al. *Helv. Chem. Acta* 1958, **41**, 2293.
35. Hugin W. and Kissling P. *Schweiz. Med. Wochenschr.* 1961, **91**, 445; Seegar R. et al. *Anaesthesist* 1962, **11**, 37; Lund L. and Stovner J. *Acta Anaesthesiol. Scand.* 1962, **6**, 85.
36. Baird W. L. M. and Reid A. M. *Br. J. Anaesth.* 1967, **37**, 775; Crul J. F. *Proc. 4th World Congr. Anaesth.* Amsterdam: Excerpta Medica, 1968, p. 418.
37. Burkett W. R. and Bonta K. L. *Fed. Proc.* 1966, **25**, 718.
38. Burkett W. R. et al *Br. J. Pharmacol.* 1968, **32**, 671.
39. Everett A. J. et al. *J. Chem. Soc. Sect. D., Chem. Commun.* 1020.
40. Durant N. N. et al. *J. Pharm. Pharmacol.* 1979, **31**, 831.
41. Crul J. F. and Booij L. H. D. J. *Br. J. Anaesth.* 1980, **52**, 495.
42. Hunt T. M. and Payne J. P. *Br. J. Anaesth.* 1980, **52**, 238P.
43. Hughes R. and Payne J. P. *Br. J. Anaesth.* 1981, **53**, 45.
44. Dale H. *Br. Med. J.* 1934, **1**, 835.
45. Dale H. et al. *J. Physiol.* 1936, **86**, 353.
46. Standaert F. G. *Clin. Anesthesiol.* 1985, **3**, 243.
47. Guy H. R. *Biophysical J.* 1984, **35**, 249.
48. Marshall I. G. and Henderson F. *Clin. Anesthesiol.* 1985, **3**, 261.
49. Singh Y. N. L. *Br. J. Anaesth.* 1982, **54**, 1295.
50. Stya M. and Axelrod D. *J. Neurosci.* 1984, **4**, 70.
51. Azar I. *Anesthesiology* 1984, **61**, 173.
52. Trautmann A. *Nature* 1982, **298**, 272.
53. Funk D. I. *Acta Anaesthesiol. Scand.* 1980, **24**, 119.
54. Jones R. M. *Anaesthesia* 1985, **40**, 964.
55. Windsor J. P. W. et al. *Anaesthesia* 1985, **40**, 146.
56. Sia R. L. and Straatman N. J. A. *Anaesthesia* 1985, **40**, 167.
57. Grob A. et al. *Bull. Johns Hopkins Hosp.* 1949, **84**, 279.
58. Churchill-Davidson H. C. and Richardson A. T. *Proc. R. Soc. Med.* 1952, **45**, 179.
59. Thesleff S. *Acta Physiol. Scand.* 1952, **25**, 348.
60. Roberts D. V. and Wilson A. *Br. J. Pharmacol.* 1968, **34**, 229; Ali H. H. et al. *Br. J. Anaesth.* 1970, **42**, 967; Lee C. M. *Anesth. Analg. Curr. Res.* 1975, **54**, 649; Zeh D. W. and Katz R. L. *Anesth. Analg. Curr. Res.* 1978, **57**, 13; Ali H. H. and Savarese J. J. *Anesthesiology* 1976, **45**, 216.
61. Miller R. D. *Anesthesiology* 1976, **44**, 318.
62. Ali H. H. et al. *Br. J. Anaesth.* 1971, **43**, 473; Ali H. H. et al. *Br. J. Anaesth.* 1975, **47**, 570.
63. Viby-Mogensen J. et al. *Anesthesiology* 1981, **55**, 458.
64. Lam H. S. et al. *Br. J. Anaesth.* 1981, **53**, 1351.
65. Norman J. *Clin. Anesthesiol.* 1985, **3**, 273.
66. Duvaldestin P. et al. *Clin. Anesthesiol.* 1985, **3**, 293.
67. Coleman A. J. et al. *Anaesthesia* 1972, **27**, 415.
68. Wong K. C. *Fed. Proc.* 1969, **28**, 420; Jones R. M. *Anaesthesia* 1985, **40**, 964.

69. Baldwin A. and Churcher M. D. *Anaesthesia* 1979, **34**, 339.
70. Miller R. D. *Can. Anaesth. Soc. J.* 1979, **26**, 83.
71. Hannington-Kiff J. G. *Anaesthesia* 1978, **33**, 931.
72. Beemer G. H. and Rozental P. *Anaesth. Intensive Care* 1986, **14**, 41.
73. Stenlake J. B. in: *Advances in Pharmacology and Therapeutics* (Stoclet J. P. ed.) Oxford: Pergamon, 1980; Hughes R. and Chapple D. J. *Br. J. Anaesth.* 1980, **52**, 238P; Kreig N. and Crul J. F. et al. *Br. J. Anaesth.* 1980, **52**, 783; Hughes R. and Chapple D. J. *Br. J. Anaesth.* 1981, **53**, 31; Payne J. P. and Hughes R. *Br. J. Anaesth.* 1981, **53**, 45.
74. Skarpa P. et al. *Br. J. Anaesth.* 1983, **55**, 275; Flynn P. J. et al. *Br. J. Anaesth.* 1984, **56**, 599.
75. Evans D. H. *Anesthesiology* 1985, **63**, 118.
76. Sokoll M. D. et al. *Anesthesiology* 1983, **58**, 450.
77. Brandom B. W. et al. *Anesthesiology* 1983, **58**, A440.
78. Hunter J. M. et al. *Br. J. Anaesth.* 1982, **54**, 1251.
79. Rowlands D. E. *Br. J. Anaesth.* 1983, **55**, 123 and 125.
80. Flynn P. J. et al. *Br. J. Anaesth.* 1984, **56**, 967.
81. Jones R. M. et al. *Br. J. Anaesth.* 1984, **56**, 453.
82. Srivastava S. *Br. J. Anaesth.* 1984, **56**, 932.
83. Scott R. P. F. et al. *Br. J. Anaesth.* 1985, **57**, 550.
84. Barnes P. K. et al. *Br. J. Anaesth.* 1984, **56**, 795P.
85. Madden A. P. et al. *Br. J. Anaesth.* 1985, **57**, 541.
86. Aldrete J. A. *Br. J. Anaesth.* 1985, **57**, 929.
87. Maharaj R. J. et al. *Br. J. Anaesth.* 1984, **56**, 459.
88. Hunter J. M. et al. *Br. J. Anaesth.* 1984, **56**, 941.
89. Baraka A. et al. *Br. J. Anaesth.* 1984, **56**, 930.
90. Pearce A. C. et al. *Br. J. Anaesth.* 1984, **56**, 973.
91. Eager B. M. et al. *Br. J. Anaesth.* 1984, **56**, 447.
92. Flynn P. J. *Br. J. Anaesth.* 1984, **56**, 599.
93. Suppan P. *Br. J. Anaesth.* 1984, **56**, 931.
94. Baraka A. et al. *Br. J. Anaesth.* 1984, **56**, 673.
95. MacDonald A. M. et al. *Br. J. Anaesth.* 1984, **56**, 651; Bell C. F. et al. *Anaesthesia* 1984, **39**, 961.
96. Buzello W. and Noldge G. *Br. J. Anaesth.* 1982, **54**, 1151.
97. Gergis S. D. et al. *Br. J. Anaesth.* 1983, **55**, 835.
98. d'Hollander A. A. et al. *Br. J. Anaesth.* 1983, **55**, 13.
99. Morganstern C. and Splinth G. *Anaesthetist* 1965, **14**, 298; Pratila M. G. and Pratilas V. *Anesthesiology* 1978, **49**, 338.
100. Casale F. E. and Farman J. V. *Br. J. Anaesth.* 1970, **42**, 65.
101. Walmsley D. A. *Lancet* 1959, **2**, 237; Evans P. J. D. and McKinnon I. *Anaesth. Intensive Care* 1977, **5**, 239; Fisher M. McD. *Anaesth. Intensive Care* 1978, **6**, 62.
102. Churchill-Davidson H. C. et al. *Anesthesiology* 1967, **28**, 540; Lowenstein E. et al. *Anesthesiology* 1970, **33**, 556.
103. Hugin W. and Kissling P. *Schweiz. Med. Wochenschr.* 1961, **91**, 455; Lund I. and Stovner J. *Acta Anaesthesiol. Scand.* 1962, **6**, 85.
104. Coleman A. J. et al. *Anaesthesia* 1972, **27**, 415.
105. Booth P. N. et al. *Anaesthesia* 1977, **32**, 320.
106. Thompson M. A. *Br. J. Hosp. Med.* 1980, **23**, 153.
107. Havill J. H. et al. *Anaesth. Intensive Care* 1978, **6**, 234.
108. Fisher M. M. et al. *Anaesth. Intensive Care* 1978, **6**, 125; Pusey J. M. et al. *Anaesthesia* 1987, **42**, 164.
109. Baird W. L. M. and Reid A. M. *Br. J. Anaesth.* 1967, **39**, 775 (reprinted in 'Classical File', *Surv. Anesthesiol.* 1981, **25**, 133).
110. Buckland R. W. and Avery A. F. *Br. J. Anaesth.* 1973, **45**, 518; Brauer S. et al. *Anesthesiology* 1978, **49**, 434.
111. Havill J. H. et al. *Anaesth. Intensive Care* 1978, **6**, 234.
112. Thompson J. N. *Anaesthesia* 1976, **31**, 219.
113. Forbes A. R. et al. *Anesth. Analg. (Cleve.)* 1979, **58**, 479.
114. Knight C. L. et al. *Anaesthesia* 1978, **33**, 139.
115. Lyons S. M. and Clarke R. S. J. *Br. J. Anaesth.* 1972, **44**, 575.
116. Coleman A. J. et al. *Anaesthesia* 1972, **27**, 415; Seed R. F. and Chamberlain J. H. *Br. J. Anaesth.* 1977, **49**, 401.
117. Pratila M. G. and Pratilas V. *Anesthesiology* 1978, **49**, 338; Smith G. et al. *Br. J. Anaesth.* 1970, **42**, 923.
118. Spiers I. and Sim A. W. *Br. J. Anaesth.* 1972, **44**, 370.

119. Duvaldestin P. et al. *Br. J. Anaesth.* 1978, **50**, 1131.
120. Somagyi A. A. et al. *Br. J. Anaesth.* 1977, **49**, 1103.
121. Miller R. D. and Rodenck L. L. *Br. J. Anaesth.* 1978, **50**, 541.
122. Cain P. A. and Ellis F. R. *Br. J. Anaesth.* 1977, **49**, 941.
123. Thompson M. A. *Br. J. Hosp. Med.* 1980, **23**, 153.
124. *See also* Simpson B. R. et al. *Lancet* 1972, **2**, 516; Brittain R. T. and Ryers M. B. *Br. J. Anaesth.* 1973, **45**, 837; Blogg C. E. et al. *Proc. R. Soc. Med.* 1973, **66**, 1023; Arora M. V. et al. *Anaesthesia* 1973, **28**, 188; Young H. S. A. et al. *Br. J. Anaesth.* 1974, **46**, 317; Blogg C. E. *Anaesthesia* 1975, **30**, 23; Young H. S. A. et al. *Anaesthesia* 1975, **30**, 30.
125. Hartley J. M. F. and Fidler K. *Anaesthesia* 1977, **32**, 14; Corrall M. and Ward M. E. *Br. J. Anaesth.* 1977, **49**, 615.
126. Collier H. O. J. et al. *Nature* 1948, **161**, 817; *Br. Med. J.* 1950, **1**, 1293.
127. Antonia R. P. et al. *Br. J. Anaesth.* 1979, **51**, 1007.
128. Aeschlimann J. A. and Reinart M. *J. Pharmacol.* 1931, **43**, 413.
129. Pal J. *Zbl. Physiol.* 1900, **14**, 255.
130. Agoston S. and Richardson F. J. *Clin. Anesthesiol.* 1985, **3**, 361.
131. Meltzer S. J. and Auer J. *J. Exp. Med.* 1909, **2**, 622.
132. Cronnelly R. *Clin. Anesthesiol.* 1985, **3**, 315.
133. Payne J. P. et al. *Br. J. Anaesth.* 1980, **52**, 69.
134. Viby-Mogensen J. et al. *Anesthesiology* 1979, **50**, 539.
135. Williams N. E. et al. *Br. J. Anaesth.* 1978, **50**, 1065.
136. Long G. et al. *Anaesth. Intensive Care* 1981, **9**, 144.
137. Cronnelly R. et al. *Anesthesiology* 1979, **51**, 222.
138. Bevan D. R. *Anaesthesia* 1979, **34**, 614.
139. Breen P. J. et al. *Anaesthesia* 1985, **40**, 844.
140. Morris R. B. et al. *Anesthesiology* 1981, **54**, 399; Cronnelly R. et al. *Anesthesiology* 1982, **57**, 261.
141. Cronelly R. et al. *Clin. Pharmacol. Ther.* 1980, **28**, 78.
142. Baird W. L. M. et al. *Br. J. Anaesth.* 1982, **54**, 375.
143. Jones R. M. et al. *Anesth. Analg. (Cleve.)* 1983, **62**, 1137.
144. Owens W. D. et al. *Anesth. Analg. (Cleve.)* 1978, **57**, 186.
145. Miller R. D. and Cullen D. J. *Br. J. Anaesth.* 1976, **48**, 253.
146. Zsigmond E. K. *Clin. Pharmacol. Ther.* 1972, **13**, 155.
147. Baraka A. *Br. J. Anaesth.* 1978, **50**, 1025.
148. Toros-Matos A. et al. *Anesth. Analg. (Cleve.)* 1980, **59**, 764.
149. Henderson R. S. and Holmes C. McK. *Anaesth. Intensive Care* 1976, **4**, 351.
150. Weinstock M. et al. *Br. J. Anaesth.* 1982, **54**, 429.
151. Weinstock M. et al. *Anesthesiology* 1983, **59**, 6.
152. Miller R. D. *Can. Anaesth. Soc. J.* 1979, **26**, 83; Burkett L. et al. *Anesth. Analg. (Cleve.)* 1979, **58**, 107.
153. Miller R. D. et al. *Anesthesiology* 1979, **50**, 416.
154. Zandastra D. F. *Br. J. Anaesth.* 1981, **53**, 865.
155. Agoston S. et al. Muscle Relaxants, Part 2. *Semin. Anesth.* Katz R. L. ed. Orlando, 1985.
156. Rosner V. et al. *Br. J. Anaesth.* 1971, **43**, 1066.
157. Bell C. M. A. and Lewis C. B. *Br. Med. J.* 1968, **3**, 587; Wilkins J. L. et al. *Br. Med. J.* 1970, **1**, 793.
158. *See also* Miller R. D. *Can. Anaesth. Soc. J.* 1979, **26**, 83.
159. Bar Z. G. *Anaesthesia* 1985, **40**, 630.
160. Fisher D. D. et al. *Anesthesiology* 1983, **59**, 220; 1984, **61**, 428; Meakin G. et al. *Anesthesiology* 1983, **59**, 316.
161. Hunt R. and Taveau R. de M. *Br. Med. J.* 1906, **2**, 1788.
162. Bovet D. et al. *R. C. 1st Sup. Sanit.* 1949, **12**, 107.
163. Castillo J. C. and de Beer E. J. *J. Pharmacol.* 1950, **99**, 458 (reprinted in 'Classical File', *Surv. Anesthesiol.* 1964, **8**, April).
164. Von Dardel O. and Thesleff S. *Nord. Med.* 1951, **46**, 1308.
165. Bourne J. G. et al. *Lancet* 1952, **1**, 1225.
166. Forbat A. et al. *Lancet* 1953, **1**, 1067.
167. Cook D. R. et al. *Clin. Pharmacol. Ther.* 1976, **20**, 493.
168. Motulsky A. G. in: *Pharmacogenetics* (Steinberg I. and Bearn D. ed.) New York: Grune & Stratton, 1964.
169. Viby-Mogensen J. *Cholinesterase and Succinylcholine.* Kobenhavn: Laegeforenningens Forlag, 1982.
170. Owen H. and Hunter A. R. *Br. J. Anaesth.* 1983, **55**, 349.
171. Evans R. T. et al. *Anaesthesia* 1980, **35**, 198.
172. Davies J. M. et al. *Anaesthesia* 1983, **38**, 1074.

173. Dean D. and Emmanuel E. R. *Anaesth. Intensive Care* 1983, **11**, 259.
174. Hilgenberg J. C. and Stoetling R. K. *Anesth. Analg. (Cleve.)* 1981, **60**, 192.
175. Viby-Mogensen J. *Anesthesiology* 1981, **55**, 429.
176. Sutherland G. A. et al. *Can Anaesth. Soc. J.* 1983, **30**, 342.
177. Donati F. and Bevan D. R. *Anesth. Analg. (Cleve.)*1985, **64**, 773.
178. Harper J. K. *Br. Med. J.* 1952, **1**, 861; Hewer C. L. *Br. Med. J.* 1952, **1**, 971; Love S. H. S. *Anaesthesia* 1952, **7**, 113.
179. Viby-Mogensen J. and Hanel H. K. *Acta Anaesthiol. Scand.* 1978, **22**, 371.
180. Lee C. et al. *Br. J. Anaesth.* 1978, **50**, 189.
181. Viby-Mogensen J. and Hanel H. K. *Acta Anaesthiol. Scand.* 1978, **22**, 371.
182. Wood G. J. and Hall J. M. *Br. J. Anaesth.* 1978, **50**, 945; Evans R. T. et al. *Anaesthesia* 1980, **35**, 198.
183. Whittaker J. P. and Wijesundera S. *Biochem. J.* 1952, **52**, 475.
184. Lehmann H. and Silk E. *Br. Med. J.* 1953, **1**, 767.
185. Zaimis E. *J. Physiol.* 1953, **122**, 238.
186. Brown E. B. and Miller F. A. *Am. J. Physiol.* 1952, **169**, 56.
187. Bauld H. W. et al. *Br. J. Anaesth.* 1974, **46**, 273.
188. Morton H. J. V. *Proc. R. Soc. Med.* 1945, **38**, 441.
189. Vickers M. D. *Br. J. Anaesth.* 1963, **35**, 528.
190. Cass N. M. et al. *Anaesth. Intensive Care* 1982, **10**, 25.
191. Bourne J. G. et al. *Lancet* 1952, **1**, 1225; von Dardel O. and Thesleff S. *Acta Chir. Scand.* 1952, **103**, 321; Churchill-Davidson H. C. *Br. Med. J.* 1954, **1**, 74.
192. Waters D. J. and Mapleson W. W. *Anaesthesia* 1971, **26**, 127.
193. Verma R. S. *Anaesthesia* 1982, **37**, 688.
194. Datta S. and Crocker J. S. *Br. J. Anaesth.* 1977, **49**, 625.
195. Capan L. M. et al. *Anesthesiology* 1983, **59**, 202.
196. Cullen D. J. et al. *Anesthesiology* 1971, **35**, 527; Freund F. G. and Rubin A. P. *Anesthesiology* 1972, **36**, 185.
197. Wig J. and Bali I. M. *Can. Anaesth. Soc. J.* 1979, **26**, 94.
198. Baraka A. *Anesthesiology* 1977, **46**, 292; Verma R. S. and Reader M. S. *Anesthesiology* 1983, **59**, 487.
199. Feingold A. and Velasquez J. L. *Br. J. Anaesth.* 1979, **51**, 241.
200. Wikinski R. et al. *Anesthesiology* 1965, **26**, 3.
201. Verma R. S. et al. *Anesth. Analg. (Cleve.)* 1978, **57**, 295; Eisenberg M. et al. *Anesth. Analg. (Cleve.)* 1979, **53**, 316.
202. Collier C. B. *Anaesthesia* 1979, **34**, 152.
203. Collier C. B. *Anaesth. Intensive Care* 1980, **8**, 26.
204. Brodsky J. B. and Ehrenwerth J. *Br. J. Anaesth.* 1980, **52**, 215.
205. Budd A. *Anaesthesia* 1985, **40**, 642.
206. Laurence A. S. *Anaesthesia* 1985, **40**, 854.
207. Youngman P. R. and Wilson J. D. *Lancet* 1983, **2**, 597.
208. Ferres C. J. et al. *Br. J. Anaesth.* 1983, **55**, 735.
209. Blitt C. D. et al. *Anesthesiology* 1981, **55**, 687.
210. Futter M. E. et al. *Br. J. Anaesth.* 1983, **55**, 947.
211. Shaw F. H. and Bentley G. A. *Med. J. Aust.* 1949, **2**, 868.
212. Cavallito C. J. et al. *Anesthesiology* 1956, **17**, 547.
213. Cordaro V. F. and Arrowood J. G. *Curr. Res. Anesth. Analg.* 1955, **34**, 112.
214. Rouse J. M. and Bevan D. R. *Anaesthesia* 1979, **34**, 608.
215. Riordan D. D. and Gilbertson A. A. *Br. J. Anaesth.* 1971, **43**, 506.
216. Krasner B. S. *Can. Anaesth. Soc. J.* 1979, **26**, 181.
217. Kay N. H. and Blogg C. B. *Anaesthesia* 1982, **37**, 1217.
218. Manser J. *Br. J. Anaesth.* 1970, **42**, 183; Magbagbeola J. A. O. *Br. J. Anaesth.* 1970, **42**, 760.
219. Stovner J. et al. *Br. J. Anaesth.* 1971, **43**, 953.
220. Graham D. H. *Anesthesiology* 1980, **52**, 74.
221. Ellis F. R. et al. *Br. J. Anaesth.* 1984, **56**, 381.
222. Paterson J. L. et al. *Br. Med. J.* 1979, **2**, 580.
223. Ganga C. C. et al. *Anaesthesia* 1982, **37**, 903.
224. *Adverse Drug Reactions Bull.* 1979, **2**, 580.
225. Booij L. H. D. J. *Br. J. Anaesth.* 1980, **52**, 1097.
226. Wenckebach K. F. *Der unregelmassige Heeztatigheit und seine klinische Bedeutung.* Leipzig: W. Englemann, 1914; Frey W. *Berl. Klin. Wochenschr.* 1918, **55**, 417; 450; Miller R. D. et al. *Anesthesiology* 1967, **28**, 1036.

227. Sher M. H. and Mathews P. A. *Anaesth. Intensive Care* 1983, **11**, 241.
228. James M. F. M. *Br. Med. J.* 1978, **1**, 442.
229. Cade J. F. J. *Med. J. Austral.* 1949, **2**, 349.
230. Havdala H. S. et al. *Anesthesiology* 1979, **50**, 534.
231. Hill G. E. et al. *Anesthesiology* 1977, **46**, 122.
232. Oh T. E. *Anaesth. Int. Care* 1977, **5**, 60.
233. Schou M. *Br. Med. J.* 1981, **283**, 1253.
234. Thornton R. J. et al. *Br. J. Anaesth.* 1976, **48**, 264; Park W. Y. and McNamara T. E. *Anesthesiology* 1979, **50**, 161.
235. Ham J. et al. *Anesthesiology* 1979, Suppl., 284.
236. Flynn P. J. et al. *Br. J. Anaesth.* 1983, **55**, 1355.
237. Norman J. et al. *Br. J. Anaesth.* 1970, **42**, 702; Dann W. L. *Br. J. Anaesth.* 1971, **43**, 959.
238. Demczuk R. J. *Anesthesiology* 1984, **60**, 69.
239. Chatterji S. et al. *Anaesthesia* 1983, **38**, 867.
240. Eielsea O. et al. *Can. Anaesth. Soc. J.* 1978, **25**, 65.
241. Holmes T. *Brody* London: T. Fischer Unwin 1898.
242. Chapple D. J. and Miller A. A. *Br. J. Anaesth.* 1987, **59**, 218.
243. Sinatra R. S. et al. *Anesth Analg. (Cleve.)* 1985, **64**, 1220.

Chapter 15　　ARTIFICIAL VENTILATION OF THE LUNGS

History
This was introduced by Arthur E. Guedel (1883–1956) and David Treweek of Los Angeles in 1934,[1] using ether. Starting off in Stage 3, Plane 2, they quickly increased the ether concentration and produced hyperventilation by bag pressure (assisted respiration) in a closed circuit with the soda-lime canister in operation. They thus caused a depression of the respiratory centre together with a lowering of the stimulant to respiration—carbon dioxide—and apnoea followed in about 4 min—the so-called 'ether apnoea'. Waters in 1936 first used the term 'controlled respiration'. It is now usually obtained by the use of muscle relaxants or narcotic analgesics.

Artificial ventilation of the lungs was used for the treatment of emphysema in 1951,[2] and in the intensive therapy unit dates from the poliomyelitis epidemic in Copenhagen in 1952.[3] (For history, *see also* Price J. L. *Med. Hist.* 1962, **6**, 67.) Rudolf Matas, (1860–1957), surgeon of New Orleans, used intralaryngeal intubation with a modified Joseph P. O'Dwyer's (1871–1897) tube in 1902.[4]

An early ventilator was described by Janeway in 1913.[5] The Stockholm surgeon, Clarence Crafoord[6] (1899–1984) reported on his spiropulsator in 1940, (the Frenkner spiropulsator was made with the help of P. Frenkner, an ENT surgeon and Andersson, an engineer in Stockholm; it was driven by compressed air), and in the following year Nosworthy's classic paper appeared.[7] The first British ventilator in commercial production was manufactured by Blease. (*See also* Woolam C. H. M. *Anaesthesia* 1976, **31**, 537, 666; Mushin W. W. et al. *Automatic Ventilation of the Lungs*, 3rd. ed. Oxford: Blackwell, 1980.)

Many accidents have occurred because of disconnection or failure of mechanical ventilators during anaesthesia. For many years IPPV was always carried out by manual compression of the reservoir bag and this technique should not be entirely discarded to-day.[8]

Apnoea can be produced during anaesthesia by:
1. Raising the threshold of the respiratory centre, as by barbiturates, narcotic analgesics, halothane, cyclopropane or a combination of these—a pharmacological method. The blood carbon dioxide no longer stimulates respiration.
2. Hyperventilation to reduce $Paco_2$ and physiological stimulus to respiration.
3. Use of a muscle relaxant to paralyse the respiratory muscles, while anaesthesia is maintained by a combination of nitrous oxide, oxygen, thiopentone, narcotic analgesics, etc.
4. A combination of the above methods.

Physiology
In positive-pressure breathing, inspiratory, intrapulmonary and intrapleural pressures are reversed from what they are during normal breathing—i.e. they become positive instead of negative. These effects are greater when the chest wall is intact than during thoracotomy.

Intrapulmonary pressure. During quiet spontaneous respiration, the difference is $2 \, cmH_2O$. During IPPV it averages 16–$20 \, cmH_2O$.

Intrapleural pressure. During spontaneous respiration, the pressure is $-5 \, cmH_2O$ at end of expiration, and during inspiration it is $-10 \, cmH_2O$. In IPPV pressure rises during inspiration from $-5 \, cmH_2O$ to $+3 \, cmH_2O$ and falls to $-5 \, cmH_2O$ during expiration.

Damage to lungs. Rupture is unlikely, as during coughing and straining pressure may rise to $100 \, cmH_2O$. It is difficult to increase pressure above $50 \, cmH_2O$ by bag pressure.

Compliance. Artificial ventilation produces about a 50% reduction in lung compliance.

Dead space. There is an increase in the ratio of physiological dead space to tidal volume (V_D/V_T ratio). This may reach values of 0.4–0.7 in ventilated anaesthetized subjects, compared to a value of less than 0.3 for spontaneous respiration. The ratio increases with: (1) Lung pathology; (2) Age; (3) Increasing respiratory frequency. Mechanical dead space may be deliberately added in certain intensive-care situations to produce normal $Paco_2$ during hyperventilation.

Respiratory alkalosis may be caused. This tends to increase the affinity of haemoglobin for oxygen, to cause cerebral vasoconstriction and to decrease cardiac output. Blood pressure is likely to fall, especially when the patient was previously in hypercapnia. Over-ventilation raises the pain threshold possibly by depressing the ascending reticular formation. Hypocapnia during anaesthesia may not be as benign as was once thought. This has been shown by an increase in postoperative reaction time. Hypocapnia, by causing vasoconstriction in normal brain tissue, directs blood flow into nearby pathological areas which have vasodilatation due to local tissue acidosis (inverse steal). Intracranial pressure is reduced. There may also be a reduced blood flow to the placenta.

Cardiovascular changes. First described by André F. Cournand.[9] (1) Abolition of thoracic pump. At the end of positive-pressure inspiration, right atrial pressure is raised and hence venous return and cardiac output are decreased. This is compensated for by a rise in the peripheral venous pressure which re-establishes venous return to its former level—due to venoconstriction; (2) Cardiac tamponade; not clinically important; (3) Interference with pulmonary blood flow. The pulmonary capillary pressure is 13 cmH$_2$O, so even slight increases in pressure in lungs may strain right heart. This may be seen even with an open chest. Retention of sodium and pulmonary oedema may be caused by long-term IPPV. Diuretics should be given when, in the absence of dehydration, sodium balance is positive for more than 3 days or when chest X-rays show signs of acute pulmonary oedema.[10]

Oxygen consumption is reduced because of the easing of the patient's muscular effort.

Technique
Tracheal intubation is extensively employed. A cuffed tube facilitates easy control of ventilation, but in the absence of an inflated cuff a pharyngeal pack, or bandaging of the lower jaw backwards to occlude the pharynx, may suffice.

Seldom should a pressure of 40 cmH$_2$O be exceeded—even though during a severe bout of coughing an intrabronchial pressure of 100 cmH$_2$O has been recorded. Rupture of the lung and its sequelae, pneumothorax, mediastinal emphysema, pulmonary interstitial emphysema and subcutaneous emphysema, are unlikely if due care is taken.

1. *Muscle relaxants.* The respiratory muscles are usually paralysed by the intravenous injection of a muscle relaxant drug in a dosage sufficient to allow IPPV to be undertaken.

2. *Intravenous agents.* Background respiratory depression with narcotic analgesic drugs facilitates IPPV. Occasionally large doses are employed to produce 'narcotic-induced apnoea'.

3. *Inhalation agents.* Those with a respiratory depressant action can be used in a similar manner, provided cardiovascular depression is avoided.

Controlled Positive Airway Pressure (CPAP)
This is a term generally used when positive pressure is applied during the expiratory phase when the patient is breathing spontaneously. It has been advocated in a variety of clinical conditions, including respiratory distress of the newborn, following cardiac surgery, etc. It is sometimes thought valuable to continue to maintain positive pressure during expiration while weaning from IPPV. In general the effects of CPAP are similar to those of PEEP.

Positive End-expiratory Pressure (PEEP)[11]
In clinical practice is has been found useful in situations where the arterial oxygen tension remains low despite high inspired oxygen concentration. It has been found useful during conditions such as fat embolism and respiratory distress of the newborn. It has proved possible to use PEEP without harmful effects on the cardiac output, though hypovolaemia should be corrected.

The importance of PEEP in intensive care situations is recognized, but there appears to be no place for it during anaesthesia for routine surgical operations. The FRC falls during anaesthesia whether respiration is spontaneous or artificial, but there is no correlation between Pa_{CO_2} and the application of PEEP.

The possible harmful effects of PEEP include:

1. Reduction of cardiac output secondary to decreased venous return to the heart.[12] Any advantage gained by increasing Pa_{O_2} may be offset if reduced cardiac output diminishes the overall oxygen delivery to the tissues.

2. It has been suggested that PEEP may cause an increase in interstitial and alveolar water in the lung, but possibly only with pressures above $16\,cmH_2O$[13] PEEP is therefore not necessarily of value in the management of patients with lung oedema.[14]

3. The increased airway pressure can result in pneumothorax and even air embolism and pneumoperitoneum.[15]

4. Renal function may be impaired.[16] Increased output of antidiuretic hormone may be stimulated with reduced urine output and water retention.

5. Rise in intracranial pressure in parallel with increase in mean intrathoracic pressure.

Indications for PEEP. These have yet to be rigidly defined. In general it may be considered to be of value:

1. In respiratory distress of the newborn.

2. A trial of PEEP may be considered whenever Pao_2 cannot be elevated to acceptable levels (say 7 kPa or 50 mmHg) with an Fio_2 of 50. PEEP may raise Pao_2 with less danger of oxygen toxicity to the lungs than if higher inspired oxygen concentrations are used. Monitoring of blood gases is essential.

Monitoring. It has been suggested that the following investigations should be performed routinely whenever PEEP is used.[17]

1. Pao_2, Fio_2 and Dao_2 at routine intervals so that PEEP will be applied only so long as it is having the desired effect.

2. Mixed venous oxygen tension and total oxygen consumption so that oxygen delivery and cardiac output can be measured.

3. Chest radiography and measurement of chest diameter to detect pneumothorax or progressive air trapping.

4. Hourly urine output and urinalysis to determine sodium excretion and glomerular filtration rate.

5. Scrupulous attention to fluid balance.

Contraindications to PEEP. These have not been established with certainty, but it is probably best avoided in the following groups of patients:

1. Those with hypovolaemia since falls in cardiac output may be severe.

2. Those with chronic bronchitis, emphysema and bronchospasm.

3. Possibly in patients with fluid retention or pulmonary oedema.

4. In the presence of fractured ribs because of the increased danger of pneumothorax.

Intermittent Mandatory Ventilation (IMV)[18]

This technique has been advocated during weaning from mechanical ventilation. The patient is allowed to breathe spontaneously, but the ventilation is augmented mechanically according to a pre-set minute volume. This can be achieved on servo-ventilators by decreasing the frequency progressively to every second or every fifth breath (f/2, f/5, etc.). It differs from the triggering devices used on earlier ventilators in that the patient cannot activate the mechanical ventilator at a high respiratory rate and the method can be used with volume-cycled as well as pressure-cycled apparatus.

It has been suggested that IMV might hasten the period of weaning from mechanical ventilation and might be of value in difficult cases. There is, however, no real evidence in the majority of patients that the technique is superior to the traditional method of allowing a patient to breath spontaneously for increasing periods under close supervision.

Mandatory Minute Volume (MMV)[19]

Mandatory minute volume is related in concept to IMV and is thought to be useful during the period of weaning from mechanical ventilation. The minute volume is pre-set, the patient breathes spontaneously as far as he is able, the remainder being delivered mechanically. (For review of methods of weaning patients from ventilators, see Barnett M. B. *Br. J. Clin. Equip.* 1980, **5**, 151.)

Hyperventilation and Hypocapnia

Hyperventilation may sometimes be necessary in the intensive care unit to obtain oxygenation, but undesirable hypocapnia may be produced. This can be overcome with the insertion of dead space, by use of the 'circle-without-absorber' system,[20] or by use of the Bain circuit.[21]

Use of IPPV in Anaesthesia

When muscle relaxants are used, controlled breathing is usually necessary in order to provide a proper interchange of gases. In thoracic surgery controlled respiration prevents paradoxical breathing, and mediastinal flap. In abdominal operations it allows good relaxation with control of the patient's oxygenation and carbon dioxide elimination. It allows surgery without deep anaesthesia and thus many anaesthetists use it during operations when muscle relaxation is not necessary. It may reduce the amount of thiopentone and relaxant required during the operation, thus contributing to the speedy recovery of consciousness and muscle tone.[22]

High-frequency Positive-pressure Ventilation (HFPPV)[23]

Three types of high-frequency low tidal volume ventilation have been used; high-frequency positive-pressure ventilation, (HFPPV) 1–2 c/s; high-frequency jet ventilation (HFJV), up to 7 c/s; and high-frequency oscillatory ventilation (HFOV), 5–40 c/s.[24]

The gas mixture is supplied intermittently through the fixed side-arm of a bronchoscope, or through a special pneumatic valve adaptor. Flow is interrupted by a solenoid valve at intervals between 55 and 800 times each minute, while high-pressure build-up is controlled by a variable orifice in the side of the tube. No air entrainment occurs so that the composition of the gases reaching the lungs can be accurately controlled. It is claimed that the high inspiratory flow of gas produces efficient pulmonary mixing of gas with minimal interference with cardiovascular function.

The technique can be applied using a narrow-bore insufflation tube down the centre of a tracheal tube, in the management of anaesthesia for resection of tracheal stenosis;[25] the tracheal tube is placed proximal to the stenosis and the insufflation tube advanced distal to it so that ventilation can be maintained while the ends of the trachea are freely mobilized. The method has also been used in the care of neonates with the respiratory distress syndrome.[26]

HFPPV has applications in the management of acute respiratory failure, though its role is controversial. It has been reported to cause improved oxygenation in infants,[27] and adults,[28] though controlled trials relating to survival are not available. Patients with large air leaks due to bronchopleural fistula may do well.[29]

See also Davey A. J. and Leigh J. M. *Anaesthesia* 1982, **37**, 670; Davey A. J. et al. *Anaesthesia* 1982, **37**, 675; Mortimer A. J. *J. R. Soc. Med.* 1983, **76**, 1073.

For the history of ventilation at high respiratory frequencies, *see* Smith R. B. *Anaesthesia* 1982, **37** 1011.

Ventilators

(For history of ventilators *see* Bendixen H. H. *Acta Anaesthesiol. Scand.* 1982, **26**, 279.)

Manually Operated Ventilators[30]

There are several simple contrivances which have been developed for ventilation of the lungs. They are portable and suitable for emergency or short-term use. Manual ventilators are useful during transfer of intensive care patients around the hospital. Desirable design features are reviewed by Gray A. J. G. *Br. J. Hosp. Med.* 1981, **25**, 173. (1) A reservoir bag with mask or tracheal tube, provided there is a source of oxygen or compressed air. (2) The Ambu Bag and the Laerdal Bag. The shape is automatically restored after compression and air is drawn in from the atmosphere. Oxygen enrichment of the air can be obtained if the bag is connected to an oxygen supply, but this is not significant unless a reservoir tube is also used.[31] (3) The Oxford Inflating Bellows.[32] (4) The Cardiff Inflating Bellows.[33] (5) The Cardiff Infant Inflating Bag.[34]

Automatic Ventilators

For a full description of many of these machines available *see* Mushin W. W. et al. *Automatic Ventilation of the Lungs*, 3rd ed. Oxford: Blackwell, 1980. Some general principles only will be noted here.

Desirable Features of an Ideal Ventilator

The ideal ventilator is compact, portable, robust, simple to operate and economical to purchase, use and maintain. Provision should be made for: (1) A maximum inspiratory flow-rate up to 80 litres/min. A tidal volume between 50 and 1500 ml at frequencies between 10 and 50/min. The I:E ratio should be variable; (2) Positive pressure during expiration, when desired. There should be continuous monitoring of airway pressure and expired minute volume; (3) Use with air, oxygen-enriched mixtures or anaesthetic gases and vapours; (4) Humidification of the inspired air; (5) Nebulization of drugs; (6) Easy to clean and sterilize. Additional systems include use of bacterial filters or disposable tubing; (7) Use with non-rebreathing or closed circuit; (8) Adaptation for paediatric use; (9) Monitoring of oxygen percentage in gases delivered to the patient, or use of a blender so that desired concentration can be set; (10) A warning system and provision for manual ventilation in an emergency. Abnormal pressure build-up, circuit disconnection or power failure should activate warning devices; (11) Gas loss in ventilator tubing due to expansion of the corrugated tube leading to the patient and to the compression of the gas in these tubes. The tubes behave in a similar manner to the respiratory airways and may produce an increase in total dead space. The volume of gas losses may amount to 140 ml/breath. To obviate these factors non-expanding tubes can be used or tidal volume measured at the catheter mount. A spirometer at the ventilator end of the expiratory limb may include gas losses in measured tidal volume. Gas loss is particularly important when volume preset ventilators are used. A dynamic method for measuring the internal compliance of ventilators has been described;[35] (12) Provision of the facility of intermittent mandatory ventilation or mandatory minute volume (*see above*).

Characteristics of Ventilators

Classification (Hunter)[36] into:

1. *Pressure preset*—build up to a preset pressure. Small leaks are automatically compensated for. Large leaks may cause the machine to stop if the preset pressure is not reached.

2. *Volume preset*—deliver a set volume of gas. Pressure will build up to overcome an obstruction. A safety blow-off is necessary, usually about $30 \, cmH_2O$.

Many machines can be used as either pressure or volume preset according to how the apparatus is employed.

Cycling. This refers to the mechanism which brings about the change from the inspiratory to the expiratory phase. (The change from expiration to inspiration is usually controlled by a timing mechanism.) Machines may be *pressure cycled, volume cycled,* or *time cycled.* In the strict sense, time cycled refers to machines with an auxiliary timing mechanism, but in the wider sense it applies to any machine in which the duration of inspiration and expiration is set by the operator.

Wave Form

1. Pressure generators. A rapid inflationary stroke to produce a square wave form. Prolongation of inspiratory phase much above 1 s does not increase filling of lungs.

2. Flow generators. Triangular wave form. Inflation pressure increases steadily throughout inspiratory phase.

Type of activation

1. Electrical—risk of explosion if flammable anaesthetic agents are in use.

2. Compressed gas. This is best supplied by pipeline though a compressor can be used.

Notes on Some Ventilators

(*See also* Review, Adams A. P. *Br. J. Clin. Equip.* 1976, **1**, 133.)

1. The Manley Ventilators.[37] A simple minute volume divider which is operated by the gas flow delivered to it. The tidal volume is set, and the machine delivers the minute volume supplied to it at an appropriate rate at a maximal inspiratory pressure of $35 \, cmH_2O$. Pressure can be varied. The authors warmly recommend it. Newer modifications include the Brompton Manley[38] and the Manley Pulmovent. The Manley Servovent is a high powered versatile apparatus, volume cycled flow generator and volume preset. The Manley Ventilator may increase the percentage of agents vaporized into the gas stream supplying it, because of back pressure. Thus a vaporizer set to deliver 1% may then deliver 1·5–2%.

2. Cape Ventilator.[39] A popular and robust apparatus which has stood the test of time. It is volume cycled. The Cape Bristol is supplied with an autoclavable patient circuit. The Cape Minor is a portable version which acts as a minute volume divider and which can be used with a 'draw-over' vaporizer.[40] It can be used with the Aga Polyvalve.

3. Bird. Developed in the USA. Automatic or patient triggered. Various models available. Incorporates a nebulizer for inhalation therapy. Can be adapted for use in anaesthesia by interposing a 'bag in bottle'. Use with the Bain circuit avoids the complexities of the various Bird modifications. Difficult to sterilize.

4. Engström Ventilator.[41] A versatile apparatus. Time cycled. Operates as an increasing-pressure generator with a volume limit during the inspiratory phase. Various models have been developed.

5. Blease Pulmoflator.[42] Various models available. Pressure preset and provided with negative phase and triggering device.

6. Oxford Penlon Ventilator.[43] Powered by compressed gas at pipe-line pressure. Flow generator, volume preset, volume cycled. The patient circuit is detachable for sterilization and can be replaced by a smaller unit and scale for paediatric use.

7. Nuffield Anaesthetic Ventilator.[44] Small and compact; convenient for use with Bain anaesthetic system. Powered by compressed gas.

8. Servo-ventilators.[45] The electronic circuits of these ventilators allow control of the various facets of IPPV by operation of simple controls. These include rate, inspiratory pressure, wave form, sighing, tiggering, control of oxygen concentration and provision for intermittent mandatory ventilation. The models in production provide autoclavable patient circuits and are generally powered by compressed air or other gas.

9. Dräger Ventilators. First Dräger ventilator constructed by Heinrich Dräger in 1907. The Narkosespiromat 656 can be used with closed or non-rebreathing systems for anaesthesia, and with oxygen enriched with air for ITU. It requires compressed air as driving gas, anaesthetic gases delivered by flow-meters and mains electricity. The Spiromat 760K and the Poliomat are designed for use in the ITU. Various models have been developed.

10. The Bourns Infant Ventilator. Time-cycled constant flow generator. Provision for F_{IO_2} between 21 and 100% PEEP and IMV. There is also a Bourns adult ventilator (Bear I) for long-term use.

11. The Loosco Amsterdam Infant Ventilator.[46] A non-return system with minimal dead space. The inspiratory time is set by an electronically regulated valve using a modified Ayre's T-piece. The minute volume is set by flow-meter, and the tidal volume delivered depends on the electronic time setting. Easily operated by hand in the event of electrical failure. Suitable for premature babies, neonates and babies up to age of 1–2 years.

12. Sheffield Infant Ventilator. This is designed for use with infants and children up to the age of 3 years. It is powered by mains electricity or battery and works on the principle of cyclical interruption of the outflow of a valveless T-piece system.

13. The MinEpac Emergency Ventilator.[47] Designed for the emergency treatment of patients with respiratory arrest. Portable and compact. Utilizes a non-return valve on the face-piece. Constant-flow generator. Time cycled. Can be adapted for use in anaesthesia. Cost moderate.

14. The Minivent.[48] Small and simple. Fits on any continuous-flow machine, and the elasticity of the distended reservoir bag provides the driving force of inspiration. A bobbin is held against a magnet except when the pressure of gases serves to force it away. The East–Freeman Automatic Vent,[48] the Microvent[49] and the Flowmaster[50] are similar.

15. Fluid logic ventilators.[51] There are no moving parts as the change of direction of gas flow depends upon pressure changes within the system. Can be made small enough for use within a hyperbaric cabinet.

16. The Carden Ventilator. Designed for use in the operating theatre; simple and flexible but its lack of sophistication requires careful and constant attention.[52]

17. A new valveless all-purpose ventilator of Chakrabarti and Whitman.[53]

For description of portable lung ventilators *see* Gray A. J. G. *Br. J. Hosp. Med.* 1981, **25**, 173.

This list is far from being comprehensive.

During anaesthesia care must be taken that air is not inadvertently admitted to the gas circuit lest patient awareness develops.

Cuirass Ventilators[54]
May still have a place for the patient with chronic respiratory failure managed outside the acute hospital.

(*See also* Payne J. P. and Bushman J. A. *Artificial Ventilation.* London: Academic Press, 1980.)

Humidification
See Chapter 38.

References

1. Guedel A. F. and Treweek D. M. *Curr. Res. Anesth. Analg.* 1934, **13**, 263 (reprinted in 'Classical File', *Surv. Anesthesiol.* 1970, **14**, 405).
2. Boutourline-Young H. J. and Whittenberger J. L. *J. Clin. Invest.* 1951, **30**, 838.
3. Lassen H. C. A. *Lancet* 1953, **1**, 37 (reprinted in 'Classical File', *Surv. Anesthesiol.* 1978, **22**, 398); Ibsen B. *Proc. R. Soc. Med.* 1954, **47**, 52.
4. Matas R. *Am. Med.* 1902, **3**, 97.
5. Janeway H. H. *Ann. Surg.* 1913, **58**, 927.
6. Andersson E. et al. *Acta Otolaryngol.* 1940, **28**, 95.
7. Nosworthy M. D. *Proc. R. Soc. Med.* 1941, **34**, 497.
8. Gilbertson A. A. *Anaesthesia* 1982, **37**, 987.
9. Cournand A. et al. *Am. J. Physiol.* 1948, **152**, 161.
10. Gett P. M. et al. *Br. J. Anaesth.* 1971, **43**, 460.
11. Cheney F. W. et al. *Anesthesiology* 1967, **28**, 670.
12. Cournand A. et al. *Am. J. Physiol.* 1948, **152**, 162; Morgan B. C. et al. *Anesthesiology* 1966, **27**, 584.
13. Noble W. H. et al. *J. Appl. Physiol.* 1975, **38**, 681.
14. Stoddart J. C. in: *Recent Advances in Anaesthesia and Analgesia—13* (Hewer C. L. and Atkinson R. S. ed.). Edinburgh: Churchill Livingstone, 1979.
15. Summers B. *Br. Med. J.* 1979, **1**, 1528.
16. Hale S. V. et al. *Anesthesiology* 1974, **41**, 452.
17. Stoddart J. C. in: *Recent Advances in Anaesthesia and Analgesia—13* (Hewer C. L. and Atkinson R. S. ed.). Edinburgh: Churchill Livingstone, 1979.
18. *See also* Downs J. B. et al. *Chest* 1973, **64**, 331; Downs J. B. et al. *Anesth. Analg (Cleve.)* 1974, **53**, 437; Desautels D. and Bartlett J. L. *Respiratory Care* 1974, **19**, 187; Lawler P. G. and Nunn J. F. *Anaesthesia* 1977, **32**, 138.
19. Hewlett A. M. et al. *Anaesthesia* 1977, **32**, 163.
20. Suwa K. and Yamamura H. *Anesthesiology* 1970, **33**, 440.
21. Henville J. D. and Adams A. P. *Anaesthesia* 1976, **31**, 247, 257; Adams A. P. *Br. J. Clin. Equip.* 1976, **1**, 133.
22. Gray T. C. and Jackson-Rees G. *Br. Med. J.* 1952, **2**, 891.
23. *See also* Gioia F. R. and Rogers M. C. in: *Recent Advances in Anaesthesia and Analgesia—15*

(Atkinson R. S. and Adams A. P. ed.) Edinburgh: Churchill Livingstone, 1985, Annotation, *Lancet*, 1986, **1**, 477.

24. McEvoy R. D. *Anaesth. Intensive Care* 1985, **13**, 178.
25. Eriksson I. et al. *Acta Anaesthesiol. Scand.* 1975, **19**, 113.
26. Heijmann K. and Sjostrand U. *Opuscular medica* 1974, **19**, 235.
27. Frantz I. D. et al. *Paediatrics* 1983, **71**, 483.
28. Schuster D. P. et al. *Chest* 1981, **80**, 682.
29. Turnbull A. D. et al. *Ann. Thorac. Surg.* 1980, **32**, 468.
30. *See also* Harber T. and Lucas B. G. B. *Ann. R. Coll. Surg. Eng.* 1980, **62**, 291.
31. Birt R. C. *Anaesthesia* 1965, **20**, 323.
32. Macintosh R. R. *Br. Med. J.* 1953, **2**, 201; Macintosh R. R. and Mushin W. W. *Br. Med. J.* 1955, **2**, 202.
33. Hillard E. K. and Mushin W. W. *Br. Med. J.* 1960, **2**, 729.
34. Mushin W. W. and Hillard E. K. *Br. Med. J.* 1967, **1**, 416.
35. Loh L. and Chakrabarti M. K. *Anaesthesia* 1971, **26**, 414.
36. Hunter A. R. *Anaesthesia* 1961, **16**, 231.
37. Manley R. W. *Anaesthesia* 1961, **16**, 317.
38. English I. C. W. and Manley R. E. W. *Anaesthesia* 1970, **25**, 541.
39. Waine T. E. and Fox D. E. R. *Br. J. Anaesth.* 1962, **34**, 410.
40. Collis J. M. *Anaesthesia* 1967, **22**, 598.
41. Engström C. G. *Br. Med. J.* 1954, **2**, 666.
42. Musgrove A. H. *Anaesthesia* 1952, **7**, 77.
43. Sugg B. R. and Prys-Roberts C. *Anaesthesia* 1976, **31**, 1234; Inkster J. S. in: *Recent Advances in Anaesthesia and Analgesia*—12 (Hewer C. L. and Atkinson R. S. ed.). Edinburgh and London: Churchill Livingstone, 1976.
44. Adams A. P. and Henville J. D. *Anaesthesia* 1977, **32**, 34.
45. Ingelstedt S. et al. *Acta Anaesthesiol. Scand.* 1972, Suppl. 47.
46. Keuskamp D. H. G. *Anaesthesia* 1963, **18**, 46; Mattila M. A. K. and Suatarinen T. *Acta Anaesthesiol. Scand.* 1971, **15**, 229; Urban B. J. and Weitzner S. W. *Anesthesiology* 1974, **40**, 423.
47. Burchell G. B. *Anaesthesia* 1967, **22**, 647.
48. Cohen A. D. *Anaesthesia* 1966, **21**, 563; Collis J. M. et al. *Anaesthesia* 1969, **24**, 81; Hawkins T. J. *Anaesthesia* 1969, **24**, 94.
49. Carden E. *Anaesthesia* 1969, **24**, 90.
50. Jones P. L. and Hillard E. K. *Anaesthesia* 1977, **32**, 619.
51. Campbell D. I. *Anaesth. Intensive Care* 1976, **4**, 7.
52. Fletcher I. R. et al. *Anaesthesia* 1983, **38**, 1089; Carden E. T. *Can. Anaesth. Soc. J.* 1974, **21**, 242.
53. Chakrabarti M. K. and Whitwam J. G. *Br. J. Anaesth.* 1983, **55**, 1005; Whitwam J. G. et al. *Br. J. Anaesth.* 1983, **55**, 1017.
54. Pinkerton H. H. *Br. J. Anaesth.* 1957, **29**, 421.

Chapter 16   # PRODUCTION OF ISCHAEMIA DURING OPERATIONS

Bleeding is due to cutting blood vessels!

Some patients bleed very little with a normal blood pressure and the relationship between BP and bleeding is not as clear as was once thought. It has even been suggested that a reduction of BP by 20–40 mmHg is sufficient to reduce bleeding (*see* Editorial, Donald J. R. *J. R. Soc. Med.* 1982, **75**, 149; Donald J. R. *Anaesthesia* 1983, **38**, 69).

History of Induced Ischaemia during Operations

In former times, chloroform was used in an effort (often very successful) to reduce bleeding. Now superseded by halothane.

Controlled arteriotomy followed by autotransfusion.[1] This is haemorrhagic hypotension (shock), and is associated with reduced oxygen availability and metabolic acidosis. It is no longer employed.

High intradural spinal analgesia by Griffiths and Gillies in 1948.[2]

High extradural spinal analgesia by Bromage in 1951.[3]

Ganglion-blocking agents. Demonstration of the ganglion-blocking effects of hexamethonium and also of pentamethonium, used to reverse the actions of decamethonium,[4] clinical hypotension shown to follow pentamethonium.[5] Hexamethonium preferred to pentamethonium by Hunter.[6] Pentolinium used by Enderby.[7] Trimetaphan used by Sarnoff[8] and by Magill and others.[9] Phenactropinium reported on by Robertson and others.[10]

Vasodilators. Sodium nitroprusside was used to control hypertensive crises in 1929[11] and in reducing bleeding during anaesthesia in 1962;[12] used in Britain in 1968.[13]

The influence of the head-up posture on the production of hypotension was early demonstrated by Enderby and was named 'postural ischaemia' by Sir Henry Dale after watching Enderby at work in 1949 (*Hypotensive Anaesthesia* (Enderby G. E. H. ed.) Edinburgh: Churchill Livingstone, 1985). The term 'physiological trespass' was coined by John Gillies of Edinburgh.[14] The plastic surgeon Sir Archibald McIndoe gave it his influential support in its early days. Halothane was advocated for hypotension in 1960.[15] Propranolol was used to control the tachycardia sometimes seen.[16]

The rubber bandage or tourniquet was introduced in 1869 by Esmarch.[17]

Increased Bleeding during Anaesthesia

Anaesthetic Causes

The production of unconsciousness results in the release of vasomotor tone at the periphery and while those vessels supplying the skin and muscles dilate, those going to the kidney and splanchnic area constrict.

Bleeding may be made worse by: (1) Respiratory obstruction; (2) Hypercapnia due to: (*a*) Inefficient carbon dioxide elimination; (*b*) Hypoventilation; (3) Coughing during induction and maintenance, especially in surgery involving the head and neck. This raises the intrathoracic pressure, venous pressure, and hence causes venous oozing; (4) Resistance in the anaesthetic system, including a tight expiratory valve causing a rise in intrathoracic pressure during expiration. (5) Unnecessary production of tachycardia by atropine and vagolytic drugs.

Non-anaesthetic Causes

(1) Venous congestion secondary to: (*a*) Posture; (*b*) Heart disease; (*c*) Lung disease; (*d*) Overtransfusion; (2) The hyperaemia of acute and chronic inflammation; (3) Conditions causing a rise in the basal metabolic rate; (4) Operations involving vascular tissues, e.g. muscle or gland; (5) A rise in blood pressure. This does not always increase bleeding; (6) Bleeding associated with systemic disease; deficiency of clotting factors, e.g. idiopathic cytopaenic

purpura, liver disease, disseminated intravascular coagulopathy, haemophilia. (*See also* Chapter 22); (7) Haemorrhagic tendency due to treatment: (*a*) Massive blood transfusion; (*b*) Citrate intoxication; (*c*) Incompatible blood transfusion: remedy—stop transfusion and give massive doses of steroids (*see also* Chapter 42); (*d*) Previous administration of anticoagulants; (*e*) Trauma to the blood in extracorporeal circulation; (8) There is no certain relationship between the degree of bleeding and the fall in blood pressure. Some patients bleed when the blood pressure is very low; (9) Bleeding due to drugs other than anticoagulants, e.g. aspirin.

A haematologist investigating a case with a history of bleeding may want to perform the following tests: (1) The examination of a stained blood film, with white cell and platelet count; (2) A one-stage prothrombin time estimation; (3) A thromboplastin generation test to help to exclude haemophilia and Christmas disease; (4) An estimation of bleeding time; (5) Whole-blood clotting time; (6) Fibrin degradation products.

(*See also* Gunning A. J. in: *Current Surgical Practice* (Hadfield J. and Hobsley M. ed.). London: Arnold, 1978, Vol. 1, Ch. 5).

Ischaemia during Operation
This may be produced by: (1) Total spinal analgesia (*see* Chapter 32); (2) High extradural block (*see* Chapter 32); (3) Ganglionic blocking agents and adrenergic blockers; (4) Drugs reducing tone of vessel walls; (5) Application of negative pressure to the lower limbs after moderate hypotension has been induced by a ganglionic blocking agent;[18] (6) Infiltration with adrenaline-saline 1–250 000 to 1–500 000; (7) Tourniquets during operations on limbs. Care must be taken that they are properly applied. Pneumatic tourniquets using a Bourdon-type pressure gauge are not always well maintained with the risk of unduly high pressures causing nerve damage.[19] Three hours is the absolute maximum. Application of tourniquets to the lower limbs raises the central venous pressure.[20]

The 'normal' blood pressure during sleep is often little above 80 mmHg.[21] Blood pressure should be monitored frequently by the most accurate method available. A systolic presure of 60–80 mmHg usually gives adequate ischaemia.

Ganglionic Blocking Agents

Pharmacodynamics
These may cause: (1) Low arterial pressure with postural sensitivity. (2) Release of autonomic tone by paralysis of ganglia at the preganglionic synapses of both sympathetic and parasympathetic systems, the former predominating. (3) Non-depolarizing myoneural block increased. (4) Respiratory depression. (5) Dilated pupils.

Hypotension and decreased haemorrhage may be due to: (1) The effects of gravity on blood distribution when the arterial pressure is low; (2) The effects of gravity on venous blood, causing it to pool in the distended veins of the lower and dependent parts of the body; (3) The reduced cardiac output consequent on the reduced venous return to the heart. As both sympathetic and parasympathetic ganglia are blocked, hypotension depends on the original balance of these two. Where there is great parasympathetic tone, its release will cause tachycardia, so that hypotension will not be maximal. Tachycardia may also be due to the hypotension stimulating the baroceptor mechanism, an example of Marey's law. Myocardial ischaemia may occur, but a reduction in peripheral resistance requires less myocardial work and oxygen consumption.

The drugs pass the placental barrier but do not cause ill effects in the fetus.

Renal blood flow. Glomerular filtration decreases with the fall in blood pressure and ceases at about 50–70 mmHg. Renal perfusion sufficient to meet the metabolic needs of the kidney does not suffer until the pressure is much lower, and as the pressure rises, function returns.

The liver. Little harm appears to result from reasonable hypotension.

Cerebral blood flow. Opinions vary about this, some investigators finding a reduced cerebral blood flow, others finding it well maintained due to decreased cerebrovascular resistance,[22] but this is influenced by blood–gas homeostasis, blood viscosity, CSF pressure and body temperature as well as by the diameter of the vessels. In cerebral atheroma, the vessels cannot dilate to decrease vascular resistance and ischaemia may therefore occur in such patients. Hypotension may cause alteration of cerebral function as shown by the flicker fusion test of Berg, while psychiatric disorders have been noticed after its use.[23]

Coronary blood flow. The state of the coronary vessels is important in the development of cardiac ischaemia when hypotension occurs, but low arterial pressure reduces cardiac work and the demand of the myocardium for oxygen so that myocardial perfusion remains adequate.[24] There is no evidence that hypotensive anaesthesia causes any permanent damage to the myocardium[25] seen on electrocardiographic evidence, although marked T of S–T wave alterations may indicate acute ischaemia.

Lung changes. The physiological dead space (adequate ventilation of under-perfused alveoli) is increased by hypotension under IPPV as it also is by the head-up position, by haemorrhage, and by the rise in the mean intrathoracic pressure associated with IPPV. Hypoventilation is to be avoided. Thus an excess of oxygen (40–50%) should always be provided.

Pharmacokinetics. The drugs are not metabolized in the body, but are excreted via the renal glomeruli, 50% of it in 2 hours and 90% within 24 hours after intravenous injection. Renal failure may delay excretion and cause accumulation of the drug. If the blood pressure drops below 50–70 mmHg glomerular filtration ceases and excretion will no longer take place.

Hexamethonium and Pentamethonium

Pentamethonium was first used as an antidote to the myoneural blocking effects of decamethonium by Organe, Paton and Zaimis in 1949,[5] while in the same year M. H. Armstrong Davison (1911–1970) of Newcastle, warned against its severe hypotensive action.[26] Cyril Frederick Scurr of London, in 1949[27] was the first deliberately to use the drug to lessen bleeding during surgery. No longer available commercially in the UK.

Pentolinium Tartrate, BP (*Pentapyrrolidinium, Ansolysen*)

Action is one of ganglion blockade. Usual dose 0·1–0·15 mg/kg given soon after anaesthesia has been induced, ranging from 8 to 10 mg in the young and sturdy patient to 1–2 mg in the elderly. Larger doses are required in those patients breathing spontaneously and smaller doses in the hypertensives. A tried and trusted drug. It is excreted in the urine. Takes about 30 min to produce a maximum fall in blood pressure.

Trimetaphan Camphorsulphonate, BP (*Arfonad*)

This compound, a thiophanium derivative, was described by Randall and others[28] in 1949. First used in the UK by Magill, Scurr and Wyman in 1953.[29] It is a ganglion-blocking agent and has a direct dilator effect on peripheral vessels. It liberates histamine. During anaesthesia it can be given as an intravenous drip in a strength of 0·1% (1 mg/ml) at a rate of 0·1–5 mg/min. With this concentration the drip starts at 60 drops/min (3–4 mg/min). The drug can be given by repeated single injections of 2·5–10 mg of a 1% solution.[30] It inhibits serum cholinesterase. Recovery is usually moderately rapid.

It causes more hypotension in arteriosclerotic patients than in those with normal blood pressure, interferes with the heat-regulating mechanism, causing hypothermia after long operations, and reduces the need for anaesthesia once a low pressure has been established. It may, however, result in tachyphylaxis, tachycardia and rather prolonged hypotension. It causes reduced coronary and renal blood flow, reduces cardiac output[31] and potentiates non-depolarizing neuromuscular block,[32] having some non-depolarizing blocking effect itself.[33] Partially excreted by the kidneys after destruction by cholinesterase although the exact mechanism is in dispute. The maximum dose should not exceed 1 g.[34] Has been used successfully with sodium nitroprusside[35] in a 10:1 mixture.[36]

Vasodilators

Sodium Nitroprusside[37]

Physical and Chemical Properties

The commercial preparation (Nipride) is freeze-dried and presented as 50 mg dry powder in a sealed ampoule. Dissolved in 500 ml 5% dextrose for clinical use (100 or 200 µg/ml). Such solutions are unstable and must be protected from light (10% decrease in potency in 3 hours, 50% in 48 hours in bright light).[38] Appearance of blue colour suggests undue breakdown and such solutions should be discarded.

The solution should be prepared immediately before use.

Pharmacodynamics

The action is a direct one on smooth muscle of blood vessels to produce relaxation and hence vasodilatation. The mode of action probably involves sulphydryl (SH) groups bound to smooth-muscle membrane.[39] There is a greater effect on arterial than on venous vessels.[40] Cardiac output is usually maintained, and here there is a major difference from the effect of other drugs. Tissue perfusion is unlikely to be compromised. Moderate tachycardia is frequent, probably due to stimulation of baroreceptor reflexes. Posture is less important than in the case of ganglion-blocking agents.[41] Renal blood flow is increased. Cerebral blood flow is maintained at arterial pressures of around 30 mmHg,[42] and intracranial pressure may rise when hypotension is only moderate or when pressure has returned to normal but autoregulation has not.[43] There is an increase in cerebral blood flow.[44] There is little effect on hepatic blood flow.

Pharmacokinetics

Sodium nitroprusside is rapidly broken down in the blood stream, probably both in the plasma and in the red cells, with the production of nitric oxide (NO) and hydrocyanic acid which is then conjugated with thiosulphate to form thiocyanate. Overdosage leads to accumulation of free cyanide ions, so that dosage must be strictly controlled. Thiocyanate levels can be measured as a monitor of toxicity during prolonged administration of nitroprusside, though it rises too slowly to be a useful index of overdose during short-term infusions. Thiocyanate is excreted in the urine. A small amount of cyanide is excreted after combination with vitamin B_{12} to form cyanocobalamin, but this is not clinically important.

Toxic reactions. There have been some case reports of cardiovascular collapse and severe metabolic acidosis after administration of large doses of sodium nitroprusside in resistant patients. It is likely that such patients have suffered acute cyanide poisoning, the metabolic acidosis being a result of histotoxic hypoxia.[45] It has been suggested that the minimal lethal dose of nitroprusside for short-term infusions is about 200–300 mg, whereas a dose of more than 20 mg is rarely necessary.[46] Nitroprusside should be avoided when normal cyanide metabolism is inhibited as in liver or renal failure, Lebers optic atrophy[82] and tobacco amblyopia.

Treatment of Overdose[46]
Fluid replacement should be adequate. If severe metabolic acidosis is confirmed, 25 ml 50% sodium thiosulphate[47] should be given intravenously over 3–5 min. If there is no improvement 20 ml (300 mg) of cobalt edetate is recommended at 1 ml/sec.[48]

Clinical Use[45,49]
A separate intravenous infusion should be set up containing 100 or 200 µg/ml in 5% dextrose. The maximum safe dose should be calculated as 1·5 mg/kg and never exceeded. An electronic drip controller or 'Dial a Flow' should be used and T-piece or two-way tap systems avoided.

An initial infusion rate of 37·5 µg/min is recommended in the healthy adult. Response is usually seen within 30 sec and thereafter arterial pressure changes determine the infusion rate; 10 µg/kg/min should not be exceeded. Arterial pressure begins to rise within one minute of the cessation of the infusion and is normally complete within 5–10 min. Blood pressure must be monitored closely throughout the operation, using a Dinamap or direct arterial method.

It has been suggested that the anaesthetic technique used should incorporate IPPV with a muscle relaxant and an inspired oxygen concentration of at least 33%.

The container of the drip solution should be protected from light by an opaque cover as the degradation products may result in toxicity.[50]

The return of normal blood pressure should take place within a few minutes of turning off the drip and, rarely, fluid loading or a pressor agent must be used.

Indications
(1) Neurosurgery.[51] Cerebral aneurysms and arteriovenous malformations. (2) Phaeochromocytoma.[52] (3) The surgery of scoliosis. (4) Aortic surgery. (5) Cardiopulmonary bypass, to decrease after-load in the immediate post-bypass period.[53] (6) Intensive care. During long-term use plasma thiocyanate levels may be monitored to avoid overdose. Levels should not exceed 1·7 mmol/litre (10 mg%). Acute hypertensive crises.[54] Cardiogenic shock to reduce cardiac work.[55] Management of ergot overdosage.[56]

(*See also* Verner I. R. in: *Hypotensive Anaesthesia* (Enderby G. E. H. ed.) Edinburgh: Churchill Livingstone, 1985, p. 138.)

Nitroglycerin (*Glyceryl trinitrate; Nitrostat*)[57]
First used for the treatment of angina by William Murrell (1853–1912) of London, in 1879.[58] The raw material of dynamite. This has been used intravenously at a rate of about 20 µg/min. Its action is similar to that of nitroprusside, but it is claimed that the course of hypotension is smoother with fewer peaks and troughs of arterial pressure. It can be used with halothane anaesthesia.

The unopened ampoules of 0·5% solution are reasonably stable but must be discarded once opened. It is rapidly destroyed in the liver. In the blood-stream methaemoglobin accumulates but this is of scant clinical importance.

Pharmacodynamics
It produces relaxation of the smooth muscle in vessel walls, especially in veins. In reasonable dosage it improves coronary perfusion. Intracranial pressure rises. Its solutions are absorbed by polyvinyl chloride containers and tubing so that polythene or glass must be used.

Clinical Use
Many workers employ a 0·01% solution with an initial drip rate of 10 µg/min. Hypotensive effects come on more slowly and last much longer than when sodium nitroprusside is infused. A power-driven infusion pump should be used for its administration. (*See also* Verner I. R. in: *Hypotensive Anaesthesia* (Enderby G. E. H. ed.) Edinburgh: Churchill Livingstone, 1985, p. 138.)

The purine, adenosine, has been successfully used to provide controllable and safe hypotension.[59]

Potentiation of Hypotension

1. Halothane
This agent can be used alone to produce hypotension but at the cost of direct myocardial depression. It can also be employed with ganglionic blocking agents: (1) Before these agents are used, or (2) It can be added to the inhaled gases in those patients in whom the blood pressure cannot be completely controlled by the classic hypotensive technique. It acts by (*a*) myocardial depression, (*b*) depression of vascular smooth muscle, (*c*) by inhibition of vasomotor reflexes.

The anaesthetist should, however, be warned against overdosage with halothane in an effort to lower systolic blood pressure. Because of its inhibitory effect on platelet aggregation halothane may not be the best agent for maximal ischaemia.[60]

2. Enflurane
Its effects on the cardiovascular system are similar to those of halothane. The dysrhythmias associated with the infiltration of adrenaline–saline are not as severe with this agent as with halothane.[61]

3. Isoflurane
Its cardiovascular effects are more benign than those of halothane or enflurane.

4. β-Blockers

Used to prevent tachycardia and its associated oozing, which may accompany ganglionic blockade, with or without halothane and IPPV,[62] e.g. propranolol 0·035 mg/kg repeated until the pulse rate is at the required rate; or practolol, 0·14 mg/kg as necessary (still available for i.v. injection). Metoprolol, a cardioselective beta adrenoceptor blocker has been used successfully to decrease arterial blood pressure and heart rate in hypertensive patients during anaesthesia, when they have received fentanyl and nitrous oxide and oxygen; in such patients, occasional bradycardia may be seen after neostigmine.[63] It is also satisfactory when used with halothane.[64]

The injections should be slow and given following the induction of anaesthesia and before the injection of the hypotensive agent. (*See also* Prys-Roberts C. in: *The Circulation in Anaesthesia*. (Prys-Roberts C. ed.) Oxford: Blackwell Scientific Publications, 1980.)

5. Labetalol

It reduces arterial pressure by reducing cardiac output and heart rate and decreases peripheral resistance. First used in anaesthesia by Scott et al. in 1976.[65] Alpha- and beta-receptors are blocked so that hypotension is produced without tachycardia in association with halothane anaesthesia; dose: 5–25 mg i.v.[66] Smaller doses are required when halothane is also administered, and even smaller doses when IPPV is employed.[65] Larger doses, up to 2 mg/kg have been given in association with a nitrous oxide, oxygen, relaxant, narcotic analgesic technique.[67] Should marked bradycardia occur, atropine may be given, though this may result in a rise of arterial pressure.[68] 10 mg of labetalol are equivalent to 2 mg of propranolol at beta-1 receptors, 0·75 mg of propranolol at beta-2 receptors, and 2 mg of phentolamine at alpha-1 receptors.[69] The half-life of labetalol given intravenously is between 3·5 and 6·3 hours, depending on the dose administered.[67,70] Deep planes of halothane anaesthesia may cause profound hypotension and bradycardia, but reversal is rapid when the concentration is reduced. Given with care, a useful agent in young and fit patients.

6. Posture

Gravity acting on the tilted patient results in blood pooling in the dilated (capacitance) veins, and this leads to decreased venous return and hypotension. Posture is also used to make the operation site ischaemic. The blood pressure is said to be reduced 20 mmHg for each 2·5 cm of vertical height above heart level, so that when the head is tilted 25° upwards, the cerebral blood pressure is likely to be about 16 mmHg less than the blood pressure at heart level. Many, but not all, experienced workers consider it reasonably safe in normal patients to allow a 25° head-up tilt with a brachial arterial blood pressure of 60–70 mmHg.

7. Intermittent Positive-pressure Ventilation[71]

This is usually employed with a high inspired oxygen concentration. Increased airway pressure is transmitted to the great veins and so venous return to the heart is decreased; this lowers the blood pressure further, depending on the pressure in the reservoir bag. Positive end-expiratory pressure (PEEP) is used as a supplement by some workers. It reduces cardiac output.[72]

There are workers of experience in the production of hypotensive anaesthesia who allow their patients to breathe spontaneously.[36]

Clinical Use of Hypotensive Agents

The technique is simple, but must be meticulous. Both the airway and the patient's ventilation must be faultless, and afferent impulses must be properly blocked. Any of the ordinary anaesthetic combinations may be used, such as thiopentone, nitrous oxide and oxygen, narcotic analgesic, relaxant or volatile agents. As full oxygenation is essential, tracheal intubation is usually employed. A labile pressure is an indication that small dosage will probably be adequate; other such indications for small dosage are increasing age and low metabolic rate. Arteriosclerotics require a small dose and little posture to get a profound effect, while young, fit patients, besides often developing tachycardia, require a steep head-up tilt and high initial dosage to ensure good ischaemia.

The arterial pressure is monitored at frequent intervals and for this an automatic recorder (Dinamap) is valuable while an oscillometer gives a clear reading at low levels of blood pressure; some workers use direct intra-arterial monitoring. Facilities for blood transfusion through an intravenous drip must be to hand as bleeding is a dangerous complication because the normal response to it, vasoconstriction, is impossible. Great care and constant attention must be given throughout the operation, and afterwards, to the patient who is taken near to the point of death. The administration of pure oxygen during hypotensive anaesthesia may contribute to the safety of the technique.

Failure to produce good ischaemia with ganglionic blocking agents may be due to: (1) Incomplete block of sympathetic ganglia; (2) Increased cardiac output due to tachycardia; (3) Presence of injected or autogenous noradrenaline or adrenaline in the circulation.

Signs of excessive hypotension include: (1) A completely dry wound; (2) Irregular respiration, if breathing is spontaneous; (3) The onset of cardiac irregularity. Measures must be taken to correct these.

To raise the blood pressure at the end of the operation, or before that if necessary, a return to the horizontal position is usually sufficient. Hypertensive drugs and also infusions may be used, e.g. ephedrine or methoxamine. Towards the end of the operation the blood pressure is allowed to rise slowly, and no patient should leave the table unless his blood pressure is 80 mmHg or more. Blood-pressure readings must be taken frequently in the postoperative period.

The results in successful cases are: (1) An ischaemic field of operation; (2) Easier surgical dissection; (3) Reduction of amount of ligatured or cauterized tissue and consequent reduction in infection; (4) Decreased oozing beneath skin flaps, less postoperative oedema and hence better healing.

Enormous experience with the employment of hypotensive anaesthesia together with great professional skill has led Enderby to state that a blood pressure of 60 mmHg can be produced in the majority of patients without complications.[73] For safe use the technique demands expertise and experience.

Hypotension in Children

This may be necessary in paediatric practice for operations such as resection of coarctation of the aorta,[74] and scoliosis surgery.[75] Sodium nitroprusside is safe in a dose up to 10 μg/kg/min.[76] High dosage can cause fatal cyanide intoxication.[77]

The Dangers

Many workers think that the technique should be confined to those cases where it makes the impossible possible. It should not be used to make the possible easy. Other workers employ it more liberally. Its advantages to the patient must be weighed against the increased risks.

Trouble has been reported from cerebral and coronary thrombosis, renal and hepatic ischaemia, reactionary haemorrhage, ileus, cerebral damage, arterial thrombosis (e.g. the carotid, central retinal artery and limb arteries), and massive atelectasis. A number of morbidity surveys have been published[78] but their validity is open to criticism. Series of cases using control groups have not shown the technique to be harmful if employed with skill.[79]

Indications

These may include the following: (1) Neurosurgery, especially in operations for vascular tumours and aneurysms. Hypotension causes shrinkage of the brain; (2) Peripheral vascular surgery, e.g. coarctation of the aorta to reduce bleeding from enlarged vessels in the chest wall; (3) Operations associated with voluminous haemorrhage, e.g. toal cystectomy, abdominoperineal resection of the rectum, panhysterectomy and pelvic exenteration; (4) Plastic surgery and operations on the nose and lacrimal apparatus;[35] (5) Microsurgery (e.g. middle ear). (6) When a patient's abnormal blood group makes transfusion difficult and in Jehovah's Witnesses who refuse blood transfusion; (7) Pelvic floor repair operations; (8) Prostatectomy; (9) To reduce uncontrollable bleeding during operation. (10) Intensive care. (11) Operations behind the eye; intraocular pressure is reduced.

Jehovah's witnesses. A sect originating near Pittsburg in 1872, whose newspaper is *The Watchtower.* Their religion proscribes blood transfusion. Autotransfusion is most useful and was first performed in 1886[80] and for clean surgery, a Bentley recirculator is useful.[81] (*See also* Findley L. J. and Redstone P. M. *Arch. Intern. Med.* 1982, **142**, 606; Coll C. E. *Anaesthesia* 1984, **39**, 497.)

Contraindications

These vary in the practice of different workers. The following conditions may increase the danger: (1) Respiratory inadequacy from any cause, especially obstructive airways disease; (2) Bronchospasm and asthma; (3) Diabetes, because ganglionic blocking agents increase the patient's response to insulin, and hypoglycaemia may result; (4) Cerebral and coronary vascular disease and atheroma; (5) Previous steroid therapy; (6) Where there is poor renal of hepatic function; (7) In Addison's disease; (8) In pregnancy; (9) *When the technical skill and experience of the anaesthetist are not of a high order*; (10) When the surgeon is not accustomed to working under hypotensive conditions.

Discussion

It would seem that in expert and experienced hands, induced hypotension in normal patients with the blood pressure reduced to 70–80 mmHg and even with 25° head-up tilt is reasonably safe. What is certain is that the technique can be lethal if its details are not fully understood and if it is not conducted impeccably.

The anaesthetist is warned against production of hypotension at the request of the surgeon where this may affect the safety of the patient.

Induced hypotension should only be employed if the anaesthetist and surgeon are in full agreement as to its desirability and are both experienced in its use.

(*See also* Symposium on Deliberate Hypotension in Anaesthesia, *Br. J. Anaesth.* 1975, **47**, 743; Tinker J. H. and Michenfelder J. D. *Anesthesiology* 1976, **45**, 340; MacRae W. R. et al. *Anaesthesia* 1981, **36**, 312; Cunningham A. J. A. *Br. J. Anaesth.* 1982, **54**, 895; Coll C. E. *Anaesthesia* 1984, **39**, 497; Enderby G. E. H. ed. *Hypotensive Anaesthesia* Edinburgh: Churchill Livingstone, 1985.)

References

1. Gardner W. J. *JAMA* 1946, **132**, 572 (reprinted in 'Classical File', *Surv. Anesthesiol.* 1969, **13**, 220); Bilsland W. L. *Anaesthesia* 1951, **6**, 20; Jackson I. *Anaesthesia* 1954, **9**, 13.
2. Koster H. *Am. J. Surg.* 1928, **5**, 554; Vehrs G. R. *NW. Med. Seattle* 1931, **30**, 256, 322; Griffiths, M. W. C. and Gillies J. *Anaesthesia* 1948, **3**, 134 (reprinted in 'Classical File', *Surv. Anesthesiol.* 1980, **24**, 342).
3. Bromage P. R. *Anaesthesia* 1951, **6**, 26.
4. Paton W. D. M. and Zaimis E. J. *Nature* 1948, **162**, 810.
5. Organe G. S. W. et al. *Lancet* 1949, **1**, 21.
6. Hunter A. R. *Lancet* 1950, **1**, 251; Shackleton R. P. W. *Br. Med. J.* 1951, **1**, 1054; Wyman J. B. *Proc. R. Soc. Med.* 1953, **46**, 605.
7. Enderby G. E. H. *Lancet* 1950, **1**, 1145; Enderby G. E. H. and Pelmore J. F. *Lancet* 1951, **1**, 663; Enderby G. E. H. *Lancet* 1954, **2**, 1097.
8. Sarnoff S. J. et al. *Circulation* 1952, **6**, 63.
9. Magill I. W. et al. *Lancet* 1953, **1**, 219.
10. Robertson J. D. et al. *Br. J. Anaesth.* 1957, **29**, 342.
11. Johnson C. C. *Arch. Int. Pharmacodyn. Thér.* 1929, **35**, 480.
12. Moraca P. et al. *Anesthesiology* 1962, **23**, 193.
13. Jones G. O. M. and Cole P. *Br. J. Anaesth.* 1968, **40**, 804.
14. Gillies J. *Ann. R. Coll. Surg.* 1950, **7**, 204.
15. Enderby G. E. H. *Anaesthesia* 1960, **15**, 25.
16. Hellewell J. and Potts M. W. *Br. J. Anaesth.* 1966, **38**, 794; Johnstone M. *Br. J. Anaesth.* 1966, **38**, 516.
17. Esmarch J. F. A. von, *Der erste Verband auf dem Schlachtfelde.* Kiel: Schwers'sche Buchhandlung, 1869.
18. Saunders J. W. *Lancet* 1952, **1**, 1286.
19. Fry D. *Br. Med. J.* 1972, **1**, 511.
20. Bradford E. *Anaesthesia* 1969, **24**, 190.
21. Richardson D. W. et al. *Clin. Sci.* 1964, **26**, 445.
22. Slack W. K. et al. *Lancet* 1963, **1**, 1082; Eckenhoff J. E. et al. *J. Appl. Physiol.* 1963, **18**, 1130; Eckenhoff J. E. *Lancet* 1964, **2**, 711.
23. Brierley J. B. and Cooper J. E. *J. Neurol. Psychiat.* 1962, **25**, 24.
24. Hickey R. H. et al. *Anesthesiology* 1983, **59**, 226.
25. Rollason W. N. and Cumming A. R. R. *Anaesthesia* 1956, **11**, 319; Rollason W. H. and Hough C. M. *Br. J. Anaesth.* 1960, **32**, 276, 286; Simpson P. et al. *Anaesthesia* 1976, **32**, 1172.
26. Davison M. H. A. *Lancet* 1950, **1**, 252.
27. Scurr C. F. *Anesthesiology* 1951, **12**, 253; Enderby G. E. H. *Lancet* 1950, **1**, 1145.
28. Randall L. O. et al. *J. Pharmacol. Exp. Ther.* 1949, **97**, 48.
29. Magill I. W. et al. *Lancet* 1953, **1**, 219.
30. Enderby G. E. H. *Postgrad. Med. J.* 1974, **50**, 572.
31. Wang H. H. et al. *Anesthesiology* 1977, **46**, 40.
32. Sklar G. S. and Lanks K. W. *Anesthesiology* 1977, **47**, 31; Graham C. W. and Walts L. F. *Anaesthesia* 1979, **34**, 1005.
33. Nakamura K. et al. *Anaesthesia* 1980, **35**, 1202.
34. Eckenhoff J. E. *Surg. Clin. North Am.* 1955, **45**, 1579.
35. MacRae W. R. et al. *Anaesthesia* 1981, **36**, 307; Boyd C. H. *Anaesthesia* 1982, **37**, 1146.
36. MacRae W. R. et al. *Anaesthesia* 1981, **36**, 312.
37. *See also* Cole P. V. in: *Recent Advances in Anaesthesia and Analgesia*—13 (Hewer C. L. and Atkinson R. S. ed.). Edinburgh: Churchill Livingstone, 1979; Verner I. F. in: *Hypotensive Anaesthesia* (Enderby G. E. H. ed.) Edinburgh and London: Churchill Livingstone, 1985.

38. Vesey C. J. and Batistoni G. A. *J. Clin. Pharmacy* 1977, **2**, 105.
39. Needleman P. et al. *J. Pharmacol. Exp. Ther.* 1973, **187**, 324.
40. Wildsmith J. A. W. et al. *Br. J. Anaesth.* 1973, **45**, 71; Styles M. et al. *Anesthesiology* 1973, **38**, 173.
41. Rowe G. G. and Henderson R. H. *Am. Heart J.* 1974, **87**, 83; Schlant R. C. et al. *Am. J. Cardiol.* 1962, **9**, 51.
42. Ivankovich A. D. et al. *Anesthesiology* 1976, **44**, 21.
43. Turner J. M. et al. *Br. J. Anaesth.* 1977, **49**, 419.
44. Ishikawa T. and McDowall M. G. *Br. J. Anaesth.* 1981, **53**, 605.
45. Cole P. V. *Anaesthesia* 1978, **33**, 473.
46. *See also* Vesey C. J. et al. *Br. J. Anaesth.* 1976, **48**, 651; Cole P. V. in: *Recent Advances in Anaesthesia and Anaglesia*—13 (Hewer C. L. and Atkinson R. S. ed.). Edinburgh: Churchill Livingstone, 1979.
47. Michenfelder J. D. and Tinker J. H. *Anesthesiology* 1977, **47**, 441.
48. Bryson D. D. *Lancet*, 1978, **1**, 92.
49. Taylor T. H. et al. *Br. J. Anaesth.* 1970, **42**, 859.
50. Arnold W. P. and Longnecker D. E. *Anesthesiology* 1984, **61**, 254.
51. Siegal P. et al. *Br. J. Anaesth.* 1971, **43**, 790; McDowall D. G. *Proc. 7th World Congress Anaes. Hamburg.* Excerpta Medica Internat. Congress Series 538, 819.
52. Csanky-Treels J. C. et al. *Anaesthesia* 1976, **31**, 60; Daggett P. et al. *Br. Med. J.* 1978, **2**, 311; Daggett P. and Verner I. R. *Br. Med. J.* 1978, **2**, 1088.
53. Benzing G. and Helmsworth J. A. *Circulation* 1976, **54**, 467; Stinson E. B. et al. *J. Thorac. Cardiovasc. Surg.* 1977, **73**, 523.
54. A.M.A. Committee on Hypertension. *JAMA* 1974, **228**, 1673.
55. Franciosa J. A. et al. *Lancet* 1972, **1**, 650.
56. Carliner N. H. et al. *JAMA* 1974, **227**, 308.
57. Fahmy N. R. *Anesthesiology* 1978, **49**, 17; Stengert K. B. et al. *Anaesthesist* 1978, **27**, 223; Chestnut J. S. et al. *J. Neurosurg.* 1978, **48**, 708.
58. Murrell W. *Lancet* 1879, **2**, 80.
59. Sollevi A. et al. *Anesthesiology* 1984, **61**, 400.
60. Fyman P. N. et al. *Br. J. Anaesth.* 1984, **56**, 1197.
61. Konchigeri H. N. et al. *Anesth. Analg. (Cleve.)* 1974, **53**, 894.
62. Hellewell J. and Potts M. W. *Br. J. Anaesth.* 1966, **38**, 794; Rollason W. N. *Br. J. Anaesth.* 1967, **39**, 183; Hewitt P. B. et al. *Anaesthesia* 1967, **22**, 82.
63. Magnusson J. et al. *Br. J. Anaesth.* 1986, **58**, 251.
64. Jakobsen C-J. et al. *Br. J. Anaesth.* 1986, **58**, 261.
65. Scott D. B. et al. *Br. J. Clin. Pharmacol.* 1976, Suppl. 817.
66. Scott D. B. et al. *Anaesthesia* 1978, **33**, 145.
67. Kanto J. et al. *Int. J. Clin. Pharmacol. Ther. Toxicol.* 1980, **18**, 191.
68. Cope D. H. P. and Crawford M. C. *Br. J. Anaesth.* 1979, **51**, 359.
69. Green D. W et al. in: *Hypotensive Anaesthesia* (Enderby G. E. H. ed.) Edinburgh: Churchill Livingstone, 1985.
70. Martin L. E. et al. *Br. J. Clin. Pharmacol.* 1976, Suppl, 695.
71. *See also* Conway C. M. *Br. J. Anaesth.* 1975, **47**, 761.
72. Eckenhoff J. E. et al. *Br. J. Anaesth.* 1963, **35**, 750.
73. Enderby G. E. H. ed. *Hypotensive Anaesthesia.* Edinburgh: Churchill Livingstone, 1985, p. 267.
74. Abbott T. R. in: *Paediatric Anaesthesia* (Rees G. J. and Gray T. C. ed.) London: Butterworth, 1981.
75. Schofield N. McC. in: *Anaesthesia for Orthopaedic Patients* (Loach A. ed.) London: Arnold, 1983.
76. Bennett N. and Abbott T. R. *Anaesthesia* 1977, **32**, 456.
77. Davies D. W. et al. *Can. Anaesth. Soc. J.* 1975, **22**, 553.
78. Little D. M. *Anesthesiology* 1955, **16**, 320; Enderby G. E. H. *Br. J. Anaesth.* 1961, **33**, 109; Bodman R. I. *Proc. R. Soc. Med.* 1964, **57**, 1184.
79. Warner W. A. et al. *Br. J. Anaesth.* 1970, **42**, 39; Hugosson R. and Hogstrom S. *J. Neurosurg.* 1973, **38**, 561.
80. Duncan J. *Br. Med. J.* 1886, **1**, 192.
81. Clarke J. M. F. *Br. J. Hosp. Med.* 1982, **27**, 497.
82. Leber T. *Arch. Ophthalmol.* 1871, **17**, 249.

Chapter 17	**HYPOTHERMIA**

Induced hypothermia is a method used to lower the metabolism of the body as a whole, and to reduce the dangers from hypoxia and the cellular damage resulting from regional occlusion of the circulation of the brain, the heart, the liver, the kidneys and the legs. Cooling enables certain specialized tissues of the body to withstand periods of hypoxia which in its absence would cause harm. It has also been used to treat hyperpyrexia during and after operation and to treat shock.

The name was first used in 1941.[1]

History

1724 G. D. Fahrenheit (1686–1736) described his scale of thermometry.

1742 A. Celsius (1701–1744), Swedish astronomer, published his work on thermometry.

1798 Dr James Currie of Liverpool published observations on the effect on man of immersion in cold water.

1848 William Thompson (Lord) Kelvin (1824–1907) described his absolute thermometric scale.

1905 S. Simpson and Perry Theodore Herring (1872–1967) coined the term 'artificial hibernation' and showed that cold—below about 28 °C—could act as a general anaesthetic.[2]

1938 Temple Fay treated carcinoma by lowering the body temperature—cryotherapy.[3]

1947 Delorme of Edinburgh showed that haemorrhagic shock was better tolerated by cooled dogs than by dogs at normal temperatures. Hypothermia used by McQuiston.[4]

1950 Wilfred Gordon Bigelow surgeon (1913–) and his colleagues from Toronto[5] showed that with progressive cooling the rectal temperature and the oxygen consumption of the body showed an almost linear relationship, that even slight shivering doubled oxygen consumption, and that no oxygen debt was incurred by the tissues. Surface cooling was the method used.

1951 Bloodstream or pervascular cooling employed by Delorme of Edinburgh[6] and by J. Boerema (1902–) of Holland.[7]

1953 Pioneer work was done by Henry Swan, Robert Virtue and their colleagues in Denver.[8]

1959 Deep hypothermia with cardiopulmonary bypass and bloodstream cooling described by C. E. Drew,[9] surgeon of London.

The so-called artificial hibernation of Laborit and Huguenard in France (1951) using chlorpromazine, etc.,[10] should not be confused with induced hypothermia.

Effects of Hypothermia

Cardiovascular System

Dysrhythmias occur at temperatures below 30 °C; spontaneous ventricular fibrillation may be seen, but is not likely above 28 °C. Factors in its causation may include: (*a*) Hypothermia; (*b*) Hyperkalaemia; (*c*) Sudden pH and P_{CO_2}

changes; (*d*) Citrate intoxication. Bradycardia not due to vagal overaction is progressive. The blood pressure, pulse rate and cardiac output fall progressively as the temperature gets lower. Stroke volume is little affected and coronary blood flow is well maintained. ECG changes include lengthening of the QRS complex and prolongation of the P–R interval.[15] Elevation of the ST segment with T-wave depression may occur. The J wave is a small positive wave on the downstroke of the R, which may appear at about 30 °C. Vasoconstriction of skin vessels occurs.

Respiratory System

Measurements of human cerebral oxygen consumption indicate that at 30 °C it is 39% and at 28 °C 35% of normal.[16] The oxygen dissociation curve is shifted to the left so that liberation of oxygen to the tissues is hindered; although more oxygen is dissolved in plasma there is reduced availability of oxygen to the tissues due to: (*a*) Depressed respiration; (*b*) Decreased cardiac output; (*c*) Vasoconstriction; (*d*) Increased blood viscosity; (*e*) Arteriovenous shunts. Tissue oxygenation may be improved by: (*a*) Controlled ventilation; (*b*) Hyperbaric oxygenation (not practical during surgery); (*c*) Controlled cooling; fall not more than 1 °C/5 min; (*d*) Controlled hypercapnia; deliberate addition of carbon dioxide to inhaled gases; (*e*) Haemodilution to reduce viscosity; use of Ringer or dextrose solutions in disposable bubble oxygenators during cardiopulmonary bypass. The respiration rate falls and breathing may cease at a temperature of 26 °C.

Acid–base Balance

Acidosis tends to be a feature of hypothermia. Factors which may produce acidosis include: (*a*) Increased solubility of carbon dioxide; (*b*) Respiratory insufficiency; (*c*) Increase in formation of lactic acid as a result of a metabolic deficit during circulatory arrest, hypoxia, shivering, surgical trauma or anaesthesia; (*d*) Decreased breakdown of lactic acid due to impaired liver function; (*e*) Depression of renal function prevents correction of acidosis.

Rapid changes of pH may be a cause of cardiac irregularities.

Measurement of pH presents some difficulties.[17] Laboratory estimations are carried out at 38 °C so a correction factor must be added of 0·0147 pH unit/1 °C fall in temperature.[18] Direct P_{CO_2} measurement presents similar problems, the equation for correction being, $P_{CO_{2(t)}} = $ antilog $[\log P_{CO_{2(38)}} - 0·021(38 - t)]$. Base excess requires no temperature correction.

Central Nervous System

The cerebral cortex can tolerate the acute hypoxia due to complete circulatory arrest for 5–10 min at a temperature of 28 °C and of 50 min at 15 °C. There is a reduction in cerebral blood flow, brain volume and cerebrospinal fluid pressure. Consciousness is usually lost between 28 °C and 30 °C. At 20 °C cardiac arrest for 20 min or less is unlikely to do serious harm to the brain.[19]

Metabolism

With each fall of 1 °C the metabolism is reduced 6–7%. The functions of the liver and kidneys are depressed during hypothermia so that intravenous agents and relaxants must be given in small amounts. Utilization of glucose is depressed, and continued intravenous infusion of glucose solution may result in a high blood-glucose level, not affected by insulin. Metabolism of substances like heparin, lactic acid and citrate is inhibited. Large transfusions of citrated blood may cause citrate intoxication; the typical ECG change of QT prolongation is an indication for the administration of calcium gluconate or chloride. Renal blood flow, glomerular filtration and selective reabsorption are diminished. Below 30°C there is a secretion of dilute urine. Following profound hypothermia (below 20°C) this water diuresis may persist into the postoperative period. Cellular damage in the liver, kidneys and adrenals has been reported.

Electrolytes

There may be a rise in serum potassium associated with acidosis, prolonged circulatory arrest, anoxia or large transfusions of stored blood. Calcium gluconate is given to cover each unit of donor blood to prevent lowering of ionized calcium. The cold heart is more sensitive to potassium, so small changes are of significance.

The Neuromuscular Junction

The duration and magnitude of block by depolarizing drugs are increased. The effect of non-depolarizing drugs is reduced. These changes are reversed on rewarming.

The Blood

Clotting mechanisms are depressed, platelet count falls rapidly, and 'sludging' may occur in capillaries at very low temperatures. Viscosity is increased. As the metabolic demand for oxygen decreases, the saturation in venous blood rises. Oxygen is more soluble in plasma at low temperatures.

Methods of Anaesthesia

The anaesthetic requirements are: (1) Light general anaesthesia; (2) Prevention of shivering; (3) Peripheral vasodilatation (with surface methods). During hypothermia minimal amounts of anaesthetic drugs are required, and their detoxication and excretion may be delayed. The actual choice of anaesthetic agents is not critical provided they are given with care. Chlorpromazine has been used in premedication or during anaesthesia to prevent shivering and promote vasodilatation and heat loss. Muscle relaxants, in conjunction with light anaesthesia, prevent shivering. Halothane has been employed to promote peripheral vasodilatation.

Monitoring of temperature, blood pressure, pulse rate, electrocardiogram and perhaps of electro-encephalogram is advisable.

Techniques of Induced Hypothermia

Surface Cooling

The original method of Bigelow.[11] The patient is anaesthetized, intubated and placed in a cold environment. The anaesthetic technique must provide: (1) Peripheral vasodilatation to promote heat exchange; (2) Absence of shivering (which prevents cooling and increases oxygen utilization). The patient may be placed between two blankets which incorporate coils of tubing. Solution containing anti-freeze is circulated through the coils after passing through a refrigerator/warming unit. Other methods include immersion of the patient in cold water,[12] the use of ice-bags[13] and air cooling.[14]

Time taken to reduce the temperature to 30–28 °C is between ¾ hour and 3 hours, depending on the size and build of the patient. It takes longer in large and obese patients, not so long in children who present a big surface area per unit mass of body weight.

Surface cooling produces extreme vasoconstriction of the peripheral vessels, even when vasodilators are administered. This delays cooling of the main body mass and hastens the development of metabolic acidosis.

After-drop. The temperature continues to fall after active cooling has been discontinued. This is due to loss of heat from the core or main body mass of the patient to the skin or superficial regions. It may be of the order of 2–6 °C. Active cooling should, therefore, cease a few degrees above the desired temperature and care taken that undue fall with its increased risk of ventricular fibrillation does not occur.

Extracorporeal Methods

Blood is taken from the circulation, cooled by means of a heat exchanger in an extracorporeal circulation, and then returned to the body. This method of cooling is faster than surface cooling. It has its main application in cardiac surgery. Profound hypothermia (15 °C) may be used. *See also* Chapter 29.

Rewarming

This must be undertaken with care as there is a danger of burning the patient if rewarming is overzealous. After surface cooling the patient can usually be allowed to regain heat normally. Rewarming can be expedited by use of a mattress with circulating fluid, by the use of warm blankets, warm water or warm air if care is taken. A temperature higher than 40 °C should not be used. In the case of direct blood cooling the heat exchanger can be used to warm up the blood passing through it.

It is usual to rewarm to 35° C or until consciousness has returned before taking the patient out of the operating theatre to the postoperative ward.

Measurement of Body Temperature

Body temperature varies slightly in different regions of the body. When hypothermia is induced different organs and tissues are cooled at varying rates according to their blood supply, the method of hypothermia, etc. Thus when the blood is cooled directly the temperature of the heart falls before that of the brain.

It is wise to place thermometers in several different situations during hypothermia. Oesophageal temperature approximates to the heart, naso-pharyngeal or tympanic membrane to the brain. Rectal temperatures may differ from both. For information on techniques of temperature measurement *see* Chapter 41.

Complications of Hypothermia

1. Ventricular Fibrillation

Causes: (1) Hypothermia below 28 °C; (2) Respiratory acidosis; (3) Physical irritation of heart; (4) Defective coronary circulation. Since the main application of hypothermia during surgery is now for cardiac procedures with cardiopulmonary bypass, resuscitative measures are not required. In other situations, appropriate treatment must be instituted.

2. Local Effects
Frostbite due to local injury. Burns due to overzealous rewarming.

Uses of Hypothermia
Hypothermia is used to protect the brain during cardiac surgery with cardiopulmonary bypass,[20] carotid artery surgery, vascular tumours in the brain and aneurysmal surgery. Surface cooling is seldom used, except in certain centres.[21] The use of hypothermia has largely been abandoned in other surgical fields. *Malignant hyperpyrexia* may require urgent surface cooling.

Profound Hypothermia[22]
The facility of cardiopulmonary bypass and rapid blood cooling allows body temperature to be reduced to around 15 °C. This affords a high degree of protection to the brain. During rewarming the heart is started by defibrillation and massage. (Cold agglutinins in profound hypothermia, *see* Leach A. B. et al. *Anaesthesia* 1983, **38**, 140.) *See also* Chapter 29.

Heat Balance in Anaesthetized Patients[23]
Heat is lost by radiation to the atmosphere and to the table from viscera and skin, by evaporation and by cold intravenous fluids. During abdominal surgery at theatre temperatures between 21 °C and 24 °C (70–75 °F) the oesophageal temperature falls about 0·7 °C during the first hour and then stops falling. With a lower theatre temperature 18–21 °C (or 65–70 °F) fall in the first hour is twice this, and continues more slowly during the second hour. Thus the critical theatre temperature is about 21 °C or 70 °F (*see* Shanks C. A. *Anaesth. Intensive Care* 1975, **3**, 104, 118; Holdcroft A. *Body Temperature Control*. London: Baillière Saunders, 1980).

As a result of heat loss, during recovery the patient may: (1) Shiver, with increased oxygen consumption, sometimes fivefold; (2) Feel uncomfortable and become restless; (3) Show peripheral vasoconstriction.

Accidental Hypothermia
This may occur during intra- or extradural block or vascular surgery with massive blood transfusion, and can be prevented by operating in a warm theatre and the use of an insulated blanket. Intravenous fluids should be warmed. It may be complicated by thrombocytopaenia.[24] Accidental hypothermia can also occur in the newborn and in the aged, and secondary to such conditions as myxoedema, hypopituitarism, adrenal failure, drug overdose, apparent drowning and as a result of coma, immobility or exposure.

Management includes: (1) Active rewarming,[25] using a radiant heat cradle, warm water-bath at 37 °C, metal foil reflective space blankets; (2) Intravenous fluid infusion; (3) Correction of hypotension; (4) Cardiac output stimulation with small doses of dopamine; (5) Correction of hypoxia with oxygen and IPPV if necessary; (6) Steroids; (7) Glucose.

Temperature Changes in Shock
Temperature gradients between core and extremities develop during shock and

these can be measured with sensitive electric thermometers, e.g. between oesophagus or rectum and the pad of the big toe.[26] It has been suggested that a toe temperature of less than 27 °C indicates a cardiac output of half normal.

Refrigeration Analgesia

Refrigeration analgesia is the application of cold to a localized part of the body to block local nerve conduction of painful impulses. It is not to be confused with induced hypothermia which is the application of cold in order to reduce the oxygen needs of the tissues during temporary interruption of the circulation.

A method of analgesia revived by F. M. Allen of New York City.[27] Very seldom used today. It involves chilling and not freezing of the tissues. It acts on all the cells of the part, not just on the nerve cells as do other anaesthetics and analgesics. It was used by Baron Dominique Jean Larrey* (1766–1862) at the battle of Preuss Eylan in 1807 and also during Napoleon's retreat from Moscow in 1812;[28] and by James Arnott (1797–1883) of Brighton in 1847.[29] Benjamin Ward Richardson (1828–1896) of London, the biographer of John Snow, used an ether spray to produce refrigeration analgesia in 1866[30] (the apparatus was later used by Joseph Lister (1827–1912) with carbolic acid in his early work on the antiseptic treatment of wounds),[31] and this gave rise to the term 'freezing' for local analgesia. The ether spray was replaced in 1890 by ethyl chloride by Redard (1841–1910)[32] of Geneva, while in 1938 Fay and Henry[33] described cryotherapy for the relief of pain and for the treatment of cancer.

The effects of chilling: (1) Interference with conduction of nerve impulses—analgesia; (2) Reduction of metabolic rate and oxygen requirements; (3) Inhibition of bacterial growth and infection; (4) Retardation of healing.

This is a practical method of pain relief. For details see the seventh edition of this Synopsis.

Cryotherapy

The destructive properties of freezing were first used by Irving Cooper,[37] and Amoils.[34] The cryolesion behaves like a burn but is almost painless. There are two ways of obtaining a subzero temperature, the open-ended spray or the closed probe. Using nitrogen in a closed probe the temperature is lowered to −20 °C. Liquid nitrogen gives a temperature of −180 °C and both nitrous oxide and carbon dioxide can be used. Nitrous oxide gives a temperature of −70 °C. These low temperatures are the result of the Joule–Thompson effect whereby the temperature is lowered as the gas passes from a higher to a lower pressure through a narrow orifice. Usually no local analgesia is necessary as cold anaesthetizes the part. Uses: (1) Surgery, e.g. haemorrhoidectomy;[35] (2) Nerve block for pain relief, e.g. ilio-inguinal[36] and intercostal nerves from inside the chest, after thoracotomy.[37] Cryoanalgesia produces prolonged but not permanent neural blockade and neuroma formation is rare. (*See also* Fay T. *N Y State J. Med.* 1940, **2**, 1351; Evans P. J. D. et al. *J. R. Soc. Med.* 1981, **74**, 804; Annotation, *Lancet* 1982, **1**, 779; Evans P. J. D. *Anaesthesia* 1981, **36**, 1013;

---

*A descendent of whose sister was Mrs Laurette McMechan a well-known anaesthetic journalist and assistant editor (1923–1970) of *Current Researches in Anesthesia and Analgesia*.

and Katz J. in: *Regional Analgesia 1884–1984*. Production ICM AB, Sweden: 1984, p. 82.)

References

1. Tablott J. H. *N. Engl. J. Med.* 1941, **224**, 305.
2. Simpson S. and Herring P. T. *J. Physiol.* 1905, **32**, 305.
3. Fay T. and Henry G. C. *Surg. Gynecol. Obstet.* 1938, **66**, 512.
4. McQuiston W. O. *Anesthesiology* 1949, **10**, 590 (reprinted in 'Classical File', *Surv. Anesthesiol.* 1968, **12**, 529).
5. Bigelow W. G. et al. *Am. J. Physiol.* 1950, **160**, 125 (reprinted in 'Classical File', *Surv. Anesthesiol.* 1968, **12**, 575); *Can. J. Med. Sci.* 1952, **30**, 185.
6. Delorme E. J. *Lancet* 1952, **1**, 1108; **2**, 914.
7. Boerema I. A. et al. *Arch. Chir. Nederl.* 1951, **3**, 25.
8. Swan H. et al. *JAMA* 1953, **153**, 1081; Katz J. *Lancet* 1982; Swan H. et al. *Ann. Surg.* 1955, **142**, 383.
9. Drew C. E. et al. *Lancet* 1959, **1**, 745.
10. Laborit H. and Huguenard P. et al. *Presse méd.* 1951, **59**, 1329.
11. Bigelow W. G. et al. *Ann. Surg.* 1950, **132**, 531.
12. Sellick B. A. *Lancet* 1957, **1**, 443.
13. Burrows M. M. et al. *Anaesthesia* 1956, **11**, 4.
14. Forrester A. C. *Anaesthesia* 1958, **13**, 289.
15. Emslie-Smith D. et al. *Br. Heart J.* 1959, **21**, 343.
16. Stone H. H. et al. *Surg. Gynecol. Obstet* 1956, **103**, 313.
17. *See* Benazon D. in: *Scientific Foundations of Anaesthesia* (Scurr C. and Feldman S. ed.), 2nd ed. London: Heinemann, 1974, p. 344.
18. Rosenthal T. B. *J. Biol. Chem.* 1948, **173**, 25.
19. Treasure T. *Ann. R. Coll. Surg.* 1984, **66**, 235.
20. Lewis F. J. *Am. J. Cardiol.* 1958, **2**, 287; Gilston A. in: *Recent Advances in Anaesthesia and Analgesia*—13 (Hewer C. L. and Atkinson R. S. ed.). Edinburgh: Churchill Livingstone, 1979.
21. Wakusawa R. et al. *Can. Anaesth. Soc. J.* 1977, **24**, 491.
22. Drew C. E. *Br. Med. Bull.* 1961, **17**, 37.
23. Hall G. M. *Br. J. Anaesth.* 1978, **50**, 39.
24. Easterbrook P. J. and Davis H. F. *Br. Med. J.* 1985, **291**, 23.
25. Ledingham I. Mc. A. and Mone J. G. *Br. Med. J.* 1980, **1**, 1102.
26. Joly H. R. and Weil M. H. *Circulation* 1969, **39**, 131. *See also* Gilston A. in: *Recent Advances in Anaesthesia and Analgesia*—13 (Hewer C. L. and Atkinson R. S. ed.). Edinburgh: Churchill Livingstone, 1979.
27. *See* Allen F. M. and Crossman L. W. *Curr. Res. Anesth. Analg.* 1943, **22**, 5 (reprinted in 'Classical File', *Surv. Anesthesiol.* 1972, **16**, 279); *Anesthesiology* 1943, **4**, 12. *See also* Furnas D. W. *Anesthesiology* 1965, **26**, 344.
28. Larrey D. J. *Mémoires de Chirugie Militaire et Campagnes* 3, **503**, Smith, Paris, 1812.
29. Arnott J. *Lancet* 1848, **2**, 98 (*see also* Bird H. M. *Anaesthesia* 1949, **4**, 10).
30. Richardson B. W. *Med. Times Gaz.* 1866, **115**, 3 February; *Dublin J. Med. Sci.* 1867, **42**, 463.
31. Lister J. *Br. Med. J.* 1871, **1**, 30.
32. Redard C. *Cong. Franç. Chir., Paris*, 1891. Paris: Germer, Baillière, et Cie, p. 431.
33. Fay T. and Henry G. C. *Surg. Gynecol. Obstet.* 1938, **66**, 512.
34. Amoils S. P. *Arch. Ophthalmol.* 1967, **78**, 201.
35. Lewis M. I. et al. *Dis. Colon Rectum* 1969, **12**, 371.
36. Wood G. J. et al. *Lancet* 1979, **2**, 479; Hannington-Kiff J. G. *Lancet* 1978, **2**, 816.
37. Katz J. et al. *Anesthesiology* 1980, **51**, Suppl., 232.

| Chapter 18 | **ACCIDENTS, COMPLICATIONS AND SEQUELAE OF ANAESTHESIA** |

Mishaps in connection with anaesthesia have been categorized as follows:[1] (1) Failure of application of existing knowledge rather than ignorance (82%); (2) Highest frequency during maintenance period; (3) Disconnections between patient and machine (20%); (4) Inadvertent gas flow change (18%); (5) Inadequate experience of anaesthetist (16%); (6) Fatigue of anaesthetist (5%).

Deaths associated with anaesthesia are responsible for about 2% of overall surgical mortality, and the causes in order of frequency are:[2] (1) Hypovolaemia; (2) Respiratory depression following myoneural blockade; (3) Complications of intubation; (4) Inadequate postoperative care and supervision. (*See also* Chapter 20).

Respiratory Difficulties During Operation

Respiratory Obstruction

The signs are: (1) Inadequate tidal exchange; (2) Retraction of the chest wall and of the supraclavicular, infraclavicular and suprasternal spaces; (3) Excessive abdominal movement; (4) Use of accessory muscles of respiration; (5) Noisy breathing (unless obstruction is absolute and complete); (6) Cyanosis; (7) The natural heave of the chest and abdomen becomes replaced by an indrawing of the upper chest and an outpushing of the abdomen because of strong diaphragmatic action.

It must be remedied in all cases, after its cause has been diagnosed. It may be due to:

1. Obstruction at the lips. Especially in edentulous patients. Remedy is use of an oro- or nasopharyngeal airway.

2. Obstruction by the tongue. First mentioned by Hall in 1856.[3] Due to approximation of the tongue to the posterior pharyngeal wall ('swallowing the tongue'). It may be especially dangerous in the recovery phase. Much less likely to occur if the patient is nursed in the lateral position. The jaw is lifted up and forwards, a manoeuvre first described in 1874.[4] At the same time the atlanto-occipital joint (the head) is extended on the vertebral column. The genioglossus on each side is important in holding the tongue away from the posterior pharyngeal wall. There is phasic activity synchronous with breathing, and tone is maximal during inspiration. It is the abolition of this tone during anaesthesia which is a major contributor to obstruction. Once the atonic tongue falls into the pharynx, obliterating the pharyngeal lumen, the suction created by inspiration pulls the tongue further back, making the obstruction worse.[5] A pharyngeal airway (size 3 for man, size 2 for women, on average) is inserted and usually restores the airway.[6] If that fails, suxamethonium is injected intravenously and the patient ventilated via tracheal tube. A nasopharyngeal tube may overcome this obstruction.

3. Obstruction above the glottis. This may be due to a swab, a tooth, a foreign body, saliva, vomitus, blood or oedema. The obstructing material must be removed by the fingers, gravity, swabbing or suction. Very rarely, dislocation of the epiglottis or cysts or tumours of the epiglottis are encountered. Treatment as for tongue obstruction. Tracheostomy rarely necessary. Work done recently in Holland[7] suggests that it is the epiglottis which is responsible for airway obstruction because it is sucked over the glottis by inspiration and this takes place before the tongue makes contact with the posterior pharyngeal wall. Extension of the head overcomes this. The hyo-epiglottic ligament levers the epiglottis around the fulcrum of the thyro-epiglottic ligament, and this anterior motion of the hyoid, as provided by neck extension, clears the airway.

4. *Obstruction at the glottis.* This is due to: (*a*) Laryngeal spasm. (*b*) Sphincter-like closure of the aryepiglottic folds. (*c*) Approximation of the ventricular ligaments or false cords. (*d*) Impaction of the epiglottis into the larynx. The remedy is visual disimpaction via a laryngoscope after ensuring proper relaxation. (*e*) Occasionally in patients who have had a large dose of relaxant which is incompletely reversed, and have been intubated, respiratory obstruction develops after extubation because the relaxed cords, instead of becoming abducted during inspiration, become sucked in by the air-stream. (*f*) Foreign bodies, e.g. teeth, vomitus; laryngoscopy or bronchoscopy required.

Peripheral stimulation causing partial or complete spasm suggests the need for deeper anaesthesia. Such stimuli occur when the cervix uteri or anal sphincter are stretched, or when the coeliac plexus or its connections are stimulated.[8] Temporary cessation of surgical stimuli may be necessary occasionally. Complete spasm leading to increasing cyanosis and hypoxia is a potentially dangerous situation. It may resolve spontaneously, and oxygen is then given to restore arterial oxygen tension rapidly.

The condition may call for active treatment. If this is considered necessary, a short-acting muscle relaxant such as suxamethonium may be given i.v. or i.m. provided that means for artificial ventilation of the lungs are available. A small dose of non-depolarizing relaxant is often sufficient to abolish partial laryngeal spasm and may even result in increased tidal exchange. The passage of a tracheal tube between the cords ensures that the condition will not recur. It is a wise precaution always to have some suxamethonium within sight at induction of any anaesthetic.

If the patient is *in extremis*, a very large needle, e.g. Tuohy, or intravenous canula (e.g. size 12G) can be inserted into the larynx through the cricothyroid membrane and oxygen given by jet technique[9] or insufflation of air, 2–3 litres/min. Mini-tracheostomy sets are now available commercially. As a 'last-ditch' airway, the spike of a 'giving-set' which enters the infusion bottle can be thrust percutaneously into the trachea through a small incision and connected an oxygen supply line.[10] The Penlon tracheotome may be used.[11] Laryngostomy may be easier and quicker and need not cause postoperative laryngeal obstruction. Tracheostomy is needed only on the rarest occasions.

5. *Bronchospasm.* It is upon the patency of the bronchiolar lumen and the quiescence of the bronchial reflexes that smooth anaesthesia largely depends (Nosworthy).[12] Intubation makes bronchospasm worse but may become necessary. Irritability is greatest at the carina. Acute infection increases sensitivity. A tendency to asthma strongly predisposes to bronchial spasm and wheezing. Pulmonary oedema also interferes with ventilation.

Management. (1) Diagnosis of cause; inadequate depth of anaesthesia, asthmatic tendency of patient, acute anaphylactic reaction. It should be differentiated from blockage of the tracheal tube and from laryngospasm. (2)

Prevention by spraying larynx and trachea with lignocaine and maintaining anaesthesia at suitable depth with halothane; theophylline premedication; aminophylline suppositories. (3) Bronchodilatation; aminophylline 250–300 mg i.v. slowly, or ephedrine 10–30 mg i.v., salbutamol 1 mg i.v. or corticosteroids, e.g. hydrocortisone, 500 mg i.v. A careful administration of ether may help in the intractable patient.

Anaesthesia is incomplete unless the threshold of irritability has been raised sufficiently to prevent the stimulus of the moment from breaking through.

6. *Faults of apparatus*.[13] (1) Kinking of the tracheal tube or breathing tube; (2) Obstruction of the tracheal tube or connections; (3) Absence of gas flow to patient due to empty cylinders or disconnection.

Management. All the anaesthetic apparatus is removed. The anaesthetist then blows down the tracheal tube. If this fails to inflate the lungs, the tracheal tube is repositioned or removed. The lungs may be ventilated with oxygen by face-mask until the situation is restored. In the last resort, the lungs should be ventilated with air, using a mask and self-inflating bag.

Respiratory Abnormalities
These include:

1. *Tachypnoea* (light anaesthesia, trichloroethylene, halothane and ether).
2. *Slow breathing* (narcotic analgesics).
3. *Shallow breathing* (deep anaesthesia, cyclopropane, halothane, muscle relaxants, etc.) The remedy is to assist or control ventilation. Idiopathic hypoventilation can occur and has been remedied by a doxapram drip 1 mg/min.[14]
4. *Irregular breathing*. Occurs in light anaesthesia and also in deep planes, heralding respiratory arrest. Cheyne–Stokes respiration may occur as a result of over-dose with narcotic analgesics, in heart failure, head injury and renal failure and after chlorpromazine.

Coughing
Occurs most commonly due to inadequate depth of anaesthesia when volatile agents are used and when patient has chemical (e.g. due to heavy smoking) or infective inflammation of the upper air passages.

Coughing may cause trouble during anaesthesia with thiopentone; this is best controlled by nitrous-oxide–oxygen and halothane or use of a muscle relaxant. It may be due to irritation of the larynx from regurgitated gastric material, from the use of artificial airways or from saliva.

Sleep Apnoea
This is an absence of inflow of air into the nose and mouth occurring for at least 10 sec, and repeated more than 30 times during a 7-hour period of sleep. It may be central, obstructive or mixed. In handicapped patients during the postoperative period such attacks may cause oxygen desaturation and prove dangerous.[5]

Respiratory Arrest
Due to obstruction of the airway or to peripheral or central respiratory depression. Ondine's curse (named from the water sprite in German mythology who killed her victims by stopping respiration) a term first used in connection with anaesthesia by Severinghaus,[15] is primary alveolar hypoventilation (unexplained

apnoea). It may follow surgery of the cervical cord.[16] Failure of automatic control of respiration for up to 10 s may occur in normal REM sleep.

Treatment. After establishing the airway, using a tracheal tube if necessary, oxygen must be carried to the alveoli. The cause is then sought and remedied.

Hiccup

This is a state of intermittent spasm of the diaphragm, accompanied by sudden closure of the glottis.

Causes. Stimulation of sensory nerve endings of phrenic, which are connected with the coeliac and other intra-abdominal autonomic plexuses. The vagus may also act as part of the afferent arc of the reflex. Thus, through these pathways, hiccup may arise from impulses in any abdominal or thoracic viscus. May occur before surgery.

Central stimulation of the medulla may be causal in, for example, alcoholic intoxication, uraemia, encephalitis.

Treatment

1. During anaesthesia: (*a*) Deepening of anaesthesia by any method; (*b*) Administration of muscle relaxant in relatively large doses; (*c*) Periodic inhalation of carbon dioxide during spontaneous respiration to produce hyperpnoea; (*d*) Intravenous injection of 4–8 mg of methylamphetamine;[17] (*e*) Inhalation of amyl nitrite; (*f*) Metoclopramide; (*g*) Ephedrine 5 mg i.v., perhaps repeated;[18] (*h*) Chlorpromazine 20–25 mg i.v.;[17] (*i*) Pouring ice-cold saline into nares with cuffed tube in position;[19] (*j*) A short sharp blast of ether to stimulate the tracheobronchial mucosa;[20] (*k*) Droperidol 5 mg i.v.;[21] (*l*) Glucagon 10 mg i.v.[22]

2. Before or after anaesthesia: (*a*) Methylphenidate, intravenous injection of 20 mg; (*b*) Block of phrenic nerves—either unilateral or bilateral: 10 ml of 0·5% bupivacaine is suitable; injection is made at a depth of 1–2 cm along a line extending 5 cm laterally from a point 2 cm above the sternoclavicular joint.

Unfortunately, even bilateral division of the phrenic nerves may fail to cure hiccup, because of the associated spasm of the intercostal and accessory respiratory muscles.

(*See also* Annotation, *Br. Med. J.* 1971, **2**, 234; Williamson B. A. W. and Macintyre I. M. C. *Br. Med. J.* 1977, **2**, 501; Nathan M. D. *Laryngoscope* 1980, **90**, 1612.)

Sweating

Eccrine sweat glands are widespread and concentrated in the skin of the palms, soles, axillae and face. They are under sympathetic cholinergic neuronal control. Apocrine glands are confined to the axillae, perineum, buttocks and external genitals. The anaesthetist usually notices sweating on the forehead or face.

Causes. (1) Patient is too hot; (2) Hypercapnia; (3) Light anaesthesia; (4) Shock; (5) Anxiety and high nervous tone.

Treatment. If excessive, infusion of normal saline, after correction of the cause. Sweating is not necessarily a call for deeper anaesthesia.

Respiratory Complications After Operation

History

For many years following the introduction of surgical anaesthesia, postoperative chest complications were ascribed to pneumonia, presumably due to the irritation of anaesthetic gases and vapours on the bronchi and lungs. In fact, postoperative atelectasis was described by Sir. W. Gairdner of Glasgow in 1850.[23] Soon after the introduction of regional analgesia, in 1900, the great German surgeon J. von Mikulicz-Radecki (1850–1905) showed that chest complications followed general and regional anaesthesia with equal frequency. The concept of atelectasis was again revived by the English physician W. Pasteur in 1908.[24] The importance of aspiration into the bronchi and the removal of the obstructing material by bronchoscopic suction was pointed out in 1925,[25] while 2 years later the reduction in the vital capacity following abdominal operations was noticed.[26] Segmental atelectasis was described and its cause was shown to be absorption of air distal to the site of obstruction by material in the bronchial lumen with superadded infection.[27] Postoperative hypoxaemia was identified in 1930 as a frequent sequel to abdominal surgery due to underventilation because of abdominal pain on breathing.[28] In 1933, D. S. King, a chest physician, spent 2 years studying the question in the wards of the Massachusetts General Hospital and thereby greatly clarified the whole question of the postoperative chest.[29]

The great increase in the incidence of postoperative pulmonary complications in smokers as compared with non-smokers was emphasized during the Second World War.[30] Mendelson's description of the acid aspiration syndrome[31] pinpointed the cause of one type of chest pathology, while the concept of the wet lung was discussed in 1945, together with a suggestion that the relief of the causal pain could be greatly improved by intercostal nerve block.[32] This later became known as the adult respiratory distress syndrome.[33] The tracheobronchial toilet was described in 1942.[34]

The inhalation of isoprenaline, postural drainage and clapping percussion of the chest wall, before and after operation in those patients with bronchial secretion, was advocated in 1953.[35] Today the concepts that hypoxaemia is due to a disturbance in the relationship of ventilation to perfusion, that is, a regional underventilation, and the importance of airway closure as a cause are regarded as important. (*See also Johns Hopkins Hosp. Bull.* 1909, April, p. 125; Morton A. *Anaesth. Intensive Care* 1975, **3**, 239; Stoddart J. C. *Br. J. Anaesth.* 1978, **50**, 695; Morton A. and Baker A. B. *Anaesth. Intensive Care* 1978, **6**, 56; Vickers M. D. *Br. Med. J.* 1982, **284**, 292.)

Incidence

Complications may be expected in 5% of all operations; in at least 10% of abdominal operations. The commonest complication is segmental atelectasis due to retention of sputum from previous infection (acute, subacute or chronic) and absorption of air distal to the block. The commonest cause of the postoperative chest in the elderly is small airways collapse. (*See also* Saady A. *Anaesth Intensive Care* 1974, **2**, 221; Hewlett A. M. and Branthwaite M. A. *Br. J. Anaesth.* 1975, **47**, 102.)

Retention of Sputum

Causes

Poor expulsive mechanism after operation due to: (1) Pain; (2) Reduced movement of diaphragm which may be due to residual myoneural block, or to pain; (3) Sedatives; (4) A tight binder or dressing; (5) Spasm of muscles of abdominal wall; (6) Abolition of the physiological sigh; (7) Prolonged inhalation of cold, dry anaesthetic gas mixtures which decrease ciliary activity.[36]

Atelectasis

Diagnosis. (1) Rapid breathing—30–60/min.; (2) Rapid heart rate; (3) Absence of pain on inspiration, unless pleural surface of lung is involved; (4) Dilatation of alae nasi and slight cyanosis; (5) Restricted movements of affected side of chest; (6) Diminution of breath sounds and perhaps decreased resonance are almost normal after abdominal operations. When the condition is established, signs of consolidation are present; (7) Lower lobes usually involved; (8) Mediastinal displacement towards affected side, in gross cases; (9) Radiographic appearance may resemble that of bronchopneumonia. Elevation of one or other side of diaphragm very common after upper abdominal operations, in absence of clinical atelectasis. In atelectasis there is contraction of lung tissue; in bronchopneumonia, swelling. Occasionally, an unresolving chest condition after operation is tuberculous. *Massive collapse* causes pain in the chest of sudden onset, dyspnoea, cyanosis, fever, tachycardia and mediastinal shift. The complications of atelectasis are bronchopneumonia, pleural effusion and bronchiectasis.

Results. (1) Inequalities of ventilation/perfusion; (2) Arterial hypoxaemia; (3) Secondary bacterial infection.

Treatment. Physiotherapy, with intelligent use of analgesics (e.g. narcotic analgesics, Entonox). The patient must attempt to clear the bronchial tree by expectoration. When problems are anticipated, continuous extradural block or other regional technique is helpful. If sputum cannot be removed, other measures must be considered such as aspiration of sputum via a tracheal tube or bronchoscope. Postoperative doxapram, and postoperative inhalation of warm humidified air have been recommended.[36] In certain patients, intermittent mandatory ventilation may be required. (*See* Chapter 15.)

Complications. (1) Arterial hypoxaemia, which may in turn cause cerebral hypoxia and restlessness; oxygen should be administered; (2) Bronchopneumonia which may need antibiotic treatment; (3) Lung abscess which should be treated initially by physiotherapy and postural drainage; (4) Respiratory failure which may need IPPV.

Prevention. Prophylactic injection of 10 ml of co-trimoxazole (Septrin) in 250 ml of normal saline, 1 h preoperatively, has been recommended.[37] Excessive sedation is to be avoided but proper analgesia is necessary. Deep breathing and coughing should take place at least once each hour, and is made less painful by the use of the Barlow belt which supports the patient's abdomen.[38] The nurse should be constantly rallying the patient, to avoid hypoventilation and hypostasis. Cough should be especially encouraged soon after a dose of narcotic analgesic; the abdomen can be held firm while the patient is coughing.

Control of pain by extradural analgesia allows free movement of the chest and good expectoration. Small volumes of analgesic solution injected at the appropriate level achieve pain relief without fall of blood pressure, as may extradural injection of a narcotic analgesic.[39] (*See* Chapter 32.)

Factors Influencing Sputum Retention and Atelectasis

Site of operation. Most common after upper abdominal operations, especially if oblique or transverse incisions are not used.[40] Fairly common following operations for hernia. Of non-abdominal operations, thyroidectomy is most often followed by chest complications. Pulmonary embolism commonest after pelvic operations.

Oral sepsis. Pulmonary suppuration may occur in patients with dental sepsis: (1)

Independently of operation; (2) Following operation under general anaesthesia; (3) Following dental extraction. The onset may be delayed for 3 weeks after operation. As a routine, dental sepsis should be eradicated 3 weeks before operation. If inhalation of a foreign body is suspected, early radiography and perhaps bronchoscopy are necessary.

Obesity. (See also Chapter 22.)

Sex. Males affected three times as frequently as females.

Age. More frequent in older age groups.

Season. More frequent in cold weather.

Respiratory muscle fatigue. This is a recently recognized entity, part of a generalized muscle fatigue after anaesthesia and operation.[41]

Smoking. By causing bronchial exudation, smoking greatly increases incidence of chest complications.

Duration of operation. (See also p. 353.)

Anaesthetic. Very little to choose between different agents and techniques, if administration is skilful. The sooner the return of the reflexes the better. Contamination of airways, tubes and lubricants may be a factor.

Pre-existing lung disease. (See also p. 109.)

The certain cause of postoperative hypoxaemia is not understood and adequate pain relief and physiotherapy, although helpful, do not always prevent this complication.

Aspiration Pneumonitis

Aspiration of stomach contents may occur before, during or after operation. Mendelson described the acid aspiration syndrome of late pregnancy in 1946[31] (*see* Chapter 27). Trouble may occur after aspiration of stomach contents of any pH, while solid material may cause obstruction. It is due to the damage to the respiratory epithelium and the vascular endothelium, resulting in leakage of fluid into the alveoli and interstitial spaces, increase of water in the lungs, reduced pulmonary compliance and acute pulmonary oedema. The clinical signs may be delayed.

Diagnosis

(1) Cyanosis, unrelieved by oxygen therapy; (2) Tachypnoea; (3) Tachycardia; (4) Prostration; (5) Coarse asthmatic rhonchi on auscultation—may not occur for some hours; (6) Chest radiograph shows area of density; (7) Cardiovascular failure may supervene. Hypotension, pulmonary oedema; usually lasts 2–4 h if the patient survives.

Management

(1) Repeated tracheal aspiration, perhaps associated with periodic intratracheal injections of up to 10 ml normal saline. Preoxygenation is advisable before suction, especially in patients with heart disease, to prevent a fall in the Pa_{O_2}; (2) Oxygen administration; (3) Treatment of cardiovascular failure; Digitalization, pressor drugs or intravenous fluids may produce pulmonary oedema (colloids are preferable to electrolytes); (4) Bronchodilator drugs; (5) Hydrocortisone may be useful; (6) Antibiotics to prevent infection, e.g. ampicillin, 500 mg 6-hourly; (7) IPPV may be required; (8) Bronchoscopy if the presence of solid material is suspected.

(*See* Zorab J. *Br. Med. J.* 1984, **288**, 1631.)

Chest physiotherapy. This may include deep breathing exercises, encouragement of coughing, postural drainage of pulmonary secretions, vibration and percussion of the chest. Routine prophylactic chest physiotherapy is said to decrease the frequency of chest infection after operation.[42]

Lung Abscess

When foreign material is introduced into the trachea, it gravitates into the dependent apex of the lower lobe with the patient lying supine, and into the dependent upper lobe with the patient on his side: these are the commonest sites of abscess. Onset may be mild, after a latent period of 2–10 days, simulating bronchitis or early bronchopneumonia. Cough, dry hacking, appears, together with wasting, chills, anorexia, etc. A leucocytosis develops, and the temperature starts to swing. Radiology in the early stages usually shows an area of consolidation. When the abscess erodes into a bronchus, foul mucopurulent sputum is coughed up and a minority of patients achieve spontaneous cure. Those who do not require postural drainage, suitable antibiotic treatment and, perhaps, operation. Occasionally, a lung abscess ruptures into the pleura, forming an empyema and a bronchopleural fistula. Such an empyema should be drained, if necessary, with the patient sitting, not lying down; local analgesia should be used; these measures prevent the patient from being drowned in his own pus.

The earliest X-ray sign is a patch of consolidation; later a fluid level may be seen.

Surgical Emphysema during Anaesthesia

This was first reported in 1912[43] during insufflation endotracheal anaesthesia. Surgical emphysema may commence as a pulmonary interstitial emphysema due to overdistension of the alveoli. The gas tracks along the sheaths of the vessels to the hilum—mediastinal emphysema, from which it may spread: (1) To the neck; (2) To the abdomen; (3) Behind the peritoneum; (4) Into the pleura (tension pneumothorax). Tension pneumothorax should always be looked for if surgical emphysema appears. Mediastinal emphysema often causes a crushing sound when the stethoscope is applied to the left border of the heart—Hamman's sign.[44] Radiologically there may be a small air space running parallel to the left or right border of the heart. Causes of mediastinal emphysema include pulmonary emphysema, asthma, pneumonia, childbirth, rupture of an air passage or of the oesophagus, penetrating wounds of the chest and tracheostomy, particularly when associated with IPPV. May be mild or very severe. Should circulatory or respiratory difficulty arise in the presence of mediastinal emphysema, an incision should be made at the root of the neck anteriorly and gas should be let out by blunt dissection.

Pneumothorax

This may occur due to malfunction of a ventilator,[45] as a result of accidental opening of the pleural cavity during operations such as cervical sympathectomy, rib resection and nephrectomy. During the operation, the lungs should be inflated to expel air as the hole is closed. Pneumothorax can also occur as a complication of anaesthetic techniques such as intercostal or brachial plexus blocks or IPPV, especially if PEEP is used. It can arise as a complication of surgical emphysema, and also during laparoscopy.

Pneumoretroperitoneum can occur.[46]

Hypoxaemia after General Anaesthesia

The Pao_2 decreases after general anaesthesia, even when respiratory function appears to be normal; the reason is often unknown. It is influenced by the site of operation, the age, the presence or absence of cardiorespiratory disease, obesity and the duration of operation[47] and the nature of the drugs used by the anaesthetist. There is an inverse correlation between age and Pao_2 before surgery in patients awaiting operation and also in the postoperative period. The Pao_2 falls with age, about 0.13 kPa for every 4 years of life, so that in old age dangerously low levels may be seen.[48] The cause of this hypoxaemia may be a mismatching of ventilation/perfusion, a shunt resulting from increase in the closing volume of the lungs (this increases also with adoption of the supine position and as a result of cigarette smoking) and perhaps to progressive inactivation of pulmonary surfactant through failure to take periodic deep breaths postoperatively. Oxygen desaturation (Sao_2) is frequent after operation under general anaesthesia, but less after regional analgesia.[49] Oxygen therapy is beneficial after operation. After abdominal operations there is a fall in functional residual capacity so that airways closure may occur in the tidal volume range. Oxygen should be given after abdominal operation to all ill patients, to those with hypoventilation from any cause, and to those having a metabolic acidosis or a fixed low cardiac output; 30–40 % oxygen is beneficial. The MC (Mary Catterall), Harris and 35 % Ventimask devices are useful. Periodic deep breathing is of the greatest importance. The maintenance of nitrogen in the alveoli during operation does not improve oxygenation either during or after surgery. Oxygen desaturation can be measured easily by pulse oximetry.

The bad effect of atropine premedication on hypoxaemia after operation is greater if it is given subcutaneously than if injected intravenously. It is said to increase the dead space, both physiological and anatomical. There is a local pulmonary alveolar vascular reflex which regulates perfusion in response to ventilation: atropine blocks this and leads to the removal of blood from the lungs into the systemic circulation. This may well be of more theoretical than practical importance. (*See also* Alexander J. I. et al *Br. J. Anaesth.* 1973, **54**, 34; Stoddart J. C. *Br. J. Anaesth.* 1978, **50**, 695; Annotation, *Br. Med. J.* 1978, **2**, 1452; Jones J. G. et al. *J. R. Soc. Med.* 1985, **78**, 1019.)

For the administration of an oxygen-enriched mixture, it has been shown that the disposable Oxygenaire mask supplied with oxygen at a flow-rate of 2 litres/min relieves desaturation and does not cause significant hypercapnia.

Extradural block may give some protection from postoperative chest complications but it is more effective after upper than after lower abdominal surgery. The injection of either a narcotic analgesic or a local analgesic solution, through an extradural catheter, is often beneficial, in the immediate postoperative period.

(*See also* Symposium, *Surg. Clin. North Am.* 1980, December, 60; Craig D. *Anesth. Analg. (Cleve.)* 1981, **60**, 46.)

Pulmonary Embolism

This is more common in medical than in surgical wards, especially in patients with heart disease and carcinoma. Massive thrombosis and embolism more frequent in old than in young patients and in septic cases and those having undergone long and difficult operations. Prolonged bed-rest, e.g. in patients with hip fractures, increases the risk. Condition usually associated with venous thrombosis in legs or pelvis. Onset may coincide with getting up or straining at stool. Sudden onset of pain in chest from second to fourteenth day after operation. Usually during second week. This may be small and ephemeral or large and fatal.

Signs
Tachycardia, a rise in the central venous pressure—distended neck veins; hypotension; cyanosis; sometimes gallop rhythm; râles and friction sounds and, later, dullness and bronchial breathing. *Radiographs of chest* may show right-sided cardiac enlargement; elevation of dome of diaphragm; shadow in the lower zone and, later, clouding in costophrenic angle due to pleural effusion. *Electrocardiograph* is abnormal in about one-half the cases and may show an S wave in limb Lead I, a Q wave in Lead III and T wave inversion in Lead III; these represent right heart strain.

Symptoms
Faintness, dyspnoea, substernal discomfort, pleural pain and haemoptysis. Pain is usually less severe than that in myocardial infarction and may be absent. Jaundice, due to haemolysis of the blood in the infarct, may be seen.

   If the embolus is massive, there is profound shock, sweating, pallor, air hunger, raised venous pressure and anxiety. Death usually follows quickly, but recoveries have been reported. Trendelenburg's operation of embolectomy has been done successfully.[50] Small emboli are often overlooked, the patient complaining only of faintness, tightness in chest; duration short, no physical signs. Non-fatal attacks are three or four times as common as fatal attacks. (*See also* Sutton P. P. *Br. J. Hosp. Med.* 1981, **25**, 144.)

Diagnosis
In typical cases after operation, there is a short period of fever suggesting thrombosis, followed by apyrexia and then the onset of embolism. Should be thought of when there is tachycardia, haemoptysis, jaundice or unilateral effusion after operation. It is often misdiagnosed as atelectasis or pneumonia. Sudden pain in the chest within 3 weeks of operation is due to embolism unless it can be proved otherwise. The condition accounts for about 6% of deaths associated with surgical operation.

   Pulmonary embolism has replaced pneumonia as the commonest type of chest disease in hospital practice and has replaced syphilis as the great imitator. The clinical, radiological and ECG features of the condition are most commonly confused with those of pleurisy, pneumonia and cardiac infarction and pulmonary embolism should be excluded in all such cases. It may also simulate cardiac asthma, bronchial asthma, pyrexia of unknown origin, atelectasis and pulmonary neoplasm. It causes pulmonary hypertension with right ventricular dilatation, engorged neck veins, enlarged liver; together with reduced left ventricular output, hypotension with impaired cerebral and coronary perfusion.

Treatment
Sedation, anticoagulants to prevent chronic pulmonary hypertension and oxygen. Streptokinase therapy is of benefit in some cases.

Pulmonary Embolism during Operation

Characterized by increasing cyanosis with adequate oxygen ventilation, good expansion of the lungs with IPPV and a falling blood pressure. The classic causes are: (1) Hypernephroma; (2) Liquor amni (in obstetric patients); (3) Detachment of a venous clot in the leg, following the application of an Esmarch bandage.[51]

See also Air Embolism (*below*).

Prevention of Pulmonary Embolism

This largely consists in the prevention, diagnosis and treatment of deep-vein thrombosis. Most thrombi occur in the calf veins, but it is only when thrombosis extends into the iliofemoral veins or originates in pelvic veins that it is likely to lead to pulmonary embolism. Deep-vein thrombosis usually occurs during or very soon after operation. There is reduced fibrinolytic activity after operation. An abrupt rise in platelet count and shortening of clotting time occurs within a few hours of the start of an operation. The mutual adhesiveness of the blood platelets increases from the fourth to the twelfth postoperative day.

Venous Thrombosis

Predisposing Factors

(1) Obesity; (2) Old age; (3) Certain operations, especially splenectomy, major operations on the hip and retropubic prostatectomy; (4) Myocardial infarction; (5) Malignant disease; (6) Patients who have been in bed for some days before operation often come to surgery with thrombophlebitis well established; (7) Oral contraceptives increase the incidence and may require low-dosage heparin therapy (*see below*); (8) History of previous thrombophlebitis.[52]

The role of platelets in the formation of haemostatic plugs and in thrombosis was first described by Giulio Bizzozero, Turin physician (1846–1901) in 1882. Antiplatelet drugs include: aspirin, sulphinpyrazone, dipyridamole, low dose heparin, ancrod and dextran.

One important factor in the complex pathogenesis of venous thrombosis is a defective fibrinolytic system. This may involve defective synthesis and release of tissue plasminogen activator and an increased concentration of the inhibitor against tissue plasminogen activator.[53]

Diagnosis

(1) Clinical examination: even when carefully done, this is very inefficient; popliteal cysts may be mistaken for thrombophlebitis; (2) Ascending phlebography; (3) The ultra-sound method; (4) Radio-immune assay;[54] (5) Use of autologous indium-111-labelled platelets;[55] (6) X-ray venography.[56]

Prevention[57]

Elimination of stasis. Reduction of coagulability of blood. Frequent movements of the ankles, feet and toes during the postoperative period and early movement. The patient should be up or in bed, and not in a chair.

Other measures which should be aggressively pursued include: (1) Early ambulation; (2) Elevation of the legs during operation; (3) Intermittent pneumatic compression of the calf, replacing the normal calf-muscle pump effect; (4) Knee-high elastic supports; (5) A heel cushion for use on the operating table, preventing pressure on calf veins; (6) Low-dose subcutaneous heparin (*see below*); (7) Electrical stimulation of calf muscles during operation; (8) Intravenous infusion of dextran 70. Infusion of 500–1000 ml (or 7–15 ml/kg) of dextran 70 has been shown to be effective in reducing the incidence of postoperative pulmonary embolism in gynaecological, general surgical operations and orthopaedic operations.[58] Dextran 70, 500 ml can be given during the operation and then daily for 2–5 days postoperatively;[59] (9) High doses of aspirin[60] (up to 1 g daily) and dipyridamole (Persantin) 100 mg four times daily, by mouth. Low-dose heparin or external pneumatic calf compression are the methods of choice in patients over 40 undergoing operations. Warfarin or antiplatelet agents may be indicated in patients undergoing total hip replacement;[61] (10) Oral contraceptives containing oestrogen may be withheld for 4–6 weeks before major surgery.[62] (*See* Chapter 24).

(*See also* Russell J. I. *Surg. Gynecol. Obstet.* 1983, **89**, 157; Buckler P. and Douglas A. S. *Br. Med. J.* 1983, **287**, 585.)

Anticoagulants
(1) Direct anticoagulant: heparin; (2) Indirect anticoagulants: the coumarins and the indanediones. These are both hypothrombinaemic agents. They reduce the synthesis of clotting factors II, VII, IX and X in the liver.

Heparin
First discovered in 1916 by a medical student in Baltimore.[63] Must be given by injection, 100–300 units being equal to 1 mg.
Action. Acts as an antithrombin. Effects come on a few minutes after injection and pass off after half-life of 2–3 h.
Prophylactic uses. 5000 units of calcium heparin can be given subcutaneously 2 h before operation and 8-hourly after operation for 7–10 days,[64] to prevent venous thrombosis. Can also be given in ultra-low dosage.[65] Low molecular weight heparin has also been recommended.[66] A single daily injection of low molecular weight heparin fraction (1850 APTT units) provides effective prevention against postoperative major pulmonary embolism.[67] (*See also* p. 376.)

Coumarins[68] and Indanediones
They act, probably , on the liver but only after being absorbed into the body and there is a delay of about 12 h before their effect takes place. Usually taken orally.
Activity of oral anticoagulants affected by: (1) Any acute illness or weight loss (increased effect); (2) Gastrointestinal upsets (reduced effect); (3) Oral anticoagulants may be potentiated by: alcohol, aspirin and its analogues, chlorpromazine, cimetidine, glucagon, metronidazole, triclofos sodium, chloral hydrate, diflunisal, certain antidepressants (tricyclics and mono-amine oxidase inhibitors), aminoglycoside antibiotics, and sulphonamides. Their effects may be inhibited by: barbiturates, antacids, antihistamines, corticosteroids and vitamins K_1 and K_2.
Control of anticoagulant effect. Heparin effect is measured by estimating the clotting time of whole blood. The oral anticoagulant drugs are assessed by the prothrombin time of Quick and by the thrombotest on capillary blood. The coagulating mechanism should be depressed so that it is two to two and a half times control value by the Quick test or 10–20% with the thrombotest.

Contraindications. History of bleeding, pregnancy, liver or kidney failure, malignant hypertension, subacute endocarditis.

Antidotes

For heparin, protamine sulphate,[69] a polycationic peptide obtained from the sperm of certain genera of fish; a strongly positive basic protein used to antagonize the negatively charged heparin[70] (*see also* p. 376) 1 mg for every 100 units given in the last dose of heparin, e.g. 5 ml of 1%, slowly. It is a myocardial depressant.[71] For oral anticoagulants, phytomenadione (vitamin K_1) 5–10 mg repeated as necessary by mouth, intramuscularly or intravenously.

Fibrinolytic Drugs

Urokinase and streptokinase which convert plasminogen to plasmin which dissolves fibrin and fibrinogen.

Surgery on Patients Taking Dicoumarol- and Indanedione-type Anticoagulant Drugs

If the prothrombin time is near the lower border of therapeutic level (e.g. one and a half to twice normal), the operation is usually safe. If it is longer than this, the operation is deferred for 48 h or, in emergency, vitamin K or K_1 10 mg is given i.v. Its action is surprisingly rapid. Fresh whole-blood transfusion also restores the prothrombin level.

Cardiovascular System

For *shock, see* Chapter 35.
For *cardiac arrest, see* Chapter 37.

Cardiac Dysrhythmias

When associated with anaesthesia and operation, were first reported in 1920.[72] May be associated with: (1) Pre-existing cardiac pathology; (2) Hypercapnia, hypoxaemia, toxaemia, drugs, etc.; (3) Electrolyte imbalance or dehydration; (4) Myocardial ischaemia or infarction.

The following may occur:

1. Sinus tachycardia: does not normally require treatment.

2. Bradycardia: usually responds to small dose of atropine (0·1 mg increments) and reduction of concentration or withdrawal of causative agent (i.e. halothane).

3. Atrial or ventricular premature contractions; usually benign and require no specific treatment other than correction of hypercapnia if present and reduction in concentration of inhalation agent.

4. Supraventricular tachycardia.

5. Ventricular tachycardia: this can be important as it can result in impairment of cardiac output and may proceed to ventricular fibrillation.

6. Nodal rhythm: common with inhalation anaesthetics; responds to intravenous atropine but seldom of serious significance.

Coronary arterial spasm may occur in non-cardiac operations, diagnosed by the ECG and relieved by infusion of nitroglycerin.[73]

Hypertension in the Immediate Postoperative Period
Possible causes are: (1) Pain; (2) Hypercapnia; (3) Emergence delirium; (4) Unsuspected phaeochromocytoma (extremely rare); (5) After coronary artery bypass grafting. A history of hypertension should be taken into consideration.

Air Embolism
This was first reported in 1821 by Magendie,[74] and by Barlow in 1830.[75]

Causes
   1. *Surgical.* Operations involving injury to veins in the neck, thorax, breast and pelvis; operations on the brain and cord in the sitting position; operations on the heart; uterine curettage and insufflation. Gas embolism may complicate irrigation of semi-closed cavities with hydrogen peroxide (e.g. the mastoid).
   2. *Diagnostic and therapeutic injection of air into:* Peritoneal cavity, pleural cavity, large joints, urinary bladder, tissue spaces, e.g. the perinephric area and nasal antra, uterus and tubes.
   3. *Surgical emphysema.*
   4. *Accidental entrance of air.* During intravenous techniques.
Factors of importance. (1) The volume of air; (2) The speed of injection; (3) The pressure in the veins; (4) Posture; (5) General condition of patient.

Signs and Symptoms
If air enters the veins in any quantity it will cause a hissing sound in the wound and it will go to the right heart and lung, causing an air-lock obstruction in the pulmonary artery. This may result in a loud precordial murmur, the so-called 'mill-wheel murmur'. It has been suggested that this term should be replaced by 'squelching gum-boot murmur' as the sound of the mill-wheel is unfamiliar to most modern anaesthetists.[76] There will also be sudden cyanosis, hypotension, engorged neck veins, tachycardia, irregular gasping respiration, progressing through tachypnoea and hypopnoea and followed by cardiac arrest.
   Early diagnosis can be made if: (1) An oesophageal stethoscope is in place;[77] (2) A Doppler ultrasonic flow detector is on the precordium;[78] (3) Monitoring of end tidal CO_2; It will fall abruptly if blood does not reach the lungs; (4) Detection by continuous infra-red CO_2 analyser; (5) The ECG shows very marked ST depression.

Treatment
(1) Prevent further entrance of air into the circulation, if necessary by compressing the neck veins to raise venous pressure locally; (2) Lower the head end of the table to keep air out of the cerebral vessels and if possible flood the wound with saline; (3) Place the patient on his left side so that bubbles are carried away from the mouth of the pulmonary artery;[79] (4) Give pure oxygen and stop administration of nitrous oxide which is more soluble in blood than nitrogen and so will increase the size of the emboli. If the lung is damaged, IPPV will require great care; (5) Insertion of a pulmonary artery catheter (Swan–Ganz) and aspiration directly from the right heart;[77] (6) If rapid improvement is not noticed, the right thorax should be opened, air aspirated from the heart and manual cardiac compression carried out. Defibrillation may be necessary, as also may the aspiration of froth from the ventricles, via a

large-bore needle. For severe cases, compression in a hyperbaric chamber has been suggested.[80]

Air in the coronary circulation may present as ST elevation or depression, or widening of the QRS complex.[81]

A patent foramen ovale can be demonstrated in 20–30% of patients, using a probe, post-mortem. Paradoxical air embolism is a danger in neurosurgical operations in the sitting position.[82]

Status Lymphaticus[83]

It is sometimes stated that sudden death during anaesthesia in children is due to status lymphaticus, whereas it may well be due to error of technique or judgement on the part of the anaesthetist and be, in fact, an anaesthetic fiction.

Posture[84]

Trendelenburg Position[85]

Experimental work has shown that tilting into a steep Trendelenburg position in young patients under light anaesthesia has no effect on the gas tension of arterial blood, and none on the pH, minute volume and respiratory rate.[86] In short stout patients, especially if there is an abdominal mass, pressure on the diaphragm from the bowel may produce cyanosis and dyspnoea and reduction of vital capacity by 15% unless IPPV is carried out. Except in very short operations, IPPV is preferable to spontaneous ventilation. Cyanosis also occurs in the face and neck of plethoric patients in this position, as a result of stagnant hypoxia due to gravity even in the presence of adequate ventilation.

If the arm is abducted, the elbow should be slightly flexed and pronated to prevent pull on the brachial plexus, and the head turned to the side of the arm, but every care should be taken to avoid this position of arm abduction with the head-down tilt.

Trendelenburg position may, however, have a harmful effect on the cardiovascular system, especially in shock where it can cause a fall in arterial pressure and cerebral perfusion. Prolonged head-down tilt can cause cerebral oedema and retinal detachment. Increased venous return can always be improved by raising the legs with the patient horizontal.

Position can be maintained by Langton Hewer's corrugated mattress.[87] Great care is needed to prevent pressure on nerves or stretching of nerve trunks.

Steep Trendelenburg position is now rarely necessary. Some degree of tilt may, however, be preferable to deepening the level of anaesthesia or the injection of an extra dose of muscle relaxant in certain patients.

Prone Position

The functional residual capacity is greater than in the supine position. In fit patients, IPPV does not significantly reduce ventilation perfusion mismatch. A pillow should be placed under each shoulder and another under the pelvis, so that breathing is not unduly interfered with and so that all pressure is completely removed from the abdomen and its large venous channels. A cuffed tracheal tube is a wise precaution in case regurgitation of stomach contents should occur. Fat subjects tolerate this position badly. The unconscious patient when moved can easily suffer skeletal injury. To prevent harm coming to heavy patients during turning, intubation can be performed in the conscious state after local analgesia and neurolept agents, so that the patient can co-operate in the movement. Retinal arterial occlusion and blindness from pressure on the eye have been reported.[88]

Lithotomy Position
When the lithotomy position is required, both legs should be moved together to avoid strain on the pelvic ligaments. If the patient is arranged while supine so that the anterior superior iliac spines are on a level with the break in the table, he will be in a good lithotomy position when the legs are supported on the stirrups and will need no further pulling about, with its risk of dislodgement of intravenous needles. The knee should be outside any metal supports.

Lateral Position
This handicaps the patient's breathing. A bridge makes it still worse, so it should be used as little as possible and for a short time only; it may be associated with hypotension. In the lateral position with the patient breathing spontaneously, both ventilation and perfusion are concentrated in the lower lung, while IPPV diverts ventilation to the upper lung, thus increasing mismatch; so spontaneous ventilation has some advantages here.

Supine Position
Pressure on and stretching of nerves of arm must be avoided by care of the arms. The following methods may be used during operation to secure the arms: (1) Each arm can be well tucked under the buttock, palm down, with the wrists held in place by a plastic J-shaped splint; (2) A draw sheet is passed under the back and over the arms, which are at the side of the body. The free ends are then firmly tucked under the buttocks, imprisoning the arms; (3) Wrist straps are firmly attached to a broad strap surrounding the table, or to the table direct; (4) Arms can be securely wrapped up at the side of the chest, with elbows flexed, in the patient's nightgown. This is useful when the gallbladder bridge is to be employed; (5) One or both arms are abducted to a right-angle *anterior* to the coronal plane of the body and secured to a padded arm-table or padded board. Arm-rests attached to the table are desirable, as they do not move with the patient; (6) Neck, knees and hip should be slightly flexed.

Firm fixation is especially necessary if light anaesthesia is to be employed or if the patient is to be operated on in the conscious state. In these cases, in addition, a padded strap should be passed just above the knees and firmly secured beneath the table.

Legs should be flat on the table, not crossed one over the other. The tendo Achillis must not rest on the unpadded edge of the table. A soft pad, raising heels from the table, avoids pressure on the calf veins, and so may lessen the incidence of thrombosis occurring at this site.

Postoperative backache is not infrequent after operations performed in the supine position. It can often be prevented by the use of an inflatable wedge, as a lumbar support.[89]

Effect of Posture on Respiration
The kidney, prone, jack-knife and Trendelenburg positions may cause reduced ventilation; lateral, reverse Trendelenburg and gallbladder positions a smaller

reduction. The lithotomy and prone positions cause no significant changes.

Effect of Posture on Blood Pressure
(1) The Trendelenburg position aids venous return to the heart. Conversely, head-up tilt may be associated with fall of blood pressure and the venous return to the heart may be diminished (with resultant hypotension); (2) Hypotension may occur during handling of organs within the abdomen; (3) Insertion of abdominal packs prior to pelvic surgery; (4) Raising of gallbladder bridge; (5) In the presence of large abdominal tumours, including the pregnant uterus, particularly when minimal external pressure is applied; (6) When the table 'break' is applied for the exposure of a kidney.

Effect of Changes of Position of Head and Neck
A patient with a decreased cardiac output, carotid artery occlusive disease, etc. may be deprived of cerebral blood supply by changes in position altering the relationships of the vertebral vessels to surrounding bony structures as by rotation of the head, hyperextension of the neck at the atlanto-occipital joint to maintain a clear airway. This can be tested for at the preoperative examination. Full extension may result in a faint.

Moving the Patient
Anaesthetized patients stand moving badly; this is especially so when the blood pressure is low. All movements should be smooth and gentle, not jerky and rough. If a canvas stretcher is not available, three people should, if possible, lift the patient, who should be rotated on to his side, face to the lifters, as soon as he is lifted from the bed or trolley.

Position in Bed
The patient should lie in the semi-prone position until his reflexes return. This is maintained by a pillow between the bed and the chest; the lower arm is placed behind the trunk; the upper knee is flexed. This helps to maintain a free airway by causing the tongue to fall away from the posterior pharyngeal wall; it also helps to prevent aspiration of vomitus into the air passages. The patient should not be placed in a head-up position until it is quite certain that his cardiovascular system is able to maintain an adequate circulation through the brain. Otherwise syncopal reactions and even death may occur.

About 20% of the deaths associated with anaesthesia occur during the first 30 min after operation.

Vomiting and Regurgitation

The practising anaesthetist is constantly faced with the problem of the aspiration of material from the alimentary canal into the air passages during induction, maintenance and immediately after anaesthesia.

The Applied Anatomy of Vomiting
The expulsion through the mouth of material from the alimentary tract by muscular action. The act of vomiting is preceded by salivation, rapid breathing, pallor, sweating, tachycardia and severe discomfort.

Like any other reflex arc, vomiting has its afferent and efferent pathways and its central connections.

Afferent Pathways

Impulses travel from many parts of the body and ascend in the visceral afferent fibres accompanying the vagus and, less importantly, the sympathetic.

Chemical changes occurring in the body do not stimulate the vomiting centre directly but reflexly by stimulating the chemoreceptor trigger zone of Borison and Wang[90] in the area postrema of the 4th ventricle which contains a mass of dopamine receptors, such chemicals being carried in the bloodstream or the cerebrospinal fluid. This stimulates the vomiting centre. Other chemical stimuli can arise from the alimentary tract (e.g. drugs, poisons, emetics, etc.).

The Vomiting Centre

This is closely related to other vital centres, e.g. the respiratory and vasomotor centres and the salivary and vestibular nuclei, in the dorsolateral border of lateral reticular formation. The chemoreceptor trigger zone lies superficial to the true vomiting centre.

The Act of Vomiting

This commences with a deep inspiration followed by closure of the glottis and nasopharynx and is immediately followed by expiration together with contraction of the muscles of the abdominal wall and descent of the diaphragm. Now, while the body of the stomach relaxes, the antrum and also the pylorus and duodenum contract. This propels stomach contents into the oesophagus and mouth, and prevents escape from the stomach via the pylorus. A pressure of $40\,cmH_2O$ is needed to lift the contents of the stomach into the mouth in the upright position. The cardia is elevated during vomiting so that the abdominal part of the oesophagus rises into the chest. While the glottis goes into spasm during the expulsive phase, it soon relaxes, so that aspiration of stomach contents into the bronchial tree is almost bound to happen in the unconscious supine patient. Predisposing factors during anaesthesia include: (1) Hypoxia; (2) Central stimulation during second stage general anaesthesia—either during induction or recovery; (3) Irritation of the base of the tongue or pharynx by airways, etc.; (4) Breath-holding and cough.

Vomiting is undesirable because: (1) It is most unpleasant; (2) It may result in aspiration into the airway; (3) It may harm the eye, skin flaps or other areas, recently operated on; (4) It may raise intraocular or intra-abdominal pressure and so interfere with healing.

Regurgitation

Being a passive act, regurgitation may be silent and unheralded, and so even more potentially dangerous than vomiting. The major mechanism preventing regurgitation is the barrier pressure; i.e. the difference between intragastric pressure and the pressure exerted by the lower oesophageal sphincter. Predisposing factors include: (1) The head-down position if the cardia is inefficient; (2) A stomach full of fluid; (3) An indwelling stomach or oesophageal tube.

Drugs favouring reflux include atropine, tricyclic antidepressants, phenothiazines, antihistamines, and ganglion-blocking agents. The tone of the lower oesophageal sphincter is increased by metoclopramide and ranitidine.[91]

The barrier pressure is increased by pancuronium and vecuronium.[92]

The Cardiac Sphincter

This is both a sphincter and a valve. It remains closed because of: (1) The presence of an anatomical muscular sphincter; (2) Folds of thickened mucosa in the oesophagus; (3) The angle at which the oesophagus meets the fundus of the stomach; (4) The pinch-cock action of the crus of the diaphragm (in two-thirds of patients the right crus only).

Integrity of the Sphincter

Its activity is controlled reflexly (vagus and sympathetic nerves). Its integrity is affected and it is made incompetent by: (1) Anatomical abnormality, e.g. hiatus hernia; (2) The presence of a stomach tube; (3) Passage of anaesthetic gas from above during attempts at IPPV; (4) Attempts at active respiration in the presence of respiratory obstruction; (5) Intravenous atropine or hyoscine—this effect may be antagonized by metoclopramide which itself increases the tone; dosage: 10 mg i.v. and by domperidone 10 mg before induction;[93] This agent is said to have fewer side-effects than metoclopramide, but on i.v. injection has caused cardiac standstill;[94] (6) Atropine 1 mg with neostigmine 2·5 mg decreases the sphincter tone, whereas atropine 1 mg with neostigmine 5 mg increases it—this larger dosage may be preferable when reversing the effects of non-depolarizing relaxants after emergency surgery, including Caesarean section;[95] (7) Cyclizine and prochlorperazine increase sphincter tone, while promethazine and droperidol decrease it.[96]

Ingesting antacid, e.g. magnesium trisilicate, 15 ml of the BPC mixture 2-hourly, may increase gastrin production and so may tighten up the sphincter. Magnesium trisilicate contains particulate matter and must be freshly prepared. Sodium citrate is stable. Both may be harmful if inhaled.[97] The citrate may be the better of the two.[98] Antacids should be given no longer than 15 min before induction of anaesthesia if the pH is to be kept greater than 3.[99] Intravenous metoclopramide doubles the basic tone of the sphincter.[100]

Thus, in normal patients under anaesthesia if the active vomiting reflex is suppressed, and the stomach is not distended no material can regurgitate from the stomach into the oesophagus, no matter what position the patient is in, so long as the valve/sphincter mechanism is not interfered with.

The Cricopharyngeal Sphincter

This is at the upper end of the oesophagus at the level of C6 and is composed of striated muscle. Its action is both voluntary and reflex. Its integrity is affected by both anaesthetics and relaxants. It acts as a sphincter normally but as a valve when paralysed. Normally it allows fluids to pass from the pharynx into the oesophagus, but not in the reverse direction. When paralysed by relaxants it tends to obstruct the passage of fluids from the pharynx to the oesophagus, but not in the reverse direction.

The lower part of the oesophagus contains plain muscle which is not affected by relaxants, but the upper part, the cricopharyngeal sphincter, behaves like striped muscle.

When considering this question, all anaesthetists should consult the first-class paper by Morton and Wylie[101] dealing with vomiting during anaesthesia and its relationship to deaths on the table in the causation of which it is one of the major factors.[102]

Causes of Vomiting

1. Vomitable material in the stomach or oesophagus; (*a*) Inadequate preoperative preparation of the patient. Gastric emptying time varies between 4 and 8 h: it is usually between 5 and 6 h; (*b*) In pyloric obstruction; (*c*) When there is peritoneal irritation (e.g. perforated peptic ulcer, acute inflammatory lesions, etc.); (*d*) Blood in the stomach, following bleeding from ulcer, tonsil beds, oesophageal varices or during gastric operations; (*e*) Gross abdominal distension; (*f*) In cases of oesophageal disease, such as pouch or obstruction.

2. Vomitable material returned into stomach from bowel, as in cases of intestinal obstruction.

3. When stomach emptying time is delayed; (*a*) In women in labour; (*b*) In cases of head injury; (*c*) When there is emotional strain associated with pain, accident and the incident of hospitalization; (*d*) In seriously ill patients; (*e*) After drugs, e.g. narcotic analgesics.

The Hydrodynamics of Regurgitation

The normal intragastric pressure is $5–7\,cmH_2O$ and double this in advanced pregnancy. This is well below the pressure required for reflux through the cardia. Even when the stomach is distended the pressure is unlikely to be greater than $18\,cmH_2O$ unless there is contraction of the abdominal muscles.

If the glottis is maintained at a height in centimetres above the cardia greater than the intragastric pressure in cmH_2O, i.e. with a head-up tilt of 40–45°, and if the abdominal muscles are prevented from contracting, then regurgitation is unlikely.

Measurements of intragastric pressure during the fasciculation following injection of suxamethonium are usually not greatly increased, but in about 12% of patients a rise greater than $19\,cmH_2O$ occurs. This evidence might suggest that suxamethonium should not be used for intubation in such patients even with a high head-up tilt, as gastric contents could be forced up to the glottis by the increase in intragastric pressure. The question needs clarification as reported pressure measurements are not in agreement.

Factors predisposing to Passive Regurgitation

1. Considerable volume of fluid in stomach which may have a pH of less than 3;[103] (*a*) In the emergency case; (*b*) The patient prepared for elective surgery has a variable amount of resting gastric juice; in the nervous patient this is increased in both quantity and acidity.

2. Incompetence of the cardia; (*a*) Hiatus hernia; (*b*) Increased vagal tone; (*c*) Presence of gastric tube.

3. Raised intra-abdominal pressure; (*a*) Posture, e.g. lithotomy position; (*b*) Suxamethonium fasciculations (this has been disputed[104]); (*c*) Pregnancy, especially where there is a high head or hydramnios.

4. Lowered intrathoracic pressure: This can occur with deep spontaneous respiration, and is exaggerated when there is respiratory obstruction as in a difficult induction of anaesthesia.

5. Obesity: There is both a raised intra-abdominal pressure and a greater

likelihood of respiratory obstruction during induction of anaesthesia, particularly in unskilled hands.

   6. Pregnancy: Incorporating several factors already mentioned.

   7. Relaxation of the cricopharyngeus by deep anaesthesia or muscle relaxants.

Time of Aspiration

(1) Before anaesthesia; (2) During induction; (3) During anaesthesia—slow insidious regurgitation; (4) In immediate postoperative period; (5) During first few postoperative days in ill patients. Gastric contents can find their way into the lungs after death.

Dangers of Vomiting during Anaesthesia

These are:

   1. The inhalation of stomach contents into the lungs, with sequelae such as pneumonitis, bronchopneumonia, atelectasis and lung abscess. Food particles and liquid vomitus with a pH of less than 3 are particularly dangerous. Liquid vomitus with a pH greater than 2·5 (e.g. bile) is less harmful.

   2. Hypoxia due to laryngeal spasm or obstruction of the air passages by solid or liquid gastric contents.

   3. Cardiac inhibition from reflexes originating in the bronchi, due to acid contamination.

   4. Reflex chemical trauma to bronchial and alveolar mucosa—acute exudative pneumonitis or Mendelson's syndrome,[31] a syndrome following the aspiration of acid gastric contents. While this is particularly likely to occur in obstetric patients, it is not confined to them. Following immediately, or after an interval of a few hours, the patient shows cyanosis, dyspnoea, bronchospasm, hypotension and tachycardia. There are rhonchi and râles in the chest with a characteristic radiographic appearance, viz. irregular mottled densities. There are no signs of massive atelectasis or mediastinal shift. Severe cases may progress to acute pulmonary oedema with rapid death, or the patient may succumb to pulmonary complication some days later.

Prevention

This involves prevention of substances entering stomach, removal of substances from stomach and prevention of substances leaving stomach in an uncontrolled manner. Metoclopramide (Maxolon) speeds the emptying of the stomach in the absence of anticholinergic premedication and also prevents vomiting. Ranitidine, 150 mg orally the night before and on the morning prior to operation, lowers the mean volume and raises the average pH of gastric contents to safe levels.[105] Cimetidine, 300 mg i.v. 2 h before induction, increases the pH of gastric juice and decreases the amount.[106] A dose of 400 mg by mouth may have a similar effect.[107] Magnesium trisilicate as a routine before general anaesthesia requiring intubation has been recommended, to reduce the dangers of aspiration. Sodium citrate (0·33 molar solution) has also been used. *Except in the gravest emergency no general anaesthetic should be given to a patient whose stomach may contain vomitable material, i.e. a patient who has not been properly prepared for anaesthesia by preliminary avoidance of food and drink. This should be an infallible rule.*

Management of General Anaesthesia
When an anaesthetic must be given for urgent reasons, a plastic Ryle's tube, e.g. size 6 gauge, should be passed from the nose into the stomach so that aspiration can take place and if necessary lavage. This should be done with the patient lying on his side to prevent soiling of lungs should he vomit. Information is thus obtained as to the amount and type of material still in the stomach. If the anaesthetist thinks that he can empty the viscus by the tube, well and good, but in all cases of doubt an oesophageal tube such as size 12 EG should be passed into the stomach, where it should remain until the patient gets his cough reflexes back at the end of the operation (although there is evidence that the presence of a tube interferes with the integrity of the cardiac sphincter mechanism, so that its withdrawal into the oesophagus before induction is recommended by some authorities). This tube will allow fairly efficient drainage of liquid and semi-solid material, and so should prevent regurgitation even if actual vomiting is not prevented.

In a patient lying supine, the long axis of the trachea is inclined at an angle of 30° downwards and backwards from the larynx so that a head-down slope of more than 30° is necessary if in fact gravity is to protect the trachea. Laryngoscopy may be difficult in this steeply inclined position.

Insertion of cuffed tube into trachea in a patient suspected of having a full stomach.
The insertion of a cuffed tracheal tube into the larynx before the onset of vomiting or regurgitation is the only safe procedure when dealing with a patient who may have vomitable material in the stomach or oesophagus. A cuffed tube should always be used when in doubt about the contents of the stomach, and before induction commences, the availability of an efficient suction apparatus, source of oxygen, laryngoscopes, tracheal tubes, airways, etc. must be checked. It is wise to induce anaesthesia in these patients on the operating table, so that tilting can be employed easily. The services of a trained assistant are invaluable.

1. The so-called 'crash-induction'. Oxygen is given for 2 min followed by the i.v. injection of thiopentone 150–300 mg, followed by suxamethonium 25–100 mg. Pretreatment with a non-depolarizer may be unwise.[108] The tube is inserted, its cuff immediately blown up and the table levelled (if it has been tilted foot-down).

Cricoid pressure. The prevention of regurgitation by occlusion of the oesophagus by backward pressure on the cricoid is recommended during induction of anaesthesia (Sellick's manoeuvre[109]) before the patient loses consciousness. The tips of the first two fingers and thumb of a helper are placed on the cricoid cartilage and press it on to the vertebral column with moderate pressure. The neck is extended and the other hand placed behind the neck to steady it. This method must not be used during active vomiting as it may lead to oesophageal rupture. It also distorts the appearance of the glottis. Cricoid pressure, to be safe, must ensure that the onset of unconsciousness, the achievement of full muscular relaxation and the application of firm cricoid pressure are timed to occur simultaneously.[110] Personnel must be properly trained in its use.[111]

2. Repeat the above method substituting vecuronium 10–15 mg for the suxamethonium. This prevents a rise in intragastric pressure following fasciculations of the abdominal muscles. Many other non-depolarizing relaxants have been recommended over the years for this technique.

3. If the condition of the patient makes the injection of thiopentone likely to be dangerous, a mixture of equal parts of cyclopropane and oxygen in a 5-litre bag may be inhaled; unconsciousness will supervene in a dozen breaths. A relaxant may be given; as above. Other inhalation agents which may be used include halothane and ether. Use of up to 5% carbon dioxide will hasten induction and discourage reflex breath holding and laryngospasm.

4. The lateral position with a head-down tilt, using a halothane–oxygen induction, 2–4% with a flow of 6 litres/min followed by suxamethonium, has its advocates.[112]

5. Topical analgesia of the upper airways and neurolept analegsia will enable a tube to be inserted into the trachea in the conscious patient. (*See* Chapter 31.)

An efficient, but not a particularly humane, method of reducing the risk of aspiration of stomach contents before induction of anaesthesia is to empty the patient's stomach by stimulating vomiting. Apomorphine 3–5 mg is dissolved in 10 ml of saline and 1 ml is injected intravenously at short intervals until the patient vomits. Apomorphine can act as a central depressant and should be followed by atropine. It has no serious effect on the fetus in labour. Its use does not guarantee an empty stomach. (*See also* Burns T. H. S. *Anaesthesia* 1982, **37**, 346.)

A further method, based on oesophageal occlusion by a balloon catheter, has been described many times, latterly by Zohairy[113] who recommends a Foley catheter number 26 Fr, which has a strong balloon of 30–100 ml capacity. This is passed with or without pharyngeal topical analgesia into the lower oesophagus before induction of anaesthesia and its cuff inflated; upward passage of stomach contents is said to be prevented during the dangerous interval between loss of consciousness and the inflation of a cuffed tracheal tube. (*See also* Mulrooney L. *Anaesthesia* 1982, **38**, 996.)

The inexperienced anaesthetist is perhaps well advised to tilt the patient's head downwards, and to induce anaesthesia with nitrous oxide, oxygen and halothane. The authors have great confidence in slow steady induction with halothane and oxygen, with or without 5% carbon dioxide, avoiding at all cost breath holding, coughing or anything causing contraction of the abdominal muscles.

Assessment of the effects of possible inhalation of gastric contents can be made following fibreoptic bronchoscopy, which is without harmful results and may show erythema around the carina. If so, early treatment can be instituted.[114]

There is no foolproof method of prevention of aspiration of gastric contents into the lungs however experienced the anaesthetist.

Heavy sedation may result in aspiration of stomach contents in the ward before or after operation.

Treatment

If vomiting occurs. The air passages must if possible be spared contamination by tilting the head downwards or turning the patient on one side. Suction must be used, and oxygen carried to the alveoli in the most efficient way that is possible under the circumstances. Tracheal intubation should only be attempted if relaxation is present and the manoeuvre likely to be quick and easy, otherwise hypoxia may be made worse rather than better. *If aspiration results.* Suction and gravity should be employed to lessen the extent of the insult to the bronchi. Tracheal suction may be sufficient in mild cases, whereas in others suction through a bronchoscope will be required. The passage of a double-lumen tube will enable bronchial lavage to be performed down each bronchus separately, while ventilation is maintained down the other, 10 ml of saline being injected and aspirated via a catheter, and repeated until the washings are clear. This should not be done immediately but after the patient has recovered from the immediate effects of the catastrophe. Bronchodilators may be helpful, while antibiotics and physiotherapy have a place too. Hydrocortisone[115] can be given intravenously and instilled into the bronchial tree, where it is said to be of more benefit than either normal saline or sodium bicarbonate solution. IPPV may be required.

To lessen the dangers of vomiting during recovery, the patient should, whenever possible, be returned to the ward with the head tilted downwards in the so-called 'tonsillar position', lying on his side. (*See* Aspiration of gastric contents, Nimmo W. S. *Br. J. Hosp. Med.* 1985 **34**, 176.)

Postoperative Nausea and Vomiting

Vomiting may be central from causes acting on the brain stem and higher centres; peripheral, from causes acting on the gut; and vestibular. It can be influenced by one or more of the following factors:

1. *Anaesthetic agent and technique.* Most likely to be produced by chloroform, ether, cyclopropane, trichloroethylene, pethidine and halothane in that order. Thiopentone, regional analgesia and myoneural blocking agents are not so frequently followed by vomiting and thiopentone induction reduces postoperative vomiting. Nitrous oxide and oxygen cause vomiting in about 15% of patients in an outpatient department. Children are more prone to vomit than adults. Intradural and extradural block usually cause less vomiting than inhalation of a volatile anaesthetic. Hypoxia predisposes to vomiting. Prolonged time of operation and depth of anaesthesia are unfavourable factors.

2. *Type of patient.* Some patients are ready vomiters, e.g. in travelling; after simple dietary indiscretions; sufferers from 'bilious' attacks. Suggestion, and the example of surrounding patients, are important factors. Suitable preoperative reassurance and 'sales talk' are important.

3. *Condition of stomach.* Vomiting is likely unless the stomach is empty. Sipping of water, soon after recovery of consciousness, may cause vomiting. Postoperative thirst should be treated by mouthwashes and dehydration by intravenous fluids. There is a group of patients in whom starvation is a cause of vomiting. They may be identified by the administration of atropine or propantheline which stops the retching or by cautious administration of spoonfuls of tea.

4. *Narcotic analgesics.* Given before and after operation, make some 30% of patients vomit. Diamorphine is said to cause less vomiting, although more respiratory depression, than morphine.

5. *Type of operation.* Vomiting is most frequent after laparotomy and especially after operation on the biliary tract.

6. *Sex.* More frequent in women than in men, and in the young than in the old.

Treatment

This consists largely in preventing the causal factors whenever possible.

The following drugs (with doses in mg) may be used in the treatment of vomiting:

1. *Anticholinergic agents.* Atropine (0·5–1); hyoscine (0·4–0·6). They inhibit the muscarinic activity of acetylcholine on the gut and may have a central action.

2. Antihistamine agents. Cyclizine hydrochloride (Marzine) (50) by deep subcutaneous injection, half an hour before and several times after operation, is free from unpleasant side-effects and reduces vomiting.[116] It can be given by suppository. It is an anticholinergic and antihistaminic. It has been added to morphine in an effort to prevent nausea and vomiting—15 mg to morphine 10 and 15 mg (Cyclimorph), but if given intravenously may cause collapse; and in a tablet with the analgesic dipipanone (Diconal). Promethazine (25), intramuscularly during operation, and (25) postoperatively for 4 doses, 4-hourly, reduces vomiting after operation quite effectively. It has antanalgesic effects, so is not the best agent for use in labour.[117] Meclozine (Ancolan) (25); Dimenhydrinate (Dramamine) (50).

3. Phenothiazine agents. Chlorpromazine (Largactil) (25–50) will also reduce the incidence of vomiting and can be given before and after operation, by mouth (25) the night before operation, repeated before and immediately after operation, by injection or per rectum as a 300 mg suppository. It is a dopamine antagonist and acts on the chemoreceptor trigger zone. Promethazine (Phenergan) (25), *see above.* Prochlorperazine (Stemetil) (12·5 intramuscularly). Perphenazine (Trifalon, Fentazin) (5 intramuscularly) at the end of the operation reduces vomiting significantly. It is occasionally followed by acute dystonic reactions.[118] Thiethylperazine dihydrogen maleate (Torecan) (5 intramuscularly) has a sedative action on both the chemoreceptor trigger zone and on the vomiting centre. Each millilitre contains 5 mg, the dose being 0·08 ml/kg bodyweight intramuscularly on return from the operating room. Effects are said to last 6 hours and hypotension, narcosis and extrapyramidal signs are seldom seen.

4. Butyrophenone derivatives. Droperidol (Droleptan) (5–10); haloperidol (Serenace) (5). These drugs have a specific effect on the chemoreceptor trigger zone.

5. Dopamine antagonists. (1) Metoclopramide acts both centrally and peripherally. It speeds gastric emptying time and increases the tone of the lower oesophageal sphincter. Will not relieve sea-sickness; (2) Domperidone; crosses the blood–brain barrier very slowly and so does not usually cause neurological or psychological side-effects.

6. Tranquillizers and sedatives

7. Chinese acupuncture. The acupuncture point is 5 cm proximal to the wrist crease, between the tendons of the palmaris longus and the flexor carpi radialis of the right forearm, 1 cm below the skin, i.e. on 'the pericardial meridian' (Dundee J. W., Chestnutt W. N. et al. *Br. Med. J.* 1986, **293**, 583).

8. Miscellaneous agents. Metoclopramide (Maxolon, Primperan), the action of which is rather short-lived. It is chemically similar to procaine-amide, but has no local analgesic or cardiac activity. It increases the tone of the lower oesophageal sphincter, speeds the rate of transit through the small gut and accelerates the emptying time of the stomach. These effects are antagonized by atropine and narcotics and are potentiated by cholinergic agents. It also depresses the vomiting centre. It may cause restlessness, drowsiness and even extrapyramidal signs if the dosage is more than 0·5 mg/kg/day (10).[119] Trimethoxybenzamide (Tigan) (400). If the patient cannot retain drugs given by mouth, the following can be given as a suppository: prochlorperazine, cyclizine, chlorpromazine, thioethylperazine.[120] (*See also* Palazzo M. G. A. and Strunin L. *Can. Anaesth. Soc. J.* 1983, **31**, 178.)

Postoperative Ileus
A troublesome complication following laparotomy. Usually self-limiting, a close
watch on fluid and electrolyte balance is necessary.

Liver Failure

May follow major surgery, cause often unknown.
   1. There is delayed recovery from the anaesthetic, merging into semicoma
and death within 48 h, preceded by hyperpyrexia. Post-mortem findings:
necrosis of liver cells.
   2. After 4 or 5 days' normal postoperative progress, patient becomes drowsy
and comatose and dies, death being preceded by oliguria. Post-mortem: liver
necrosis and kidney tubule necrosis.

Effect of Anaesthetic Agents
(1) Halothane: *See* Chapter 10; (2) Chloroform: Considered by many to be a
true hepatotoxin. Others believe that the dangers have been magnified and that
many older studies are invalid because of inadequate control of conditions
surrounding the administration;[121] (3) Other inhalation agents: Transient
changes in liver function tests have been reported but there is no evidence of
serious toxic effects.

Other Factors
(1) Hypoxia: The oxygen consumption of the liver is normally one-third that of
the entire body, or $40 \, ml/min/m^2$ body surface; (2) Hypercapnia is a factor
in producing liver damage; (3) Hypotension: The normal value for hepatic blood
flow in man in 1·5–1·8 litres/min of which 20–40% is from the hepatic
artery, the remainder from the portal vein. The portal vein is loaded with
absorbed materials, has an oxygen saturation of 60–75% and a pressure of
8–10 mmHg; (4) Nutritional status; (5) Blood transfusion: *See* Chapter 42; (6)
Non-anaesthetic drugs; (7) Viral hepatitis: It is estimated that about 100
patients/million may develop coincidental viral hepatitis in the weeks following
anaesthesia; (8) Other infective processes; (9) The nature and site of surgical
trauma.

Postoperative Jaundice
This may be due to either a conjugated or an unconjugated hyperbilirubinaemia,
the former the more common and possibly due to shock, septicaemia, type-B
hepatitis virus, drugs, e.g. phenothiazines, sulphonamides, erythromycin or
intravenous tetracycline. May also be due to halothane.
   Jaundice due to the unconjugated fraction may result from haemolysis
following transfusion, particularly after long-stored blood, or to Gilbert's
syndrome,[122] familial unconjugated hyperbilirubinaemia (deficiency of hepatic
UDP-glucuronosyl transferase activity; B-GTA). This is asymptomatic and
benign and is associated with neither liver disease nor anaemia. The plasma
unconjugated bilirubin is usually less than 6 mg/100 ml.
   Postoperative jaundice is not uncommon and is likely to be due to bilirubin
overload consequent on blood transfusion, resorption of haematoma or
haemoperitoneum and inability of the liver to excrete it due to disturbed cellular

metabolism associated with surgery and anaesthesia. It may be related to shock (causing hepatic cellular hypoxia), sepsis or heart failure.

Rarer causes include infection and damage to the biliary tract. Jaundice may follow anaesthesia in the absence of halothane.

(*See also* Axon J. T. R. *Br. J. Hosp. Med.* 1979, **21**, 464; Strunin L. *Anaesthesia and the Liver*. Oxford: Blackwell, 1979; *See also* Chapter 22.)

Urological Problems

Failure to pass Urine

There is a normal oliguria for the first 24 h after operation. The daily urine volume is not a safe guide to postoperative renal function. Pathological oliguria may be due to:

1. Prerenal. Fall in blood pressure, hypovolaemia, haemorrhage, loss of intestinal fluids and severe sepsis are possible causes. A raised level of antidiuretic hormone during anaesthesia and surgery contributes to a decreased urine secretion.

2. Renal. Damage to renal tubules by: (*a*) Hypoxia; (*b*) Toxins—(i) bacterial; (ii) products of tissue autolysis. Clinically, acute glomerulonephritis; bilateral cortical nephrosis and acute tubular necrosis are described; (*c*) Mismatched blood; (*d*) Hypotension.

3. Postrenal. Ureteral obstruction, bladder-neck obstruction, etc. ligation of ureters in pelvic surgery, neurological conditions, following the injection of ephedrine.

(*See also* Annotation, *Br. Med. J.* 1980, **1**, 2.)

Difficulty in Micturition

Occurs more frequently after central neural blockade than after other methods of anaesthesia. Occurs in about 10% of cases following general anaesthesia. It is influenced by:

1. Type of patient. Most common in anxious, apprehensive type. Patients with an enlarged prostate may develop retention after operation.

2. Type of operation. Most common after abdominal and pelvic operations, including haemorrhoidectomy. A rectal tube predisposes to difficulty with micturition.

3. Attitude of sisters and nurses. Incidence of condition differs from hospital to hospital. In some wards it is expected and so is frequently encountered.

4. Deep sedation. By removing desire for micturition.

Treatment

(1) Encouragement and suggestion; (2) Sit patient up in bed, if possible with legs over side of bed; hot bath; (3) Catheterization should not be left too long, otherwise stretching of bladder wall occurs making natural micturition less likely.

Neurological Complications and Sequelae

Convulsions[123]

Several types of abnormal muscular action may occur during anaesthesia: (1) Deep ether convulsions (*see* Chapter 10); (2) Clonus—usually occurring in light anaesthesia and disappearing when anaesthesia is deepened. Commonly seen in the legs and may be stopped by raising thighs, leaving legs unsupported or by injecting a small dose of muscle relaxant; (3) Epilepsy—intubation may be required to ensure oxygenation; (4) Convulsions due to hypoxia; (5) Convulsions due to local analgesic drugs, e.g. lignocaine, bupivacaine. Treat with intravenous thiopentone and oxygen inhalations and/or suxamethonium. Diazepam may also be used; (6) Tremor associated with the intravenous injection of barbiturate, usually a pronator spasm of the arm receiving the injection. Muscle movements are more common with the newer intravenous induction agents, e.g. etomidate; (7) Enflurane, methohexitone and Althesin cause increased activity on EEG and epileptiform seizures have been reported.

Severe myoclonus (wrongly called shivering) after halothane may be taken for a convulsion. It can be treated by methyl phenidate[124] or by orphenedrine 60 mg i.v.[125]

Delayed Recovery from Anaesthesia

This may be due to: (1) *Drugs used during operation* in relative overdosage, e.g. phenothiazine derivatives, narcotic analgesics, thiopentone, volatile agents. Unconsciousness associated with prolonged apnoea; (2) *Disturbances of physiology resulting from anaesthesia*, e.g. hypercapnia, a hypoxic episode during anaesthesia, electrolyte and acid–base disturbances, fainting (especially in the dental chair), induced hypotension, hypothermia in infants; (3) *Disturbances resulting from surgery*, e.g. shock, metabolic acidosis, fat embolism, air embolism, operative trauma in brain surgery; (4) *Incidental disease*, e.g. cerebral embolism, thrombosis or haemorrhage, cardiac infarction, thrombosis or haemorrhage occurring during operation, myxoedema, hypopituitarism, hypoglycaemia, hyperglycaemic coma with ketosis, adrenal deficiency, uraemia, liver failure, an occult and undiagnosed meningioma.[126] The patient may have been unconscious before operation or may be moribund; (5) *Drugs given before operation*, e.g. mono-amine oxidase inhibitors (with pethidine during operation), sedatives; (6) *The central anticholinergic syndrome*—may be treated with physostigmine salicylate, 1–2 mg (*see* Chapter 8); (7) Early postoperative septicaemia.

Delayed Post-anoxic Encephalopathy[127]

The neuropathological changes at death following acute anoxia are degeneration of nerve cells in the deeper layers of the cerebral cortex, in the Ammon's horn area of the hippocampus and in the globus pallidus. A form of encephalopathy which may often be fatal has been described which may follow some days or weeks after apparent clinical recovery from the anoxic episode due to either cardiac standstill or carbon monoxide poisoning. It is recommended that all patients who have recovered from severe anoxia should be treated by complete bed-rest for at least 10 days, where they can be kept under close observation.[128]

Brain Death[129]

This may result from surgical mishaps, severe hypoxia, cardiac standstill or peripheral circulatory failure. (*See* Chapter 37.)

Peripheral Nerve Injuries[130]

First recognized by Budinger[131] (1894) as being due to malposition of the patient with consequent stretching and compression of nerves. Brachial plexus damage may occur when the arm is abducted during surgery if care is not taken. (*See also* Parks B. J. *Surgery* 1973, **74**, 1973.)

Aetiology

1. Stretching and compression of nerves may occur as a result of muscle relaxation which allows adoption of unphysiological positions. This is combined with abolition of pain and discomfort which would otherwise act as a warning.

2. Injection of substances into or around nerves. Irritation may be chemical, as a result of direct needle trauma, or due to bacterial contamination or haematoma. Can occur as a result of intravenous or intramuscular injection.

3. Use of tourniquets, if excessive pressure is allowed over a nerve trunk.[132] (The pneumatic tourniquet was introduced by Harvey Cushing of Boston to minimize bleeding from the scalp.[133]) It is essential to check the accuracy of the anaeroid gauge against a mercury column.[134] Pressure for upper-limb ischaemia need only exceed arterial blood pressure by 50–75 mmHg. Should not be left inflated for more than 3 h.[135]

4. As a result of hypotension, causing ischaemia.

5. Toxicity due to degradation products of anaesthetic agents (e.g. trichloroethylene).

6. Hypothermia, when minimal pressure may cause injury.

Specific Neuropathies

1. Brachial plexus. Stretching can occur as a result of: (*a*) Dorsal extension and lateral flexion of head to opposite side; (*b*) Abduction, external rotation and dorsal extension of the arm; (*c*) Suspension of the arm from a bar when the patient is in lateral position; (*d*) Extreme abduction of the arms above the head with the patient supine; (*e*) Suspension by wrists to prevent slipping of patient in Trendelenburg position. *Compression* can occur: (*a*) When shoulder braces are used with Trendelenburg position. If placed too medially the clavicle may be depressed so that the plexus has to traverse a longer and more devious course; (*b*) With the arm abducted and Trendelenburg position the plexus may be depressed and stretched over the head of the humerus. Shoulder braces, placed too laterally, may further depress the head of the humerus and with it the plexus; (*c*) The plexus may be deviated posteriorly by the tendon of pectoralis minor or by the tip of the coracoid process in the obese patient undergoing cholecystectomy with gallbladder bridge inserted. Various *congenital anomalies* may render plexus more vulnerable, e.g. hypertrophy of scalenus anterior or scalenus media, cervical rib, anomalous derivation of the plexus and abnormal slope of the shoulder.

The entire plexus may be injured or the upper roots only. It is less common for the lower roots to be affected alone. Involvement may be restricted to one cord.

To avoid stretching the plexus, the following measures should be taken: (*a*) Shoulder braces must be padded and must make contact with acromion as far laterally as possible, but they are better avoided, the patient being supported on a non-slip mattress (Langton Hewer[136]); (*b*) Arm-board must be built-up with pads to prevent backward displacement of arm; (*c*) Hyperextension and external rotation of elbow must be avoided; (*d*) Intravenous injections should be given with the arm at the patient's side or folded across the chest. Prognosis is good, but recovery may take months. The deltoid, biceps and brachialis are the muscles usually affected.

2. Radial nerve. Can be injured due to stretching if the arm is allowed to sag over the side of the table. Can be compressed by use of a vertical screen support. Wrist-drop results.

3. Ulnar nerve. Can occur if the elbow is allowed to fall over the sharp edge of the table so that the nerve is compressed against the medial epicondyle of the humerus. Injury has also been reported as a result of acute flexion of the elbow when the arm is placed in front of the chest. The nerve is stretched around the medial epicondyle of the humerus. Weakness of ulnar side of fist results and later 'claw hand'. Relatively minor trauma to the ulnar nerve may cause severe disability.[137]

4. Median nerve. May be damaged as a result of technically perfect intravenous injections in the cubital fossa, as a result of direct needle trauma or extravasation of drugs. Results in inability to oppose thumb and little finger.

5. Lateral popliteal nerve. Compression between the head of the fibula and a lithotomy pole badly placed damages the nerve and may result in foot-drop. This is the most frequently damaged nerve in the lower limb.

6. Saphenous nerve. Compression can occur between lithotomy pole and medial tibial condyle, when the leg is suspended lateral to the pole. Sensory loss results along the medial side of the calf.

7. Sciatic nerve. Can be traumatized by intramuscular injections in the buttock. It may be damaged in emaciated patients, lying on a hard table with opposite buttock elevated, as for hip-pinning. Paralysis of all muscles below knee, and perhaps of hamstrings results, with sensory loss.

8. Pudendal nerve. Can be compressed against a poorly padded perineal post during hip-pinning with traction to legs. The nerve is pressed against the ischial tuberosity. Result is loss of perineal sensation and faecal incontinence.

9. Femoral nerve. Can be damaged by use of a self-retaining retractor during lower laparotomy. Result is loss of flexion of hip and loss of extension of knee. Sensation is lost over the anterior thigh and anteromedial aspect of the calf.

Damage to nerves may be caused by a tourniquet (*tourner* = to turn) or compression bandage.[138]

10. Supra-orbital nerve. Can occur due to compression by a metal endotracheal connector or tight head-harness. Result is photophobia, numbness of the forehead and pain in the eye.

11. Facial nerve. Can be compressed between fingers and ascending ramus of mandible.[139] Result is facial paralysis. *Buccal branch* has been injured by tight harness. Result is paralysis of orbicularis oris.

12. Abducens nerve with other cranial nerves. Can follow spinal analgesia. *See* Chapter 32.

13. Trigeminal nerve. Toxic damage has followed use of trichloroethylene with soda-lime. *See* Chapter 10.

(*See also* Britt B. A. and Gordon R. A. *Can. Anaesth. Soc. J.* 1964, **11**, 514.)

Postanaesthetic Excitement

Most common in children; after operations for cataract and in the strong and fit. Made worse by premedication with sedative but non-analgesic drugs, operations causing great pain or a full bladder. Analgesics should be given in adequate dosage for pain, while apomorphine (which is a direct dopamine receptor stimulant), 1–2 mg i.v., may quell gross restlessness. Psychic abnormalities may be the cause. (*See also* Drummond G. B. *Br. J. Anaesth.* 1975, **47**, 130.)

Paralysis following Intra- or Extradural Analgesia
See Chapter 32.

Neurological Complications following General Anaesthesia
Neurological complications can follow general as well as spinal analgesia. A case of diplopia following thiopentone, curare and cyclopropane;[140] a case of ascending spinal paralysis under nitrous-oxide–oxygen, ether and gallamine,[141] peroneal nerve palsy and meningitis have all been reported.[142]

Postoperative convulsions.[123] Possible causes include: hypoxia, cerebral oedema, alkalaemia, embolus (blood clot, fat or air), deep ether, local analgesics, hyperpyrexia, hypoglycaemia, hypocalcaemia due to massive blood transfusion, cerebrovascular accident, uraemia or eclampsia.

Postoperative headache. About 40% of patients get headache after operation and over 80% in the headache prone.[143] Migraine can often be prevented by avoiding anxiety (e.g. by haloperidol) and hypoglycaemia (by i.v. glucose). For management of migraine attacks *see* Fell R. H. *Anaesthesia* 1980, **35**, 1006.

Postoperative decrease in mental function. This may last for up to 6 weeks after prolonged surgery under general anaesthesia. Habitual caffeine consumption may be related to this. Regional analgesia is not associated with such problems.[144] It has been suggested that mental function in the days immediately following a general anaesthetic lasting more than 45 min, is less efficient than it would have been, had a general anaesthetic not been given.[144]

Awareness During Surgery

Some patients, anaesthetized with nitrous-oxide–oxygen, IPPV and muscle relaxants, have reported awareness during anaesthesia.[145] The signs of awareness include restlessness, sweating, reactive pupils, irregular respiration (if breathing is spontaneous), hypertension, tachycardia and lacrimation. It is possible if hypnosis is used that memory may be recalled for incidents occurring during operation. It is surely a strange outlook of our speciality which, in an effort to spare patients the undoubted harm of too deep anaesthesia, subjects them to the no less undesirable trauma of awareness, a euphemism for inadequate anaesthesia. Intravenous analgesics (e.g. fentanyl) may help to obtund pain (which is seldom complained of), but will not prevent awareness. For this purpose, volatile agents are preferable, e.g. 0·5% halothane.

Patients lightly anaesthetized for dental and orthopaedic operations can often remember conversations which have taken place during the operation.[146]

Dreams during Anaesthesia. (*See also* Harris T. J. B. et al. *Br. J. Anaesth.* 1971, **43**, 172; Wilson S. L. et al. *Anesth. Analg. (Cleve.)* 1975, **54**, 609; Famewo C. E. *Can. Anaesth. Soc. J.* 1976, **23**, 636; Utting J. E. in: *Recent Advances in Anaesthesia and Analgesia*—14 (Hewer C. L. and Atkinson R. S. ed.), Edinburgh: Churchill Livingstone, 1982.)

Anaesthetists may be sued for causing psychological trauma due to awareness during operation.[147]

Extrapyramidal Side-effects

Drugs causing Extrapyramidal Effects
Phenothiazines, butyrophenone derivatives, metoclopramide,[148] large doses of

methyldopa and rauwolfia alkaloids, levodopa.

Signs and Symptoms of Extrapyramidal Disorders
Acute dystonia, painless spasmodic contractions; akathesia, uncontrolled restlessness; pseudoparkinsonism; persistent tardive dyskinesia, grimacing, pulling faces, etc.

Treatment
Withdraw drug. For acute dystonic states, promethazine 25 mg i.v., procyclidine (Kemadrin) 10 mg i.v. or diazepam 10 mg i.v.

Other agents: benzhexol (Artane), benztropine mesylate (Cogentin), orphenadrine HCl (Disipal).

Malignant Hyperpyrexia

First put on a scientific basis by Denborough et al. in 1962.[149]

Definition
A specific condition in which heat production exceeds heat loss in the body to cause a rise of temperature of at least 2 °C/h. First described in 1960 in Australia.[150]

It is inherited as an autosomal dominant with incomplete penetrance and generation skipping. It is characterized by cyanosis, mottled rash, muscle rigidity (after suxamethonium), hypercapnia, hyperventilation, dysrhythmias and pyrexia (a relatively late sign). Exhaustion and cardiac failure cause death in 70%. The condition can be diagnosed quite early on by the recognition of an abnormally high end-tidal CO_2 as measured by capnography or by mass spectrometry.[151]

Cause
Drug administration, particularly anaesthetics but also mono-amine oxidase inhibitors, phenothiazines, amide local analgesics (lignocaine) and tricyclic antidepressants. The most commonly implicated anaesthetics are suxamethonium and halothane.

Incidence
About 1 in 14 000 unselected population. Age distribution: 19 months to 70 years. It becomes more severe after puberty. The affected patient is commonly a young athletic male. In Denmark there was one case of fulminant hyperpyrexia in 250 000 anaesthetics but there was suspicion of it in 1:16 000 patients who received all types of anaesthetics and in 1:4200 when both suxamethonium and a potent inhalation agent were employed. Of those who received suxamethonium, 1:12 000 developed spasm of the masseters.[152]

Biochemistry
The primary lesion is in the skeletal musculature, probably in the sarcoplasmic reticulum which contains an intergral enzyme system controlling movement of calcium ions. There is also a suggestion that massive uncoupling of oxidative phosphorylation in the mitochondria could account for the rapid rise in

temperature. The site of action of dantrolene[153] remains to be positively identified. The following parameters may be monitored: hypoxia, hypercapnia, hyperkalaemia, respiratory and metabolic acidosis, hypocalcaemia, hypomagnesaemia, hyperphosphataemia, diffuse intravascular coagulation, haemolysis, raised creatine phosphokinase (e.g. 80 000 units) and transaminases. Heat production is up to 2000 kJ/h.

Conditions with which it is Particularly Associated
Arthrogryposis multiplex congenita, osteogenesis imperfecta, congenital ptosis and strabismus, hernias, kyphoscoliosis, cleft palate and 'malignant hyperpyrexia myopathy'.

Management
(1) The anaesthetic mixture is withdrawn and the patient hyperventilated with oxygen. The severity of the condition is dose related, so early cessation of the anaesthetic is of the utmost importance; (2) The patient is cooled with ice, wet sheets, fan, cold water gastric and peritoneal lavage; (3) Blood–gas estimation, serum electrolytes, temperature measurement. Acidosis is corrected with bicarbonate; (4) Glucose 50%, 1 litre and insulin 100 units is infused; (5) Diuresis is promoted; (6) Dantrolene 100–300 mg is injected i.v.; (7) Dexamethasone 20 mg or other steroid is given i.v.; (8) Procaine 100 mg may be given i.v. up to 30 mg/kg.

An emergency pack for this condition may be kept in the theatre refrigerator. It contains procaine, isoprenaline, dopamine, methylprednisolone, 8·4% sodium bicarbonate, 50% glucose, dantrolene and insulin.

Prognosis
Is worse with late identification, increased dose of halothane or suxamethonium in attempt to abolish rigidity, temperature greater than 44 °C, high level of rigidity (which persists after death). Successful treatment brings about reversal of effects in ½–1 h. Reappearance of symptoms some hours after successful treatment has occurred.[154]

Management of Subsequent Anaesthesia in a Known Case
Preoperative oral dantrolene is given for 24 h, 4 mg/kg divided into three or four doses. The following anaesthetics are considered safe: thiopentone, opiates, diazepam, pancuronium and probably nitrous oxide. Some doubt exists about Althesin and phenothiazines. Lignocaine and atropine should be avoided. Bupivacaine may be safe.[155] Procaine is allowable. A vaporizer-free anaesthetic machine with new hoses is used. Full monitoring, cooling and treatment facilities are to hand. Pancuronium, if used, is not reversed with neostigmine and atropine, but IPPV is maintained until it wears off.

Investigation of Patient and Relatives
Muscle biopsy with measured exposure in vitro (Univ. Dept of Anaesthesia; University of Leeds; Malignant Hyperthermia Unit). Affected persons may wear bracelets with the name of the disease stamped on.

Dantrolene
Dantrolene is a muscle relaxant acting by uncoupling excitation–contraction

sequence by reduction of calcium release from the sarcoplasmic reticulum. Dose: 1 mg/kg, repeated if necessary, i.v. Over-dose effects may be seen in amounts above 4 mg/kg i.e. weakness. Reversal, if necessary, by germine monoacetate 0·5 mg/kg and transiently by neostigmine 0·04 mg/kg. 4-Amino-pyridine may produce a slow, incomplete reversal.[156]

(*See also* Denborough M. A. et al. *Lancet* 1960, **2**, 45 (for history); Gronert G. A. *Anesthesiology* 1980, **53**, 395; Ellis F. R. and Heffron J. J. A. in: *Recent Advances in Anaesthesia and Analgesia*—15 (Atkinson R. S. and Adams A. P. ed.) Edinburgh: Churchill Livingstone, 1985.)

Endocrine Effects

Acute Adrenocortical Deficiency
This usually shows itself during the first day or two after operation as acute circulatory collapse with hypotension, tachycardia, pallor and sometimes pyrexia and unconsciousness. The state of adrenocortical deficiency may arise in those patients who have been treated for some time with steroids and from whom the drug has been suddenly withheld before operation. The treatment is intravenous hydrocortisone in full doses.[157] Metabolic and endocrine responses to surgery can be influenced by: (1) Central neural blockade with its associated afferent block; (2) Large doses of opioids i.v. to block hypothalamopituitary function; (3) Changing the humoral status of the patient by inhibition of catabolic hormones, or by the induction of anabolic hormones, such as insulin.

Central neural blockade reduces or prevents a rise in catecholamines and cortisol. Its effects are greater in lower than in upper abdominal surgery.

General anaesthesia has little effect in suppressing endocrine response to surgical trauma. (*See* Kaufman L. in *Anaesthetic Review*—1 Edinburgh and London: Churchill Livingstone, 1982, Ch.4.; *Adverse Reactions* (Fisher M. M. ed.) *Clin. Anesthesiol.* 1984, **2**, 3.)

Miscellaneous Complications

Ophthalmological Complications
1. *Corneal abrasion*. This should be prevented by tulle gras, adhesive tape sealing the lids or drops of oil into the conjunctival sac before anaesthesia. It can be diagnosed if a drop of 0·5% amethocaine is put into the eye, followed by fluorescein, when the abraded cornea will take up the stain. Treatment consists of a firm pad and bandage.

2. *Acute glaucoma* (closed angle) in susceptible patients who will complain of pain in and around the eye of a different nature to that due to foreign bodies or abrasions. On examination the eye is red, the cornea cloudy and the pupil dilated on the affected side. There may be nausea and vomiting. Treatment in emergency: acetazolamide 500 mg or a drip of 10% mannitol intravenously; eserine or pilocarpine drops, 1%, into the conjunctival sac. Skilled ophthalmic help needed urgently.

3. *Vitreous haemorrhage*. This has followed hypotensive techniques.

4. *Retinal infarction* from pressure of an anaesthetic mask on the eyeball. The blindness may be transient.

5. *Retinal emboli.*

6. *Transient cortical blindness*. Due to spasm of basilar arteries.[158]

7. *Ocular displacement*. This has occurred during IPPV in the head-down position; due to increased venous pressure.[159]

Local Complications of Intravenous Therapy

When infusions are taken down within 12 h, thrombophlebitis is rare, but the incidence rises steeply thereafter. In-line filters reduce this complication. Following single injections or use of an indwelling needle for serial injections during anaesthesia a significant number of patients have signs of a haematoma afterwards and some have pain at the injection site for several weeks. The incidence of these complications is less when veins in the antecubital fossa are used than for veins in the back of the hand. An increased incidence of thrombophlebitis (not in the upper limb) has been reported to follow intravenous saline infusions.[160] *See also* Chapter 42.

Complications of Low Environmental Temperature

Operating rooms should be kept at a temperature of 21–23 °C. If it is below 21 °C the normal lightly anaesthetized patient (without a major body cavity open) loses heat and if the oesophageal temperature falls below 36 °C postoperative shivering with increased oxygen consumption and circulatory stress may occur. The temperature of very young, the old, ill and the cachectic patient is still more important, as is that of those receiving large volumes of cold infusions. More heat is lost if the abdomen or the thorax is open. It has been suggested that all patients should have the nasopharyngeal and the oesophageal temperatures continuously recorded to warn against both hypo- and hyperthermia.[161] (*See also* p. 315.)

Shivering after Operation

This can follow cyclopropane, ether, thiopentone, halothane or any combinations of these, but it is most common after halothane when some type of spasticity is seen in 70% of patients. It need not be due to heat loss and there is no significant difference in body temperature between shivering and non-shivering patients. It is often accompanied by a positive Chvostek sign. The rise in the metabolic rate with increased oxygen consumption up to 500% with increased cardiac work and fall in Pao_2 may be prevented by ventilation with warmed humidified anaesthetic gases during operation.[161] Intravenous pentazocine 30 mg[162] and methyl phenidate[124] have been recommended to control shivering. Diazepam, 20 mg by mouth before operation has also been recommended.[163]

Postoperative Parotid Swelling

See Reilly D. J. *Anesth. Analg. (Cleve.)* 1970, **49**, 560.

Spontaneous Rupture of Tympanic Membrane

This has been reported in a previously fit patient receiving nitrous oxide and oxygen.[164]

Hospital Associated Viral Infections

Anaesthetists can both give and receive serious viral infections, the commonest being hepatitis B and herpes simplex. Thorough and frequent hand washing is important while the wearing of gloves may protect both doctor and patient.[165]

Unfavourable Effects of Prolonged Anaesthesia

May include: (1) Accumulation of anaesthetic agents in depots with slow subsequent elimination; (2) Development of shock; (3) Blood volume may be diminished; (4) Postoperative respiratory difficulties; (5) Effect on fluid and electrolyte balance; (6) Metabolic disturbances, e.g. reduced BMR, hyperglycaemia; (7) Subsequent mental changes; (8) Higher infection rate; (9) Nitrous oxide may enter air spaces within the body; effect on bone marrow after prolonged use.

In the authors' opinion the good fast surgeon obtains better results than the good slow surgeon.

Minor Sequelae[166]

These are often the cause of considerable discomfort to the patient. They include trauma to lips, gums and teeth, sore throat, corneal, pharyngeal or laryngeal abrasions, superficial phlebothrombosis and simple ecchymosis following intravenous injections, backache following lithotomy position, nausea and vomiting and an occipital bald spot following pressure during prolonged surgery and for which a special pillow may be preventive. They occur in a disappointingly high proportion of patients and are only to be avoided by greater care in the handling of the unconscious. Minor sequelae following day-case surgery can cause considerable distress to an otherwise healthy subject.

Persistent Priapism

This can not only be embarrassing but may make operations such as cystoscopy undesirable. All surgical stimulation should be temporarily halted and general anaesthesia deepened. Should this fail, propranolol 1 mg or practolol 3·5 mg may be given i.v. and nitrous oxide discontinued.[167]

Postoperative Pyrexia

Among the causes of this may be wound infection, haematoma formation, deep-vein thrombosis, bronchopulmonary infection or atelectasis, Gram-negative urinary-tract infection, blood-transfusion reactions, intraperitoneal infections, Gram-negative septicaemia (*see* Chapter 35), halothane anaesthesia. The wisdom of antibiotic cover in clean cases is controversial. (*See also* Fraser I. and Johnstone M. *Br. Med. J.* 1981, **283**, 1299.)

Conversation in the operating theatre may be a cause of airborne infection of the patient. Most masks allow bacterial contamination round their sides so that a mask covered by a full head and neck hood is advocated. There is a positive correlation between bacterial contamination of a wound and the amount of conversation taking place during an operation. So for all the surgical team, 'silence is golden'.[168]

Postoperative Hypotension

Causes may be: (1) Cardiovascular; (2) Respiratory; (3) Pharmacological; (4) Neurogenic; (5) Haemorrhage; (6) Endocrine; (7) Postural. The commonest cause is hypovolaemia, requiring infusion; other causes may be the injection of a narcotic-analgesic drug; vagal overactivity, requiring atropine to combat bradycardia; adrenal insufficiency, requiring a corticosteroid; prolongation of central neural blockade.

Immunological Sequelae[169]

1. Immune reaction to anaesthetic vapours or to intravenous agents, or their metabolites of the antigen/antibody type, or complement C_3 cleavage type, occurs with immediate (anaphylactic) or delayed response. Histamine, serotonin, vasoamines, kinins and prostaglandins are among the final mediators of these responses. Treatment includes steroids, plasma expanders, IPPV with oxygen and circulatory support.

2. Depression of the immune competence of the host. This is due simply to the stress of operation and involves: (*a*) Secretion of steroids which depress leucocyte phagocytosis, lymphocyte reactivity and immunoglobulin production. (*b*) Secretion of catecholamines which reduce leucocyte activity. However, the half-life of IgG antibodies is 24 days, which outlasts any temporary depression due to operative stress.

In addition, prolonged exposure to nitrous oxide and hydrocarbon anaesthetics causes leucopenia.[170]

Hazards to Medical and Nursing Staff[171]

There have been a number of surveys suggesting that the anaesthetist and other theatre staff are exposed to hazard as a result of their occupation. Anaesthetists are thought to be more prone to coronary artery disease and suicide than their fellows in other occupations. Other hazards include liability to renal calculi, exposure to radiation (though the average exposure has been calculated as 13 mR/week against a maximum allowable exposure of 100), muscular and ligamentous strains as a result of lifting patients, the possibility of exposure to hepatitis B antigen (*see below*), and fatigue (which may result in slow reaction time in an emergency and inability to form judgements). Many individual anaesthetists work long hours. Chronic intermittent exposure to nitrous oxide may interfere with vitamin B_{12} metabolism[172] and rarely causes polyneuropathy.[173]

Reproduction
Interest has been aroused in the possible effects of working conditions in operating theatres in respect to increased rates of spontaneous abortion,[174] an increased incidence of congenital abnormalities in children born, and in a higher than normal proportion of female to male births in the wives of male anaesthetists.[175] Mutagenic changes are unlikely in operating theatre personnel.[176] There is no proof of any causal relationship between the data obtained[176] and any anaesthetic agent present in the atmosphere of operating rooms, but there is general agreement that all reasonable steps should be taken to reduce contamination. Some recent work tends to be reassuring.[193]

Malignant Disease
Variable results have been obtained from surveys made. The finding of an increased incidence of malignancy in the lymphoid and reticular systems in anaesthetists has not been confirmed by a more recent study[177] and it does not appear that British anaesthetists suffer from cancer more than their fellows.[175]

Measures to Reduce Pollution
(*See also* Smith W. D. A. *Br. J. Clin. Equip.* 1978, **3**, 49.)

1. Room ventilation. The air-conditioning systems of modern theatres are designed to prevent bacterial contamination and are ineffective in removing anaesthetic waste. The pattern of air flow in any operating room depends on many factors which vary at different times.[178]

2. Disposal of waste gases to outside air. (*a*) *Passive removal:* A special expiratory valve (e.g. Enderby[179]) or gas-tight hood over an existing valve is needed. Expired gases must be led along a widebore tube and the resistance to flow should not exceed $0.05\,kPa$ ($0.5\,cmH_2O$) at a flow-rate of 30 litres/min. This is provided by 50 m of unbent smooth-bore metal piping, but resistance is increased if bends are incorporated or if corrugated anaesthetic hose is used. (*b*) *Assisted passive systems:* Passive ducting into the non-recirculating operating theatre ventilating system. The preferred outlet is above a flat roof using a T-termination with a downward right-angle bend at each end, perhaps covered with a wire mesh. (*c*) *Active scavenging:* An appropriate device is essential to prevent negative pressure being transmitted to the patient circuit. The hospital piped medical vacuum system has also been used, perhaps combined with the Cardiff Aldasorber.[180] It should be noted that tubing used in scavenging systems has no anti-static properties.[181]

3. Activated charcoal can be used to adsorb organic anaesthetic vapours, but nitrous oxide is not removed. The Cardiff Aldasorber is available commercially. The canister will be exhausted after a time as measured by the gain in weight which results from adsorption of vapour.

4. The use of low-flow (e.g. 1 litre/min) rebreathing systems or completely closed systems reduces the amount of anaesthetic agent which is discharged into room air and reduces cost.

5. Total intravenous anaesthesia with avoidance of inhalation agents. Drugs used[182] include thiopentone, fentanyl, pentazocine and ketamine.

6. The use of regional analgesia combined with intravenous sedation.

7. Special problems exist in dental anaesthesia in the outpatient department,[183] but an effective gas collecting and disposal system has been described.[184] The design of pharyngeal and oral packs is also important.

8. Filling of vaporizers causes discharge of significant amounts of a volatile liquid to the atmosphere. It may be wise to charge vaporizers at the end of the day when few people are in the room, rather than at the beginning of a list.

Trace Concentrations and Performance[185]
Many studies have been made on the effects of trace concentration of anaesthetic agents on the anaesthetist; though much of the experimental evidence is based on amounts higher than the 600 ppm nitrous oxide and 10 ppm halothane commonly found. It is doubtful whether contamination of this degree has any effect on the anaesthetist's performance. The aim of scavenging is to reduce concentrations to about 30 ppm for nitrous oxide and 1 ppm for halothane.

The Hazards to Theatre Personnel from Blood of Hepatitis B Carriers
Hepatitis B antigen (HBAg), Australia antigen, serum hepatitis (SH) antigen, was first described by Blumberg in 1965 (for which he received the Nobel prize).[186] The incidence of the carrier state is about 0.2% in UK, 5% in the eastern Mediterranean countries and 10% in those of SE Asia. The carrier state in a patient is an indication for very careful safeguards and not a contraindication to surgical or obstetric care. The virus is transmitted not only by shed blood and body

secretions but also by close physical contact. Patients with the antigen in their bloodstream range from those with jaundice (serum B hepatitis) to symptomless carriers, but all are potentially infective. If adequate hygienic measures are scrupulously observed by all contacts there need be no danger during surgical, obstetrical or medical investigation and treatment, nor need a carrier give up the practice of medicine.

Patients under high suspicion of being hepatitis B carriers include the following: (1) All patients with liver disease, both acute and chronic; (2) Patients undergoing haemodialysis or who have received a renal transplant; (3) All patients suffering from leukaemia, reticuloses, polyarteritis nodosa or polymyositis; (4) Patients being treated by radiotherapy or immunosuppressive drugs; (5) Immigrants or visitors from countries with a high background of carriers; (6) Patients who have been transfused in, or have recently returned from, areas with a high background of incidence; (7) Patients who have ever received blood from paid donors; (8) Inmates of prisons or institutions for the mentally defective; (9) Drug addicts, prostitutes and homosexuals; (10) Those with tattoos.

Carriers can be divided into two groups:[187] (1) Simple carriers who have anti-HBe and a low level of HBsAg in their blood; (2) Super-carriers who are HbsAg positive have higher titres of HBsAg and DNA polymerase in their blood and tend to have mildly raised serum liver transaminase levels. These latter are more infective. A super-carrier may convert to a simple carrier, perhaps after several years. To be certain of the carrier state, two or more blood specimens should be tested over a period of months.

The virus is killed by autoclaving and by ionizing radiation and probably does not survive immersion for at least 3 h in a hypochlorite–detergent mixture (e.g. Domestos or Chloros 10% with an ionic detergent) which corrodes metal, or in 10% formaldehyde, which does not. Glutaraldehyde is also effective.

Prevention of infection spread from carriers presenting for operation requires most diligent care to be taken:
1. Before operation. Prevention of contamination of nurses, assistants and porters, the anaesthetic trolley and its coverings, dressings, suction tubes and swabs. Disposables should be disinfected and incinerated. The number of individuals handling the patient must be kept to a minimum and all must be protected by gowns, gloves, overshoes. Buckets containing plastic bags partially filled with hypochlorite–detergent can receive swabs, used syringes, needles, gloves and overshoes which are then discarded.
2. During operation. Theatre linen, if possible, should be burnt, if not it should be disinfected as above. Instruments are to be disinfected before they are cleaned and autoclaved. Biopsy specimens and blood, etc. must be sent to the laboratory in sealed containers suitably labelled.
3. After operation. In the theatre, where possible everything should be washed down with hypochlorite–detergent and instruments soaked in 10% formalin. Used syringes and needles are to be disinfected for at least 3 hours and, in plastic bags, sent for destruction. Particular care must be taken to render needles harmless. Face-masks, tracheal tubes, reservoir bags, sucker tubing, etc. should be disinfected, then destroyed, while laryngoscope blades are to be soaked for at least 3 hours in 10% formaldehyde. The anaesthetic machine should be well washed down with the recommended antiseptic solution and the ventilator decontaminated with formaldehyde. Infusion apparatus must be destroyed and

not sent back to the blood bank. When possible, patients likely to be high risk should be operated on at the end of the list.

Patients found to be 'Australia antigen positive' (surface antigen HBsAg) should be tested for 'e' antigen (HBeAg) and its antibody (anti-HBe). Patients positive for HBeAg should be regarded as infectious and all precautions taken to avoid contamination with the patient's blood. The patient who is HBsAg positive but HBeAg negative may require further investigation but is non-infectious for practical purposes, though he is not acceptable as a blood donor.

Anyone at special risk, as after a prick from a needle contaminated with infected blood, may require an intramuscular injection of 500 mg of anti-HBAg serum.

(*See* detailed description in Waterson A. P. *Br. J. Hosp. Med.* 1973, **10**, 520; Waterson A. P. *Br. J. Anaesth.* 1976, **48**, 21. For recommendations on taking blood from patients who have hepatitis B *see* Welsby P. D. *Br. Med. J.* 1981, **1**, 1052; Callender M. F. et al. *Br. Med. J.* 1982, **284**, 324.)

Because of the high incidence of serological markers of hepatitis B in anaesthetic personnel, they should be considered at higher risk than some other doctors and should (perhaps) receive immunization against hepatitis B infection.[188]

AIDS
See Chapter 22.

Addiction and the Anaesthetist
(*See* Spielleman W. G. et al. *Anesthesiology* 1984, **60**, 335.)

Suicides in Anaesthetists in Training
The incidence is rather high but there is no evidence that it has any relationship to the training or professional life style of the young doctor.[189]

Other Hazards[190]
1. Electrical. Electrocution is a hazard unless proper precautions are observed and frequent testing of plugs and appliances carried out (*see* DHSS Hospital Technical Memorandum, No. 8). The use of conductive footwear and flooring increases the risk. Particular care is necessary during electrical defibrillation. (*See also* Hull C. J. *Br. J. Anaesth.* 1978, **50**, 647.)

2. Fires and explosions (*see* Chapter 5). All theatre personnel should be aware of the procedure to be followed in the case of fire. Electrical lifts will cease to function and patients may have to be evacuated by towing them inside a special sheet. (*See also* Vickers M. D. *Br. J. Anaesth.* 1978, **49**, 659.)

(*See also* DHSS, *Code of Practice for the Protection of Persons against Ionizing Radiations from Medical and Dental Use.* HMSO, 1972; Cooper J. B. et al. *Anesthesiology* 1978, **49**, 399; Utting J. E. et al. *Can. Anaesth. Soc. J.* 1979, **26**, 472; Craig J. and Wilson M. E. *Anaesthesia* 1981, **36**, 933.)

Responsibility for Deaths or Misadventure Associated with Anaesthesia[190]

Before and during every operation the anaesthetist has the following rights: (1) The right to be informed by the surgeon as to the nature and extent of the proposed operation; (2) The right to encourage his surgeon; (3) The right to warn; (4) The right to decline.

In the case of a death on the operating table, legal responsibility will exist only if either the surgeon or the anaesthetist has failed in the proper execution of his functions and duties as a person of professional skill. Neither the surgeon nor the anaesthetist is legally responsible if death has resulted from a genuine error of judgement, but he is expected to exercise care, skill and judgement in all that has to do with the anaesthetic procedure, including the assessment of the fitness of the patient to withstand the strain of anaesthesia successfully. The actual decision to operate, together with the choice of operation, is the responsibility of the surgeon. The anaesthetist is always free to state whether or not the patient is fit for general anaesthesia, the degree of risk involved, and to refer difficult cases to experienced colleagues. In England and Wales, deaths are reported to HM Coroner, in Scotland to the Procurator Fiscal,[191] if the death: (1) Takes place on the operating table during operation or anaesthesia; (2) Is clinically attributable to the anaesthetic; (3) Occurs up to 12 h after operation, so that the cause of death can be determined.

Careful notes in all cases are most important.

Consent Forms
If used, are read to the patient and explained if requested. Jehovah's Witnesses and members of some other sects may wish to add special clauses (e.g. concerning blood transfusion), limiting some areas of treatment.[192]

Identification of Patients
This and the exact site and nature of the operation require a clearly defined system, a high level of discipline and great vigilance. A patient may give the wrong name and agree to the wrong operation. The very old, the very young and the mentally ill may be unable to verify these details at all. The enemies of correct management at this point are: (1) Too much haste; (2) Too much work; (3) Too little sleep (for the anaesthetist); (4) Change in the operating list after it is typed out.

Morbidity and Mortality in Association with Anaesthesia
(*See* Macintosh R. R. *Br. J. Anaesth*. 1948, **21**, 7; Lunn J. N. and Mushin W. W. Mortality associated with anaesthesia. Nuffield Provincial Hospitals Trust, 1982; Anaesthesia-related surgical mortality. Lunn J. N. et al. *Anaesthesia* 1983, **38**, 1090; Anaesthetic deaths. Payne J. P. *Br. J. Hosp. Med.* 1983, **30**, 411; Factors affecting mortality in hospital. Farrow S. C. et al. *Br. J. Anaesth.* 1982, **54**, 811 and 819.)

Misadventure
'A doctor is not liable for mischance or misadventure, nor is he liable for an error of judgement. He is not liable for choosing one course out of two which may be open to him, or following one school of thought rather than another. He is only liable if he falls below the standard of a reasonably competent practitioner in his field, so much so that his conduct may be held to be, I will not say deserving of censure, but at any rate, inexcusable, (Lord Denning: Hucks v. Cole, 1968, Bar Library Transcript No. 181). Again, 'A physician is not required to exercise the highest degree of skill and care possible, but only that degree ordinarily employed

by members of good standing in the same community' (Medico-legal Abstracts, *JAMA* 1955, **158**, 777). (*See also* Symposium, *J. R. Soc. Med.* 1980, **73**, 288.)

Damage to teeth
It is inevitable that on occasions, teeth will be damaged during the course of safe anaesthetic practice.

Recognition of Hazard
The risk is mainly to front teeth. Mishaps to posterior crowns are unlikely to be due to anaesthetic manoeuvres. Preoperative questioning of the patient may reveal the existence of frontal crowns or other teeth at risk. The patient may be warned of the risk of damage, and in extreme cases, specific informed consent obtained for anaesthesia. The mouth is examined for: (1) Frontal crowns (not always easy to recognize); (2) Loose teeth; (3) Buck uppers and inwardly-pointing lowers; (4) Awkward gaps between teeth. *Hazards should be recorded in the anaesthetic sheet.*

Prevention
1. Preoperative dental treatment.
2. Avoidance of the use of oral airways if possible. Nasal airways should be considered, even in the presence of partly blocked nasal passages, or following nasal surgery.
3. Blind nasal intubation if possible. Failing this, tooth-guards and special laryngoscope blades (e.g. Bowen–Jackson) are used.
4. Where the patient's life is at risk because of inability to maintain the airway, maintenance of respiration takes absolute priority over all other considerations, and teeth or crowns may require removal to facilitate this. (Damage to teeth does not imply negligence.) Any such event should be fully documented. At nasal operations, the tracheal tube is best placed well away from any crowns, while acknowledging the risk. After operation, nasopharyngeal airways offer a reasonable solution.

Management of the 'Damaged Tooth Event'
The broken fragments are all accounted for and retained. *The event is recorded in the notes.* The patient is informed of the full circumstances.

A particular risk exists during *electroconvulsive therapy*, where the electrical stimulus is applied directly to the muscles of mastication, producing maximal contraction, even in the presence of full neuromuscular blockade. Further, depressed patients often have neglected teeth. A rubber bite-block is used to spread the force across all the teeth, but occasionally damage is inevitable. Nasal airways may be used in the recovery phase if necessary.

See Wright R. B. and Manfield F. F. V. *Damage to Teeth During the Administration of General Anaesthesia.* Medical Protection Society.

References

1. Cooper J. B. et al. *Anesthesiology* 1978, **49**, 399; Annotation, *Br. Med. J.* 1979, **1**, 703; Rowland D. J. *Br. J. Hosp. Med.* 1976, **16**, 310.
2. Harrison A. A. *Br. J. Anaesth.* 1978, **50**, 1041.

3. Hall M. *Lancet* 1856, **1**, 393.
4. Heiberg J. *Med. Times Gaz.* 1874, Jan. 10th.
5. Nunn J. F. *J. R. Soc. Med.* 1985, **78**, 983.
6. Guedel A. E. *JAMA* 1933, **100**, 1862.
7. Boidin M. P. *Br. J. Anaesth.* 1985, **57**, 306.
8. Brewer N. et al. *Curr. Res. Anesth. Analg.* 1934, **13**, 257.
9. Jacobs H. B. *JAMA* 1972, **222**, 1231; Pottecher T. et al. *Ann. Francaise d'Anaes. Reani.* 1984, **3**, 54.
10. Fisher J. A. *Can. Anaesth. Soc. J.* 1979, **26**, 225.
11. Hayes B. *Br. Med. J.* 1978, **1**, 254.
12. Nosworthy M. D. *Anaesthesia* 1948, **3**, 86.
13. *See also* Thompson P. W. in: *Recent Advances in Anaesthesia and Analgesia—12* (Hewer C. L. and Atkinson R. S. ed.). Edinburgh: Churchill Livingstone, 1976.
14. Hunter A. R. *Anaesthesia* 1984, **39**, 726.
15. Severinghaus J. W. and Mitchell R. A. *Clin. Res.* 1962, **10**, 122.
16. Vella L. M. et al. *Anaesthesia* 1984, **39**, 108.
17. Fry E. N. S. *Br. Med. J.* 1977, **2**, 704.
18. Sohn Y. Z. et al. *Can. Anaesth. Soc. J.* 1978, **25**, 431.
19. Ravindran R. S. *Anesth. Analg. (Cleve.)* 1981, **60**, 121.
20. Bateman D. V. *Anaesthesia* 1985, **40**, 917.
21. Kumar C. and Mehta M. *Anaesthesia* 1984, **39**, 1035.
22. Gardner A. M. N. *Br. Med. J.* 1985, **290**, 822.
23. Gairdner W. T. *Mon. J. Med. Sci.* 1850, **11**, 122, 230.
24. Pasteur W. *Lancet* 1908, **2**, 1351; Lee J. A. *Anaesthesia* 1978, **33**, 362.
25. Jackson C. and Lee W. E. *Ann. Surg.* 1925, **82**, 327.
26. Chirchill E. D. and McNeil D. *Surg. Gynecol. Obstet.* 1927, **44**, 483.
27. Coryllos J. *JAMA* 1929, **93**, 98; *Surg. Gynecol. Obstet.* 1931, **50**, 795.
28. Overholt R. H. *JAMA* 1930, **95**, 1484.
29. King D. S. *Surg. Gynecol. Obstet.* 1933, **57**, 43; *Curr. Res. Anesth. Analg.* 1933, **12**, 243.
30. Morton H. J. V. *Lancet* 1944, **1**, 368.
31. Mendelson C. L. *Am. J. Obstet Gynec.* 1946, **52**, 191.
32. Burford T. H. and Burbank B. *J. Thorac. Surg.* 1945, **14**, 415.
33. Harley H. E. S. *Proc. R. Soc. Med.* 1961, **54**, 558.
34. Waters R. M. *Br. J. Anaesth.* 1942, **18**, 1.
35. Palmer K. N. V. and Sellick B. A. *Lancet* 1953, **1**, 114.
36. Gawley P. H. and Dundee J. W. *Br. J. Anaesth.* 1981, **53**, 1073.
37. Morran C. and McArdle C. S. *Br. J. Surg.* 1980, **67**, 464.
38. Barlow D. *Lancet* 1964, **2**, 736.
39. Graham J. L. et al. *Anaesthesia* 1980, **35**, 158.
40. Ali J. and Ali-Khan T. *Surg. Gynecol. Obstet.* 1979, **148**, 863.
41. Rose E. A. and King. T. C. *Surg. Gynecol. Obstet.* 1978, **147**, 97.
42. Mocran C. G. et al. *Br. J. Anaesth.* 1983, **55**, 1113.
43. Woolsey W. C. *N.Y. St. J. Med.* 1912, **12**, 171.
44. Hamman L. *Trans. Assoc. Am. Physicians* 1937, **52**, 311.
45. Hilton P. J. and Clement J. A. *Anaesthesia* 1983, **38**, 342.
46. Hillman K. M. *Anaesthesia* 1983, **38**, 136.
47. Marshall B. E. And Wyche M. W. *Anesthesiology* 1972, **37**, 178.
48. *See* Editorial, *Br. J. Anaesth.* 1971, **43**, 229.
49. Jones J. G. et al. *J. R. Soc. Med.* 1985, **78**, 1019.
50. Trendelenburg F. *Arch. klin. Chir.* 1908, **86**, 686.
51. Pollard B. J. et al. *Anesthesiology* 1983, **58**, 373; Lee J. Alfred *Region. Anesth.* 1985, **10**, 99.
52. Simpson F. G. et al. *Lancet* 1980, **1**, 331.
53. Nilsson I. et al. *Br. Med. J.* 1985, **290**, 1453.
54. Kakkar V. V. *Br. J. Hosp. Med.* 1977, **18**, 32; Mitchell J. R. A. *Br. Med. J.* 1979, **1**, 1523.
55. French A. et al. *Br. Med. J.* 1981, **1**, 1020.
56. Ramsay L. E. *Br. Med. J.* 1983, **286**, 698.
57. Calnan J. S. and Allenby F. *Br. J. Anaesth.* 1975, **47**, 151; Annotation *Br. Med. J.* 1981, **281**, 1341.
58. Johnson R. et al. *Clin. Orthop.* 1977, **127**, 123.
59. Gruber U. F. et al. *Br. Med. J.* 1980, **280**, 69.
60. McKenna R. et al. *Br. Med. J.* 1980, **1**, 514.

61. Davies G. C. and Salzman E. W. *J. R. Soc. Med.* 1981, **74**, 177.
62. Vessey M. P. et al. *Br. Med. J.* 1970, **3**, 123.
63. McLean J. *Am. J. Physiol.* 1916, **41**, 250.
64. Kakkar V. V. *Proc. R. Soc. Med.* 1975, **68**, 263.
65. Negus D. et al. *Lancet* 1980, **1**, 891.
66. Kakkar V. V. et al. *Br. Med. J.* 1982, **284**, 375.
67. Kakkar V. V. and Murray W. J. G. *Br. J. Surg.* 1985, **72**, 786.
68. Discovered by Karl Paul Link, *Harvey Lect.* 1943, **39**, 162.
69. Waters E. T. et al. *Science* 1938, **87**, 582.
70. Barrow J. C. *Anesth. Analg. (Cleve.)* 1985, **64**, 348.
71. Marin-Neto J. A. et al. *Br. J. Anaesth.* 1978, **50**, 1079.
72. Levine S. *JAMA* 1920, **75**, 795.
73. Baird C. et al. *Anaesthesia* 1983, **38**, 467.
74. Magendie F. *J. Physiol. Exp. (Paris)*, 1821.
75. Barlow J. *J. Med. Chir. Trans* 1830, **16**, 19.
76. Thomas D. and van der Wetden C. *Anaesthesia* 1983, **38**, 1005.
77. Marshall W. K. and Bedford R. F. *Anesthesiology* 1980, **52**, 131.
78. Edmonds-Seal J. et al. *Proc. R. Soc. Med.* 1970, **63**, 831; Maroon J. C. and Albin M. S. *Anesth. Analg. (Cleve.)* 1974, **53**, 399.
79. Durrant T. M. et al. *Am. Heart. J.* 1947, **33**, 269.
80. Khalil S. N. et al. *Br. J. Anaesth.* 1979, **51**, 461.
81. Spencer F. C. et al. *J. Thorac. Cardiovasc. Surg.* 1965, **49**, 615.
82. Clayton D. G. and Evans P. *Anaesthesia* 1985, **40**, 981.
83. Medical Research Council (Status Lymphaticus Commission), *Br. Med. J.* 1931, **1**, 468.
84. Healy T. E. J. and Wilkins R. C. *Ann. R. Coll. Surg.* 1984, **66**, 56.
85. Friedrich Trendelenburg (1844–1924) first used his tilt in 1880 when Professor of Surgery at Rostock to facilitate urological operations. This was popularized by his pupil Willy Meyer in 1884 in the US. Trendelenburg later occupied the surgical chairs at Bonn and Leipzig. He described a tracheotomy tube with inflatable cuff in 1869. (*See also* Lee J. Alfred *Region. Anesth.* 1985, **10**, 99.)
86. Scott D. B. et al. *Br. J. Anaesth.* 1966, **38**, 174; Scott D. B. and Slawson K. B. *Br. J. Anaesth.* 1968, **40**, 103.
87. Hewer C. L. *Lancet* 1953, **1**, 522.
88. Lincoln J. P. and Sawyer N. P. *Anesthesiology* 1966, **22**, 800.
89. O'Donovan N. et al. *Br. J. Anaesth.* 1986, **58**, 280.
90. Borison H. L. and Wang S. C. *Pharmacol. Rev.* 1953, **5**, 193.
91. Brock-Utne J. G. et al. *Anaesth. Intensive Care* 1984, **12**, 140.
92. Hunt P. C. W. et al. *Anaesthesia* 1984, **39**, 412.
93. Brock-Utne J. G. *Anesth. Analg. (Cleve.)* 1980, **59**, 921.
94. Roussak J. B. et al. *Br. Med. J.* 1984, **289**, 1579.
95. Brock-Utne J. G. et al. *Anesth. Analg. (Cleve.)* 1978, **57**, 171.
96. Brock-Utne J. G. et al. *Br. J. Anaesth.* 1978, **50**, 295.
97. Bond V. et al. *Anesthesiology* 1979, **51**, 452.
98. Wrobel J. et al. *Anaesth. Intensive Care* 1982, **10**, 116.
99. Crawford J. S. and Potter S. R. *Anaesthesia* 1984, **39**, 535.
100. Heitman P. and Möller N. *Scand. J. Gastro-enterol.* 1970, **7**, 621; Annotation, *Br. Med. J.* 1971, **3**, 205.
101. Morton H. J. V. and Wylie W. D. *Anaesthesia* 1951, **6**, 190.
102. Edwards G. et al. *Anaesthesia* 1965, **11**, 194.
103. Ong B. Y. et al. *Can. Anaesth. Soc. J.* 1978, **25**, 36.
104. Smith G. et al. *Br. J. Anaesth.* 1978, **50**, 1137.
105. Andrews A. D. et al. *Anaesthesia* 1982, **37**, 22.
106. Maliniak K. and Vakil A. B. *Anesth. Analg. (Cleve.)* 1979, **58**, 309; Dobb G. et al. *Br. J. Anaesth.* 1979, **51**, 967.
107. Husemeyer R. P. et al. *Anaesthesia* 1978, **33**, 773.
108. Jenkin J. G. *Anesthesiology* 1984, **61**, 346.
109. Sellick B. A. *Lancet* 1961, **2**, 404.
110. Sellick B. A. *Anaesthesia* 1982, **37**, 213.
111. Howells T. H. et al. *Anaesthesia* 1983, **38**, 457.
112. Bourne J. G. *Anaesthesia* 1962, **17**, 379.
113. Zohairy A. F. M. *Br. Med. J.* 1967, **1**, 546; Cucchiana R. F. *Anesth. Analg. (Cleve.)* 1976, **55**, 816.

114. Campinos L. et al. *Br. J. Anaesth.* 1983, **55**, 1103.
115. Coriat P. et al. *Anaesthesia* 1984, **39**, 703.
116. Dundee J. W. *J. R. Soc. Med.* 1980, **73**, 231.
117. Vella L. et al. *Br. Med. J.* 1985, **290**, 1173.
118. Dundee J. W. et al. *Br. J. Clin. Pharmacol.* 1975, **2**, 81.
119. Howard F. A. and Sharp D. S. *Br. Med. J.* 1973, **1**, 446.
120. *Drugs and Therapeutic Bulletin* 1983, **21**, 53.
121. Davidson M. H. A. *Anaesthesia* 1959, **14**, 127; Poe M. F. and Mayfield J. R. *Anesthesiology* 1960, **21**, 508.
122. Gilbert A. and Lereboullet P. *Sem. Méd.* 1901, **71**, 241; Taylor S. *Anaesthesia* 1984, **39**, 1222.
123. Jones D. F. *Anaesthesia* 1980, **35**, 50.
124. Brichard G. and Johnstone M. *Br. J. Anaesth.* 1970, **42**, 718.
125. Fry E. N. S. *Anaesthesia* 1983, **38**, 128.
126. Fraser A. I. C. and Goat V. A. *Anaesthesia* 1983, **38**, 128.
127. Annotation *Lancet* 1962, **2**, 546.
128. Adams J. H. *Br. J. Anaesth.* 1975, **47**, 121.
129. Searle J. F. *Hosp. Update* 1980, **6**, 359; Beecher H. K. and Todd D. P. *Ann. Surg.* 1954, **140**, 2.
130. Britt B. A. and Gordon R. A. *Can. Anaesth. Soc. J.* 1964, **11**, 514.
131. Budinger K. *Arch. klin. Chir.* 1894, **47**, 121.
132. Mullick S. *Surg. Gynecol. Obstet.* 1978, **146**, 821; Gilliatt R. W. *Mayo Clinic Proc.* 1981, **56**, 361; Durkin M. A. P. and Crabtree S. D. *J. R. Soc. Med.* 1982, **75**, 658.
133. Cushing H. *Med. News* 1904, **84**, 577.
134. Klenerman L. *J. Bone Jt Surg. (U.K.)* 1983, **65**, 374.
135. Klenerman L. *The Hand* 1980, **12**, 231.
136. Hewer C. L. *Anaesthesia* 1953, **8**, 198.
137. Medicine and Law, *Lancet* 1984, **1**, 1306.
138. Esmarch J. F. A. *Chirurgie* 1873, **19**, 373.
139. Nightingale P. J. and Longreen A. *Anaesthesia* 1982, **37**, 322.
140. Norman J. E. *Anaesthesia* 1955, **10**, 88.
141. Sinclair R. N. *Anaesthesia* 1954, **9**, 286.
142. Lett Z. *Br. J. Anaesth.* 1964, **36**, 266.
143. Hannington-Kiff J. G. *Br. J. Anaesth.* 1969, **41**, 401; McDowell S. A. et al. *Anaesthesia* 1970, **25**, 334.
144. Flatt J. R. et al. *Anaesth. Intensive Care* 1984, **12**, 315.
145. Winterbottom E. H. *Br. Med. J.* 1950, **1**, 247; Hutchinson R. *Br. J. Anaesth.* 1961, **33**, 463; Waters D. J. *Br. J. Anaesth.* 1968, **40**, 259; Utting J. E. *Anaesth. Intensive Care* 1975, **3**, 334; Mainzer J. *Can. Anaesth. Soc. J.* 1979, **26**, 381; Blacker R. S. *JAMA* 1975, **234**, 67; Blacher B. S. *Anesthesiology* 1984, **61**, 1.
146. Bennett H. L. et al. *Br. J. Anaesth.* 1985, **57**, 174.
147. Medicine and Law, *Lancet* 1984, **1**, 1249.
148. Bateman D. N. et al. *Br. Med. J.* 1985, **291**, 930.
149. Denborough M. H. et al. *Br. J. Anaesth.* 1962, **34**, 395.
150. Denborough M. H. and Lovell R. R. H. *Lancet* 1960, **2**, 45.
151. Neubauer K. R. and Kaufman R. D. *Anesth. Analg. (Cleve.)* 1985, **64**, 837.
152. Ording H. *Anesth. Analg. (Cleve.)* 1985, **64**, 700.
153. Harrison G. G. *Br. J. Anaesth.* 1977, **49**, 315; Freisen C. M. et al. *Can. Anaesth. Soc. J.* 1979, **26**, 319.
154. Matthieu A. et al. *Anesthesiology* 1979, **51**, 454.
155. Willatts S. M. *Anaesthesia* 1979, **34**, 41.
156. Lee C. et al. *Anesthesiology* 1981, **54**, 61.
157. Lundy J. S. *Anesthesiology* 1953, **14**, 376.
158. Johnson R. C. and Moss P. J. *Anaesthesia* 1981, **36**, 954.
159. Hardy P. A. J. *Anaesthesia* 1982, **37**, 317.
160. Janvrin S. B. et al. *Br. J. Anaesth.* 1980, **52**, 690.
161. Pflug A. E. et al. *Can. Anaesth. Soc. J.* 1978, **25**, 43.
162. Fry E. N. S. and Desphande S. *Br. J. Anaesth.* 1978, **50**, 80.
163. Goold J. E. *Anaesthesia* 1984, **39**, 35.
164. White P. F. *Anesthesiology* 1983, **59**, 369.
165. Du Moulin G. C. and Hedley-Whyte J. *Anesthesiology* 1983, **59**, 51.
166. Riding J. E. *Br. J. Anaesth.* 1975, **47**, 91.

167. Fry E. N. S. *Br. J. Anaesth.* 1985, **291**, 974.
168. Lettrs R. M. and Doermer E. *J. Bone Jt Surg.* 1983, **65A**, 357.
169. Watkins J. *Br. J. Hosp. Med.* 1980, **23**, 583; Symposium, *Br. J. Anaesth.* 1979, **51**, 1; Watkins J. *Br. J. Anaesth.* 1987, **59**, 104.
170. Sturrock J. E. and Nunn J. F. *Anesthesiology* 1975, **43**, 21.
171. *See also* Cohen E. N. *Anesthetic Exposure in the Workplace.* New York: MTP Press, 1980.
172. Amess J. A. L. *Lancet* 1978, **2**, 339; Layzer R. B. *Lancet* 1978, **2**, 1227.
173. Layzer R. B. et al. *Neurology* 1978, **28**, 504; Brodsky J. B. et al. *Anesth. Analg. (Cleve.)* 1981, **60**, 297.
174. Mehta S. and Burton P. *Anaesthesia* 1977, **32**, 924; Vessey M. P. *Anaesthesia* 1978, **33**, 430; Vessey M. P. and Nunn J. F. *Br. Med. J.* 1980, **2**, 696.
175. Cohen E. N. et al. *Anesthesiology* 1974, **41**, 321; Knill-Jones R. P. et al. *Lancet* 1975, **2**, 807; Salo M. and Vapaavuori M. *Br. J. Anaesth.* 1976, **48**, 877.
176. Baden J. M. *Br. J. Anaesth.* 1979, **51**, 417.
177. Bruce D. L. et al. *Anesthesiology* 1974, **41**, 71.
178. *See* Smith W. D. A. in: *Recent Advances in Anaesthesia and Analgesia*–12 (Hewer C. L. and Atkinson R. S. ed.). Edinburgh: Churchill Livingston, 1976.
179. Enderby G. E. H. *Anaesthesia* 1972, **27**, 334.
180. Vaughan R. S. et al. *Anaesthesia* 1977, **32**, 339.
181. Spence A. A. and Smith W. D. A. *Anaesthesia* 1979, **34**, 823.
182. Savege T. M. in: *Recent Advances in Anaesthesia and Analgesia*–13 (Hewer C. L. and Atkinson R. S. ed.). Edinburgh: Churchill Livingstone, 1979; Jago R. H. and Restall J. *Anaesthesia* 1977, **32**, 904.
183. Hillman K. M. et al. *Anaesthesia* 1981, **36**, 1257.
184. Parbrook G. D. and Monk I. B. *Br. J. Anaesth.* 1975, **47**, 1185.
185. *See also* Smith G. and Shirley A. W. *Br. J. Anaesth.* 1977, **49**, 65; Ferstandig L. L. *Anesth. Analg.* 1978, **57**, 328; Smith G. and Shirley A. W. *Br. J. Anaesth.* 1978, **50**, 701.
186. Blumberg B. S. et al. *JAMA* 1965, **191**, 541; Blumberg B. S. et al. *Ann. Intern. Med.* 1967, **66**, 924.
187. Tedder R. S. *Br. J. Hosp. Med.* 1980, **23**, 266.
188. Berry A. J. et al. *Anesthesiology* 1984, **60**, 6.
189. Helliwell P. J. *Anaesthesia* 1983, **38**, 1097.
190. Cooper J. B. et al. *Anesthesiology* 1978, **49**, 399.
191. Gillies A. M. et al. *Br. Med. J.* 1979, **1**, 1246; Annotation, *Br. Med. J.* 1979, **1**, 703.
192. Casale F. *Br. Med. J.* 1979, **1**, 1796. For specimen consent forms *see* Thornton J. A. and Levy C. J. *Techniques of Anaesthesia*, 2nd ed. London: Chapman and Hall, 1981, Appendix 1.
193. Spence A. A. *Br. J. Anaesth.* 1987, **59**, 96.

Chapter 19	**DRUGS USED IN ASSOCIATION WITH ANAESTHESIA**

Analeptics and Antagonists

The chief action of these drugs is to stimulate respiration, to reverse narcotic activity of sedative drugs, to restore blood pressure and reflex activity and to elevate mood. When given in large doses they are mostly convulsants. Their stimulating action on respiration is greatest in non-anaesthetized or lightly anaesthetized patients. In conditions of respiratory arrest their use comes far behind that of oxygen and IPPV.

Vanillic Acid Diethylamide (*Ethamivan*)
This is a central and reflex (carotid body) respiratory stimulant. Well absorbed from mucosa of mouth and tongue in neonates in a dose of 0·5 ml. For

neonates the dose is 0·2 ml of 5% solution intramuscularly. Adult dose 100 mg repeated.

Tetrahydroaminacrine (*Tacrine hydrochloride, THA, Romotal*)
This was first synthesized in 1945 by Albert and Gledhill and was used by Shaw and Bentley in 1949. It is a partial antagonist to morphine, in contradistinction to naloxone, a complete antagonist.

It is used to potentiate and prolong neuromuscular block produced by suxamethonium[1] and reduces likelihood of biphasic block.

Doxapram Hydrochloride (*Dopram, Stimulexin*)
First described in 1962. A non-specific respiratory stimulant acting on peripheral chemoreceptors. Clinical doses do not reduce the analgesic effects of morphine and pethidine,[2] but reverse the depressant respiratory effects.[3] Can be given i.m., dose 1·0–1·5 mg/kg, or as a drip i.v. at the rate of 100 ml/min, 2 mg/ml in 5% dextrose (about 3 mg/min).[4] May be useful in treatment of barbiturate overdosage.[5] The hyperpnoea produced may aid blind nasal intubation[6] and may speed recovery from general anaesthesia due to a volatile agent[7] and perhaps due to a barbiturate.[8] May reduce postoperative respiratory complications.[9] It should be used with great care in patients with hypertension, status asthmaticus, coronary heart disease and thyrotoxicosis.

In a double-blind trial doxapram was found to be the most efficient respiratory stimulant of five tested (nikethamide, prethcamide, amiphenazole and ethamivan). Ethamivan came second.[10] Issued in 5-ml ampoules and 500-ml containers for intravenous infusion.

Methyl Phenidate (*Ritalin*)
This was first used in Germany in 1954.[11] It is a psychomotor stimulant with activity between that of caffeine and amphetamine and a non-specific respiratory stimulant which can be given intravenously, intramuscularly or by mouth. Dose: 0·1–0·2 mg/kg i.v. up to 20 mg. Has been used to alleviate hiccups and 'shivering' after halothane. (For details *see* eighth edition of this Synopsis.)

Pressor Agents

Pressor drugs may act: (1) By liberating catecholamines; (2) Peripherally, on vessels; (3) Centrally, on the heart. Drugs of this nature should not be used routinely, but only when a severe fall of blood pressure is anticipated or actually occurs.

The pressor drugs related to adrenaline may be used after intradural or extradural block and during general anaesthesia. These sympathomimetic amines may be grouped in several ways, none of them completely satisfactory.

Classification[12]
A. Naturally occurring catecholamines which stimulate α- and β-receptors directly: adrenaline, noradrenaline and dopamine.
B. Sympathetic amines which act directly, as well as indirectly by releasing catecholamines and stimulate both α- and β-receptors, e.g. ephedrine, metaraminol and mephentermine.

C. Sympathomimetic amines which act directly on α-receptors, e.g. phenylephrine and methoxamine.

D. Sympathomimetic amines which act directly on β-receptors, e.g. isoprenaline.

The three naturally occurring catecholamines are adrenaline, noradrenaline and dopamine; they all contain the group 3:4 dihydroxybenzene (catechol).

Table 19.1. Adrenergic receptors

Organ	Receptor type	Effect of stimulation
Heart	β_1	Increased rate, force of contraction and acceleration of conduction
Bronchi	β_2	Dilatation
Arterioles	β_2	Dilatation
	α	Contraction
Gut	α	Reduction of motility
Liver	β_1	Glycogenolysis
Muscle	β_1	Glycogenolysis

Adrenaline, BP (*Epinephrine, USP*)

History

The adrenal glands were described by Bartholomaeus in 1563 and modern knowledge of adrenal physiology started with the description by Thomas Addison (1793–1860) of London in 1855 of the disease which bears his name. Adrenaline was isolated by George Oliver (1841–1915), a practitioner in Harrogate, and J. J. Abel of the Johns Hopkins Hospital and Sir Edward Schäfer (1850–1935) in 1894[13] from the adrenal medulla, who showed that it contained a pressor agent. Produced in crystalline form by Takamine (1854–1922)[14] (who determined its constitution and patented it under the name of 'adrenaline'),[15] and Aldrich,[16] independently, in 1901; the first hormone to be synthesized, by Friedrich Stolz (1860–1936) in 1904.[17] (The word 'hormone' (Greek = I excite) was introduced by E. H. Starling (1866–1927) of London in 1905.[18]) It is derived from noradrenaline which is synthesized in the body from tyrosine; dopa and dopamine being intermediate stages.

Pharmacodynamics

Stimulates both α- and β-receptors. It is formed in the adrenal medulla where it is stored in intracellular granules (and at adrenergic nerve endings) and is liberated by acetylcholine (humoral transmitter) by impulses from the sympathetic preganglionic fibres supplying the medullary cells. Ampoules of adrenaline can be autoclaved once or twice without loss of potency.

Cardiovascular system. Increases the stroke volume, rate and cardiac output. It increases the incidence of dysrhythmias, by making the automatic conducting system more irritable. The systolic blood pressure rises, but the diastolic falls. Vessels in different situations react to adrenaline in different ways. While the vessels of the skin, mucosae, subcutaneous tissues, splanchnic area and kidneys are constricted (α-effects), those in muscles are relaxed after physiological doses (β-effects), constricted after large doses. While the cerebral and pulmonary arteries are constricted blood pressure in the coronaries is likely to rise. Angina pectoris may be precipitated in patients with coronary disease, because of the augmentation of cardiac work on top of narrowed vessels. The peripheral venous pressure is increased. It is the most potent drug known to stimulate an arrested heart, but its transient and rather violent effect and the danger of ventricular dysrhythmias limit routine use as a pressor agent. Increases platelet stickiness and reduces clotting time, leading to shorter bleeding time. The cardiovascular effects of adrenaline are reduced by acidosis.[19]

The renal blood flow. This is decreased. Secretion of urine is reduced.

The respiratory system. Bronchial tone decreased, following both topical (1–100 solution in atomizer) and systemic administration. Depth of respiration slightly increased, and irregular breathing sometimes seen.

The alimentary canal. While the muscle of the gut is relaxed, the pyloric and ileocolic sphincters are contracted (both α- and β-effects) leading to ileus. The spleen contracts and empties its cells into the circulation. The secretion of the intestinal glands is inhibited.

Sweating and pilomotor activity not much stimulated in man. Dilates the pupil when carried to the eye in the bloodstream.

Glycogen is mobilized from the liver, giving rise to an increase in the blood-sugar level; anti-insulin effect. Rise in metabolic rate, lipolysis, and muscle catabolism. Large doses stimulate, small clinical doses inhibit uterine tone in labour. It elevates the pain threshold.

Following injection, untoward reactions may include anxiety, restlessness from mild cerebral stimulation, throbbing headache, vertigo, pallor and palpitations; hyperthyroid and hypertensive patients are specially liable to these effects.

It must be used with the greatest care when the patient is inhaling chloroform, trichloroethylene, halothane or cyclopropane or receiving mono-amine oxidase inhibitors or tricyclic antidepressants, because of the risk of the production of ventricular fibrillation. In the presence of thyrotoxicosis and of hypertension, it must be given with great caution. Should not be used with local analgesics in ring block of the digits or penis or of the external ear.

Pharmacokinetics
It is mostly degraded by conjugation with glycuronic and sulphuric acids and excreted in the urine. A smaller part is oxidized by amine oxidase and inactivated by *o*-methyl-transferase.

Clinical Uses
(1) To produce vasoconstriction in local analgesia thereby reducing toxicity and prolonging analgesic effect; (2) To provide ischaemia in the skin and subcutaneous tissues before incisions, e.g. in thyroidectomy (1–200 000 to 1–500 000); (3) In the treatment of cardiac arrest. Given i.v., adrenaline may cause severe myocardial ischaemia.[20] Total dose should not exceed 0·5 mg (i.e. 0·5 ml 1–1000 solution); (4) In the treatment of anaphylactic shock an i.v. bolus dose of 0·1 mg should not be exceeded, but may be repeated; (5) As a bronchodilator.

Noradrenaline Acid Tartrate, BP (*l-Arterenol, Norepinephrine, Levophed*) (*nor = Nitrogen ohne Radikol*—German)
Clinically it is used for its vasopressor effects only (α-adrenergic

receptor stimulant). It is the neurohumoral transmitter for sympathetic nerve endings.

History
Humoral transmission of nerve impulses described by Elliott in 1905 and proved by Otto Loewi (1873–1961) of Berlin, in 1921.[21] Properties of racemic noradrenaline described by George Barger (1878–1939) and Henry Hallett Dale (1875–1968) in 1910.[22]

Pharmacodynamics
A powerful α-receptor-site stimulator. Probably the major pressor amine found at postganglionic adrenergic nerve-endings responsible for reflex vascular effects, adrenaline being mainly responsible for metabolic activities.

Indications
Seldom used now. It is of value immediately after removal of a phaeochromocytoma[23] in patients in whom the peripheral resistance is very low because of tissue acidosis; in the patient whose heart has been poisoned by β-adrenergic blockade; in intra-aortic balloon pumping to raise the diastolic blood pressure.[24] An i.v. infusion of 500 ml of dextrose containing 2–4 mg can be given until the effects are obtained. Its addition to solutions of local analgesics is not recommended as it may cause hypertension. Nor is it suitable for the treatment of hypotensive shock states.

Ephedrine, BP
A direct α- and β-adrenergic stimulator and a releaser of catecholamines from receptor sites. Introduced into Western medicine in 1924 by Schmidt and Chen.[25] The active principle (isolated in 1885 by Yamanash and named by N. Nagai (1844–1929) in 1887)[26] of ma huang, a Chinese plant. Chemically allied to adrenaline. Manufactured synthetically. Its adrenaline-like properties were described by Japanese pharmacologists in 1917.[27]

Pharmacodynamics
The laevo-rotatory form is more active. It delays the destruction of adrenaline and noradrenaline and so maintains a high blood catecholamine level. Releases stored noradrenaline from nerve endings in the vessel walls.[28] (1) A potent sympathetic stimulant. The rate and force of cardiac contraction are increased and blood pressure raised. Arterioles are constricted. The duration of effect is some 30–40 min but repeated doses are not so effective (tachyphylaxis); (2) Relaxation of smooth muscle of bronchi; (3) Dilates pupil; (4) Stimulation of cerebral cortex and medulla with subjective feeling of apprehension, trembling and discomfort; (5) Probably dilates coronary arteries; (6) Increases bladder-neck tone; (7) A local analgesic effect.

Uses
First used to control hypotension during spinal analgesia in 1927.[29] The drug has the advantage that cardiac output and venous return are increased. Has been used in states of hypotension, bronchospasm, heart block, carotid sinus syndrome, urticaria, narcolepsy, enuresis and myasthenia.

Put up in ampoules of 30 mg. Dose: 15–30 mg by injection; up to 50 mg by mouth.

Methylamphetamine Hydrochloride, BP
Its use has been discontinued in many hospitals for social (not pharmacological) reasons. *See* Eighth Edition of this Synopsis.

Metaraminol Bitartrate (*Aramine*)
An α-stimulator with slight β-stimulating effects. Pharmacologically similar to ephedrine. Introduced in 1951,[30] and first used in spinal analgesia 3 years later.[31] Unlike noradrenaline and ephedrine it is not readily destroyed by tissue enzymes. It stimulates the myocardium without producing dysrhythmia. It raises both the systolic and diastolic blood pressures. Its action is partly direct on the vessel walls and partly due to the liberation of noradrenaline from stores in nerve endings or chromaffin cells. No influence on mental state. May cause reflex bradycardia which can be abolished by atropine. After intramuscular injection, 10 min elpase before its action is seen; after intravenous injection, 2 min. Duration of effect 20–60 min.

Dosage: intramuscularly 2–10 mg; intravenously 0·5–5 mg; by infusion, 15–100 mg in 250–500 ml as a substitute for the noradrenaline drip.

Supplied in 1-ml ampoules of 1% solution.

Methoxamine Hydrochloride, BPC (*Vasoxine*)
This is a synthetic vasopressor. It was synthesized in 1942.[32] It can be autoclaved, is non-irritating and is a potent agent with a rather prolonged effect which comes on 2 min after intravenous injection and may last up to 1 h. First used to maintain blood pressure in spinal analgesia in 1950.[33]

It has no effect on cardiac output, and causes increased peripheral resistance, and a rise in the right atrial and ventricular pressure and in peripheral venous mean pressure. Its action is peripheral on the arteries and veins (α-stimulator). Pulse rate slowed, an effect blocked by atropine. Gives rise to no cardiac dysrhythmias and seems to be safe in the presence of halothane. Does not stimulate the higher centres. Pilomotor effect marked and causes desire to empty bladder. It reduces the urinary volume by depressing the glomerular filtration rate and constricting the renal artery. Must be used carefully in cases of hypertension, cardiac disease and hyperthyroidism. Large doses can act as a partial β-stimulator and induce ectopic beats.

Dosage: 5–20 mg intramuscularly; 2 mg intravenously.

Phenylephrine Hydrochloride, BP (*Neosynephrine, Neophryn*)
An α-stimulator and in large doses a β-stimulator. First described in 1910 by Barger and Dale[34] and in 1931 by Kuschinsky and Oberdisse.[35] First used as a pressor agent in spinal analgesia in 1938.[36] Chief effect is to cause vasoconstriction by direct action on vessel walls, and so can be used in place of adrenaline, together with local analgesics for infiltration or intradural block. Effect lasts 10–15 min. Has no effect on conducting tissue of heart, but may cause bradycardia from vagal stimulation, so that bradycardia, together with heart block, are contraindications to its use. Dilates the pupil; relieves nasal congestion. Sensitizes the heart to catecholamines so that if cyclopropane or

halogenated volatile anaesthetics are being used, initial dose should not exceed 2–5 mg intravenously.

Felypressin (*Octopressin*)
This is 2-phenylalanine-8-lysine vasopressin, a synthetic derivative of the octopeptide hormone vasopressin from the posterior pituitary. Causes contraction of all smooth muscle—including coronaries—but has little oxytocic or antidiuretic effect. On injection causes local vasoconstriction without secondary vasodilatation as adrenaline does. Little effect on cardiac rhythm and may be relatively safe in patients receiving tricyclic antidepressants, mono-amine oxidase inhibitors, halogenated volatile anaesthetics or cyclopropane. Dose: up to 5 pressor units. Available in combination with prilocaine to prolong the effects and increase the efficiency of dental analgesia.

If pressor agents are required in patients inhaling halogenated vapours or cyclopropane, methoxamine or ephedrine would appear to be reasonably safe.

Adrenergic Beta Stimulants

Dopamine (Intropin)
A physiological derivative of noradrenaline occurring naturally and having the following actions: (1) Improves cardiac contractility without increasing its rate and hence myocardial oxygen consumption, a β-adrenergic effect. Effects blocked by β-antagonists, e.g. propranolol. In high dosage has α-adrenergic stimulating effects which can be abolished by vasodilators, e.g. phenoxybenzamine; (2) Increases renal blood flow by vasodilatation and stimulation of 'dopamine receptors' in the renal artery; this results in diuresis and saluresis. Effects blocked by dopamine antagonists, e.g. haloperidol.[37] Clinical effects are thus increase in cardiac output, renal blood flow and rise in arterial pressure. Can be used to treat exacerbations of chronic cardiac failure and acute reduction of cardiac output, as after cardiac surgery; it may be useful in septicaemia. Urine flow, blood pressure and cardiac output should be monitored. It is inactivated by alkalis and *patients should be normovolaemic before its use*. It is postulated that there are two types of dopamine receptors, D1 which is mainly inhibitory, and D2, mainly stimulant. Side-effects are dose-dependent and include nausea and vomiting, dyspnoea, headache, angina, hypertension and dysrhythmia. It is given intravenously in an infusion of normal saline, Ringer-lactate or 5% dextrose, the dose being 2 µg/kg/min to increase renal blood flow; 5 µg/kg/min to stimulate cardiac β-receptors; higher dosage, e.g. 15–25 µg/kg/min stimulates α-receptors, causing decreased blood flow in all organs. Has been used in the management of kidney donors. (Renal effects of dopamine, *see* Editorial, *Anesthesiology* 1984, **61**, 487.) Each 5-ml ampoule contains 40 mg/ml.

Dobutamine
A derivative of dopamine with α- and β-stimulating effects, a synthetic catecholamine, has no specific effect on the kidney vasculature. May be useful when dysrhythmias are a problem.

Isoprenaline Sulphate, BP (*Isoproterenol, USP*)
A powerful β-adrenergic stimulant drug, a synthetic catecholamine. Has

inotropic and chronotropic effects on the heart and causes peripheral vasodilatation. The drug is used in cardiogenic shock to increase cardiac output and improve tissue perfusion. It may be given by intravenous drip, 1–5 mg in 500 ml 5% glucose at a rate of 2–4 μg/min or in a bolus dose of 1–2 μg. It also causes bronchodilatation and in the treatment of asthma may be administered by sublingual tablets, 10 or 20 mg, or by inhalation of 1% spray. Heart block is sometimes treated by 30 mg sustained-action tablets 4-hourly or 5-mg suppositories 3–4-hourly. May increase myocardial oxygen demand and cause subendocardial ischaemia.

Salbutamol (*Ventolin*)
A selective β-stimulant with little or no β_1 (cardiac) stimulant action. Administered by metered aerosol inhaler, 100 μg per time or intravenously. In high doses, however, it does stimulate the heart and is a vasodilator. Has been used during cardiac surgery, 10–15 mg in 500 ml of 5% dextrose, i.v. Maximal bronchodilatation occurs within 5 min and the duration of effect is about 4 hours. Can be given by mouth 2–4 mg 6–8-hourly. Used to treat asthma, bronchospasm and premature labour.

Terbutaline (*Bricanyl*)
Also a selective β-stimulant used in the treatment of bronchospasm. Peak action occurs 30 min after subcutaneous injection or 2–3 h after oral administration. Oral dose is 2–4 mg 8-hourly.

Gross hypertension may follow the use of *ergot* preparations given intravenously if the patient has already received a sympathomimetic amine, as ergometrine (ergonovine), ergotamine and ergotoxin may cause contraction of the muscular wall of blood vessels.

Following intra- or extradural sympathetic blockade, hypotension is best treated by posture, oxygen, intravenous fluid and either ephedrine or methylamphetamine.

Influence of Other Drugs on Patients Given Pressor Amines

1. Monoamine Oxidase Inhibitors
These may potentiate the hypertensive effects of sympathomimetic amines, leading to hypertensive crises and dysrhythmias.

2. Tricyclic and Quadricyclic Antidepressants
These may increase the cardiovascular effects of catecholamines, leading to dysrhythmias and hypertension.

3. Anaesthesia with halogenated vapours and cyclopropane
These may sensitize the heart to the dysrhythmic effects of catecholamines.

4. Chlorpromazine and Promethazine
These cause the pressor activity of injected adrenaline to be reversed. They do not greatly affect the pressor activity of noradrenaline. They reduce the pressor activity of methoxamine and phenylephrine.

5. Guanethidine (*Ismelin*)

Its hypotensive effects are probably achieved in the same way as those following reserpine except that it does not deplete the catecholamines in the brain or adrenal gland. In a limb isolated by a tourniquet has been used to release sympathetic tone.[38]

6. Reserpine

Patients under its influence show a diminished response to those pressor amines which act by releasing stores of noradrenaline in the vessel walls. This effect may last for 2 weeks after reserpine has been discontinued.

Use of Pressor Drugs in Anaesthesia

In modern anaesthetic practice, pressor drugs are used with decreasing frequency, but the following are relative indications: (1) In hypotension produced by drugs, e.g. ganglionic blocking agents, opioids, barbiturates, halothane, droperidol, etc.; (2) In hypotension due to a threatened coronary circulation. Vasopressin and angiotensin, coronary constrictors both, should not be used; (3) Following removal of phaeochromocytoma; (4) To maintain renal function and urinary output (along with generous fluid replacement). Dopamine increases renal blood flow; (5) In hypotension following intradural and extradural block, rarely; (6) Following incompatible blood transfusion; (7) After heart surgery; (8) In hypotension due to diminished circulatory volume, pressor drugs are harmful, reducing tissue perfusion and increasing acidosis; may also result in renal iscahemia and cardiac overload.

Tachyphylaxis often causes trouble when pressor agents are used, e.g. the bad reputation of the noradrenaline drip (embalming fluid!).

Adrenergic Blocking Agents

α-Blockers

These can be separated into the following groups:

1. The Imidazolines

(*a*) Tolazoline, BP (Priscol) antagonizes the vasoconstrictive effects of the catecholamines and in addition has a direct vasodilating effect on blood vessels. Can be injected into an artery to relieve spasm (25–30 mg). (*b*) Phentolamine methane-sulphonate and hydrochloride, BP (Regitine, Rogitine).[39] This drug has an atropine-like effect on the heart and is a direct stimulant of cardiac muscle. Short duration of action, so best given as continuous intravenous drip 1–2 mg/min. Acts as a competitive inhibitor at the receptor site and can be promptly reversed by use of α-stimulants. Dose for adrenaline over-dose: 5–10 mg intravenously.

2. The Chloro-ethylamines

(*a*) Phenoxybenzamine hydrochloride BP (Dibenyline, Dibenzyline). The blocking effects of this agent take about 30 min to develop with a duration of action of several hours until the drug is excreted. Used in phaeochromocytoma surgery and to antagonize the vasoconstriction associated with shock (together with fluid replacement). Can be given either by mouth or by drip intravenously, 1 mg/kg in 500 ml 5% glucose; (*b*) Dibenamine.

3. The Ergot Alkaloids
Ergotamine and certain dehydrogenated derivatives have a feeble anti-adrenaline action but may potentiate the effects of other pressor agents especially in hypertensive patients, e.g. during labour. Their vasoconstrictor effects are due to α-adrenergic stimulation.[40]

4. The Phenothiazines
Chlorpromazine and certain other related compounds have an α-blocking effect.

5. The Butyrophenone Derivatives
Droperidol and haloperidol.

6. Thymoxamine
Dose 0·1 mg/kg by bolus intravenous injection 2–4 hourly. Complications: severe hypotension, hypoglycaemia.

Use of α-blockers in the shocked patient is dangerous unless adequate volume replacement has been achieved by rapid intravenous infusion and there is monitoring of central venous and arterial pressures. With these safeguards, α-blockers often produce a rise in arterial and venous Pa_{O_2}.

β-Blockers
β-Blockers competitively block the positive inotropic effect of isoprenaline but are without effect on the similar actions of calcium and digitalis glycosides—$β_1$- effects: cardiac, renin release; $β_2$-effects: bronchial, vascular, insulin release, uterine receptors.

Propranolol[41]
Propranolol is a crystalline solid soluble in water and alcohol. The L-isomer has the following effects:
Cardiovascular system
1. Slows the heart by direct action on cardiac sympathetic-β-receptors. Abolishes the tachycardia caused by isoprenaline injection. Does not depress the vagus.
2. Decreases contractile force and blocks positive inotropic effects of isoprenaline, but not those of digitalis or calcium.
3. Peripheral vascular resistance first temporarily decreased, then increased for a prolonged period.[42]
4. Reduction of blood pressure.
5. Causes slight prolongation of A–V conduction but has no effect on intraventricular conduction.
6. Propranolol is liable to precipitate and intensify heart failure.
Nervous system. The D-isomer is a powerful local analgesic. This is the 'membrane-depressant effect' or 'quinidine effect'. Sympathetic system—no stimulation. Propranolol reduces the sensation and physical effects of fear and anxiety.
Myoneural junction. Augments action of depolarizing and reduces action of non-depolarizing agents.

Respiration. Blocks sympathetic bronchial dilatation and may cause severe bronchospasm, especially in asthmatic and bronchitic patients—an effect reversed by isoprenaline and atropine. May delay time of effective fetal respiration by effect on fetal chemoreceptors.

Metabolism. Blocks lipolysis, muscle glycogenolysis, insulin release and, when combined with an α-blocker, the raised metabolic rate due to adrenaline (β_2-effect). Inhibits plasma renin activity (β_1-effect).

Clinical uses in anaesthesia. Protects the heart from adrenergic stimulation associated with anxiety, atropine, surgical stimulation, injected adrenaline, thyrotoxicosis, postoperative thyroid crises, phaeochromocytoma and hypercapnia, and so reduces dysrhythmias, but also cardiac output. Has been used to abolish dysrhythmias associated with the use of halothane, cyclopropane and chloroform, and hypothermia. To potentiate hypotension caused by ganglion-blocking agents: it prevents tachycardia in patients with chronic myocardial ischaemia. Dose in adults: 0·5–10·0 mg i.v.

Practolol

Introduced in 1968.[43] No local analgesic effect. Used in anaesthesia intravenously in doses up to 20 mg. Unwanted side-effects only occur with long-term treatment.

Uses of β-Blockers

1. To lower arterial pressure and control angina pectoris.
2. To control sinus tachycardia and prevent dysrhythmias due to injected adrenaline or phaeochromocytoma removal (with α-blockers).
3. To control thyrotoxicosis before surgery.
4. In obstructive cardiomyopathy.

Table 19.2. Some current β-blocking drugs

Cardioselective		Non-cardioselective	
No intrinsic sympathomimetic activity	With intrinsic sympathomimetic activity	No intrinsic sympathomimetic activity	With intrinsic sympathomimetic activity
Metoprolol	Practolol	Propranolol	Aprenolol
Atenolol	Acebutolol	Sotalol	Oxprenolol
		Timolol	Pindolol
		Labetalol	
		Nadolol	

Dangers of Beta-blockers

1. Bronchospasm in asthmatics (with non-selective blockers.) Atenolol, practolol and metoprolol are relatively free from this defect.
2. The non-selective blockers may cause hypoglycaemia in diabetics and mask its effects.
3. May precipitate cardiac failure in patients with decompensation.
4. Prolonged administration of practolol may cause corneal damage, psoriatic

kyperkeratotic skin reactions, deafness, sclerosing peritonitis and systemic lupus erythematosus.

    5. Intermittent claudication and Raynaud's phenomena may be aggravated.

    6. Diminished reflex response to haemorrhage.

    7. Atrioventricular conduction defects may occur.

    8. Fatigue, dizziness, depression, hallucinations, vivid dreams, somnolence, insomnia, myasthenic syndrome, dyspepsia, low birth weight of offspring, delayed spontaneous respiration of offspring born by Caesarean section.

    9. Reduced cardiac output in patients receiving cyclopropane anaesthesia.

    10. Effects prolonged and potentiated by liver disease.

(*See also* 'Which beta-blocker?' Breckenridge A. *Br. Med. J.* 1984, **286**, 1085.)

Calcium Antagonists

These drugs cause blockade of the slow calcium ion influx into the contractile and conducting myocardial cells, resulting in slow conduction, prolonged refractory period and depression of contractility.[44] The different drugs in this group vary in their electrophysiological effects on the fast and slow inward currents which accounts for the differences in their pharmacological effect.

Verapamil (Isoptin)

A synthetic papaverine derivative. May be given orally or intravenously, but larger doses are needed by mouth because of considerable first pass elimination in the liver. Doses orally 80–160 mg 8-hourly; onset in 2 h, peak effect in 5 h, or intravenously, 75–150 µg/kg, onset in 2 min, duration of action 10–15 min. There is preferential uptake and binding in the AV node so that action there is longer lasting than elsewhere. Ninety per cent is bound to plasma proteins.

    Its main use is the termination and prevention of paroxysmal ventricular tachycardia. Great caution should be used if given in association with β-blockers since negative chronotropic and inotropic effects may be augmented. Contraindications include pre-existing hypotension, sinus node dysfunction, A–V block and marked left ventricular dysfunction. May be of use in refractory ventricular fibrillation during cardio-respiratory resuscitation.[45]

Nifedipine (Adalat)

A dihydropyridine. Oral or sublingual dose 10–20 mg 4–8-hourly. Onset after oral ingestion 15–20 min but only 2 min when given intranasally as a spray. Little first pass liver extraction. Main clinical use as coronary and peripheral vasodilator. Antagonizes intracellular calcium which is the necessary trigger for excitation-contraction coupling in vascular smooth muscle. Less effect on A–V node than verapamil. Dilates coronary arteries in dosage which does not depress myocardial contractility. Valuable in variable (Prinzmetal) angina due to myocardial spasm as well as classic angina. Can be used in association with β-blockers, nitrates, frusimide, anticoagulants and anti-hypertensives.

Diltiazem (Tildiem)

A benzothiazepine. Intermediate pharmacological position between verapamil and nifedipine. Oral administration 60–90 mg 8-hourly, with extensive first pass hepatic extraction; onset in 15 min with peak effect in 30 min. Intravenous dose 75–150 µg/kg.

Use with Volatile Anaesthetic Agents
General anaesthetic agents have a non-specific calcium antagonist action which is the cause of myocardial depression and vascular dilatation. Calcium antagonists may cause a hypotensive response during general anaesthesia with volatile agents. This may occur with halothane[46] and other volatile supplements.[47] In animals, MAC values may be decreased.[48] Cessation of therapy with nifedipine prior to cardiac surgery may result in post bypass hypertension.[49]

Other Effects
(1) Use with muscle relaxants. The effects of non-depolarizing drugs may be potentiated.[50] A monitor should be used to regulate relaxant dosage; (2) Cerebral blood flow. This may increase as a result of vascular dilatation.[51] (*See also* Jones R. M. in: *Recent Advances in Anaesthesia and Analgesia—15* (Atkinson R. S. and Adams A. P. ed.) Edinburgh: Churchill Livingstone, 1985.) For history of their development, *see* Fleckenstein A. *Circ. Res.* 1983, **52** (Suppl. 1) 3.

Antacids and Other Agents

Magnesium Trisilicate and Sodium Citrate
See Chapter 27.

Magnesium Hydroxide (8·3%; Milk of Magnesia)
Used in obstetrics and intensive care. Dose: 10–20 ml oral.

Dimethicone with Aluminium Hydroxide (*Asilone*)
Reduces foaming in the stomach during gastroscopy. Dose: 5–10 ml oral.

Cimetidine (*Tagamet*)
Does not affect acid already in the stomach, but raises the pH above 2·5 in about half an hour. This histamine H_2-receptor antagonist has also been used in anaphylactic reactions. Dose: 200 mg by mouth or i.m.

Ranitidine (*Zantac*)
An H_2 receptor blocker which reduces the production of gastric acid. Like cimetidine it is used to reduce the acidity of gastric contents before induction of anaesthesia. Dose 150 mg by mouth, by slow injection (50 mg, every 6–8 h), or by infusion (25 mg/h).

Hyoscine N-butyl Bromide (*Buscopan*)
Used in gastroscopy to reduce gastric motility. Dose: 10–20 mg i.v.

Metoclopramide (*Primperan; Maxolon*)
Speeds gastric emptying; anti-emetic; sometimes effective against hiccup; increases tone of cardiac sphincter, an effect counteracted by atropine. Dose averages 10 mg. Overdosage, seldom seen by anaesthetists, may cause extrapyramidal effects.[52] A dopamine receptor antagonist.

Domperidone (*Motilium*)
It inhibits the chemoreceptor trigger zone (like metoclopramide), has a relaxing effect on the lower oesophageal sphincter and the gut, including the pylorus. When given i.v. inhibits postoperative vomiting and also that due to cytotoxic drugs.[53]

Anticoagulants

Used for the prophylaxis of venous thrombosis and for anticoagulation during arterial and cardiac surgery.

Heparin
Rapidly effective. Prepared from the liver and lungs of animals; it carries a strong electronegative charge. Part destroyed by heparinase, and partly excreted in the urine. Dose: 1000–5000 units subcutaneously 6–12 hourly for 3 days perioperatively to prevent thrombophlebitis; 100 units/kg in arterial surgery; 100–300 units/kg in extracorporeal circuits. Best given (for prolonged effect) by continuous i.v. infusion; otherwise at intervals of not more than 6 h, i.v. Dose controlled by the activated partial thromboplastin time. May be reversed by protamine sulphate, 1 mg for every 100 units of heparin remaining in the circulation, i.v. The half-life of heparin is about 1 h, but this may be prolonged for 4–8 h during surgery or after trauma. With aspirin the risk of bleeding is increased.

Coumarins
Preoperative dosage adjustment to an acceptable prothrombin time (e.g. one and a half to twice normal) is essential. There may be a reduced anticoagulant effect associated with barbiturates, due to increased metabolism and increased bleeding, with aspirin. Reversal of the coumarins by vitamin K analogues, in an emergency, may be monitored by the anaesthetist by placing serial blood samples in glass containers and timing the clotting process. Normal is 3–5 min. Duration of coumarins in common use is 6–48 h.

Antifibrinolysins

Unwelcome fibrinolysis after cardiopulmonary bypass and in the prostatic bed after prostatectomy is antagonized by ε-aminocaproic acid: 4 g i.v. An overdose may lead to disseminated intravascular coagulation.

Diuretics

Mannitol (*Osmitrol*)
This acts within minutes and last for 1–4 hours. Circulatory overload may be a problem. Mannitol is filtered by the glomeruli but none is reabsorbed by the tubules. Used for forced diuresis as after mismatched transfusions, and to reduce cerebral oedema. It remains extracellular and is inert in the body. Used as 10 or 20% solution, 0·5–1 g/kg by infusion. Extravenous leakage causes a sore arm.

Urea
Used to treat cerebral oedema. Contraindicated in renal and hepatic failure and in cerebral haemorrhage. Given as a 30% solution in 5 or 10% glucose solution, 40–80 g (3–4 ml/min).

Sodium Excretors
These cause water, sodium and potassium loss by inhibiting reabsorption from the renal tubules. They include frusemide (Lasix), thiazides and ethacrynic acid. They act very rapidly and potentiate antihypertensive drugs. Massive doses of frusemide may increase gentamicin-induced renal failure. Ethacrynic acid may cause hyperuricaemia, raise the blood urea level, produce diarrhoea and potentiate the actions of both warfarin and lithium salts. The hypokalaemia produced by the sodium excretors may potentiate the action of digoxin.

Aldosterone Antagonists
(*Spironolactone, Aldactone*)
These have a potassium-sparing effect; diuresis commences after 2–3 h. Dose of spironolactone: 150 mg by mouth; of soldactone: 200 mg i.v. which acts more slowly.

Digoxin

Used to control atrial fibrillation and improve ventricular filling and ejection. Dose: 0·05–0·25 mg by mouth. Some preparations are absorbed much more completely than others. Absorption after intramuscular injection is very slow. Great care is necessary before injecting the drug intravenously to partially digitalized patients. Toxicity potentiated by hypokalaemia which may be produced by diuretics. Toxic effects during operation include extreme brady-cardia with coupled ventricular ectopic beats and slight depression of the ST segment. Very rarely, tachycardia may occur. Overdose may require dialysis.

Antibiotics

Penicillins
These are frequently used for the treatment of major infections and for prophylaxis of bacterial endocarditis. Penicillins are bacteriocidal. Benzyl penicillin, 0·5–4 g 4-hourly, is usually effective against streptococci which cause bacterial endocarditis. Ampicillin is also active against gram-negative bacteria. Cloxacillin has activity against staphylococci. Meclocillin is a recent addition to the ever-growing range of penicillins. Patients with penicillin allergy may often be given erythromycin 250–1000 mg instead.

Erythromycin
This is similar to penicillin but is active against Legionnaire's disease.

Aminoglycosides
This group includes streptomycin, gentamicin and neomycin. They share the following disadvantages: (1) In large doses they cause non-depolarizing neuro-muscular block resistant to neostigmine, but partly reversed by intravenous

calcium; (2) They may be nephrotoxic, especially when combined with some other drugs, e.g. gentamicin with cephaloridine, gentamicin with frusemide or when given with methoxyflurane (*See also* Atkinson R. S. et al. *Handbook of Intensive Care*. London: Chapman and Hall, 1981, Ch. 25.)

Perioperative antibiotics
(*See* Keighley M. R. B. *Br. Med. J.* 1983, **286**, 1844.)

Aminophylline

A bronchodilator. May cause gastric irritation and headache. Can be given as a suppository. Has been used for nocturnal cardiac asthma and left ventricular failure. Dose, by mouth 100–300 mg; i.v. 5 mg/kg, slowly (in patients not taking xanthine drugs). Has been used to reverse the respiratory depressant effects of morphine;[54] dose 2 mg/kg. i.v.

Dantrolene Sodium

Used for the treatment of malignant hyperpyrexia and in medicine for muscle spasticity. Interferes with the release of calcium from sarcoplasmic reticulum. Supplied in an ampoule containing dantrolene 20 mg, mannitol, 13 g, buffered to a pH of 9·5 with sodium bicarbonate. Dose 1 mg/kg, repeated carefully up to 10 mg/kg (*see also* Chapter 18).

Corticosteroids

These are used for steroid cover in patients who have been treated with steroids, in the emergency treatment of anaphylaxis including mismatched blood transfusion, to reduce the antigen–antibody reaction, and in the intensive care unit for various specific conditions.

The effects of corticosteroids are: (1) Glucocorticoid: Hyperglycaemia, nitrogen loss, osteoporosis, peptic ulceration; (2) Mineralocorticoid: Sodium retention, hypertension, oedema; (3) Androgen: Hirsutism and aggressive behaviour; (4) Other: Anti-inflammatory, suppression of immune antigen–antibody response, delayed wound healing, reduced response to infections, tendency to thrombo-embolism, reduction of intracranial pressure.

Commonly used corticosteroids include hydrocortisone hemisuccinate 100 mg, prednisone 20 mg and dexamethasone 4–100 mg. (For steroid cover, *see* Chapter 22.)

References

1. Gershon S. et al. *J. Pharm. Pharmacol.* 1958, **10**, 638; Gordh T. and Wahlin A. *Acta Anaesthesiol. Scand.* 1961, **5**, 55; Buley R. and Morgan M. S. *Afr. Med. J.* 1975, **49**, 85.
2. Dundee J. W. et al. *Br. J. Pharmacol.* 1973, **48**, 326P.
3. Gairola R. L. et al. *Anaesthesia* 1980, **35**, 17.
4. Gupta P. K. and Dundee J. W. *Anaesthesia* 1974, **29**, 40.
5. Dundee J. W. et al. *Anaesthesia* 1974, **29**, 710.
6. Davies J. A. H. *Br. J. Anaesth.* 1968, **40**, 361.
7. Robertson G. S. et al. *Br. J. Anaesth.* 1977, **49**, 133.

8. Riddell P. L. et al. *Br. J. Anaesth.* 1978, **50**, 921.
9. Gawley T. H. et al. *Br. Med. J.* 1976, **2**, 122.
10. Edwards G. and Leszcynski S. O. *Lancet* 1967, **2**, 226.
11. Meier R. et al. *Klin. Wochenschr.* 1954, **32**, 445.
12. Aviado D. M. *Sympathomimetic Drugs*, Springfield, Ill.: Thomas, 1970, p. 7.
13. Oliver G. and Schäfer E. A. *J. Physiol.* 1895, **18**, 230.
14. Takamine J. *Therapeutic Gaz.* 1901, **27**, 221.
15. Takamine J. *Am. J. Pharmacol.* 1901, **73**, 523.
16. Aldrich T. B. *Am. J. Physiol.* 1901, **5**, 457.
17. Stolz F. *Berl. Chem. Ges.* 1904, **37**, 4149.
18. Starling E. H. *Lancet* 1905, **2**, 339.
19. Stutzman J. W. and Allen C. R. *Proc. Soc. Exp. Med. Biol.* 1941, **47**, 218.
20. Horak A. et al. *Br. Med. J.* 1983, **286**, 519.
21. Loewi O. *Pflugers Arch.* 1921, **189**, 239.
22. Barger G. and Dale H. H. *J. Physiol.* 1910, **41**, 19.
23. Pratilas V. and Pratila M. G. *Can. Anaesth. Soc. J.* 1979, **26**, 253.
24. Gilston A. in: *Recent Advances in Anaesthesia and Analgesia*—13 (Hewer C. L. and Atkinson R. S. ed.). Edinburgh: Churchill Livingstone, 1979, Chap. 3.
25. Chen K. K. and Schmidt C. F. *J. Pharmacol. Exp. Ther.* 1924, **24**, 339.
26. Nagai N. *Pharm. Zeit.* 1887, **32**, 700.
27. Amatsu H. and Kubota S. *Kyoto Igakhai Zasski* 1917, **14**, 77.
28. Burn J. H. and Rand M. J. *Lancet* 1958, **1**, 673.
29. Ockerblad N. F. and Dillon T. G. *JAMA* 1927, **88**, 1135.
30. Beyer K. H. et al. *Fedn Proc. Fedn Am. Socs Exp. Biol.* 1951, **10**, 281.
31. Poe M. F. *Anesthesiology* 1954, **15**, 547.
32. Baltzly R. and Buck J. S. *J. Am. Chem. Soc.* 1942, **64**, 3040.
33. King B. D. and Dripps R. D. *Surg. Gynecol. Obstet.* 1950, **9**, 695.
34. Barger G. and Dale H. H. *J. Physiol.* 1910, **41**, 19.
35. Kuschinsky G. and Oberdisse K. *Arch. Exp. Path. Pharmak.* 1931, **162**, 46.
36. Lorhan P. H. and Oliverio R. M. *Curr. Res. Anesth. Analg.* 1938, **17**, 44.
37. Breckenridge A. M. et al. *Eur. J. Clin. Pharmacol.* 1971, **3**, 131.
38. Hannington-Kiff J. C. *Lancet* 1974, **1**, 1019; *Br. Med. J.* 1979, **2**, 367.
39. Taylor S. H. et al. *Circulation* 1965, **31**, 741.
40. Wassef M. R. et al. *Br. J. Anaesth.* 1974, **46**, 473.
41. Black J. W. et al. *Lancet* 1964, **1**, 1080; *Br. J. Pharmacol.* 1965, **25**, 547.
42. Johnsson G. *Acta Pharmacol. Toxicol. (Copenh.)* 1975, **36**, Suppl. 59.
43. Dunlop D. and Shanks R. G. *Br. J. Pharmacol.* 1968, **32**, 201.
44. Durant N. N. et al. *Anesthesiology* 1984, **60**, 298.
45. Kapur P. A. et al. *Anesth. Analg. (Cleve.)* 1984, **63**, 460.
46. Fahmy N. R. and Lappas D. G. *Anesthesiology* 1983, **59**, A39.
47. Skarran K. *Anaesthesiology* 1983, **59**, 362.
48. Maze M. et al. *Anesthesiology* 1983, **59**, 327.
49. Casson W. R. et al. *Anaesthesia* 1984, **39**, 1197.
50. Bikhaz G. B. et al. *Anesthesiology* 1982, **57**, A268 and 1983, **59**, A269; Lawson N. W. et al. *Anesth. Analg. (Cleve.)* 1983, **62**, 50; Carpenter R. L. and Mulroy M. F. *Anesthesiology* 1983, **59**, A392.
51. Lynch C. and Bedford R. F. *Anesthesiology* 1983, **59**, A392.
52. Hughes R. L. *Anaesthesia* 1984, **39**, 720.
53. Brogden R. N. et al. *Drugs* 1982, **24**, 360; *Drug Ther. Bull.* 1983, **21**, 47.
54. Stirt J. A. *Anaesthesia* 1983, **38**, 275.

Chapter 20   # POSTOPERATIVE OBSERVATION ROOM[1]

The anaesthetist is responsible for the well-being of his patient until the patient is conscious (some forms of surgery are exceptions, e.g. neurosurgery), and his vital functions are stable and can be preserved without assistance.[2]

After the anaesthetic, this period is normally spent in the postoperative observation room, the patient being supervised by nurses, and the anaesthetist carrying medical responsibility for the postanaesthetic aspects of the case.

Problems of the Immediate Postoperative Period[3]

History
Advocated by A. L. Flemming, President of the Anaesthetic Section of the Medical Institute of Birmingham in 1921.[4] The first Postoperative Observation Room (Recovery Ward) was opened in the UK in 1955,[1] although Lundy at the Mayo Clinic had organized such a facility in 1942.

Problems may include, among others: pain, respiratory obstruction, hypoxia, hypovolaemia, residual neuromuscular block, nausea and vomiting, hypotension, abnormalities of the rate or rhythm of the heart, shivering and restlessness, ventilation/perfusion abnormalities.

Control of Postoperative Pain[5]

Two main problems exist in this area (*see also* Chapter 8).

1. Management of pain on return to consciousness. Since the introduction of postoperative observation units into European anaesthesia 30 years ago, this situation has been improved. The dose of an analgesic required to prevent pain is only a fraction of that required to control it once it has become severe.

2. Management of the return of pain when the first postoperative dose of analgesic has worn off. At this point the largely unsupervised patient may suffer unnecessarily. Several approaches have been made to solve this problem. (*a*) The use of long-acting regional blocks where appropriate; (*b*) The use of continuous infusion or 'on-demand' injections of opioids. This is effective but very expensive; (*c*) The use of 'as-required' doses of the very long-acting opioids, e.g. methadone, dextromoramide, and levorphanol, which give up to 12 hours of analgesia, especially useful at night. (If the first dose fails to control pain, it may be reinforced with one intravenous dose of a medium-duration opioid, e.g. pethidine.) Levorphanol, in particular, has very few side-effects within its therapeutic range. Buprenorphine is fairly long-acting, has frequent side-effects, and many patients are either over-sensitive or over-resistant to it.

The postoperative observation rooms, which should be close to the operating theatre, and supervised by members of the departments of anaesthesia and surgery, serve a most useful purpose. Respiratory and circulatory depression are detected early and efficiently treated by the skilled nursing sister in charge of the room, which is suitably equipped with oxygen therapy equipment, ventilators, self-inflating resuscitation bags and monitoring appliances, intravenous drip apparatus, beds which can be easily tipped, proper lighting and suction apparatus. There should be equipment for intubation and bronchoscopy.

In the postoperative room the nursing and medical staff must observe, check and, if necessary, remedy: (1) The comfort of the patient, including relief of pain, restlessness, nausea, vomiting and shivering; (2) The airway and respiratory activity; (3) The pulse and blood pressure; (4) The temperature; (5) The intravenous drip; (6) The surgical drain, catheter, etc.; (7) The urine output.

The advantages are obvious: it prevents duplication of equipment, economizes skilled nursing staff and saves lives. It must be remembered in this connection that almost half the deaths occurring in the immediate postoperative period are due to inadequate nursing care including respiratory obstruction.

Monitoring (*See* Chapter 41.)

The classic sign of haemorrhage, i.e. tachycardia and restlessness, is often absent in the postoperative ward. Measurement of the actual loss, if possible, or the CVP, assumes greater importance. Increasing girth is of no help in the diagnosis of intra-abdominal haemorrhage.

Postoperative Restlessness
After hypoxaemia, pain, haemorrhage and full bladder have been corrected, this usually responds to a small dose of benzodiazepine. (*See also* Chapter 18.)

Position of Patient
The lateral position is the safest for the airway, with one or other knee drawn up to prevent rolling. After some orthopaedic and other procedures, it may be impossible to place the patient on the side, and he is then at greater risk of airway obstruction or inhalation of vomit. (*See also* p. 332.)

The postoperative observation room should be staffed for 24 h each day, three beds being sufficient for one busy operating theatre, on average.

The patient is discharged back to his ward when he is conscious, is able to maintain an adequate ventilation and when his cardiovascular condition is in a stable state.

(*See also* Farman J. V. *Br. J. Hosp. Med.* 1978, **19**, 606; Symposium on Recovery from Anaesthesia, *J. R. Soc. Med.* 1979, **72**, 270; 'Patient flow patterns in a recovery room and implications for staffing' Bell M. et al. *J. R. Soc. Med.* 1985, **78**, 35; *Recovery Room Care* (Frost E. M. and Andrews A. C. ed.), *Int. Anesthesiol. Clin.* 1983, 2. Springfield, Ill.: Little, Brown; *Postanaesthetic Recovery*, Eltringham R. J. et al. Berlin & Heidelberg: Springer-Verlag, 1984. For postoperative scoring system, *see* Thomas D. and Davis A. C. *Anaesth. Intensive Care*, 1984, **12**, 125.)

References

1. Jolly C. and Lee J. A. *Anaesthesia* 1957, **12**, 49; Discussion, *Proc. R. Soc. Med.* 1958, **51**, 151; Atkinson R. S. in: *Recent Advances in Anaesthesia and Analgesia*—13 (ed. Hewer C. L. and Atkinson R. S.), Edinburgh: Churchill Livingstone, 1979.
2. Green R. A. *Anaesthesia* 1986, **41**, 129.
3. Asbury A. J. *Br. J. Hosp. Med.* 1981, **25**, 159.
4. Flemming A. L. *Lancet* 1923, **2**, 227.
5. Weiss O. F. et al. *Anesth. Analg. (Cleve.)* 1983, **62**, 70.

Chapter 21   RECORDS, CLINICAL TRIALS AND
STATISTICS

Anaesthetic Records

Pioneers in anaesthetic record keeping include Harvey Cushing in 1895[1] and
Ralph Waters in 1936.[2]

A record should be kept of all administrations of anaesthesia. Record charts
enable the anaesthetist to assess accurately the condition of the patient during
the operation and they are invaluable for reference, both clinical and possibly
medicolegal.

Nosworthy's cards[3] enable the sex, age, physical state, preoperative complications, anaesthetic techniques, complications during anaesthesia, plane of
anaesthesia, site of operation, duration of operation, premedication, anaesthetics used, postoperative complications, etc., to be accurately charted, while they
allow for a 5-min record of the pulse and blood-pressure readings. By converting
a series of circles into notches, rapid sorting is possible with the aid of a knitting
needle. (*See also* Seed R. F. and Welsh E. A. *Anaesthesia* 1976, **31**, 1199; Lunn
J. N. and Vickers M. D. *Anaesthesia* 1982, **37**, 651; Middleton H. and Hales S.
Anaesthesia 1982, **37**, 1121; Norman J. *Anaesthesia* 1985, **40**, 1238.)

Some types of record combine preoperative assessment with a record of vital
signs during operation. Other record systems incorporate carbon copies which
may be retained as departmental records when the originals are filed in the case
notes. Computers are used to store information in some centres.

*In every case, the agents, doses, and methods of administration should be
written in the operation book, followed by the anaesthetist's signature.*

A record of all intravenous fluids given during operation should be entered on
the case-sheet, including the identification numbers of any bottles of blood.

A clean sheet of paper and a pencil are still the best tools for collecting
worth-while data which will be useful in the future.

Clinical Trials

Clinical trials of new drugs offer considerable challenges. It is very difficult to
ensure that there is similarity between two or more groups of patients, except for
the factor under investigation. Observer or operator bias must be eliminated as
far as possible. The very fact that clinical trials are performed in a controlled
environment limits the application of the knowledge gained in its relevance to
situations outside that environment.

Some factors which must be considered when trials are planned include.[4]

1. Sex. For example, females are more prone to postanaesthetic nausea and
vomiting than males.

2. Accompaniments of anaesthesia, such as hypercapnia, passive hyperventilation, posture, etc., may affect observations.

3. Dosage and route of administration of drugs are important. The results
obtained in a clinical trial may not be valid for a different dose or method of
administration in clinical practice.

4. Persons carrying out trials often possess greater than average skills with the technique, e.g. local blocks.

5. The small numbers involved in a trial may not reveal uncommon side-effects. This is especially true if the operator is not looking for, or is unaware of, a particular effect.

There is a difference between statistically significant and clinically significant observations. When large numbers of cases have been required to demonstrate a statistically significant effect, the clinician must use judgement in deciding whether it is sufficient to affect clinical practice.

Investigation of a Drug[5]

Before a new drug is released for clinical use it must pass through various stages of investigation:

1. Chemical tests of purity and, where appropriate, tests for bacterial sterility.

2. Investigations in animals. Pharmacologists test the activity and potency and look for side-effects. Routine tests include estimation of minimum lethal dose on large populations of small animals, investigations into effects on cardiovascular, respiratory, central and autonomic nervous systems, hepatotoxicity, nephrotoxicity and teratogenic hazards.

Such investigations are limited by the wide occurrence of species variation. This may result in lack of appreciation of dangers in the human, but may also cause lack of further investigation of drugs which would be valuable therapeutic agents.

3. Trials in humans. The use of healthy volunteers has limitations. Small numbers are generally available and it is not possible to investigate effects on disease processes. In the UK the Committee on the Safety of Medicines looks continuously at new drug submissions. Doctors wishing to conduct trials on their own responsibility can apply for the Committee's approval. Payment of volunteers, or the use of volunteers from prisons or mental institutions, is also suspect on ethical grounds in Britain.

Clinical trials on patients are generally required. Such trials should be planned to obtain the maximum amount of unbiased information from the minimum number of patients in the shortest time with the least potential hazard and inconvenience. Protocols must be sanctioned by the appropriate ethical committee. It is not possible to submit patients to known hazards, while the use of invasive techniques for measurement may not be justified. The patient's informed consent should be obtained.

(*See also* 'Statement by the Medical Research Council', reproduced in *Br. J. Anaesth.* 1967, **39**, 283; Annotation, *Br. Med. J.* 1977, **1**, 1238; Dundee J. W. *J. R. Soc. Med.* 1980, **73**, 695.)

Blind Trials

In obtaining data it is necessary to eliminate observer bias as far as possible. A *single-blind trial* is carried out when the patient is unaware which of various methods of treatment is being applied. A *double-blind trial* is carried out when the physician or other observers are also unaware. It is often difficult or impossible to carry out blind trials. This may be because of some obvious difference in physical or pharmacological properties of substances under test. Observer bias is likely unless identical preparations of active drug and placebo are prepared and administered in random fashion using a number code which is not broken until all data have been obtained. Bias may still occur if the observer is aware that one particular property (e.g. duration of action) is being examined.[6]

(*See also* Hamilton M. *Br. J. Anaesth.* 1967, **39**, 287; Dundee J. W. *Proc. R. Soc. Med.* 1974, **67**, 586; Bulpitt C. J. *Br. J. Hosp. Med.* 1975, **13**, 611.)

Statistics

Defined as numerical facts systematically collected, on a given subject. The pioneer of vital statistics was W. Farr (1807–1883), who wrote his classic *Vital Statistics*. London: Stanford, 1885. It is interesting that he agreed with John Snow, following the cholera epidemic in Newcastle upon Tyne in 1853, that the disease was due to contaminated water (after first opposing the theory).

The data obtained from any clinical trial must be subjected to statistical analysis to determine the likelihood that results obtained from a small sample of patients are applicable to a large population.

Average. The *arithmetic mean* is the sum of observations divided by the number of observations. The *median* is the central value when all values are listed in order from lowest to highest. The *mode* is the most frequent observation—the value at which the ideal curve to which the observations conform reaches its highest point.

Variability. The *range* is the distance between the smallest and greatest observation.

Standard deviation (SD or sigma, σ). This is a measure of the scatter of observations around their mean. *Mean deviation* is the sum divided by the number of deviations. Standard deviation uses squares. This renders all deviations from the mean with a positive sign. The sum of the squares divided by the number of observations gives the value, *variance*. The *standard deviation* is the root of this value. When using a number of observations to estimate the variability in the general population, better estimates are obtained by dividing by one less than the total number of observations (i.e. $n-1$). This is more important when samples are small. The *coefficient of variation* is the standard deviation expressed as a percentage of the mean of the distribution.

It is more important to think in terms of 'frequency distribution' than of average. With a measurement that follows a normal distribution, nearly one-third of the values observed differ from the mean value by more than once the standard deviation. In a normal distribution, values that differ by more than twice the standard deviation are fairly rare. Values that differ by more than three times the standard deviation are very rare (1 in 370).

Standard error ($\sigma/\sqrt{n}$) (standard error of the mean) (SE). Not applicable to less than 20 individuals and with caution to less than 100. (*See also* Horan B. F. *Anaesth. Intensive Care* 1982, **10**, 297.)

Proportion or Percentage. The SE can be calculated for samples of different sizes. The relation of the difference between an expected percentage and an observed percentage to this standard error shows whether the difference is likely or unlikely to have arisen by chance. As a convention $2 \times$ SE is taken as a criterion. If the difference is more than $2 \times$ SE it is said to be *significant* (i.e. unlikely to have arisen by chance). If less than $2 \times$ SE it is not significant.

Caution is needed if numbers are less than 50. Any such test indicates probability and not proof, and gives no indication of the origin of the difference beyond saying that chance is unlikely.

Differences between proportions. The standard error of a difference between proportions. In reasonably large samples this may be taken to be the square root of the sum of the squares of the two individual standard errors of values in the two samples.

Note that 'significant' and 'important' are not synonymous.

Differences between averages. With reasonably large numbers of observations (25–30) the standard error of the difference between two means may be taken to be the square root of the sum of the squares of the two individual standard errors of the separate means in the two samples. A difference of more than twice this SE may be accepted as significant, a figure of twice indicating a probability of 1 in 20. With smaller numbers the *t*-test is the more appropriate measure.

Student's t test.[7] This may be applied when the observations are 25 or less. A calculation of standard deviation of the observations available is made, and standard error calculated of the observed difference between means, and the ratio calculated of the actually observed difference to the standard error. A special table of *t* values is then used. The value of *P*, that is the probability of getting that value by chance, is read off.

χ^2 *or chi-square test.* This is a method for testing the presence or absence of an association between different characteristics. It is a measure of the likelihood or unlikelihood of such an association being the result of chance. χ^2 equals the sum of all the values of the square of the difference between the observed number and the expected number divided by the expected number. It is important to consider both the value of χ^2 itself, and the number of sub-groups contributing to it. Tables of χ^2 are used to determine *P*. A value of *P* of 0·05 or less is usually taken as significant. The smaller the value of *P*, the less likely are the observations made to be due to chance.

Sequential analysis.[8] Special charts are used. It can only be applied when there is a simple investigation between two alternatives. It is of most value in comparing two drugs or procedures with respect to a single outcome. The chart is drawn on squared paper. Beginning in the bottom left-hand corner a line of crosses can be made proceeding vertically if the first alternative occurs and horizontally if the second applies. If the drugs or procedures are carried out in random variation of matched pairs, the line of crosses will gradually extend across the graph. When the line crosses pre-drawn limits representing probabilities at various values for *P*, the result of the trial may be considered significant to that value of *P*. If the line crosses other pre-drawn limits the result is not significant.

The linear analogue.[9] The patient is asked to mark a point on a linear scale to assess the severity of a symptom such as pain. The scale ranges from a zero (no pain at all) to a maximum (as much as can be imagined) and meaningful results can be obtained in statistical studies of analgesic techniques.

(*See also* Hill A. B. *Principles of Medical Statistics*, 9th ed. London: The Lancet Ltd, 1972; Armitage P. *Statistical Methods in Medical Research*. Oxford: Blackwell, 1972; Swinscow T. D. V. *Statistics at Square One*, 7th ed. London: Macmillan, 1983; Sykes M. K. et al. *Principles of Clinical Measurement* 2nd ed. Oxford: Blackwell, 1981; Gore S. M. and Altman D. G. *Statistics in Practice* London, British Medical Association, 1982; Goldstone L. A. *Understanding Medical Statistics*. London: Heinemann, 1983.)

References

1. Beecher H. K. *Surg. Gynecol Obstet.* 1940, **71**, 689.
2. Waters R. M. *J. Indiana State Med. Assoc.* 1936, **29**, 110.
3. Nosworthy M. *Curr. Res. Anesth. Analg.* 1945, **24**, 221; and *St. Thomas' Hosp. Rep. (London)*, 1937, **2**, 54; Nosworthy M. D. *Anaesthesia* 1963, **18**, 209.
4. Editorial, *Br. J. Anaesth.* 1967, **39**, 272.
5. Gray T. C. *Br. J. Anaesth.* 1967, **39**, 279.
6. Hoffer A. *Can. Med. Assoc. J.* 1967, **97**, 123; Watt M. J. et al. *Anaesthesia* 1968, **23**, 331.
7. Gosset W. S. *Biometrica* 1908, **6**, 1; Swinscow T. D. V. *Br. Med. J.* 1976, **2**, 291, 358, 408; Malt R. A. *N. Engl. J. Med.* 1977, **296**, 626; Kirkwood B. R. *Br. J. Clin. Equip.* 1980, **5**, 233.
8. *See* Armitage P. *Sequential Medical Trials*, Oxford: Blackwell, 1960.
9. Revill S. I. et al. *Anaesthesia* 1976, **31**, 1191.

4

Chapter 22   **MEDICAL DISEASES**
            INFLUENCING ANAESTHESIA

Anaesthesia is now a very safe procedure in the fit healthy patient. The risk is increased when systemic disease is present. In a study where patients were classified according to physical status (*see* Chapter 7), 16 000 cases of physical status I were operated on without any death attributable to anaesthesia. In patients of physical status V, there was a 10% mortality rate.[1] Recent audit[2] has shown that the overall 6-day mortality after surgery is around 0·6%, but the figure of deaths possibly related to anaesthesia is of the order of 0·25%. (*See also* Gray T. C. *J. Med. Defence Union* 1985, **1**, 9.)

The Geriatric Patient

Assessment of the Anaesthetic Risk in the Elderly Patient
  1. What is the *prognosis*? i.e. the chance of surviving the operative period? e.g. Female, 80–90 years, fractured neck of femur, one systemic disease, one operation, survival = 80–87%. Female, 80–90 years, second fractured neck of femur, one systemic disease, second operation, survival = 70%.
  2. What *problems* does the patient have?
  3. How can the *preparation* of the patient for surgery be matched to these problems?
  The elderly patient presents two distinct sets of problems, which affect each other:
  1. An increased incidence of concurrent diseases. The elderly patient is likely to have more than one concurrent disease, and to be taking many drugs (*see below*).
  2. The state of being elderly, which incorporates:
  Taking longer to recover from both trauma and surgery, both physically and mentally.
  Slower wound healing, weaker tissues, weaker muscles, poorer balance. Tendency to bedsores.
  Slower metabolic rate, making it easier to severely overventilate mechanically, slower metabolism of drugs, prolonging the action of muscle relaxants, increased target organ sensitivity, e.g. the reduced MAC percentages for the elderly, and the smaller doses of thiopentone required.
  Poorer memory, especially for recent events, making history-taking difficult.

(Memory assessment by the Camden Scale: what is your name? when were you born? where do you live now? who is the reigning monarch? who is the prime minister? what is the date/day of the week today?)

More complaining about trivial and fabricated events.

More confusion resulting from the upheaval of hospital admission.

Less renal function. (Declines 1% per year after 40 years.)

Less homeostasis in fluid balance, thus more easily dehydrated or overloaded.

Reduced body water.

Less homeostasis in temperature control.[3]

Less homeostasis in arterial and venous pressure control.

Greater tendency to urinary retention and constipation (exacerbated by anticholinergics and opioids respectively).

Deafness with resulting difficulty in communication.

Reduction of functional capabilities progressively with age, e.g. breathing capacity, vital capacity, cardiac index (1% per year decline over 40 years of age).

Poor adaptation to hospital diet.

Malnutrition, e.g. relative starvation, obesity, anaemia, vitamin deficiency, hypoproteinaemia.

'Hidden pathology', e.g. painless peritonitis,[4] apyrexial septicaemia,[5] silent myocardial infarction. The clinical examination reveals less of the abnormalities than in the young, hence the need for routine tests of full blood count, urine test, electrolytes, chest X-ray and ECG. These results may call for further monitoring. Only 13·5% of patients over 65 years had normal cardiorespiratory function in a series.[6]

Silent aspiration of gastric contents in very sick patients.

Osteoporosis, loss of teeth and jaw substance.

A difference between chronological age and biological age, e.g. a 90-year-old may appear as healthy and resilient as an ordinary 70 year old. Such a person will probably react to anaesthesia like a 90 year old.

Lowering arterial pressure produces more side-effects than in the young.

A tendency to die, either of the state itself, or of one of the concurrent diseases. The idea of assessment is to estimate how near they are to this point. Three questions emerge here: first, what is the severity of the risk? secondly, how quickly can that risk be reduced? thirdly, should the operation be postponed for medical treatment to improve the patient?

Assessment of Risk Severity (for all age groups)

Several systems are in use,[6] and although lack of fitness is not exactly synonymous with risk, it is closely parallel, when added to the severity of the operation.[7]

1. A.S.A. Classification (*see also* p. 109)

ASA 1. The patient has no organic, physiological, biochemical or psychiatric disturbance. The pathological process for which operation is to be performed is localized and does not entail a systemic disturbance.

ASA 2. Mild to moderate systemic disturbance caused either by the condition to be treated surgically or by other pathophysiological processes. Mild organic heart disease, diabetes, mild hypertension, anaemia, old age, obesity, mild chronic bronchitis.

ASA 3. Limitation of life-style. Severe systemic disturbance or disease from whatever cause, even though it may not be possible to define the degree of disability with any finality, e.g. angina, healed myocardial infarction, severe diabetes, cardiac failure.

ASA 4. Severe systemic disorders that are already life-threatening, not always correctable by operation, e.g. marked cardiac insufficiency, persistent angina, active myocarditis, advanced pulmonary, renal endocrine or hepatic insufficiency.

ASA 5. Moribund. Little chance of survival, but submitted to operation in desperation. Little if any anaesthesia is required.

If the operation is an emergency, the letter E is placed beside the numerical classification, and the patient is considered to be in poorer physical condition (*see* Goldstein A. and Keats A. S. *Anesthesiology* 1970, **33**, 130).

The ASA scheme is the most comprehensive system, but ignores the risk of the asymptomatic patient who, for example, may have severe coronary artery disease. It also ignores the inherent risks of a particular operation.

2. *The Goldman Cardiac Risk Factor Index*[8]

The following items carry scores: S3 sound or gallop rhythm, 11; Any dysrhythmia, 7; Age over 70 years, 5; Myocardial infarction within last 6 months, 10; 5 or more ventricular ectopic beats per min, 7; Emergency surgery, 4; Aortic stenosis, 3; Abdominal or thoracic operation, 3; Poor general condition, 3; A total over 13 gives a poor prognosis (11% life-threatening complications) and a cardiology consultation is advisable. Above 26, the perioperative mortality rate is over 50%, and only life-saving operations are considered. Angina, hypertension and prolonged surgery were added to this list by Peter.[9]

3. *Multivariate Risk Index*

The following have positive risk value: Increasing age over 70, male sex, history of smoking, obesity, bedsores, incontinence, concurrent infection, potassium depletion, anaemia, recent trauma, repeat surgery,[10] organ failure, e.g. cardiac (previous myocardial infarction, angina, cardiomegaly on chest X-ray, congestive cardiac failure, ECG abnormalities, untreated moderate or severe hypertension), respiratory, hepatic, renal and endocrine failure score likewise). House-boundness puts the patient in a higher risk category.

4. *The Cooperman Scheme*[11]

Can the Patient be Made any Fitter than he is Now?
Many elderly patients fall into three groups:

1. Normal (13·5% of total) ——→ accept for general anaesthesia

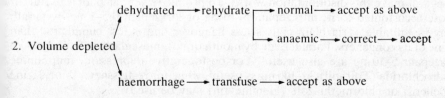

dysrrhythmia ──► correct ──► accept as above

3. Abnormal left ventricle ──► fluid retention ──► diuretics ──► accept

hypertensive ──► correct ──► accept

ischaemia ──► acute ──► postpone if possible

chronic:

a. mild → accept if the patient appreciates risk
b. severe → inoperable except for life-saving surgery

After history and examination, non-invasive tests of organ function are performed. Some of these (e.g. for geriatric dysautonomia) may be difficult in a patient bedridden with fractured neck of femur. A compromise test for this example is a change of arterial pressure or ECG between supine and sitting, or a slowing of pulse or ECG changes on deep breathing indicating poor control by the autonomic system.[12]
The anaesthetist's responsibility is to recognize risk factors and to advise surgeons and others that they should be corrected before elective surgery. The anaesthetist may be asked to help in this process if he has the time and facilities. This is more important in the case of emergency surgery where time is short and speedy correction is necessary. If the patient asks about risk, the anaesthetist must give an accurate and honest answer and therefore needs current morbidity and mortality figures at his disposal (*see* 'Mortality associated with Anaesthesia' (Lunn J. N. and Mushin W. W. ed.) London: Nuffield Provincial Hospitals Trust, 1982). It is not the anaesthetist's responsibility to push prognostic data at a patient who does not ask to know them. *Common sense is an invaluable tool in interpreting these situations.*

(*See also Anaesthesia and the Geriatric Patient* (Krechel S. W. ed.) New York: Grune & Stratton, 1985; Mohr D. N. *J. Am. Geriatr. Soc.* 1983, **31**, 99; *Anaesthesia in the Elderly*, Davenport H. T. Edinburgh: Churchill Livingstone, 1986.)

Pre- and Postoperative Sedation
Old people may become confused; a common cause for this being cerebral hypoxia due to cardiovascular or respiratory abnormality, and deafness. Sedatives will make this disorientation worse. To produce sleep, alcohol is useful for those accustomed to it; nitrazepam 5–10 mg or lorazepam 0·5–1 mg by mouth may be suitable. Triazolam causes less hangover and is less cumulative than some of its congeners. Paraldehyde by mouth or intramuscularly in 5-ml doses or diazepam 5–10 mg are also useful. For postoperative depression, imipramine hydrochloride (Tofranil) 30–100 mg is useful, while for restlessness, thioridazine (Melleril) or chlormethiazole (Heminevrin) may be used.

For severe pain, the authors find small doses of diamorphine, 1–2·5 mg, satisfactory, repeated if necessary.

Anaesthesia

There is a reduction in anaesthetic requirements in old age.[13] Thiopentone is well tolerated as a rule, if dosage is kept low, but its metabolism and excretion are slowed down. Non-depolarizing relaxants not as well reversed (especially in hypothermic individuals) as in the young.

Early postoperative ambulation is usually desirable, to prevent the development of phlebothrombosis, while rapid recovery of the cough reflex is important in the prevention of postoperative atelectasis. A common cause of death is pulmonary embolism.

In old people with emphysema, general anaesthesia, maintaining spontaneous respiration, has given good results and for abdominal surgery thiopentone, nitrous oxide and oxygen may well be combined with small doses of relaxants, and volatile agents. Good speedy operating is valuable at all times and is especially to be desired in elderly people. Postoperative hypoxaemia increases with age and after major surgery. Oxygen should be given in the immediate postoperative period.

Extra- and intradural analgesia is often very suitable for operations below the umbilicus.

(*See also* Sewell I. A. *Hosp. Update*, 1979, **5**, 791, 889; Palmberg S. and Hirsjarvi E. *Gerontology* 1979, **25**, 103; White D. *Br. J. Hosp. Med.* 1980, **24**, 145.)

Pregnancy

(*see also* Chapter 27)

Some drugs may be harmful to the fetus, e.g. norethisterone, antithyroid drugs, tetracycline, streptomycin, sulphonamides, salicylates, and cytotoxic drugs.

The following drugs may, if given to the mother, harm the suckling: phendindione, narcotic analgesics, benzodiazepines, chlorpromazine.

General anaesthetics given in early pregnancy may cause damage to the developing fetus. Simple menstrual history-taking can often identify women at risk. Non-urgent surgery should be postponed if early pregnancy is suspected. Hypoxia and hypotension must be avoided. The operative event may cause miscarriage or premature labour, and general anaesthesia should be avoided if at all possible. In extreme emergency, however, if anaesthesia is necessary the following should be avoided: hypoxia, acidosis, severe maternal alkalosis, teratogenic drugs (anaesthetics are not teratogenic in the clinical situation).[14]

Threatened premature labour may be controlled by selective β_2-adrenergic agonists, terbutaline and salbutamol. Their side-effects are dysrhythmias, hypokalaemia, increased secretion of insulin, and pulmonary oedema.

In advanced pregnancy the hypotensive supine syndrome of late pregnancy must be borne in mind and many such patients are better anaesthetized in the lateral position or with a pad under the right buttock.[15] Middle trimester safest time for surgery.

(*See also* comprehensive review in *Br. J. Hosp. Med.* 1976, **15**, April; Pedersen H. and Finster M. *Anesthesiology* 1979, **51**, 439.)

Hiatus Hernia

The presence of this abnormality, often unknown or unsuspected, may result in regurgitation during induction or maintenance of anaesthesia. It is most likely to occur in middle-aged obese patients or those in advanced pregnancy and is fostered by a pressure differential between the stomach and the oesophagus.

If there is a history suggestive of hiatus hernia with complaints of pyrosis with retrosternal pain and reflux into the oesophagus induced by gravity, then such patients should be treated by the anaesthetist as if they are suffering from acute intestinal obstruction in order to reduce the likelihood of regurgitation and subsequent aspiration of gastric contents into the lungs. Among other measures preoperative administration of an H_2 antagonist or an antacid mixture may be used.

Anaemia

A condition in which there is a reduced concentration of haemoglobin in peripheral blood in the presence of a normal blood volume. There is an oxygen lack in the circulating blood—a reduction in oxygen content, not in oxygen tension. It should, when possible, be treated medically before operation and it is doubtful if major elective surgery should be performed in patients with a haemoglobin concentration of less than 8 g%. Anaemia results in a shift of the oxygen dissociation curve to the right.[16] If haemoglobin is less than 10 g%, a transfusion should normally be given if possible at least 24–48 h before surgery, to allow time for the oxygen dissociation curve to return to the left (2,3-diphosphoglycerate deficiency), and smoking should be prohibited, to reduce the carboxyhaemoglobin level, which may represent 10–15% of the available haemoglobin, but which is useless for oxygen transport. Anaemia causes atony of muscles including myocardium. In anaemia, grave hypoxia may not be accompanied by cyanosis.

Sickle-cell Anaemia and Sickle-cell Trait (Drepanocytosis)[17]

First described by J. B. Herrick of Chicago (1861–1954)[18] (who gave the first modern description of coronary thrombosis in 1912). A hereditary haemolytic anaemia, transmitted by both sexes. Only a small proportion of patients carrying the gene have sickle-cell anaemia. This is a recessive disease not infrequently seen in patients of tropical African or West Indian descent, all of whom must be considered to be at risk, and commonest in children. May also occur in patients from certain parts of Italy or Greece. It is due to the replacement of normal haemoglobin A by abnormal haemoglobin S, which was first described by Pauling in 1949.[19] In *sickle-cell anaemia* 90% of the haemoglobin is of the S variety, and patients are homozygotes, genotype SS; in the *trait* haemoglobin S represents 30–40% of the total haemoglobin, the remainder being of the normal type. Such patients with the *trait* are usually (but not always) symptomless and present no special anaesthetic risks. They are heterozygotes, genotype AS. Haemoglobin S is vulnerable to reduction in Po_2 of blood (first described in 1917).[20] Should this be less than 5·5 kPa the reduced haemoglobin forms liquid crystals called 'tactoids' which distort and finally rupture the red cells. These altered cells cause capillary and venous thromboses and later infarction, and their destruction results in anaemia. In the trait, sickling occurs at a Po_2 of 2·7 kPa. Increasing the Po_2 does not reverse the changes. Acute crises may interrupt the chronic state.

Normal adults have haemoglobin A. The neonate has haemoglobin F at a level of 70%. Trouble may occur when the red cells contain haemoglobin S, haemoglobin C (also a predominantly Negro variant), or in β-thalassaemia (found in a population band through the Mediterranean to China, and in some West African and West Indian Negroes).

Patients may present for surgery because of: (1) Abdominal pain due to vascular lesions; (2) Osteomyelitis; (3) Priapism; (4) Leg ulcers; (5) Gallstones; (6) General surgical diseases.

Management

Patients with the trait (haemoglobin AS), when well managed, do not present much anaesthetic risk[21] except in major interventions such as thoracotomy. All Negroes should be tested for anaemia and sickling before operation (including dental), even if this means postponement of operation. About 10% of British Negroes are at risk. If the haemoglobin is less than 11 g% and the sickling-test positive, sickle-cell anaemia is probable.

The *Sickledex test* is a commercial macroscopic test. A positive test does not differentiate between the disease and the trait and the laboratory must then proceed to genotyping. However, if the haemoglobin estimation is normal and a blood film shows no cell abnormalities it is likely that the trait is present. It should be noted that anaemia can be masked by dehydration and that HbSC and HbS Thal may not show anaemia.

In those affected the following must be avoided: (1) Hypoxia; (2) Hypothermia; (3) The use of tourniquets (this may rule out intravenous regional analgesia); (4) Acidosis and circulatory stasis.

Trait. Preoxygenation, at least 30% oxygen during operation, postoperative oxygen therapy and good hydration are recommended as essential. Sequelae, e.g. infarction, can also occur in patients with the trait.

Disease. These patients are at high risk and demand attention to detail, full oxygenation and avoidance of cardiorespiratory depression.

A transfusion of packed cells should be given if haemoglobin is less than 8 g% and major surgery is contemplated. For the management of open heart surgery in patients with homozygous sickle-cell disease, *see* Reithmuller R. et al. *Anaesthesia* 1982, **37**, 324. In life-saving operations exchange transfusions may be required.[22] Unnecessary transfusion is harmful as it may result in increased blood viscosity. Administration of alkali before and during operation is controversial. Before operation sodium bicarbonate may be given 0·5–1 g/kg daily, or in emergency 0·3 mmol/kg intravenously. During surgery isotonic sodium bicarbonate may be infused intravenously at a rate of 0·3 mmol/kg/h.

Sickling is more likely to occur in the presence of acidosis but the shift of the dissociation curve to the left with alkalinization means that less oxygen is available to the tissues at any given Pa_{O_2}.

Regional analgesia, with the exception of Bier's block, should be preferred to general anaesthesia where suitable. General anaesthesia must include the administration of at least 30% of oxygen and preoxygenation before induction. Sickling can occur in what seems to be a faultless anaesthetic procedure. Postoperative hypoxaemia must be prevented and anticoagulants may be required after surgery to prevent pulmonary embolism, especially if thrombosis, or pain in the bones is present.

Blood from a patient with sickle-cell trait can be safely donated for transfusion but not that from patients with other haemoglobinopathies.

(*See also* Davies S. C. and Hewitt P. E. *Br. J. Hosp. Med.* 1984, **31**, 440.)

Thalassaemia

Similar considerations apply as in sickle-cell anaemia. Such patients may possess no haemoglobin A and sickling is likely to occur when the HbS concentration is high. The patient with *homozygous* β-*thalassaemia* (Cooley's anaemia, Mediterranean anaemia or T disease) has fetal haemoglobin in the red cells in significant amounts. Continuous haemolysis results in anaemia and blood transfusion is likely to be needed. *Heterozygous* β-*thalassaemia* is of different types and it is necessary to have precise identification. HbC thalassaemia is relatively mild, but HbS thalassaemia gives rise to serious problems. HbE thalassaemia is associated with severe anaemia.

(*See also* Howells T. H. in: *Recent Advances in Anaesthesia and Analgesia*—12 (Hewer C. L. and Atkinson R. S. ed.). Edinburgh: Churchill Livingstone, 1976.)

Polycythaemia[23]

Operations on patients with uncontrolled polycythaemia carry a high risk of reactionary haemorrhage, e.g. after dental extractions, due to clotting defects, as well as postoperative thrombosis of arteries and veins. It is rare in patients under 40 and is twice as common in males as females. It may be suspected in patients with a ruddy cyanosis and injected conjunctivae, especially if there is splenomegaly and pruritis. There is an increased haemoglobin level and packed-cell volume. In primary polycythaemia the patient should be treated before operation by myelosuppressive drugs or radiotherapy, while a normal blood picture and blood volume should have been present for several months before the proposed surgery. In emergency cases, repeated and voluminous phlebotomies may be helpful. There is a risk of postoperative cardiac infarction. Patients with a PCV over 50% are at risk of thrombosis. Below 45%, there is no greater risk than usual. Between 45 and 50% lies an area of uncertainty where prophylaxis is wise.

Idiopathic Myoglobinuria (Idiopathic Recurrent Rhabdomyolysis)

Rhabdomyolysis may follow the use of suxamethonium.[24]

Methaemoglobinaemia

Methaemoglobin (ferric haemoglobin) is derived from normal ferrous haemoglobin when the iron in the haem group is oxidized. If a patient appears cyanosed in the absence of heart or lung disease, the blood should be spectroscopically examined for abnormal pigments. Cyanosis is seen if 1·5 g/100 ml of blood is converted to methaemoglobin. It can be reconverted to haemoglobin by reducing enzymes, ascorbic acid, glutathione or methylene blue. Symptoms rarely occur unless 20% methaemoglobin is present. At levels above this, fatigue, dyspnoea, tachycardia, headache, dizziness and even coma and death can occur. The condition can be idiopathic or secondary to exogenous agents, e.g. nitrites, sulphonamides, phenacetin, *prilocaine*, bizarre poisons, etc. Methaemoglobinaemia can be dangerous during anaesthesia as the oxygen-carrying capacity of the blood is reduced, the oxygen dissociation curve being shifted to the left. The condition is treatable by the intravenous injection of 1% solution of methylene blue (1–2 mg/kg given over 5 min) which specifically converts methaemoglobin to normal haemoglobin. In extreme cases exchange transfusion may be considered.

Haemophilia[25]

First described by J. C. Otto (1774–1844) in 1803[26] and in this century by Bullock and Fildes in 1911.[27] There are between 1500 and 2000 male haemophiliacs in Britain and 1 in every 3000–4000 live male births is affected. It is a sex-linked recessive disorder, although about 30% of males with the disease have no history of blood abnormality in previous generations. If a female carries the haemophilia gene she is herself unaffected but has a 1:2 chance of passing the disorder on to her sons, or a carrier state to her daughters. Female obligatory carriers of Factors VIII or IX deficiency may have postoperative bleeding problems.[28] Diagnosis may be difficult but the thromboplastin-generation test will detect almost every case. There is no such thing, surgically, as a mild haemophiliac. With good pathological backing, most patients with this disorder can withstand necessary operations. About 88% of coagulation defects are due to haemophilia A, 8% being due to haemophilia B or Christmas disease. Estimation of the amounts of these factors requires attendance at a haemophilia centre. Once diagnosed, an official Haemophilia Card is issued to the patient. In this disease the Factor VIII may vary from 0 to 20% (normal is 100%). For safe surgery 25% is required. A small number of haemophiliacs have, in addition, a circulating anticoagulant which destroys all AHG injected and so makes them unsuitable for surgery. It is now possible to detect in utero the carrier state in female children of haemophiliac men. Haemophiliac patients may carry the AIDS virus due to receiving infected blood or blood products.

Christmas Disease (Factor IX deficiency)

This has the same mode of inheritance and clinical features as haemophilia, but the Christmas factor is more stable than anti-haemophilic globulin and is present in stored normal blood.

Operation Regime

Haemophilia A (Factor VIII) and Haemophilia B (Factor IX or Christmas Disease)
There may be spontaneous bleeding, e.g. into knee, ankle or elbow joints. Treatment requires the transfusion of materials rich in the deficient factor until a haemostatic level is reached and the maintenance of this level until healing is well advanced. The biological half-life of Factor VIII is 8–12 h, of Factor IX, 18–24 h. The available materials are dried Factor VIII fraction, porcine Factor VIII, cryoprecipitate and dried Factor IX fraction. Before operation patients should have their blood tested for Factor VIII antibody and if this is present, operation, unless life threatening, must be postponed. A transfusion of Factor VIII is given just before the operation, then twice daily for 5–10 days and then daily for 1–3 weeks. Factor VIII must be kept above 50 i.u./dl. Daily assessment of the patient's Factor VIII before and after treatment must be made.

In surgery called minor such as dental extraction, Desmopressin (DDAVP) a vasopressin analogue may be used. Before extraction, 25–30 i.u./kg followed by intravenous tranexamic acid 10 mg/kg is given, and after the extractions, this acid is taken by mouth thrice daily for 10 days. Penicillin V should be given to prevent or inhibit infection of the sockets (*see* Rizza C. R. *Prescriber's J.* 1984, **24**, 71). (*See also* Chapter 25.) (*See also*[149])

(*See also* Rudowski W. J. *Ann. R. Coll. Surg.* 1981, **63**, 111; Rizza C. R. and Spooner R. J. D. *Br. Med. J.* 1983, **286**, 929.)

AIDS (Acquired Immune Deficiency Syndrome)

Patients with this condition present a hazard to staff. Barrier nursing, isolation and extreme caution in handling body fluids and excreta is advised. Gloves and a disposable apron or gown are worn, and samples are collected into hazard-labelled disposable units, the outsides of which are free from contamination and destroyed after use. Specimen containers are sealed (but not with pins, staples or metal clips) and kept separate from the request forms. Luer fittings should ideally be lockable.

It is important to recognize the infected patient, with symptoms of prolonged anorexia, weight loss, fever, lymphadenopathy, opportunistic infections and neoplasms such as Kaposi's sarcoma. Definitive serum testing for HIV or LAV antibody is diagnostic.[29]

The mortality of the definitive disease is high and these patients are severely immunosuppressed.

The majority of infected individuals are asymptomatic carriers. The incubation period is 15–58 months.

(*See also* AIDS and Anaesthesia, Lee K. G. and Soni N. *Anaesthesia* 1986, **41**, 1011.)

Myasthenia Gravis[30]

The *myasthenic state* may be present as follows:

1. Myasthenia gravis: (*a*) Classic; (*b*) Undiagnosed; (*c*) During remission. First described by Thomas Willis (1621–1675)[31] in 1672 and Samuel Wilks (1824–1911) in 1877[32] and named pseudoparalytica myasthenica by Friedrich Jolly (1844–1904), the German neurologist, who also described its electrodiagnosis.[33] Name changed to myasthenia gravis in 1900.[34]

The treatment of myasthenia by the anticholinesterase drug physostigmine was first described by Remen of Münster in 1932[35] and M. Walker in 1934 in Greenwich.[36] It appears to be a condition in which the response of the motor end-plate to acetylcholine no longer gives a short depolarizing block, but results in a more prolonged dual block and consequent muscular weakness.

The first thymectomy for myasthenia gravis was performed by F. Sauerbruch (1845–1951) in 1911[37] and the operation was further developed by Blalock[38] in 1936. Geoffrey Keynes did the first such operation in Britain in 1942.[39]

2. Associated with other diseases: (*a*) Thyrotoxicosis; (*b*) Collagen diseases: (*c*) Carcinoma, especially of the bronchus; (*d*) Thymoma.[40]

3. Caused by drugs: antibiotics of the aminoglycoside group, neomycin, streptomycin, gentamicin, kanamycin, polymyxin, etc.

A mild myasthenic state can exist, causing muscular weakness and tiredness, not thought to be significantly pathological, and diagnosed by the injection of edrophonium.

Myasthenia gravis is a chronic disease of disputed aetiology, possibly an auto-immune reaction of the motor end-plate,[41] commonly in young adults, characterized by exacerbations and remissions. It may occur at any period of life including childhood and old age, and while severe cases are easily diagnosed, mild ones can be overlooked and may cause anaesthetic difficulties. Some of the muscles of the head and neck are usually involved and may give rise to ptosis, dysphagia and easy fatigue of the jaw muscles. Muscle weakness comes on after exercise and improves following rest. The myoneural block which is present may be non-depolarizing in some end-plates (and so reversible), but depolarizing in others. Regular plasmapheresis may maintain reasonable remissions.

A cholinergic crisis due to an excess of acetylcholine consists of a state of muscle weakness and fasciculation, lacrimation, sweating and abdominal colic, due to relative over-dosage with anticholinesterase drugs.

Both myasthenic and cholinergic crises are medical emergencies which may require IPPV in an ITU.

A type of defect of muscarinic-receptor function has been described in which, instead of supersensitivity to cholinergic drugs, there is a lack of response to cholinergic drugs and also to anticholinesterases. This may be an auto-immune disease resembling myasthenia, in which there is a post-junctional defect.

Tests for Myasthenia Gravis

1. Electromyography. Reduction in response to a single twitch in rested

muscles. During repetitive stimuli at both high and low frequencies, myasthenic muscle gives a decreased response.

2. Edrophonium. In myasthenics there is a full but temporary return of muscular power. In normal patients and myasthenics who are adequately treated there may be muscular fasciculations, colic, salivation and diarrhoea, but muscular power is unaffected.

3. Acetylcholine receptor antibody estimation.[42]

Preoperative Preparation

The serum potassium should be estimated as hypokalaemia aggravates myasthenia. A chest radiograph is desirable. Neostigmine can be given by mouth until the optimum dosage is reached but should be slightly reduced just before operation to avoid anticholinesterase excess. A nasogastric tube may well be in place for swallowing problems.

Sedative premedication should be minimal. Opiates and barbiturates should be avoided. Steroid cover is required for those receiving it regularly.

Use of Relaxants in Myasthenia Gravis

1. Non-depolarizing relaxants cause hypersensitivity of affected muscles only. Other muscles behave normally. In myasthenia successfully treated with steroids and not requiring anticholinesterases, there is still sensitivity to muscle relaxants.

2. Decamethonium and suxamethonium are normally well tolerated in mild cases but cause hypersensitivity in severe cases, but the block is a non-depolarizing one, preceded by a brief depolarizing block, i.e. it is a phase II block.

Anaesthetic Management

The chief concern is to ensure adequate respiration both during and after the operation, while the special difficulties to be borne in mind are muscular weakness and bronchial secretion from neostigmine. Regional analgesia which does not depress respiration, e.g. intra- or extradural block to T.10, may be suitable. Anaesthetic agents which are rapidly eliminated are the drugs of choice. Relaxants are better avoided, but if necessary, small doses of suxamethonium or atracurium with monitoring of the neuromuscular block, may be considered.[43] Tracheal intubation may well be advisable, both to ensure a perfect airway and to facilitate tracheobronchial aspiration. Neostigmine should be administered with care as problems may arise with overdosage. Where possible, the advice of a neurologist should be sought and elective procedures carried out in a hospital which provides intensive care facilities. In elective minor surgical procedures spontaneous respiration is usually adequate, e.g. dental conservation in children. Mandatory minute volume ventilation may be beneficial in the postoperative period.

For anaesthesia for trans-cervical thymectomy, *see* Girnar D. S. and Weinrich A. I. *Anesth. Analg. (Cleve.)* 1976, **55**, 13.

For management of myasthenia gravis, symptomatic and immunological, *see* *Lancet* Leading article, 1984, **2**, 135.

Neonatal myasthenia has been described.

Myasthenic Syndrome Complicating Bronchial Carcinoma (Pseudomyasthenia)

A condition of muscular weakness developing at the periphery in a patient with bronchial carcinoma, usually in older males. A small minority of patients with bronchial carcinoma, less than 1%, may develop prolonged apnoea after anaesthesia. The condition was first described as a distinct entity by Eaton and Lambert in 1957 (the Eaton–Lambert Syndrome).[44] The latent myasthenic response may also be seen in patients with thyroid disease, polyarteritis nodosa, polymyositis, dermatomyositis, systemic lupus erythematosus; symptoms of muscular weakness should be inquired about and liver function assessed if such patients are to receive relaxants. It differs from myasthenia gravis as follows: (1) It involves the proximal muscles of the limbs rather than the bulbar and extra-ocular muscles; (2) The presence of aching muscular pains in the limbs; (3) Diminished tendon reflexes; (4) A poor response of the myoneural block to neostigmine; (5) A very marked sensitivity to tubocurarine, even 5 mg sometimes causing prolonged apnoea; (6) Electromyographic characteristics: (*a*) Low-voltage action potentials at twitch rates of supramaximal stimulation, i.e. reduced response. (*b*) Growth of potentials with tetanic rates of stimulation, i.e. increased response. Guanidine (250 mg t.d.s) and calcium may have therapeutic value, but cholinesterase inhibitors are of little benefit. Patients under anaesthesia being treated with thiotepa may have prolonged impairment of neuromuscular function, refractory to neostigmine.[45] Temporary improvement of the muscle weakness may follow surgical removal of the carcinoma. (*See also* Croft P. *Br. J. Hosp. Med.* 1977, **17**, 356.)

Management of Myasthenic Emergencies (impaired ventilation)
These may be related to, or unassociated with, anaesthesia and surgery. The first and most important factor is to ensure a clear airway and adequate respiratory exchange, using intermittent positive pressure. The emergency may be due to: (1) Myasthenia in exacerbation: (2) Cholinergic crisis; (3) A less clear-cut entity associated with insensitivity of the neuromuscular junction to acetylcholine. It is advisable to withhold all drugs until the nature of the emergency has been diagnosed.

The patient should be nursed in an intensive care unit and will require full monitoring facilities. The reactions of the end-plates to neostigmine may be complex and require expert evaluation. Plasma electrolytes, particularly potassium, should be restored to normal values.

Plasma exchange will produce temporary benefit.[46]

Rheumatoid Arthritis

First described in 1880; a disease of modern times; may be associated with vasculitis in various organs, heart and lung involvement and peripheral neuropathy and Sjogren's syndrome (keratoconjunctivitis sicca). Potential difficulties may arise from (1) Flexion deformity of cervical vertebrae and involvement of temporomandibular joints making laryngoscopy difficult; (2) Involvement of small joints of larynx and neuropathy of laryngeal muscles causing stridor; (3) Amyloidosis of kidneys; (4) Tendency to respiratory depression and interstitial pneumonia after operation; (5) Steroid therapy; (6) Fragility of veins; (7) Heart involvement; (8) Enlarged liver; (9) Cervical cord and vertebral artery compression; (10) Atrophy of skin, making intravenous therapy difficult. Thus there may be difficulty in intubation together with the need for great care after operation. Preoperative chest radiography may be required.

Ankylosis of Jaw

This may be part of a generalized arthritis and may render laryngoscopy difficult. It must be diagnosed before induction, and sometimes blind intubation is of service. The production of apnoea before intubation is not recommended unless the anaesthetist is sure he can inflate the lungs.

Ankylosing Spondylitis

First described by B. Connor in 1693. The lungs in this condition perform efficiently, and sufferers from it may undergo operation on the lungs, heart or abdomen without pulmonary complications as the diaphragm provides good compensation for the reduced chest movement. Great care must be taken to ensure that efficient ventilation returns after operation. Extradural block for hip surgery may be technically easier via the sacral than the lumbar approach.

Stiffness of the cervical spine and of the atlanto-occipital joint may cause difficulty during tracheal intubation, and have led to spinal fractures. Ankylosis of the temporomandibular or crico-arytenoid joints may cause problems so that occasionally the blind technique must be employed or awake intubation, translaryngeal retrograde intubation or tracheostomy may be required.

Unexpected cardiac death has been reported following operation in patients suffering from this condition.[47] (*See also* Sinclair J. R. and Mason R. A. *Anaesthesia* 1974, **39**, 3; Lloyd E. L. *Anaesthesia* 1984, **39**, 722; Whittmann F. J. and Ring P.A. *J. R. Soc. Med.* 1986, **79**, 457.)

Scoliosis

May be associated with congenital heart disease. Usually idopathic but may be due to neuromuscular disorders, myotonia, muscular dystrophy, etc. Malignant hyperpyrexia has been seen in these patients. A narcotic, nitrous oxide, oxygen, IPPV technique is usually satisfactory. For Harrington rod surgery,[48] it may be necessary to waken the patient during the operation, to prevent paraplegia. Fears concerning dropping the blood pressure (e.g. by extradural block) have been expressed because of the risk of reducing the blood supply to the cord.[49] These patients are likely to have reduced vital capacity so their tidal volume is limited and cannot increase, e.g. as a result of premedication which may slow the breathing rate. Airway obstruction is seldom a feature. Fluoroscopic assessment of diaphragmatic movement is helpful in estimating operative risk. Underventilation in these patients is a danger even before anaesthesia is induced and may be present also after operation, when they may require most careful observation and if necessary IPPV. They show respiratory handicap and may have a lowered blood oxygen saturation and an abnormal ventilation perfusion ratio. The resulting hypoxia and hypercapnia eventually lead to fluid retention and to pulmonary hypertension as the result of pulmonary vasoconstriction. Right heart failure may follow as in chronic obstructive lung disease.

(*See also* Abbott T. R. and Bentley G. *Anaesthesia* 1980, **35**, 298.)

Ehlers–Danlos Syndrome[50]

A congenital connective tissue disease with hypermobility of joints and excessive elasticity of skin. For anaesthesia, *see* Dolan P. et al. *Anesthesiology* 1980, **52**, 266.

Achondroplasia

First described in 1791 by Sommering (1755–1830), Polish–German physician, in 1791, and by M. H. Romberg (1795–1873) in 1817. There may be difficulties with tracheal intubation, due to abnormalities at the base of the skull. For Caesarean section, extradural block, although perhaps technically difficult, has been safely used.[51]

Porphyria

(from the Greek *porphyros* = purple)

First described by Schultz in 1874 and named by B. J. E. Stokvis (1834–1902), a Dutch physician, in 1889.[52] Rare in England, prevalent in South Africa and Scandinavia. There are three hepatic porphyrias in which acute porphyria can be precipitated by barbiturates or sulphonamides, and all are inherited by Mendelian dominance, the affected patients being heterozygous; (1) Intermittent acute porphyria (seen in Sweden); (2) Porphyria variegata, not uncommon in white South Africans; (3) Coproporphyria, in which the predominant porphyrin in the urine and faeces is coproporphyrin; (4) Cutaneous porphyria (porphyria cutanea tarda) which may be acquired or hereditary. The first is the most common type seen in the UK. Cutaneous porphyrias are little if at all sensitive to barbiturates. Acute intermittent porphyria, porphyria variegata and hereditary coproporphyria are known as 'irreducible porphyrias' as clinical and biochemical manifestations may be induced by certain drugs or clinical conditions.[53] Porphyria is a congenital metabolic defect and is characterized in its active phase by the passage or urine which turns red or brown on standing. If the condition is suspected the urine should be tested for the characteristic pigment by spectroscopy and the stool tested for coproporphyria.

Acute attacks may arise *de novo* or may be associated with infection, pregnancy or the ingestion of such drugs as barbiturates, alcohol, steroids, phenytoin and sulphonamides. *Clinical features* are: (1) Gastrointestinal: acute abdominal pain and vomiting; (2) Neurological: lower motor neuron lesions, sensory disturbance, epilepsy, mental symptoms, rarely coma; (3) Cardiovascular: tachycardia and raised blood pressure when disease active; (4) A photosensitive disease of the skin. *Diagnosis* is by measurement of porphyrins or their precursors in the urine or faeces.

Barbiturates as premedication and thiopentone and its congeners are absolutely contraindicated as their administration may be followed by lower motor neuron paralysis, mental disturbances or even death. Thiopentone stimulates the enzyme delta-ALA-synthetase, increasing the formation of porphobilinogen, leading to progressive neuropathy. In clinical attacks there is an accumulation of delta-aminolaevulinic acid and porphyrobilinogen. In the acute phase, artificial ventilation may be required. If intravenous induction is planned, etomidate and ketamine[54] can be given. For pain, aspirin, morphine, pethidine or methadone is suitable but pentazocine, chlordiazepoxide and phenylbutazone should be avoided. For sleep chloral hydrate or trichloroethyl phosphate is suitable. Nitrous oxide, oxygen, volatile agents, relaxants and their reversal agents need not be withheld.

Medicolegal rather than scientific reasons make some workers avoid regional analgesia in these patients.

Probably King George III and some of his descendants suffered from this condition (Malcapine I. and Hunter R. *Br. J. Med.* 1966, **1**, 65).

(*See also* Parish R. K. and Moore M. R. *Br. J. Anaesth.* 1978, **50**, 1099; Yeung Laiwah A. C. et al. *J. R. Soc. Med.* 1983, **76**, 386; Drugs and Porphyria. Magnus I. A. *Br. Med. J.* 1984, **288**, 1474.)

Liver Disease

Blood Supply
About 30% of total blood flow is provided by the hepatic artery which supplies 70% of oxygen requirements. Blood perfusion from the portal vein is about 70% but it carries only 30% of oxygen requirements. Total blood supply is in excess of 1·5 l/min. Anaesthesia causes changes in hepatic blood flow but there is little information concerning any harmful effects which may ensue, but *see* p. 187.

Liver Function Tests
These are imprecise indicators of liver function; they have a place in pre- and postoperative assessment, but no role in intraoperative monitoring. Examples of important biochemical estimations include: (1) Serum bilirubin. This may be elevated as a result of hepatocellular damage, excess formation (haemolysis), or extrahepatic biliary obstruction. If direct bilirubin is greater than 15% of the total, there is likely to be hepatic dysfunction; (2) Transaminases. These are present in liver cells and may leak into the bloodstream when damage occurs. Other tissues such as heart, lung and skeletal muscle also contain transaminases, so elevation of blood levels is not specific for liver pathology; (3) Serum alkaline phosphatase. The enzyme is present in bile duct cells. Blood levels are raised in the presence of biliary obstruction, but also in hepatocellular disease. Also found in other tissues; (4) Serum albumin. Normal value is 3·5–5·5 mg%. The half-life is about 3 weeks, so falls do not occur for some time following liver damage. Albumin levels less than 3·5 mg% usually point to significant disease. The production of globulin is unaffected by liver disease.

Liver Function
When this is abnormal, problems may arise related to anaesthetic practice: (1) Protein. The liver is the principal site for the synthesis of important proteins, including albumin, prothrombin and fibrinogen. Coagulation problems may arise; (2) Lipid. Impaired lipoprotein synthesis may result in the accumulation of fat in the liver; (3) Carbohydrate. In advanced liver disease, hypoglycaemia may occur; (4) Bio-transformation of drugs. The liver is the site for many metabolic processes including the synthesis, conjugation, oxidation, reduction and hydrolysis. Drug elimination may therefore be impaired in advanced liver

disease. Low levels of serum albumin may lead to changes in protein binding, thus leaving greater quantities in the unbound form to exert their pharmacological effects.

The Effects of Anaesthetic Drugs on Liver Cells
Anaesthetic agents can affect events at subcellular level. For example 2% halothane vapour almost totally arrests cell division in the broad bean after 8 hours exposure.[55] Chromosomes become contracted and thickened but the process is reversible. It is likely that any effects on cells of the human liver such as depression of mitochondrial utilization, conjugation of bilirubin and biotransformation of drugs will be short-lasting. For the possible mechanisms of hepatotoxicity in man, due to halothane, *see* Chapter 10.

Anaesthesia in the Presence of Overt Liver Disease
Factors to be considered include: (1) Low protein albumin. A level of below 3·2 g% has been held to contraindicate surgical intervention for the relief of portal hypertension.[55] The use of intravenous drugs such as barbiturates, muscle relaxants or local analgesic agents may have to be re-evaluated in the light of possible effects on protein binding; (2) Serum cholinesterase. The level must be depressed to at least half the normal before any effects on suxamethonium elimination are seen. Problems are unusual in clinical practice; (3) Clotting factors. These may be abnormal due to: (*a*) Decreased synthesis which may or may not be vitamin K dependent. Levels of thrombin or prothrombin may be low; (*b*) The half-life of coagulation factors may be shortened as a result of increased utilization (e.g. disseminated intravascular coagulation, loss into extravascular compartments, excessive bleeding); (*c*) Abnormal coagulation factors can be produced (dysfibrinogenaemia); (*d*) Thrombocytopaenia; (*e*) Impaired platelet function; (4) Encephalopathy. Advanced liver disease leads to altered consciousness, often preceded by intellectual changes, psychiatric and personality disorders, leading eventually to coma and death. Factors leading to encephalopathy include: (*a*) Hypnotic drugs and sedatives. These should be avoided whenever possible in patients with marked cirrhosis. Diazepam, 5 mg i.v. has been suggested as the most suitable agent; (*b*) Gastrointestinal haemorrhage; (*c*) Misuse of diuretics with disturbance of electrolyte balance; (*d*) Presence of infection; (*e*) Progression of underlying disease; (5) There is a risk of precipitating hepatorenal failure in jaundiced patients. Urine production should be maintained at 30 ml/h, at least, and diuretics administered if necessary.

Risk Factors
Scoring systems have been devised in order to grade the severity of operative risk. Coma can be graded from 1 to 5 according to the mental state and the EEG.[56] Coma level, bilirubin level, albumin level, prothrombin time etc. can be scored to produce a scale of operative risk.[57]

Australia Antigen

See Chapter 18.

Polyarteritis Nodosa

First described in 1866 by Kussmaul (1822–1902).[58] In this disease there may be an abnormal response to suxamethonium because of associated liver dysfunction. Before depolarizing relaxants are used in this condition, investigation of liver function may be prudent. The same response may occur in the presence of polymyositis, dermatomyositis and systemic lupus erythematosus.

Hyperthyroidism

First use of antithyroid drugs in 1943 (thiourea).[59] The anaesthetist, noticing an enlarged thyroid, should inquire about the existence of thyrotoxicosis, and if it is severe, right heart failure, atrial fibrillation and liver damage may be present. The patient should be euthyroid before operation. For details *see* Chapter 24. Hyperthyroidism without an enlarged thyroid may be present. When postoperative hypothyroidisim is suspected, a thyroid-stimulating hormone test will aid diagnosis.

Hypothyroidism

The word 'myxoedema' was introduced by Ord in 1878.[60] In this condition, the metabolism of drugs, especially sedatives used in premedication, and narcotics, is likely to be delayed, and respiratory depression is easily produced. There may be secondary changes in the pituitary gland and the adrenal cortex which may impair the normal response to stress. There may also be hypothermia, hypoglycaemia, muscular weakness, hydropericardium and even coma. Reversal is necessary before operation otherwise the prognosis is likely to be bad. Postoperative hypotension should be treated by intravenous hydrocortisone. Mild, undiagnosed hypothyroidism in patients undergoing surgery may postoperatively result in myxoedema with coma, and respiratory obstruction may occur, requiring intravenous T.3 thyroid replacement therapy and airway support.[61]

Oral thyroxine takes 10 days to exert its effect. To correct hypothyroidism before operation 25 µg of tri-iodothyroxine (T.3) can be given intravenously in a drip or a solution of 0·1 mg/l in 5% dextrose at 20 drops per min with ECG control (look for flattened T-waves or ST depression), using special caution in those patients over 50 and those suffering from angina. Intravenous hydrocortisone is also beneficial.

The nitrous oxide, oxygen, volatile agent, relaxant sequence with IPPV is perhaps the most suitable anaesthetic technique.

Anaesthesia in Patients with Impaired Renal Function

Most patients with mild abnormality do well under anaesthesia, unless more than 50% of the nephron mass is damaged. Depression of renal function is due to humoral and vascular changes, shown by oliguria and reduced excretion of solutes, and many anaesthetics cause this. Patients with pre-existing renal impairment may be put at risk if subjected to: (1) Hypovolaemic hypotension; (2) Hepatic failure or obstructive jaundice; (3) Major vascular surgery; (4) Major trauma; (5) Sepsis; (6) Patients over 50 subjected to major surgery with massive blood transfusion; (7) Toxaemia of pregnancy and amniotic fluid embolism; (8) The use of certain antimicrobial drugs e.g. gentamicin.

Renal blood flow, blood volume and renal perfusion pressure must be maintained. Intravenous mannitol, frusemide and dopamine may be useful, with maintenance of blood volume. These patients are unduly sensitive to narcotics, although diazepam is well tolerated. Suxamethonium may be safe unless the serum potassium is more than 5 mmol/l. Gallamine and alcuronium are better avoided. Regional block may be suitable provided the BP is maintained. (*See* Maddern P. *Anaesth. Intensive Care* 1983, **11**, 321; Symposium on the Kidney. *Anaesth. Intensive Care* 1983, **11**, November.)

There are problems in the following areas: (1) Drug intolerance. Renally excreted drugs are of course greatly potentiated and prolonged, e.g. gallamine. A complete and up-to-date list is found in the *British National Formulary*; (2) Fluid balance. Dialysis patients are on sodium and water restriction and should not be overloaded by the anaesthetist! A few renal failure patients are 'salt losers'; (3) Diet. Parenteral nutrition is tailored to restrict protein while providing essential amino acids; (4) Hypertension (*see below*); (5) Anaemia. Lower levels of haemoglobin than normal may have to be accepted. Transfusion (though unpopular with nephrologists) is likely to be required. Erythrocytosis may follow transplantation; (6) Osteodystrophy and hypercalcaemia; (7) Aluminium toxicity. Derived from aluminium in dialysis water, this may be associated with severe dementia.

The principles of anaesthesia in renal failure are to be found in Chapter 24.

Cardiovascular Disease[62]

Implications for Anaesthesia

Possible cardiovascular pathology includes (1) Myocardial infarction; (2) Progressive myocardial ischaemia; (3) Dysrhythmias; (4) Congestive cardiac failure; (5) Stroke. Aggressive monitoring, and systematic prevention and treatment of abnormalities likely to cause myocardial ischaemia are required. The following conditions carry a progressively increasing risk: (1) Emergency operations; (2) Intrathoracic or abdominal operations; (3) Poor general condition; (4) Tight aortic stenosis; (5) Age over 70; (6) Ventricular premature beats (more than 5/min); (7) Cardiac rhythm other than sinus; (8) Cardiac infarction during the last 6 months; (9) Third heart sound or increasing jugular venous pressure; (10) Tachycardia. Both hypo- and hypertension are to be avoided. The ASA classification of physical status was not designed to estimate postoperative risk, but the multifactorial index of cardiac risk was.[63]

Anaesthesia may affect the heart:

1. By causing dysrhythmias, including ventricular fibrillation and alterations in cardiac rate.

2. By direct depressant effect on the myocardium, causing reduced cardiac output and even asystole.

3. As a result of hypotension, especially when the heart cannot compensate by increasing the cardiac output (tight valvular stenosis, constrictive pericarditis).

4. As a result of hypoxia and hypercapnia.

In general, patients with compensated heart disease tolerate anaesthesia well, provided it is carefully administered and overdosage, hypoxia and hypotension avoided.

1. Hypertension and Arteriosclerosis

Some problems associated with anaesthesia in the hypertensive patient: increased tendency to constriction of vascular smooth muscle in response to stress and to some drugs; tendency to thrombosis in atheromatous coronary and cerebral vessels; associated renal failure; left ventricular hypertrophy and tendency to heart failure if the arterial pressure falls.

The vast majority of moderately hypertensive patients are managed success-fully provided due care is taken with the anaesthetic. The untreated hypertensive patient has a reduced blood volume, and reacts to anaesthesia like any other hypovolaemic patient. Minimal doses of anaesthetic agents are indicated, with infusion of plasma expander, e.g. dextran 70, immediately preoperatively. If possible, operation is delayed for a week until adequate antihypertensive treatment has had effect. The risks are then reduced. The diastolic blood pressure should be below 110 mmHg.[64]

Preoperative Assessment.[65] The cause of the hypertension should be sought (essential, malignant, endocrine, drug-induced, coarctation, etc.). The effects of the condition are also elicited: on the heart (ischaemia, failure), on the brain (transient ischaemic episodes), on the kidneys (uraemia, oedema), on the liver (failure); on the eyes and on the extremities. Chest X-ray, ECG and the appropriate blood tests are performed.

Management. Priority is given to maintenance of blood flow to coronary, cerebral and renal circulations. Adequate blood pressure is maintained since normal autoregulation may be diminished. Tracheal intubation may raise the blood pressure, an effect which, though normally thought of as dangerous, may be very welcome if the pressure is uncomfortably low following induction. This effect of intubation is reduced by spraying the larynx and trachea with lignocaine. This also inhibits dysrhythmias as does fentanyl. The nitrous-oxide–oxygen–relaxant technique, trichloroethylene and neuroleptanalgesia have their place. Opinions about ketamine here vary widely. It keeps the blood pressure up (sometimes dangerously so) at the expense of increased cardiac work. Hypertensive patients react badly to rapid changes of position.

Postoperatively. Severe rises of blood pressure may be seen, as an inappropriate response to pain. Even a small haemorrhage may cause severe hypotension. (*See also* Murkin J. M. *Anesth. Analg. (Cleve.)* 1982, **61**, 371 and The Experts Opine. *Surv. Anesthesiol.* 1983, **27**, 56.)

2. Cardiac Failure with Decompensation[65]

These cases present serious risks. Preoperative diagnosis of the cause and correction of the failure are required. Most anaesthetic agents make cardiac failure worse, whereas opioids, benzodiazepines and phenothiazine premedicants are well tolerated by the patient. Local analgesic techniques are sometimes to be preferred. If operation cannot be delayed and general anaesthesia is necessary, the following points should be borne in mind: (*a*) The tachycardia normally seen on induction may be absent in these cases. Transient asystole due to suxamethonium is sometimes seen. Atropine reduces this possibility; (*b*) Existing pulmonary oedema increases respiratory work, so intubation, relaxation and IPPV may be indicated. Nitrous oxide (one of the safest agents in this condition) and oxygen may then be sufficient for analgesia; (*c*) Hypoxia must be avoided; (*d*) Cyclopropane is useful because of its easily reversible abdominal relaxation. Gentle IPPV may be required; (*e*) Ketamine, while maintaining blood pressure, increases left ventricular work and myocardial oxygen demand; (*f*) Central venous and pulmonary artery wedge pressure monitoring (PAWP) are useful. They may have to be kept as high as the preoperative values; (*g*) If the patient's blood pressure and flow are decreasing steadily, adrenergic drugs may be indicated, e.g. ephedrine 10–30 mg i.v., dopamine infusion 5–15 µg/kg/min; (*h*) Fully monitored alpha-adrenergic blockade may help by reducing afterload.

3. Cardiac Infarction
First premortem diagnosis by Adam Hammer (1818–1878) in 1878,[66] and classic description by W. P. Obrastow in 1910[67] and J. B. Herrick (1861–1954) in 1912.[68] Operation within 3 months of cardiac infarction carries a 35% risk of reinfarction, most likely to occur on the third postoperative day. Upper abdominal and thoracic operations carry the highest risk. The incidence is not related to the type of general anaesthetic used. Operation 3–6 months after infarction carries a 16% risk of reinfarction, while operation 6 months or more after infarction carries about a 5% chance of reinfarction. These considerable risks must be balanced against those of not undertaking the operation proposed. Occasionally a treatable cause of myocardial infarction may be found, e.g. polycythaemia. Full oxygenation and prevention of either hypoxia or hypotension are of course most important. (*See* 'Coronary Artery Grafts', Chapter 29.)

4. Coronary Atheroma
Preoperative assessment by resting ECG, exercise ECG, (the maximal degree of S–T depression relative to increase in heart rate),[69] angiography, thallium scan, cardiac catheterization,[70] and existence of angina. Monitoring has not affected the incidence of cardiac complications and the risk of reinfarction persists for up to a week after operation. Control of hypertension, dysrhythmias and cardiac failure are required in addition to good analgesia.[71] However, in one series, aggressive therapy and invasive monitoring reduced the perioperative reinfarction rate to 7·8% after recent infarction, and 3·4% after old myocardial infarction. Anoxia of the heart muscle must be avoided by maintaining good tissue perfusion and an adequate diastolic blood pressure, as coronary flow depends on the diastolic pressure. A turbulent induction should be avoided. The mechanics of respiration must be safeguarded to ensure adequate filling of the right heart. Reduction of preload by use of vasodilators and β-blockers has been recommended to reduce risks of further heart attacks.[72] A balance must be struck between keeping the diastolic pressure up, to ensure adequate coronary filling, and keeping systolic pressure down to reduce after-load and thus myocardial oxygen demand. Nifedipine and nitroglycerin are useful as coronary vasodilators.[73] Isosorbide, nifedipine and nitroprusside, but not verapamil, reduce afterload and control postoperative hypertension. In a series,[74] 28% of patients with known coronary artery disease had intraoperative S–T segment depression on ECG (best seen in lead CM_5), during increases in blood pressure and pulse rate, following intubation. Control of the cardiac rate–systolic pressure product (upper acceptable limit 20 000 in normal patients, 15 000 in those with coronary disease) was advised, with halothane, nitroglycerin or mild β-blockade. The rate-pressure product is thought by some workers to be important in the management of

patients with actual or possible heart disease with coronary insufficiency undergoing surgery (or exercise),[72] but its usefulness has been challenged.[75] Full oxygenation is again mandatory. Tachycardia due to atropine may decrease coronary filling time by shortening diastole. Halothane is well tolerated in patients with myocardial ischaemia who are not in failure and have good ventricular function.[76] (*See also* Gilston A. in *Recent Advances in Anaesthesia and Analgesia*—13 (Hewer C. L. and Atkinson R. S. ed.) Edinburgh: Churchill Livingstone, 1979.)

5. Heart Block

A term introduced by W. H. Gaskell (1847–1914), first described in 1691 by Gerbezius. Stokes-Adams attacks described by W. M. Stokes (1804–1878)[77] and R. Adams (1791–1875).[78] In complete atrioventricular dissociation the idioventricular rate is about 35 beats/min. This constitutes a fixed output state, the heart being unable to increase output in response to stress.

Preoperative assessment. Exercise tolerance, ECG and chest X-ray. The block may be due to ischaemia, valvular disease, previous cardiac surgery, myocarditis or may be congenital. A trial of atropine may detect and treat some patients whose block is vagal. Ephedrine or sublingual isoprenaline or salbutamol may increase the cardiac rate usefully.

Second-degree block may proceed to complete block under anaesthesia. Right bundle branch block is of little significance, whereas left bundle branch block limits cardiac output.

In complete heart block, general anaesthesia is seldom indicated until a pacemaker has been inserted. (*See* 'Intravenous Techniques', Chapter 42.) It is important to avoid reduction in cardiac output, to maintain full oxygenation, avoid blood loss, sudden postural change and damage to pacemaker. ECG should be monitored continuously. Safety precautions include a standby external pacemaker and drugs such as procaine amide, lignocaine, vasopressors and isoprenaline. Anaesthetic technique should include preoxygenation, careful use of intravenous anaesthetics and intubation.

6. Atrial Fibrillation

A term (auricular) first used by Sir James McKenzie (1853–1925) in 1908.[79] Should, if possible, be controlled preoperatively by digitalization until the ventricular rate is reasonably slow. Other methods of control include β-blockers, procaine amide, quinidine, verapamil, diphenylhydantoin, cardiac pacing and cardioversion.

7. Ventricular Ectopic Beats

If necessary, controlled by lignocaine, isoflurane, verapamil and IPPV.

8. Myocarditis[80]

General anaesthesia may be dangerous, especially in older patients.

9. Congenital and Rheumatic Heart Disease

Patients require careful supervision and smooth anaesthesia. It is wise to administer antibiotic cover if there is danger of subacute bacterial endocarditis.

Mitral incompetence: Antibiotic cover is usual. Mild reductions of systemic vascular resistance are helpful. Severe tachycardia and bradycardia are to be avoided. *Mitral stenosis*: Antibiotic cover is usual. The patient may be on anticoagulants for arterial and venous thromboembolism, and digoxin for atrial fibrillation. The left ventricle requires a longer diastolic filling time, so tachycardia is undesirable, whether due to atropine or anxiety. Mild reductions of systemic vascular resistance are beneficial (with relief of pulmonary hypertension) but great reductions lead to severe hypotension due to fixed cardiac output. Minimal doses of anaesthetic are desirable. Hypotension may require dopamine or other adrenergic drug. Volume overload is a risk, especially postoperatively, with resultant pulmonary oedema made worse by respiratory failure and hypoalbuminaemia. *Aortic stenosis*: antibiotic cover may be required. Preservation of normal sinus rhythm is very important. Lignocaine for ventricular ectopic beats, atropine for bradycardia, practolol for tachycardia, and defibrillation for supraventricular tachycardia may be required. PAWP may underestimate LVEDP by up to 7 mmHg. *Aortic incompetence*: improved by mild tachycardia and vasodilatation with moderate fluid loading to maintain the diastolic pressure. Antibiotic cover may be required. Spinal blockade has not proved helpful because of destabilization of the circulation.

10. Constrictive Pericarditis[81]
Thiopentone has a bad reputation in this disease. The heart is unable to compensate for sudden changes in haemodynamics such as may occur when peripheral resistance is altered.

11. Presence of a Pacemaker
During endoscopic prostatectomy there is electromagnetic interference from the diathermy apparatus, using the 'cutting' current, not when using the 'coagulation' current. For all operations the diathermy plates and electrodes should be sited well away from the pacemaker (*See also* Chapter 5.) When diathermy is used there is a risk of damage to the pacemaker by the high currents which can be induced in the pacemaker via its pacing lead which acts as an aerial. A further theoretical danger is the induction of ventricular fibrillation in the patient's heart by these currents. While diathermy is best avoided in patients carrying a pacemaker, an operation may be undertaken safely provided that the active diathermy electrode is kept at least 15 cm from the pacemaker and the indifferent diathermy plate placed as far away from the pacemaker as possible and in a direction which ensures that the diathermy dipole will be at right angles to that of the pacemaker system. AC and DC electric motors may also cause problems, but in practice this is unusual.[82]

12. Sick Sinus Syndrome[83]
A dysrhythmia originating in the atrium which may go on to cardiac standstill and may be seen during anaesthesia. It has been suggested that before anaesthesia, patients should have a temporary transvenous pacing wire inserted under local analgesia, if the condition is uncontrollable.[84,85]

General Discussion
Patients with organic heart disease who can carry on their daily jobs usually tolerate anaesthesia and operation well.

The following conditions should be detected before anaesthesia as they may lead to sudden death, especially if hypoxia or sudden alteration in the blood pressure should occur: (1) Recent cardiac infarction; (2) Angina pectoris; (3) Aortic stenosis; (4) Aortic reflux and aortitis with involvement of the orifices of the coronary arteries; (5) Complete heart-block with Stokes–Adams attacks.

Suxamethonium, in patients with valvular incompetence, takes longer to act—up to 2 min—and may have to be given in larger doses (e.g. 100 mg) than in normal patients before intubation, due to a slow time of onset consequent on a reduced circulation time. In the digitalized patient dysrhythmias may occur following suxamethonium.

Gallamine may so increase the cardiac rate as to initiate decompensation, so it must be used most carefully in heart conditions associated with tachycardia. A pulse rate about 70/min is ideal. Above 100 beats/min, the shortened diastolic interval reduces coronary perfusion time.

Congestive heart failure occurring as a postoperative complication may be difficult to diagnose. The appearance of triple rhythm or atrial fibrillation may be significant, while orthopnoea may precede signs of pulmonary congestion in early left heart failure. Increase in venous filling in the neck heralds right heart failure. Measurement of central venous pressure may be useful (*see* Chapter 41).

The production of cardiac dysrhythmias should of course be avoided if possible (e.g. by the avoidance of hypoxia and hypercapnia).

Anaesthesia for the Patient in Shock

(*see also* 'Resuscitation' Chapter 38)

Operation should not be undertaken, except in cases of grave emergency, until the patient is resuscitated. Full fluid replacement before use of vasodilator drugs is imperative. Acidosis is corrected with sodium bicarbonate. Once improvement has occurred, with filling of jugular veins, and hands and feet becoming warm and pink, the operation need not be delayed. The blood pressure should, if possible, be restored to at least 100 mmHg and the clinical condition should show signs of improvement. A systolic blood pressure above 100 mmHg indicates that blood volume is probably not less than 70% of normal.

Shocked and recently resuscitated patients require much smaller amounts of anaesthetic agents than do normal patients. Vomiting may occur at this light plane as shock is an important cause, along with fear and anxiety, of delayed gastric emptying. Hypoxia must be avoided most carefully.

Premedication should be given intravenously, just before induction of anaesthesia, atropine alone being usually sufficient.

Induction. A full stomach may complicate induction, and aspiration of gastric contents must be prevented (*see* Chapter 18).

Maintenance. Light general anaesthesia is the method of choice. Cyclopropane is well tolerated and does not cause a further fall in blood pressure, but prolonged administration in shock may be harmful as among other effects it reduces renal blood flow. Volatile agents must be used carefully as hypotension may be potentiated but renal and cerebral blood flow tends to be enhanced. Ether is also a useful agent in shock, as blood pressure is usually well maintained in light planes, associated with an adrenergic effect. Anaesthesia protects against brain damage in shock.

A cuffed tracheal tube is often desirable both to minimize the chances of underventilation and to guard against aspiration of gastric contents.

Regional analgesia may be very satisfactory if hypotension is avoided. (*See* Bridenbaugh L. D. and Moore D. C. in: *Clinical Management of the Patient in Shock* (Orkin L. ed.). Oxford: Blackwell, 1965, Chap. 5.)

The blood pressure and pulse rate should be charted regularly.

The Treatment of Shock during Operation

1. Raise the patient's legs.
2. Lighten anaesthesia if necessary and see that oxygen in plenty is reaching the alveoli. IPPV may be beneficial.
3. Arrange for blood, dextran, plasma or electrolyte intravenous infusion.
4. Consider the use of hydrocortisone.
5. Circulatory monitoring. As shock deepens, first peripheral pulses disappear, then central pulses, then pupils dilate, then the cardiac impulse disappears, then the heart sounds fade out. Last of all, the ECG shows cardiac arrest.

Diabetes

Insulin was isolated and treatment of diabetics commenced with it in 1922.[86] Diabetes is a disease affecting the metabolism of fat and glucose and may cause problems due to:

1. A rising blood sugar—polyuria, thirst, pruritus, etc.
2. Ketosis, i.e. metabolic acidosis causing hyperventilation, multisystem organ failure, loss of extracellular sodium and water, dehydration leading to circulatory collapse and coma; exacerbated by anaesthesia.
3. Peripheral vascular disease. A disproportionate number of operations in diabetic patients are for the treatment of vascular disease, either myocardial or of the legs.
4. Diabetic nephropathy.
5. Neuropathy. Autonomic neuropathy can present problems including cardiorespiratory arrest, postural hypotension and postoperative retention of urine. Sleep apnoea in diabetic patients with autonomic neuropathy[87] may have serious consequences when additional factors such as the administration of respiratory depressant drugs in anaesthesia or hypoxia are present. Such patients may die suddenly during pneumonia or in association with anaesthesia.
6. Poor wound healing in major surgery.[88]

Most anaesthetic agents cause a slight rise in blood sugar, but this is seldom significant. Ether causes a pronounced rise and is to be avoided.

Schemes of Control for Operation Period

There is no single scheme to cover all cases. Generally speaking, it is wiser to have a slightly increased blood sugar than to risk hypoglycaemia. The aim is to keep blood glucose around 10 mmol/l and to maintain the flow of glucose into the cells. The greatest danger is hypoglycaemia, especially in the cells of the central nervous system. Another great danger is electrolyte disorder due to shortage of insulin, with acidosis and hyponatraemia.

Avoiding general anaesthesia solves most of the perioperative problems of the diabetic. However, even for local analgesia, the patient may have to be starved.

Symptoms of hypoglycaemia: shaking and trembling, sweating, pins and needles in tongue and lips, hunger, palpitations, diplopia, slurring of speech, confusion, truculence, restlessness, epileptic fits, unconsciousness.

Symptoms of keto-acidosis: dehydration, over-breathing, acetone in the breath, hypotension, glycosuria and ketonuria; usually high serum potassium. Ketostix ++ or +++.

1. Diabetes controlled by diet. Control may be upset as a result of surgery. Hyperglycaemia and glycosuria persisting beyond the first postoperative day may require insulin.

2. Patients receiving oral hypoglycaemic drugs (type 2 or maturity-onset insulin-independent diabetes). Most of these agents have a duration of action not exceeding 12–16 h. Chlorpropamide, however, has a half-life of 36 h and a duration of action up to 60 h. Fasting hypoglycaemia may occur, and the drug should be stopped at least 24 h preoperatively. Phenformin increases lactic acid production by stimulating anaerobic metabolism.

3. The well-controlled diabetic on insulin (type 1 or juvenile-onset insulin-dependent diabetes). The aim is: to prevent ketoacidosis, and to avoid hypoglycaemia. An elective operation should preferably be carried out in the early morning. The patient should be stabilized on soluble insulin, twice daily, for 2–3 days before operation. Various regimes have been recommended for the operative period: (*a*) The Alberti regime.[89] 16 units of insulin are added to 500 ml of 10% glucose, with 20 mmol of potassium chloride. This is infused intravenously, 100 ml/h. Many personalized versions of this regime exist. The important features are that the insulin is given continuously, without absorption problems, and that it is balanced with the correct amount of glucose. Earlier doubts about adsorption of insulin into the plastic of the container appear to have been unfounded. Blood glucose is estimated at the start of the operation and in the postoperative room. The Alberti regime may be continued, with blood glucose monitoring, until the patient starts to eat again. Much depends on the size of the operation and the duration of starvation. (*b*) Other physicians prefer to administer half of the normal dose of soluble insulin in the morning with 500 ml 5% glucose intravenously 6-hourly. Operation is carried out in the morning and at midday the remainder of the morning insulin dose is given unless blood glucose is less than 6 mmol/l (108 mg %). Bolus intravenous injections of 10 g glucose can be given if necessary. The evening dose of insulin can be given as usual unless blood glucose is below the level quoted above. (*c*) The normal insulin dosage may be administered and glucose solution infused intravenously to maintain requirements. This approach can be used when there is no time for preoperative stabilization with soluble insulin, but if long-acting insulin has been given there is lack of flexibility. Blood glucose and plasma potassium are checked before the infusion starts and after 2–3 h.[90] Appropriate changes can then be made.

If surgery has to be delayed until late in the day prolonged fasting may present a threat to the diabetic patient. The preoperative regime should then include both carbohydrate and insulin.

4. The poorly controlled diabetic. The sign of inadequate control is *ketosis* accompanying glycosuria. This is a medical emergency requiring the assistance of an experienced physician. Elective and non-urgent surgery must be postponed, but operations such as drainage of abscesses or treatment of infected gangrene are necessary to achieve control. After partial correction of acidosis with sodium bicarbonate (50 mmol if $pH > 7.1$; 100 mmol if $pH < 7.0$), the *Alberti regime* offers a scheme for rapid control of the situation (*see above*), or hourly i.v. injections of 5 units of soluble insulin.[91] Hypokalaemia is corrected with potassium chloride 10–20 mmol/h, if the urine flow is greater than 1 ml/min. Phosphate deficiency in acute ketoacidosis averages 1 mmol/l. There is a real danger of vomiting during induction in the diabetic with ketosis.

5. *Diabetic coma.*[92] The following abnormalities require treatment: (*a*) Lack of insulin; (*b*) Dehydration; (*c*) Loss of sodium and potassium ions; (*d*) Metabolic acidosis; (*e*) Precipitating diseases. Insulin has a short half-life (5 min) in the blood and it is advantageous to administer small doses frequently. Sodium bicarbonate should be administered in small quantities of isotonic solution; there is a danger that overzealous dosage may cause rapid changes in potassium level with perhaps cardiac arrest. The following regimen has been recommended: (*a*) Blood analysis for sugar, urea, electrolytes, haemoglobin and packed-cell volume; (*b*) Urinalysis and insertion of urinary catheter; (*c*) Administer oxygen to maintain Pao_2 above 10 kPa; (*d*) Nasogastric tube and stomach aspiration; (*e*) Monitor electrocardiogram; (*f*) *Insulin:*[93] May be given as 6 units/h by continuous infusion (mechanical pump or burette). Addition of human albumin prevents adsorption to walls of container. Otherwise soluble insulin 10 units i.m. plus perhaps 10 units i.v. immediately; then 5 units i.m. hourly, doubled if blood sugar does not fall. Blood sugar is measured 2-hourly. When the level falls below 11–14 mmol/l (200–250 mg %) insulin may be given according to a sliding scale. (*g*) *Fluid and electrolytes*: Average deficit—water 6 litres, sodium 500 mmol, chloride 400 mmol, potassium 350 mmol. Rate of infusion recommended 1000 ml normal (0.9%) saline in 30 min, 500 ml in next 30 min, then 1000 ml every 2–3 h. Electrolytes measured 2-hourly and change to 0.45% saline if serum sodium rises above 155 mmol/l. Potassium should be added, 13 mmol (1 g) in the first hour then 26 mmol hourly. Five per cent dextrose may be given when blood sugar falls below 11–14 mmol/l. (*h*) *Sodium bicarbonate*: Given only if acidaemia is severe, $[H^+]$ greater than 100 nmol/l (pH less than 7.0). It should be given in isotonic (1.4%) solution to a maximum of 100 mmol. (*i*) Treatment of any underlying cause (e.g. antibiotics for bacterial infection) should be commenced early. For management of diabetic crisis in children, *see* Moseley J. *Br. Med. J.* 1975, **1**, 59.

It should be remembered that coma can occur in a diabetic patient without ketoacidosis. Differential diagnosis may include: (*a*) *Hyperosmolar, non-ketoacidotic diabetic coma:*[62] The patient is dehydrated with high blood sugar but no ketonuria. Sodium bicarbonate is contraindicated and hypotonic solutions (0.45% saline) are required; (*b*) *Lactic acidosis:*[94] May occur in patients treated with phenformin. Blood lactic acid levels should be determined, but the condition may be suspected when the 'anion gap' (difference between sum of sodium and potassium ions and sum of chloride and bicarbonate ions) is greater than 20. Large amounts of bicarbonate may be needed intravenously; (*c*) *Cerebral oedema*: May occur as complication of prolonged hypoglycaemia or when intravenous fluids have been given too rapidly; (*d*) Causes of coma unconnected with diabetes.

6. *Emergency Surgery*. Factors to consider are: (*a*) Good hydration; (*b*) Freedom from keto-acidosis; (*c*) Possible hypoglycaemic effect of drugs already administered; (*d*) Importance of treating predisposing infection, e.g. abscess.

Postoperative Control of Diabetes

There is a tendency towards hyperglycaemia, with a peak at 4 h after operation (even more marked in cardiopulmonary patients). The subsequent daily insulin requirement will probably be raised by 10% for 2 days.[95]

The Alberti regime is claimed to produce good control. Those patients who received subcutaneous insulin (half dose of their usual preparation) with a 5% glucose drip, may require further insulin later that day (s.c. or i.v.) as dictated by blood or urinary glucose monitoring 4-hourly on the day of operation, less often thereafter, if stable. A return to the patient's usual regime is made as soon as he is eating normally. The *'sliding scale'* still has practical value: 2% urine glucose or blood glucose 20 mmol/l—20 units insulin; 1% urine glucose or blood glucose 10 mmol/l—10 units insulin. Patients receiving oral hypoglycaemic control can usually be managed without the hypoglycaemic drugs until normal eating is resumed. In the complicated surgical case, such patients may require a temporary period of control by the Alberti regime, e.g. in the intensive therapy unit, where resistance to insulin is commonly seen. Special care should be taken following Caesarean section in a diabetic patient and after amputation of a gangrenous leg since insulin requirements may fall rapidly.

Duration of action of some agents: soluble insulin 6–8 h; lente insulin 20–24 h; chlorpropamide 60 h; glibenclamide 12–16 h; phenformin 6–8 h. A constant infusion of 5% glucose guards against hypoglycaemia. Hartmann's solution is probably best avoided in diabetic patients, as the lactate may be metabolized with resultant hyperglycaemia.[96]

Glucose should never be given by mouth as a preoperative measure because of the risk of vomiting or regurgitation.

Hexamethonium and β-blocking agents may enhance the action of insulin and cause hypoglycaemia. Glucocorticoids may result in carbohydrate intolerance. The diuretic thiazides, ethacrynic acid and frusemide, may inhibit insulin secretion. Diabetic patients sometimes develop a syndrome simulating an acute abdomen. Hyperglycaemic coma takes time to develop whereas *hypoglycaemia* can come on during an operation and may be characterized by sweating, pallor, tachycardia, dilated pupils, abnormal eyeball tension, etc. It should be treated by intravenous glucose 25%. It may be the cause of a delayed return to consciousness. Normal diet should be restored as soon as possible in the diabetic after operation.

Should the diabetes become unstable in the postoperative period, it is a good plan to prescribe soluble insulin according to 4-hourly urine testing.

Surgical Treatment of Hyperinsulinism

When a tumour is to be removed a preoperative glucose load should be given and a 25% solution should be infused via a central line during the surgical procedure.

Chronic Alcoholism

Because of the likelihood of both intraoperative and postoperative problems, early recognition with very careful preoperative assessment is required. Chronic alcoholism causes liver damage. Alcohol is eliminated in the liver by conversion to acetaldehyde with the aid of the enzyme cytosol dehydrogenase. Chronic alcoholism leads to induction of drug-metabolizing enzymes so that if the liver is not seriously damaged, the patient may be less sensitive to drugs, e.g. thiopentone and diazepam.[97] Hepatic cirrhosis may be associated with hyperventilation and arterial oxygen desaturation, the latter due to shunting of blood from peri-oesophageal and mediastinal veins to pulmonary veins. There is increased peripheral blood flow and vasodilatation and this may result in cardiac hypertrophy. There may be cardiomyopathy and congestive failure and diminished adrenocortical response.

Anaesthesia

Alcohol should not be withdrawn while awaiting operation.[98] Diazepam and chlordiazepoxide are useful sedatives. Regional analgesia should be considered but associated hypotension may harm a damaged liver. Cyclopropane and halothane both reduce hepatic blood flow, the former by vasoconstriction, the latter by hypotension. There may be a decreased tolerance to suxamethonium and an increased tolerance to tubocurarine due to the decreased cholinesterase content of serum and to protein binding due to the increased gamma-globulin seen in this condition. In acute alcoholism, patients withstand shock and trauma badly perhaps due to vasodilatation. Postoperative decreased adrenocortical response to stress occurs.[98]

To prevent withdrawal symptoms 8–10% alcohol in saline i.v. 500 ml over several hours may be helpful.[98] (*See also* Edwards R. and Mosher J. B. *Anaesthesia* 1980, **35**, 476; Edwards R. *Br. Med. J.* 1985, **291**, 423.)

Obesity

Julius Caesar said 'let me have men about me that are fat!' (Shakespeare, W. Julius Caesar, Act. I, Sc. 2). Back to base Julius! This proves that he was no anaesthetist! This condition, usually the result of superalimentation, is perhaps the most common abnormality present in patients who require surgical operations. It is a serious handicap to surgeon and anaesthetist alike. 'Whatever the quantity that a man eats, it is plain that if he is too fat, he has eaten more than he should have done' (Samuel Johnson, 1709–1784).

The Disadvantages of Obesity

1. The respiratory system. Reduced vital capacity, inspiratory capacity, expiratory reserve volume, functional residual capacity and increase in closing volume, increased work of breathing, hypoxaemia, diaphragmatic splinting. Some parts of lungs are underventilated, causing an increase of shunting and hypercapnia and hypoxaemia. Increased incidence of postoperative chest complications. Hypoxic pulmonary arterial constriction with right ventricular strain.

The Pickwickian syndrome.[99] Somnolence due to chronic hypercapnia.

2. The cardiovascular system. Total blood volume increased with increase in cardiac work. Tendency to hypertension and coronary disease. Increased risk of postoperative thrombosis. In obesity there is less water per unit of body weight and dehydration is badly tolerated. Varicose veins are common.

3. Miscellaneous. Tendency to hiatus hernia. Increased incidence of burst abdomen. Possibility of endocrinopathies. Shorter life expectancy. Possibility of diabetes, hypertension, cholelithiasis, gout.

4. Technical. Difficult to move and to lift and to nurse. Spontaneous breathing handicapped. Need for tracheal intubation increased and because of short thick neck this may be troublesome. Awkward venesection and placement of needles for regional analgesia. Less tolerance of Trendelenburg and lithotomy positions. Induction of anaesthesia usually much more tiresome. Difficulty to maintain patent airway during induction and after operation. Difficulty of access for the surgeon in the abdomen, chest and mouth. It is reported that the morbidly obese do well under thoracic extradural block together with light general anaesthesia with IPPV.[100] For arterial pressure monitoring an intra-arterial cannula gives more accurate results than a cuff on an obese arm.

This condition is usually preventable but seldom prevented. Preoperative dietetic guidance should be more common. (*See also* Bromage P. R. and Fox G. S. *Anaesthesia* 1976, **31**, 557; Strauss R. J. and Wise L. *Surg. Gynecol. Obstet.* 1978, **146**, 286; Symposium on Obesity, *Surg. Clin. North Am.* 1979, **59**, December; Obesity Symposium, *J. R. Coll. Physicians, Lond.* 1983, **17**, 5; The perioperative management of morbidly obese patients (a surgeon's perspective). Ramsey-Stewart G. *Anaesth. Intensive Care* 1985, **13**, 399.)

Pulmonary Disease

In chest disease functional defects may be in: (1) Gas transport; (2) Gas mixing; (3) Blood distribution; (4) Regional gas distribution.

Acute Infection

Acute coryza is seldom a contraindication to minor surgery[101] provided the patient is apyrexial and without abnormal physical signs in the chest. Blocked nostrils may require the early use of an oropharyngeal airway. For major elective operations, especially those on the thorax or abdomen, postponement will usually be the rule because of the risk of ensuing bronchial infection. Patients at particular risk include those on immunosuppressive drugs and those with valvular disease of the heart (risk of bacteraemia).

Chronic Infection[102]

Chronic bronchitis is a condition with chronic or recurrent increase in the volume of mucoid bronchial secretion sufficient to cause expectoration. Sputum should be coughed up before anaesthesia, by postural drainage for 2 h, if necessary. Induction should be smooth to avoid stimulation of cough and laryngeal reflexes. Rapid induction with tracheal intubation in light anaesthesia may provoke coughing, straining and bronchospasm. Pre- and postoperative physiotherapy may be required.[103]

Emphysema

Emphysema is a condition of the lungs characterized by increase beyond the normal in the size of air spaces distal to the terminal bronchiole, either from dilatation or from destruction of their walls. This causes dyspnoea because of defective chest mechanics; the stretch receptors are overstimulated and ventilation is thereby limited. There may be a horizontal flattened diaphragm which pulls the lower ribs inwards during inspiration, and early use of the sternomastoids and scalene muscles. The arterial P_{CO_2} rises and the respiratory centre becomes less sensitive, although some chemoreceptors still respond to oxygen lack. When a chest infection is superadded, hypoventilation is made worse. Such patients are a problem and the following points merit attention: (1) Hypersensitivity of respiratory reflexes (bucking, bronchospasm, etc.) to irritant vapours, thiopentone, secretions and intubation; (2) Piston-type respiration where diaphragm moves up and down like a piston in a cylinder, while the thoracic cage fails to expand. This can seriously impede the abdominal surgeon in his work if respiration is spontaneous; (3) Dependence on chronic hypoxia for the respiratory drive, via the aortic and carotid bodies. This is impaired if the patient breathes an oxygen-rich atmosphere during or after anaesthesia. The pink colour due to this hyperoxaemia may mask hypoventilation so that carbon dioxide narcosis goes unnoticed; (4) Undue sensitivity to such respiratory depressants as opiates and barbiturates; (5) During controlled ventilation there may be difficulty in inflation, necessitating the use of high pressure, with adverse effects on the circulation, and reduced elastic recoil leading to inefficient expiration; (6) Patient may be accustomed to a relatively high $P_{a_{CO_2}}$ and low $P_{a_{O_2}}$.

General anaesthesia is associated with impairment of pulmonary ventilation/perfusion ratios, shown clinically as relative hypoxaemia, and increased alveolar-arterial tension difference. The peak expiratory flow rate is a simple indicator of respiratory function and can be measured by a Wright Peak Flow Minimeter.

Anaesthetic Management

Preoperative care. This should include amelioration of bronchospasm and infection, reduction in body weight and physiotherapy.

Premedication. Trimeprazine, diazepam, promethazine and atropine are well tolerated. Opiates and barbiturates may cause undue respiratory depression. Ephedrine and aminophylline may be helpful.

Anaesthesia. Regional block, e.g. extradural for lower abdominal operations or brachial plexus, when suitable. Good reasons can be advanced for preferring either spontaneous or controlled respiration. If no relaxation is required, spontaneous respiration with a smooth induction and perhaps a volatile agent.

The use of relaxants. When relaxation is required or when piston respiration makes conditions difficult, controlled respiration will be necessary following the use of a relaxant. This need not be followed by difficulty in restarting respiration if curarization is properly reversed, even if the $P_{a_{CO_2}}$ is lower than the patient's normal level. Postoperative IPPV may be beneficial, especially in obese patients.

Postoperative care. Oxygen may be needed and ventilation may require stimulation: (1) Chemically, by nikethamide 10 ml well diluted, ½-hourly or as a continuous intravenous drip, or dichlorophenamide (Daranide) 50 mg 4-hourly which is also a carbonic anhydrase inhibitor. Doxapram hydrochloride

0·4–5 mg/min as an infusion may also be useful.[104] (2) Mechanically, by IPPV perhaps through a tracheostomy.

For clinical assessment of respiratory function *see* Rigg J. R. A. and Jones N. L. *Br. J. Anaesth.* 1978, **50**, 3; Loh L. et al. *Br. J. Anaesth.* 1978, **50**, 63.

Asthma (*see also* Chapter 38.)

A disease characterized by variable dyspnoea due to widespread narrowing of peripheral airways in the lungs, varying in severity over short periods of time, either spontaneously or as a result of treatment, and not being due to cardiac asthma. The term 'bronchospasm' was first used by T. Willis (1621–1675). Various treatments first used: subcutaneous adrenaline, 1898; ephedrine, 1925; corticosteroids, 1952; disodium cromoglycate, 1967; selective β_2-adrenergic stimulant, 1968. Drugs which may cause bronchoconstriction in atopic patients include penicillins, antisera, iodine-containing contrast media, relaxants, thiopentone. These effects may be the result of IgE-mediated histamine release; by a non-allergic mechanism, e.g. prostaglandin F_2 alpha, used for induced abortions, non-cardioselective β-blockers, etc.

Preoperative Treatment of Patients With Severe Bronchial Asthma

Except in emergency, patients with asthma should not be operated on until their lung condition is as near normal as possible—the incidence of lung complications after operation in asthmatics is high. (1) Bronchodilators. (2) Steroids—to reduce oedema and relieve spasm. (3) Physiotherapy.

Anaesthetics well tolerated, ether and halothane, being bronchodilators. Nebulized isoprenaline can be given during the operation. The following may make the asthma worse: intravenous thiopentone; clumsy induction of general anaesthesia with a volatile agent; tracheal intubation, especially in light planes of anaesthesia or with incomplete relaxation; stimulation of the upper respiratory tract by acid gastric contents; blood, mucus, etc. Acute bronchospasm following intubation may be treated with aminophylline, 5 mg/kg, i.v. given slowly; also hydrocortisone. Salbutamol, 0·2 mg, may be given slowly by the same route. β_2-blockade must be avoided.

(*See also* Symposium on Anaesthesia and Respiratory Dysfunction. *Br. J. Anaesth.* 1982, **54**, 701.)

Disease of the Nervous System

Spinal analgesia and extradural block are usually inadvisable because future symptoms and signs may be blamed (unjustly) on these methods of analgesia. A history of frequent headaches may also make spinal analgesia undesirable. But *see also* Crawford J. S. et al. *Anaesthesia* 1981, **36**, 821.

Epilepsy

Patients with epilepsy should be kept on anticonvulsants before, during and after operation. In susceptible patients, epilepsy may be triggered off by cholinergic drugs, methohexitone, mono-amine oxidase inhibitors, phenothiazines, tricyclic antidepressants, enflurane, and sudden withdrawal of barbiturates, diazepam and hypocapnia.

Narcotic Addiction
These patients may manufacture symptoms to earn an operation in order to obtain morphine afterwards. *Withdrawal symptoms* may include cramp, vomiting and diarrhoea, while intestinal obstruction is often simulated. There may be multiple abscesses from unhygienic injections, with thombophlebitis, so that the external jugular veins remain the only usable channels for intravenous therapy. Frequent history of viral hepatitis and asthma. Sedative premedication may require large doses of drugs to be effective. Hypotension is common in the operating theatre. The patient may interfere with the wound to prolong stay in hospital, so that great care and discipline are required from the operation. Tetrahydrocannibol in the blood stream, from cannabis, causes atropine to have a pressor effect, while anticholinergic drugs and local analgesic drugs with added adrenaline can potentiate cannabis-induced tachycardia.[105] Amphetamine addiction may increase the required doses of anaesthetic agents.[106] (*See also* Geelhoed G. W. and Joseph W. G. *Surg. Gynecol. Obstet.* 1974, **139**, 749.) Addicts may be HIV positive.

Paraplegia[107]
Patients with *transection of the cord* at or above T.5 may get severe hypertension after certain visceral stimuli, e.g. distension of the bladder or rectum. Ganglionic blockade may be required to relieve this as also may extradural block.[108,109] About 40% of such patients about to undergo operation will require anaesthesia as it is difficult to be sure that the lesion of the cord is complete. Suxamethonium may be dangerous in the period of 14–28 days after onset of paraplegia. This is because of the raised serum potassium which may be associated with cardiac dysrhythmias when suxamethonium is given.

The following factors must be borne in mind: (1) Excitability of autonomic reflexes; (2) Psychiatric difficulties; (3) Chronic infection; (4) Nutritional difficulties; (5) Disturbed temperature regulation; (6) Problems of pain; (7) Problems of respiration; (8) Problems of position on the operating table; (9) Dangers of suxamethonium with paraplegia of recent onset. Little rise in blood pressure is likely if patients are anaesthetized with thiopentone, nitrous oxide, tubocurarine, a volatile agent and IPPV.

Autonomic hyperreflexia. Due to a lesion in the spinal cord. The arterial pressure may rise following visceral stimulation, such as distension of the bladder. Pentolinium tartrate has been used to control this.[109]

Dystrophia Myotonica
First described by Déléage in 1890 and again in 1909.[110] This is a hereditary disease. Patients may show one or more of the following characteristics: (1) Expressionless face; (2) Sternomastoid wasting; (3) Limb weakness with inability to let go after a handshake or to relax previously contracted muscles; (4) Cataract; (5) Frontal baldness; (6) Atrophy of gonads; (7) Thyroid adenomata; (8) Percussion myotonia; (9) Involvement of external muscles of the eye;[111] (10) Familial incidence.

It is a primary disorder of muscular fibres and not of the myoneural junction. The sufferer may have respiratory muscle weakness giving rise to reduced pulmonary ventilation and an increased Pa_{CO_2}. There may be cardiovascular impairment and adrenal cortical dysfunction.

Anaesthetic Management

Lung function should be investigated by: (1) Measurement of VC; (2) FEV_1; (3) Fluoroscopy of chest to see if there is myotonia of the diaphragm.

Respiratory depressants should be avoided before, during and after operation. Thiopentone has no specific peripheral depressant effect as it has in porphyria but if it is used it should be given in 50-mg doses while its effects are watched. Cardiovascular depression, including dysrhythmia and heart block, may occur during anaesthesia.[112] Assisted respiration may be required during operation, while IPPV perhaps through a tracheostomy may be necessary in the immediate postoperative period. Intubation is usually possible without the use of relaxants.

Spinal analgesia does not relax myotonia but injection of local analgesic solution into the muscle may do so. Non-depolarizing relaxants do not abolish myotonia but may be given very sparingly. Atracurium has been used successfully.[113] Dantrolene has been used for muscle relaxation.[114] Extradural block may be satisfactory.[115] Anticholinesterase drugs should not be used. Depolarizing relaxants may be hazardous and may increase the myotonia. The increased muscle tone may represent an exaggerated fasciculation which gives place to ordinary depolarizing relaxation with injection of additional doses of the drug. The possibility of this disease, also of diabetes, should be borne in mind in anaesthetizing young patients with cataracts. (*See also* Mudge B. J. et al. *Anaesthesia* 1980, **35**, 492; Aldridge L. M. *Br. J. Anaesth.* 1985, **57**, 1119.)

Huntington's (1850–1916) Chorea[116]

It is suggested that inhalation agents are the most suitable. Thiopentone may cause prolonged apnoea and should be avoided,[117] or used with great care,[118] and because the serum cholinesterase may be abnormal, the action of suxamethonium may be increased. On the other hand, some cases respond normally to suxamethonium.[119] Other workers have used thiopentone safely, and non-depolarizing relaxants.[120] (*See also* Lamont A. S. M. *Anaesth. Intensive Care* 1979, **7**, 189; Browne M. G. and Cross R. *Br. J. Anaesth.* 1981, **53**, 1367; Lamont A. S. M. *Anaesthesia* 1983, **38**, 295.)

Hypokalaemic Familial Periodic Paralysis

Thiopentone may cause temporary peripheral paralysis while muscle relaxants may cause residual muscle weakness.[121]

Multiple Sclerosis

Disseminated sclerosis, a term used by German pathologists in 1882, was changed to multiple sclerosis in 1946. Description systematized by J. M. Charcot (1825–1893) in 1868,[122] and by Cruveilhier in 1842. In the past it has been suggested that general anaesthesia may exacerbate the symptoms and thiopentone, non-depolarizing relaxants and methoxyflurane have been questioned, but firm conclusions cannot be drawn. Central neural blockade is better avoided on medicolegal grounds, although it has been suggested that the relapse rate is no greater following intradural block than after general anaesthesia.[123] Postoperative deterioration is likely to be associated with pyrexia secondary to surgical complications rather than anaesthetic agents used.[124] Special anaesthetic care is not usually necessary. (*See also* Jones R. M. and Healy T. E. J. *Anaesthesia* 1980, **35**, 879.)

Motor Neurone Disease
First described by Erb (1840–1921)[125] in 1884 and by Gowers (1845–1915) in 1902.[126] This disease causes changes not only in striated muscle but also in cardiac muscle and in the smooth muscle of the alimentary tract.

Premedication
These patients have a tendency to tachycardia, so excitement must be avoided and atropine may be less suitable than hyoscine.

Anaesthesia
Intravenous barbiturates should only be given in small doses, their effects being carefully watched. The disease does not involve the myoneural junctions but both types of relaxant should only be given in small doses and their effects assessed before additional amounts are injected. Inhalation agents may be suitable but the concentration of halothane should be increased with care. Postoperative respiratory depression has been reported so that respiratory depressant drugs and relaxants must be given very cautiously.

Complications
As the myocardium may be involved in the disease process, tachycardia is frequent and should not be made worse by the anaesthetic; preoperative digitalis may be desirable. Acute dilatation of the stomach may be seen after operation and may be due to a disorder of the smooth muscle of the wall of the viscus, it should be preventable by parenteral fluid therapy during the first day or two after operation and by assumption of the prone position for periods during the first 24 or 48 h. If these measures fail, then a Ryle's tube must be passed. Postoperative dysphagia may occur.

Duchenne Muscular Dystrophy
Sudden cardiac arrest may occur during anaesthesia.[127] Suxamethonium should be avoided and some patients may develop malignant hyperthermia. Temperature and the ECG should be monitored throughout the operation.[128]

Diseases of the Adrenal Glands

Primary Adrenal Failure
May be seen following: (1) Removal, i.e. adrenalectomy; (2) Destruction, e.g. Addison's disease; adrenal apoplexy; (3) Exhaustion, e.g. starvation and toxaemia; (4) Dysfunction, virilizing hyperplasia.

Secondary Adrenal Failure
This may occur as a result of: (1) Removal of the pituitary gland (hypophysectomy); (2) Destruction of the pituitary gland, e.g. tumours; Simmonds' disease; (3) Inhibition of the pituitary gland due to steroid therapy. Death due to circulatory failure may occur in patients who, having been on doses of cortisone for long periods, are suddenly deprived of it before the stress of anaesthesia and operation.[129] (*See also* p. 423.)

Addison's Disease
Described by Thomas Addison (1793–1860) of Guy's Hospital.[130] Patients with

this complaint are susceptible to infection, to loss of sodium chloride and to narcotics. They are likely to be debilitated, hypotensive and perhaps tuberculous. They are bad anaesthetic risks as Addisonian crises are easily precipitated. These start with loss of sodium chloride in the urine and so of large amounts of water. The circulating fluid is reduced, while diarrhoea and vomiting make the plasma volume smaller. Dehydration and circulatory collapse follow, and, in addition, there is often autonomic imbalance. If such a patient is operated on and Addison's disease not diagnosed, severe postoperative collapse may occur. If the disease, however, is recognized, adequate preoperative treatment greatly lessens the risk, although postoperative hypotension is likely. If it occurs it should be treated by infusion and the intravenous injection of hydrocortisone. Preoperative management consists in giving sodium chloride and fluid, dextrose and cortisone to maintain the circulating blood volume as near normal as possible. Hypotension and anoxia should be avoided. Thiopentone may cause a serious fall in blood pressure. For anaesthesia in Addisonian crisis, *see* Smith M. G. and Byrne A. J. *Anaesthesia* 1981, **36**, 681.

Waterhouse–Friderichsen Syndrome[131]
This is usually fatal and is often associated with meningococcal septicaemia, first described by Voelcker (1861–1946) in 1894.[132] Hyperpyrexia and circulatory collapse are the usual modes of death. Rarely the condition comes to operation because of associated arterial embolism or peritonitis. Hydrocortisone is indicated.

Diseases of the Pituitary Gland

Hyperpituitarism
In adults acromegaly, in children and adolescents gigantism. (*See* Chapters 24 and 26.)

Acromegaly
First described by Saucerotte (1741–1812)[133] in 1801 and by Pierre Marie (1853–1940) in 1886.[134] Due to an eosinophilic and chromophobe cell tumour of the pituitary forming after the epiphyses have fused. Slow onset with bony changes in the jaws, enlarged tongue, thickening of the mucosa of the pharynx, enlarged larynx with elongation and thickening of the cords. There may be laryngeal stenosis[135] and the cricoid may be narrowed, so making intubation difficult. Diligent postoperative observation is required. The use of a fibreoptic laryngoscope has been suggested.[136] (*See also* Recent developments in acromegaly, Jadresic A. *J. R. Soc. Med.* 1983, **76**, 947.) The hands become 'spade-like' and there may be kyphosis, diabetes and an enlarged thyroid. May present as carpal tunnel syndrome. There may be difficulty in intubation, and the wise anaesthetist being forewarned will be forearmed. Blind nasal intubation may have a place here. Sleep apnoea is common and may be central, obstructive or mixed.[137]

Postoperatively, there may be airway obstruction from pathological narrowing of the small airways,[138] and resultant acute pulmonary oedema[139] so that relatively prolonged intubation or even tracheostomy may have to be considered. Careful postoperative observation is very important. An impaired ulnar artery circulation in one or both hands may occur in acromegaly, so arterial cannulation of the dorsalis pedis may be safer than use of the radial artery.[140]

For *hypophysectomy*, the ordinary technique for supratentorial operations is employed. Steroid cover must be commenced before the operation and continued. Thyroxine may be required for the first 10 postoperative days, as thyroid deficit takes some days to develop. When the operation is performed for metastatic cancer, preoperative attention to anaemia, pleural effusions and bony secondaries making movement dangerous because of the possibility of fractures, must be borne in mind. For yttrium-90 implantation, *see also* Whitwam J. G. et al. *Br. J. Anaesth.* 1973, **45**, 1121.

Hypopituitarism (Simmonds' Disease)[141]

Morris Simmonds (1855–1925). Chronic hypopituitarism is most commonly due to ischaemic necrosis of the anterior lobe of the pituitary following haemorrhage or shock in labour (Sheehan's syndrome).[142] It may also be due to tumours in surrounding tissues. There may be results of the interference of secretion of any of the hormones produced by the gland: growth hormone, corticotropin (ACTH), thyrotropin, gonadotropin and antidiuretic hormone. Substitution therapy may be required. It may be suspected if there is absence of a palpable thyroid, absence of pubic hair and genital hypoplasia with loss of sexual function, amenorrhoea and low BMR. There may be additional suprarenal deficiency requiring steroids, and an increased sensitivity to barbiturates and narcotic analgesics. General anaesthesia is liable to precipitate coma in these patients. Cortisone may be helpful.

Recent Steroid Therapy

Adrenal cortical hormones: (1) Glucocorticoids: hydrocortisone sodium succinate. Hydrocortisone (cortisol) is a naturally occurring substance and, in addition, there are a number of synthetic substances with largely the same effects. During and after anaesthesia the main sign of deficiency of hydrocortisone is hypotension. This influences the metabolism of carbohydrate and opposes the action of insulin. It has anti-inflammatory effects and in large dosage promotes the excretion of nitrogen and causes muscle wasting, skin atrophy and osteoporosis; (2) Mineralocorticoids: aldosterone. This is secreted in response to a reduction in extracellular fluid volume, and promotes retention of sodium and excretion of potassium by the kidneys; (3) Sex hormones.

Steroid therapy suppresses the formation of ACTH by the anterior pituitary with resultant adrenocortical atrophy. The cortex is then unable to secrete extra hormones in response to the stress of anaesthesia, operation or trauma. The first death from this cause was reported in 1952 following therapeutic doses of cortisone.[143]

Adrenocortical reserve is *diminished*: (1) In Addison's disease, whether treated or untreated; (2) After bilateral adrenalectomy; (3) During steroid therapy; (4) When a patient has received steroids in the past. It may be that adrenocortical reserve is sufficient to meet the ordinary needs of life, but that the reserve is inadequate to meet the extra burden of anaesthesia and operation.

As short a course as 1 week may produce depression of the cortex. Depression may last as long as 1–2 years, and in some cases of prolonged therapy the cortex may never regain its full functional reserve.

There are no satisfactory simple tests for adrenocortical reserve. The response of the cortex to ACTH given intravenously over 8 h is reflected as a fall of eosinophils in peripheral blood and a rise in corticoids and 17-ketosteroids in the 24-h urine. Such tests are cumbersome and unsuited to routine use. Where facilities for blood-cortisol estimation are available, a preoperative stress test can be carried out. A small dose of insulin is given, and frequent estimations of blood sugar and blood cortisol carried out. A fall in blood sugar indicates a successful test, a rise of blood cortisol a satisfactory response indicating the presence of adrenocortical reserve, and steroid cover is not required.

In the absence of such testing it is best to assume that there is some diminution of reserve whenever a course of steroids has recently been given. Collapse is unlikely to occur more than 2 months after cessation of treatment. It is generally safer to give cortisone cover than to omit it in cases of doubt. The normal adult secretes 20–30 mg of hydrocortisone daily and this may reach 400 mg daily in response to surgery and anaesthesia.

Spinal analgesia is the only form of pain relief which does not cause a rise in blood-cortisol levels during anaesthesia, though the effects of stress are evident in the postoperative period when the local analgesic effect is over. Under general anaesthesia there is a rise during abdominal surgery, but not much rise during neurosurgical operations. Anaesthesia itself causes only a mild stress reaction.

Cortisone cover can be provided by intramuscular injection of hydrocortisone hemisuccinate 100 mg 6-hourly. This can be commenced at the time of premedication and continued for 3 days in the case of major surgery, for 24 h following minor operations such as hernia repair, and restricted to a single injection prior to endoscopy or other brief procedure. Further doses can be given if complications ensue. Intramuscular injections give more satisfactory plasma levels than the intravenous route. The latter produces sharp peak blood levels and is indicated in emergency situation (e.g. 100 mg as a bolus dose). Depot preparations have also been used as a single injection.[144]

Other steroid derivatives include prednisone and prednisolone (3 to 5 times as potent as cortisone), triamcinolone (15 times as potent), betamethasone and dexamethasone (35 times as potent).

Corticosteroids are often contraindicated in patients with tuberculosis, local or systemic infection unless controlled by antibiotics, active peptic ulcer, psychosis, osteoporosis, renal dysfunction, diabetes mellitus, glaucoma, hypertension, myasthenia gravis, thrombotic disorders, congestive heart failure and those who are pregnant.

Ill-effects of steroids: (1) Increased susceptibility to infection; (2) Retarded healing; (3) Gastrointestinal bleeding and perforation; (4) Impaired electrolyte balance.

Carcinoid Tumours

First described by Merling in 1838 and named by Obendorfer[145] in 1907 because less malignant than carcinoma. Arise from argentaffin Kultschitzky cells of the crypts of Lieberkuhn of the gastrointestinal tract; 50–90% originate in the area of the appendix, and these tumours neither metastasize nor secrete. Extra-appendicular tumours are often malignant and about 25% of malignant carcinoids produce and secrete serotonin (5-hydroxytryptamine) and other hormones including bradykinin.

Malignant carcinoid syndrome. There are big variations in the clinical manifestations. The syndrome does not occur unless there are hepatic secondaries with secretion of bradykinin and serotonin into the hepatic veins. It may be characterized by: (1) A growing intra-abdominal malignancy; (2) Cutaneous flushes; (3) Other symptoms may include: profuse perspiration, nausea and vomiting, abdominal distension and cramps, diarrhoea; (4) Dyspnoea, respiratory stridor, asthmatic attacks; (5) Tachycardia and fall in blood pressure; (6) Long-term manifestations: valvular fibrosis of the right side of the heart which may require surgery, arthritis, sclerodermic changes, telangiectasia of the face, dependent oedema.

Problems associated with serotonin dysfunction may be: (1) Delayed awakening from anaesthesia; (2) Attacks of tachycardia and/or hypertension; (3) A raised blood sugar; (4) Hypoproteinaemia; (5) Hyperpnoea.

Those associated with bradykinin dysfunction may include: (1) Flushing of the skin progressing to hypotension and shock; (2) Bronchospasm.

Attacks may be precipitated by: (1) Palpation of the tumour; (2) Hypotension; (3) Fear; (4) Eating, drinking, defaecation.

Diagnosis is confirmed by measuring urinary secretion of 5-hydroxyindole acetic acid. Normal 2–9 mg/24 h, greater than 25 mg/24 h is diagnostic. Up to 1000 mg/24 h have been secreted.

Medical treatment with antiserotonin drugs, aprotinin, EACA, corticosteroids, adrenergic blockers and cytotoxic agents has been disappointing. Surgical treatment may be directed towards removal of the primary tumour, removal of secondary deposits or replacement of heart valves since progression of the disease is slow. Preoperative treatment may include aprotinin (Trasylol) if clinical features suggest bradykinin secretion (e.g. infusion of 200 000 units started 1 h before surgery). Methotrimeprazine may be used to control serotonin effects (2·5–5·0 mg i.v. depending upon response). Cyproheptadine may be used before operation, having antiserotonin effects.

Any preoperative hypotension or hypokalaemia will require treatment. Anaesthesia may be uneventful, but may provoke an attack of the syndrome with an acute flushing and severe bronchospasm. This is particularly likely if hypotension is allowed to occur and so spinal techniques are not recommended. Morphine may cause serotonin release. Smooth induction of anaesthesia is to be desired. Pancuronium is recommended as the relaxant of choice.[146] Halothane may cause unwanted hypotension. Neurolept agents are controversial. Vasopressors are contraindicated as they may cause release of tumour hormones. Careful monitoring should continue into the postoperative period. Treatment of an attack during anaesthesia is to avoid reflex responses and to maintain ventilation of the lungs using high inflation pressures if necessary. Aprotinin and steroids have both been recommended during anaesthesia.[147]

The serotonin blood level is also increased in argentaffinoma of the lung, non-tropical sprue and intestinal lipodystrophy.

(*See also* Miller R. et al. *Can. Anaesth. Soc. J.* 1978, **25**, 240; Kleine J. W. et al. *Anesthesiology* 1978, **49**, 55; Rawlinson W. A. L. et al. *Anaesthesia* 1980, **35**, 585; Fleming F. *Anaesthesia* 1980, **35**, 589; Eisenkraft J. B. et al. *Anaesthesia*

1981, **36**, 881; Fletcher I. R. and Carson J. *Anaesthesia* 1983, **38**, 510; Tornebrandt K. et al. *Anaesthesia* 1983, **38**, 957; Perioperative management of carcinoid syndrome using ketanserin, *see* Houghton K. and Carter J. A. *Anaesthesia* 1986, **41**, 595.)

Homocystinuria[148]

An inborn error of metabolism due to deficiency of the enzyme cystothionine synthetase. Precautions to be considered in the event of a surgical operation include heparinization to prevent thrombosis and pulmonary emboli (especially after operations for dislocated lens), and a low methionine diet. Perioperative hypoglycaemia may occur.

References

1. Dripps R. D. et al. *JAMA* 1961, **178**, 261.
2. Lunn J. N. and Mushin W. W. *Mortality associated with Anaesthesia* Nuffield Provincial Hospitals Trust, London, 1982; *Proc. Eur. Acad. Anaesthesiol* (Vickers M. D. and Lunn J. N. ed.) Berlin: Springer-Verlag, 1982.
3. Emslie-Smith D. *Br. J. Hosp. Med.* 1981, **26**, 442.
4. Vowles K. *Br. J. Hosp. Med.* 1981, **26**, 454.
5. Leeming J. T. *Br. J. Hosp. Med.* 1981, **26**, 459.
6. Del Guerico L. R. M. and Cohn J. D. *JAMA* 1980, **243**, 1350.
7. Foëx P. in: *Recent Advances in Anaesthesia and Analgesia*—14 (Atkinson R. S. and Hewer C. Langton ed.) Edinburgh: Churchill Livingstone, 1982).
8. Goldman L. et al. *N. Engl. J. Med.* 1977, **297**, 845.
9. Peter K. et al. *Anesthesiologie und Intensivmedizin*, 1980, **9**, 240.
10. Galasko C. S. B. et al. *Injury* 1985, **16**, 398; Boston D. A. *Injury* 1982, **14**, 207.
11. Domaingue C. M. et al. *Anaesth. Intensive Care* 1982, **10**, 324.
12. Duke P. C. et al. *Can. Anaesth. Soc. J.* 1976, **23**, 111.
13. Munson F. S. and Hofmann J. C. *Anesth. Analg. (Cleve.)* 1984, **63**, 998.
14. Report of the Committee on Drugs of the American Colleges of Pediatrics and Obstetricians and Gynecologists. *Pediatrics* 1978, **62**, 402.
15. White D. G. *Br. J. Hosp. Med.* 1980, **24**, 145.
16. Richards D. W. and Strauss M. L. *J. Clin. Invest.* 1927, **4**, 105.
17. *See also* Lehmann H. and Huntsman R. G. *Man's Haemoglobins*, 2nd ed. Amsterdam: North Holland Publishing Co., 1974.
18. Herrick J. B. *Arch. Intern. Med.* 1910, **6**, 517.
19. Pauling L. et al. *Science, N.Y.* 1949, **110**, 543.
20. Emmel V. E. *Arch. Intern. Med.* 1917, **20**, 586.
21. Searle J. F. *Anaesthesia* 1973, **28**, 48; Oduro K. A. and Searle J. F. *Br. Med. J.* 1972, **4**, 596.
22. Van der Pette J. E. W. et al. *J. R. Soc. Med.* 1982, **75**, 777.
23. Barabas A. P. *Br. J. Hosp. Med.* 1980, **23**, 289.
24. Gibbs J. M. *Anaesth. Intensive Care* 1978, **6**, 141; Hool G. J. et al. *Anaesth. Intensive Care* 1984, **12**, 360.
25. Biggs R. *Br. J. Hosp. Med.* 1971, **6**, 343.
26. Otto J. C. *Med. Reposit., N.Y.* 1803, **61**, 1.
27. Bullock W. and Fildes P. *Haemophilia.* London: Dulau Co., 1911.
28. Inwood J. and Meltzer D. B. *Can. Anaesth. Soc. J.* 1978, **25**, 266.
29. Davis K. C. et al. *Ann. Intern. Med.* 1983, **98**, 284; Curran J. W. et al. *N. Engl. J. Med.* 1984, **310**, 69; Hirsch M. S. et al. *N. Engl. J. Med.* 1985, **312**, 1; Bayer W. L. et al. *Clin. Haematol.* 1984, **13**, 253.
30. Scadding G. K. and Havard C. W. H. *Br. Med. J.* 1981, **283**, 1008.
31. Willis T. *The London Practice of Physick.* London: T. Cassell, 1685.
32. Wilks S. *Guy's Hosp. Rep.* 1877, **3** (Series 27), 7.
33. Jolly F. *Neurol. Zbl.* 1895, **14**, 34.

34. Campbell H. and Bromwell E. *Brain* 1900, **23**, 277.
35. Remen L. *Dtsch. Z. NervenHeilk.* 1932, **128**, 66.
36. Walker M. *Lancet* 1934, **1**, 1200.
37. Sauerbruch E. F. *Mitt. Grenzgeb. Med. Chir.* 1912–13, **25**, 746.
38. Blalock A. et al. *Ann. Surg.* 1939, **110**, 544.
39. Keynes G. *Br. J. Surg.* 1946, **33**, 201.
40. Weigert C. *Arch. Psychiat. Nerv. Krankh.* 1901, **34**, 1063.
41. Engel A. G. et al. *Mayo Clin Proc.* 1977, **52**, 267.
42. Wojciechowski A. J. P. et al. *Anaesthesia* 1985, **40**, 882.
43. Ward S. and Wright D. J. *Anaesthesia* 1984, **39**, 51.
44. Eaton M. L. and Lambert E. H. *JAMA* 1957, **163**, 1117.
45. Clement J. G. *Anesthesiology* 1976, **46**, 220; Bennett E. J. et al. *Anesthesiology* 1977, **47**, 317.
46. Newsom-Davies J. et al. *Neurology (Minneapolis)*, 1978, **28**, 266.
47. Bromley I. M. and Hirsch N. P. *Anaesthesia* 1984, **39**, 723.
48. Harrington P. R. *J. Bone Jt Surg.* 1962, **44A**, 591.
49. Purnell R. J. *Anaesthesia* 1982, **37**, 1115.
50. Ehlers E. *Derm. Zeit.* 1901, **8**, 173; Danlos H. *Bull. Soc. Franç. Dermatol. Syph.* 1908, **19**, 70.
51. Cohen S. E. *Anesthesiology* 1980, **52**, 264.
52. Stokvis B. J. E. *Ned. Tijdschr. Geneesk.* 1889, **25**, 409.
53. Mustajoki P. and Heinonen J. *Anesthesiology* 1980, **53**, 15.
54. Rizk S. F. et al. *Anesthesiology* 1977, **46**, 305.
55. Hunt A. H. *A Contribution to the Study of Portal Hypertension.* London: Churchill Livingstone, 1958; Bowen R. A. *Anaesthesia* 1960, **15**, 3.
56. Kennedy J. et al. *Q. J. Med.* 1973, **42**(NS) 549; Trey C. et al. *N. Engl. J. Med.* 1966, **274**, 473.
57. Pugh R. N. H. et al. *Br. J. Surg.* 1973, **60**, 646.
58. Kussmaul A. and Maier R. *Dtsch. Arch. Klin. Med.* 1866, **1**, 484.
59. Astwood D. E. *JAMA* 1943, **122**, 78.
60. Ord W. M. (1834–1902), *Med. Chir. Trans.* 1878, **43**, 57.
61. Sherry K. M. and Hutchinson I. L. *Anaesthesia* 1984, **39**, 1112.
62. Gerich J. E. et al. *Diabetes* 1971, **20**, 228.
63. Goldman L. and Caldera D. L. *Anesthesiology* 1979, **50**, 285; Foëx P. *J. R. Soc. Med.* 1983, **76**, 760.
64. Editorial, *Anesthesiology* 1979, **50**, 284.
65. Foëx P. *Br. J. Anaesth.* 1978, **50**, 15.
66. Hammer A. *Wien. Med. Wochenschr.* 1878, **28**, 97.
67. Obrastow W. P. and Strascheskow N. D. *Zeit. Clin. Med.* 1910, **71**, 116.
68. Herrick J. B. *JAMA* 1912, **59**, 2015.
69. Elamin M. S. et al. *Br. Heart J.* 1982, **48**, 311.
70. Epstein S. E. et al. *N. Engl. J. Med.* 1982, **307**, 1487.
71. Goldman L. *Ann. Intern. Med.* 1983, **98**, 504.
72. Jones R. M. et al. *Anaesthesia* 1980, **35**, 1010.
73. Forman R. et al. *Circulation* 1983, **67**, 1200.
74. Roy W. L. et al. *Anesthesiology* 1979, **51**, 393.
75. Coelho E. M. et al. *Angiology* 1982, **33**, 685.
76. Hilfiker O. et al. *Br. J. Anaesth.* 1983, **55**, 927.
77. Stokes W. M. *Dubl. Q. J. Med. Sci.* 1846, **2**, 73.
78. Adams R. *Dubl. Hosp. Rep.* 1827, **4**, 353.
79. McKenzie J. *Diseases of the Heart.* London: Froude, 1908.
80. Fenoglio J. J. et al. *N. Engl. J. Med.* 1983, **308**, 12.
81. Chevers N. *Guy's Hosp. Rep.* 1842, **7**, 387.
82. Gold R. G. *Prescriber's J.* 1984, **24**, 115.
83. Ferrer M. I. *JAMA* 1968, **38**, 560.
84. Burt D. E. R. *Anaesthesia* 1982, **37**, 1108.
85. Reid D. H. *Br. J. Hosp. Med.* 1984, **31**, 341.
86. Banting F. G. and Best C. H. *J. Lab. Clin. Med.* 1922, **7**, 25.
87. Rees P. J. et al. *J. R. Soc. Med.* 1981, **74**, 192.
88. Casey J. et al. *Surgery* 1983, **93**, 822.
89. Thomas D. J. B. et al. *Anaesthesia* 1984, **39**, 629.
90. Alberti K. G. M. M. and Thomas D. J. B. *Br. J. Anaesth.* 1979, **51**, 693.

91. Alberti K. G. M. M. and Hockaday T. D. R. *Clin. Endocrinol. Metab.* 1977, **6**, 421.
92. *See also* Hockaday T. D. R. and Alberti K. G. M. M. *Br. J. Hosp. Med.* 1972, **7**, 183; Page M. McB. et al. *Br. Med. J.* 1974, **2**, 687; Semple P. F. et al. *Br. Med. J.* 1974, **2**, 694; Atkinson R. S. Hamblin J. J., and Wright J. E. C. *Handbook of Intensive Care* 1981, London: Chapman and Hall.
93. *See also* Alberti K. G. M. M. et al. *Lancet* 1973, **2**, 515.
94. Watkins P. J. et al. *Br. Med. J.* 1969, **1**, 744; Woods H. F. *Br. J. Hosp. Med.* 1971, **6**, 668.
95. Thomas D. J. B. et al. *Anaesthesia* 1983, **38**, 1047.
96. Thomas D. J. B. and Alberti K. G. M. M. *Br. J. Anaesth.* 1975, **50**, 185.
97. Annotation *Br. Med. J.* 1980, **1**, 507.
98. Haxholdt O. St. and Johansson G. *Anaesthesia* 1982, **37**, 797; Haxholdt O. St. et al. *Anaesthesia* 1984, **39**, 240.
99. Named for Mr Wardle's fat boy in Charles Dickens's (1812–1870) *The Pickwick Papers*, 1837; *see* Burwell C. S. *Am. J. Med.* 1956, **21**, 84 (reprinted in 'Classical File', *Surv. Anesthesiol.* 1977, **21**, 477).
100. Buckley F. P. et al. *Anaesthesia* 1983, **38**, 840; Whalley D. G. et al. *Anaesthesia* 1981, **53**, 811.
101. Ellis G. H. *Anaesthesia* 1955, **10**, 78.
102. For X-ray assessment *see* Kerr I. H. *Br. J. Anaesth.* 1974, **46**, 558.
103. Cowan K. A. *Ann. R. Coll. Surg.* 1979, **61**, 366.
104. Gupta P. K. and Dundee J. W. *Anaesthesia* 1974, **29**, 33.
105. Beaconsfield F. et al. *N. Eng. J. Med.* 1972, **287**, 209.
106. Michel R. and Adams A. P. *Anaesthesia* 1979, **34**, 1016.
107. Guttmann L. and Whitteridge D. *Brain* 1947, **70**, 36.
108. Watson D. W. and Downey G. O. *Anesthesiology* 1980, **52**, 259.
109. Basta J. W. et al. *Br. J. Anaesth.* 1977, **49**, 1087.
110. Steinert H. *Dtsch. Z. Nerven Heilk.* 1909, **37**, 58; Batten F. E. and Gibbs H. P. *Brain* 1909, **32**, 187.
111. Kiloh L. G. and Nevin S. *Brain* 1951, **74**, 115.
112. Ellis F. R. *Br. J. Anaesth.* 1980, **52**, 153.
113. Nightingale P. et al. *Br. J. Anaesth.* 1985, **57**, 1131.
114. Phillips D. C. and Ellis F. R. *Anaesthesia* 1984, **39**, 568.
115. Harris N. E. M. *Anaesthesia* 1984, **39**, 1032.
116. Huntington G. *Med. Surg. Reporter (Philadelphia)* 1872, **26**, 317.
117. Blanloeil Y. et al. *Anaesthesia* 1982, **37**, 695.
118. Browne G. M. *Anaesthesia* 1983, **38**, 65.
119. Costarino A. and Gross J. R. *Anesthesiology* 1985, **63**, 570.
120. Farina J. and Ranscher L. A. *Br. J. Anaesth.* 1977, **49**, 1167.
121. *See also* Foëx P. *Br. J. Anaesth.* 1978, **50**, 15; Foëx P. *Br. J. Anaesth.* 1981, **53**, 731; Foëx P. in *Recent Advances in Anaesthesia and Analgesia*—14 (Atkinson R. S. and Hewer C. L. ed.) Edinburgh: Churchill Livingstone, 1982.
122. Charcot J. M. *Gaz. Hôp. civ. milit., Paris*, 1868, **41**, 554; C. R. Soc. Biol. (Paris) 1868, **20**, 16.
123. Bouchard P. et al. *Ann. Fr. Anaesth. Reanim.* 1984, **3**, 195.
124. Siemkowicz E. *Anaesthesia* 1976, **31**, 1211.
125. Erb W. H. *Dtsch. Arch. Klin. Med.* 1884, **34**, 467.
126. Gowers W. R. *Br. Med. J.* 1902, **2**, 89.
127. Seay A. R. et al. *Pediatrics* 1978, **93**, 88.
128. Smith C. L. and Bush G. H. *Br. J. Anaesth.* 1985, **57**, 1113.
129. Fraser C. G. et al. *JAMA* 1952, **149**, 1542.
130. Addison T. *Lond. Med. Gaz.* 1849, **48**, 517.
131. Waterhouse R. *Lancet* 1911, **1**, 577; Friderichsen C. *Jb. Kinderheilk.* 1918, **87**, 109.
132. Voelker A. R. *Middx Hosp. Rep. Med. Surg. Path. Regist.* 1894, 278.
133. Saucerotte N. *Mélang. de Chirurg. (Paris)* 1801, **1**, 407.
134. Marie P. *Med. Rev. Paris* 1886, **6**, 297.
135. Chappell W. F. *J. Laryngol.* 1896, **10**, 142.
136. Ovassapian A. *Anaesthesia* 1982, **37**, 1136.
137. Perks W. H. et al. *Br. Med. J.* 1980, **1**, 894.
138. Harrison B. D. W. *Q. J. Med.* 1978, **47**, 517.
139. Goldhill D. R. et al. *Anaesthesia* 1982, **37**, 1200.
140. Campkin V. *Anaesthesia* 1980, **35**, 1008.
141. Simmonds M. *Dtsch. Med. Wochenschr.* 1914, **40**, 322.
142. Sheehan H. L. *Am. J. Obstet. Gynecol.* 1954, **68**, 202.

143. Fraser C. G. et al. *JAMA* 1952, **149**, 1542.
144. Gran L. and Pahle J. A. *Anaesthesia* 1978, **33**, 59.
145. Obendorfer S. S. *Frankf. Z. Path.* 1907, **1**, 426.
146. Lippmann M. and Cleveland R. J. *Anesth. Analg. (Cleve.)* 1973, **52**, 768.
147. Nielsen M. S. and Manners J. M. *Anaesthesia* 1979, **34**, 494.
148. Carson N. A. J. *Br. J. Hosp. Med.* 1969, **2**, 439.
149. Ah Pin P. J. *Br. Dent. J.* 1987, **162**, 151.

Chapter 23	**DICTIONARY OF RARE DISEASES OF IMPORTANCE TO THE ANAESTHETIST**

An anaesthetist faced by problems which may arise in his patient due to an unusual disease may find the following list useful in his choice of anaesthetic.

Achalasia of the cardia—increased regurgitation risk.

Achondroplasia—intubation difficult, *see* p. 401.

Acromegaly—airway very difficult, intubation difficult, narrow cricoid ring diabetes, post-hypophysectomy. Steroids required, *see* p. 422.

Addison's disease—hypovolaemia, hyponatraemia, hypoglycaemia. Steroids required, *see* p. 421. T. A. Addison (1793–1860) London physician.

Adrenogenital syndrome—may be mistaken for pyloric stenosis. Fludrocortisone cover may be required for salt loss. Preoperative electrolyte check required. (Bongiovanni A. M. and Root A. W. *N. Engl. J. Med.* 1963, **268**, 1283, 1342, 1391.)

Agranulocytosis—susceptible to infections.

AIDS. See AIDS and anaesthesia. Lee K. G. and Soni N. *Anaesthesia* 1986, **41** 1011. (*See also* p. 396.)

Albers-Schonberg disease—brittle bones, risk of fractures while moving or positioning patient. Anaemia, splenomegaly. Heinrich Ernst Albers-Schonberg (1865–1921) Hamburg physician.

Albright–Butler syndrome—renal calculi with renal failure, acidosis, hypokalaemia. (Morris R. C. *N. Engl. J. Med.* 1969, **281**, 1405.)

Albright's osteodystrophy (pseudohypoparathyroidism)—ectopic calcification, hypocalcaemia, neuromuscular excitability, convulsions. F. Albright (1900–1969), Boston physician.

Alcoholism—resistance to anaesthetic, cirrhosis, cardiomyopathy, perioperative withdrawal crisis (delirium tremens), *see* p. 415.

Alport syndrome—conduction deafness and renal failure in adult life.

Alström syndrome—obese, deaf and blind by 7 years of age. Diabetes and renal failure in adult life. C. H. A. Alstrom (1903), Stockholm geneticist.

Amoebiasis—anaemia, dehydration, liver abscess with pulmonary complications.

Amyloidosis—unexpected cardiac or renal failure may occur. (Welch D. B. *Anaesthesia* 1982, **37**, 63).

Amyotonia congenita (Kugelberg–Welander disease, Werdnig–Hoffmann disease). Spinal muscular atrophy with anterior horn cell degeneration. Very sensitive to thiopentone, respiratory depressants and muscle relaxants. (Ellis F. R. *Br. J. Anaesth.* 1974, **46**, 605.)

Amyotrophic lateral sclerosis (motor neuron disease)—very sensitive to thiopentone, curare and respiratory depressants. Suxamethonium causes dangerous hyperkalaemia. (Rosenbaum K. J. et al. *Anesthesiology* 1971, **35**, 638.) *See* p. 421.

An-albuminaemia—sensitivity to protein-bound drugs, e.g. thiopentone curare, bupivacaine.

Andersen's disease (glycogen storage disease IV)—hypoglycaemia under anaesthesia. Dorothy H. A. Andersen (1901–1963), New York pathologist.

Anhidrotic ectodermal dysplasia (Christ–Siemens–Touraine syndrome)—difficult intubation, heat intolerance, recurrent chest infections. (Beahrs J. O. et al. *Ann. Intern. Med.* 1971, **74**, 92.)

Ankylosing spondylitis—difficult intubation sometimes. *See* p. 400.

Anorexia nervosa—hypothermia, hypotension, hypokalaemia, anaemia.

Apert's syndrome (craniosynostosis)—difficult intubation, raised intracranial pressure, other congenital defects, e.g. heart disease. (Andersson H. and Gomes S. P. *Acta Paediatr. Scand.* 1968, **57**, 47.) Eugene Apert (1868–1940), Paris paediatrician.

Arthrogryphosis (congenital contractures)—difficult veins, difficult airway, sensitive to thiopentone, associated congenital heart disease of 10% of patients. Possibility of malignant hyperpyrexia. (Baines D. B. et al. *Anaesth. Intensive Care* 1986, **14**, 370.)

Asbestosis—pulmonary fibrosis. May be on steroids, may have tuberculosis.

Asplenia syndrome—associated congenital heart disease with failure.

Ataxia-telangiectasia—immunoincompetence (IgA and IgE). Recurrent infections.

Atrial fibrillation (acute)—procainamide infusion has been recommended. (Fulham M. J. and Cookson W. O. C. *Anaesth. Intensive Care* 1984, **12**, 121.)

Atrial septal defect (ASD)—antibiotic cover is usual. Decreasing systemic vascular resistance decreases the shunt, as does IPPV.

Atrio ventricular block (1st degree)—there may be severe bradycardia during anaesthesia. (Hayward R. et al. *Anaesthesia* 1982, **37**, 1190.)

Auto-immune anaemias—may be on steroids. Respiration may be difficult to restart after IPPV.

Autonomic hyper-reflexia, see Hutchinson R. C. *Anaesthesia* 1986, **41**, 663.

Barlow's syndrome (click-murmur mitral valve prolapse)—bradycardia resistant to atropine, dysrhythmias responding to B blockade, and thromboembolism occur. Excessive tachycardia and anxiety should be avoided. Antibiotic cover is usual.

Beckwith syndrome (infantile gigantism)—macroglossia with airway problems, severe hypoglycaemia. (Filippi G. and McKusick V. A. *Medicine (Baltimore)* 1970, **49**, 279.)

Beri-beri—cardiomyopathy with failure, muscular weakness.

Berylliosis—pulmonary fibrosis. May be on steroids.

Blackfan–Diamond syndrome (congenital red-cell aplasia)—on steroids, thrombocytopenia, anaemia.

Bowen's syndrome (cerebrohepatorenal syndrome)—renal failure, hypoprothrombinaemia, sensitivity to muscle relaxants. J. T. Bowen (1857–1941) Boston dermatologist.

Bronchiolitis fibrosa obliterans—pulmonary fibrosis. May be on steroids.

Buerger's disease—bronchitis and emphysema, peripheral vascular insufficiency. Indirect arterial pressure measurements may be inaccurate.

Bullous cystic lung disease. (For suggested technique of anaesthesia *see* Normandale J. P. and Feneck R. O. *Anaesthesia* 1985, **40**, 1182.)

Burkitt's lymphoma—may be difficult to intubate. Denis P. B. Burkitt (1911–), of Dublin, London and Uganda.

Burns—hypovolaemia, lung burns, hyperkalaemia with suxamethonium, intubation problem sometimes, *see* p. 477.

Carcinoid syndrome—tricuspid valve malfunction, sudden bronchospasm, especially with cyclopropane and hypotension, *see* p. 424.

Cardiac tamponade—low cardiac output, high venous pressure, anaesthesia and IPPV may worsen the failure.

Carpenter's syndrome (cranial synostosis with small mandible, congenital heart disease)—intubation problems. (Andersson H. and Gomes S. P. *Acta Paediatr. Scand.* 1968, **57**, 47.) George C. Carpenter (1859–1910), London paediatrician.

Chagas disease (American trypanosomiasis)—hepatic failure, cardiomyopathy. (Barretto J. C. *Br. J. Anaesth.* 1979, **51**, 1189.) Carlos Chagas (1879–1934) Brazilian physician.

Chediak–Higashi syndrome (immunodeficiency, with some albinism)—recurrent infections, thrombocytopenia. May be on steroids. (Blume R. S. and Wolff S. M. *Medicine (Baltimore)*, 1972, **51**, 247.)

Cherubism—oral airway obstruction, intubation may be impossible, urgent tracheostomy may be required. Corrective surgery very haemorrhagic.

Choanal atresia—nasal obstruction.

Chotzen syndrome (craniosynostosis)— difficult intubation, sometimes renal failure. (Andersson H. and Gomes S. P. *Acta Paediatr. Scand.* 1968, **57**, 47.) F. C. Chotzen, Breslau psychiatrist.

Christmas disease, see p. 396.

Cleft palate—difficult intubation, respiratory obstruction with heavy sedative premedication, *see* p. 561.

Cockayne's syndrome (Cockayne E. A. *Arch. Dis. Child* 1936, **11**, 1)—an inherited autosomal recessive disorder with progressive mental and physical retardation, deafness, blindness, bony malformations etc. Intubation may be very difficult. (Cook S. *Anaesthesia* 1982, **37**, 1104.)

Congenital analgesia—sedation or general anaesthesia may be required and abnormal responses to drugs may be present. (Layman P. R. *Anaesthesia* 1986, **41**, 395.)

Congenital trophoblastic disease—patients have a low plasma cholinesterase level and elevated chorionic gonadotrophin. (Davies J. M. et al. *Anaesthesia* 1984, **12**, 1074.)

Conn's syndrome—hypertension, hypokalaemia, oedema. J. C. Conn (1907–), Ann Arbor internist. (*See also* p. 456.)

Conjoined twins (Siamese twins)—intubation difficulties sometimes, adrenal failure, one infant may exsanguinate the other at operation, multiple anaesthetics required. Slow gas induction due to wider distribution of the agents, *see* p. 563.

Conradi's syndrome (chondrodystrophy and mental deficiency)—renal and congenital heart disease sometimes.

Cretinism—intubation difficulties, sensitivity to anaesthetic drugs.

Creutzfeldt–Jacob disease—for anaesthesia *see* MacMurdo S. D. et al. *Anesthesiology* 1984, **60**, 590.

Cri-du-chat disease (microcephaly, micrognathia)— difficult airway, difficult intubation, associated congenital heart disease.

Crohn's disease—anaemia, toxaemia, hypoproteinaemia. May be on steroids. B. B. Crohn (1884–1983), New York physician.

Crouzon's disease (Craniosynostosis)—difficult intubation, postoperative respiratory obstruction. Corrective operations very haemorrhagic. (Andersson H. and Gomes S. P. *Acta Paediatr. Scand.* 1968, **57**, 47.)

Cushing's syndrome—diabetes, hypertension, hypokalaemia, sodium retention, obesity, thin skin. Harvey Cushing (1869–1939), Boston neurosurgeon.

Cutis laxa (elastic degeneration)—fragile skin, blood vessels, lung infections and emphysema common. Pendulous laryngeal and pharyngeal mucosa may obstruct breathing. (Wooley M. W. et al. *J. Pediatr. Surg.* 1967, **2**, 325.)

Cystic fibrosis—Atropine may inspissate secretions. (Lamberty J. M. and Rubin B. K. *Anaesthesia* 1985, **40**, 448.) Nasal polypectomy may be required and children withstand anaesthesia well. Due to exocrine gland dysfunction. May have chronic obstructive lung disease, airway obstruction, malnutrition and bleeding tendency. There is a risk of respiratory problems but careful management will usually avoid these.

Cystic hygroma—respiratory obstruction after induction, corrected by nasal airway, difficult intubation sometimes. (*See* p. 562.)

Dermatomyositis—mouth opening restricted, chest infections, anaemia, hypersensitivity to non-depolarizing relaxants (Eisele J. H. in: *Anesthesia for Uncommon Diseases* (Katz E. and Kadis M. ed.). Philadephia: Saunders, 1973.)

Diaphragmatic hernia—often an emergency, dyspnoea, hypoxia, acidosis, cardiac failure, pneumothorax, postoperative respiratory failure. (*See* p. 392.)

DiGeorge syndrome (immune deficiency, athymia)—chest infections, stridor, aortic arch obstruction with cardiac failure, hypoparathyroidism, tetany. Fresh donor blood is irradiated to prevent graft-versus-host reaction.

Disseminated sclerosis (multiple sclerosis)—deterioration may follow pyrexia, *see* p. 420.

Down's syndrome (Mongolism)—difficult to sedate, large tongue, small mouth, intubation and airway difficult. Risk of extubation stridor, especially after cardiac surgery. Associated congenital heart disease. Extubation laryngeal spasm may occur. The eye is sensitive to atropine but large doses of hyoscine may be required for hypersalivation. Asymptomatic atlanto-axial instability may be a problem so that radiological assessment of the cervical spine should be undertaken before operation. (Gallamnaugh S. C. *Br. Med. J.* 1985, **291**, 117.) *See* Chapter 28. J. Langdon Down (1826–1896), London physician.

Duchenne muscular dystrophy—muscular weakness with frequent cardiac involvement. Atropine, opiates and non-depolarizing relaxants may well be avoided. A volatile agent may give adequate relaxation. Has been associated with malignant hyperpyrexia. (Ellis F. R. *Br. J. Anaesth.* 1974, **46**, 605; Lintner S. P. K. and Thomas P. R. *Br. J. Anaesth.* 1982, **54**, 1331; Rosenberg H. Heiman-Patterson T. et al. *Anesthesiology* 1983, **59**, 362.) G. B. D. Duchenne (1806–1895), French neurologist. (*See* p. 421.)

Dysautonomia (Riley–Day syndrome) reduced autonomic stability, hypersalivation, regurgitation, poor temperature control, sensitive to respiratory depressants, IPPV usually required while anaesthetized, due to CO_2 insensitivity. Dopamine hydroxylase is deficient, hypersensitivity to dopamine and other adrenergic and cholinergic drugs. Reduced sensitivity to pain. (Meridy A. W. and Greighton R. E. *Can. Anaesth. Soc. J.* 1971, **18**, 563; Cox R. G. and Sumner E. *Anaesthesia* 1983, **38**, 293; Foster J. M. G. *Anaesthesia* **38**, 391; Stenquist O. and Sigurdsson J. *Anaesthesia* 1982, **37**, 929; Sweeney B. F., Jones S. et al. *Anaesthesia* 1985, **40**, 783.) Conrad M. Riley (1913–) Denver paediatrician; R. L. Day (1905–), Pittsburg physician. (*See* p. 564.)

Dystrophia myotonica—respiratory failure and infections, hypertonic muscles, cardiac involvement. Prolonged muscle spasm after suxamethonium, neostigmine and shivering. Hypersensitivity to respiratory depressants and non-depolarizing relaxants (which in some cases may *not* relax the myotonia). Associated with malignant hyperpyrexia. Regional and inhalation techniques are recommended. Prolonged apnoea may follow the injection of normal doses of thiopentone, *see* p. 419. Dystrophia in babies (*see* Bray R. J. and Inkster J. S. *Anaesthesia* 1984, **39**, 1007.)

Ebstein's abnormality (tricuspid valve disease)—supraventricular tachycardia during induction. W. E. Ebstein (1836–1912), Göttingen physician.

Edward's syndrome (trisomy 18)—congenital heart disease, micrognathia, renal failure.

Ehlers–Danlos syndrome (collagen abnormality)—fragile skin, veins, arteries and tracheal mucosa. Intubation may cause severe tracheal bruising. Spontaneous rupture of cerebral and other vessels, may be associated with aneurysms, spontaneous pneumothorax. (Wooley M. W. et al. *J. Ped. Surg.* 1967, **2**, 325.) (*See* p. 401.)

Eisenmenger's complex—vasoactive agents should not be administered unless specially indicated. (Bird T. M. and Strunin L. *Anaesthesia* 1984, **39**, 48; Lumley J. et al. *Anesth. Analg. (Cleve.)* 1977, **56**, 543; and Foster J. M. G. and Jones R. M. *Ann. R. Coll. Surg.* 1984, **66**, 153.)

Ellis–Van-Creveld disease (chondro-ectodermal dysplasia)—respiratory failure, congenital cardiac septal lesions.

Epidermolysis bullosa—skin and mucous membranes easily blistered with scarring. The no-touch technique is called for! May be on steroids; may be associated with porphyria. Sticky tape may damage skin. Ketamine has been recommended. (Fox W. T. *Lancet* 1979, **1**, 766; Kubota Y. et al. *Anesth. Analg. Curr. Res.* 1961, **40**, 244; Reddy A. R. R. and Wong D. H. W. *Can. Anaesth. Soc. J.* 1972, **19**, 536; Frost P. M. *Anaesthesia* 1980, **35**, 918; James I. G. and Wark R. *Anesthesiology* 1982, **56**, 323; Tomlinson A. A. *Anaesthesia* 1983, **38**, 495; James I. G. *Anaesthesia* 1983, **38**, 1106.)

Epilepsy—convulsions from perioperative drug withdrawal and enflurane. Loose teeth, *see* p. 418.

Erythema multiforme—post-intubation laryngeal oedema. (Cucchiara R. C. and Dawson B. *Anesthesiology* 1971, **35**, 537.)

Exomphalos and gastroschisis—post-correction respiratory failure.

Fabry's syndrome (lipidosis)—myocardial ischaemia in early adult life, renal failure.

Familial periodic paralysis—the hyperkalaemic type is associated with paralysis after general anaesthesia, especially thiopentone and relaxants. (Streeten D. J. in: *Metabolic Basis of Inherited Disease* (Stanbury J. B. ed.). New York: McGraw-Hill, 1972.) (For anaesthesia, *see* Fozard J. R. *Anaesthesia* 1983, **38**, 294.)

Fanconi syndrome (renal tubular acidosis)—acidosis, dehydration, hypokalaemia, renal failure. (Morris R. C. *N. Engl. J. Med.* 1969, **281**, 1405. Guido F. Fanconi (1903–), Zurich paediatrician.

Farber's disease (lipogranulomatosis)—cardiac and renal failure. Granulomas may exist in the larynx. (Gilbertson A. A. and Boulton T. B. *Anaesthesia* 1967, **22**, 607.)

Farmer's lung—pulmonary fibrosis. May be on steroids.

Fat embolism—respiratory failure. (*See* 'Adult respiratory distress syndrome', Chapters 8 and 38.)

Favism (glucose-6-phosphate-dehydrogenase deficiency)—anaemia; haemolysis may result from sulphonamides and aspirin. (Gilbertson A. A. and Boulton T. B. *Anaesthesia* 1967, **22**, 607.)

Felty's syndrome (a form of idiopathic thrombocytopenic purpura)—anaemia, neutropenia, infections. May be on steroids. Augustus R. Felty (1895–), US physician.

Fetal surgery—for anaesthesia, *see* Spielman F. J. et al. *Anaesthesia* 1984, **39**, 756.

Fibrodysplasia ossificans (myositis ossificans)—difficult to intubate; reduced thoracopulmonary compliance.

Fibrosing alveolitis (Hamman–Rich syndrome)—cyanosis, left heart failure. May be on steroids.

Friedreich's ataxia—myocardial degeneration with failure and dysrhythmias, respiratory failure, diabetes, and peripheral neuropathy. Cases may be treated like those with amyotrophic lateral sclerosis. Non-depolarizing relaxants, carefully monitored, especially atracurium can be used (Bell C. F. et al. *Anaesthesia* 1986, **41**, 296 and *see* Bird T. M. and Strunin L. *Anesthesiology* 1984, **60**, 377). An autosomal recessive inherited disease causing progressive ataxia and usually additional myopathy. For anaesthesia, *see also* Bell C. F., Kelly J. M. et al. *Anaesthesia* 1986, **41** 296. Nicolas Friedreich (1825–1882). Heidelberg physician.

Gardner's syndrome (multiple polyposis)—no specific difficulties.

Gargoylism—respiratory obstruction after induction, very difficult intubation, cardiomyopathy and valve lesions.

Gaucher's disease—thrombocytopenia, neutropenia, anaemia.

Gilbert's disease (Familial unconjugated hyperbilirubinaemia.)—jaundice (for which the anaesthetist may be blamed!) (*see* p. 343.) Nicholas A. Gilbert (1858–1927), Paris physician.

Glanzmann's disease (thrombasthenia)—abnormal haemorrhage, platelet infusion rarely effective. May be on steroids.

Glomus jugulare tumours—for anaesthesia, *see* Mather S. P. and Webster N. R. *Anaesthesia* 1986, **41**, 856; Braude B. M., Hockman R. et al. *Anaesthesia* 1986, **41**, 861.

Glucagonoma—for anaesthetic management of glucagonoma, *see* Nicoll J. M. V. and Catling S. J. *Anaesthesia* 1985, **40**, 152.

Glue-sniffing—unstable circulation due to grossly increased catecholamines.

Glycogenoses—Type I (Von Gierke's disease)—perioperative acidosis and hypoglycaemia. Diazoxide has been recommended. *Type II (Pompe's disease)*—heart failure and neuromuscular weakness, macroglossia. Rarely survive infancy (McFarlane H. J. and Soni N. *Anaesthesia* 1986, **41** 1219.). *Type III*—perioperative hypoglycaemia. *Type IV*—perioperative hypoglycaemia. *Type V (McArdle's disease)*—muscle weakness, cardiac failure. (*See* Cox J. M. *Anesthesiology* 1968, **29**, 1221.)

Goldenhar syndrome (oculoauriculovertebral syndrome)—difficult intubation and airway. Associated congenital heart disease; small mandible.

Golz–Gorlin syndrome (focal dermal hypoplasia)—difficult airway due to frequent facial asymmetry.

Goodpasture's syndrome—severe repeated intrapulmonary haemorrhage with fibrosis. Hypertension, anaemia, renal failure. May be on steroids. E. W. Goodpasture (1886–1960), Boston pathologist.

Gorlin syndrome (skeletal abnormalities with multiple naevi)—no specific problems.

Gout—dehydration, uricaemia may be worsened by methoxyflurane, ethanol and lactate.

Groenblad–Strandberg disease (pseudoxanthoma elasticum)—fragile blood vessels with frequent rupture and bruising and displacement of i.v. infusions.

Guillain–Barré disease (acute idiopathic polyneuritis)—may require IPPV in intensive care, circulation sometimes unstable due to autonomic dysfunction, usually self-limiting in up to 6 weeks. Suxamethonium may cause dangerous hyperkalaemia for up to 3 months after onset. (Smith R. B. *Can. Anaesth. Soc. J.* 1971, **18**, 199; Perel A. et al. *Anaesthesia* 1977, **32**, 257.) G. C. Guillain (1876–1961), Paris neurologist. J. A. Barré (1880–), Strasbourg neurologist.

Haemochromatosis and severe haemosiderosis—hepatic cirrhosis, diabetes and later cardiac failure.

Haemorrhagic telangiectasia (Rendu–Osler–Weber syndrome)—post-intubation laryngeal bruising and obstruction. Risk of epistaxis.

Haemophilia—see p. 395.

Hallermann–Streiff syndrome—difficult intubation, brittle teeth, hypoplastic nares.

Hallervorden–Spatz disease (Elejalde B. R. and de Elejalde M. M. J. *Clin. Genet.* 1979, **16**, 1.) A rare progressive disorder of the basal ganglia which occurs in late childhood and leads to death. The patients are demented and show various types of myotonia and muscular rigidity. Halothane induction and maintenance relieve the dystonic posturing which returns after operation, as with other basal ganglion disorders. (Roy R. C. et al. *Anesthesiology* 1983, **58**, 382.)

Hamman–Rich syndrome—acute diffuse interstitial lung fibrosis.

Hand–Schuller–Christian disease (histiocytic granulomata)—diabetes insipidus, hepatic failure, pancytopenia, respiratory failure, laryngeal involvement. May be on steroids. (Lieberman P. H. et al. *Medicine (Baltimore)* 1969 **48**, 375.)

Hare lip—see Cleft palate and see p. 561.

Henoch–Schönlein purpura—bruising tendency.

Hepatolenticular degeneration (Kinnier–Wilson disease)—defect in copper metabolism, hepatic failure, epilepsy, trismus, weakness.

Hermansky syndrome (thrombasthenia, albinism)—bruising, platelet infusion may be required.

Holt–Oram syndrome (hand–heart syndrome)—congenital heart disease. (Lewis M. et al. *JAMA* 1965, **193**, 1080.)

Homocystinuria—see p. 426.

Hunter syndrome (mucopolysaccharidosis II)—thoracic skeletal abnormalities with respiratory failure, cardiac failure, stiff joints, laryngeal and pharyngeal involvement with obstruction. (Gilbertson A. A. and Boulton T. B.

Anaesthesia 1967, **22**, 607.) C. H. Hunter (1872–1965), English paediatrician.

Huntington's chorea—see p. 420. G. H. Huntington (1850–1916), New York neurologist.

Hurler syndrome ((Gargoylism) mucopolysaccharidosis I)—as above and below, death before puberty from cardiac involvement. Difficult intubation, chest infections, heart failure. (Gilbertson A. A. and Boulton T. B. *Anaesthesia* 1967, **22**, 607.)

Hydatid disease—pulmonary, hepatic, cardiac, renal and cerebral cysts may cause local problems.

Hydrocephalus—if there is a ventriculo-atrial valve in place antibiotic cover is often advised before dental treatment. The large occiput may make intubation difficult so that the body should be raised on a pillow or mattress.

Hyperparathyroidism—may be associated with hypercalcaemia with danger of cardiac arrest. Risk temporarily diminished by potassium infusion. For anaesthesia *see* The experts opine. *Surv. Anesthesiol.* 1985, **29**, 72. *See also* p. 456.

Hyperpituitarism—see p. 422.

Hypokalaemic familial periodic paralysis—see p. 420.

Hypoparathyroidism (*see also* Albright's osteodystrophy)—hypersensitivity to sedatives and anaesthetics; hypocalcaemia with muscular weakness.

I cell disease (mucopolysaccharidosis VII)—hernias, thick secretions, airway obstruction.

Ichthyosis—a congenital condition in which there may be difficulty in fixing an extradural catheter to the skin, if adhesives are used. (Smart G. and Bradshaw E. G. *Anaesthesia* 1984, **39**, 161.)

Idiopathic myoglobinuria—see p. 395.

Idiopathic thrombocytopenic purpura—bruising, haemorrhage. Heparin and aspirin are avoided. May be on steroids. Platelet infusions for surgery, rebound thromboses after splenectomy.

Infective mononucleosis—airway obstruction due to enlarged tonsils may prove fatal. (Catling S. J. et al. *Anaesthesia* 1984, **39**, 699; Carrington P. and Hall J. I. *Br. Med. J.* 1986, **292**, 195.)

Insulinoma—for removal of, *see* Muir J. J. et al. *Anesthesiology* 1983, **59**, 371. *See* p. 449.

Jaw, congenital fusion of in a neonate—Seraj M. A. et al. *Anaesthesia* 1984, **39**, 695.

Jervell–Lange–Nielsen syndrome—deafness with cardiac dysrhythmias, long Q–T interval and enlarged T wave. Risk of cardiac arrest. Pacemaker insertion may help. (Jarvell A. et al. *Am. Heart J.* 1957, **54**, 59.) For anaesthesia, *see* Medak R. and Benumof J. L. *Br. J. Anaesth.* 1983, **55**, 361; Freshwater J. V. *Br. J. Anaesth.* 1984, **56**, 655.

Jehovah's Witnesses—blood transfusion refused. For anaesthesia, *see* Clarke J. F. M. *Br. J. Hosp. Med.* 1982, **27**, 487; Wickham N. W. R. and Hardy R. N. *Hosp. Update* 1982, **8**, 1433; Harris T. J. B. et al. *Anaesthesia* 1983, **38**, 989 and in heart surgery, Henderson A. M., Maryniak J. K. et al. *Anaesthesia* 1986, **41**, 748.

Kaposi's sarcoma—pigmented sarcoma of the skin (M. K. Kaposi (1837–1902), Austrian dermatologist.) May be associated with AIDS.

Kartagener's syndrome—dextrocardia, sinusitis, bronchiectasis (due to defective ciliary function), immunoincompetence. (Miller R. D. et al. *Chest* 1972, **62**, 130.)

Kasabach–Merritt syndrome—rarely survive more than a few weeks from birth, enlarging haemangioma with haemorrhage and thrombocytopenia. May be on steroids.

Kearns–Sayer syndrome—the reaction to muscle relaxants is normal, but complete and sudden heart block may develop during anaesthesia. (D'Ambra M. N. et al. *Anesthesiology* 1979, **51**, 343.)

Kelly–Paterson syndrome (Plummer–Vinson syndrome, sideropenic dysphagia)—in the very advanced case, regurgitation on induction.

Klinefelter syndrome—crush fractures of osteoporotic vertebrae. H. K. Klinefelter (1912–), Baltimore physician.

Klippel–Feil syndrome (congenital fusion of cervical vertebrae)—difficult intubation; other congenital abnormalities may coexist (Katz J. and Kaddis E. B. *Anesthesia and Uncommon Diseases*. Philadelphia: Saunders, 1973.) (Klippel M. and Feil A. *Soc. Anat. Paris Bull. et Memb.* 1912, **14**, 185.) For anaesthesia *see* Naguib M. et al. *Canad. Anaesth. Soc. J.* 1986, **33**, 60.

Klippel–Trenaunay syndrome (angio-osteohypertrophy)—high output failure, thrombocytopenia, cleft palate, short wide neck and inability to extend neck.

Kwashiorkor—difficult to intubate due to pterygoid fibrosis. Low serum electrolytes and serum cholinesterase.

Larsen's syndrome (multiple joint dislocations)—difficult intubation, pulmonary infections. (Wooley M. W. et al. *J. Ped. Surg.* 1967, **2**, 325.)

Laryngotracheo-oesophageal cleft—*see* Armitage E. N. *Anaesthesia* 1984, **39**, 706.

Laurence–Moon–Biedl syndrome—obesity, polydactyly, mental retardation; associated congenital heart disease, renal failure.

Leber's disease—congenital optic atrophy. There may be idiopathic hypoventilation with sensitivity to diazepam and mild analgesics. *See* Hunter A. R. *Anaesthesia* 1984, **39**, 781.

Leopard syndrome—multiple leopard skin spots, hypertelorism, severe pulmonary stenosis. (*Scott. Med. J.* 1983, **28**, 300.)

Leprechaunism—abnormal endocrine state, mentally defective; hyperinsulinism, hypoglycaemia, renal failure.

Leprosy—leprosy patients are often on steroids. Some parts of the body may be analgesic.

Lesch–Nyhan syndrome (hyperuricaemia)—renal failure before puberty.

Letterer–Siwe disease (histiocytosis)—as for leukaemia; gingivitis with very loose teeth.

Leukaemia—anaemia, thrombocytopenia, veins may be difficult. May be on steroids.

Lipodystrophy—liver failure, renal failure, diabetes.

Lowe syndrome (oculocerebrorenal syndrome)—renal failure, hypocalcaemia, acidosis.

McArdle's disease—glycogenosis V, a hereditary myopathy causing glycogen to accumulate in muscle. Atracurium appears to be a safe agent for the production of muscle relaxation in short procedures (Rajah A. and Bell C. F. *Anaesthesia* 1986, **41**, 93.)

Macroglossia, Acute—Holmes W. and Ball I. M. *To-day's Anaesthetist* 1986, **No. 2**, 26.

Mafucci syndrome (enchondromas and haemangiomas)—anaemia, sensitivity to vasodilator drugs, fragile bones, labile blood pressure.

Mandibulofacial dysostosis (Treacher–Collins syndrome)—micrognathia, difficult intubation. Coexistent congenital heart disease sometimes. Tracheal ventilation via a 16 G needle has proved useful. (Smith R. B. et al. *Br. J. Anaesth*. 1974, **46**, 313; Collins E. and Treacher J. *Trans. Ophthal. Soc. UK*. 1900, **20**, 190.)

Maple syrup urine disease (branched-chain ketonuria with neuropathy)—a metabolic disease of children involving an accumulation of keto-acids and amino-acids in the blood and urine, with abnormalities of blood sugar. *See* Delaney A. and Gal T. J. *Anesthesiology* 1976, **44**, 83.

Marchiafava–Michaeli syndrome (auto-immune haemolytic anaemia with paroxysmal nocturnal dyspnoea)—venous thromboembolism. May be on steroids.

Marfan's syndrome (arachnodactyly, congenital connective tissue disorder)—emphysema, cataracts, high arched palate, pneumothorax, coronary thrombosis, dissecting aneurysms, easily dislocated joints, aortic and mitral regurgitation, kyphoscoliosis. (Wooley M. W. et al. *J. Ped. Surg*. 1967, **2**, 325.) Young patients with this syndrome are a high anaesthetic risk group (Verghese C. *Anaesthesia* 1984, **39**, 917). *See also* Annotation, *Br. Med. J*. 1982, **285**, 464. B. J. A. Marfan (1858–1943), Paris paediatrician— (1896).

Maroteaux–Lamy syndrome mucopolysaccharidosis IV)—cardiac failure, respiratory failure, anaemia, thrombocytopenia. (Gilbertson A. A. and Boulton T. B. *Anaesthesia* 1967, **22**, 607.)

Meckel's syndrome (microcephaly, micrognathia, congenital cardiac disease) —difficult intubation, renal failure. J. F. Meckel (1781–1833), anatomist from Halle.

Meig's syndrome (ovarian cyst with embarrassing pleural effusion)—the effusion may be tapped before anaesthesia. J. V. Meig (1892–1963), Boston gynaecologist.

Methaemoglobinaemia—made worse by prilocaine (*see* p. 395.)

Mikulicz's syndrome (salivary and lachrymal gland enlargement)—difficult airway and intubation sometimes, due to glandular enlargement. It has been suggested that atropine and hyoscine are best avoided. J. von Mikulicz-Radecki (1850–1905), Breslau surgeon.

Moebius' syndrome—a rare congenital abnormality of the cranial nerves. For anaesthetic problems *see* Krajcirik W. J. et al. *Anesth. Analg. (Cleve.)* 1985, **64**, 371.

Mongolism—see Down's syndrome.

Morquio's syndrome (mucopolysaccharidosis IV)—kyphoscoliotic dwarfs with atlanto-axial instability. Respiratory and cardiac failure by early adult life. Aortic incompetence. (Gilbertson A. A. and Boulton T. B. *Anaesthesia* 1967, **22**, 607; Birkinshaw K. J. *Anaesthesia* 1975, **30**, 46.)

Moschkowitz disease (a form of thrombocytopenic purpura)—renal damage. May be on steroids.

Motor neuron disease—hypersensitivity to all muscle relaxants. Laryngeal incompetence. Lung cancer may be present. *See also* p. 421 and Amyotrophic lateral sclerosis.

Moya-moya disease—a rare abnormality of the cerebral circulation with narrowing or occlusion of the anterior and middle cerebral arteries, first described in Japan in 1961. For anaesthesia *see* Bingham R. M. and Wilkinson D. J. *Anaesthesia* 1985, **40**, 1198.

Mucopolysaccharidosis—a hereditary connective-tissue disorder with deposition of abnormal amounts of mucopolysaccharides in body tissues. May be difficulties with airways and intubation because of secretions. Preoperative tracheostomy may occasionally be required. Other problems—very slow recovery; with breath holding, bronchospasm and frequent cyanosis, postoperative dehydration and chest infection. A light premedication with oral diazepam and glycopyrronium, and antibiotics for those with valvular lesions has been described. (Baines D. and Keneally J. P. *Anaesth. Intensive Care* 1983, **11**, 198; Kempthorne P. M. and Brown T. C. K. *Anaesth. Intensive Care* 1983, **11**, 203; King D. H. et al. *Anaesthesia* 1984, **39**, 126; Brown T. C. K. *Anaesth. Intensive Care* 1984, **12**, 178.)

Multiple myelomatosis—pathological fractures, especially of vertebrae, care needed in positioning, hypercalcaemia, anaemia, hyperviscosity, renal failure, coagulopathies.

Multiple sclerosis—see p. 420.

Muscular dystrophy—weak flaccid skeletal and eventually cardiac muscles. Sensitivity to atropine, opiates and non-depolarizing relaxants, may not reverse after anticholinesterase drugs. May be confined to ocular muscles (Robertson, J. A. *Anaesthesia* 1984, **39**, 251). May be associated with malignant hyperpyrexia. (Ellis F. R. *Br. J. Anaesth.* 1974, **46**, 605.)

Myasthenia gravis and myasthenia congenita—see p. 397 (Dalal F. Y. *Anaesthesia* 1972, **27**, 61.)

Myositis ossificans—difficult intubation sometimes. In severe cases, reduction of thoracic compliance with respiratory failure.

Myotonia congenita (Thomsen's disease)—*see* Dystrophia myotonica. (Ravin M. et al. *Anaesth. Analg.* 1975, **54**, 216.) A. J. T. Thomsen (1815–1896), Danish physician.

Neurofibromatosis—fibromas may occur in larynx or heart, excessive response to relaxants, rarely associated with phaeochromocytomas. (*See* von Recklinghausen's disease.) F. D. von Recklinghausen (1833–1910), German pathologist.

Neuromuscular syndromes (associated with malignant disease). (Croft P. *Br. J. Hosp. Med.* 1977, **17**, 356.)

Niemann–Pick disease (sphingomyelin infiltration, xanthomatosis)—anaemia, thrombocytopenia, respiratory failure.

Noack's syndrome (craniosynostosis)—sometimes difficult to intubate (Andersson H. and Gomes S. P. *Acta Paediatr. Scand.* 1968, **57**, 47.)

Noonan syndrome (micrognathia, heart disease, renal failure)—congenital cardiac lesion problems.

Opitz Frias syndrome—the hypospadias dysphagia syndrome; the G syndrome. Rare congenital condition with genital and craniofacial abnormalities. (Opitz J. M. et al. *Birth Defects* 1969, **5**, 95.) For anaesthesia *see* Bolsin S. N. and Gillbe C. *Anaesthesia* 1985, **30**, 1189.

Osler–Weber–Rendu syndrome—see Haemorrhagic telangiectasia. W. Osler (1849–1919), physician, Baltimore and Oxford; F. Parkes Weber (1863–1962), London physician; H. J. Rendu (1844–1902), French physician.

Osteogenesis imperfecta (fragilitas ossium)—fragile bones, teeth easily damaged, excessive haemorrhage during surgery. (Robinson C. and Wright D. J. *To-day's Anaesthetist* 1986, **1**,*No. 2*, 22; Cunningham A. J. et al. *Anesthesiology* 1984, **61**, 91.)

Pancreatitis—severe toxaemia and shock, hypocalcaemia, relaxant reversal difficulties.

Paraplegia—autonomic instability, liability to bed-sores. Hyperkalaemia may follow suxamethonium *see* p. 419.

Patau syndrome (trisomy 13)—micrognathia, difficult to intubate, congenital heart disease.

Pellagra—neuropathy and difficult intubation.

Pemphigus vulgaris—for anaesthesia in an acutely traumatized patient, *see* Vatashshy E. and Aronson H. B. *Anaesthesia* 1982, **37**, 1193.

Pharyngeal pouch—regurgitation of contents, not controlled by cricoid pressure.

Phenylketonuria—sensitivity to opioids and barbiturates, so inhalation induction is recommended. Epileptic fits, hypoglycaemia.

Pierre Robin syndrome—*see* p. 564.

Plummer–Vinson syndrome—*see* Kelly–Paterson syndrome. H. S. Plummer (1874–1936), Mayo Clinic physician; P. P. Vinson (1890–1959), US surgeon.

Pneumatosis cystoides intestinalis—nitrous oxide is contraindicated. *See* Sutton D. N. and Ooskitt K. R. *Anaesthesia* 1984, **39**, 776.

Pneumoconiosis—pulmonary fibrosis and emphysema, excessive sputum, reduced compliance, cyanosis. May be on steroids.

Polyarteritis nodosa—*see* p. 403.

Polycystic kidneys—renal failure, pulmonary cysts may coexist with danger of pneumothorax; 1 in 7 have cerebral aneurysms. Polycystic liver may coexist.

Polycythaemia—*see* p. 394.

Polymyositis—*see* dermatomyositis.

Polysplenia—associated congenital heart disease.

Pompe's disease—*see* Glycogenoses

Porphyrias—paralytic crises precipitated by barbiturates, hydroxydione, diazepoxide, anticonvulsants, nikethamide and other non-anaesthetic drugs *see* p. 401.

Potter's syndrome (Potter E. L. *Am. J. Obstet. Gynecol.* 1946, **51**, 855 and 559; Potter E. L. *Obstet. Gynecol.* 1965, **25**, 3.)—oligohydramnios in the mother and renal agenesis, typical facies and pulmonary hypoplasia in the baby. In spite of intubation, ventilation may be impossible (Van der Weyden, *Anaesth. Intensive Care* 1982, **10**, 90).

Prader–Willi syndrome—(after the neonatal phase) extreme obesity, polyphagia, dental caries. Blood glucose should be maintained during fasting. (Dunn H. G. *Acta Paediatr. Scand.* 1968, Suppl. 186; Attlee J. L. *Anesthesiology* 1976, **44**, 161; Mayhew J. F. and Taylor B. *Canad. Anaesth. Soc. J.* 1983, **30**, 565; Yamashita M. et al. *Canad. Anaesth. Soc. J.* 1983, **30**, 179.) A. P. Prader, H. Willi (1900–71), Zurich paediatricians. (*See* p. 564.)

Progeria (premature ageing)—myocardial ischaemia, hypertension, cardiomegaly.

Progressive external ophthalmoplegia (PEO)—all induction agents used intravenously should be given slowly and in small dosage (James R. H. *Anaesthesia* 1986, **41**, 216).

Progressive muscular dystrophy—*see* p. 439.

Prolonged Q–T syndrome—an inherited condition causing attacks of dysrhythmia leading to syncope. Should be treated with β-blockers. *See* O'Callaghan A. C. et al. *Anaesth. Intensive Care* 1982, **10**, 50.

Prune belly syndrome (pseudoxanthoma elasticum), (congenital absence of abdominal muscles)—inability to cough causes postoperative respiratory problems. (Hannington Kiff J. G. *Br. J. Anaesth.* 1970, **42**, 649; Karamanian

A. et al. *Br. J. Anaesth.* 1974, **46**, 897; Krechel S. L. W. *Anesth. Anal.* 1981, **60**, 344; Henderson A. M. et al. *Anaesthesia* 1987, **42**, 54.)

Pulmonary cysts—increase in size with possible rupture during anaesthesia.

Pulmonary hypertension (primary)—for extradural analgesia in, *see* Davies M. J. and Beavis R. *Anaesth. Intensive Care* 1984, **12**, 165.

Reiger's syndrome—as for Dystrophia myotonica.

Rheumatoid arthritis and Still's disease—difficult intubation, difficult veins, poor spontaneous respiration. May be on steroids. *see* pp. 399 and 442.

Rickets—kyphoscoliotic respiratory limitation, difficult spinal analgesia, hypocalcaemia.

Riley–Day syndrome—*see* Dysautonomia.

Romano–Ward syndrome (Romano C. et al. *Clin. Pediatr.* 1963, **45**, 656 and Ward O. C. *J. Irish Med. Assoc.* 1964, **54**, 103)—congenital delay of depolarization and recovery of the Q–T interval. May cause sudden death at any age during induction of anaesthesia; *see* Ponte J. and Lund J. *Br. J. Anaesth.* 1981, **53**, 1347.

Rubinstein syndrome (microcephaly, chronic lung disease)—associated congenital heart disease.

San Filippo syndrome (mucopolysaccharidosis III)—no specific problems. (Gilbertson A. A. and Boulton T. B. *Anaesthesia* 1967, **22**, 607.)

Sarcoidosis—pumonary and laryngeal fibrosis, cardiac failure, dysrhythmias, hypercalcaemia. May be on steroids.

Scleroderma (diffuse thickening of skin, fibrosis leading to muscle degeneration in the diaphragm which may contribute to respiratory problems. Blood pressure is difficult to measure, poor lung compliance)—difficult intubation due to restricted mouth opening, difficult veins, regurgitation, respiratory failure, hypovolaemia, hypotension, renal failure, prolonged action of local analgesics in the peripheries. May be on steroids. (Birkhan J. et al. *Anaesthesia* 1972, **27**, 89; Sweeney B. *Anaesthesia* 1984, **39**, 1145; Iliffe G. D. and Pettigrew N. M. *Br. Med. J.* 1985, **286**, 337.)

Scurvy—anaemia, bruising, loose teeth.

Sheie disease (mucopolysaccharidosis V)—hernias, joint stiffness, aortic incompetence in adult life.

Shy–Drager syndrome (Shy G. M. and Drager G. A. *Arch. Neurol.* 1960, **2**, 511; King D. H. et al. *Br. J. Anaesth.* 1984, **39**, 126.) (central nervous and autonomic degeneration)—highly labile blood pressure, ephedrine suitable for hypotensive crises. It has been suggested that methoxyflurane, cyclopropane and ether be avoided (Cohen C. A. *Anesthesiology*, 1971, **35**, 95; Simpson E. W. *Anaesthesia* 1980, **35**, 1020. For anaesthesia, *see* Hutchinson R. C. and Sugden J. C. *Anaesthesia* 1984, **39**, 1229.)

Siamese twins—*see* Conjoined twins.

Sick sinus syndrome (Reid D. S. *Br. J. Hosp. Med.* 1984, **31**, 341). *See also* p. 409.

Simmonds' syndrome and Sheehan's syndrome (post-partum pituitary necrosis)—as for Addison's disease. *See* p. 423 M. S. Simmonds (1855–1925), Hamburg pathologist; Sheehan H. L. (1900–), British pathologist.

Sickle-cell disease—*see* p. 392.

Silver syndrome (dwarfism, micrognathia)—difficult intubation sometimes.

Sipple syndrome (multiple endocrine adenomatosis)—as for phaeochromocytoma (*see* p. 456.)

Sjogren's syndrome (keratoconjunctivitis sicca)—worsened by atropine and hyoscine, improved by humidification. H. S. Sjogren (1899–), Stockholm ophthalmologist.

Smith–Lemli–Opitz syndrome (micrognathia, mentally defective, hypoplasia of thymus)—difficult intubation, infection problems.

Spinal muscular atrophy (Seddon S. J. *Anaesthesia* 1985, **40**, 821.)

Stevens–Johnson syndrome—*see* Erythema multiforme. A. M. Stevens (1844–1945), US paediatrician; F. C. Johnson (1897–1934), US paediatrician.

Stickler's syndrome—(progressive arthro-ophthalmopathy)—progressive myopia, retinal detachment, secondary glaucoma, pain and stiffness of joints, kyphosis, maxillary hypoplasia, deafness, possible intubation problems. (*See* Stickler G. B. et al. *Proc. Mayo Clin.* 1965, **40**, 433; Stickler G. B. and Pugh D. G. *Proc. Mayo. Clin.* 167, **42**, 495.)

Still's disease (juvenile chronic polyarthritis)—Airway maintenance may be difficult because of limited movement of the jaws and of the cervical spine. Atlanto-axial subluxation due to erosion of the odontoid process may be present. Blind nasal intubation, or the use of the fibreoptic laryngoscope may be necessary. (Smith B. L. Abstr. 8th World Congress, Manila, 1984, **2**, A 114 and D'Arcy J. et al. 1976, *Anaesthesia* **31**, 624.) G. F. Still (1868–1941), London paediatrician. Ketamine is a useful drug here.

Sturge–Weber syndrome (cavernous angioma of face with intracranial involvement)—epilepsy and hemiparesis may occur. W. A. Sturge (1850–1919), F. Parkes Weber (1863–1962), English physicians.

Syringomyelia—occasional respiratory failure.

Systemic lupus erythematosus—anaemia, bruising, renal and respiratory failure, nasal skin involvement. May be on steroids.

Takayasu's disease (ITA)—*see* Thorburn J. R. and James M. F. M. *Anaesthesia* 1986, **41**, 734.

Tangier disease (analphalipoproteinaemia)—sensitivity to muscule relaxants, ischaemic heart disease, anaemia, thrombocytopenia.

Thalassaemia—haemolytic anaemia, intubation difficulties have been described. Homozygous form fetal Hb, heterozygous forms HbC, HbE, HbS with sickling problems (*see* p. 394.)

Total body irradiation—in children, with high dosage, *see* Lo J. N. and Buckley J. J. *Anesthesiology* 1984, **61**, 101.

Tourette syndrome—for anaesthetic implications *see* Morrison J. E. and Lockhart C. H. *Anesth. Analg. (Cleve.)* 1986, **65**, 200.

Tracheo-oesophageal fistula—milk aspiration into lungs, stomach full of air, causing respiratory embarrassment. IPPV difficult with low fistula. For anaesthesia in adults, *see* Chan C. S. *Anaesthesia*, 1984, **39**, 158. (*See* p. 561.)

Treacher Collins syndrome—*see* Mandibulofacial dysostosis. E. Treacher Collins, British ophthalmologist. (*See* Chapter 28.)

Tricuspid incompetence—antibiotic cover is usual. Afterload reduction and preload increases have proved helpful. (Stone J. G. et al. *Anesth. Analg. (Cleve.)* 1980, **59**, 737.)

Trisomy 13—*see* Patau syndrome.

Trisomy 18—*see* Edwards' syndrome.

Trisomy 22—severe hypoglycaemia during perioperative starvation.

Tuberous sclerosis—renal failure, cardiac dysrhythmias, lung cysts, which may rupture.

Turner's syndrome (XO chromosome with micrognathia, congenital heart disease and renal anomalies)—difficult intubation, prolonged effects from renally excreted drugs. (Strader E. A. et al. *J. Pediatr.* 1971, **79**, 473.)

Urbach–Wiethe disease (mucocutaneous hyalinosis)—difficult intubation.

Von Gierke's disease (glycogen storage problems with hepatic and renal failure)—severe perioperative starvation, hypoglycaemia and acidosis. (Cox J. M. *Anesthesiology* 1968, **29**, 1221.)

Ventricular septal defect (VSD)—'the louder the murmur, the smaller the defect'. Antibiotic cover is usual. Mild reduction of systemic vascular resistance is desirable. Hypovolaemia is to be avoided.

Von Hippel–Lindau syndrome (haemangioblastomas)—associated with phaeochromocytoma; hepatic and renal failure. (Steiner A. C. et al. *Medicine* 1968, **47**, 371.)

Von Recklinghausen's disease (neurofibromatosis)—may have fibromas of larynx and heart; may have phaeochromocytoma, kyphoscoliosis, multiple lung cysts and renal failure. There is an excessive response, sometimes, to non-depolarizing relaxants and suxamethonium. (Manser J. *Br. J. Anaesth.* 1970, **42**, 183; Brasfield R. D. and Das Gupta T. R. *Ann. Surg.* 1972, **175**, 86; Baraka A. *Br. J. Anaesth.* 1974, **46**, 701; Fisher M. M. *Anaesthesia* 1975, **30**, 648; Van Aken H. et al. *Anaesthesia* 1982, **37**, 827.)

Von Willebrand's disease (pseudohaemophilia)—defective platelet adhesiveness with Factor VIII deficiency. Controlled by tranexamic acid, 1 g, and desmopressin (DDAVP), 24 µg, given slowly, i.v., 1 h before operation, 4 h after operation, and 24 h after operation. Tranexamic acid is then continued, 1 g orally, 8-hourly, for a week. Cryoprecipitate is considered if this treatment fails to correct coagulopathy. Salicylates are avoided. E. A. von Willebrand (1870–1949), physician, Finland.

Weaver's syndrome—rare developmental condition with unusual craniofacial appearance and other abnormalities which may cause airway problems. (Weaver D. D. et al. *J. Pediatr.* 1974, **84**, 547.) *See* Turner D. R. and Downing J. W. *Br. J. Anaesth.* 1985, **57**, 1260.

Weber–Christian disease (global fat necrosis)—adrenal failure, occasional constrictive pericarditis. Subcutaneous fat is carefully protected at operation. (Spirak J. L. et al. *Johns Hopkins Med. J.* 1970, **126**, 344.)

Wegener's granuloma (ulceration of midline structures of face)—possible airway involvement causes difficulties, also renal failure. May be on steroids. F. Wegener (1907–), Berlin pathologist.

Welander's muscular atrophy (peripheral muscular atrophy)—very sensitive to thiopentone, relaxants and opiates. (Ellis F. R. *Br. J. Anaesth.* 1974, **46**, 605.)

Werdnig–Hoffman disease (infantile muscular atrophy)—respiratory failure, worsened by relaxants and opioids. (Ellis F. R. *Br. J. Anaesth.* 1974, **46**, 605.) G. W. Werdnig, Graz neurologist; J. Hoffman (1857–1919), Heidelberg neurologist.

Werner syndrome (type I endocrine adenomatosis)—renal failure, severe hypoglycaemia, bronchial carcinoid tumours, hypercalcaemia. (Werner P. *Am. J. Med.* 1963, **35**, 205.)

Werner syndrome (premature ageing) (cf. Hutchinson Gilford syndrome—progeria)—myocardial ischaemia, diabetes. (McKusick V. A. *Heritable Disorders of Connective Tissue*, 4th ed. St. Louis: C. V. Mosby Co., 1972.)

Wilson's disease (hepatolenticular degeneration from copper deposits)—hepatic and renal failure. (Gilbertson A. A. and Boulton T. B. *Anaesthesia* 1967,

22, 607.) S. A. Kinnear Wilson (1877–1937), London neurologist.

Wolff–Parkinson–White syndrome—ECG shows prolonged QRS and short P–R interval due to various cardiac disorders; worsened by neostigmine. Tachycardia produces S–T depression, so hyoscine preferred to atropine for premedication. Paroxysmal supraventricular tachycardia may accompany induction. Termination of paroxysmal supraventricular tachycardia with phenylephrine (Jacobson L. et al. *Anaesthesia* 1985, **40**, 657). Gallamine should be avoided. (Starre P. J. A. *Anesthesiology* 1978, **48**, 369.) L. W. Wolff; J. P. Parkinson; Paul Dudley White, US cardiologists.

(*See also* Morton L. T. *A Medical Bibliography*, 3rd ed. London: Deutsch, 1970; Magalini S. I. *Dictionary of Medical Syndromes*. Philadelphia: Lippincott, 1971; Jones A. E. P. and Pelton D. A. *Can. Anaesth. Soc. J.* 1976, **23**, 207; Stoetling P. *Anesthesia and Coexisting Disease*. Philadelphia: Saunders, 1982.)

Chapter 24　　**SURGICAL OPERATIONS AND CHOICE OF ANAESTHETIC**

Abdominal and General Surgery

History

The abdomen was seldom opened before the 1880s; McBurney did an appendicectomy in New York in 1898, Billroth performed a partial gastrectomy in Vienna in 1881; Dean sutured a perforated duodenal ulcer in 1894 at the London Hospital, Lawson Tait did a cholecystectomy in Birmingham in 1879, Conrad Ramstedt did a pyloromyotomy in Münster in 1911 and Dragstedt performed a vagotomy in 1943 in Chicago. Reginald Fitz (1843–1913) described the surgical treatment of acute appendicitis in Boston in 1886.

Requirements for General Anaesthesia

1. Unconsciousness (unless regional analgesia is employed), with complete absence of awareness.

2. Prevention of gastric contents entering the glottis.

3. Suppression of reflex responses to surgical stimuli.

4. Good relaxation of the anterior abdominal wall.

5. Reasonably rapid return of consciousness and of the upper respiratory tract reflexes.

(For Vomiting and Regurgitation; Prevention and Treatment, *see* Chapter 18. For Management of the Acid Aspiration Syndrome, *see* Chapter 27.)

Pharmacology

Halothane increases the blood supply of the gut, and hypocapnia due to hyperventilation reduces it. Morphine increases the tone of the bowel especially in diverticular disease. Diazepam inhibits the tone of the gut and may even cause ileus. β-blockers may decrease the lumen of the bowel. Metoclopramide increases the tone of the small bowel, an action opposed by atropine.

Pretreatment by glycopyrronium may enable neostigmine to be given without causing too much bowel constriction,[1] but this has been contradicted.[2] The use of opioid drugs does not appear to interfere with the radiological interpretation of operative cholangiography, nor to increase spasm of the sphincter of Oddi.[3]

Central neural blockade increases blood flow in the colon.

Outline of the Authors' Technique of General Anaesthesia for Abdominal Surgery

1. Intravenous induction, using 2·5% thiopentone or alternative agent.

2. Injection of a non-depolarizing relaxant in a dose sufficient to allow easy intubation, giving time for maximal neuromuscular block to occur (3 min), during which the lungs are gently inflated with a nitrous-oxide–oxygen mixture (if there is a risk of vomiting or regurgitation and consequent aspiration of stomach contents, suxamethonium may be preferred, to allow more rapid intubation).

3. Tracheal intubation after optional spraying of the larynx with no more than 3 ml of 4% lignocaine solution, followed by careful inflation of the tracheal cuff.

4. Maintenance with a nitrous-oxide–oxygen mixture and IPPV, supplemented with either a narcotic analgesic drug, or minimal concentrations of a volatile agent, to ensure complete unconsciousness. Additional doses of the non-depolarizing relaxant may be given as required, such doses being monitored by clinical response or a nerve stimulator.

5. At the termination of the operation, an anticholinesterase is injected to overcome neuromuscular block, preceded by atropine or glycopyrronium to counteract its muscarine-like effects. The nerve stimulator may be used to gauge the adequacy of reversal.

6. When spontaneous respiration is established, tracheobronchial suction and oesophageal toilet, deflation of the cuff and removal of the tracheal tube can be effected. The patient is then transferred to his bed to receive oxygen by catheter or mask. He will normally be turned on to his side to facilitate nursing.

7. Monitoring throughout the perioperative period may include arterial blood pressure, ECG, capnography, temperature, oximetry, etc.

Capnography may show that the end-expiratory P_{CO_2} after a long operation under hyperventilation at 10 litres/min can be as low as 3·5 kPa and the addition of 5% CO_2 to the gas mixture at the end of the operation will raise this back to normal and will help to restore normal breathing.[4]

Alternative Techniques

These include:

1. Use of volatile agent as the main drug to provide anaesthesia and relaxation of the abdominal wall, e.g. halothane, enflurane, isoflurane, ether, or cyclopropane; small doses of a relaxant in a subsidiary role.

2. Regional block with or without general anaesthesia to provide unconsciousness, e.g. extra- or intradural, abdominal field block.

3. Muscle relaxant drugs may be given by infusion.

4. Neurolept anaesthesia with muscle relaxant drugs and IPPV, avoiding awareness.

Hiccup is a troublesome reflex, too often associated with present-day methods of light anaesthesia. Its exact cause is ill understood, but it is likely to be associated with a high nervous tone, and light anaesthesia. The best method of prevention and treatment is the use of *adequate* amounts of a relaxant drug. It may also yield to: (1) Increase in analgesia, e.g. by injection of a narcotic analgesic drug; (2)

Inhalation of concentrated ether vapour for a few breaths; (3) Increased depth of general anaesthesia; (4) Block of vagus nerves near cardia. This also has prophylactic value; (5) Intravenous injection of methyl phenidate (Ritalin), 20 mg or metoclopramide;[5] (6) Intravenous ephedrine, 5 mg perhaps repeated once;[6] (7) Instillation into the nose of 5 ml of ice-cold water.[7]

Preparation for Emergency Operations
Fluid and electrolyte balance must be corrected when possible.

The problem of regurgitation and vomiting is not confined to obstetrical and emergency abdominal operations, and if there is suspicion that the stomach is not empty a nasogastric tube (6–12 gauge, 4–7 mm diameter) should be passed through the nose[8] or an oesophageal tube (gauge 12) passed through either the nose or mouth (*see* Chapters 18 and 27). The stomach should then be aspirated with the patient supine and on each side in turn. When there is retroperistalsis, e.g., in acute intestinal obstruction, the stomach may refill from the duodenum between the time of emptying and the introduction of the tracheal tube with the risk of the inhalation of intestinal contents (*see also* Chapter 18).

The Hydrodynamics of Regurgitation
See Chapter 18.

Rapid Induction and Intubation
The technique to induce anaesthesia followed almost immediately by tracheal intubation (so-called 'crash induction') is designed to forestall the dangers of vomiting, regurgitation and aspiration of stomach contents. Following pre-oxygenation, the induction dose of thiopentone is immediately followed by an intubating dose of suxamethonium. Pre-curarization is probably unwise. An assistant who must be properly trained, applies cricoid pressure as the patient loses consciousness, while the anaesthetist proceeds to tracheal intubation and inflation of the cuff. Cricoid pressure is released and the tube tested for correct positioning. When suxamethonium is contraindicated, an alternative technique is to inject vecuronium or alcuronium immediately before the thiopentone; this gives reasonable intubating conditions earlier than when any other non-depolarizing agent is used.

Perforated Peptic Ulcer
The operation[9] is usually short and the patient may be shocked; he is very liable to postoperative chest complications. His stomach is likely to contain vomitable material. Precautions must be taken to prevent aspiration of gastric contents during induction of anaesthesia. Most workers prefer the pre-oxygenation, thiopentone, relaxant, nitrous oxide, oxygen hyperventilation technique described above with a volatile supplement if necessary.

Operations for Peptic Ulcer
First gastrectomy by Theodore Billroth (1825–1897) in 1881 in Vienna;[10] first gastrojejunostomy in 1884 by Anton Wolfler (1850–1907)[11] first vagotomy in 1943.[12] Before operation, many surgeons like the patient to swallow a nasogastric tube, so that the stomach can be aspirated and kept empty. This is a most unpleasant experience for the patient. Other workers favour the passage of an oesophageal or nasogastric tube after anaesthesia has been induced.

Passage of Nasogastric Tube

In the conscious patient. The nasogastric tube has three markings on it corresponding to the average distance between the upper teeth and the pylorus, the fundus, and the cardia, respectively. A more efficient tube is the semi-stiff oesophageal tube (e.g. size 12, 7 mm diameter), through which can be sucked a larger volume of fluid, together with small solid particles. Gastric aspiration does not guarantee an empty stomach. Plastic tubes are usually preferable to those made of rubber. The patient sits up and a well-lubricated tube (glycerin or liquid paraffin) is inserted into a patent naris, which has been cocainized. The patients sips water while the tube is advanced with each act of swallowing. It should be inserted until the third mark is at the naris. A tube which is too soft should be discarded, as it must not collapse when subjected to the negative pressure of the sucker. Distance from incisor teeth to cardia averages 43 cm (17 in). A nasogastric tube may be in the trachea without either the patient or the anaesthetist being aware of it.

In the unconscious patient. A plastic tube can frequently be introduced into the stomach 'blind'. If this is not possible a well-lubricated nasogastric tube is inserted into a No. 6 Magill nasotracheal tube so that its tip is just within the lumen of the larger tube near the bevelled end. This is then passed blindly or with the aid of a finger or laryngoscope into the oesophagus from the nose. The oesophageal opening is slightly to the left of the midline. The nasogastric tube is now inserted well into the stomach through the Magill tube. It is often helpful to slit the Magill tube lengthwise prior to use so that it can be easily separated from the nasogastric tube on withdrawal. When aspiration of stomach contents (on auscultatory evidence of bubbling on both injection and aspiration of 5 ml of saline followed by 5 ml of air[13]) shows its correct position, the Magill tube is withdrawn and the nasogastric tube held firmly against the posterior wall of the pharynx as the larger tube leaves the nose. Intermittent suction is kept up during the operation. It must not be accidentally caught in the surgeon's gastric clamp.

Acute Intestinal Obstruction

Factors to be considered are:

1. The degree of circulatory collapse.

2. The presence or absence of regurgitation or vomiting. The former is a passive process requiring no muscular force: the latter is a muscular reflex act. The former is aided by a head-down tilt and rendered less likely if the head is tilted upwards 45°.

3. The degree of distension

4. The degree of electrolyte and fluid imbalance. This must be controlled with infusion of Hartmann's or other appropriate solution. The moderately dehydrated patient has lost 6% of total body fluids. The severely dehydrated patient has lost 10% of total body fluids, and shows loss of skin elasticity, sunken eyes, dry tongue and oliguria.

5. In all bowel operations except those of the shortest duration, nitrous oxide inhaled into the lungs may be partially excreted into the gut, causing distension.[14]

In both normal people and those with intestinal obstruction, much fluid is excreted by the proximal small intestine, only to be reabsorbed lower down. In high obstruction, this subsequent reabsorption is prevented. Low obstruction gives rise to distension. Vomiting causes loss of chlorides and alkalosis, and consequently great fluid loss and dehydration. Distension causes interference with circulation of the bowel wall, and pressure on the great veins results in reduced venous return to the heart, hypotension and interference with cardiac action due to increased intra-abdominal pressure. If this cannot be relieved, PEEP may be beneficial.[15]

Biochemical changes in intestinal obstruction include: (1) Haemoconcentration; (2) Metabolic acidosis; (3) Diminution of serum chlorides; (4) Increased blood urea and non-protein nitrogen; (5) Increase in carbon-dioxide combining power of serum; (6) Acid urine, with perhaps ketone bodies and low urinary chloride; (7) Abnormalities of potassium metabolism.

The stomach should always be emptied by either a nasogastric or a wider bore oesophageal tube, preferably the latter. Grave illness does not make this any less necessary. The tube should be taken out before induction of anaesthesia but may be reintroduced after induction and retained until the return of the reflexes. A patient with increasing cyanosis, tightly clenched jaws and faeculent material issuing from the nose is a truly terrifying sight, and one which carries a bad prognosis. That which cannot be easily treated had better be prevented.

General anaesthesia is safer in ill subjects. The actual agents and techniques used to produce general anaesthesia vary with different workers.

Intra- and extradural analgesia (with or without a light general anaesthetic) produce good relaxation, contract the bowel and do not interfere with the cough reflex (when used alone). They produce hypotension and are questionable in shocked and debilitated patients, e.g. where systolic blood pressure is below 100 mmHg.

Burst Abdomen

This may be caused by poor surgical technique, indifferent anaesthesia, the nature of the patient's disease and his nutritional state. It is a serious complication and carries a high mortality from acute peritonitis, atelectasis, intestinal obstruction, renal or cardiac failure. Prolapse of a small piece of bowel or omentum into the wound is usually only the tip of the iceberg so that only too frequently the whole incision must be examined and completely resutured. This can only be done successfully with full relaxation. Care must be taken to protect the lungs from stomach contents during induction and from atelectasis after operation.

Operations on the Colon and Rectum[16]

Maximal relaxation is necessary and contracted intestines an advantage. Extra- or intradural analgesia with light general anaesthesia, or light general anaesthesia with a muscle relaxant are suitable. Adequate intraoperative fluid replacement must be maintained during colon resection and anastomosis which is a prerequisite for successful healing.[17]

The authors prefer either a combination of thiopentone, volatile agent, relaxant and nitrous-oxide–oxygen, given through a large orotracheal tube with controlled respiration, or a continuous or single injection extradural block combined with light general anaesthesia and spontaneous (or occasionally assisted) respiration. This avoids the use of neostigmine.[18] There is evidence that patients operated on for colorectal cancer survive longer if they are not given blood transfusions during their operations.[19] Both halothane and central neural blockade increase colon blood flow whereas the hypocapnia which may be associated with hyperventilation, decreases it.

Neostigmine may contribute to a breakdown of an intestinal anastomosis by the production of early and intense peristalsis. Neither atropine nor glycopyrronium effectively abolish the increase in intraluminal pressure of total colon activity after neostigmine given to reverse a non-depolarizing relaxant.[2] Halothane given towards the end of the operation may prevent this. For preoperative preparation *see* Reid D. J. *Br. J. Hosp. Med.* 1976, **15**, 405.

Biliary Tract Surgery

First successful cholecystectomy by Lawson Tait (1845–1899) in Birmingham in 1879[20] and Carl Johan August Langenbuch (1876–1901) of Berlin in 1882.[21] First cholecystogram by Evarts Ambrose Graham (1883–1957) of St Louis in 1924.[22] First exploration of common duct for stone by Thornton in 1891.[23] Vitamin K analogue may be necessary before operation. Anaesthetic technique is similar to that used for gastric operations. High elevation of a gallbladder bridge may cause hypotension by interfering with venous return by obstructing the vena cava. The dynamics of the biliary ducts must be considered in connection with pre- and postoperative pain relief in patients with biliary disease. Normally the increase in intrabiliary pressure required to overcome the tone of the sphincter of Oddi does not cause pain. Analgesics (e.g. morphine and pethidine) may, by stimulating this sphincter to contract, increase the intrabiliary pressure up to $20\,cmH_2O$ and thus produce pain. Fentanyl raises intrabiliary pressure but the effect wanes within 25 min. Cholinergic drugs have a similar effect. The use of opioid drugs does not appear to interfere with the radiological interpretation of operative cholangiography, nor to increase the low incidence of spasm of the sphincter of Oddi.[3] To relieve biliary colic, therefore, the dose of analgesic must be great enough to cause cerebral depression. The following drugs lower intrabiliary pressure by relaxing the sphincter: (1) Amyl nitrate; (2) Nitroglycerin 1 mg; (3) Papaverine 30 mg. Atropine, even up to 2 mg, is disappointing in this respect. With biliary obstruction gallamine is often suitable.[24]

If a choledochogram is required, apnoea for up to 30 s may be necessary. To relax spasm of the sphincter of Oddi during cholecystography, glucagon 1 ml may be helpful (in the absence of insulinoma or phaeochromocytoma).[25]

The usual techniques for pain relief in operations in the upper abdomen are employed postoperatively.

Cases of *acute haemorrhagic pancreatitis* are bad anaesthetic risks no matter what agent and method are used; thus obscure abdominal emergencies should have serum amylase tests done so that operation can be avoided. Hypocalcaemia may complicate pancreatitis and may result in difficult reversal of non-depolarizing relaxants.[26] Intravenous aprotinin (Trasylol), an inhibitor of kallikrein, has been recommended. For description of anaesthesia for *excision of islet-cell tumour of pancreas, see* Chari P. et al. *Anaesthesia* 1977, **32**, 261; Lamont A. S. M. and Jones D. *Anaesth. Intensive Care* 1978, **6**, 261. (*See also* Chapter 22.)

(For history of choledochoscopy *see* Ashby B. S. *Ann. R. Coll. Surg. Engl.* 1985, **67**, 279.)

Portal Hypertension

For history of portocaval shunt, *see* Donovan A. J. et al. *Surg. Gynecol. Obstet.* 1978, **147**, 423.

Liver Transplantation[27]

First successful orthotopic liver transplant by Thomas Earl Starzl of Denver in

1963.[28] This presents complex problems. The anaesthetic technique recommended consists of nitrous oxide, oxygen, relaxant and IPPV with occasional analgesic supplements. Atracurium is the relaxant of choice. Large blood transfusions are required and metabolic acidosis is likely to occur. Rises in serum potassium are common during operation but hypokalaemia may be a feature later on. Transplantation of an ice-cold liver produces a fall in body temperature. (*See also* Carmichael F. J. et al. *Anesth. Analg. (Cleve.)* 1985, **64**, 107; Borland I. M. et al. *Anesth. Analg. (Cleve.)* 1984, **64**, 117.)

Haemorrhoidectomy
Surgical assault on the anal region results in severe pain, reflex response, e.g. movement of body muscles, reflex laryngeal spasm (Brewer–Luckhardt reflex). To overcome these, pain requires surgical anaesthesia; muscle movement requires deep anaesthesia or a relaxant, laryngeal spasm requires a tracheal tube, deep anaesthesia, or a relaxant. All can be controlled by regional analgesia. Light general anaesthesia alone has no place here. Some surgeons require maximal relaxation of the anal sphincter while others prefer a certain amount of tone to be retained. The choice is between:
   1. *Deep general anaesthesia.* Thiopentone (0·25–1 g), nitrous oxide and oxygen, in addition to the use of a volatile inhalation agent.
   2. *Extradural sacral block.* 15–20 ml of 1·5% lignocaine or 5–10 ml of 0·5% bupivacaine[29] with adrenaline (*see* Chapter 32). Extradural injection into the sacral canal (0·5% bupivacaine) at the conclusion of the operation greatly reduces postoperative discomfort. It can be given by anaesthetist or surgeon.
   3. *Low intradural block* (S.4–5), e.g. lignocaine 50–75 mg or 0·5% bupivacaine plain, or heavy solution, 2 ml between L.4 and L.5 with patient sitting.
   4. *Local infiltration* with lignocaine or bupivacaine. From a point 2·5 cm (1 in) posterior to the anus, with the index finger of the left hand in the rectum, 1·5% lignocaine–adrenaline solution is injected: total amount, 25 ml. Only one site of injection used, and anus and anal canal are ensheathed by a cylinder of solution.[30]
   Cryotherapy for haemorrhoids has been performed without anaesthetic.[31] All regional techniques can be combined with light general anaesthesia.
   The first postoperative bowel action can be made more tolerable by the self-administration of nitrous oxide (Entonox) or trichloroethylene (in air). Xyloproct suppositories can also be used. For the relief of postoperative pain a combination of morphine and bupivacaine given into the sacral extradural space may be used.[32] For lateral sphincterotomy, local analgesia and general anaesthesia give equally good results.

Hernia
A pioneer surgeon was Edoado Bassini (1844–1924) of Italy.[33] General anaesthesia is usually employed, e.g. thiopentone, nitrous-oxide–oxygen analgesic and relaxant. Other workers use a volatile inhalation agent. Ilio-inguinal nerve block, with infiltration of the neck of the sac as an adjunct to general anaesthesia allows lighter planes of anaesthesia and also provides postoperative pain relief. It can also be used without general anaesthesia. Intra- and extradural block are suitable in fit patients and must be carried to T.10; if the cord is to be

under tension, to T.7 and if the peritoneum is to be under tension, to T.5. For extradural block, 25–30 ml of 1·5% lignocaine or 12–15 ml of 0·5% bupivacaine. For intradural block, 1·4–1·6 ml of 5% lignocaine hyperbaric solution or 3–4 ml of hyperbaric bupivacaine 0·5%. For regional field block, *see* Chapter 31. Bupivacaine, 0·25% solution, infiltrated 30–45 min before the incision, gives efficient and prolonged postoperative analgesia.[34] Very suitable for day-stay surgery.[35]

Postoperative chest complications frequently follow these operations, especially in fit young men who smoke cigarettes, no matter what anaesthetic agent is used. They should, consequently, be advised to avoid smoking for the month preceding operation, and be taught how to breathe deeply and how to cough effectively. In addition, they will require vigorous 'shake-up' treatment after operation.

Operations for incisional hernia require profound relaxation.

The chief danger in operation for *strangulated hernia* is from aspiration of stomach contents into the chest during induction of anaesthesia.

See also under Acute Intestinal Obstruction, p. 447.

Ventral Hernia

General anaesthesia, together with a muscle relaxant, is suitable. Bucking and coughing on the tracheal tube during extubation, with consequent strain on suture lines, should be prevented.

For fit adult patients, extra- or intradural analgesia can be used, to facilitate wound closure by contracting the bowels. Giant ventral hernia repair may embarrass postoperative respiration. This is managed either by elective postoperative mechnical ventilation or by performing a two-stage operation.

Jejuno-ileal Shunts

First performed in 1954.[36] *See* McKenzie R. et al. *Anesth. Analg. (Cleve.)* 1975, **54**, 65.

Mastectomy

First radical mastectomy performed by Willian Stewart Halsted (1852–1922) of Baltimore in 1891.[37] A faultless airway coupled with adequate ventilation minimizes oozing as also does a table tilted upwards (although the risk of air embolism is increased in this position). Only light general anaesthesia is required and many anaesthetists avoid intubation for local removal of breast tumours. Nitrous oxide and oxygen, with minimal intermittent thiopentone and a narcotic analgesic, is a good combination, with or without the addition of a little volatile agent and spontaneous breathing. Others prefer the intravenous barbiturate, relaxant, intubation and nitrous-oxide–oxygen by the IPPV technique.

Breast biopsy can be successfully performed under infiltration analgesia.[38]

Anaesthesia in Varicose Vein Surgery

Ligation was proposed by Friederich Trendelenburg (1844–1927) in 1890.[263,266] Charles Mayo (1865–1939) of Rochester, Minn. described the removal of the long saphenous vein in 1906.[264] The malleable wire stripper first used in 1954.[265]

A head-down tilt reduces blood loss. The anaesthetic technique should enable the patient to move his legs as soon after operation as possible. Ligation of the short saphenous venous system can often be carried out with the patient in the lateral position. Maintenance of a free airway in a patient in the prone position may require tracheal intubation. The anaesthetist must guard against boredom during this operation.

Day-stay Surgery

History
Extensively practised in Belfast and in Glasgow during the first decade of this century.[39] Also in the US.[40]

Indications
For patients whose operation lasts up to 30 min, is not likely to be associated with severe postoperative pain or the use of drains or catheters, who is otherwise generally fit and whose domestic arrangements are suitable. Surgery in children.[41]

Precautions
A preoperative history and general examination in the surgical clinic, anaesthetic clinic or at domiciliary visit is performed. Co-operation with the family doctor is important. Preoperative standardized check-lists,[42] which the patient or his relatives fill in, are useful. Preoperative instructions should be in writing and easy to understand. Particular care is necessary before accepting patients for this type of surgery with the following conditions: Ischaemic heart disease, unstable diabetes, those on steroid medication, those living more than 1 hour's journey from the hospital, those living alone or who are over 70 years of age, those with acute respiratory infection or chronic respiratory failure. Oral temazepam suitable for premedication if required.[43] Some prescribe oral antacids.[44]

Technique
In the ideal technique the requirements are those for any general anaesthetic; rapid painless induction, adequate anaesthesia and analgesia without depression of the cardiovascular or respiratory systems, rapid smooth recovery with a peaceful pain-free postoperative period from the completion of the surgical procedure until the termination of the effects of the anaesthetic agents.[45] Ideally the day-stay theatre should be adjacent to the day-stay ward and the postoperative observation room. Operations should be performed early in the day. Premedication should be minimal or avoided completely. Infants should be put first on the list to prevent hypoglycaemia from starvation. The anaesthetic is only started when the surgeon and operating team are ready and the anaesthetic should be the lightest compatible with safety. Only agents which are rapidly eliminated should be used, e.g. nitrous oxide, halothane, isoflurane or enflurane.[46] All three inhalation agents, halothane, enflurane and isoflurane appear to be satisfactory for day-stay surgery, with similar rates of recovery.[47] Suxamethonium may cause muscle pains the following day unless precautions are taken. Tracheal intubation is not contraindicated. Diazepam and fentanyl have a rebound effect 4–8 hours after administration which although not greater than the initial effect, may be dangerous.[48] Local analgesia on its own or combined with light general anaesthesia has the advantage of excellent

postoperative pain relief. In suitable patients both intra- and extradural block may be employed.[49] Cryo-analgesia has also been described.[50] Propofol has been recommended for induction of anaesthesia though the authors find thiopentone satisfactory in reasonable dosage.

For local analgesia in day-stay surgery, *see* Wildsmith J. A. W. *Hosp. Update* 1982, **8**, 559.

Assessment of Recovery and Fitness to go Home[51]

Usually undertaken by an experienced nurse: (1) Awakening; ability to answer questions and obey commands;[52] (2) Fitness to walk to the bathroom; Romberg's test and stabilometry;[53] (3) Fitness to return home; reaction time tests; Maddox wing (*see* Chapter 14); (4) Fitness to go out alone, usually allowed the day after anaesthesia. Research tools include the EEG, the track tracer, psychomotor tests, choice reaction tests;[54] (5) Fitness to go to work; this depends on the surgery involved; usually the following day. *See also* Thompson P. W. *Proc. R. Soc. Med.* 1975, **68**, 415; Ogg T. W. *Br. Med. J.* 1980, **2**, 212; Davenport H. T. in: *General Anaesthesia* 4th ed. (Gray T. C. and Utting J. E. ed.) London: Butterworths, 1980; Atkinson R. S. in: *Recent Advances in Anaesthesia and Analgesia*—14 (Atkinson R. S. and Hewer C. L. ed.) London: Churchill Livingstone: 1980; Loder R. E. *Anaesthesia* 1982, **37**, 1037; Burn J. M. B. *Br. Med. J.* 1983, **286**, 492; Symposium on Day-stay Surgery. *Can. Anaesth. Soc. J.* 1983, **30**, 541; Review article on supplemental medication for day-stay patients undergoing surgery under regional analgesia, Philip B. A. *Anesth. Analg. (Cleve.)* 1985, **64**, 1117; Commission on the provision of surgical services; guidelines for day-stay surgery. *R. Coll. Surg. Engl.* 1985.

Assessment of Fitness to Drive

Views differ. The drugs used, their amounts and timing are important in assessment. An interval of 48 hours has been suggested[55] while others think a shorter time safe.[56] Perhaps a median time is 24 hours. Following the injection of local analgesics, one hour after the return of normal function.[57]

Surgery of Endocrine Glands

Thyroid Operations

The great pioneer of surgery of the thyroid was Theodore Kocher (1841–1917) of Bern. For this he received the Nobel Prize in 1909, the first, and only surgeon for many years subsequently, to be so honoured. Antithyroid drugs were first used in medical treatment in 1943 (thiourea).[58]

Thyroid Function

Clinical assessment can be supplemented by: (1) Thyroid radioactive iodine uptake after 20 min and 48 h; (2) Thyroid scan; (3) Estimation of triiodothyronine; (4) Triiodothyronine suppression test; (5) Serum cholesterol (high in myxoedema).

Preoperative Preparation

Toxic patients can be treated medically or surgically. When surgery is advised the patient should first be rendered euthyroid by medical treatment, although β-blockade has been used as it controls the hyperdynamic circulation more rapidly.[59] Iodine was used to treat goitre in 1821 by J. F. Coindet (1774–1834), Swiss physician, and is used today in the immediate preoperative period. Lugol's iodine (iodine 5% in 10% potassium iodide) (Jean G. A. Lugol, 1786–1851, of Paris) has largely been replaced by the tablet of potassium iodide (e.g. 60 mg three times daily). Carbimazole causes vascularity of the thyroid gland and a change to potassium iodide is usually made 7–10 days preoperatively. Propranolol (e.g. 40 mg four times daily) does not affect the size and vascularity of the gland, but since it does not infuence the thyrotoxicosis itself (only the effects on the cardiovascular system) it may be combined with potassium iodide before and perhaps immediately following operation. (*See also* Greene R. *Prescribers J.* 1980, **20**, 73.) It is important to check the possibility of respiratory obstruction from retrosternal goitre, compression of the trachea or its deviation by examination of the radiographs.

Anaesthetic Agents
All the commonly used agents have their advocates, and respiration may be spontaneous or controlled. Coughing must be prevented by a volatile agent, topical analgesia or by muscular paralysis.

Airway
A tracheal tube is usually employed to maintain the airway in thyroid surgery.

One is *essential* when: (1) The trachea is deviated or compressed; (2) Goitre is retrosternal; (3) Malignancy is suspected; (4) The vocal cords are functioning abnormally when viewed through a laryngeal mirror in husky, stridulous patients.

Stimulation of the recurrent laryngeal nerve causes spasm of the corresponding cord, with a high-pitched crowing sound, when patient is not intubated. If nerve is divided, the cord first becomes abducted and flaccid; later it assumes the cadaveric position between abduction and adduction. Later still, some voluntary control is gained.

A cuffed tube is likely to cause more postoperative tracheitis than an uncuffed one and in the absence of IPPV is usually quite unnecessary.

Techniques for intubation under regional analgesia. See Chapters 12 and 31.

Conduct of Anaesthesia
In very large goitres, difficulties are more likely to be surgical rather than anaesthetic.[60] The eyes should be protected from the mask, towels, etc. Hyperextension of the neck is unnecessary and should be avoided. A head-up tilt is said to reduce venous oozing. Infiltration of the skin and subcutaneous tissues in the zone of the incision reduces oozing in the skin flaps. Injection of 1–200 000 to 1–500 000 adrenaline–saline (if thought desirable) should precede the incision by 15 min but the addition of bupivacaine to the adrenaline does not relieve postoperative pain.[61] Cardiac dysrhythmia can be greatly reduced by maintaining blood-gas equilibrium or by β-blockers.

The trachea and pharynx should be aspirated with a sucker at the conclusion of the operation, but vigorous coughing immediately after operation is to be avoided as it may contribute to reactionary haemorrhage. If 20–50 mg of suxamethonium are given before extubation and the patient then inflated with oxygen, the cords can be examined at the time when respiration returns, to see that they move normally.

The tracheal tube can otherwise remain in situ postoperatively until it is resented by the patient or removed by the anaesthetist.

Respiratory Obstruction after Thyroidectomy

The causes may be:

1. Reactionary haemorrhage. This may cause pressure on the trachea and requires immediate evacuation of the haematoma and restoration of the airway.

2. Oedema of the larynx, which is usually seen on the second or third day after operation. Diagnosis is by indirect laryngoscopy and if stridor becomes troublesome a tracheal tube or tracheostomy will be required. Oedema of the pharynx may also be a cause of obstruction.[62]

3. Recurrent laryngeal nerve injury.[63] Injury to the recurrent laryngeal nerve may be transient or permanent. The former is not uncommon and even if bilateral need not be serious unless there is, in addition, oedema causing obstruction. Permanent injury to one nerve may be symptomless and is not serious unless the patient earns his living with his voice as the opposite cord compensates for the immobile cord. Permanent injury to both cords is very serious because both voice and airway are impaired owing to the narrow glottis. Either a permanent tracheostomy or an operation to widen the glottis is required. Even slight obstruction may prove fatal in handicapped patients, e.g. cardiac cases, and tracheostomy is always better done early than late. Its delay is the most frequent cause of death after thyroidectomy.

4. Collapse of trachea. This can occur due to erosion of the tracheal cartilages by a large goitre, but is rare unless the actual tracheal cartilage is removed in malignant cases. The unsupported walls of the trachea may collapse inwardly so causing partial or even total obstruction when the tube is removed. Immediate reintubation must be done at once. Tracheostomy may be necessary.

5. Injury to the superior laryngeal nerve. This is rare but can be suspected if there is: (*a*) A change in the voice; (*b*) Difficulty in swallowing. The former is due to cricothyroid paralysis, the latter to sensory paralysis. The condition soon improves. In a series of over 300 thyroidectomy operations, the operation carried a hazard to the voice in 5% of patients, with permanent damage, measured by sophisticated methods, in 3%. There is as great a need for care of the external laryngeal nerve as for the recurrent branches, by the surgeon.[64]

6. Mucus or blood in the airway

See Wade J. S. *Ann. R. Coll. Surg. Engl.* 1980, **62**, 15.

Obstruction to respiration severe enough to cause insomnia requires either tracheostomy or intubation.

Routine examination of the larynx before and after thyroidectomy has shown that one-third of cases of unilateral paralysis resulting from trauma to the recurrent nerve are symptomless and in nearly all of these a normal voice is re-established whether the paralysis disappears or not: treatment is unnecessary.

Other Complications

1. Thyroid crisis. Now rarely seen. The patient may complain of abdominal pain, fever, diarrhoea, gross nervousness and restlessness with tachycardia and dysrhythmias. An acute abdomen may be suspected. A sudden crisis in an unsuspected thyrotoxic patient after operation requires administration of a β-blocker, e.g. propranolol 80 mg 4-hourly by mouth or serial doses of 1 mg to a maximum of 10 mg i.m., together with potassium iodide and hydrocortisone. Mild tachycardia or pyrexia during the first few postoperative days may indicate a lesser degree of thyroid overactivity and may be abolished or prevented by oral potassium iodide.

2. *Postoperative hypoparathyroidism.* A low serum calcium (normal 4·5–5·5 mmol/l) requiring calcium gluconate 10%, up to 20 ml slowly i.v. There may be tetany, and Chvostek's and Trousseau's signs may be present. *See also* Chapter 22.

Postoperative Care

Fowler's position; analgesics when required; aspirin for the muscular pain in the neck. Nausea and vomiting should be prevented by anti-emetic drugs.

Hyperparathyroidism

The parathyroids help to maintain a normal serum calcium level (2·2–2·6 mmol/l), together with diet, kidney function and calciferol. Hyperparathyroidism results from excessive secretion, usually due to an adenoma, occasionally to diffuse hypertrophy of the glands. It may be associated with renal stones, bone pain progressing perhaps to osteitis fibrosa, loss of appetite, nausea and thirst. After parathyroidectomy the serum calcium falls and there may be tetany, requiring intravenous calcium gluconate. In advanced cases of hyperpathyroidism there may be dehydration, sodium depletion from polyuria and renal failure. Fluids and oral (or intravenous) phosphates may be required.

Primary Aldosteronism (Conn's Syndrome)

Described by Conn in 1955.[65] Tumours of the adrenal cortex occur in two-thirds of cases and require surgical removal. Clinical features include hypertension, hypokalaemic alkalosis and hypokalaemic nephropathy.[66] Preoperative management includes correction of metabolic disturbances and potassium depletion (spironolactone and potassium supplements). Anaesthetic management is likely to be complicated by large swings of blood pressure and control may be difficult. Temporary hypoaldosteronism can occur after operation and may require fludrocortisone 0·1–0·5 mg daily. (*See* Shipton E. A. & Hugo J. M. *Anaesthesia* 1982, **37**, 933.)

Phaeochromocytoma

First reported by Frankel in 1886[67] and named by Ludwig Pick (1868–1935), of Berlin.[68] This is a tumour of the adrenal medullary cells of chromaffin origin, which, although it may be histologically benign, may be dangerous because of excessive secretion of adrenaline and noradrenaline. The growth may not be confined to the adrenal but may occur wherever chromaffin tissue is found, e.g. in the paravertebral space, near the great vessels of the abdomen, in the organ of Zuckerkandl near the aortic bifurcation, and in the coeliac plexus. The patient exhibits hypertension, either paroxysmal or continuous, hyperhidrosis and elevated basal metabolic rate with some fever and reduced blood volume. Some cases of hypotension have also been described. The condition is diagnosed by clinical examination; estimation of urinary catecholamines which may be 100–300 µg daily (normal 20–40); certain radiological investigations, and by pharmacological agents, e.g. phentolamine, 5 mg i.v., causing a fall in blood pressure, or histamine 0·05 mg, causing a rise (this may be dangerous).

Preoperative Care[69]

Alpha-adrenergic blockade prevents dangerous elevation of blood pressure during surgery, e.g. phenoxybenzamine 10 mg by mouth, 8-hourly, increased by 10 mg increments until the recumbent diastolic pressure is 90–100 mmHg without postural hypotension. Therapy should continue for 1 week preoperatively. Beta-adrenergic blockade is indicated in the presence of tachycardia or dysrhythmia, e.g. propranolol 40 mg orally, 8-hourly.

Anaesthetic Technique

The effects of excess adrenaline or noradrenaline during operation when the tumour is manipulated may cause a problem. Careful monitoring is advised and continuous intra-arterial blood pressure recording may be useful. Premedication should include sedatives to reduce anxiety. General anaesthesia is usually employed, but agents which cause sympathetic stimulation are to be avoided. Intravenous agents with nitrous oxide, oxygen and relaxants are recommended. Excessive hypertension may be controlled by the use of sodium nitroprusside; further rise when the infusion is discontinued may indicate the presence of more chromaffin tissue.[70]

(*See also* Bingham W. et al. *Anaesthesia* 1972, **27**, 49; Cousins M. J. and Rubin R. B. *Br. J. Anaesth.* 1974, **46**, 78; Stamenkovic L. and Spierdijk J. *Anaesthesia* 1976, **31**, 941; Desmonts J. M. et al. *Br. J. Anaesth.* 1977, **49**, 991; Dagget P. et al. *Br. Med. J.* 1978, **2**, 311; Hull C. J. *Br. J. Anaesth.* 1986, **58**, 1453.)

Management of the Condition in Children

See Black G. W. et al. *Br. J. Anaesth.* 1969, **41**, 185.

Neuroblastoma

This is a catecholamine-secreting malignant tumour arising from the sympathetic nervous system in infants and children, situated in the retroperitoneal or retropleural region. It may secrete catecholamines during surgery and should be managed like a phaeochromocytoma with α-adrenergic blocking agents, e.g. phentolamine, and blood transfusion.

See also Whitwam, J. G. *Anaesthesia* 1977, **32**, 829.

Gynaecology

First successful removal of an ovarian cyst in 1817 by Ephraim McDowell (1771–1830), of Kentucky,[71] and first successful closure of a vesicovaginal fistula in 1852 by James Marion Sims (1813–1883), of New York.[72] First successful surgical treatment of ruptured ectopic pregnancy by Lawson Tait of Birmingham (1845–1899).[73]

Main problems—haemorrhage, postoperative vomiting and deep vein thrombosis.

Abdominal operations call for profound relaxation to prevent damage to muscles and the upper abdominal peritoneum from abrasion by packs. They can be performed under spinal analgesia, either intradural or extradural (which the authors warmly advocate) (*see* Chapter 32), or under general anaesthesia.

For Wertheim's hysterectomy[74] (Ernst Wertheim, 1864–1920, of Vienna) the authors employ extradural block up T.5 with light tracheal general anaesthesia.

The Trendelenburg position is unphysiological and should be maintained for as short a time as possible. It may lead to headache, regurgitation[75] and a steep rise in CVP.[75] The less steep it is the better for the patient's respiratory and cardiovascular function. Levelling of the table should be gradual, with a watch on venous and arterial blood pressure. The leg veins contain 500 ml or more of blood each side. Investigations have shown that in patients undergoing major gynaecological surgery under extradural lumbar block and light general anaesthesia, and operated on in either the horizontal, head-down or lithotomy positions, no significant effects of posture were detected as measured by minute volume and blood-gas estimations,[76] but the lithotomy position may give rise to postoperative backache if a lumbar support is not used.

Vaginal operations can be performed under extradural lumbar or sacral block (*see* Chapter 32) or general inhalation anaesthesia. Stretching of the cervix or trauma to the perineum may produce laryngeal spasm, requiring a deeper plane of anaesthesia or a small dose of a muscle relaxant. The authors prefer intradural or lumbar extradural block for vaginal repair operations. It combines afferent block, muscular relaxation and moderate hypotension and ischaemia. The dosage of 1·5% lignocaine solution used for extradural block is 20–30 ml, of 0·5% bupivacaine, 10–20 ml.[77] Light thiopentone sleep can be employed if thought desirable, or heavy premedication may suffice. Some workers prefer to use induced hypotension by ganglionic blockade for vaginal surgery. Other surgeons infiltrate the tissues with adrenaline-saline (1–250 000 to 1–500 000). *For dilatation and curettage*, thiopentone, with nitrous oxide and oxygen, or nitrous oxide, oxygen, volatile agent or muscle relaxant. While suxamethonium may occasionally be necessary, its routine employment is unwarranted because of the muscular after-pains which sometimes develop. In problem patients, a small dose of a long-acting relaxant or diazepam may help to smooth out difficulties. The barbiturate should be in the bloodstream at the exact time that the surgical stimulus is applied.

Anaesthesia for laparoscopy.[78] Laparoscopy was first employed in 1910, using a cystoscope.[79] It is not a minor procedure and is accompanied by an increase in blood glucose, plasma cortisol, prolactin and growth hormone.[80] The patient is usually in a steep Trendelenburg position. A distended stomach may be injured by the operator; it must be prevented, or if present, deflated.[81] The injected gas, usually CO_2, may cause cardiovascular disturbances due to the raised intra-abdominal pressure. These include rise or fall of arterial pressure, central venous pressure and heart rate. Hypercapnia causes increase in circulating catecholamines, peripheral vascular resistance and sometimes hypokalaemia.[82] Peak levels of $Paco_2$ may not arise until after completion of the operative procedure. CO_2 embolus has been reported.[83] Recent studies[84] using impedance cardiography suggest that a moderate fall in stroke volume and cardiac output is related to the volume of gas used for peritoneal insufflation. If the operation is performed soon after delivery, smaller doses of suxamethonium will be required than in normal women due to a lowering of serum cholinesterase activity.[85]

The gas may accidentally be injected into aorta, inferior vena cava, retroperitoneal tissues causing caval compression, hollow viscera or abdominal wall. The intra-abdominal pressure should probably not exceed 30 cmH$_2$O, a pressure adequate for good surgical exposure. The gas is absorbed but can be removed from the bloodstream by hyperventilation and IPPV. These changes are less frequent if N_2O is substituted for CO_2, although the risk of explosion from diathermy is introduced. The risk will be increased if gas from an injured viscus enters the peritoneal cavity.[86] Light general anaesthesia through a tracheal tube, with IPPV and relaxants, is a suitable combination and preferable to techniques of spontaneous respiration when the incidence of dysrhythmia is high, although nitrous oxide, oxide and enflurane, with spontaneous respiration is stated to give good results.[87] The operation can be done under infiltration analgesia[88] as a day-stay case. A generous volume of 0·5% lignocaine solution should be infiltrated into the puncture sites. Gross obesity, marked anxiety, the presence of peritoneal adhesions and the proposed application of Fallopian rings are relative contra-indications. It is safe, and in skilled hands, without discomfort.[89] The gas must be let out at the end of the operation or shoulder pain may result, lasting several days.[90]

Pneumothorax has been reported, presumably due to the passage of gas through congenital defects in the diaphragm.[91] Other complications reported include brachial plexus palsy (poor positioning) and regurgitation of gastric contents. Magnesium trisilicate before induction has been recommended for this.[92] (*See also* Neufeld G. R. *Surg. Gynecol. Obstet.* 1978, **147**, 705.)

Termination of Pregnancy. It is most important to check in these patients that the stomach is empty before induction. For the vaginal operation, thiopentone with nitrous oxide and oxygen, and perhaps trichloroethylene, diazepam or neurolept agents, is usually satisfactory. Halothane relaxes the uterus, but halothane 0·5% is a suitable agent for termination in the first trimester.[93] Light general anaesthesia with IPPV and a relaxant is suitable for the abdominal operation. Ergotamine tartrate, intravenously, raises venous as well as arterial tone and in patients with pre-existing heart disease may result in angina or acute pulmonary oedema. It may cause bronchospasm, nausea and vomiting. Oxytocin, 5 units, may be preferable.

This can also be done under paracervical block with heavy sedation,[94] using the vaginal route, or under ketamine-dissociative anaesthesia.

For anaesthesia for operations during pregnancy, *see* p. 391.

Ophthalmic Surgery

In intraocular surgery, a sudden rise in intraocular tension from the normal 15–25 mmHg following coughing, vomiting, contraction of the orbicularis oculi or straining may cause displacement of iris or vitreous into the wound, and so in the past these operations have been usually performed under local analgesia. (It was, in fact, the poor quality of the general anaesthesia available in Vienna in the 1880s that stimulated Carl Koller to seek practical means of producing local analgesia of the eye, and to employ cocaine for this purpose—so initiating the whole concept of local analgesia in surgery.) Now, following modern improvement in general anaesthetic technique, cataract operations in the younger patients are usually done under careful general anaesthesia, taking great pains to avoid coughing and similar disturbances. Ocular ischaemia is aided by a flawless anaesthetic technique, a tilted table and the instillation of adrenaline into the conjunctival sac.

Extraction of the lens nucleus for cataract was first described by Jacques Daviel, French oculist (1696–1762), in 1753. The ophthalmoscope was invented in 1851 by H. L. F. von Helmholtz (1821–1894).

Tone of Pupil

Dilatation—drops of 0·5% tropicamide with maximum effect in 40–60 min, wearing off in a few hours. Effects of atropine last many days. It is parasympatholytic and weakens the sphincter muscles of the pupil; both are potentiated by phenylephrine 10%. Effects reversed by 0·5% pilocarpine which stimulates muscle fibres of the pupillary sphincter. Thymoxamine reverses the action of phenylephrine. The risks of causing acute closed-angle glaucoma is very small.[95]

Innervation of the Eye

(1) Motor. Superior oblique muscle from 4th cranial nerve. Lateral rectus from 6th. All other extra-ocular muscles from the 3rd nerve. Orbicularis oculis from the 7th; (2) Sensory. Optic nerve conveys vision. Other sensation from ophthalmic division of the 5th nerve; (3) Parasympathetic. Fibres arise from the Edinger–Westphal nucleus and run with the 3rd nerve to synapse in the ciliary ganglion, then via the short ciliary nerves. Stimulation of the parasympathetic causes constriction of the pupil and of the ciliary muscle; (4) Sympathetic. Fibres from T.1 synapse in the superior cervical ganglion and travel via the carotid plexus to join the long and short ciliary nerves. Stimulation produces dilatation of the pupil.

Local Analgesia

See Loan W. B. and Johnston S. S. in: *Anaesthesia for Eye, Ear, Nose and Throat Surgery* (Morrison J. D., Mirakhur R. K. and Craig H. J. L. ed.). Edinburgh: Churchill Livingstone, 1975; Allen E. D. and Elkington A. R. *Br. J. Anaesth.* 1980, **52**, 689.

Advantages. (1) Safer; (2) Less postoperative nausea and vomiting; (3) Early ambulation and feeding; (4) Less bleeding; (5) Less risk of pulmonary embolism; (6) Less upset of biochemical processes; (7) Less postoperative restlessness; (8) Less postoperative lung pathology; (9) Less postoperative coronary or cerebral thrombosis;[96] (10) Loss of memory function in the elderly after cataract extraction under general anaesthesia is no worse than after regional analgesia plus sedation,[97] but regional analgesia often preferred.

Disadvantage. Lack of control of the patient. Difficulty in controlling intra-ocular pressure.

Technique of analgesia of cornea and conjunctival sac. Drops of 4% lignocaine should be instilled into the conjunctival sac every 2 min on five occasions: 2–4% cocaine may be used when prolonged intense analgesia is required. This will given analgesia and vasoconstriction of the cornea and conjunctiva, but not of the iris or ciliary body; nor will it produce analgesia in a glaucomatous eye. Cocaine has the disadvantage that it produces dilatation of the pupil (bad in glaucoma), slight cloudiness of the cornea, while it irritates and dries the corneal epithelium. Amethocaine 0·5 or 1%, which lasts longer, does not have these effects and can also be used for tonometry. If the local analgesic drug is dissolved in methyl cellulose, stinging of the eye will not result when instillation into the conjunctival sac takes place. Adrenaline can be added to these local analgesics to produce ischaemia. Oxybuprocaine has been used for local analgesia.

Infraorbital block (*see* Chapter 31) from the infraorbital canal below the eye produces analgesia of the central part of the lower lid; lacrimal block, its lateral part; supra- and infratrochlear block, its medial part; these can all be reached as they emerge from the skull.

The lacrimal, supraorbital, supra- and infratrochlear nerves together supply the upper lid, the upper part of the lacrimal fossa, and the upper canaliculus.

Akinesia or facial nerve block is necessary before all intraocular operations under local analgesia, to prevent blepharospasm.

1. Van Lint's technique,[98] the first method for producing akinesia in operations for cataract extraction. From a point 1 cm behind the lateral margin of the orbit at the level of the inferior margin, solution is injected first upwards and then horizontally between the muscles and the bone.

2. O'Brien's technique.[99] From a weal just in front of the tragus, below the zygomatic process, a needle injects solution over the condyloid process of the mandible.

Retro-ocular block. This must be done before operation under local analgesia on the globe of the eye. After topical analgesia of the cornea and conjunctival sac, the long and short posterior ciliary nerves and ciliary ganglion are blocked within the muscle cone. These supply the uveal tract and cornea and reduce the tone of the extraocular muscles. Retro-ocular block dilates the pupil, causes exophthalmos, reduces intraocular pressure and makes prolapse of the vitreous less likely. Hyaluronidase (6–10 turbidity-reducing (TR) units to each millilitre of solution) aids spread. The injection should also paralyse the extraocular muscles. Two per cent lignocaine or prilocaine is a suitable solution, 2 ml (4 ml for enucleation).

1. Superior,[100] through the superior rectus, with the patient looking downwards, from a weal just above the middle of the tarsal plate. A 5-cm needle is used and is inserted 3–4 cm backwards, slightly inwards and downwards. During movement of the needle, injection is continuous as a safeguard against injuring veins.

2. Inferolateral, from a weal at the inferolateral margin of the orbit. A 5-cm needle is inserted backwards along the floor of the orbit, until its tip is posterior to the eye at the apex of the orbit: 1–2 ml of solution are injected. A transconjunctival approach may also be employed. Deposition of a little solution is also necessary in superior rectus.

Retrobulbar haemorrhage. This is likely to follow puncture of a vessel by the needle used for retrobulbar block. It results in a rise in intraorbital pressure with proptosis and requires postponement of the operation.

Retro-ocular block using bupivacaine has been reported as resulting in brainstem anaesthesia with apnoea, needing IPPV and intubation.[101]

General Anaesthesia

Intraocular pressure.[102] Ideally the eye should be soft before the anterior chamber is opened, as a sudden decompression may produce stresses which can in turn result in haemorrhage. General anaesthesia should not cause a rise in intraocular pressure. Pressure can be measured, using the indention tonometer of Schiotz or the applanation tonometer. Anaesthesia should aim at reduction of choroidal vascular congestion, which in turn causes reduction in intraocular tension. Choroidal blood flow is affected by Pa_{CO_2} (similar in effect to the cerebral circulation).

Intraocular pressure is lowered by: (1) Hypocapnia; (2) Hypotension; (3) Reduction of central venous pressure; (4) Hyperoxaemia; (5) Acetazolamide; (6) Intravenous anaesthetics and narcotic analgesics; (7) Volatile anaesthetic agents; (8) Mannitol, up to 1·5 g/kg; (9) Sucrose, 50% solution, 1 g/kg; (10) Non-depolarizing relaxants.

It is raised by: (1) Hypoxaemia; (2) Hypercapnia; (3) Coughing, sneezing, straining and other causes of raised central venous pressure; (4) Suxamethonium; (5) Atropine (in narrow-angle glaucoma only); (6) Local steroids.

When the blood pressure rises, the intraocular pressure does not greatly alter but when it is less than 85 mmHg the intraocular pressure falls.[103]

Drainage of the anterior chamber is increased by contraction of the ciliary muscle, e.g. eserine; decreased by relaxation, e.g. atropine. (*See* review on anaesthesia and intraocular pressure. Murphy D. F. *Anesth. Analg. (Cleve.)* 1985, **54**, 520.)

Advantages. (1) Co-operation of patient ceases to become a problem; (2) No risk of retrobulbar haematoma from injection of local analgesic drug; (3) Less of an ordeal for the patient; (4) Quiet atmosphere in theatre facilitates delicate surgery.

Anaesthetic Drugs in Ophthalmic Surgery

Premedication. Drugs used must not contribute to postoperative vomiting. Narcotic analgesics are better avoided for this reason. Suitable agents include phenothiazine derivatives, diazepam and lorazepam. The authors currently favour lorazepam, 5 mg in healthy young adults, 1–2·5 mg in older patients, by mouth. Oral diazepam causes no change in intraocular pressure.[104]

Atropine. This with other mydriatics raises the intraocular pressure only in the presence of glaucoma with a narrow angle between the cornea and iris, a genetically determined state. Atropine may precipitate an acute attack of glaucoma in these patients, but dilatation of the pupil is without risk in the majority of patients with glaucoma.[105] Sensitivity to atropine drops into the conjunctival sac does not contra-indicate intramuscular or intravenous atropine. Pilocarpine drops, 1%, overcome this danger by constricting the pupil.

Adrenaline. Does not dilate the pupil if instilled into the conjunctival sac. Adrenaline is rapidly absorbed from the conjunctival sac and may cause systemic effects. One drop of 1–100 solution contains 1·4 mg!

Morphine. Contracts the pupil from stimulation of the 3rd cranial nerve nucleus.

Suxamethonium. This increases intraocular tension but the rise is probably confined to the period of apnoea and so is no reason for banning this useful aid to intubation. The average rise is 7–8 mmHg.[106] It comes on in 30 s, is maximal at 2 min and has disappeared in 6 min after injection.[107] It should not be used during an operation when the eye is already open, for fear of precipitating vitreous prolapse, e.g. in penetrating injury.[108] Fazadinium, 1 mg/kg or alcuronium 0·3 mg/kg may be a useful alternative for rapid intubation.[109]

The mechanism of the rise in intraocular pressure is not fully understood. It may be that contraction of the extraocular muscles is important, but there is evidence that pressure rises even when these muscles have been detached from their insertions.[110]

These effects can be prevented by the injection, 3–5 min beforehand, of a small dose of a non-depolarizing relaxant (but this view has been disputed).

The intravenous injection of *acetazolamide*, 500 mg immediately before induction of anaesthesia, largely prevents rise in intraocular pressure due to suxamethonium. It is a carbonic anhydrase inhibitor and interferes with the secretion of aqueous. Its other effects includes diuresis, depression of the central nervous system, potassium loss, metabolic acidosis and alteration of the response of the respiratory centre to carbon dioxide. It has no effect on either the pupil size or the drainage from the eye.

Non-depolarizing relaxants. Reduce the tone of extraocular muscles and produce apnoea. Gallamine blocks the oculocardiac vagal reflexes. IPPV has the advantage that rise in the $Paco_2$ with associated rise in intraocular pressure can be prevented. It allows light planes of anaesthesia to be maintained with rapid recovery on completion of surgery.

Intravenous and intramuscular agents. Thiopentone is popular for the induction of anaesthesia and for maintenance of anaesthesia. It reduces the tension in normal and glaucomatous eyes.

Chlorpromazine, promazine, promethazine, perphenazine, droperidol and haloperidol reduce incidence of vomiting.

Inhalation agents. *Halothane, isoflurane* and *enflurane* given to supplement nitrous oxide and oxygen, or with oxygen alone, in a non-rebreathing, partially rebreathing or closed system, offer good conditions, with quiet respiration and minimal postoperative nausea and vomiting. Intraocular pressure falls, even when arterial pressure is maintained, but is more certain when hypotension occurs. The $Paco_2$ can be prevented from rising if muscle relaxants and IPPV are used to maintain the $Paco_2$ at normal levels.[111] *Trichloroethylene* is a useful alternative when undesirable arterial pressure falls in association with halothane or enflurane and it may be used with IPPV. Intraocular pressure falls if $Paco_2$ remains normal.[112]

Ecothiopate iodide (phospholine iodide, an organophosphate derivative of choline). Low levels of serum cholinesterase amounting to a twofold reduction in one-third of patients can occur within a few days of commencing the use of drops of this agent in the treatment of glaucoma.[113] Although a 50% reduction in enzyme activity should not prolong apnoea with suxamethonium for more than 10–15 min, smaller amounts than usual of the relaxant should be used. The effects of these drops on the enzyme level lasts 2–4 weeks after the cessation of treatment.

Hypotensive anaesthesia in ophthalmic surgery. Hexamethonium has been recommended for bloodless field surgery and also in the treatment of haemorrhage following non-perforated eye injuries.

Some Suitable General Anaesthetic Techniques

1. *Squint*. Intravenous thiopentone, suxamethonium, tracheal tube, and nitrous-oxide–oxygen–halothane with spontaneous respiration or muscle relaxant and IPPV. The oculocardiac reflex is discussed below.

2. *Intraocular operations*. Intracapsular extraction, removal of the lens with its capsule, is the operation now usually done for cataract. The binocular microscope for operating was first used as a colposcope in 1953 and first used in ophthalmology at Tübingen, its employment having been stimulated by Julius Lempert in otology in 1938.[114] Lysis of the zonule supporting the lens was described by Joaquin Barraquer of Barcelona in 1958. Extraction of the lens by first touching it with a cryoprobe (temperature −30°C) was described by T. Krawitz of Poland in 1961. Standard techniques are satisfactory with use of a tracheal tube to ensure the airway. Coughing on the tube is to be avoided, and if the eye is open this complication may be disastrous as vitreous can be extruded and eyesight may be lost. The techniques should aim at enabling extubation to be carried out without the production of coughing, and so topical analgesia of the larynx and trachea with 4% lignocaine is in most cases helpful. Postoperative

tracheal suction is better avoided in most patients for the same reason. There are workers of experience who only insert a tracheal tube in especially difficult patients in both children and adults. The lower jaw may need support and an oropharyngeal airway can be connected to the gas supply by a Charles airway adaptor[115] in the absence of a tracheal tube.

Some suitable techniques are: (1) Thiopentone, suxamethonium, halothane with nitrous oxide and oxygen or oxygen alone; with spontaneous respiration. Enflurane and isoflurane are alternatives to halothane,[116] and trichloroethylene is a useful substitute, should arterial pressure fall too much; (2) IPPV, thiopentone, nitrous oxide, oxygen, non-depolarizing muscle relaxant; halothane, enflurane, isoflurane or trichloroethylene may be used as a supplement. The Bain circuit is convenient as it is non-obtrusive in the surgical field and allows normocapnia when the total gas flow is appropriate;[117] (3) A combination of local analgesia with heavy sedation, e.g. neurolept analgesia.[118]

Corneal Grafts. The first corneal[119] graft was carried out in 1906 in Austria. Tudor Thomas of Cardiff was a pioneer in the 1920s in the UK. Operations to restore eyesight after damage to the front of the eye require anaesthesia as for intraocular operations.

Anterior Chamber Implants. Harold Ridley used the first intraocular lens implant in 1948,[120] a technique developed by D. P. Choyce.[121] The principles of anaesthesia are the same as for other intraocular procedures.

Vitriectomy. Diseased and fibrosed vitreous is removed and replaced by a balanced salt solution. General anaesthesia is required with complete immobility of the patient for several hours. A microscope and a small fibreoptic light source are used, in a darkened theatre. Sulpha-hexafluoride is employed to fill the vitrectomized eye to prevent retinal detachment. Nitrous oxide can diffuse into the eye with considerable increase in its volume and must be discontinued at this stage and alternative drugs employed to maintain anaesthesia. Repeated operations at short intervals may be required. Non-depolarizing relaxants, IPPV and full monitoring techniques are recommended.[122]

Retinal Detachment. Meticulous anaesthesia is required and a smooth and quiet emergence and postoperative period are wanted in order to reduce the likelihood of further detachment.

Glaucoma. Patients have often received medical treatment with drugs such as cholinergics and anticholinesterases (e.g. ecothiopate). Acetazolamide can cause dehydration and metabolic acidosis. Systemic atropine is not contra-indicated in normal dosage. The anaesthesist should avoid agents and techniques which cause a rise in intraocular pressure. (*See also* Adams A. P. and Jones R. M. *Br. J. Anaesth.* 1980, **52**, 663.)

3. *Examination of the eyes in small children.* Spontaneous breathing without a treacheal tube using a small mask for halothane with nitrous oxide and oxygen is satisfactory. Ketamine has been suggested (e.g. 2 mg/kg i.v. or 10 mg/kg i.m.)

4. *Tonometry in infants.* This is required when buphthalmos is suspected. Nitrous-oxide–oxygen–halothane is satisfactory. Ketamine has also been advocated.

5. *Laser treatment.* When applied to the retina, this can be carried out without general anaesthesia; a few drops of local analgesic solution in the conjunctival sac allows treatment without major discomfort.

Special Points
(1) All disturbances causing movement, cough or contraction of the orbicularis

oculi must be avoided as they may increase the intraocular tension with resulting iris prolapse or vitreous prolapse; (2) Postoperative vomiting and coughing should be minimized for the same reason; (3) Postoperative restlessness may be due to a full bladder; (3) Congenital cataract may be associated with dystrophia myotonica or with diabetes; (4) *Oculocardiac reflex* (Aschner's reflex), first described in 1908.[123] A variety of stimuli arising in or near the eye may cause abnormalities of the rate or rhythm of the heart. Anaesthesia appears to make the heart vulnerable to increased vagal tone, especially in the young. It is suggested that patients with blue or grey eyes are less likely to develop an oculocardiac reflex dysrhythmia than similar patients with brown or hazel eyes.[124] Cardiac standstill is the danger, preceded by bradycardia, especially following traction on the internal rectus, or pressure on the eyeball, so that adequate cardiac monitoring should accompany these interventions. Gallamine and atropine intravenously are useful preventatives, though they carry a risk of ventricular ectopic beats as a result of unopposed adrenergic stimulation. Alcuronium has been reported to provide greater protection against bradycardia than pancuronium, tubocurarine or vecuronium.[125] Glycopyrronium has a similar effect but causes less tachycardia.[126] Hyoscine butyl bromide, 10–20 mg i.v. (Buscopan) has been recommended.[127] Retrobulbar injection of local analgesic solutions is not as efficient. The oculocardiac reflex may also be seen during operations for the correction of facial fractures[128] in patients with the Marcus Gunn syndrome[129] and in operations on the empty orbit.[130]

Perforating eye injuries.[131] Smooth anaesthesia is mandatory as there is a risk of vitreous extrusion and possible loss of sight if intraocular pressure rises as a result of coughing or straining. Suxamethonium is seldom justified because of its effects on intraocular pressure. Surgery is rarely very urgent and intubation with a large dose of non-depolarizing relaxant is preferred. (*See* Symposium on Eye Surgery, *Br. J. Anaesth.* 1980 (July).)

Prochlorperazine is a useful drug for the prevention of nausea and vomiting after eye operations.[132]

Recently, workers of experience report many hundreds of cases intubated with suxamethonium with no trouble from vitreous prolapse, especially when the patient is at risk of aspirating gastric contents.[133] Vecuronium given before the thiopentone has also been used.

(*See also* Elliott J. and Morrison J. D. in: *Anaesthesia for Eye, Ear, Nose and Throat Surgery*, 2nd ed. (Morrison J. D., Mirakhur R. K. and Craig H. J. L. ed.) Edinburgh: Churchill Livingstone, 1985.)

Orthopaedic Operations

Orthopaedics, a term introduced in 1741 by Nicolas Andre, professor of medicine in Paris in a book entitled *Orthopaedia, or the Art of Correcting Deformities in Children*. First performance of:

Open plating of fractures by Sir Wm Arbuthnot Lane in 1903; The intermedullary nail (Gerhard Kuntscher of Hamburg, 1967); The Smith-Petersen nail, 1939; the Charnley arthroplasty, 1970.

Plaster of Paris bandages first used by Anthonius Mathijsen (1805–1878), a Flemish surgeon, in 1852.

Manipulations, requiring good relaxation for a short time, are conveniently done under thiopentone or methohexitone, a relatively large dose being given just before the surgeon is ready to produce his trauma. A relaxant can be added if required. Pre-oxygenation is beneficial.

The application of a tourniquet or Esmarch bandage[134,266] (Johan Friedrich August von Esmarch, 1823–1908, of Kiel) to the lower limb causes a rise in central venous pressure and arterial pressure, which may be serious in handicapped patients, with actual or potential congestive cardiac failure. The pressure in a pneumatic tourniquet should be the arterial pressure plus 30–50 mmHg in the arm and plus 50–70 mmHg in the leg; duration of inflation in the arm should not exceed 1 hour and in the leg, 1½ hours, and should be used with the greatest care in patients with ischaemic vascular disease and if sickle-cell trait is present. Application of an Esmarch bandage may cause the release of a blood clot causing pulmonary embolism.[135] The acidosis resulting from ischaemia in the limb may precipitate a crisis in a patient with sickle-cell disease (*see* Chapter 22). A tourniquet may also be associated with postoperative deep vein thrombosis.[136,137] The pressure gauges of tourniquets used for surgery and anaesthesia, especially if IVRA is used (Chapter 31), should be tested at least monthly to ensure that their measurements are reasonably accurate.[138] The Esmarch bandage should not be used as a tourniquet.

Leg amputations may be done under unilateral intradural spinal analgesia, a method well tolerated in old people undergoing amputation for gangrene: care must be taken, hopefully to keep the block unilateral, by maintaining the lateral position for 20–30 min after subarachnoid injection with the diseased side down. Because of the possibility of phantom limb pain, in amputees this may not be the first choice.[139] Otherwise thiopentone, nitrous-oxide–oxygen with or without a relaxant, a narcotic analgesic, a tracheal tube, or volatile agent. Refrigeration analgesia can be used (*see* Chapter 17). Meticulous preoperative preparation and postoperative care together with low-dose heparin can improve the prognosis of this potentially dangerous operation.[140]

For operations on the limbs, more use should be made of various techniques of regional analgesia including intravenous regional analgesia, sciatic nerve, lumbar plexus compartment block[141] and wrist and finger block, etc. particularly for prolonged postoperative pain relief.[142] (*See also Practical Regional Analgesia* (Lee J. A. and Bryce-Smith R. ed.). Amsterdam: Excerpta Medica Foundation, 1976.)

Internal Fixation of Hip Fractures

A pioneer of the surgery of fracture of the neck of the femur was the Norwegian, Marius Nygaard Smith-Petersen (1886–1953), working in Boston.[143]

Main problems. The patient is usually elderly and often handicapped by cardiovascular and respiratory conditions, diabetes, anaemia, dehydration, mental deterioration and sometimes hypothermia. Many will be suffering from hypoxaemia, perhaps due to fat embolism, and this will be made worse by operation. Abnormalities should be detected and if possible treated before surgery; postponement of the fixation for a few days after injury will not increase morbidity or mortality. A femoral nerve block will ease the pain during movement of the patient.[144] Extradural methadone may have a place.[170]

Anaesthesia. Any reasonable method of pain relief, if carefully applied and if dosage is kept low, is usually safe on the operating table, but postoperative morbidity and mortality may be influenced by the technique employed.[145,146] There are arguments for and against most of the commonly employed procedures, including spontaneous respiration with minimal halothane, narcotic analgesic or trichloroethylene, and IPPV with barbiturate, nitrous oxide, oxygen and a relaxant; hypocapnia must be avoided. Patients in poor condition may be managed by a combination of femoral nerve block, i.v. ketamine and diazepam.[147] Intermittent ketamine, with or without diazepam, is reported to give better results than IPPV with relaxant.[146] Extradural block has been used, while intradural analgesia has been shown to give good results[145] and to reduce postoperative hypoxaemia[148] and even mortality.[149] Postoperative analgesia may be satisfactorily obtained by lateral cutaneous nerve block.[150]

Sequelae and complications. Mortality is said to be more than 27% in patients over 80[151] and is chiefly due to chest infections and to pulmonary embolism. Oxygen therapy and plasma volume expanders may be necessary in the postoperative period. Mortality at 4 weeks following general anaesthesia was 2·7% in a series of patients undergoing operations for fixation of the neck of the femur.[152]

Arthroplasty of the Hip Joint[153]

Problems. The age and size of some patients; bleeding during and after operation; possible lateral position of the patient. The use of polymethyl methacrylate cement to fix the prostheses to the bone, first used in 1953,[154] has been followed by hypotension and even by cardiac standstill, probably due to vasodilatation caused by the systemic absorption of the monomer. The prior infusion of 500 ml of a suitable plasma volume expander will go a long way to counteract this, and a head-down tilt of the table may be helpful. When this cement is used for arthroplasty of the knee joint, the tourniquet prevents absorption of the monomer and consequent blood pressure fall. The surgical contortions may cause injury to leg veins leading to thrombophlebitis. Cardiovascular collapse during this operation may also be due to air embolism. An attempt to prevent this by flushing the marrow cavity of the femoral shaft with CO_2[155] has been made.

Anaesthesia. Many agents and techniques are described,[156] including spontaneous respiration with a volatile agent, and IPPV with relaxant and nitrous oxide and oxygen and narcotic analgesic which may inhibit the hormonal response to surgery. Tracheal intubation is usual and an intravenous drip mandatory. Bleeding is always a problem and is not lessened by neurolept anaesthesia. Some workers advocate hypotensive anaesthesia[157] and if this technique is used, sodium nitroprusside may be preferable to trimetaphan[158] and normovolaemic haemodilution has been employed.[159] Central neural blockade by lowering the blood pressure reduces bleeding and may reduce the incidence of thrombophlebitis. Maintenance of blood pressure by ephedrine, under spinal analgesia does not necessarily increase bleeding.[159] Intradural block has its advocates[160] e.g. 2 ml of hyperbaric 0·5% bupivacaine,[161] and so has extradural analgesia.[162,163] Hypothermia must be prevented. Before the prosthesis is inserted into the femoral shaft, pure oxygen may be given for a few minutes. In high risk patients with cardiovascular conditions, a right atrial catheter may be inserted so that air bubbles can be aspirated.[164]

Complications and sequelae. Thrombophlebitis occurs in about 20% of patients after operation[165] and every method of prevention deserves attention (*see* Chapter 18). It may lead to pulmonary embolism. With extradural block there is improved fibrinolysis and so less tendency for clot formation than if a general anaesthetic is given.[166] Fat embolism is not infrequent and may account for some cases of postoperative hypoxaemia. Air embolism may occur.[167] Fluid must be replaced and if necessary blood, bearing in mind postoperative oozing. Infection, if it occurs, is a very serious sequel and to prevent it the Charnley clean air enclosure has been used successfully.[168]

Acrylic cement was popularized by Sir John Charnley[169] but originated by Haboush.[154] In hip surgery, both pulse rate and ECG monitoring should be routine.

Spinal Fusion
Hypotensive anaesthesia has been recommended to reduce bleeding.[171] The anterior approach in the neck may result in vocal cord paralysis.[172]

Fractures of the Cervical Spine
The patient should be intubated and placed on the operating table with the cervical collar and traction still in place so that the position is not altered. This may be difficult, but the patient usually adopts the position providing the clearest airway. Intubation may be difficult and may require great care.[173] Fixation interferes with the anaesthetist's manoeuvres. Correction of severe flexion deformity of the cervical spine may cause difficulty with intubation. This may be accomplished by passing a nasal tube over a fibreoptic bronchoscope, under topical analgesia.[174] *See also* Chapter 12.

Manipulation and Plaster-of-Paris in Children.
Ketamine has a place in the management of small children who require repeated manipulation and application of plaster-of-Paris.

Arthroscopy
General anaesthesia avoids damage to the instrument from movement. Air embolism has been reported. Arthroscope designed in 1960.[175] For history, *see* McGinty J. B. *J. Irish Coll. Phys. Surg.* 1981, **11**, 63.

It can be successfully done on a 'day-stay' basis.[176]

Operations for Kyphoscoliosis[177] (*See also* p. 400.)
The main problems are prolonged surgery, heat loss, blood loss, poor access to the patient who will be on a Toronto Frame, pre- and postoperative respiratory failure, metabolic acidosis before and after operation, postoperative ileus and severe postoperative pain. In addition, some surgeons may request a 'wake-up test' in which the patient is woken up in the middle of the operation and asked to move his toes, to exclude possible cord compression.[178] At the end of the operation, during which a narcotic, relaxant, nitrous oxide and oxygen technique, with IPPV is usually satisfactory, the muscle relaxant is reversed after the patient is placed supine, to prevent coughing while being moved. A rapid wake-up allows early assessment of toe movement. For postoperative pain, a morphine drip has proved useful.[178] Light general anaesthesia with extradural block has also been recommended.

Laminectomy
First classic description of a prolapsed disc in 1934.[180] Surgery of the thoraco-
lumbar spine demands scrupulous anaesthetic technique and careful positioning
to avoid an increase in pressure in the extradural veins; the main problem is to
produce an ischaemic field. Some workers infiltrate the skin incision and
interspinal region with adrenaline–saline solution to aid haemostasis. Extradural
lumbar block has also been used with success and this we recommend in suitable
patients.

Anaesthesia for *bone-marrow harvest*, for transplantation, *see* Filshie J. and
Pollock A. N. *Anaesthesia* 1984, **39**, 480.

Pain after *Keller's operation* for hallux valgus can be relieved by infiltration of
the pseudarthrosis with bupivacaine.[179]

For more detailed information, *see Anaesthesia for Orthopaedic Patients.*
Loach, A. London: Arnold, 1983.

Otorhinolaryngology

In throat and nose surgery, the problems of anaesthesia are related to the fact
that the operations are carried out on the upper respiratory tract. The
anaesthetist must preserve a clear airway, while allowing the surgeon adequate
access, and must take steps to prevent soiling of the trachea and bronchial tree
with blood and debris. The problems are most evident during operations on the
larynx itself.

The following factors should be considered when surgery is to be carried out
on the upper respiratory tract:

1. Premedication must be adequate, but not heavy enough to cause a sluggish
cough reflex after operation.

2. Smooth induction will reduce the incidence and degree of haemorrhage.

3. No topical analgesic should be applied to the larynx or trachea, as the
cough reflex must be brisk after operation.

4. Entrance of blood and debris into the chest must be prevented by the use of
an inflatable cuff on a tracheal tube and/or efficient pharyngeal packing.

5. The use of a slight reversed Trendelenburg position minimizes venous
oozing.

Induction with thiopentone, intubation using a relaxant, and maintenance
with nitrous oxide, oxygen and a volatile agent, with or without narcotic
analgesic, can usually be relied on to provide a safe and smooth technique.

Intranasal Operations
If topical or regional analgesia is not used, general anaesthesia should be
maintained through an orotracheal tube sealed off with a cuff or a pharyngeal or
nasopharyngeal pack. These packs should not be removed until the return of the
patient's cough reflex. Forgetfulness to remove a pharyngeal pack, on the other
hand, is one of the easiest mistakes for an anaesthetist to make and it can readily
prove fatal. Connections to the tube can conveniently be led down over the
patient's chest. In this position, particularly if the surgeon asks for flexion of the
neck, there is a liability for the tube to kink—a non-kinking tube, such as a
nylon-reinforced or Oxford tube, is advantageous. Muscle relaxants will aid
intubation, but care must be taken to see that the cough reflex is active at the

end of the operation. General anaesthesia may be combined with topical application of vasoconstrictors to the nose (e.g. cocaine 1–10%) to reduce bleeding, or injection into the nasal septum of octopressin and prilocaine[181] (*see* Chapter 31) and block of the sphenopalatine ganglion which carries the vasodilator fibres to the nasal blood vessels.

Anaesthesia for Manipulation of Fractured Nasal Bones
The safe technique involves tracheal intubation with cuff and/or pack to prevent aspiration of blood should haemorrhage occur. The anaesthetic agents should permit rapid return of protective reflexes. If plaster-of-Paris is applied, the closed eyes may be protected with adhesive tape. Minor manipulation can sometimes be carried out under intravenous anaesthesia in the head-down position. Anaesthesia for rhinoplasty, *see* Scott D. L. *Anaesthesia* 1982, **37**, 464.

Tonsillectomy in Children

Premedication
Provision of the right psychological atmosphere is of the greatest value in obtaining smooth induction of anaesthesia without tears. Both preoperative crying and tachycardia are reported to increase bleeding in these operations.[182] Sedative premedication must be given carefully because of possible depressant effect on the cough reflex. When the facilities of a postoperative observation room are available and the nursing supervision before and after operation is skilled and alert, heavy basal narcosis can be prescribed so that the child arrives in the anaesthetic room asleep. Oral trimeprazine (Vallergan) 3 mg/kg body weight given 2 h preoperatively, or, on a weight basis, part of the ampoule containing papaveretum 20 mg and hyoscine 0·4 mg in 1 ml (*see* p. 127). The technique associated with minimal vomiting is premedication with trimeprazine and atropine orally, with relief of postoperative pain by dihydrocodeine.[183] Ketamine 3 mg/kg intramuscularly has been recommended.[184]

Atropine or hyoscine can be given by injection once oral sedative medication has had its effect. Many prefer hyoscine 0·2 mg intramuscularly. Otherwise hyoscine 0·4 mg can be given by mouth.

Where skilled nursing facilities do not exist it is safer to avoid all sedative premedication and use atropine or hyoscine alone for premedication. This is especially true before guillotine tonsillectomy when rapid return of reflexes is essential.

Dissection Tonsillectomy
Many anaesthetists prefer a tracheal tube which may be nasal or oral (if adenoids are to be curetted). An oral tube may be kept clear of the operative field if a Doughty blade on the Boyle–Davis gag is used.[185] The use of a tube allows the plane of anaesthesia to be more easily maintained, reduces oozing and obviates respiratory obstruction. IPPV can be combined with it or the patient allowed to breath a volatile anaesthetic spontaneously. The alternative is endopharyngeal insufflation using the B–D gag, in which case the patient should be taken well down into Plane 3 before the mouth is opened and the operation commenced. If this is not done it may be difficult to maintain adequate anaesthesia until the end of the operation.

Nitrous oxide, oxygen and a volatile agent, or thiopentone and relaxant are satisfactory techniques. The aim should be to have the patient coughing within a minute or two of the completion of the operation. A nasal tube is very satisfactory for *adult tonsillectomy*. Topical application to the tonsillar fossae of 10% lignocaine, used carefully in a spray, is reported to reduce postoperative pain, without interfering with protective reflexes.[186]

Adenoids can be curetted either with the tracheal tube in situ or after its withdrawal when the cough reflex has been re-established.

The patient should be returned to the ward in the tonsil position (semi-prone, prevented from rolling on to his face by a pillow beneath the chest, and prevented from rolling supine by bringing the lower arm behind the body) and remain in this position until full consciousness is regained. Aspirin, because it interferes with blood clotting, should not be used for one week before operation, or for the relief of postoperative pain.

Guillotine Tonsillectomy
A technique popularized in 1910 in the USA and in the UK[187] and still used occasionally.

Premedication is atropine alone. The teeth are examined and any loose ones noted: if these are disturbed they must be accounted for. A Doyen gag is inserted and if possible opened while the child is conscious and he is then anaesthetized with nitrous oxide, oxygen and a volatile agent such as halothane. The tonsils are removed in the supine position with the child breathing air and he is then immediately turned on to his side while the adenoids are curetted. He returns to his bed in the tonsil position, a welter of blood, sweat and tears, but in skilled surgical and anaesthetic hands the results can be good.

Anaesthesia for Post-tonsillectomy Haemorrhage
This can be a grave responsibility. It may be due to platelet dysfunction following aspirin therapy; this can be controlled by a platelet transfusion. It is wise that experienced anaesthetists should be in charge of such difficult cases. The patient is likely to have a stomach full of blood clot and to be shocked. Visible blood loss is only a fraction of total haemorrhage. Blood loss is replaced by transfusion, before reinduction of anaesthesia. After atropine premedication anaesthesia may be induced by the thiopentone, suxamethonium rapid intubation ('crash') technique (*see* p. 446). Some workers prefer induction with an inhalation agent with the patient in the lateral position, initially. Orotracheal intubation is usually employed, but cuffed tubes are not usually recommended in small children. Perioperative suction is likely to be necessary while vomiting of blood after operation must be expected and care taken to prevent its aspiration into the trachea. Aspiration via a gastric tube passed before leaving theatre is advisable. It gets rid of *some* of the blood.

Mortality of tonsillectomy in children varies from about 1 in 1800[188] to 1 in 10 000.[189]

Anaesthesia in Upper Respiratory Tract Obstruction
This may occur: (1) At the lips; (2) In the mouth; (3) In the nose; (4) In the pharynx; (5) In the larynx; (6) In the trachea.
Signs: Stridor; dilating alae nasi; rib and intercostal retraction; use of accessory

muscles, e.g. scalenes and sternomastoids; indrawing over clavicles; perhaps cyanosis.

Symptoms: Dyspnoea; anxiety, restlessness; inability to sleep.

Diagnosis: Inspiratory stridor suggests obstruction at or above cords; expiratory stridor suggests obstruction in bronchial tree; inspiratory with expiratory stridor suggests tracheal obstruction. Soft tissue X-rays of the neck may be useful.

These cases present difficulties because of possible

1. Trismus, e.g. in Ludwig's angina which may not relax with suxamethonium.

2. Voluntary use of accessory muscles of respiration to overcome respiratory obstruction associated with the lesion; if this is present, fatal hypoxia may follow loss of consciousness. Thus tracheostomy under local analgesia may be necessary before the induction of general anaesthesia. Blind nasal intubation in the conscious patient after spraying the nares and larynx with local analgesic solution (cocaine 4% in the nares) may be the method chosen by experienced workers in some cases. The inhalation of a mixture of helium 79% and oxygen 21% has a density of 330 as against 1000 for air. A volatile agent, or cyclopropane, can be added to this mixture and fairly readily inhaled with much less distress to the patient than he experiences with air. Premedication must not depress respiration.

A peritonsillar abscess can be opened under lignocaine or cocaine topical analgesia with the head low. Light general anaesthesia in the same position, with a mouth gag and sucker to hand, is permissible in patients without severe respiratory obstruction.

In severe upper respiratory obstruction, tracheostomy may be necessary before induction of general anaesthesia, or even during induction in an emergency.

When inducing general anaesthesia in a patient with an acute infection of the neck or chronic laryngeal obstruction, who is hypoxic, apnoea must not be produced until it is certain that the lungs can be inflated. One hundred per cent oxygen should be given for 10 min, followed by a smooth nitrous-oxide–oxygen–halothane induction. Early passage of a nasopharyngeal tube will remove any respiratory obstruction due to trismus, or the presence of a bulky or oedematous tongue or pharynx. Blind nasal intubation can then be carried out. A rather small tube, e.g. size 6·5 or 7, is easier to insert than a larger one, and is permissible for short operations.

Laryngectomy

First performed by Theodor Billroth (1829–1924) in Vienna in 1874.[190] The available methods are:

1. With no pre-existing tracheostomy. A cuffed tracheal tube is passed, and a tracheostomy performed towards the end of the operation.

2. Tracheostomy performed immediately before the operation under general or local analgesia—the insertion of a cuffed tube through the opening.

3. Anaesthesia through a pre-existing tracheostomy opening.

Anaesthetic Management

It is important to assess the likelihood of narrowing of the laryngeal aperture by growth clinically (stridor, indirect laryngoscopy), by peak flow meter and from soft-tissue X-rays of the neck. When there is obvious respiratory difficulty, it is wise to intubate or to perform a preliminary tracheostomy under local analgesia. If there is any doubt, it is better to omit respiratory depressant drugs and give atropine or hyoscine alone for premedication.

During induction of anaesthesia care must be taken that control of the airway is maintained. In some cases where there is respiratory obstruction it is difficult to inflate the lung using a bag and mask. Distortion of the normal anatomy by tumour or oedema may render intubation difficult. In these circumstances the authors prefer to give a sleep dose of thiopentone through an indwelling needle. Nitrous oxide and oxygen are given, and ability to inflate the lungs tested by manual compression of the reservoir bag. If this is readily achieved suxamethonium follows, the larynx sprayed with 4% lignocaine, and a large-sized cuffed tracheal tube passed. (Occasionally it is only possible to pass a small tube, and a range of tubes should be available.) Anaesthesia is continued with nitrous oxide and oxygen, supplemented by a volatile agent. The aim is to secure quiet respiration with laryngeal reflexes obtunded. Obstructed inspiration may lead to a negative pressure in neck veins with the danger of air embolism. Construction of a tracheostomy early in the operation simplifies the airway management.

When the larynx is severed from the trachea, the tracheal tube is removed. The surgeon inserts a sterile tube via the tracheostome. The authors have found a cuffed nylon-reinforced latex tube useful for this purpose. It can be led down over the sternum and the connections kept clear of the surgical field. A relaxant/IPPV technique has the disadvantage that the patient is at risk if a pipe connection is dislodged, or from delay during the change of the tracheal tube.

An intravenous drip should be set up. Blood transfusion may be required, particularly if block dissection of the neck is undertaken. After laryngectomy, parenteral nutrition may be undertaken until the suture lines are healed. *See* Chapter 40.

For *laryngofissure*, a cuffed tube is inserted from the mouth before the early dissection is done. After a planned tracheostomy a tube is placed in the trachea by the surgeon and connected to the anaesthetic machine.

Carotid sinus syndrome shown by either or both bradycardia and hypotension may follow dissection round the carotid bulb. Should these signs not disappear following the cessation of surgical stimulus, atropine may be required. This may also be associated with other operations in the neck, e.g. thyroidectomy.

Pharyngolaryngectomy[191]

Cancer of the hypopharynx treated by simple pharyngolaryngectomy to be followed by multi-stage plastic repair causes few anaesthetic problems other than those encountered in laryngectomy. But the more recently developed one-stage operations using colon or stomach as replacement are lengthy and pose additional problems:

1. Space around the patient is restricted, and it is important that the anaesthetist has adequate access.

2. Hypotension and cardiac dysrhythmias can occur during mobilization of the oesophagus and transference of stomach or colon to the neck.

3. Rupture of the trachea has occurred.[192] Should this happen, it becomes impossible to ventilate the lungs until an endobronchial tube is passed below the site of rupture.

4. Total thyroidectomy is also performed. Thyroxine will be required as replacement therapy. Calcium metabolism may be disturbed due to removal of the parathyroids.

5. Postoperative intravenous feeding will be necessary.

(For anaesthetic management of reconstruction of the lower part of the trachea, *see* Kahvyssi D. et al. *Br. J. Anaesth.* 1975, **47**, 82.)

Laryngoscopy[193]

Problems include: (1) Need for relaxation of the jaw and cords; (2) Facility to observe cord movement in some cases; (3) Rise of blood pressure and dysrhythmias associated with manipulation of the larynx; (4) Quick recovery of laryngeal reflexes with absence of spasm; (5) The possible presence of lesions which cause obstruction to the airway. *Local analgesia* (as for Bronchoscopy, *see* Chapter 29). *General anaesthesia* using nitrous oxide, oxygen and a volatile agent. A long plastic 5- or 6-mm cuffed tracheal tube is inserted through the nose so that the tube lies between the arytenoids. Suxamethonium, either in repeated doses or by continuous drip, and IPPV allow early return of reflexes. Awareness must be avoided. A ventilating laryngoscope, employing Sanders insufflation technique for bronchoscopy, can be used.[194] A fibreoptic instrument may be helpful to visualize the larynx and to act as an introducer to facilitate tracheal intubation in difficult cases.

Microsurgery of the Larynx

First use of operating microscope for microsurgery of larynx by Scalco in 1960.[195] This demands meticulous anaesthetic management to provide a relaxed patient who is absolutely immobile with full return of the protective reflexes at the end of the procedure. The following techniques have been recommended:

1. Thiopentone, nitrous oxide, oxygen and non-depolarizing relaxant or volatile agent. Topical analgesia helps to ensure smooth quiet resumption of respiration. An oral or nasal tracheal cuffed tube of 5–6 mm internal diameter is used.[196,197] Its use allows adequate pulmonary ventilation using IPPV without encroaching on the surgical field. The cuff prevents blood from trickling down the trachea. The patient is placed in the lateral position before extubation.

2. Neuroleptanalgesia has been recommended. Arterial blood pressure rises during microlaryngoscopy but can be prevented from so doing by i.v. fentanyl.[198] A tracheal tube is not used. *See* Chapter 13. The Kleinsasser laryngoscope can also be modified to carry a side-tube which can be used to administer oxygen and anaesthetic gases into the laryngeal lumen at any stage.

3. Deep halothane anaesthesia followed by nasopharyngeal insufflation of halothane has been recommended in children. Spontaneous respiration is maintained, and the tube does not reach the larynx. Topical lignocaine spray is helpful.

4. The Sanders oxygen injector, as used to maintain pulmonary ventilation during bronchoscopy, can be modified for attachment to the laryngoscope used for microsurgery. If the injector is placed below the cords there is little risk of blowing blood clot down the tracheobronchial tree. This can be achieved by puncture of the cricothyroid membrane and passage of an intravenous catheter which replaces the jet.[199] Alternatively, the thin catheter can be passed via the mouth.[200] An injector device can also be made for insertion in to the trachea through the cords.[201] There is a risk of hyperinflation of the lung and surgical emphysema if upper airway obstruction prevents free exhalation.[202] The problem is that during expiration, blood and mucus may shoot up all over the surgeon!

Laser Surgery to the Larynx

The surgeon, using the operating microscope, guides the laser beam to excise lesions of the larynx. It is necessary that the target should remain quiescent, but when regular movements occur (as with the use of the Sanders injector), the surgeon can time his manipulations to coincide with the rhythm produced by the anaesthetist. When a tracheal tube is used, there is a danger of ignition of the tube by the laser in the presence of a nitrous-oxide–oxygen mixture, with results likely to be fatal. Techniques to maintain ventilation, using a full relaxant technique include:

1. Use of a metal tube which will not ignite.[203]

2. Protection of the tube by wrapping it in aluminium tape.

3. Avoidance of a tube, ventilation being maintained by a Sanders injector attached to the surgeon's laryngoscope.

4. Use of a respiratory mixture made non-explosive by dilution with nitrogen or helium, to keep the percentage of oxygen below 30%.[204] Nitrous oxide also supports combustion.

5. Patients with a pre-existing tracheostomy are best managed by retaining the silver tracheostomy tube in position.

The Medical Laser

The laser is a light beam (*L*ight *A*mplification by *S*timulated *E*mission of *R*adiation) of radiation which can be focused on to a very small spot. The CO_2 surgical laser vaporizes tissue on this spot but surrounding tissue is hardly affected by the temperature rise; coagulation damage is therefore closely confined. It is sufficient for the control of bleeding, with minimal oedema formation and good healing. These are attractive features in surgery of the larynx. Lasers can also be focused into an optical fibre for endoscopy work.

All surgical lasers present potential hazard to both patients and staff. The eyes and skin of the former must be protected. Lasers can also ignite combustible materials.

Injuries to Larynx and Trachea (including Cut Throat)[205]

These may occur as a result of accident or attempted suicide. The wound may be open and clear or there may be considerable tissue destruction. Closed injuries may cause haematoma or surgical emphysema. First-aid treatment includes hemostasis by digital pressure or surgical clip. Intravenous fluids may be required. A clear airway must be established and pneumothorax excluded or if necessary treated. Spinal cord lesions can occur. The patient should be nursed in head-down position to prevent air being sucked into an open vein.

Anaesthesia may be hazardous due to blood and debris in the airway and a full stomach. Gastric tubes or cricothyroid pressure may be contra-indicated if there is a risk of increasing tissue damage. The first priority is maintenance of the airway and, if necessary, a tracheal tube must be passed in the awake patient. The method of anaesthesia will depend upon assessment of the individual case. Local analgesia is sometimes indicated. Muscle relaxants must not be used unless the anaesthetist is confident of maintaining ventilation. Tracheostomy is occasionally necessary. The fibreoptic laryngoscope has proved useful when obstruction is due to a damaged epiglottis.[206] (*See also* Flood I. M. and Astley B. *Br. J. Anaesth.* 1982, **54**, 1339.)

Tracheostomy
P. F. Bretonneau (1778–1962) of Tours performed a tracheostomy (for diphtheria) in 1825.

General Anaesthesia
Patients in the intensive therapy unit may well have a tracheal tube in place already. If not, an orotracheal tube is inserted after induction of light general anaesthesia with muscle relaxants if necessary. The cuff of the tracheal tube should not be deflated before the trachea is opened and the tube should not be withdrawn through the cords until the tracheostomy tube is satisfactorily in place. This allows ready replacement of the original tube should difficulties arise. Care should be taken when patients are already on mechanical ventilation or when muscle relaxants are used so that there is a rapid and smooth transfer of anaesthetic connections from one tube to the other. (*See also Br. J. Hosp. Med.* 1976, **16**, 78.)

Local Analgesia
Emergency tracheostomy under local analgesia is rarely justified today as tracheal intubation to ensure a clear airway throughout the procedure offers a positive advantage. It should be undertaken only when respiratory obstruction prevents introduction of a tracheal tube. Extension of the neck to facilitate surgical access may actually increase the degree of obstruction in some cases.

Anaesthesia for Tracheal Resection
Anaesthesia for resection of tracheal stenosis can be performed using high-frequency jet ventilation.[207]
See Mounir N. et al. *Can. Anaesth. Soc. J.* 1979, **26**, 26 and Harrison, M. J. *Anaesthesia* 1985, **40**, 708; Baraka A. *Anesth. Analg. (Cleve.)* 1977, **56**, 429.

Anaesthesia for Excision of Pharyngeal Pouch
Pharyngeal pouch first described by Ludlow of Bristol in 1764.[208] The anaesthetist may be asked to pack the pouch with gauze, after induction, to help with its identification. Contents of the pouch may spill into the pharynx during induction.

Excision of Pharyngeal Pouch
The patient may have undergone recurrent chest infections due to aspiration of pouch contents. The anaesthetist should be aware of this possibility associated with induction of anaesthesia. Cricoid pressure does not prevent regurgitation from the pouch. Endoscopy may be carried out to identify the pouch and pack it with gauze prior to neck exploration. This can be removed by the anaesthetist when it is no longer required. Sometimes operative treatment may be carried out endoscopically when the 'carina' between pouch and oesophagus is removed by diathermy.

Operations on the Middle and Inner Ear
A. F. von Troeltsch (1829–1890) invented the otoscope in 1860 and performed the first mastoid operation for suppurative otitis media in 1861. Julius Lempert, New York otologist pioneered fenestration in 1938.[114]

Myringotomy

For all patients other than young children, an aerosol spray of 10% lignocaine can be directed towards the upper wall of the auditory canal, so that the solution runs downwards on to the drum and so avoids pain and coldness on the drum head. Otherwise general anaesthesia is required. When the operating microscope is used, a tracheal tube helps to avoid airway obstruction and provides a still field. Vagal cardiac arrest may occur if the 'vagal' area of the tympanic membrane (supplied by the auricular branch) is incised. Atropine will prevent this.

Mastoid Operations

Some surgeons like to be able to observe facial twitching should the facial nerve be stimulated by manipulations in the vicinity. Immediate steps can then be taken for decompression should injury be demonstrated. For this reason some surgeons and anaesthetists avoid the use of muscle relaxants. The operations of *myringoplasty, tympanoplasty* and *stapedectomy* are greatly facilitated by the provision of an ischaemic field.[209] This may be provided by the use of standard techniques (*see* Chapter 16). The authors prefer the use of oxygen–halothane, using a non-kinking tube, with or without IPPV. Blood pressure must be monitored and the use of a pulse monitor and ECG is helpful (*see* Chapter 41). Some workers use direct intra-arterial measurements.[210]

In all ear operations there are theoretical considerations which may arise due to diffusion of nitrous oxide into the middle ear if that agent is used for anaesthesia.[211] Nitrous oxide will cause increased pressure within the middle ear with bulging of the intact drum. When the patient is breathing a nitrous oxide mixture spontaneously, middle ear pressure can increase by $39\,mmH_2O$ per minute; with IPPV it may increase by $63\,mmH_2O$ per minute, and these pressures can be reached within 5 min.[212] This may be important during operations such as myringoplasty. The problem is avoided if nitrous oxide is discontinued 30 min before anticipated placement of the graft. Anaesthesia may be maintained with intravenous agents or combinations such as oxygen and halothane until surgery is completed. Air may be used for IPPV.[213]

Anaesthesia for removal of inhaled foreign bodies in children *see* Baraka A. *Br. J. Anaesth.* 1974, **46**, 124.

Plastic Surgery and Burns

For history of the treatment of burns, *see* Wallace A. F. *Hosp. Update* 1980, **6**, 375; McGinty J. B. *J. Irish Coll. Phys. Surg.* 1981, **11**, 63.

Burned patients require relief from pain and the maintenance of a free airway. Burns can often be cleaned and dressed under a narcotic analgesic, given slowly by intravenous injection so that the minimal effective dosage can be ascertained. Alternatively, neurolept analgesia can be used. Yet another technique combines Entonox with intravenous droperidol 0·2 mg/kg, and phenoperidine 0·03–0·05 mg/kg. Antibiotics, antipseudomonas vaccine (PEVOI) and multiple skin-grafting operations may be required.

General anaesthesia is often carried out using thiopentone, non-depolarizing muscle relaxant, nitrous-oxide–oxygen, with analgesic supplement.[214] Large tidal volumes are advocated as alveolar ventilation should be high. Controlled hypotension has been advocated[215] to reduce blood loss during tangential excision when removal of layers of burnt tissue is associated with considerable haemorrhage.

The danger of suxamethonium used for tracheal intubation in anaesthesia for burns has been pointed out. Cardiac arrest, perhaps due to increased serum potassium, would seem to be a definite danger in such cases, especially if the initial burns occurred between 3 and 7 weeks before the anaesthesia. Intravenous atropine should reduce the risk of cardiac arrest. Serum cholinesterase may be low.

Ketamine has been recommended for treatment of burns, especially where scarring of the neck makes airway maintenance difficult. Dose about 2 mg/kg i.v. or 10 mg/kg i.m. Small doses, 4 mg/kg i.m., have been used for tangential excision[216] or even 1·5 mg/kg with or without diazepam.[217] It is not a suitable technique for repeated burns dressings in an effort to maintain normal feeding, as the larynx does not always protect the lungs from soiling, during ketamine anaesthesia. It is useful for setting up drips in burned children.

The Respiratory Injury in Burns
This may be due to inhalation of hot gas, smoke or poisonous fumes from burning plastics. Inhalation of carbon monoxide is also an occasional problem. Raised carboxyhaemoglobin levels have been found in the blood of victims dying in house fires.[218] In survivors, raised levels are associated with clinical evidence of inhalation of smoke;[219] oxygen therapy is therefore of value. Cyanide levels are also increased in those with raised carboxyhaemoglobin.[219]

Assessment
(1) Clinical—coughing, the nature of the sputum (e.g. carbon-stained), pulmonary oedema, cyanosis, dyspnoea; (2) Blood gases, chest X-ray.

Management
(1) Oxygen inhalation; (2) High-humidification, nebulized-water droplet inhalation; (3) Steroid therapy; (4) IPPV if necessary. Respiratory obstruction may occur in the glottic region and nasotracheal intubation is advocated in cases of doubt.[220] The use of a fibreoptic bronchoscope, in skilled hands may be useful in diagnosis.[221] Tracheostomy is to be avoided if possible because of the risk of infection.

Lower airways obstruction occurs due to toxic fumes. Respiratory failure may be delayed until the 4th to the 10th day. The clinical picture which develops may be of adult respiratory distress syndrome.

The burned patient may be hypovolaemic with loss of water and protein from the circulation. Intravenous infusion may be necessary with plasma administration as indicated by frequent microhaematocrit estimation. Size of the burn may be assessed by the 'rule of nines' in which the head is assessed as 9% of body surface area, arms 9% each, thorax 18%, abdomen 18% and legs 18% each.

Renal failure, associated with either haemoglobinuria or myoglobinuria, may occur. In the presence of dark brown or coloured urine, urine output should be increased to prevent renal damage. Alkalinization of the urine is also protective.

Hypercatabolism is frequently a problem (*see also* Davies J. W. L. *J. R. Soc. Med.* 1982, **75**, Suppl. 1, 20). The rise in metabolic rate following burns is greater than after other forms of trauma. There is loss of body heat, disturbance of the vasoconstrictor mechanism, and a reset of the hypothalamic thermostat, all made worse by pain and apprehension. There is a rise in plasma catecholamines, cortisol and glucagon.[222] Hyperglycaemia is common and there is probably enhanced degradation of insulin. Energy requirement may be as high as 17 MJoules/24 h (4000 Kcal). Palatable food is best but will often need to be supplemented by enteral tube feeding and sometimes parenteral nutrition if alimentary function is disturbed. During anaesthesia, hypermetabolism is reflected in the need for increased alveolar ventilation. Hyponatraemia is a frequent complication. A urinary catheter may be necessary. A rapid load of salt-containing fluid is recommended, diminishing over 48 h or when urine secretion has been achieved (*see also* Settle J. A. D. *J. R. Soc. Med.* 1983, **72**, Suppl. 1, 6). Plasma protein fraction has also been used to maintain normal central venous pressure and urine output. In war or disaster situations, a mixture of Hartmann's solution and gelatin solution has been used.[223] (*See also* Diamond A. W. et al. *Anaesthesia* 1975, **30**, 791. The Experts Opine *Survey of Anesthesiology* 1978, **22**, 89; Hackett M. E. J. *Hospital Update* 1980, **6**, 963; Modern Trends in Burns Care; Symposium *J. R. Soc. Med.* 1982, Suppl. 1, 75; Brown J. and Ward D. J. *Br. J. Hosp. Med.* 1984, **31**, 360; Brown J. in: *Recent Advances in Anaesthesia and Analgesia*—15 (Atkinson R. S. and Adams A. P. ed.) Edinburgh: Churchill Livingstone, 1985; Martyn J. *Anesthesiology* 1986, **65**, 67.)

Plastic Surgery

History

For history of plastic surgery, *see* Bennett J. P. *J. R. Soc. Med.* 1983, **76**, 152.

First described in Europe by Tagliacozzi (1546–1599) in 1586.[224] Thiersch graft described in 1874;[225] Wolfe's full-thickness grafts in 1875;[226] and the split-skin graft in 1929.[227] It was in connection with the development of plastic surgery at the Queen's Hospital, Sidcup, by Sir Harold Gillies[228] that Magill and Rowbotham developed insufflation, then inhalation endotracheal anaesthesia in the UK.[229]

Skin grafts can often be removed painlessly from the thigh after block of the lateral femoral cutaneous and, if necessary, the femoral nerves, or by intradermal and subcutaneous infiltration of skin of anterior part of thigh. Work has also been done on superficial freezing of donor areas by ice-bags. The main problems in anaesthesia for plastic surgery are: (1) Access—this may be restricted because of facial injuries, scars, cleft palate, or because of bizarre positions requested by plastic surgeons; (2) Provision of ischaemic skin to facilitate the work of the surgeon—this may conflict with the priority for cerebral perfusion, e.g. during mammoplasty with the patient in the sitting position.

For anaesthetic management of patients undergoing operations for free flap transfer it is important to prevent vasoconstriction in the skin with: sodium nitroprusside; light general anaesthesia; maintenance of arterial blood pressure above 100 mmHg; maintenance of normal P_{CO_2} and P_{O_2}; adequate circulatory volume and avoidance of cooling; good postoperative analgesia and avoidance of bradycardia with its possibility of diminished cardiac output. Central neural blockade does not prevent arterial muscle spasm.[230]

The anaesthetist in the plastic unit needs to have a strong feeling for the theatrical and a good sense of humour.

(For an early history of plastic surgery in the UK *see* Bodenham D. C. *Ann. R. Coll. Surg. Eng.* 1981, **63**, 233.)

Radiology

(*See Proc. R. Soc. Med.* 1975, **68**, 765; *also* Chapters 26 and 30.)

General Considerations

An increasing number of diagnostic and therapeutic procedures are now taking place in X-ray departments. Many of these do not require surgical incision or general anaesthesia. Interventional radiology has applications in biopsy procedures, decompression and drainage of abnormal collections of fluid, extraction of stones and vascular procedures. Coronary angioplasty allows treatment of some cases of coronary artery occlusion, though facilities must be available for cardiopulmonary by-pass procedures if required. Those working in the radiology department must be competent to treat cardiopulmonary collapse. Balloons can also be employed in the carotid artery in selected cases.[231]

Carotid angiograms frequently require IPPV to reduce the Pa_{CO_2} to 3·5 kPa (*see also* Chapter 26).

Lumbar Aortograms. IPPV is not necessary. The patient lies prone. Immobilization of children for various scanning procedures may be achieved by heavy premedication (including rectal ketamine)[232] or general anaesthesia. Adults may occasionally require general anaesthesia, e.g. spontaneous respiration using either enflurane or isoflurane is satisfactory.[233]

Systemic reactions to intravascular contrast media.[234] Patients undergoing this procedure should have ECG and BP monitoring. There should be regular cardiopulmonary resuscitation drills for the Radiology staff together with the availability of respiratory care equipment, oxygen, plasma volume expander, suction, atropine, diphenhydramine, steroid and adrenaline. Reactions are not uncommon and may occur in young healthy patients but are more likely to occur in patients with strong allergic, asthmatic, atopic or cardiac histories. Reactions may be of five types, single or multiple; vasomotor, vasovagal, dermal, osmotic or anaphylactic.

To prevent pain during intra-arterial injection of contrast media, lignocaine can be used.[235] Bupivacaine may also be employed.[236]

All varieties of arteriography, including aortography, cerebral, femoral and brachial are rendered virtually painless by the use of the newer low osmolar contrast media iohexol, iopamidol, iogalate and, to a less extent, metrizamide. They are much more expensive however.[237]

Urology

Max Nitze of Germany (1848–1906) developed the first electrically illuminated cystoscope in 1879. Sir Peter Freyer (1852–1921) developed suprapubic prostatectomy in London in 1901. Millin's retropubic operation first performed in 1945.

Main problems. Normal operative procedures cause little change in the renal circulation, but often result in oliguria and fluid retention. Under anaesthesia the blood pressure is a poor guide to the renal circulation but function is seriously impaired with pressures below 60 mmHg. Total renal ischaemia of more than 30-min duration is likely to result in damage to the tubules.

Uraemia. Many patients undergoing urological operations are old, atheromatous, and suffering from disease of the kidneys and cardiovascular system. A high blood urea may be associated with a decreased tolerance towards intravenous barbiturates and narcotic analgesics, which should be used carefully. Uraemia, which is due to renal failure, may be associated with the passage of too little, too much or a normal volume of urine. The patient may complain of nausea, vomiting or diarrhoea. There may be electrolyte imbalance, elevation of the serum potassium, metabolic acidosis, anaemia, cardiac failure, halitosis from ammoniacal decomposition of the salivary urea, drowsiness, convulsions and coma. The blood urea seldom rises above normal until the glomerular filtration rate has fallen to about 25% of normal. Symptoms due to uraemia are rare until the blood urea approaches 15 mmol/l. Vomiting, if severe and persistent, may result in hypokalaemia and hyponatraemia. Old patients are usually more placid and philosophical than young patients, so are often good subjects for regional analgesia, which may be especially suitable in uraemia. Premedication should be minimal and, when necessary, atropine should be used in all patients over the age of about 60, rather than hyoscine.

Nephrectomy
First performed by Gustav Simon (1824–1913) of Heidelberg, in 1870.
Nerve supply to kidney, ureter and bladder—All arise in the 10th, 11th, 12th thoracic and 1st lumbar segments. Abnormal peristalsis of the ureter, causing pain, may be relieved by atropine, probanthine, hyoscine-n-methyl bromide (Buscopan) and the narcotic analgesics. The bladder, lower ends of the ureters and the prostate are supplied by filaments of the inferior hypogastric plexus. This is formed from: (1) The sympathetic T.11 to L.2 roots; (2) The parasympathetic— S.2, S.3 and S.4.

Lateral position throws strain on respiratory efficiency of patient, for although perfusion of the alveoli in the lower lung is increased, ventilation is decreased. Nevertheless, oxygen uptake from the lower lung is always greater. A reduction of minute volume of 9% occurs in the lateral position with spontaneous breathing. Use of kidney bridge increases this strain, and further predisposes to postoperative atelectasis of dependent lower zone. Occlusion of the inferior vena cava may occur with the use of the kidney bridge in the lateral position, leading to sudden severe hypotension. A tracheal tube is usually required.

When the patient is turned on his back at the end of the operation the opportunity to expand the lower lung fully should be taken.

Nitrous-oxide–oxygen, with thiopentone and a relaxant and perhaps a narcotic analgesic, makes a useful combination with IPPV, and so does a volatile agent with either spontaneous or assisted respiration.

Intradural analgesia is useful when the patient is fit and muscular, and extradural block gives good results. Owing to the discomfort of the lateral position, light general anaesthesia is often a useful supplement. Analgesia must ascend to T.8. Neither method greatly influences the tone of the ureters.

Rarely, the pleura is damaged during kidney operations; the resulting collapse of the upper lung may, in association with the handicapped lower lung, prove dangerous unless IPPV is employed. An underwater drain in the early postoperative period may be required.

Transplantation of the ureter requires maximal relaxation, obtained either by extradural analgesia or by a muscle relaxant with light general anaesthesia.

Patients who have undergone a ureterosigmoidostomy may develop a hyperchloraemic acidosis due to reabsorption of chloride from the bowel, and a hypokalaemia, the latter giving rise to muscular weakness, and even respiratory paralysis. Serum electrolytes should be checked daily and normal saline infusions avoided. Treatment includes potassium replacement and, if necessary, assisted respiration. These electrolyte changes do not occur with transplantation into an ileal loop.

Tumour embolus causing collapse and cardiac arrest is an occasional complication of operations for carcinoma of the kidney.

Transurethral Resection of the Prostate (TURP)
Thiopentone–nitrous-oxide–oxygen and an analgesic supplement with or without a relaxant are suitable. Low intradural spinal block is very satisfactory, e.g. bupivacaine, 0·5% solution, 2–4 ml.[238] Lumbar or sacral extradural block may also be used.

Water may be absorbed into the vascular system (transurethral prostatectomy TURP syndrome) and result in: (1) Haemolysis with subsequent renal damage; (2) Water intoxication which results when a greatly increased volume of water enters the circulation. It causes a dilutional hyponatraemia which may lead to prolonged action of non-depolarizing relaxants, cerebral or pulmonary oedema, raised blood pressure, acute left ventricular failure, cardiac arrest,[242] nausea, vomiting, headache, and possibly convulsions and coma. Postoperative hyponatraemia must be sought for and treated.[239] Water intoxication may lead to bradycardia, rise in both systolic and diastolic arterial pressure, cerebral agitation and depression. The resulting hyponatraemia may cause a widening of the QRS complex and T-wave inversion. Treatment is up to 100 ml of 5% sodium chloride i.v. with an osmotic diuretic.[240] The TURP syndrome may give rise to pulmonary oedema, cerebral and cardiac problems, is difficult to predict and to manage if fully developed. If possible it should be prevented by monitoring the sodium in the serum during the operation and treating any patient with a concentration of less than 120 mmol/l with frusemide 20 mg i.v. and 500 ml of 1·8% sodium chloride.[241] Normal serum sodium is 131–140 mmol/l and it may be decreased to about 120 mmol/l. Intravenous sodium chloride 5% solution and a loop diuretic[242] may be helpful in treatment. Normal saline, used for irrigation, partly dissipates the electric current of the diathermy. Cold irrigating solutions may cause hypothermia.[243]Glycine 1·5% at an optimal pressure of 70 cm H_2O, used for irrigation, may result in excretion of large amounts of oxalate and glycolate which may be dangerous if the urinary flow rate is allowed to drop during the first 10 days or so after operation. The use of glycine does not always prevent over hydration and ECG monitoring is desirable when irrigating fluid is used. Glycine 1·5% is hypotonic. Its non-electrolytic nature prevents dissipation of diathermy current during prostatic resection.

Oozing during this operation may be increased by anything raising the central venous pressure, e.g. straining, vascular over-load with irrigating fluid, over-transfusion; by pressor drugs and by prolonged operation time. If the blood pressure can be maintained at a steady 80 mmHg, oozing is minimized. Blood loss is usually less with central neural blockade than with general anaesthesia. It increases with duration of operation and the weight of tissue removed.[244]

For anaesthetic and perioperative management of insertion of peritoneovenous shunt, *see* Bettaney D. A. M. et al. *Anaesth. Intensive Care* 1982, **10**, 108.

Abdominal Prostatectomy[245]

Sir Peter Freyer (1852–1921) was a pioneer of the suprapubic, Terence Millin of the retropubic operation. Relaxation is required and considerable haemorrhage may occur. *Extradural analgesia* using 7–20 ml of 1·5% lignocaine or 7–15 ml of plain bupivacaine 0·5%, with or without light general anaesthesia, gives good results, especially if emphysema and bronchospasm are also present. *Intradural spinal analgesia* to T.10, obtained by bupivacaine, prilocaine or lignocaine, provides relaxation and reduces haemorrhage. The blood pressure can, in these cases, be maintained by intravenous infusion and suitable drugs, e.g. ephedrine, should this be thought necessary. (*See also* Chapter 32.)

Many workers prefer for prostatectomy a *general anaesthetic*, e.g. thiopentone with nitrous-oxide–oxygen, relaxant, IPPV technique, with or without an analgesic or volatile supplement. Blood should be available for transfusion to replace the measured amount lost. To reduce the incidence of clot retention intravenous mannitol 10%, 1 litre in 4 hours, has been found to be superior to frusemide.[246] During transvesical prostatectomy there is considerable heat loss, so intravenous fluids should be warmed.[247]

Hypotensive Anaesthesia

Good results are obtained in experienced hands, with low morbidity and mortality. *See also* Chapter 16.

Prostatic Biopsy

This may be performed under general anaesthesia, local analgesia or sedation with diazepam and a narcotic analgesic.[248]

Transurethral resection of a bladder tumour may result in movement of the patient's legs due to stimulation of the obturator nerve. Muscle relaxants or obturator nerve block will prevent this.[249]

Cystoscopy

The first electrically illuminated cystoscope was introduced in 1879 by Max Nitze (1848–1906) of Berlin.[250] If a *general anaesthetic* is used for cystoscopy, the anaesthetist must provide: (1) Complete loss of sensation; (2) Relaxation of bladder sphincters and abdominal wall; (3) Quiet breathing through a patent airway; (4) Freedom from hazard of explosion. In the authors' opinion, this anaesthetic procedure can be difficult to accomplish smoothly, e.g. in emphysematous old men with bronchitis. It should never be undertaken lightly and may require tracheal intubation. Even in experienced hands, anaesthesia for cystoscopy is often inelegantly given. Halothane and oxygen with or without nitrous oxide or other volatile agents is an excellent choice, while an i.v. narcotic analgesic may be a useful addition. Repeated cystoscopy may be required.

Topical analgesia is fairly satisfactory, e.g. lignocaine 1 or 2% jelly, but should not be used after recent instrumentation or in the presence of bleeding from the urethra (*see* Chapter 31). Cases with gross cystitis are often unsuitable for local analgesia as the distension of the bladder with irrigating fluid causes painful spasm. Women will frequently tolerate this examination without general anaesthesia if topical analgesia and simple sedatives are used, e.g. diazepam. *Extradural sacral block* is very satisfactory as is low *intradural* spinal analgesia.

Circumcision

In babies and children nitrous-oxide–oxygen and volatile agent, e.g. halothane. Induction can be carried out with nitrous-oxide–oxygen halothane, cyclopropane, or intravenous agent. Babies easily develop laryngeal spasm, sometimes necessitating interruption of the operation until the airway is patent again. Adequate depth of anaesthesia before the infliction of surgical trauma will usually prevent what may be a very dangerous complication. Other workers, experienced in infant anaesthesia, prefer intravenous barbiturate, suxamethonium, intubation and nitrous oxide–oxygen given by IPPV with a volatile agent and narcotic analgesic. *In adults*, thiopentone, with nitrous oxide and oxygen, and perhaps a volatile agent or a narcotic analgesic,[251] extradural sacral block, or regional block (*see* Chapter 31). Extradural sacral injection of bupivacaine (0·5%) will control postoperative pain in children[251] (*see* Chapter 32). In adults the injection of 1·5 ml of 1% lignocaine or 0·5% bupivacaine into each dorsal nerve of the penis will achieve the same result. Smaller doses can be used for children. Postoperative phenobarbitone or β-blocker medication for 3 days helps to prevent painful erections after operation.

Vasectomy

Innervation of the scrotum and its contents is derived from T.10 and T.11 (splanchnic) and L.1 and L.2 together with S.2 and S.3 somatic. While most of these operations can be done under local infiltration analgesia,[252] many surgeons of experience prefer general anaesthesia as it reduces the incidence of haematoma formation. This may be partly due to the pre- and postoperative sedation and the short bed-rest required. Traction on the cord may result in cardiac arrest; preoperative atropine is desirable.[253]

Renal Transplantation

First transplantation of a kidney by Richard H. Lawler (1935–1982) in 1950. For history, *see* Starzl T. E. *Surg. Clin. North Am.* 1978, **58**, 552. Immunological basis of tissue rejection described by Medawar in 1944.[254] Patients awaiting renal transplantation have usually suffered from chronic renal failure for some time and have had repeated haemodialysis. The oxygen pathway to the tissues may be compromised by the presence of pulmonary oedema, lung infections and anaemia. Transfusions should not be given except to replace blood loss as they may lead to haemosiderosis and the stimulation of cytotoxic antibodies. Hypertension is commonly present and this may be treated with methyldopa, while digoxin may be indicated in the presence of heart failure. Neurological complications may develop in cases of long-standing renal failure and may take the form of tremor, convulsions, coma, peripheral neuropathy and myopathy. Diabetic patients may present a particular hazard associated with hyperkalaemic peaks related to hyperglycaemia.[255]

Haemodialysis

Insertion of a Scribner shunt involves the insertion of an arterial and venous cannula with connecting link, in either the arm or leg. General anaesthesia and local infiltration with lignocaine have been used but are not always satisfactory.

Regional analgesia with bupivacaine has been advocated; axillary brachial plexus block with 10–15 ml 0·5% solution for the arm; sciatic and femoral block for the leg (15–20 ml and 10 ml solution).

When anaesthetizing a patient on renal dialysis, the following points must be kept in mind: preoperative preparation must be thorough; anaemia is usually present; there may be impaired excretion of some of the drugs used; intravenous infusions must not be given into the arm with the fistula; blood loss must be monitored and replaced as necessary; because of its renal excretion, gallamine is not the first choice of relaxants; suxamethonium should be avoided where possible because of the raised serum potassium.

Preoperative Preparation
Adequate correction of anaemia, acidosis, electrolyte imbalance, etc. is seldom possible as renal transplantation is carried out as an emergency procedure when a suitable donor is available. The stomach may not be empty. Veins may be difficult. Preoperative preparation should include tissue typing, provision of 2 units of matched blood, and estimation of haemoglobin, urea and electrolytes.

Technique
Oral magnesium trisilicate 30 ml has been advocated to reduce stomach acidity in case of regurgitation. Premedication may be with atropine only. Inhalation induction spares veins. A suitable technique is preoxygenation, cyclopropane induction, tracheal intubation after suxamethonium, and maintenance with nitrous oxide–oxygen, a volatile agent or fentanyl, muscle relaxants and IPPV. Atracurium is the preferred relaxant as recovery of muscular tone does not depend on renal function. The use of suxamethonium is feared by some because of the elevation of serum potassium which may occur in a patient who already has hyperkalaemia. The rise is likely to be less than 0·7 mmol/l with a single dose of 1 mg/kg but may be greater when repeated doses are given or in the presence of peripheral neuropathy.[256] There may be a rise in blood pressure on release of renal clamps. Other techniques which have been advocated for renal transplantation include intradural or extradural spinal block and neuroleptanalgesia. Fluid overload is to be avoided and intravenous fluids containing potassium should not be used. Blood transfusion is recommended when 10% of the blood volume has been lost. (*See also* Farman J. V. in: *Recent Advances in Anaesthesia and Analgesia*—12 (Hewer C. L. and Atkinson R. S. ed.). Edinburgh: Churchill Livingstone, 1976.) Following five years' experience of renal transplantation anaesthesia in 270 patients, intravenous induction, suxamethonium and intubation, tubocurarine, IPPV with narcotic and halothane supplements, with reversal of the relaxant by atropine and neostigmine is recommended as a good and safe technique.[257]

Percutaneous Lithotripsy
Stones in the genitourinary tract can now be dispersed without operation in many cases by extracorporeal shock-wave lithotripsy (ESWL). Although non-invasive, the technique causes pain and this can be relieved by either central neural blockade up to T.6, by intercostal block and local infiltration.[267] or by routine general anaesthesia.[258]

Helmstein Balloon[259]

The balloon is placed inside the bladder and inflated. The aim is to cause necrosis of tumour cells which are susceptible to ischaemia by pressure from the inflated balloon. It is necessary to maintain this system for periods of about 6 h.

An extradural block up to T.10 is carried out with an extradural catheter, providing pain relief and reduction of systolic blood pressure below 100 mmHg, i.e. below the pressure in the balloon.[260] Some workers use two catheters, the lower one at L.4–5 to control pain and an upper one at T.12–L.1 to control arterial pressure.

Vascular Surgery

Anaesthesia for Peripheral Vascular Surgery

The blood pressure should be well maintained. Muscular relaxation is not necessary unless the operation proceeds into the abdomen. The patient is placed on a warming mattress. A large-bore drip cannula is inserted and blood warmer used. Some workers employ an extradural catheter to enable local analgesic drugs or narcotic analgesics to be injected in the postoperative period. The general condition of patients is often poor as they have other manifestations of arterial disease.

Main problems—poor cardiovascular reserve, with tendency to vascular accidents, massive transfusion, clotting problems, high blood viscosity. The haemoglobin level and red cell count are often high, and abnormal fibrinogens contribute to this viscosity. Haemodilution with dextran 70 or other colloid is often beneficial. Peripheral vascular disease; non-invasive physiological measurements (*see* Clifford P. C. *Br. J. Hosp. Med.* 1984, **32**, 82).

Anaesthesia for Carotid Artery Surgery
See Chapter 26.

Anaesthesia for Leaking Aortic Aneurysm

First resection of an aortic aneurysm performed in 1951.[261] This condition carries a high mortality. Patients are usually in poor general condition and may be suffering from shock, ileus due to retroperitoneal haematoma, or haematemesis from leakage into the duodenum from the aneurysm. Large volumes of blood may be required with the usual risks which may follow massive transfusion, such as a failure of clotting mechanism, accidental hypothermia, and calcium and potassium imbalance requiring intravenous calcium. Blood filters and warmers are used. Autotransfusion may be required. Several large-bore drips may be needed. Metabolic acidosis may occur.

If the lesion is above the origin of the renal arteries the outlook is especially grave as the application of an aortic tourniquet is likely to cause renal and spinal cord ischaemia with irreversible damage.

The technique of general anaesthesia should provide tracheal intubation free from the risk of aspiration of stomach contents with induction preferably in the head-down position because of the associated shock. Reduction of intra-abdominal pressure by anaesthesia may lead to renewed bleeding, so induction should take place in the operating room, so that an aortic clamp can be applied rapidly. Maintenance should be light general anaesthesia with non-depolarizing relaxants as required. The patient may be in a critical shocked condition. It may be necessary to proceed with operation without waiting for resuscitative measures. Blood transfusion should be started as quickly as possible. Coughing and straining are to be avoided lest the aneurysm should rupture. It may therefore be wise to avoid preoperative passage of an oesophageal tube, and to use a muscle relaxant to prevent coughing on the tracheal tube. The blood supply to the cord may be compromised during aortic surgery. Infrarenal cross clamping of the aorta may produce profound and sustained changes in renal haemodynamics and if prolonged, cause harm.[262] During operation arterial pressure, ECG, central venous pressure and urine output should be monitored. *Postoperatively* it is convenient to nurse the patient in an intensive care unit so that observation can be continued and cardiorespiratory support maintained. In appropriate cases elective IPPV can be carried out.

Anaesthesia for Ruptured Thoracic Aorta
This may be required for surgical repair following trauma in road traffic accidents. Cardiopulmonary bypass may be necessary.

Anaesthesia for Aortograms. See p. 480.

The Ultimate Choice
Choice of anaesthetic is always dependent on the skill and experience of the anaesthetist and on the preferences of the surgeon and the patient. Every form of anaesthesia has its disadvantages and complications and is responsible for a certain morbidity and mortality. To everything there is a season.

It is relatively easy to acquire techniques, but judgement in their use is the reward of clinical experience, carefully garnered (Walsh).

There is no general anaesthetic which can be called 'the best', and an anaesthetist is likely to benefit his patient most when he uses the technique and drugs with which he is familiar.

Skilfully managed, any one of a number of agents and techniques can usually be applied, the final solution often being a matter of individual preference.

For practical advice on anaesthetic technique in various types of operation the reader is referred to Stark D. C. C. *Practical Points in Anesthesiology.* New York: Medical Examination Publishing Co. Inc., 2nd ed. 1980.

References

1. Kaufman L. *J. R. Soc. Med.* 1983, **76**, 693.
2. Child C. S. *Anaesthesia* 1984, **39**, 1083.
3. Chisholm R. J. et al. *Anaesthesia* 1983, **38**, 689.
4. Ivanov S. D. and Nunn J. F. *Br. J. Anaesth.* 1969, **41**, 28.
5. Vasiloff N. *Can. Anaesth. Soc. J.* 1965, **12**, 306.
6. Sohn Y. Z. et al. *Can. Anaesth. Soc. J.* 1978, **25**, 431.
7. Milo E. M. et al. *Abst. 8th World Congress, Manila* 1984, **2**, A412.
8. Tucker A. and Lewis J. *Br. Med. J.* 1980, **2**, 1128.
9. First performed in the UK by Dean H. P. *Lancet* 1894, **1**, 1191.
10. Billroth T. (1829–1894) *Wien. Med. Wochenschr.* 1881, **31**, 162.
11. Wolfler A. (1850–1917), *see* Dagensheim G. A. *Surg. Clin. North Am.* 1978, **58**, 927.
12. Dragstedt L. and Owen F. M. *Proc. Soc. Exp. Biol. Med.* 1943, **53**, 152.
13. Fry E. N. S. *Br. Med. J.* 1978, **1**, 110.

14. Eger E. I. and Saidman L. J. *Anesthesiology* 1965, **26**, 61; Lewis G. B. H. *Br. J. Anaesth.* 1984, **56**, 1370 (correspondence).
15. Burchard K. W. and Ciombor D. M. *Surg. Gynecol. Obstet.* 1985, **161**, 313.
16. Kraske P. (1851–1930) *Dtsch. Ges. Chir.* 1885, **14**, 445; Miles E. *Lancet* 1908, **2**, 1812.
17. Foster M. E. et al. *Br. J. Surg.* 1985, **72**, 831.
18. McLaren A. D. *Br. Med. J.* 1981, **2**, 675.
19. Blumberg L. et al. *Br. Med. J.* 1985, **290**, 1037; Fielding L. P. *Br. Med. J.* 1985, **291**, 842.
20. Lawson Tait R. *Med. Times Gaz.* 1879, **2**, 594.
21. Langenbuch L. K. (1864–1901) *Berl. Klin. Wochenschr.* 1882, **19**, 725.
22. Graham E. and Cole W. *JAMA* 1924, **82**, 613.
23. Thornton J. *Lancet* 1891, **1**, 525.
24. Ramzan I. M. et al. *Anesth. Analg. (Cleve.)* 1981, **60**, 289.
25. Bordley J. K. and Olson J. E. *Surg. Gynecol Obstet.* 1979, **149**, 583.
26. McKie B. D. *Br. J. Anaesth.* 1969, **41**, 1091.
27. Farman J. V. in: *Recent Advances in Anaesthesia and Analgesia*—12 (Hewer C. L. and Atkinson R. S. ed.). Edinburgh: Churchill Livingstone, 1976.
28. Starzl T. E. et al. *Surg. Gynecol. Obstet.* 1963, **117**, 659.
29. Watt M. J. et al. *Anaesthesia* 1968, **23**, 2, 331.
30. Feeley M. et al. *J. Irish Coll. Phys. Surg.* 1974, **3**, 83.
31. Thompson J. P. S. *Br. J. Hosp. Med.* 1978, **20**, 600.
32. Pybus D. A. et al. *Anaesth. Intensive Care* 1983, **11**, 27.
33. Bassini B. E. (1846–1924) *Arch. Klin. Chir.* 1890, **40**, 429; Halsted W. S. (1852–1922) *Johns Hopkins Hosp. Bull.* 1893, **4**, 17; Tanner N. C. *Br. J. Surg.* 1942, **29**, 285.
34. Kingsnorth A. N. et al. *Ann. R. Coll. Surg. Engl.* 1979, **61**, 451.
35. Flanagan L. and Bascom J. U. *Surg. Gynecol. Obstet* 1981, **153**, 557.
36. Kremen A. J. et al. *Ann. Surg.* 1954, **140**, 349.
37. Halsted W. S. *Johns Hopkins Hosp. Rep.* 1891, **2**, 255; *Ann. Surg.* 1894, **20**, 497; 1907, **46**, 1.
38. Dixon J. M. and Crofts T. J. *J. R. Coll. Surg. Edinb.* 1983, **28**, 292.
39. Calwell H. G. *Br. Med. J.* 1980, **1**, 115; Nicholl J. H. *Br. Med. J.* 1909, **2**, 753.
40. Waters R. M. *Am. J. Surg.* (Anesth. Suppl.), 1919, **33**, 71.
41. Kay B. *Acta Anaesth. Scand.* 1966, suppl 25, 421; Davenport H. T. et al. *Canad. Anaesth. Soc. J.* 1971, **105**, 498; Atwell J. D. et al. *Lancet* 1973, **2**, 895; Armitage E. N. *Lancet*, 1975, **2**, 21.
42. Ogg T. W. *Br. Med. J.* 1976, **1**, 82; Knight R. F. in: *Clinics in Anaesthesiology* Preparation for Anaesthesia 1986, **4**, 509. (Stevens A. J. ed.), Pitman, Kent, 1980; Rollason W. N. and Hems G. *Ann. R. Coll. Surg. Engl.* 1981, **63**, 45.
43. Beechey A. P. C. et al. *Anaesthesia* 1981, **36**, 10.
44. *See* Brown B. R. ed. *Outpatient Anaesthesia*, Davis, Philadelphia, 1978.
45. Goold J. E. *J. R. Soc. Med.* 1983, **76**, 415.
46. Padfield A. and Mullins S. R. C. *Anaesthesia* 1980, **35**, 508.
47. Carter J. A. and Dye A. M. *Anaesthesia* 1985, **40**, 545.
48. Adams A. P. and Pybus D. A. *Br. Med. J.* 1978, **1**, 278.
49. Atkinson R. S. and Lee J. A. *Anaesthesia* 1985, **40**, 1059.
50. Wood G. J. et al. *Lancet* 1979, **2**, 479; Wood G. J. et al. *Anaesthesia* 1981, **36**, 603.
51. *See also*, Korttila K. *Anaesthesia* 1976, **31**, 724; Fahy A. and Marshall M. *Br. J. Anaesth.* 1969, **41**, 433; Ogg T. W. *Br. Med. J.* 1972, **4**, 573; Ogg T. W. *Proc. R. Soc. Med.* 1975, **68**, 414; Brindle G. F. and Soliman M. G. *Can. Anaesth. Soc. J.* 1975, **22**, 613; Smith B. L. and Young P. W. *Anaesthesia* 1976, **31**, 181.
52. Steward D. G. *Can. Anaesth. Soc. J.* 1975, **22**, 111.
53. Steward D. G. *Can. Anaesth. Soc. J.* 1978, **25**, 4.
54. Doenicke A. et al. *Can. Anaesth. Soc. J.* 1967, **14**, 567.
55. Havard J. *Br. Med. J.* 1978, **1**, 1595; Routh G. S. *Br. Med. J.* 1979, **1**, 673.
56. Baskett P. J. F. and Vickers M. D. *Lancet* 1979, **1**, 490.
57. Seppala J. et al. *Drugs* 1979, **17**, 389; Ashton H. *Adverse Drug Reactions* 1983, Feb. 98.
58. Askwood E. B. *JAMA* 1943, **122**, 78.
59. Trench A. J. et al. *Anaesthesia* 1978, **33**, 535.
60. Singh H. and Rao Y. N. *Anaesthesia* 1978, **33**, 555; Swadia V. N. et al. *Br. J. Anaesth.* 1981, **53**, 963.
61. Park G. R. et al. *J. R. Coll. Surg. Edin.* 1983, **28**, 295.
62. Bexton M. D. R. and Radford R. *Anaesthesia* 1982, **37**, 596; Wade H. *Ann. R. Coll. Surg.* 1980, **62**, 15.

63. *See also* Mountain J. C. et al. *Surg. Gynecol. Obstet.* 1971, **133**, 1; Stewart G. R. et al. *Br. J. Surg.* 1972, **59**, 379.
64. Kark A. E. et al. *Br. Med. J.* 1984, **289**, 1412.
65. Conn J. W. *J. Lab. Clin. Med.* 1955, **45**, 6.
66. *See* Black G. W. and Montgomery D. A. D. in: *Medicine for Anaesthetists* (Vickers M. D. ed.). Oxford: Blackwell, 1977.
67. Frankel F. *Virchow Arch. Path. Anat.* 1886, **103**, 244.
68. Pick L. *Berl. Klin. Wochenschr.* 1912, **19**, 16.
69. Black G. W. and Montgomery D. A. D. in: *Medicine for Anaesthetists* (Vickers M. D. ed.). Oxford: Blackwell, 1977.
70. Csánky-Treels J. C. et al. *Anaesthesia* 1976, **31**, 60.
71. McDowall E. *Elect. Rep. Analyt. Rev.* 1817, **7**, 242.
72. Sims J. M. (1813–1883) *Am. J. Med. Sci.* 1852, **23**, 59.
73. Tait L. *Med. Times Gaz.* 1881, **2**, 654.
74. Wertheim E. (1864–1920). *Archs f. Gynaek.* 1900, **61**, 627.
75. Taylor J. and Weil R. H. *Surg. Gynecol. Obset.* 1967, **124**, 1005.
76. Scott D. B. and Slawson K. B. *Br. J. Anaesth.* 1968, **40**, 103.
77. Watt M. J. et al. *Anaesthesia* 1968, **23**, 2.
78. *See also* Atkinson R. S. in: *Recent Advances in Anaesthesia and Analgesia*—12 (Hewer C. L. and Atkinson R. S. ed.). Edinburgh: Churchill Livingstone, 1976; Nuefeld J. S. et al. *Surg. Gynecol. Obstet.* 1978, **147**, 705; Cuschieri A. *Br. J. Hosp. Med.* 1980, **24**, 252.
79. Jacobeus H. C. *Münch. Med. Wochenschr.* 1910, **57**, 2090.
80. Cooper G. M. et al. *Anaesthesia* 1982, **37**, 266.
81. Chiu H. H. and Ng J. H. *Anaesth. Intensive Care* 1977, **5**, 169.
82. Hassan H. and Tomlin P. J. *Anaesthesia* 1979, **34**, 897.
83. Clark C. C. et al. *Anaesth. Intensive Care* 1977, **5**, 650.
84. Lenz R. J. et al. *Anaesthesia* 1976, **31**, 4.
85. Ganga G. et al. *Anaesthesia* 1982, **37**, 903.
86. Cameron A. E. et al. *J. R. Soc. Med.* 1983, **76**, 1015.
87. Harris M. N. E. et al. *Br. J. Anaesth.* 1984, **56**, 1214.
88. Seed R. F. et al. *Anaesthesia* 1970, **25**, 223; Scott D. B. *Anaesthesia* 1970, **25**, 590; Friedman I. H. et al. *Surg. Gynecol. Obstet.* 1977, **144**, 906; Steptoe P. C. *Br. Med. Bull.* 1970, **26**, 60.
89. Gordon A. G. *J. R. Soc. Med.* 1984, **27**, 540.
90. Dodson M. E. *Br. J. Anaesth.* 1978, **50**, 169.
91. Calverly R. K. and Jenkins L. C. *Can. Anaesth. Soc. J.* 1973, **20**, 679.
92. Tay H. S. and Chiu H. H. *Anaesth. Intensive Care* 1978, **6**, 134; Duffy B. C. *Br. J. Anaesth.* 1979, **51**, 1089.
93. West S. L. et al. *Anaesthesia* 1985, **40**, 669.
94. Loring K. C. et al. *Br. Med. J.* 1971, **4**, 477; Guillebaud J. *Br. Med. J.* 1979, **1**, 1148.
95. Phillips C. I. *Br. Med. J.* 1984, **288**, 1779.
96. Backer C. L. et al. *Anesthesiology* 1979, **51**, Suppl. 61; Backer C. L. et al. *Anesth. Analg. (Cleve.)* 1980, **59**, 257.
97. Karkunen U. and John G. *Acta Anaesth. Scand.* 1982, **26**, 294.
98. Van Lint A. *Ann. Oculist.* 1914, **151**, 420.
99. O'Brien C. S. *Arch. Ophthalmol.* 1929, **1**, 447.
100. Macintosh R. R. and Ostlere M. *Local Analgesia. Head and Neck*, 2nd ed. Edinburgh: Livingstone, 1967, p. 121.
101. Editorial, *J. Neuro-ophthalmol.* 1981, **1**, 172; Smith J. L. *Ann. Ophthmol.* 1982, **14**, 1005; Chang J. L. et al. *Anesthesiology* 1984, **63**, 789.
102. *See also* Jay J. L. *Br. J. Anaesth.* 1980, **52**, 649; Le May M. *Br. J. Anaesth.* 1980, **52**, 655; Holloway K. B. *Br. J. Anaesth.* 1980, **52**, 671; Rose N. M. and Adams A. P. *Anaesthesia* 1980, **35**, 569.
103. Schreuder M. and Linssen G. A. *Anaesthesia* 1972, **27**, 165.
104. Trew C. T. et al. *Anaesthesia* 1982, **37**, 339.
105. Foulds W. S. *Br. J. Anaesth.* 1980, **52**, 643.
106. Katz R. L. *Anesthesiology* 1968, **29**, 70.
107. Pandey K. et al. *Br. J. Anaesth.* 1972, **44**, 191.
108. Feneck R. O. and Cook J. H. *Anaesthesia* 1983, **38**, 120.
109. Eltringham R. J. *Abst. 8th World Congress, Manila*, 1984, **2**, A327.
110. Craythorne N. W. B. et al. *Anesthesiology* 1960, **18**, 44.
111. Adams A. P. et al. *Br. J. Ophthalmol.* 1979, **63**, 204.

112. Adams A. P. et al. *Anaesthesia* 1979, **34**, 526.
113. McGavi D. D. M. *Lancet* 1965, **2**, 272.
114. Lempert J. *Arch. Otolaryngol.* 1938, **28**, 42.
115. Charles H. *Br. Med. J.* 1937, **1**, 449.
116. Eisele G. et al. *Anaesthesist* 1978, **27**, 322.
117. Adams A. P. et al. *Br. J. Ophthalmol.* 1979, **63**, 204; Adams A. P. et al. *Anaesthesia* 1979, **34**, 526.
118. Bryn Thomas K. *Proc. 2nd Eur. Cong. Anaes. (Vienna)* 1966, **2**, 229.
119. Zirn E. A. *von Graefes' Arch. Ophth.* 1906, **64**, 580.
120. Ridley H. *Lancet* 1952, **1**, 118.
121. Choyce D. P. *Intraocular Lenses and Implants.* London: Lewis, 1964.
122. Mirakhur R. K. *Ann. R. Coll. Surg. Engl.* 1985, **67**, 34.
123. Aschner S. *Wien. Klin. Wochenschr.* 1908, **21**, 1529; Dagnini G. *Bol. della Sc. Med.* 1908, **8**, 380.
124. Fry E. N. S. and Hall-Parker B. J. P. *Br. Med. J.* 1974, **4**, 659.
125. Karkunen U. et al. *Br. J. Anaesth.* 1985, **57**, 1209.
126. Myers E. F. *Anesthesiology,* 1979, **51**, 350.
127. Fry E. N. S. *Anaesthesia* 1975, **30**, 549; Fry E. N. S. and Hall-Parks B. J. P. *Br. J. Ophthalmol.* 1975, **59**, 529.
128. Robideaux V. *Anesthesiology* 1978, **49**, 433.
129. Gunn M. *Trans. Ophthalmol. Soc. UK* 1883, **3**, 283; Kwik R. S. H. *Anaesthesia* 1980, **33**, 46.
130. Kerr W. J. and Vance J. P. *Anaesthesia* 1983, **38**, 883.
131. *See also* Ellingham T. R. *Anaesthesia* 1976, **31**, 433; Elliott J. and Morrison J. D. in: *Anaesthesia for Eye, Ear, Nose and Throat Surgery.* Edinburgh: Churchill Livingstone, 1975; Adams A. K. and Jones R. M. *Br. J. Anaesth.* 1980, **52**, 663.
132. Van den Berg A. A. *Anaesth. Intensive Care* 1985, **13**, 95.
133. Libonati M. M. et al. *Anesthesiology* 1985, **62**, 637; Bourke D. L. *Anesthesiology* 1985, **63**, 727.
134. Esmarch J. F. A. von (1823–1908), *Der erste Verband auf dem Schlaftfelde.* Kiel, 1869.
135. Mihic D. N. *Anesthesiology* 1984, **60**, 526; Pollard P. J. et al. *Anesthesiology* 1983, **58**, 373.
136. Zahavi J. et al. *Lancet* 1980, **2**, 663.
137. Klenerman L. *J. R. Soc. Med.* 1982, **75**, 31.
138. Klenerman L. *J. Bone Joint Surg.* 1962, **44B**, 937; Klenerman L. *J. R. Soc. Med.* 1982, **75**, 31; Hallett G. *Br. Med. J.* 1983, **286**, 1267.
139. Murphy J. P. and Anandaciva S. *Anaesthesia* 1984, **39**, 188.
140. Mann R. A. M. and Bissett W. I. K. *Anaesthesia* 1983, **38**, 1185.
141. Edmonds-Seal J. et al. *J. R. Soc. Med.* 1980, **73**, 111.
142. Brands E. and Callanan V. I. *Anaesth. Intensive Care* 1978, **6**, 256.
143. Smith-Petersen M. N. et al. *Ann. Surg.* 1931, **23**, 715; *Surg. Gynecol. Obstet.* 1937, **64**, 287.
144. Berry F. R. *Anaesthesia* 1977, **32**, 576; Brands E. and Callanan V. I. *Anaesth. Intensive Care* 1978, **6**, 256.
145. McLaren A. D. et al. *Anaesthesia* 1978, **33**, 10; McKenzie P. J. et al. *Br. J. Anaesth.* 1980, **52**, 49; Sikorski J. M. et al. *Br. Med. J.* 1985, **290**, 439.
146. Spreadbury T. H. *Anaesthesia* 1980, **35**, 208.
147. Howard C. B. et al. *Anaesthesia* 1983, **38**, 993.
148. McKenzie P. I. et al. *Br. J. Anaesth.* 1980, **52**, 49.
149. Davis F. M. et al. *Br. Med. J.* 1980, **2**, 1528.
150. Jones S. F. and White A. *Anaesthesia* 1985, **40**, 682.
151. Gallanaugh S. C. et al. *Br. Med. J.* 1976, **2**, 1496.
152. Goucke C. R. *Anaesthesia* 1985, **40**, 578.
153. Thompson F. R. et al. *N. Engl. J. Med.* 1952, **52**, 3011; McKee G. K. *Proc. R. Soc. Med.* 1958, **31**, 883; Charnley C. J. *J. Bone Joint Surg.* 1960, **42B**, 28; Charnley C. J. *Lancet* 1961, **1**, 1129.
154. Kiaer S. *C. R. du 5ième Cong. Internat. de Chir. Orthop.* 1953, p. 534; Haboush J. J. *Bull. Hosp. Joint Dis., N.Y.* 1953, **14**. 242.
155. Harvey P. B. and Smith J. A. *Anaesthesia* 1982, **37**, 714.
156. Alexander J. P. and Barron D. W. *Anaesthesia* 1978, **33**, 748.
157. Barbier-Böhm G. et al. *Br. J. Anaesth.* 1980, **52**, 1039.
158. Vazeery A. K. et al. *Br. J. Anaesth.* 1983, **55**, 783.
159. Thorburn J. *Br. J. Anaesth.* 1985, **57**, 290.

160. McLaren A. D. et al. *Anaesthesia* 1978, **33**, 10; Bridenbaugh L. D. *Survey of Anesthesiology* 1974, **18**, 178.
161. Chambers W. A. et al *Br. J. Anaesth.* 1982, **54**, 75.
162. Hole A. J. et al. *Acta Anaesth. Scand.* 1980, **24**, 279; Modig J. et al., *Acta Anaesth. Scand.* 1980, **24**, 305.
163. McKenzie P. J. et al. *Br. J. Anaesth.* 1980, **52**, 49; Nightingale P. J. and Marstrand T. *Br. J. Anaesth.* 1981, **53**, 369.
164. Andersen K. H. *Anaesthesia* 1983, **38**, 1195; *see also* Correspondence, *Anaesthesia* 1983, **38**, 68 and 69.
165. Harris W. H. et al. *J. Bone Joint Surg.* 1974, **56A**, 1552.
166. Modig J. et al. *Br. J. Anaesth.* 1983, **55**, 625.
167. Michel R. *Anaesthesia* 1980, **35**, 858.
168. Lidwell O. M. et. al. *Br. Med. J.* 1982, **285**, 10.
169. Charnley J. *J. Bone Joint Surg.* 1960, **42B**, 28.
170. Nyska M. et al. *Br. Med. J.* 1986, **283**, 1347.
171. Cole P. V. in: *Recent Advances in Anaesthesia and Analgesia*—13 (Hewer C. L. and Atkinson R. S. ed.) London: Churchill Livingstone, 1979, Chapter 6.
172. Heeneman H. *Laryngoscope* 1973, **83**, 17.
173. Doolan L. A. and O'Brien J. F. *Anaesth. Intensive Care* 1985, **13**, 319.
174. Ovassapian A. et al. *Anesthesiology* 1983, **58**, 370
175. *See* Bedford A. et al. *J. R. Soc. Med.* 1979, **72**, 6.
176. Hadden W. A. and Nichol R. O. *J. R. Coll. Surg. Edinb.* 1982, **27**, 19.
177. Harrington H. *J. Bone Joint Surg.* 1962, **44A**, 591; Kafer E. R. *Anesthesiology* 1980, **52**, 339.
178. Abbott T. R. and Bentley G. *Anaesthesia* 1980, **35**, 298.
179. Porter K. M. and Davies J. *Ann. R. Coll. Surg. Engl.* 1985, **67**, 292.
180. Mixter W. J. and Barr J. S. *N. Engl. J. Med.* 1934, **211**, 210.
181. Taylor S. et al. *Anaesthesia* 1984, **39**, 520.
182. Haq I. U. and Dundee J. W. *Br. J. Anaesth.* 1968, **40**, 972.
183. Smith B. L. and Manfold M. L. M. *Br. J. Anaesth.* 1974, **46**, 373.
184. Ryhanen P. et al. *Laryngoscope* 1980, **90**, 494.
185. Doughty A. G. *Lancet* 1957, **1**, 1074.
186. Williams A. and Hamilton A. *Anaesthesia* 1986, **41**, 222.
187. Whillis S. S. and Pybus F. C. *Lancet* 1910, **2**, 875; Sluder G. *JAMA* 1911, **56**, 867.
188. Alpert J. J. et al. *Lancet* 1968, **1**, 1319.
189. Tate N. *Lancet* 1963, **2**, 1090.
190. Gussenbauer C. *Arch. f. Klin. Chir.* 1874, **17**, 343.
191. Campkin T. V. *Br. J. Anaesth.* 1970, **42**, 1073; Condon H. A. *Br. J. Anaesth.* 1971, **43**, 1061; Plant M. *Anaesthesia* 1982, **37**, 1211.
192. Loach A. B. *Anaesthesia* 1974, **29**, 448.
193. Atkinson R. S. in: *Recent Advances in Anaesthesia and Analgesia*—12 (Hewer C. L. and Atkinson R. S. ed.). Edinburgh: Churchill Livingstone, 1976.
194. Sanders R. D. *Del. State Med. J.* 1967, **39**, 170; Albert S. N. *Br. J. Anaesth.* 1971, **43**, 1098; Lee S. T. *Br. J. Anaesth.* 1972, **44**, 874.
195. Scalco A. N. et al. *Ann. Otol. Laryngol.* 1960, **69**, 1134.
196. Koo M. K. T. *Anaesth. Intensive Care*, 1980, **8**, 469.
197. Pollard B. J. *Anaesthesia* 1968, **23**, 534; Atkinson R. S. in: *Recent Advances in Anaesthesia and Analgesia*—12 (Hewer C. L. and Atkinson R. S. ed.). Edinburgh: Churchill Livingstone, 1976; Coplans M. P. *Anaesthesia* 1976, **31**, 430; Benjamin B. and Gronow D. *Anaesth. Intensive Care* 1979, **7**, 258.
198. Magnusson J. and Werner O. *Anaesthesia* 1983, **38**, 103.
199. Spoerel W. E. et al. *Br. J. Anaesth.* 1971, **43**, 932; Smith R. B. *Anesth. Analg. (Cleve.)* 1974, **53**, 225.
200. Carden E. and Ferguson G. B. *The Laryngoscope* 1973, **83**, 691; Smith R. B. et al. *Br. J. Anaesth.* 1974, **46**, 313.
201. Norton M. L. et al. *Am. J. Otol. Rhinolaryngol.* 1976, **85**, 656; Rontal M. et al. *Laryngoscope* 1980, **90**, 1162.
202. Chakrabarti K. et al. *Br. J. Anaesth.* 1973, **45**, 733; Spoerel W. E. and Greenway R. E. *Can. Anaesth. Soc. J.* 1973, **20**, 369.
203. Hunton J. and Oswal V. H. *Anaesthesia* 1985, **40**, 1210
204. Chilcote R. T. et al. *Anesthesiology* 1983, **59**, 258.
205. Clarke R. S. J. in: *Anaesthesia for Eye, Ear, Nose and Throat Surgery* (Morrow W. F. K. and Morrison J. D. ed.). Edinburgh: Churchill Livingstone, 1975; Davies J. R. *Br. J. Anaesth.*

1978, **50**, 511; Dash H. H. and Gale G. R. *Br. J. Anaesth.* 1983, **55**, 1271.
206. Davies J. R. *Br. Med. J.* 1979, **2**, 610.
207. Rogers R. C. et al. *Anaesthesia* 1985, **40**, 32; Selby D. G. et al. *Anaesth. Intensive Care* 1982, **11**, 166.
208. Ludlow A. quoted by Hunter W. *Med. Observations and Enquiries*, 1767, **3**, 85.
209. Condon H. A. *Clin. Otolaryngol.* 1979, **4**, 241; Eltringham R. J. et al. *Anaesthesia* 1982, **37**, 1028; Rollason W. N. et al. *Anaesthesia* 1983, **38**, 590.
210. Kerr A. R. *Br. J. Anaesth.* 1977, **49**, 447.
211. Davis I. et al. *Anaesthesia* 1979, **34**, 147.
212. Casey W. F. and Drake-Lee A. B. *Anaesthesia* 1982, **37**, 896.
213. Perreault L. et al. *Canad. Anaesth. Soc. J.* 1981, **28**, 136.
214. Brown J. M. in: *Recent Advances in Anaesthesia and Analgesia*—15 (Atkinson R. S. and Adams A. P. ed.) Edinburgh: Churchill Livingstone, 1985.
215. Szyfelbein S. K. *J. R. Soc. Med.* 1982, **75**, Suppl. 1, 26.
216. Demling R. H. et al. *J. Trauma* 1978, **18**, 269.
217. Slogoff S. et al. *Anesth. Analg. (Cleve.)* 1974, **53**, 354.
218. Birky M. M. et al. *Fires and Materials* 1979, **3**, 211.
219. Clark C. J. et al. *Lancet* 1981, **1**, 1332.
220. Bartlett R. H. et al. *Arch. Surg.* 1976, **111**, 744.
221. Clark C. J. et al. *Anaesthesia* 1983, **38**, 35.
222. Batstone G. F. *J. R. Soc. Med.* 1982, **75**, Suppl. 1, 12.
223. Williams J. G. et al. *Br. Med. J.* 1983, **286**, 775.
224. Mercuriali G. *De decoratione* 2nd ed. Frankfurt, 1586.
225. Thiersch C. *Arch. Klin. Chir.* 1874, **17**, 318.
226. Wolfe J. R. *Br. Med. J.* 1875, **2**, 360.
227. Blair V. P. and Brown J. B. *Surg. Gynecol. Obstet.* 1929, **49**, 82.
228. Gillies H. D. *Plastic Surgery of the Face.* Oxford: Oxford Medical Publications 1920.
229. Bodley P. *Proc. R. Soc. Med.* 1978, **71**, 839.
230. Apt C. et al. *Ann. R. Coll. Surg. Engl.* 1985, **67**, 177.
231. Debum G. et al. *J. Neurosurg.* 1978, **49**, 635.
232. Edge W. G. and Morgan M. *Anaesth. Intensive Care* 1977, **5**, 153.
233. Smith M. et al. *Anaesthesia* 1985, **40**, 680.
234. Goldberg M. *Anesthesiology* 1984, **60**, 46.
235. Widrich W. C. et al. *Radiology* 1977, **124**, 37; Gordon I. J. and Westcott J. L. *Radiology* 1977, **124**, 43.
236. Selby D. G. *Anaesth. Intensive Care* 1982, **10**, 167.
237. Grainger R. G. *Br. Med. J.* 1984, **289**, 144.
238. Axelsson K. H. et al. *Br. J. Anaesth.* 1984, **56**, 271.
239. Taylor R. O. et al. *J. Urol.* 1958, **79**, 490; Rose G. A. et al. *Br. Med. J.* 1981, **232**, 317.
240. Thomas D. and Hales P. *Anaesth. Intensive Care* 1984, **12**, 366; Pierce J. M. *J. Urol.* 1962, **87**, 181.
241. Dodson M. E. *Br. Med. J.* 1985, **291**, 1577.
242. Charlton A. J. *Anaesthesia* 1980, **35**, 804.
243. Rawstron R. E. et al. *Anaesth. Intensive Care* 1981, **9**, 43.
244. Abrams P. H. et al. *Anaesthesia* 1982, **37**, 71.
245. Freyer P. (1852–1921) *Lancet* 1900, **1**, 774.
246. Leaper D. J. et al. *J. R. Coll. Surg. Edinb.* 1977, **22**, 412.
247. Jenkins J. et al. *Anaesthesia* 1983, **38**, 748.
248. Rhind J. R. *Br. Med. J.* 1980, **2**, 722.
249. Yoshikawa K. et al. *Anaesthesia* 1983, **38**, 70.
250. Nitze M. *Wien. Med. Wochenschr.* 1879, **29**, 779, 806.
251. Lunn J. N. *Anaesthesia* 1979, **34**, 552.
252. Regan N. A. *Br. Med. J.* 1971, **3**, 283.
253. Blandy J. P. *Br. J. Hosp. Med.* 1979, **21**, 520.
254. Medawar P. B. *J. Anat.* 1944, **78**, 879.
255. Charters P. *Anaesthesia* 1981, **36**, 199.
256. Walton J. D. and Farman J. V. *Anaesthesia* 1973, **28**, 626.
257. Marsland A. R. and Bradley J. P. *Anaesth. Intensive Care* 1983, **11**, 337.
258. Webb D. B. et al. *Ann. R. Coll. Surg. Engl.* 1985, **67**, 337; Frank M. et al. *Ann. R. Coll. Surg. Engl.* 1985, **67**, 341; Abbott M. A. et al. *Anaesthesia* 1985, **40**, 1065; Wickham J. E. A. et al. *Br. Med. J.* 1985, **290**, 1188; Peterson G. N. et al. *Anaesthesia* 1985, **40**, 460.

259. Helmstein K. *Br. J. Urol.* 1972, **44**, 434.
260. Brown P. R. et al. *Anaesthesia* 1974, **29**, 422; Lahiri S. K. and Boys J. E. *Br. J. Anaesth.* 1973, **45**, 1162; Coombs G. B. *Br. J. Urol.* 1975, **47**, 177.
261. Dubost C. et al. *Arch. Surg.* 1952, **64**, 405.
262. Gamulin Z. et al. *Anesthesiology* 1984, **66**, 394.
263. Trendelenburg, Friedrich (1844–1924) *Beitr. Klin. Chir.* 1890, **7**, 195.
264. Mayo C. H. *Surg. Gynecol. Obstet.* 1906, **2**, 385.
265. Myers T. T. and Cooley J. C. *Surg. Gynecol. Obstet.* 1954, **99**, 733.
266. Lee J. Alfred *Regional Anesthesia* 1985, **10**, 99.
267. Malhotra V. et al. *Anesth. Analg. (Cleve.)* 1987, **66**, 85.

Chapter 25　　　　**DENTAL ANAESTHESIA**

History

For the early uses of nitrous oxide *see* Chapter 10. After the introduction of ether and chloroform, nitrous oxide fell into disfavour, until interest was revived in its use for dental extractions over 100 years ago by G. Q. Colton and T. W. Evans. The latter demonstrated his method in London on 31 March 1868.[1] Other pioneers of nitrous oxide anaesthesia include Edmund Andrews (1824–1904) who used it with oxygen, Sir F. Hewitt, who advocated sound teaching and practice in the use of anaesthetics in the dental surgery and designed an apparatus,[2] and E. I. McKesson (1881–1935) whose demand-flow machine is still in use.[3] Nasal administration became commonly used in dentistry about the turn of the century[4] although Clover and Alfred Coleman had used it in 1868.[5] In modern times there has been a reappraisal of dental anaesthesia, formerly carried out with nitrous oxide, and oxygen or air alone, aimed at the prevention of hypoxia and the provision of better operating conditions for the surgeon. Improved anaesthestic technique allows the surgeon more time and increases the range of procedures which can be undertaken in the dental chair. The eugenol derivative, oil of cloves, was first used as a local analgesic in 1890.[6]

Modern practice includes the use of halothane as a volatile supplement,[7] the use of intravenous techniques,[8] diazepam,[9] and the use of tracheal intubation,[10] while the dangers of fainting when the patient is held in the sitting position have been pointed out by Bourne.[11] The Society for the Advancement of Anaesthesia in Dentistry has been active since 1958.[12] It is now possible to offer 'ultra-light' intravenous anaesthesia for conservative work in the dental chair employing, e.g. methohexitone,[13] propanidid[14] or diazepam.[12] Diazepam first used in dental surgery in 1966.[15] General anaesthetics administered to ambulatory patients is declining in the UK and largely abandoned elsewhere. In the UK about one and a half million administrations take place yearly.[16] The first local dental block was given by R. J. Hall,[17] Halsted's assistant in New York's Roosevelt Hospital in 1884; in the UK by W. A. Hunt of Yeovil.[18]

Ambulatory Patients

The addition of oxygen to nitrous oxide in dental anaesthesia was popularized by Frederick Hewitt.[2] In the first 50 years of the century if pure nitrous oxide was administered, the patient would pass through the stages of analgesia and excitement until the stage of surgical anaesthesia was reached. Oxygen was then added to prevent hypoxia, but the amount was carefully regulated as the margin between too light anaesthesia and dangerous hypoxia is small. Skilled administration was necessary if smooth anaesthesia was to be given consistently, and some degree of hypoxia had to be accepted. The signs are those of analgesia, excitement and light surgical anaesthesia and the signs of hypoxia must be considered. The classic signs of nitrous-oxide–oxygen anaesthesia (McKesson) are described elsewhere.[19]

The modern view is that at least 30% of oxygen should be given routinely and supplements used as necessary.

A patient over 16 years of age can give his own permission for anaesthesia in the UK.

Apparatus

For many years, intermittent-flow machines have been favoured for dental anaesthesia. Most popular have been the five Walton models[20] (the first dates from 1925) and the McKesson apparatus.[3] Since they operate on the demand system, reservoir bags are not necessary (except in so far as a reservoir is an integral part of the machine itself, e.g. McKesson). The Bain circuit should not be used with intermittent-flow apparatus, because of the increased inspiratory resistance; rebreathing is likely to occur. Accurate oxygen percentages below 20% are no longer required, and doubt has been cast on the accuracy of many intermittent-flow machines in general use. The Walton V and the AE machines are no longer manufactured but the McKesson is. Another development is the use of premixed gas cylinders[21] (50% of each gas), together with a halothane vaporizer. Provision for scavenging of gases can easily be provided. Equipment is now available which utilizes flow-meters but there is also provision for dialling an oxygen percentage between 30 and 100% (Quantiflex).

Vaporizers for attachment to anaesthetic machines include the Rowbotham, Goldman, McKesson and AE. Since they are intended for use over short periods no provision is made for temperature compensation. Incorporation of a blotting-paper wick in the Goldman vaporizer increases the maximum vapour concentration and enhances clinical efficiency.[22] Normally it gives halothane vapour between 0·1 and 2·5%.

Uptake and Elimination of Nitrous Oxide[23]

During dental anaesthesia peak inspiratory flow-rates may be between 30 and 200 l/min, tidal volumes between 300 and 3000 ml, and respiratory minute volume between 11 and 50 l/min. The arterial blood concentration of nitrous oxide reaches an initial plateau within 10 min. In this time, depending upon factors such as inhaled concentration, alveolar ventilation and cardiac output, the arterial tension will be over 90% of the inhaled tension. On discontinuing, blood levels fall rapidly over 10 min.

Four 'zones' of nitrous oxide anaesthesia have been described:

1. Moderate analgesia (6–25% N_2O inhaled); 25% N_2O is more potent than 10 mg morphine.

2. Dissociation analgesia (26–45%); 30% gives rise to psychological symptoms and lack of ability to concentrate. This is more severe at 45%.

3. Analgesic anaesthesia (46–65%). Near complete amnesia. Patient may respond to commands.

4. Light anaesthesia (66–80%). Complete analgesia and amnesia. Not possible to communicate with patient.

Posture
The supine position for dental anaesthesia is favoured by an increasing number of anaesthetists because of the dangers of hypotension and inadequate cerebral perfusion (fainting) (*see* p. 499). Others feel that the sitting position discourages regurgitation of stomach contents and helps to prevent soiling of the pharynx with blood and debris. Some dental surgeons find extraction of teeth easier in the sitting position. The subject is controversial. The dependent position of the legs is to be avoided since blood may pool in them. A faint is vasovagal syncope.[24] (*See also* Tomlin P. J. and Roberts J. F. *Br. Dent. J.* 1981, **150**, 312.)

Selection of Patients for General Anaesthesia in Dental Surgery
Whenever possible, local techniques are to be preferred but general anaesthesia may be required: In small children, especially when removal of teeth in different quadrants of the mouth is planned; in adults when multiple extractions are to be performed on a single occasion; in the presence of acute sepsis; following failed local analgesia, for any reason; when the patient is too apprehensive to co-operate, when local methods would normally suffice.

When the patient has valvular disease of the heart he may be at risk from bacteraemia during extractions, so antibiotics should be administered, e.g. procaine penicillin 600 000 units with penicillin G, 200 000 units 1 h preoperatively and once daily for 2 days postoperatively.

Some Abnormal Types of Patient
1. Patients who are frightened and have a poor command of themselves. These are difficult to control and may need premedication. Intravenous induction is often beneficial.
2. Patients who resist all anaesthetics. Chronic alcoholics; vigorous young men. Intravenous induction may avoid prolonged excitement stage.
3. Children under 4. Premedication is helpful. A sympathetic but firm approach should be used. The authors favour nitrous-oxide–oxygen and halothane, using a face mask for induction. Above the age of 12, most children can be treated as adults. At the age of about 7, intravenous induction can be offered.
4. Obesity. Difficult veins; difficult airway.
5. Patients who have missed periods and may be pregnant. Elective general anaesthesia is undesirable during the first 3 months and the last 3 months of pregnancy.
6. Patients who are anaemic. Oxygen-rich mixtures should be used.
7. Patients with decompensated heart disease. These are best managed in the hospital environment. It is a good plan to precede anaesthesia by the inhalation for 10 min of 100% oxygen. In the presence of valvular lesions, antibiotic cover should be given to prevent subsequent development of subacute bacterial endocarditis. Antibiotics also necessary in patients with hip prostheses.
8. Patients with hypertension. With good oxygenation and careful management these do well.
9. Diabetics. If receiving insulin, they can often be given a short anaesthetic

with safety just before a meal is due. They should be kept under observation until they have received some nutriment by mouth in case hypoglycaemia should develop. Diabetic autonomic neuropathy presents a hazard (*see* Chapter 22).

10. Steroid therapy. For simple extractions steroid cover is not usually required. If there is doubt, the patient should take an extra tablet that day. Otherwise 100 mg hydrocortisone may be given intravenously just prior to anaesthesia.

11. Mono-amine oxidase inhibitors. These drugs are contraindications to the use of pethidine and related compounds. Nor should pressor drugs be used in patients taking antidepressants.

12. The physically or mentally handicapped require careful mnagement. It may be necessary to administer general anaesthesia for conservation with tracheal intubation. Premedication is important and combinations such as nitrazepam 10 mg and droperidol 20 mg (in adults) orally 2 h before induction have been recommended. Sedation by diazepam before local analgesia or general anaesthesia is also useful. Initial dose in children up to the age of 10 years is 1 mg/year, i.v. In older patients 15–20 mg.

Relative Contraindications to General Anaesthesia in the Dental Chair

1. Patients whose stomachs may not be empty.

2. Patients with acute infections or tumours in the region of the upper airways which cause or may cause obstruction.

3. Special care will be required in patients with the following conditions: (*a*) sickle-cell disease; (*b*) severe coronary disease; (*c*) extreme obesity; (*d*) severe chronic bronchitis and obstructive airways disease; (*e*) spastic states; (*f*) haemophilia; (*g*) patients on medication with certain drugs.

It is unwise to allow patients who have received intravenous anaesthetics to return home alone, to drive a car or to cook on the day of the anaesthetic.

Clinical Administration in the Dental Surgery

The stomach and bladder should be empty, the nose should be blown and dentures should be removed. The anaesthetist must be sure that the patient is fit for the proposed operation and tight garments must be loosened in obese patients. Premedication is not given, but the patient should be treated sympathetically and the procedure explained to him. It is easy to suggest that pain and discomfort will ensue, and this is to be avoided. Dental forceps and other instruments should be prepared unobtrusively and an atmosphere of calm confidence adopted.

The patient should lie in the horizontal position or be seated comfortably in the chair, with the head rest adjusted to allow surgical access. The hands may be placed in the trouser pockets or arms comfortably folded. A restraining lap belt may be valuable in the robust individual. Saliva must be swallowed before consciousness is lost to prevent it irritating the larynx and causing cough.

After insertion of a mouth prop, anaesthesia is induced by intravenous injection or the patient is instructed to breathe through his nose while the inhalation mixture (usually nitrous-oxide–oxygen and halothane) is administered by nasal mask; 30% oxygen is recommended in the mixture. Some administrators prefer to induce anaesthesia with a face-mask, substituting a nasal inhaler when the patient has lost consciousness. Surgical anaesthesia is marked by loss of eyelash reflex, eyeball movements and then fixation, relaxation of the jaw. The hiss of the expiratory valve is good evidence of free nasal respiration.

The anaesthetist has several duties which he must perform simultaneously during the dental operation. These include: (1) Maintenance of a clear airway. This may be difficult during operations on the lower jaw when there is a tendency to flex the head and obstruct respiration; (2) Provide counter-pressure, if required by the dental surgeon, and hold the head and jaw securely; (3) See that a dental pack is used to prevent inhalation of blood and debris and to discourage mouth breathing; (4) Observe the vital signs, pulse and respiration, and take early action should untoward reactions (e.g. fainting) occur. Pulse monitors seldom function well during the conditions of outpatient anaesthesia, but a finger can usually palpate the superficial temporal artery; (5) The anaesthetist must sometimes assist in the insertion of mouth gags, particularly when extractions on both sides of the mouth are necessary; (6) He must observe the dials and gauges of the anaesthetic apparatus at all times and make sure that connections are maintained and that cylinders do not run empty unnoticed. *Unobstructed breathing through the nose is essential.*

As soon as the operation is complete, anaesthesia should be discontinued and the patient allowed to recover consciousness. The anaesthetist should anticipate surgical procedures so that agents such as halothane are switched off before completion of extractions. Recovery will not then be prolonged. Pure oxygen may be given with advantage for a few minutes before removal of the mask. The patient must be carefully observed at this stage, to ensure that blood clot or debris is expelled from the mouth and not inhaled, and to control any signs of excitement during the recovery. Fainting can also occur *after* the operation is completed, and the anaesthetist must be prepared to level the chair and elevate the legs.

Volatile Agents

These may be added to a nitrous-oxide mixture.

1. Halothane. Usually given from the Goldman or similar simple vaporizer. A popular and potent supplement to nitrous oxide and oxygen with smooth rapid recovery. Associated with a high incidence of cardiac dysrhythmias. *Enflurane* causes fewer dysrhythmias, but is less satisfactory in use.[25] *Isoflurane*[63] can be used.

2. Trichloroethylene. Less potent than halothane but may be used as an analgesic supplement.

Tracheal intubation has been advocated for the ambulant patient. Tube may be inserted blindly, nasally, or through the mouth, following suxamethonium or halothane, but requires a degree of skill. Useful in long conservation procedures.

Intravenous Agents[26]

May be given for induction prior to nitrous-oxide–oxygen anaesthesia, as a sole agent for simple extractions, or in intermittent doses for more prolonged procedures.

1. Barbiturates. First used in dental surgery in 1932 (hexobarbitone).[27] Methohexitone is thought to have a quicker recovery than thiopentone and so is preferred by many for the ambulant patient. Given as a 1% solution, about 1·5 mg/kg being an average dose. Methohexitone followed by nitrous oxide and oxygen has been recommended as the method of choice for dental extractions.[28] A sleep dose of thiopentone can be used, continuing with nitrous-oxide–oxygen. Larger doses (up to 4 mg/kg) may be used as a sole agent for extractions provided undue difficulty is not anticipated, though it may be wise to lie the patient flat in case hypotension should occur.

2. Diazepam. (Diazemuls) This has been used as a sedative cover in dental surgery and conservation. First used for this purpose in 1966 and 1968.[29] The cardiac output and stroke volume are decreased. The patient should be prepared as for general anaesthesia and should be supine. The drug is given at a rate of about 2·5 mg each half minute until drowsiness, slurred speech and drooping eyelids make their appearance: usual dose between 12 and 20 mg. At this point either light general anaesthesia or local analgesia is administered. Atropine premedication reduces troublesome salivation, while amnesia is usually present. Local burning or even thrombosis at the injection site may be seen. Complete recovery may take several hours, although long before this the patient may sit up in the dentist's waiting room. The combination of diazepam with methohexitone may cause cardiovascular depression.

3. Narcotic Analgesics, e.g. pethidine or pentazocine, can be given intravenously before nitrous oxide anaesthesia or to supplement diazepam. Grave respiratory depression must be avoided.

Tracheal intubation with either spontaneous respiration or IPPV ventilation gives good results, in experienced hands.[30]

Complications of Anaesthesia in the Dental Chair[31]

1. Hypoxia. Even when 30% oxygen is given during dental anaesthesia arterial hypoxia is likely to occur unless a perfect airway is maintained. This can be difficult when the surgeon exerts pressure during extractions in the lower jaw. Obstruction can occur as a result of malposition of packs and it is possible for the nasal mask to obstruct the nasal openings. There is evidence that some deaths in the dental surgery may result from hypoxia.

2. Excitement. A quiet calm commentary by the anaesthetist helps to allay fears and allows the patient to know that the anaesthetist is aware that the patient is still awake. Struggling during the excitement stage is less common when potent supplements such as halothane are used. In sturdy and frightened patients intravenous induction is usually indicated as surgical anaesthesia is then achieved rapidly and supplementary doses can be given if necessary.

3. Mouth-breathing. This dilutes the mixture delivered from the anaesthetic apparatus by nasal masks. In frightened or difficult patients and in small children the full face-mask should be used for induction. Mouth-breathing may occur due to premature insertion of mouth gags or faulty positioning of a mouth pack. The oropharyngeal barrier formed by apposition of the dorsum of the tongue and the palate may be broken by mouth gags, operator's fingers, packs or anything which depresses the tongue.

4. Airway Obstruction. This can be caused by the tongue, enlarged tonsils and adenoids, and laryngeal spasm. The latter may be due to irritation by foreign material such as blood, saliva or dental debris, as well as by anaesthetic vapours. Proper use of mouth packs is important in prevention. A nasopharyngeal airway may sometimes be helpful and bilateral nasopharyngeal tubes have been advocated.[32]

5. Contamination of the Trachea. Regurgitation of digested material can occur in the presence of hiatus hernia, achalasia of the cardia or pharyngeal pouch. Actual vomiting can occur in light planes of anaesthesia. Precautions must be taken to prevent inhalation of blood or tooth fragments. Lung abscess may result.[33] Prevention may include use of throat pack, unhurried surgery, tranquil anaesthesia, efficient and reliable suction, vigilance, careful postoperative positioning. Tracheal soiling may also occur in conscious patients sedated with diazepam. A powerful sucker should always be available.

6. *Respiratory arrest*. This may be due to: (*a*) Respiratory obstruction—and is treated accordingly; (*b*) Breath-holding in light anaesthesia—treatment usually unnecessary; (*c*) Apnoea due to severe hypoxia—treatment is by inflation of the lungs with oxygen; (*d*) Grave cardiovascular depression—rarely.

7. *Cardiac dysrhythmias*. There is evidence of increased sympathetic activity during dental anaesthesia,[34] shown by tachycardia and an increase in circulating catecholamines. Parasympathetic responses can also occur. Ventricular dysrhythmias have been reported during dental anaesthesia in the ambulant patient.[35] The incidence may be up to 38% when halothane is given, but does not occur with intravenous methods.[36] Atropine increases the incidence of dysrhythmias during nitrous-oxide–oxygen and halothane anaesthesia in children.[37] Practolol premedication produces a significant reduction[38] as does local analgesia. Patients who have abnormalities of rhythm are likely to have delayed recovery. Pulse monitors are not reliable detectors of ectopic beats in the dental chair, due to movements of the patient. Dysrhythmias have been reported in patients receiving tricyclic antidepressants.[39] Gingival retraction cord, used to produce ischaemia, is impregnated with 8% racemic adrenaline and so may cause severe dysrhythmias in patients under halothane; a death has been reported from this cause.[40] Cord impregnated with either zinc chloride or aluminium sulphate can be used instead to reduce bleeding. Enflurane is associated with a lesser incidence of dysrhythmias in dental patients than halothane[25] but is less convenient to use. (For the ECG in dental anaesthesia, *see* Rollason W. N. *SAAD Digest* 1983, **5**, 112.)

8. *Fainting and hypotension*. Bourne has drawn attention to the possibility of fainting during the administration of nitrous oxide in the dental chair.[11] The pulse should be frequently monitored, e.g. the carotid, superficial temporal or facial artery, in both the semi-recumbent and the sitting postures. Should the patient suddenly become pale, he must be immediately tilted into the horizontal position to prevent cerebral ischaemia. If this is neglected, delayed recovery from anaesthesia, permanent cerebral damage from hypoxia or even death may result. It is an arguable proposition that all dental operations should be performed with the patient in the horizontal position.[41] Collapse and death has also followed local analgesia.[42]

Causes of hypotension during dental anaesthesia may include: (*a*) Emotional factors, operative before or during early stages of anaesthesia; (*b*) Hypoxia. Some subjects faint when given hypoxic mixtures (10% oxygen), in the absence of anaesthesia; (*c*) Pressure on the carotid sinus area when supporting the jaw; (*d*) Bradycardia and hypotension due to surgical stimulation of vagal reflexes; (*e*) Cessation of anaesthesia. Anaesthesia may protect against syncopal reactions, which become manifest at the end of the procedure.

9. *Nausea and vomiting*. This can be reduced if hypoxia is scrupulously avoided, or if droperidol 0·25 mg i.v. is given. This does not delay recovery.[43]

10. *Deaths*. Some 7–12 deaths associated with general anaesthesia for dental operations occur annually in the UK. It is often difficult to determine the true cause of death, but hypoxia and pulmonary oedema feature in a number of reports. Cardiomyopathy presents a special risk and diabetic autonomic neuropathy is important (*see* Chapter 22). The need for general anaesthesia in the dental chair in the UK is rapidly declining because of the success of modern methods of prevention of dental caries.[44]

11. Following extraction under local or general anaesthesia there is a high incidence of morbidity due to such factors as sore lips, inability to open mouth and eat normally, drowsiness, nausea, vomiting, giddiness and headache.[45]

12. Pain. Intravenous aspirin (lysine acetyl salicylic acid, 1·8 g in 10 ml saline) immediately prior to induction of general anaesthesia may be of use for the relief of postoperative pain in outpatient dental anaesthesia.[46]

13. Hazards to dental and nursing staff. Occupational exposure to nitrous oxide may cause depression of vitamin B_{12} activity resulting in measurable changes in bone marrow secondary to impaired synthesis of deoxyribonucleic acid (DNA).[47]

Mouth Packs
These perform vital functions: (1) To soak up blood and saliva; (2) To discourage mouth-breathing; (3) To prevent soiling of the lower respiratory tract. They may be: (1) Moist cellulose flange packs[48] (one for each side of mouth). Placed by the operator; (2) Gauze, 12-fold, 8 cm by 120 cm (at least 14 cm outside the mouth at all times) or a strip of gamgee tissue.

Packs need to be inserted carefully and may need to be changed during the course of operation. A pack should be inserted into the retromolar space between the underside of the tongue and the teeth on the side to be operated on, with its free end on the opposite side.[49] The tongue should be displaced upwards and medially so that it makes apposition with the soft palate, not the posterior pharyngeal wall; this discourages mouth-breathing.

(*See also* Deaths and dental anaesthetics. Lewis B. *Br. Med. J.* 1984, **286**, 3; Deaths associated with dentistry. Coplans M. P. and Curson I. *Br. Dent. J.* 1982, **153**, 357.)
Regional Analgesia See Chapter 31.

Conservative Dentistry
Cavity fillings may be painful and require analgesia or even anaesthesia for their completion. General anaesthesia is a controlled state of unconsciousness accompanied by partial or complete loss of protective reflexes. Deep sedation is a depressed level of consciousness with some blunting of protective reflexes, although it remains possible to arouse the patient. Conscious sedation is a light level of sedation with full activity of protective reflexes and ability to respond to verbal command.

1. Local analgesic injection. Infiltration or inferior dental nerve block. The most frequently employed method.

2. 'Ultra-light' anaesthesia with methohexitone. A cannula is inserted in a convenient arm vein and connected to a syringe. Anaesthesia is induced and intermittent supplementary injections given as required. Scrupulous attention must be paid to the airway and the insertion of a pack to prevent inhalation of water or tooth powder. This technique has been criticized on the grounds that clinical studies have shown respiratory obstruction, arterial hypoxaemia, tachycardia, fall in peripheral resistance, and unsatisfactory operative conditions and patient tranquillity in an unacceptable proportion of patients.[50] This is a highly controversial method. The case for the defence is well put in *Drummond-Jackson's Dental Sedation and Anaesthesia* (Sykes P. ed.). London: SAAD, 1979.

3. Intravenous diazepam, 10–20 mg slowly over 2 min. A suitable end-point has been described as occurring when a degree of ptosis is observed.[51] Local

analgesia is required in addition. Diazepam may be painful on injection and may cause venous thrombosis. The competence of the laryngeal closure reflex is impaired for 5–10 min following intravenous diazepam. Combination with pentazocine has been recommended; dose 30 mg.[52] Midazolam has advantages over diazepam, with faster onset of sedation, quicker recovery and fewer sore arms. Average dose, 2–3 mg, given slowly, so minimizing hiccups and respiratory depression. The solution contains 10 mg in 5 ml.[53]

4. Full general anaesthesia with tracheal intubation. The anaesthetist has full control of the patient's airway while a throat pack can be used to prevent tracheal soiling. This is a satisfactory technique in selected healthy ambulant patients, though they may suffer complications such as muscle pains, if suxamethonium is used, and sore throat. They must have a period of rest before being escorted home in a motor vehicle and should continue to rest at home for the remainder of the day. Some workers prefer to intubate under halothane, with or without vercuronium, so lessening muscle pains and possible dysrhythmias. Intravenous atropine, barbiturate and short-acting relaxant may be followed by nitrous oxide, oxygen and halothane from a Magill circuit (Mapleson A).

5. The Jorgensen technique[54] (The Loma Linda Dental School, Univ. of California). The aim is to provide good sedation while work is carried out under local analgesia.

6. Relative analgesia.[55] the Quantiflex apparatus has been used to provide inhalation of sub-anaesthetic concentrations of nitrous oxide during conservation under local analgesia. Nitrous oxide 25% with oxygen 75% gives inhalation analgesia.[56]

Dihydrocodeine, although effective in the relief of pain in labour, after operation, and of skeletal origin, is reported to act as an anti-analgesic when given after dental extraction.[57]

There appears to be little difference in morbidity between general and regional analgesia in the dental chair.[58]

(*See also* Matthews R. A. *Dental Local Analgesia*. Bristol: Wright, 1982.)

Anaesthesia for Inpatients

Dental patients are admitted to hospital and treated as inpatients when either the dental procedure or anaesthetic facilities exceeds the scope of the outpatient department, or when the general condition of the patient contraindicates outpatient anaesthesia.

Inpatients should receive a full general examination. Premedication can be prescribed. The anaesthetic technique usually involves tracheal intubation with a throat pack to prevent aspiration of blood and debris. Two tampons (Tampax) tied together, lying one each side of the nasotracheal tube in the pharynx, give a reasonably watertight seal. A nasotracheal tube is usually preferred, but an orotracheal tube is sometimes more acceptable to the surgeon, as when the site of operation is the upper incisor area (apicectomy, dental cysts, etc.).

Complications and hazards include:

1. Epistaxis and nasal trauma due to passage of a nasal tube. Can be minimized by prior spraying of the nasal mucosa with a vasoconstrictor (e.g. cocaine 4%).

2. Sore throat. Due to the insertion of a throat pack, when bruising and abrasion of the mucus membrane of the palate and fauces can readily occur.

3. Muscle pains. When suxamethonium is used to facilitate intubation, postoperative muscle pains can be very distressing, since the patients are ambulant early ('the body all aching and racked with pain' syndrome). These pains can be abolished if other means are used to facilitate intubation; for example: (1) Use of gallamine, 20 mg 3 min before the injection of suxamethonium; (2) Use of deep anaesthesia with halothane; (3) Blind intubation after use of carbon dioxide to produce hyperventilation; (4) Use of non-depolarizing relaxants for intubation. All these methods have their disadvantages also, and many anaesthetists prefer suxamethonium because of the quick and smooth intubation which can be undertaken in light planes of anaesthesia.

4. Ventricular dysrhythmias have been reported as a result of surgical stimuli during dental extractions.[59] These are, however, transient, and it would appear that their significance is not great provided the anaesthetic technique is impeccable. An ECG may be useful to indicate their occurrence. Premedication with a β-blocker reduces the incidence. Less common if halothane avoided.

The types of patient who present for inpatient operation because of their general physical condition include:

1. Mental defectives and spastics, who are difficult to manage in the dental chair under local analgesia.[60]

2. Cardiac patients, who require careful anaesthetic management, and may require antibiotic cover. (*See* Report on Working Party for Antimicrobial Chemotherapy. *Lancet* 1982, **2**, 1323.) At least 30% oxygen should be administered.

3. Cases of chronic respiratory disease, particularly where there is gross derangement of ventilation–perfusion relationships.

4. Those with a haemorrhage disorder, e.g. haemophilia, Christmas disease, thrombocytopenia, or where there is a history of severe post-extraction haemorrhage. The blood should be examined for coagulation defects preoperatively and, if necessary, appropriate treatment arranged.

The Haemophiliac Patient

For details of management *see* Chapter 22. Extreme gentleness is required during anaesthesia to avoid trauma. An oral tube is preferred to a nasal, and throat packs are not used. Surgery should include meticulous haemostasis. *See* Voke J. et al. *Haemophilia Centre Handbook*. London: Immuno Ltd, 1980.

Faciomaxillary Operations

For history of faciomaxillary surgery and anaesthesia, *see* Ward T. *Ann. R. Coll. Surg. Engl.* 1975, **57**, 67.

Fractured Jaw

This may be part of a grave emergency complicated by intraoral haemorrhage, obstructed airway and associated injuries (including head injury and loss of consciousness). In these very severe cases the protective laryngeal reflexes may be obtunded with danger of aspiration of blood, teeth and other debris. Unstable fractures can allow the tongue to fall back and obstruct the airway. Such patients demand urgent treatment. Most mandibular fractures are unilateral and do not require urgent treatment. In others trismus may be a feature. The jaw injury is usually less serious and operative treatment can be carried out as an elective procedure. Fractures of the maxillae can be classified according to the Le Fort scheme.[61] There may be associated periorbital oedema and epistaxis, and cerebrospinal rhinorrhoea is not infrequent. Diplopia may occur with orbital fracture. Respiratory problems occasionally arise if the mobile maxilla approximates to the posterior pharyngeal wall or the dorsum of the tongue.

The anaesthetist who is asked to deal with a fractured mandible and/or maxilla should look out for: (1) Associated injuries, especially: (*a*) Head injuries—loss of consciousness, depressed fractures, raised intracranial tension; (*b*) Chest injuries—pneumothorax or haemothorax; (*c*) Abdominal injuries—ruptured viscera; (*d*) Major bone fractures. The presence of associated injuries results in increased haemorrhage and shock; (2) Presence of blood and debris in the pharynx, larynx and trachea. There may be respiratory obstruction and the laryngeal reflexes may be obtunded. Occasionally it is necessary to bronchoscope the patient for tracheobronchial toilet. (3) Possibility of swallowed blood which may be regurgitated as anaesthesia is induced. It is seldom practical to ask the patient to swallow an oesophageal tube. (4) The possibility of food in the stomach if the operation is an emergency.

First-aid treatment may include: (1) In the unconscious patient, it may be wise to pass a tracheal tube, usually via the nose. Rarely a tracheostomy may be required; (2) Temporary fixation with dental wire of large displaced fragments of bone; (3) Pharyngeal (or tracheobronchial) toilet; (4) Treatment of shock, if present, by blood transfusion, etc.

Anaesthetic technique

Premedication. In the emergency case it is wise to restrict premedication to atropine or hyoscine. Respiratory depressants are to be avoided. An anti-emetic drug is used to prevent postoperative vomiting (when the jaws have been wired together).

Induction. This should only be commenced when the anaesthetist is satisfied that arrangements have been made to deal with any emergency that may arise and that he has adequate help. The anaesthetist should place the patient on an operating table or trolley that can be instantly tipped. Suction should be available and switched on. Rarely bronchoscopy may be indicated. The usual precautions to prevent regurgitation of stomach contents should be taken.

Induction is usually carried out with thiopentone and short-acting relaxant. Visualization of the larynx may be rendered difficult if blood and debris are present—but the shattered tissues do not resist introduction of the laryngoscope and intubation can usually be performed without difficulty. The anaesthetist should be as gentle as possible in order to avoid further mobilization of the fracture.

A nasotracheal tube is usually preferred. This may be cuffed.[62] A pharyngeal pack can also be inserted—but should be removed and pharyngeal toilet performed immediately before the jaws are wired together.

Maintenance is by inhalation anaesthesia. Smooth anaesthetic technique is desirable, with rapid return of reflexes at the end of operation and absence of vomiting, coughing and straining. Anti-emetic drugs may be used with advantage in premedication or postoperatively.

When the jaws have been wired together the patient should leave theatre with a nasopharyngeal airway in situ. A pair of wire cutters should remain near the patient, so that they can be used in an emergency to free the jaws, and the mouth and pharynx can be sucked out. The nursing attendants should know how to use the instrument and which wires to cut. In fact on occasion it may be life-saving, in the presence of severe respiratory obstruction. (*See also* Langdon J. D. and Rapidis A. D. *Br. J. Hosp. Med.* 1982, **28**, 589.)

(*See also* Hughes G. in: *General Anaesthesia*, 4th ed. (Gray T. C. et al. ed.) London: Butterworth, 1980; *Anaesthesia and Sedation in Dentistry* (Coplans M. P. and Green R. A. ed.) Amsterdam: Elsevier, 1983.)

References

1. Evans T. W. *Br. J. Dent. Sci.* 1868, **11**, 196, 318.
2. Hewitt F. W. *Anaesthetics and their Administration*. London: Griffin, 1893; Hewitt F. W. *The Administration of Nitrous Oxide and Oxygen for Dental Operations*. London: Ash, 1897.
3. McKesson E. I. *Br. Med. J.* 1926, **2**, 1113.
4. Coleman F. *Dent. Rec.* 1942, **62**, 143, 167.
5. Clover J. T. *Br. Med. J.* 1868, **2**, 491; Coleman A. *Br. J. Dent. Sci.* 1868, **11**, 128.
6. Redman in Hollander-Schneidermühl's *Handbuch der Zahnartzl.* 1890, p. 149.
7. Walsh R. S. *Br. J. Anaesth.* 1958, **30**, 578.
8. Drummond-Jackson S. L. *Dental Cosmos* 1935, **77**, 130; Howells T. H. *Br. J. Anaesth.* 1968, **40**, 182.
9. Peabody J. B. *Texas Dent. J.* 1965, **83**, 12.
10. Danziger A. M. *Br. Dent. J.* 1962, **113**, 426.
11. Bourne J. G. *Lancet* 1957, **2**, 499.
12. *Drummond-Jackson's Dental Sedation and Anaesthesia* (Sykes P. ed.). London: SAAD, 1979.
13. Green R. A. and Jolly C. *Br. J. Anaesth.* 1960, **32**, 593.
14. Goldman V. and Kennedy P. *Anaesthesia* 1964, **19**, 424.
15. Davidau A. *Rev. Stomatol.* 1966, **67**, 589.
16. Dinsdale R. C. W. and Dixon R. A. *Br. Dent. J.* 1976, **144**, 271.
17. Hall R. J. *N.Y. Med. J.* 1884, **40**, 643.
18. Hunt W. A. *Br. Dent. J.* 1886, Jan.
19. Clement F. W. *Nitrous Oxide–Oxygen Anaesthesia*, 3rd ed. London: Kimpton, 1951; Lee J. A. and Atkinson R. S. *Synopsis of Anaesthesia*, 7th ed. Bristol: Wright, 1973.
20. Smith W. D. A. *Br. J. Anaesth.* 1961, **33**, 440.
21. Latham J. and Parbrook G. D. *Anaesthesia* 1966, **21**, 472; 1967, **22**, 316.
22. Young T. M. *Br. J. Anaesth.* 1969, **41**, 120.
23. *See also* Green R. A. and Coplans M. P. *Anaesthesia and Analgesia in Dentistry*. London: Lewis, 1973.
24. Lewis T. *Br. Med. J.* 1932, **1**, 873.
25. Wright C. J. *Anaesthesia* 1980, **36**, 775; Ryder W. and Wright P. A. *Anaesthesia* 1981, **36**, 532; Barker G. I. and Briscoe C. E. *Br. J. Anaesth.* 1981, **53**, 1079.
26. Coplans M. P. and Green R. A. *Anaesthesia and Sedation in Dentistry*. Amsterdam: Elsevier, 1983.
27. Drummond-Jackson S. L. *Dent. Cosmos* 1935, **77**, 130.
28. Young T. M. *Anaesthesia* 1974, **29**, 614.
29. Davidau A. *Rev. Stomatol.* 1966, **67**, 589; Brown P. R. H., Main D. M. G. and Lawson J. I. M. *Br. Dent. J.* 1968, **125** (2), 498.
30. Sale J. P. et al. *Anaesthesia* 1985, **40**, 3.
31. *See also* Love S. H. S. in: *General Anaesthesia for Dental Surgery* (Hunter A. R. and Bush G. H. ed.). Altrincham: Sherratt, 1971, p. 104; Love S. H. S. *Br. J. Anaesth.* 1968, **40**, 188.
32. Doctor N. H. *Anaesthesia* 1977, **32**, 273.
33. Brock R. C. *Guy's Hosp. Rep.* 1947, **96**, 141.
34. Edmondson M. D. et al. *Br. Med. J.* 1972, **2**, 47; Taggart P. et al. *Br. Med. J.* 1976, **2**, 787; Al-Khishali T. et al. *Anaesthesia* 1978, **33**, 184.
35. Kaufman L. *Proc. R. Soc. Med.* 1966, **59**, 731; Ryder W. *Anaesthesia* 1970, **25**, 46.
36. Ryder W. *Proc. R. Soc. Med.* 1971, **64**, 82; Ryder W. and Townsend D. *Br. J. Anaesth.* 1974, **46**, 760; Bradshaw E. G. *Anaesthesia* 1976, **31**, 13.
37. Thurlow A. C. *Anaesthesia* 1972, **27**, 429; Whalley D. G. et al. *Br. J. Anaesth.* 1976, **48**, 120.
38. Ryder W. et al. *Anaesthesia* 1971, **26**, 508.
39. Plowman P. E. and Thomas W. J. W. *Anaesthesia* 1974, **29**, 576.

40. Hilley M. D. et al. *Anesthesiology* 1984, **60**, 587.
41. Bourne J. G. *Studies in Anaesthetics*. London: Lloyd-Luke, 1967, p. 131.
42. Tomlin P. J. *Anaesthesia* 1974, **29**, 551; Coplans M. P. and Curson I. *Br. Dent. J.* 1976, **141**, 255.
43. O'Donovan N. and Shaw J. *Anaesthesia* 1984, **39**, 1172.
44. Parbrook G. D. *Br. J. Anaesth.* 1986, **58**, 369.
45. Muir V. M. J. *Anaesthesia* 1976, **31**, 171.
46. Foster J. M. G. and Cashman J. N. *Anaesthesia* 1985, **40**, 576.
47. Sweeney B. et al. *Br. Med. J.* 1985, **291**, 567.
48. Drummond-Jackson S. L. *Br. Dent. J.* 1964, **116**, 15.
49. Coplans M. P. and Barton P. R. *Br. Dent. J.* 1964, **116**, 209.
50. Wise C. C. et al. *Br. Med. J.* 1969, **2**, 540; Mann P. E. et al. *Anaesthesia* 1971, **26**, 3; Thornton J. A. *Proc. R. Soc. Med.* 1971, **64**, 83.
51. Verrill P. *Br. Dent. J.* 1969, **127**, 85.
52. Sykes P. *Br. Med. J.* 1977, **2**, 832; Corrall I. M. et al. *Anaesthesia* 1979, **34**, 850.
53. Rosenbaum N. L. *Br. Dent. J.* 1985, **158**, 139.
54. Jorgensen N. B. and Leffingwell F. *Dent. Clin. North Am.* 1961 (July), p. 299; Jorgensen N. B. et al. *J. Soc. Cal. Dent. Clins.* 1963, **31**, 7; *see also* Bourne J. G. *Studies in Anaesthetics*. London: Lloyd-Luke, 1967, p. 116; Jorgensen N. B. and Hayden J. Sedation; local and general anesthesia in dentistry. 3rd ed. Philadelphia: Lea & Febiger, 1980.
55. Langa H. *Relative Analgesia in Dental Patients*. Philadelphia: Saunders, 1976; Young T. M. et al. *Br. Dent. J.* 1976, **141**, 34.
56. Edmunds D. H. and Rosen M. *Anaesthesia* 1984, **39**, 138.
57. Seymour R. A. et al. *Lancet* 1982, **1**, 1425.
58. Muir V. M. J. et al. *Anaesthesia* 1976, **31**, 171.
59. Kaufman L. *Proc. R. Soc. Med.* 1966, **59**, 731.
60. Diamond D. W. and Cochrane D. F. *Anaesthesia* 1976, **31**, 190.
61. McGregor I. A. *Fundamental Techniques of Plastic Surgery*. Edinburgh: Churchill Livingstone, 1972.
62. Davies J. A. H. *Anaesthesia* 1967, **22**, 153.
63. Cripps T. P. and Edmondson R. S. *Anaesthesia* 1987, **42**, 189.

(*See also* Editorial. General anaesthesia in dentistry. *Br. Dent. J.* 1981, **151**, 357; Report of Working Party on Training in Dental Anaesthesia (Wylie W. D.) *Br. Dent. J.* 1981, **151**, 385. Report of the Interfaculty Working Party (Seward) formed to consider the implementation of the Wylie Report. *Br. Dent. J.* 1981, **151**, 389.)

Chapter 26   NEUROSURGICAL ANAESTHESIA[1]

History

First successful diagnosis and surgical removal of a cerebral tumour took place in 1885.[2] Sir Victor Horsley (1857–1917) of London removed an extradural spinal cord tumour for the first time in 1884. He began to develop neurological surgery as a separate specialty, having been appointed surgeon to the National Hospital for Nervous Diseases, Queen's Square in 1886, and this influenced Harvey Cushing (1869–1939) of Boston (who introduced the silver clip to arrest haemorrhage in 1911 and pioneered the use in surgery of the high-frequency current (diathermy) in 1928[3] and whose anaesthetist in Boston was Dr Walter M. Boothby), and Walter Dandy (1886–1946) of Philadelphia (who described ventriculography in 1918[4] and air encephalography in 1919[5]). Egas Moniz of Lisbon used cerebral angiography in 1927.[6] A pioneer British neurosurgical anaesthetist was Zebulon Mennell (1876–1959).[7] The first planned operation for cerebral aneurysm took place in 1932[8] and the first localization of a cerebral tumour by EEG was reported in 1936[9] and by radio-isotopes in 1948.[10] In the early days of anaesthesia for neurosurgery, chloroform and ether both had their advocates and gradually chloroform, up to 2% of vapour, given, for example, by means of the Vernon Harcourt (1834–1919) apparatus[11] or the Junker bottle or one of its many modifications (Junker F. A. (1818–1901)[12]) won the day. Harvey Cushing, later to become a pioneer neurosurgeon had a death under anaesthesia in 1893 at the Massachusetts General Hospital and this stimulated him to introduce the ether chart, a record of BP, pulse rate and respiration rate during all major administrations.[13] Early pioneers of neurosurgical anaesthesia in the UK, many of them part-time general practitioners, included Zebulon Mennell (appointed to the staff of the National Hospital in 1911[14]) Maxwell Brown and John Gillies in Edinburgh, Noel Gillespie and John Challis at the London Hospital, Olive Jones in Oxford, and Harry Brennan and Andrew Hunter in Manchester. As the use of tracheal intubation spread in the 1930s and 1940s, workers eagerly adopted it for neurosurgery, usually along with a Magill system (Mapleson-A), but experience soon showed that bleeding from inside the cranium was unacceptable, due, as it proved to be, to a combination of hypercapnia and increase in the venous pressure associated with resistance to expiration. This gave place in 1957 to the use of relaxants to enable IPPV with its consequent hypocapnia and absence of tone in the anterior abdominal wall and hence lower CVP to be employed by Furness in Australia.[15]

Over the years general anaesthesia with inhalation agents has been the most popular method of anaesthesia for these operations, including trichloroethylene in 1941. Local analgesia has had its advocates while sedation produced by the rectal administration of bromethol in the late 1920s and ether-oil[16] enabled some workers to solve their problems. (*See also* Dott N. *Proc. R. Soc. Med.* 1971, **64**, 1051; Hunter A. R. *Ann. Roy Coll. Surg. Engl.* 1981, **63**, 316; Hunter A. R. in: *Anaesthesia; Essays on its History* (Rupreht J. et al. ed.) Berlin: Springer-Verlag, 1985, p. 148.)

Special Problems Involved
(1) Raised intracranial tension; (2) The poor general condition of some patients; (3) The length of operation; (4) Maintenance of the airway. Inaccessibility of the tracheal tube and connections during long operations, coupled with the strict necessity of maintaining an absolutely free airway with absence of straining or coughing. The need to suck out the trachea in some patients; (5) Posture. Head-up, sitting, lateral or prone positions may be required throughout a lengthy operation. There may be great danger to the patient through imperfect positioning; (6) Surgical trauma may produce haemorrhage and/or cerebral ischaemia. Vital structures are often very near the area of surgical manipulation. The anaesthetist must keep a close watch on the vital signs using efficient monitoring; (7) Use of diathermy requires non-explosive technique; (8) Air embolism may occur in head-up positions.

A smooth induction, absence of straining and normal blood-gas tensions are essential in neurosurgical anaesthesia. A short period of straining, accompanied by the inevitable hypoxia and hypercapnia may cause oedema of the brain which may persist for some time after the patient's respiration has settled down; this may cause surgical difficulty.

Cerebral Haemodynamics
Though cerebral blood flow, cerebral vascular resistance and cerebral metabolic

rate are factors which can be measured, their relationship and significance are not fully understood. The brain should probably be regarded as several organs within a compact structure with separate functional needs and separate patterns of regional blood flow, not necessarily reflected in total measurements.

Intracranial contents may be considered as comprising: solids in brain tissue 24%, water in brain tissue 60%, cerebral blood volume 3–5%, cerebrospinal fluid 11–13%. The intracranial contents are restricted inside a rigid indistensible chamber, the skull, although some volume changes can occur via the foramen magnum to the spinal cord, subarachnoid and extradural spaces.

Cerebral Blood Flow is Regulated by

1. *The blood CO_2 tension*. A Pa_{CO_2} of 8–11 kPa increases cerebral blood flow by 100%, while a decrease to 3·5 kPa reduces blood flow by 30%.
2. *Venous Pressure*. This may be influenced by: (*a*) Gravity; (*b*) Intrathoracic pressure; (*c*) Intra-abdominal pressure; (*d*) Blood volume; (*e*) Circulatory efficiency; (*f*) Venous tone; (*g*) Venous obstruction in the neck.
3. *Arterial blood pressure*. If the other factors controlling cerebral blood flow are kept within normal limits, cerebral blood flow does not alter greatly with blood pressures between 90 and 180 mmHg. In the supine position the healthy brain receives between 750 and 900 ml of blood per min or about 15% of the left ventricular output.
4. *Extracellular pH*. Rise in hydrogen ion concentration dilates cerebral arteries and arterioles. This probably accounts for P_{CO_2} change effects.
5. *Cerebrospinal fluid pressure*.
6. *Oxygen tension*. Inhalation of high oxygen tension reduces cerebral blood flow by no more than 10%. A reduction of oxygen inhalation to 10% increases cerebral blood flow by 30%. This may be mediated via carotid body chemore-ceptors.[17]
7. *Neurogenic factors*. Thought to have little effect on cerebral blood flow, but some workers believe that extraparenchymal small arteries and veins are under neurogenic control so that the dilatation of vessels due to hypercapnia may be opposed at least partially.
8. *Temperature*. Heat causes cerebral vasodilatation while cold has the reverse effect.
9. *Drugs*. Cerebral vasodilatation is produced by all inhalation agents, probably excluding light levels of isoflurane, and ketamine. Hyperventilation can to some extent counteract the vasodilator effect, though not reliably. The rise in intracranial pressure produced by anaesthetic agents like halothane is greater in patients who already have a space-occupying lesion than in the normal individual. Intracranial pressure may be increased more in a compartment of the brain containing a space-occupying lesion than elsewhere with resultant 'shift' at the level of the tentorium or foramen magnum. Other drugs produce a reduction in cerebral blood flow, including neurolept analgesia (droperidol and fentanyl), thiopentone, methohexitone and diazepam.

About two-thirds of the blood flow to the brain arrives via the carotid and one-third by the vertebral arteries.

Prostaglandins (present in platelets) cause cerebral vasoconstriction and may be a mechanism in spasm secondary to intracranial haemorrhage.

The anaesthetist can reduce bleeding during intracranial operations by strict attention to blood-gas homeostasis and to intracranial venous pressure.

(*See also* Shapiro H. M. *Anesthesiology* 1975, **43**, 445.)

The critical value for cerebral flow-rate is 30 ml/100 g brain/min (normal 53 ml/100 g/min). Where cerebrovascular disease and marginal cerebral blood flow pre-exist, abrupt rises in venous pressure during straining or coughing may produce symptoms of insufficiency, especially if there is an associated fall in arterial pressure (e.g. during induction of anaesthesia).

Intracerebral Steal and Counter-steal
Local brain pathology associated with local acidosis may have produced maximal local vasodilatation. In these circumstances rise of Pa_{CO_2} dilates vessels in normal brain tissue so that blood is 'stolen' from the pathological area. The converse happens in hypocapnia with the result that hyperventilation may divert blood to abnormal parts of the brain. This may be important following trauma.

Cerebrospinal Fluid
See Chapter 2.

Intracranial Pressure[18]
Normal intracranial pressure is about 130 mm of CSF, measured in the horizontal position with the spine and external occipital protuberance in the same line. Raising the head 20 cm above the horizontal reduces the intracranial pressure by 20 cmH$_2$O.[19]

Decreased Intracranial Pressure
This may occur: (*a*) Following blood loss; (*b*) Following dehydration; (*c*) Postoperatively, after removal of a space-occupying lesion. Its significance to the anaesthetist is not great. Occasionally, following removal of a subdural or extradural haematoma it may be desirable to lower the head of the table and infuse fluid intravenously in order to re-expand the brain.

Raised Intracranial Pressure
This may occur physiologically as a result of coughing, sneezing, straining at stool, etc. Pathologically raised intracranial tension may occur: (1) By pressure from outside. A bony tumour or craniostenosis; (2) By presence of a space-occupying lesion, neoplasm, abscess or haematoma; (3) In hydrocephalus; (4) With venous obstruction; (5) With arterial dilatation, e.g. secondary to hypercapnia; (6) With cerebral oedema, which in turn may be due to inflammation, neoplasm, trauma, hypoxia, venous obstruction, etc.; (7) With head-down position.

With an intact skull, a rise in intracranial pressure may not cause immediate harm, but if the skull is opened, there is the risk of herniation of brain tissue through the craniotomy wound.

Anaesthetic Technique

Local Analgesia
The added risks of general anaesthesia in the presence of raised intracranial

tension, coupled with the insensitivity of most of the intracranial structures to painful stimuli, suggest the advantages of local techniques.

The skin and scalp may be infiltrated with 0·25–0·5% lignocaine. Adrenaline should be added in strength of between 1–250 000 and 1–500 000 to cut down oozing.

The bone is only slightly sensitive and drilling, though uncomfortable, is usually tolerable. The contents of the cranium are insensitive with a few exceptions. Sensitive regions are: (1) The dura mater at the base of the skull; (2) The area around the middle meningeal artery; (3) The nervus spinosus; (4) The trigeminal ganglion.

During operation careful watch on the patient's general condition is mandatory, just as in general anaesthesia. Alterations in levels of consciousness may also be observed. Sometimes a patient will need restraint. Oxygen blown under the towels near the mouth will prevent a feeling of suffocation. The anaesthetist should be prepared to intervene to provide an artificial airway should the level of consciousness deteriorate.

Advantages of Local Analgesia
1. Avoidance of further rise of intracranial pressure which may occur with general anaesthesia, especially if coughing or straining is allowed.
2. The airway is well maintained in the conscious patient and respiration is often quieter than can be obtained with general anaesthesia.

Disadvantages of Local Analgesia
1. Unsuitable for children.
2. Unsatisfactory for uncooperative adults. If there is impairment of consciousness, restraint will be needed to prevent movements of the limbs and head.
3. Long operations are a strain for the conscious patient.

Indications for Local Analgesia
1. The presence of raised intracranial pressure where the operative intervention is relatively slight, e.g. ventriculography, burr-hole biopsy, etc.
2. When the patient's co-operation is required at some stage in the operation, e.g. localization of subjective phenomena.
3. For some emergencies, where a rapid rise of intracranial tension may make general anaesthesia particularly hazardous, e.g. middle meningeal haemorrhage.
4. Where facilities for skilled administration of general anaesthesia are not available.
5. When the general condition of the patient is a contraindication to general anaesthesia.

General Anaesthesia

Premedication
Sedative drugs, particularly narcotic analgesics, should be withheld in the presence of: (1) Raised intracranial pressure; (2) Head injury; (3) The prone, sitting or steep head-up position with spontaneous respiration.

Atropine or hyoscine should be given in sufficient dosage to prevent salivation. This is particularly important as tracheal suction is not easy once the operation has begun.

Induction
Induction should be smooth to avoid coughing or straining or undue central depression. After an episode of coughing, it may take half an hour for the central venous pressure to return to normal.

The Airway
Intubation is essential to ensure a clear airway in intracranial surgery or in laminectomy but every effort must be made to reduce the rise in intracranial pressure associated with it. The cords and trachea should be sprayed with topical analgesic and the tube lubricated with analgesic ointment to help to prevent coughing. The tube should be of the largest size consistent with atraumatic introduction—usually 8–12 mm internal diameter. Precautions should be taken to prevent kinking. It is helpful to remove the soft bevel of a reinforced nylon tube so that it cannot cause respiratory obstruction by impinging on the tracheal wall.[20] An Oxford tube is also suitable. A cuffed tube is normally used as it prevents aspiration of stomach contents, protects the lungs in case of haemorrhage into the nasal airways (e.g. from open frontal sinus, fractured base of skull, etc.) and facilitates IPPV. When spontaneous respiration is allowed there should be no resistance to respiration and T-piece systems have been recommended, especially in children.

The Course of Anaesthesia
Muscle-relaxant drugs facilitate IPPV so that Pa_{CO_2} can be lowered. Light planes of anaesthesia allow rapid recovery of consciousness at the end of the operation. Topical analgesia helps to prevent coughing and straining in the patient who breathes spontaneously. An intravenous drip is necessary for all major cases.

Monitoring[21]
Readings of blood pressure, pulse rate and respiratory rate should be taken at least every 10 min. Any changes not obviously related to anaesthesia should be reported to the surgeon as they may be caused by intracranial manipulations or by a sudden rise in intracranial pressure. The electrocardiogram acts as an excellent pulse monitor and is of particular value in posterior fossa surgery when irregularities may occur due to air embolism. An oesophageal or precordial stethoscope may also be useful as the typical murmur of air in the heart may be heard. End-tidal carbon dioxide tension may fall when air blocks part of the pulmonary vasculature and a rapid response analyser provides early warning. Ultrasound detectors[22] can also be used over the jugular veins. (*See also* Buckland R. W. and Manners J. M. *Anaesthesia* 1976, **31**, 633.) Some anaesthetists who favour hyperventilation techniques perform hourly estimations of blood gases. Direct monitoring of intracranial pressure can be undertaken via a catheter placed in the lateral ventricle or by use of implanted extradural transducers.[23] This is more important in intensive therapy than during operation. Where much bleeding is expected, a central venous line is

often used and if the patient is in the sitting position, the tip may be inserted into the right side of the heart to aid the management of air embolism.

Air Embolism[24]

Many of the veins in the fibro-fatty tissues of the back of the neck do not collapse readily after they have been divided, but are held open. The mastoid emissary vein is a particularly common site for air entry. Portals of entry within the dura are relatively uncommon. For signs, diagnosis and treatment *see* Chapter 18.

Agents and Techniques

Effect of Anaesthetic Agents[25]

1. Narcotic analgesic agents. Little effect on cerebral blood flow unless Pa_{CO_2} rises. Neuroleptanalgesia produces a reduction when used in high dosage with controlled ventilation.

2. Intravenous barbiturates. Cerebral blood flow is reduced when they are given in dosage sufficient to produce anaesthesia. This may amount to 30% in light and 50% in deep thiopentone anaesthesia. The use of thiopentone (1 g in 500 ml of dextrose–saline) or methohexitone (500 mg in 500 ml) as a drip to supplement nitrous-oxide–oxygen anaesthesia, together with a relaxant and IPPV, has been recently recommended. The use of a bolus injection reduces intracranial pressure when it is acutely elevated but not when it is normal.[26] Thiopentone may protect the brain cells from the effects of ischaemic damage (e.g. after cardiac arrest).[27] This has been disputed.

3. Ketamine. Causes rise in cerebral blood flow with marked regional variations. Its other advantages, however, make it popular for use in small children undergoing radiodiagnostic procedures.

4. Nitrous oxide. Little effect on cerebral blood flow, but causes a significant depression of cerebral metabolic activity so that venous oxygen saturation is higher than normal. Nitrous oxide may diffuse into gas-filled cavities resulting in a rise of intracranial pressure during air encephalograms. It causes a rise in intracranial pressure in patients with a pre-existing intracranial lesion.

5. Halothane. A cerebral vasodilator in all clinical concentrations. The rise in intracranial tension produced is greater when pressure is already high due to a space-occupying lesion. Cerebral blood flow may be reduced if severe hypotension occurs. Halothane depresses cerebral metabolic activity so that oxygen saturation of cerebral venous blood is raised. It is possible that halothane might cause intracerebral stealing of blood from ischaemic to normal areas of brain. (*See also* Greenbaum, R. *Br. J. Anaesth.* 1976, **48**, 773.)

6. Enflurane increases cerebral blood flow and it has been shown to produce increase in intracranial pressure in patients with space-occupying lesions, even during hypocapnia. It remains to be seen whether the convulsive and EEG activity are important clinically but concentrations up to 1% are well tolerated.

7. Isoflurane may be better than either halothane of enflurane in preventing rise in the intracranial pressure during neurosurgical operations.[28,29] It has little effect on intracranial pressure in patients with intracranial tumours and in low concentration can be used safely in intracranial operations.[30]

8. Trichloroethylene. A cerebral vasodilator. Also produces rise in cerebral venous blood oxygen saturation. Increase in intracranial tension, accentuated when pressure already raised due to space-occupying lesion.

9. Chloroform, ether, methoxyflurane and cyclopropane. Similar effects to halothane.

The vasoconstrictive effect of hypocapnia due to IPPV often overcomes the vasodilatory effects of a volatile agent.

10. Muscle relaxants. Suxamethonium produces a mild, short-lived rise in cerebral blood flow and intracranial pressure. Other muscle relaxants have no direct effect. Reduction in tone of abdominal wall promotes a fall in central (and therefore cerebral) venous pressure.

11. Diazepam does not increase cerebral blood flow.

Hyperventilation Causing Hypocapnia[31]

Relaxants and IPPV were first used in 1957.[15] IPPV with hyperventilation is a standard technique during intracranial surgery and, providing the blood pressure is maintained, in the sitting or head-up position. The advantages are: (1) Cerebral vasoconstriction leads to an excellent surgical field; (2) The moderate rises of arterial P_{CO_2} (over 7 kPa) which are common in light general anaethesia with spontaneous respiration are avoided; (3) Minimal quantities of anaesthetic agents are required.

The anesthestic agents used are thiopentone, nitrous-oxide–oxygen, muscle relaxant and full topical analgesia to the larynx and trachea. Volatile supplements, halothane or enflurane are sometimes given in the initial stages. Hyperventilation may counteract the vasodilator effect of inhalation agents, but this cannot be relied upon. It is, however, common practice to add 0·5% halothane intermittently to nitrous-oxide–oxygen. This helps to prevent rise of blood pressure and awareness. The relaxant is given in full doses to increase overall compliance which allows ventilation with minimal elevation of mean airway pressure. A mechanical ventilator ensures that ventilation is uniform. It may be combined with a negative phase. In some units blood gases are monitored and ventilation adjusted accordingly. There is no indication for lowering $P_{a_{CO_2}}$ below 3·5 to 4·0 kPa, at which level the cerebral blood flow has been reduced to about 50%. Levels below 2·6 kPa may lead to EEG changes and an increase of anaerobic metabolism of glucose in the brain.[32]

Other workers have used the neurolept agents. Premedication with droperidol and atropine, then intravenous phenoperidine, 5 mg, after which the patient must be reminded to breathe. Then thiopentone, suxamethonium, intubation, nitrous oxide, oxygen, IPPV with a non-depolarizing relaxant to reduce inflation pressures to a low level.

Controlled Ventilation with Normal $P_{a_{CO_2}}$

Respiratory alkalosis may be undesirable: (1) In the sitting position, when hypotension may occur; (2) During hypothermia, when there is likelihood of cardiac dysrhythmias.

In these circumstances, it may be desirable to keep $P_{a_{CO_2}}$ within normal limits. This can be accomplished if serial blood-gas estimations are made.

Spontaneous Respiration

This is now less popular than formerly, since, even with impeccable technique, small rises of $P_{a_{CO_2}}$ occur with resultant increase in cerebral blood flow and intracranial pressure. Spontaneous respiration may have advantages in posterior fossa explorations, when the surgeon is working near the brain stem. Sudden changes in respiratory pattern may then indicate ischaemia of the vital centres and serve as a warning mechanism to the surgeon.

Techniques include: (1) Thiopentone (sleep dose), nitrous-oxide–oxygen, halothane or trichloroethylene. Suxamethonium for intubation. Small doses of narcotic analgesic to control tachypnoea; (2) A thiopentone or methohexitone infusion may be used to supplement nitrous oxide and oxygen; Barbiturates cause a reduction in cerebral blood flow;[33] (3) Neuroleptanalgesia. Useful where retention of consciousness and patient co-operation are desired, e.g. stereotaxic surgery for Parkinsonism, electrocorticography, carotid artery ligation and some radiodiagnostic procedures.[33] Droperidol and fentanyl cause a reduction in cerebral blood flow.

Summary
There is general agreement that IPPV, with or without the use of volatile agents, is the most advantageous technique for supratentorial lesions, and in the prone position. For posterior fossa explorations some anaesthetists use IPPV. Others prefer to maintain spontaneous respiration, finding it helpful as a monitor during surgical manipulations close to the brain stem. Despite the theoretical objections to halothane, it has been used successfully in neurosurgery by experienced anaesthetists, especially in the spontaneously breathing patient.[34]

Reduction of Intracranial Tension
A raised intracranial tension produces a tight dura and brain and makes exploration difficult. There are various methods of reducing intracranial tension: (1) Ventricular tap. The surgeon needles the lateral ventricle and removes fluid until the pressure falls; (2) Spinal drainage. Controlled withdrawal of CSF via a catheter put into the subarachnoid space in the lumbar region. Fluid is not withdrawn until the dura is open to prevent coning. Drainage has also been recommended for some operations where the brain itself is normal, e.g. repair of traumatic CSF leak and hydrocephalus; (3) Use of hypertonic solutions intravenously: (*a*) *Mannitol* ($C_6H_{12}O_6$) is a hexahydric alcohol closely related to the hexose sugars and isomeric with sorbitol. Solutions can be sterilized by autoclaving. Dose of the intravenous solution, 20%, is about 0·5 mg/kg over 5–10 min, which may be preceded by *frusemide* 1 mg/kg.[35] Causes a brisk osmotic diuresis, and small 'rebound' increase in brain volume; (*b*) *Urea*, 30% solution in 10% invert sugar in water, run in intravenously over 1–2 hours at a rate of 60 drops/min; it is eventually distributed to the brain and owing to the reverse osmotic gradient results in a rebound increase in brain volume; (*c*) 100 ml 50% *sucrose*; (*d*) *Triple strength plasma*, 1–1·5 g/kg bodyweight. Osmotic dehydration should be begun at the optimal time. During the first hour there are likely to be the effects of increased blood and intracranial pressure with increase in cerebral blood flow and bleeding. It should therefore be started at the time of induction of anaesthesia, or preferably earlier; (*e*) *Oral glycerol* may also be used 0·5–2 g/kg. These agents also have a diuretic effect, so it is important to watch out for bladder distension. An indwelling urethral catheter is valuable in long operations. Failure to produce diuresis may necessitate cessation of this type of therapy; (4) Increasing head-up tilt; (5) Lowering blood pressure. Use of ganglionic-blocking drugs and sodium nitroprusside; (6) Hypothermia; (7) Hyperventilation (*see above*); (8) Use of muscle relaxants to reduce intra-abdominal pressure and hence venous pressure (*see above*); (9) Use of agents such

as thiopentone, methohexitone, droperidol and fentanyl which cause a reduction in cerebral blood flow;[36] (10) Use of steroids. Dexamethasone has been advocated for the prophylaxis and treatment of postoperative oedema. Steroids should be started at least 24 h and perhaps for 2–4 days before surgery and tapered over a few days postoperatively. Dose 10 mg i.v. or i.m. followed by 4 mg i.m. 6-hourly. Treatment takes 12–24 h to become effective; (11) At the end of the operation before extubation and suction, 1·5 mg of lignocaine/kg i.v. prevents a rise in intracranial tension without lowering arterial pressure.[37]

Use of Hypothermia in Neurosurgery
This is now rarely used.[38] Advantages: (1) It allows important vessels to be temporarily occluded during removal of vascular tumours or aneurysms; (2) It produces a reduction in CSF pressure; (3) It may make hypotensive techniques safer. The technique used is almost always surface cooling. Surgical repair of intracranial aneurysms has been performed under profound hypothermia (15 °C) with extracorporeal circulation.

Elective cardiac arrest[39] has also been used together with moderate hypothermia (31 °C), in treatment of intracranial aneurysms and angiomata. This is achieved for periods up to 8 min by intracardiac pacing and placement of a balloon catheter in the ascending aorta, allowing adequate coronary perfusion. Cerebral metabolism is depressed by the combination of barbiturates and hypothermia.[40]

Controlled Hypotension
This is particularly useful in the removal of haemorrhagic tumours (e.g. meningioma) and in the surgery of intracranial aneurysms. It also produces a reduction in intracranial tension. Autoregulation may then be impaired for some hours and postoperative IPPV has been suggested following induced hypotension in patients with raised intracranial pressure. The technique of controlled hypotension is discussed in Chapter 16. *See also Br. J. Anaesth.* 1982, **54**, 253P; *Anaesthesia for Neurosurgery*. Marshall M. *Hosp. Update* 1981, October, 1057.

Posterior Fossa Craniotomy
This may be performed in the prone, lateral or sitting position. Careful attention to positioning is required. Flexion of the head on the neck aids surgical access but may cause a rise in intracranial tension. Surgical manipulations near the brainstem may interfere with the vital centres causing respiratory or pulse irregularities. Removal of an *acoustic neuroma*, which lies in the cerebellopontine angle, may cause a rise in blood pressure during dissection of the upper pole of the tumour from the 5th nerve root, and vagal effects during separation of the lower pole which is adjacent to vagal rootlets.[42] Air embolism is a particular hazard in the sitting position and so is hypotension. Some workers advocate that all posterior fossa surgery should be performed in the prone position to avoid the dangers of air embolism.[43] Hypotension may be counteracted by (1) Pressor drugs; (2) Bandaging of the lower extremities to prevent venous pooling; (3) Simple elevation of the thighs until they are at a right angle to the body with full extension of the knees on a slightly tilted table. The sitting position may also be employed for operations on the cervical spine. Many anaesthetists do not employ controlled respiration which would mask respiratory signs. Others believe that the improved surgical field obtained by IPPV outweighs this disadvantage.[41] As 25–35% of

normal people have symptomless patent foramina ovale,[45] it may be wise to avoid PEEP in seated patients because of the risk of paradoxical air embolism as well as of impaired haemodynamic performance.[46] Massive swelling of the face and tongue may complicate posterior fossa surgery in the sitting position and may require prolonged intubation.[47] Cardiovascular instability may be associated with the sitting position.

A pneumatic cuff around the neck[44] has been suggested as a substitute for bilateral jugular venous occlusion to prevent air embolism during operations in the sitting position.[48] Air embolism has been successfully treated by hyperbaric oxygen.[49]

Trans-sphenoidal Surgery
For anaesthetic technique *see* Messick J. M. et al. *Anaesth. Analg. (Cleve.)* 1978, **57**, 206; Mounir R. A. et al. *Can. Anaesth. Soc. J.* 1980, **27**, 491.

Intracranial Aneurysms[41]
Surgical treatment may be difficult and carry a high risk depending on the general condition of the patient, the level of consciousness, the site of the aneurysm and its relation to adjacent structures. Preoperative management may include analgesics to treat headache (but not potent respiratory depressants) and the use of hypotensive agents (e.g. hydralazine) to treat hypertension. Angiography is necessary to locate the site of the aneurysm. Anaesthesia usually consists of intravenous induction, tracheal intubation, muscle relaxation, nitrous-oxide–oxygen and IPPV. Deliberate hypotension is often desirable to facilitate surgical access. Standard methods of hypotension are used, but it may be necessary to lower systolic pressure to 50–60 mmHg for short periods. Injection of thiopentone, pentobarbitone or amylobarbitone has been suggested to protect the brain during a period of severe hypotension. The operating microscope is now often used by the surgeon. Postoperative care may include measures to treat spasm of cerebral arteries. Cerebral hypoxia is less likely if systolic pressure is at least 110 mmHg and β_1 agonists may produce some relaxation of spasm (e.g. isoprenaline).[50] Patients who have been given ganglion-blocking drugs may have fixed, dilated pupils for some hours after operation.

Operations on the Vertebral Column
The first operative cure of ruptured disc was in 1934.[51] Tumours of the spinal cord may interfere with intercostal nerve supply or even the phrenic nerve roots. Operations for prolapsed intervertebral disc may be carried out in the lateral, prone or 'Muslim praying position'; sometimes the sitting position is employed for cervical and upper thoracic operations.

Bleeding from the extradural veins is the chief problem. Pressure on the chest or abdomen, coughing and straining squeeze blood out of the abdominal and thoracic veins into the vertebral veins, so distending them. The ideal position (if the surgeon cannot be persuaded to operate with the patient on his side) is the jack-knife position with the prone patient's pelvis supporting his weight. This allows the extradural veins to collapse. The field of operation should then be the highest point on the operating table. A head-down position is contraindicated if a myelogram has been recently performed. A muscle relaxant, by reducing intra-abdominal pressure, will reduce bleeding. Adrenaline 1–250 000 in saline can be infiltrated into the skin and subcutaneous tissues.

For explorations in the lumbar region, a light general anaesthetic given through a tracheal tube is usually employed, otherwise an extradural spinal analgesic can be used. The authors recommend this technique in suitable cases which may require the injection of large volumes of solution, e.g. lignocaine 1·5% solution with adrenaline, 35–40 ml in young fit patients, if bleeding is to be reduced.[52] If a general anaesthetic is given and the operation performed with the patient prone, a stomach tube should be passed to avoid aspiration of stomach contents into lungs, as regurgitation may follow pressure on the patient's abdomen. In these cases, a well-padded rest should be placed beneath each shoulder, and beneath the pelvis, so that a small space separates the patient's chest from the table. This will aid respiration and reduce bleeding by preventing an increase in the abdominal and hence in the extradural venous network. Also it will prevent circulatory depression resulting from pressure on the inferior vena cava. The Toronto frame may also be used. In the prone position IPPV should be considered. During high spinal surgery, cardiac dysrhythmias may occur, requiring cholinergic or adrenergic therapy, or both.[53] Cervical cord surgery may be followed by sleep apnoea (Ondine's curse).[54]

When the surgeon places special value on wound ischaemia, hypotension can be produced by: (1) Intradural block; (2) Extradural block; (3) Ganglion-blocking agents or sodium nitroprusside; (4) Halothane, with or without IPPV.

Anaesthesia and Spinal Cord Injury

If the patient's lowest functional root is C.5 he is totally dependent on others; if it is C.7 he can become independent. In *autonomic hyper-reflexia*, nitrous oxide, oxygen and halothane give good control of possible hypertension. Because of the dangers of possible hyperkalaemia, suxamethonium may be undesirable.[55] (*See also* Chapter 14).

Anaesthesia for Carotid Artery Surgery

See also Fitch W. *Br. J. Anaesth.* 1976, **48**, 491.

Problems present themselves in these cases: (1) The prevention of anoxic brain damage during periods of arterial occlusion: (2) The management of a group of patients, many of them elderly with generalized arterial disease; (3) The difficulty in recognizing ischaemic damage if general anaesthesia is used; (4) The possibility of reflex bradycardia from manipulations near the carotid sinus (prevented by infiltration of local analgesic, or intravenous atropine). Postoperative hypertension can be controlled by repeated doses of hydralazine, 10 mg.[56]

A careful study of arteriograms may assist in the assessment of possible collateral circulation.

Surface cooling to 30 °C with nitrous-oxide–oxygen and halothane in a semi-closed system has been employed. Hypercapnia has been used to promote blood flow to the brain through collateral vessels during occlusion of the carotid artery. Cervical plexus block has also been advocated.[57] Shunts can be used to take blood from the femoral to the carotid artery or to bypass the segment of artery clamped. When they are used direct blood cooling can be instituted. *See also* Cerebral perfusion and cerebral protection during carotid end-arterectomy (McMeniman W. J. and Kam P. C. A. *Anaesth. Intensive Care* 1983, **11**, 228.)

Anaesthesia for Thermocoagulation of the Roots of the Trigeminal Nerve[58]
This may be accompanied by hypertension, so that remedies for this should be at hand.[59]

Anaesthesia for Diagnostic Procedures (*See also* Chapter 24)

Cerebral Angiography
This was popularized by Egon Moniz,[60] of Portugal—of leucotomy fame—in 1927. It is usually done through the intact skin, when contrast medium is injected into a carotid artery; average dose about 30 ml. The femoral artery may be used. Local analgesia may be used, though there may be subjective symptoms of flushing, heat and retrobulbar pain. Some favour general anaesthesia for all cases, believing that the vasodilatation produced is of value.

Hyperventilation with IPPV results in increase in cerebrovascular resistance and improves the quality of carotid angiograms by allowing a relatively greater concentration of contrast medium in the cerebral arteries and veins (though this is disputed);[61] a $Paco_2$ of 4 kPa is probably optimal.[62] Transit time is slowed. Hyperventilation may be disadvantageous in cases of subarachnoid haemorrhage with arterial spasm. Arterial cannulation carries a risk of spasm and thrombosis afterwards and pretreatment with dextran-70 has been recommended to reduce its incidence[61] (e.g. 6 ml/kg of 6% dextran-70). The quantity of saline used to keep the needle patent between injections of contrast medium may become significant in children and in patients with cardiac insufficiency.

Ventriculography
First performed by Dandy (1886–1946) in 1918.[63] Local analgesia is satisfactory in adults, unless it is anticipated that craniotomy will follow radiography. The ventricle should be tapped at the conclusion of the investigation if general anaesthesia becomes necessary, particularly if nitrous oxide is to be used as it may diffuse into the cavity with further rise of intracranial pressure. The danger of this is probably small.[64] General anaesthesia is required in children from the start. The patients must be carefully watched for several hours after completion of the investigation.

Pneumo-encephalography
Pioneered by Dandy in 1919.[65] Air is introduced to the ventricular system from below. There is a danger of herniation of the medulla and air embolism. The investigation should not be carried out in the presence of raised intracranial pressure. The patient is placed in a sitting position. (1) Cisternal injection: With neck flexed, a needle is introduced into the cisterna magna; fluid removed; and air introduced; (2) Lumbar injection: Lumbar puncture; fluid removed; air introduced. Seldom required today.

When the air has reached the ventricular system, radiographs are taken. These investigations are often very unpleasant when performed under local analgesia. Symptoms include headache, nausea, vomiting, sweating, while hypotension and bradycardia may occur. Headache may last for hours or days and may be relieved by DOCA 5 mg t.d.s.[66] General anaesthesia is usually preferred.

Anaesthetic Technique

The principles of technique do not differ from those of neurosurgical operations in general. IPPV may prevent reduction in size of lateral ventricles due to increase of intracranial blood volume as a result of rise of Pa_{CO_2}, but may be associated with fall in arterial pressure in patients in the upright position. Nitrous oxide will diffuse into any air-containing cavity. If the ventricles are outlined with air, nitrous-oxide administration may result in a further rise in intracranial pressure. A nylon-reinforced latex tube is recommended to ensure a clear airway at all times. Local analgesia to the larynx together with a sufficient depth of anaesthesia to prevent coughing on the tube is advisable. The head and neck may be moved for radiographs. The anaesthetic connections must not block the radiological field; if necessary the patient may be disconnected from the machine during exposure.

Ketamine has been recommended for neurodiagnostic procedures in small children. It may be injected prior to pneumo-encephalography, ventriculography, myelography or lumbar puncture. It renders the child unconscious and analgesic without the need for tracheal intubation. This is helpful during positioning of the patient, as the airway seldom becomes obstructed. Dose about 2 mg/kg i.v. or 10 mg/kg i.m.

Myelography[67]

General anaesthesia with tracheal intubation may be necessary in children. Examination takes place in the dark and careful monitoring is required. Because of the occasional complication following injection, written request by the consultant in charge of the patient should always be obtained by the anaesthetist, if he is to do the lumbar puncture and inject the contrast medium.

Computerized Tomography (CT Scanning)[68]

Described in 1974.[69] It is vital that the head is kept completely still for the duration of the investigation and general anaesthesia is required in restless or unco-operative subjects and young children.[70] Since general anaesthesia may itself affect intracerebral blood flow and pressure it must be conducted with as much care as for a major neurosurgical intervention.

Anaesthesia in Head Injuries

Anaesthesia may be required for elevation of a depressed fracture, suture of widespread lacerations, etc. These may be associated with considerable blood loss. Pain relief may also be required for treatment of some other surgical conditions in the presence of a head injury.

Each case needs individual assessment. Look for: (1) Evidence of an acute rise of intracranial pressure (e.g. middle meningeal haemorrhage, dilated fixed pupil on one side, slow breathing or apnoea, hypertension, bradycardia, etc.); (2) Level of consciousness and maintenance of airway; (3) Evidence of bleeding into airway (e.g. fracture base of skull); (4) Associated injuries (e.g. pneumothorax, ruptured spleen, fractured femur); (5) Shock; (6) Full stomach.

A cuffed tracheal tube is usually indicated especially in comatose patients, when it may be passed after the injection of suxamethonium and topical analgesia. The operation can then be performed under local analgesia or light general anaesthesia. Tracheostomy may be required. Careful observation is necessary. Blood transfusion may be indicated. Cerebral damage may follow an additional rise in intracranial injuries in the intensive therapy unit, *see* Chapter 39.

For treatment of head injuries in the intensive therapy unit, *see* Chapter 39.
See also Severe Head Injuries; the First Hour. Richards P. Editorial, *Br. Med. J.* 1986. **293**, 643.

Problems of Intensive Care after Neurosurgery
See Campkin T. V. and Turner J. M. *Neurosurgical Anaesthesia and Intensive Care*. 2nd ed. London: Butterworths, 1986.

Electroconvulsive Therapy (Electroplexy)
Convulsions were first used in psychiatry in 1934 by Meduna of Budapest, who employed a relative overdose of cardiazol.[71] Fluothyl (Indoklon) as an inhalation agent was used for the same purpose.[72] Cerletti and Bini induced them electrically in 1938;[73] Bennett used curare in 1940[74] before its use in anaesthesia, to modify cardiazol-induced convulsions; Huguenard and Boué employed gallamine for ECT in 1948; and Holmberg and Thesleff used suxamethonium in 1951.[75]

Atropine premedication is usually given but may not be necessary.[76] Thiopentone (1 mg/kg) or methohexitone (0·5–1 mg/kg) or other induction agent (e.g. etomidate)[77] is given intravenously, followed by suxamethonium 25–40 mg. When the twitching ceases and the chest has been inflated with oxygen, the patient is given the shock therapy. The lungs are again inflated until the effect of the relaxant drug has worn off. Damage to the teeth and lips is a real danger and is likely to occur during the passage of the current rather than during the modified convulsion. When teeth are present, they should be separated by firm rubber tubing or other suitable bite block. In the absence of limb movements, a modified convulsion is likely if: (1) There is a pilomotor reaction (seen in half the patients);[78] (2) The pupil fails to contract when inspected or hippus is seen.

There is evidence that patients suffering from depression with anxiety, one of the chief indications for this treatment, have an abnormally high cholinesterase level. Post-suxamethonium pain is rare. Cardiac arrest has been reported following this treatment. The difference between high and low energy ECT has been pointed out by Robin.[79] (For ECT machines, *see* Mikhail W. I. et al. *Br. J. Hosp. Med.* 1984, **31**, 369.) Prolapsed disc and fracture of a long bone are the main dangers, although ruptured urinary bladder has been reported.[80]

Ventricular dysrhythmia and hypertension may be serious complications of ECT. If pretreatment with i.v. lignocaine is used it may prevent the electric stimulus from producing a convulsion. If instead 0·5 mg of propranolol, i.v. is used 2 min before anaesthesia is induced, this failure of response will not occur.[81] (*See also Handbook of Neuroanaesthesia; Clinical and Physiologic Essentials*. (Newfield P. ed.) Boston: Little Brown, 1983.)

Circulatory Changes in ECT
In modified ECT (i.e. ECT performed under anaesthesia), atropine accelerates the heart rate; thiopentone and methohexitone cause a slight fall in BP; suxamethonium may have no effect at all or may result in bradycardia and rise in BP; oxygen inflation causes a fall in BP and pulse pressure, as after a Valsalva manoeuvre and like the latter, when the intrathoracic pressure due to the anaesthetist's bag pressure falls, there is a slight overshoot with reflex rise in BP and pulse pressure.

With the onset of the fit, if atropine 1 mg has been given, both systolic and diastolic pressures rise, but if atropine is omitted the shock causes asystole for 3–5 s with consequent fall in BP. But the heart restarts and there is a progressive rise in BP. During recovery, BP and pulse rate return to normal. These circulatory changes, no worse than those following defaecation or coughing, are usually well tolerated, even in hypertensives and other patients with heart disease, so that the treatment need seldom be proscribed for these reasons.

Relative Contraindications

(1) Cardiac infarction or major cardiovascular accident within 3 months; (2) Congestive cardiac failure; (3) Aneurysm of a major vessel; (4) Severe osteoporosis; (5) A major fracture; (6) A brain tumour.[82] As both the systolic and diastolic blood pressures and the heart rate rise and as the catecholamines are increased during the treatment, patients with hypertension or cardiac hypertrophy will need careful assessment before being subjected to this heroic but effective form of treatment[83] but usually do well. In mid pregnancy, ECT does not appear to harm the fetus.[84] Well tolerated in old age. Postictal confusion may occur. The omission of atropine may result in a period of asystole for up to 5 sec but also lessens the risk of regurgitation (because of its relaxing effect on the lower oesophageal sphincter).[85] (*See also* Rich C. L. and Ty-Smith N. *Can. Anaesth. Soc. J.* 1981, **28**, 153.)

ECT for Patients with a Pacemaker
(*See* Jauhar P. et al. *Br. Med. J.* 1979, **1**, 90.)

References

1. Hunter A. R. *Neurosurgical Anaesthesia*, 2nd ed. Oxford: Blackwell, 1976; McDowall D. G. in: *Recent Advances in Anaesthesia and Analgesia*—12 (Hewer C. L. and Atkinson R. S. ed.). Edinburgh: Churchill Livingstone, 1976; Frost E. A. M. *Clinical Anesthesia in Neurosurgery*. Stoneham MA: Butterworth, 1984; Cotterell J. E. and Turndorf H. *Anesthesia and Neurosurgery*. St. Louis: Mosby, 1980; Campkin T. V. and Turner J. M. *Neurosurgical Anaesthesia and Intensive Care*, 2nd ed. London: Butterworth, 1986.
2. Bennett A. H. and Godlee R. J. *Med. Chirurg. Trans.* 1885, **68**, 243.
3. Cushing H. (1869–1939) *Surg. Gynecol. Obstet.* 1928, **47**, 751.
4. Dandy W. *Ann. Surg.* 1918, **68**, 5.
5. Dandy W. *Ann. Surg.* 1919, **70**, 397.
6. Moniz E. *Rev. Neurol.* 1927, **2**, 72.
7. Hunter A. R. *Anaesthesia* 1983, **38**, 1214.
8. Dott N. M. (1897–1974) *Trans. Med.-chir. Soc. Edinb.* 1932, n.s. **47**, 219.
9. Walter W. G. *Lancet* 1936, **2**, 305.
10. Moore G. E. *J. Neurosurg.* 1948, **5**, 392.
11. Vernon Harcourt A. G. *Br. Med. J.* **2**, July 18.
12. Junker F. A. *Med. Times Gaz.* 1867, Nov. 30th.
13. Cushing. H. *Boston Med. Surg. J.* 1903, **148**, 250; Beecher H. K.: *Surg. Gynecol. Obstet.* 1940, **71**, 689.
14. Hunter A. R. *Anaesthesia* 1983, **38**, 1214.
15. Furness D. N. *Br. J. Anaesth.* 1957, **29**, 415; Mortimer P. L. F. *Br. J. Anaesth.* 1957, **29**, 528; Galloon S. *Anaesthesia* 1959, **14**, 79.
16. Gwathmey J. T. *N.Y. Med. J.* 1913, **98**, 1101.
17. Ponté J. and Purves M. J. *J. Physiol.* 1974, **237**, 315.
18. *See also* Turner J. M. and McDowall D. G. *Br. J. Anaesth.* 1976, **48**, 735; Jones R. F. C. et al. *Anaesth. Intensive Care* 1981, **9**, 336.

19. Marshall M. *Hosp. Update* 1981, Oct. 1057.
20. Ballantine R. I. W. and Jackson I. *General Anaesthesia for Neurosurgery.* London: Churchill, 1960.
21. *See also* McDowall D. G. *Anesthesiology* 1976, **45**, 117; Marshall M. *Current Topics in Anaesthesia Series*—3, London: Arnold, 1979.
22. Maroon J. C. et al. *J. Neurosurg.* 1969, **31**, 196; Edmonds-Seal J. and Maroon J. C. *Anaesthesia* 1969, **24**, 438; Michenfelder J. D. et al. *Anesthesiology* 1972, **36**, 164.
23. Schettini A. et al. *J. Neurosurg.* 1971, **34**, 38.
24. Buckland R. W. and Manners J. M. *Anaesthesia* 1976, **31**, 663.
25. *See* McDowall D. G. in: *General Anaesthesia* (Gray T. C. and Nunn J. F. ed.), 3rd ed. London: Butterworths, 1971, Vol. 1, Chap. 18; Greenbaum R. *Br. J. Anaesth.* 1976, **48**, 773.
26. Shapiro H. M. et al. *Br. J. Anaesth.* 1973, **45**, 1057.
27. Rockoff M. A. and Shapiro H. M. *Anesthesiology* 1978, **49**, 385; Bleyaert H. L. et al. *Anesthesiology* 1978, **49**, 390.
28. Adams R. W. et al. in: *Proc. 2nd Int. Symposium on Intracranial Pressure* (Lundberg N. et al. ed.). Berlin: Springer-Verlag.
29. Campkin T. V. *Br. J. Anaesth.* 1984, **56**, 1083.
30. Moss E. et al. *Br. J. Anaesth.* 1983, **55**, 1083.
31. *See also* Gilbert R. G. B. et al. *Anaesthesia for Neurosurgery.* London: Churchill, 1966; Hunter A. R. *Neurosurgical Anaesthesia*, 2nd ed. Oxford: Blackwell, 1976.
32. Wollman H. *Anesthesiology* 1965, **26**, 329; Alexander S. C. et al. *Anesthesiology* 1965, **26**, 624.
33. McCormish P. B. and Bodley P. O. *Anaethesia for Neurological Surgery*, London: Lloyd-Luke, 1971, p. 95.
34. *See* Correspondence, Johnston M. and Foster B. et al. *Br. J. Anaesth.* 1969, **41**, 561.
35. Marshall M. *Current Topics in Anaesthesia Series*—3. London: Arnold, 1979.
36. *See also* Smith A. L. *Anesthesiology* 1977, **47**, 285.
37. Donegan M. F. and Bedford R. F. *Anesthesiology* 1980, **52**, 516; Bedford R. F. et al. *Anesth. Analg. (Cleve.)* 1980. **59**, 435.
38. McDowell D. G. *Br. J. Anaesth.* 1971, **43**, 1084; Marshall M. *Current Topics in Anaesthesia Series*—3. London: Arnold, 1979.
39. Campkin T. V. and Dallas S. H. *Br. J. Anaesth.* 1968, **40**, 527.
40. Lafferty J. J. and Keykhah M. M. *Anesthesiology* 1978, **49**, 159.
41. Marshall M. *Current Topics in Anaesthesia Series*—3. London: Arnold, 1979.
42. Hunter A. R. in: *General Anaesthesia* (Gray T. C. and Nunn J. F. ed.), 3rd ed. London: Butterworths, 1971, Vol. 2. Chap. 23.
43. Walters F. and Torrens F. *Br. J. Anaesth.* 1982, **54**, 363.
44. Sale J. P. *Anaesthesia* 1984, **39**, 795.
45. Thompson T. and Evans D. C. *Q. J. Med.* 1930, **23**, 135.
46. Perkins N. A. K. and Bedford R. E. *Anesth. Analg. (Cleve.)* 1984, **63**, 429.
47. Tattersall M. P. *Anaesthesia* 1984, **39**, 1015.
48. Pfitzner J. and McLean A. G. *Anaesthesia* 1985, **40**, 624.
49. Ireland A. et al. *Br. Med. J.* 1985, **291**, 106.
50. Sundt T. M. et al. *Surg. Neurol.* 1977, **7**, 259.
51. Mixer W. J. and Barr J. S. *N. Engl. J. Med.* 1934, **211**, 210.
52. Thorne T. C. and Watt M. J. personal communication.
53. Rayner P. R. *Br. Med. J.* 1983, **287**, 182.
54. Vella L. M. et al. *Anaesthesia* 1984, **39**, 108.
55. Fraser A. and Edmonds-Seal J. *Anaesthesia* 1982, **37**, 1084.
56. Davies M. J. and Cronin K. D. *Anaesth. Intensive Care* 1980, **8**, 190.
57. McCrory C. B. et al. *Proc. 2nd Eur. Cong. Anaesth.* 1966, **2**, 43; Erwin D. et al. *Anaesthesia* 1980, **35**, 246.
58. Lowe S. S. et al. *Anaesthesia* 1983, **38**, 152.
59. Kehler C. H. et al. *Neurosurgery* 1982, **10**, 2; Samuel S. I. and Brodsky J. B. *Anaesthesia* 1983, **38**, 91.
60. Moniz E. *Rev. Neurol.* 1927, **2**, 72.
61. Marshall M. *Current Topics in Anaesthesia Series*—3. London: Arnold, 1979.
62. du Boulay G. H. and Symon L. *Proc. R. Soc. Med.* 1971, **64**, 77.
63. Dandy W. E. *Ann. Surg.* 1918, **68**, 5.
64. Moseley I. F. et al. *J. Neurol. Neurosurg. Psychiat.* 1977, **40**, 1033.
65. Dandy W. E. *Ann. Surg.* 1919, **70**, 397.

66. Wolfson B. et al. *Anaesthesia* 1970, **25**, 328.
67. Whitby J. D. *Anaesthesia* 1971, **26**, 36; Bull J. *Br. Med. J.* 1973, **1**, 280.
68. *See* McDowall D. G. in: *Recent Advances in Anaesthesia and Analgesia*—12 (Hewer C. L. and Atkinson R. S. ed.). Edinburgh: Churchill Livingstone, 1976.
69. New P. F. J. et al. *Radiology* 1974, **110**, 109.
70. Ferrer-Brechner T. and White J. *Anesth. Analg. (Cleve.)* 1977, **56**, 344; Aidinis S. J. et al. *Anesthesiology* 1976, **44**, 420.
71. Major R. H. *History of Medicine*. Springfield, Ill.: Thomas, 1954, Vol. 2.
72. Krantz J. C. et al. *Science* 1957, **126**, 353.
73. Cerletti U. and Bini L. *Boll. Atti Acad. Med.* 1938, **64**, 136.
74. Bennett A. E. *JAMA* 1940, **114**, 322.
75. Holmberg A. G. and Thesleff S. *Nord. Med.* 1951, **46**, 1567.
76. Wyant G. M. and MacDonald W. B. *Anaesth. Intensive Care* 1980, **8**, 445.
77. O'Carroll T. M. et al. *Anaesthesia* 1977, **32**, 868.
78. McCleave D. J. and Blakemore W. B. *Anaesth. Intensive Care* 1975, **3**, 750.
79. Robin A. *Br. Med. J.* 1982, **285**, 441; Robin A. and Tissera S. A. *Br. J. Psychiatry* 1982, **141**, 314.
80. Irving A. D. and Drayson A. M. *Br. Med. J.* 1984, **288**, 194.
81. Hood D. D. and Mecca R. S. *Anesthesiology* 1983, **58**, 379.
82. Freeman C. P. L. *Br. J. Hosp. Med.* 1979, **21**, 281.
83. Jones R. M. and Knight P. R. *Anaesthesia* 1981, **36**, 295.
84. Views, *Br. Med. J.* 1984, **288** 1239; *Obstet. Gynecol.* **63**, Suppl. 39.
85. Verheecke G. and Troch E. *Anaesth. Intensive Care* 1982, **11**, 166.

Chapter 27   # OBSTETRICAL ANAESTHESIA AND ANALGESIA

History

Non-pharmacological methods. Hypnosis has been used periodically since Anton Mesmer first wrote about it in 1777, and childbirth without pain, employing *relaxation and a naturalistic* approach, is an old and frequently revived technique (Grantley Dick-Read, 1890–1959).[1]

The *decompression suit* was proposed in 1959.[2]

Sedatives and analgesics. When the senior author of this book was an undergraduate student of midwifery, *chloral hydrate* (Liebreich, 1869), *tincture of opium* and *bromide* formed a popular analgesic mixture, designed to encourage sleep, rather than to relieve pain. This gave place to *barbiturates* in the years following the introduction of barbitone by Emil Fischer and von Mering in 1903. Phenobarbitone appeared in 1912,[3] Pernocton[4] and pentobarbitone[5] came later, and Somnifaine in 1924.[6]

Morphine has been used with success in labour[7] since its isolation by Serturner in 1806; fetal respiratory depression is its chief disadvantage. It was hoped, in vain, that *papaveretum* would be without this stigma.[8] It was first used in obstetrics by Jaeger in 1910.[9]

Morphine and hyoscine were used in the technique of Dammerschlaf (twilight sleep) by von Steinbuchel of Graz[10] and by Carl Joseph Gauss of Freiburg, later of Würzburg,[11] following the use of the mixture as a true anaesthetic.[12] *Hyoscine* alone was used in large doses in 1928,[13] but it produced far too much restlessness (the central anticholinergic syndrome[14]). *Pethidine* was used by

Benthin in Germany in 1940. Naloxone, a major advance in the treatment of respiratory depression in mothers and infants, was first used by Clark in 1971.[15]

Ketamine was first used in obstetrics by Akamatsu in 1974.[16]

Agents introduced into the rectum to relieve the pains of labour started in 1847[17] when *ether and air* were employed. *Ether and oil* had a vogue;[18] *bromethol* was first used in 1927 and was closely followed by paraldehyde.[19] Various drugs of the *phenothiazine group* have been used, and promazine was for a time popular. Synergistic prescriptions of drugs, such as rectal oil ether, morphine and magnesium sulphate, were at one time warmly recommended.[20] *Diazepam* was investigated by Bepko.[21]

(*See also* Gaton D. *Anesthesiology* 1977, **46**, 132.)

Regional techniques. Soon after Bier gave the first *intradural spinal block* in 1898, it was used in labour.[22] The so-called 'controlled spinal' was used in 1928.[23] Saddle block was described in 1946.[24] *Sacral extradural block* was described for use in labour by Stoeckel,[25] *paracervical block* by Gellert[26] and *paravertebral block* of T.11 and T.12 by Cleland.[27] Eugen Bogdan (1899–1975) of Bucharest worked out the afferent pathways of labour pains[28] and gave continuous extradural sacral cinchocaine in 1931.[29] This work was independent of that of Cleland. Lumbar *extradural analgesia* was described in 1928[30] and *continuous caudal* (sacral extradural) block in 1938.[31] This was ably popularized by R. A. Hingson.[32] *Continuous lumbar extradural* block was reported some time later.[33] *Pudendal block* was first described by Müller in 1908.

Inhalation methods. *Ether* was the first and was given by J. Y. Simpson on 19 January 1847.[34] The following year, Walter Channing, Professor of Obstetrics at Harvard, published his book *A Treatise on Etherisation in Childbirth*, illustrated by 581 cases.

Chloroform was proposed as a substitute for ether, also by Simpson[35] and he gave it for the first time on 8 November 1847. When Scottish Calvinists objected on moral[36] and scriptural grounds to the relief of pain in labour (Genesis, 3, 17: 'In sorrow shall thou bring forth children'), Simpson quoted to them, knowing his Bible, Genesis, 2, 21: 'And the Lord God caused a deep sleep to fall on Adam, and he slept, and He took one of his ribs and closed up the side instead, thereof.' Simpson thus yielded up the pride of place as the first obstetric anaesthetist to God. Pain relief in labour only became really respectable when John Snow gave chloroform to Queen Victoria during the birth of her eighth child, Prince Leopold, in 1853 (*narcose à la reine*), a technique described in his book *On Chloroform and Other Anaesthetics* (*see also* the 7th edition of this Synopsis). The most common way of administration was the open drop method or by blowing air over chloroform vapour.[37,38] The drug was first used in the USA by A. K. Gardner in 1848. *Divinyl ether* was used by Wesley Bourne in 1935.[39] *Cyclopropane* had a short popularity in obstetrics just as it had in general surgery, especially in Montreal and Madison.[40] *Trichloroethylene* was found to be a useful analgesic in labour soon after its first use in surgery[41] and early reports came from Barnet[42] and from London.[43] *Nitrous oxide* has had a long reign and is still a valuable analgesic today. First used in 1880[44] it was revived in 1915.[45] A method of self-administration was described by that pioneer of anaesthesia, Guedel.[46] Yet another advance was the introduction of the gas air machine by R. J. Minnitt (1890–1974) of Liverpool[47] and its modifications.[48] This method of self-administration held the field in the UK for some years but was given up because it could well cause fetal hypoxia. *Nitrous oxide with oxygen* was used in 1949[49] and the *pre-mix of nitrous oxide and oxygen* in equal volumes (Entonox) was advocated by Tunstall in 1961[50] and is extensively used today. *Methoxyflurane* has been found to be safe when given in a low concentration for short periods.[51] The Leboyer technique calls for calm, and soft music at delivery.[52]

First Caesarean section, with a surviving mother, in England took place in Lancashire by James Barlow, in 1793.

Important concepts in the history of obstetric analgesia include the description of the *hypotensive supine syndrome*,[53] the description of the *acid aspiration syndrome*[54] and one easy way of reducing the effects of this by routine administration of an antacid mixture before anaesthesia.[55]

Safe and pain-free childbirth is a dream for the future rather than a reality today. This long catalogue of worthy effort, extending back for more than a hundred and forty years, will surely be added to in the days to come.

Fetoscopy was first performed by Scrimgeour in 1973.[56] Amniocentesis was done as early as 1930.[57] *See also* Poppers P. J. The history and development of obstetric anaesthesia, in: *Anaesthesia; Essays on its History*. (Rupreht J. et al. ed.) Berlin: Springer-Verlag, 1985.

Pregnancy

Pregnancy and labour produce remarkable physiological and psychological changes in the mother.

1. Circulatory system. The enlarged uterus pushes the diaphragm upwards. This results in a change in position of the heart which is lifted upwards, shifted to the left and anteriorly, and rotated towards a transverse position. The electrocardiogram may show a large Q-wave and inverted T-waves in Lead III. Heart rate increases during pregnancy, reaching a peak between 28 and 36 weeks to about 10–12 beats above normal. There is a significant increase in cardiac output which reaches a peak 30–50% above normal at term.[58] Whereas the healthy heart compensates well for these changes, the diseased heart may be severely taxed. Peripheral resistance is reduced in pregnancy, and mean blood pressure reaches its lowest point at the time of maximal cardiac output. Venous pressure is normal, except where the gravid uterus may compress the inferior vena cava. Blood volume is increased, plasma volume more than red cell volume, so that haematocrit falls, and uterine blood flow is markedly increased.

2. Respiratory system. Upward displacement of the diaphragm results in decrease of vertical diameter of the thorax and increase in transverse diameter. X-rays show increased lung markings probably due to an increase of blood volume in the pulmonary vessels. Minute ventilation rises to levels of 50% above normal. Both the diaphragmatic and the thoracic excursion is increased, at least in the upright position. Functional residual capacity is decreased from the 20th week. Closing volume is greater than functional residual capacity in about half of women in late pregnancy.[59] Pa_{CO_2} falls by the 12th week of pregnancy to about 4 kPa (30 mmHg) and stays low until term. Pa_{O_2} is sometimes reduced at term and may be higher in the sitting than in the supine position.[60] Oxygen consumption rises during the last trimester due to the metabolic needs of the uterus, placenta and fetus. Basal metabolic rate is increased by about 15%. Smoking during pregnancy is associated with smaller babies and higher perinatal mortality.[61] Carboxy-haemoglobin may be a factor.

3. Fluids and electrolytes. Water and salt retention occur. Probably related to the secretion of steroids by the placenta.

4. Endocrine glands. There is hyperplasia of the anterior pituitary, thyroid and adrenal cortex.

5. Pyschology. The impact of pregnancy and parturition may have a considerable emotional effect.

For discussion of the altered pharmacokinetics and adverse reactions to drugs used in pregnancy, *see Br. J. Hosp. Med.* 1982, **28**, 559 et seq.

There is no evidence that nitrous oxide should not be given in early pregnancy.[179]

Supine Hypotensive Syndrome of Late Pregnancy[62]

This is a condition of circulatory depression due to diminished venous return caused by the gravid uterus pressing on the inferior vena cava and perhaps the aorta. Most patients compensate by blood flowing through the azygos system via the paravertebral veins. It is relieved by a pillow under one side or the adoption of the lateral position.

Analgesia in Vaginal Delivery

The unprepared and untreated patient will feel pain during uterine contractions which occur in normal uncomplicated labour. The belief that primitive woman had no fear, no tension and a painless labour is not founded on fact. The intensity of the pain is related to: (1) The severity and duration of uterine contractions; (2) The degree of dilatation of the cervix, and how rapidly this is achieved with each contraction; (3) The distension of perineal tissue; (4) Other factors including age, parity, the size of the fetus in relation to the birth canal, etc.

The ideal procedure should: (1) Produce efficient relief from pain, with consciousness between pains and good co-operation from the patient; (2) Not depress the respiration of the fetus; (3) Not depress the uterus, causing prolonged labour; (4) Be non-toxic; (5) Be safe for mother and child.

No agent at present in use fulfils all these conditions. Analgesia is not necessary in every case of labour and sympathetic explanation may be all that is required.

I. Non-pharmacological Methods

Since drugs administered may cross the placenta to depress the fetus, any method which avoids or restricts their use deserves attention.

1. 'Natural childbirth'. A naturalistic approach with emphasis on the attainment of relaxation of muscles. Patients are taught the art of relaxation and given exercises in a course of lectures and demonstrations.[63] Psychoprophylaxis in labour (Lamaze preparation).[64]

2. Similar work in France and in the USSR (Velkowski) in 1947 involves a psychosomatic approach.

3. Hypnosis. This makes considerable demands on time for both patients and staff. Only about 25% of patients can be successfully treated in this way. The method has, therefore, not proved popular for general use.

4. Decompression suit. Decompression of the abdomen and lower part of the thorax to 1–2 lb/sq in below atmospheric pressure allows the uterus to become more spherical and to act at a greater mechanical advantage. It facilitates labour, shortens the first stage, and gives considerable pain relief.[65]

5. Transcutaneous nerve stimulation is beneficial in about 20% of patients.[66]

II. Sedatives and Analgesics

Placental Transfer of Drugs

All drugs found in maternal blood cross the placenta to some extent unless they are altered or destroyed in passage, especially those with a high lipid solubility and low degree of ionization.[67] Placental vascular activity and metabolism also play a part.

1. Simple oral sedatives. Chloral hydrate, a soporific and mild analgesic, is excreted by the kidneys. A safe dose is 2 g. Can be given in tablet form as dichloralphenazone (Welldorm) or as trichlorethyl phosphate (Triclofos) and, if necessary, with *tincture of opium* (1 ml).

2. Pethidine hydrochloride, BP (*see also* Chapter 8). The English National Board for Midwifery allow it to be used by midwives acting alone if certain rules are observed.

As it depresses fetal respiration it should not be given within 3 h of delivery. There is increased uterine activity and relaxation of spasm of the cervix. It is very useful in cases with a rigid, slowly dilating os.

Dosage. Initial dose 100–150 mg when labour is well established. Should not be given too soon, as then it may abolish pains. Usually given by intramuscular injection, when effects comes on in 15 min and is maximal 1–1½ h after injection, in both mother and fetus (respiratory depression). Additional similar amounts are injected when required, e.g. every 2–3 h. Maximum dosage allowed for a midwife working alone is 200 mg in any one labour. Fetal depression due to pethidine can be reversed by intramuscular injection of naloxone 200 µg.[68]

3. Morphine (*see also* Chapter 8). Dose 10 mg i.m. Analgesic action maximal at 90 min. Fetal respiratory depression maximal at 2 h. In small doses, morphine increases the intervals between pains; in larger doses it may depress contractions.

4. Hyoscine (*see also* Chapter 8). (1) Does not increase pain threshold; (2) Alters patient's reaction to pain by producing amnesia, excitement and sometimes delirium resembling acute mania[69] (the central anticholinergic syndrome). It should not be given late in labour as then it may cause restlessness and lack of co-operation. It passes the placental barrier.

Twilight sleep. Morphine and hyoscine.[70] Today the technique is seldom used. *See* fifth edition of this Synopsis, 1964.

5. Bromethol, BP (Avertin) (*see also* Chapter 8). The usual dose per rectum is 75 mg/kg, after deducting 6 kg for the weight of the uterus and its contents. This method is not recommended as an anaesthetic in labour but has its place in the treatment of eclampsia.

6. Diazepam.[21,71] Rapidly crosses the placenta. Produces amnesia and reduces maternal apprehension without causing untoward effect on the fetus. Dose: 0·3 mg/kg i.m., not normally exceeding 30 mg.[72] Dose: 5–10 mg i.v. It is not an analgesic drug. *Lorazepam* has been used in patients with hypertension in pregnancy and may cross the placenta to affect the neonate. It should be used only when there are facilities for neonatal intensive care.

(*See also* Morgan C. A. and Paull J. *Anaesth. Int. Care* 1980, **8**, 278.)

III. Regional Analgesia[73]

Autonomic Nerve Supply of Uterus

1. Sympathetic (motor to upper uterine segment). The middle thoracic segments from T.6 downwards, perhaps as low as L.2, via splanchnic nerves and coeliac, aortic, renal and hypogastric plexuses, and thence with blood vessels to the great cervical ganglion of Frankenhäuser. In addition, some of the motor supply of the body of the uterus may come from below the sensory supply, i.e. T.11, L.2.

2. Visceral afferent (sensory from uterus).[27,74] Block of these eases pain of the first stage of labour, with the exception of those near the end of this stage. Eleventh and 12th thoracic (and possibly 1st lumbar). Fibres go from uterus (ganglion of Frankenhäuser) via sympathetic nerves to pelvic, hypogastric and aortic plexuses, enter the sympathetic chain at the level of L.5 and ascend in the chain, entering the cord via the white rami of T.11 and T.12, and the 11th–12th posterior thoracic roots and thence up posterior columns of cord. Block of the sympathetic chain between L.5 and T.12 gives the same freedom from first-stage labour pains as block of the 11th–12th thoracic ganglia.

3. Visceral afferent and efferent parasympathetic (inhibitory to uterus; sensory and motor to cervix). Second, 3rd and 4th sacral nerves, directly to great cervical ganglion of Frankenhäuser.

Somatic Afferent Nerves of Lower Birth Canal

The inferior rectal, perineal and dorsal nerve of the clitoris—from the pudendal nerve (S.2, 3, 4). The ilio-inguinal (L.1) and the genitofemoral (L.1, 2). There are twenty nerves transmitting labour pains, viz.: (1) The visceral afferents of the 11th and 12th thoracic—pain of uterine contraction; (2) The posterior roots of the 2nd, 3rd and 4th sacral nerves, carrying pelvic afferents (Henry Head, 1861–1940)—pain of cervical dilatation; (3) The rectal, perineal and pudendal branches of the sacral plexus—pain of perineal stretching; (4) The ilio-inguinal and genitofemoral branches of the lumbar plexus.

With all forms of regional block, blood pressure fall must be avoided because of the risk of fetal hypoxia, and to prevent this the patient should be nursed in the lateral position or a wedge used to prevent caval compression. If it occurs the legs should be elevated, plasma-volume expander infused and oxygen administered. Pressure should not be allowed to fall below 90 mmHg. The initial and most useful treatment of hypotension is the rapid infusion of a plasma-volume expander. Pressor drugs do not necessarily improve the blood flow to the uterus. It is best to avoid the α-stimulating pressor drugs. Recommended are ephedrine 12–25 mg i.v. or metaraminol as an intravenous drip. Intravenous injection of ergometrine soon after a patient has received a vasopressor may cause dangerous hypertension.

The postpartum uterus contracts well. Obstetric paralysis due to pressure of the fetal head or the forceps on the lumbosacral trunk may occur even with intradural or extradural analgesia! Neuropathy if due to the block itself is likely to be bilateral and to have a segmental (radicular) rather than a peripheral distribution.

1. Subarachnoid Block (Intradural) (*see also* Chapter 32).

Can be used for mid or low forceps extraction, for Caesarean section or for normal delivery. For normal delivery or for outlet forceps with episiotomy, block should extend to S.1 (saddle block, to denote a zone of analgesia of the perineum and perianal region, without involvement of the legs). Uterine muscle can function without neural control and may have its own intrinsic pacemakers. Successful uterine activity leading to delivery can occur in the presence of a total spinal block.[75]

Hyperbaric 5% lignocaine or hyperbaric amethocaine (dose: 1 ml) is injected between L.4 and L.5 in either the sitting position or in the lateral position with the vertebral canal inclined caudally, and after an interval of a minute or so the patient is turned to the supine position with lateral tilt. The onset of analgesia takes about 5 min.

Isobaric 0.5% bupivacaine in a dose of 3 ml is also satisfactory[76] with the patient in the lateral position for the injection, and immediately placed in the supine position with a wedge under the loin.

For high forceps or intrauterine manipulation, block should reach T.10 to abolish the traction pain associated with a high forceps delivery which will result if the sacral nerves alone are blocked. Spinal analgesia does not influence the course of established labour provided the level of block is not above T.10 and blood pressure is maintained.

Perineal analgesia removes the bearing-down reflex but saddle block does not greatly delay normal labour if, when the cervix is fully dilated, the patient is encouraged to bear down during the pains.

In both subarachnoid and extradural block, a given dose of local analgesic solution may ascend higher in pregnant than in non-pregnant patients, so doses should be given with care.

Advantages of intradural block: (1) No fetal respiratory depression; (2) Excellent relaxation of pelvic floor muscles; (3) Absence of aspiration of stomach contents and risk of asphyxia, Mendelson's syndrome, pneumonia, etc.; (4) Delivery of patient while she is conscious; (5) Can be quickly performed and has a rapid onset.

If used in congestive heart failure, for forceps delivery, to help spare the mother the exertion of pushing out the baby, subarachnoid injection should be made immediately the cervix is fully dilated, and forceps applied.

Postoperative headaches are rather frequent (*see* Chapter 32).

2. Extradural Lumbar Block (*see also* Chapter 32).

An excellent method of pain relief for normal labour or operative delivery, usually achieved by serial injections of bupivacaine through an indwelling catheter.[77] The English National Board for Midwifery has approved that midwives be allowed to give top-up injections, always provided the first top-up dose has been given by the anaesthetist and with no untoward result. The midwife must receive training in the technique.

Indications. The aim is to relieve pain, prevent exhaustion and preserve morale. Indications are not absolute, but may be placed in an order of priority; (1) Pre-eclamptic toxaemia; (2) Slow, painful labour; (3) Cardiac and respiratory distress; (4) Premature or high-risk fetus; (5) Multiple pregnancy; (6) Breech delivery; (7) Diabetes; (8) Incoordinate action of uterus; (9) Recent laparotomy; (10) Trial of labour; (11) Operative labour—especially with full stomach; (12) Failure of conventional analgesia; (13) Fear of repetition of painful labour; (14) Express wish of patient to have painless labour; (15) As a local policy for all women, unless contraindicated.

Contraindications. Near-absolute contraindications are: (1) Patient unwilling; (2) Haemorrhagic disease or anticoagulant therapy; (3) Local sepsis; (4) Lack of experience of anaesthetist and inadequate supervision; (5) Inade quate facilities (apparatus or personnel) for immediate resuscitation should untoward events occur. Other contraindications are *relative*: (6) Shock, hypotension, hypovolaemia; (7) Neurological disease; (8) Previous spinal surgery, or difficult anatomy; (9) Previous Caesarean section, as it is feared that analgesia may prevent recognition of a rupture of the uterus—some workers disagree; (10) Severe heart disease and hydramnios; (11) Existing supine hypotension.

Technique. The catheter may be introduced in the L.2–3 or L.3–4 interspace. It should not be advanced more than a short distance into the extradural space as it may take an undesired direction. The markings on needle and catheter are useful here.[78] Head-down tilt may aid spread to T.10. Drugs used include:

1. Bupivacaine 0·5%, 0·375%, 0·25% or even 0·125%. The 0·75% solution should not be used in labour. There is evidence that risks to the fetus, if they exist, are less than with lignocaine.[79] There is no advantage to be gained by adding adrenaline, which does not prolong duration of the block, and does not protect against maternal toxicity unless the dosage is large.[80] Tachyphylaxis does not occur. Effective duration of action of a single injection about 3 hours. A dose 6–8 ml of 0·375% solution has been recommended for normal labour, 8–10 ml for forceps delivery and 15–20 ml for Caesarean section.[72] A continuous infusion of bupivacaine following an initial dose of 7–10 ml of 0·25% solution has been recommended, rate approximately 10 ml/h.[81] A mechanical infusion pump has been used.[82]

2. Lignocaine 1·0 or 1·5%. Lignocaine is rapidly carried from the extradural space to fetal blood, and is present there in high concentration (in relation to the maternal plasma concentration) within 15 min of injection. Maternal plasma concentration at delivery is directly related to total dose of lignocaine. Carbonated lignocaine solutions have given better results in clinical practice.[82]

3. Mepivacaine 1·5% More likely to give rise to side-effects in the mother.

4. Prilocaine. Not recommended in obstetrics as it may cause methaemoglobinaemia and a blue baby.

5. Chloroprocaine has a rapid onset of action but is of short duration. It may be used for the initial injection to obtain analgesia quickly. Its analgesic effects may wear off suddenly. (*See* Chapter 32.)

6. Etidocaine, 1% solution, is a good agent for Caesarean section,[83] but is not favoured for normal delivery because it causes a high degree of motor block.

7. Opioids, diluted in 5–10 ml of saline. Morphine 2 mg, diamorphine 1 mg, buprenorphine 0·15 mg or pethidine. Solutions without preservatives should be used. Cardiovascular effects are minimal. Maternal respiratory depression and nausea may occur if the above doses are exceeded. Duration of action 6–48 h. The method does not always give good results.

Dose. Whatever agent is used, in whatever strength, a volume of 5–8 ml is sufficient to produce analgesia in the desired segments, though this has been challenged.[84]

The free end of the catheter may be attached to a bacterial filter (Millipore) or a 50-ml syringe charged with analgesic fluid and enclosed in a sterile polypropylene bag.

Effects on the fetus. The progressive fetal acidosis which occurs during delivery under conventional analgesia is abolished when extradural analgesia is effective. Neurobehavioural responses of newborn infants may be affected when ligno-caine of mepivacaine have been used.[85] This does not occur with bupivacaine,[86] probably because it is bound to protein and has a very low fetal to maternal blood ratio. Chloroprocaine does not affect the fetus because it is rapidly hydrolysed.

Difficulties and complications. All reported series report failure to achieve complete pain relief in a proportion of cases. This may take the form of unblocked segments. A high success rate is achieved only by scrupulous attention to detail, slow injection of analgesic solution and readiness to withdraw partially or even replace the catheter when necessary. Other measures which may be needed include injection of a supplementary dose with change of posture. Extradural block may increase the need for instrumental delivery.[87]

Posture is also important in the prevention of caval compression and the supine position is to be avoided or a wedge used if the patient has to be put in the lithotomy position or if Caesarean section is necessary.

Horner's syndrome has been reported as a sequel.[88]

Spinal headache is a distressing complication which may result from inadvertent dural puncture. *See* Chapter 32 for details of management.

Advantages and disadvantages. The need for fetal resuscitation is reduced. *Neurological complications* are not unknown following normal delivery without regional block. Electromyographic and careful neurological examinations usually enable an accurate diagnosis to be made.[89]

3. Extradural Sacral Block—Continuous Caudal Block[90]

Whatever the merits or demerits of continuous caudal block throughout labour, there is no doubt about the excellence of a single injection given for forceps delivery. Continuous caudal block is relatively safe for mother and child, gives superlative relaxation of the lower birth canal and good analgesia. Lignocaine 1–1·5% solution 16–20 ml or bupivacaine 0·5% 10–15 ml are the recommended agents and doses. Should continuation of the analgesia be decided upon, topping-up doses of 10 ml can be given when necessary. The method should only be used when every means of resuscitation is to hand. High spread can occur following sacral injection as evidenced by reports of meiosis and ptosis.[91] It is not without its disadvantages and is accompanied by a high forceps rate and increased frequency of anomalies of rotation, e.g. persistent occipito-posterior position and mid-transverse arrest of the head. The third stage is short and post partum blood loss minimal. The method is useful in uterine inertia and in cervical dystocia. The pain following episiotomy can be relieved by sacral extradural morphine, 4 mg dissolved in 20 ml of saline, relief lasting up to 12 hours.[92]

The dangers are: (1) Accidental subarachnoid block; (2) Infection; (3) Broken needle; (4) Intrafetal injection.

For relief of first-stage pain, block must reach T.11 and T.12: for painless delivery, block of the sacral nerves is necessary.

Technique. With patient in the lateral, knee–elbow or knee–chest position, a plastic catheter or a malleable spinal needle is inserted into the sacral canal for 2·5–3 cm. To this is attached a closed system comprising a length of fine-bore, plastic tubing, a filter, a syringe and sometimes a reservoir containing the analgesic solution. The needle or catheter is taped between the buttocks and the patient turned on her side. Injections are not begun until labour is well established.

Solutions used:

1. Bupivacaine (0·5%): for first-stage pains, 16–20 ml injected with the patient horizontal; for second-stage, 5–10 ml with patient sitting for 10 min, to block sacral nerves.

2. Lignocaine, 1–1·5% 20 ml. This gives a block up to T.11 in most cases, patients in labour show a higher level of analgesia than in normal women using the same dose. Repeated injections have decreasing effect.

4. Pudendal Nerve Block and Local Infiltration

This may be used for: (*a*) Normal delivery—the sensory nerve supply of the vulva comes from the ilio-inguinal nerve anteriorly and from the perineal branch of the posterior cutaneous nerve of the thigh posteriorly; (*b*) Episiotomy; (*c*) Outlet forceps; (*d*) Repair of lacerations.

Indications may include fetal distress, delayed second stage, assisted breech delivery and multiple pregnancy. It can be used for forceps delivery because it is associated with less danger, both for the mother and for the baby, than general anaesthesia. This block is usually carried out by the obstetrician. For details of technique *see* eighth edition of this Synopsis.

5. Paracervical Nerve Block

Seldom performed today, and then usually by the obstetrician. For further information *see* eighth edition of this Synopsis.

Administration of Analgesia by Midwives

The English National Board for Midwifery lays down rules relating to analgesia in labour administered by midwives working alone. A practising midwife must not, on her own responsibility, administer an inhalation analgesic unless:

1. She has received special instruction in the essentials of obstetric analgesia at an institution approved by the Board, and has satisfied the institution or Board that she is thoroughly proficient in the use of the apparatus.

2. The patient has at some time during the pregnancy been examined by a registered medical practitioner who has signed a certificate that he finds no contraindication to the administration of analgesia by a midwife. Should the patient subsequently contract an illness requiring medical attention, the onus is on the midwife to obtain confirmation that the certificate remains valid. In Scotland, the patient must be examined by a registered medical practitioner within 1 month of confinement and a certificate signed that the patient is fit for the administration of analgesic agents.

3. One other person, acceptable to the patient, who in the opinion of the midwife is suitable for the purpose, is present at the time of the administration, in addition to the midwife.

The following apparatus are approved by the Board for the use of midwives: The Entonox Apparatus (approved in 1965) for administration of premixed nitrous-oxide–oxygen (50% of each). Emotril Trichloroethylene Automatic Inhaler (0·5 or 0·35% in air). Tecota Mark 6 Trichloroethylene Inhaler (0·5 or 0·35% in air). The trichloroethylene inhalers must be tested by the National

Physical Laboratory before use and rechecked at 12-monthly intervals. The responsibility for checking devolves on the owner of the vaporizer.

Since 1970 a midwife has been allowed to top-up extradural catheters, always provided that: (*a*) She has been trained in the technique; (*b*) The first top-up dose has been given by the anaesthetist; (*c*) Analgesia obtained is satisfactory and no obstetric complications have arisen. Even so, competent help should be readily available should maternal collapse occur. This will often be the anaesthetist.

Pethidine can be administered by the midwife in doses of 100 mg; not more than 200 mg may be given to any one patient.

The midwife can also administer the following drugs: chloral hydrate, syrup of chloral, potassium bromide, tincture of opium, pil. opii, Dover's powder, pentazocine, ergotamine maleate, naloxone, oxytocin, and promazine.

IV. Inhalation Analgesia[93]

1. Nitrous Oxide

Nitrous oxide does not interfere with uterine contractions, nor has it any effect on the fetus. In rats nitrous oxide has been shown to decrease both maternal and fetal methionine synthetase activity,[94] but this is without clinical significance in obstetric practice. Authority for the use of nitrous oxide and air by midwives in the UK was withdrawn by the Central Midwives Board in 1970. Nitrous-oxide–air, hitherto administrated from the Minnitt Gas–Air Machine,[95] (R. J. Minnitt (1890–1974), Liverpool anaesthetist), a modification of McKesson's oxygen apparatus, introduced in 1933, but delivers a hypoxic mixture.[96]
Premixed nitrous-oxide–oxygen.[97] The mixture is very acceptable to the patient if given from a mouth-piece, rather than from a mask.

It is important to check that the machine is working well, that cylinders contain gas and that dentures are removed. Inhalation must begin some seconds before the onset of the pain. If the patient holds her own mask, it will fall from her hand, should unconsciousness supervene: this is a safety factor. Nitrous oxide 50% and oxygen 50% (Entonox) is used. Self-administration in labour has been shown to increase maternal Pa_{O_2} at the time when placental flow is greatest.[98]

Late second-stage pains are fairly regular, and it is often possible to commence inhalation a minute before the pain is expected and to continue until the pain is maximal, followed by bearing down. In this way, the blood is saturated with nitrous oxide during the most agonizing phase of the contraction.

2. Trichloroethylene

(*See* Chapter 10.) This has been given from: (*a*) The Emotril Automatic Inhaler[99] (*E*pstein, *M*acintosh, *O*xford, *Tril*ene) which delivers 0·5% trichloroethylene in air and is compensated for changes in environmental temperature: it will also give a weaker vapour (0·35%) should the patient become too drowsy with the higher concentration. (*b*) The Tecota Inhaler Mark 6 (*t*emperature *c*ompensated *t*richloroethylene *a*ir).

General Anaesthesia

There is a definite maternal death rate for which the anaesthetist must take some blame.[100] (*See Report on Confidential Enquiries into Maternal Deaths in*

England and Wales 1970–72 and 1973–75; *Report on Health Social Subjects*, No. 14, 1979. London: HMSO.[101,102,103] Latest confidential enquiry into maternal deaths in England and Wales is for the years 1979–81 and was published in 1986. Commonest causes of death were hypertensive states including eclampsia, anaesthesia, and pulmonary embolism. Separate reports for Scotland have been published by the Scottish Home and Health Department, 1978.) Deaths are associated with: (1) Aspiration of stomach contents; (2) Hypoxia associated with difficulty in tracheal intubation; (3) Hypotension from any cause, including accidental subarachnoid injection; (4) Inadequate blood transfusion, too little, and too late.

Equipment

Apparatus for the administration of general anaesthesia should be accompanied by (1) Laryngoscopes and tracheal tubes; (2) Efficient suction; (3) A table which can be rapidly placed in the head-down position; (4) The means to produce a lateral tilt; (5) Resuscitation equipment including provision for the administration of oxygen and appropriate drugs; (6) Intravenous cannulae and infusion sets, with appropriate fluids.

Prevention of Vomiting during Anaesthesia in Labour

(*See also* Chapter 18.) Vomiting is always a real danger during labour as the patient may not be suitably prepared, while the gastric emptying time is delayed. There may, too, be associated hiatus hernia. Promethazine, because of its antanalgesic effect, should not be given as an anti-emetic in labour.[104]

Diet. A satisfactory regimen must be instituted to lessen the likelihood of acid stomach contents being present should general anaesthesia be required. It has been suggested[105] that patients be classified as 'normal' or 'high-risk' cases:

1. *'Normal' Cases.* Unlikely to require general anaesthesia. The aim is to provide a light, easily digestible diet and to avoid large pieces of meat or vegetables with a high-fibre content. Fried food should be avoided and the ingestion of milk curtailed. Sieved foods are allowed. Drinks should not contain more than 5% glucose as stronger solutions delay gastric emptying. Small meals 3-hourly are preferable to large meals.

2. *'High-risk' Cases.* In these cases the obstetric history suggests that operative delivery may be required. Patients should be placed in the 'high-risk' category even if it is planned to use regional analgesia. Aspiration of vomitus can occur during spinal analgesia for Caesarean section. In these patients, once active labour is established, they should be given nothing by mouth except for antacids. They should received intravenous fluids, 500 ml 5% dextrose, 4-hourly. Both pethidine and diamorphine delay gastric emptying time,[106] and so does maternal fatigue and exhaustion. Normal labour does not retard gastric emptying time,[107] but food and drink should be of the low residue, low fat type.

3. *The Use of Antacids.* Antacids, such as magnesium trisilicate mixture, BPC, which also contains sodium bicarbonate and must be freshly prepared,[108] or sodium citrate (20 ml of 0·3 Molar) should be given 2-hourly to reduce gastric acidity, 30 ml of the former is recommended immediately before induction of anaesthesia. The same amount of Milk of Magnesia can also be given.[109] There is evidence that the antacid may 'layer' in the stomach unless the patient is rolled from side to side to ensure mixing. Oral cimetidine, 300 mg 2 or 3 h before anaesthesia, may contribute to safety.[110] Ranitidine is now widely used.[111]

Before induction of anaesthesia, a No. 10 oesophageal tube may be passed if the anaesthetist cannot guarantee safety from aspiration of gastric contents without it. Trouble may arise from: (1) *Gross obstruction* by solid or liquid material. (2) *Mendelson's or the acid pulmonary aspiration syndrome*.[54] This is a serious condition which may follow the aspiration of gastric contents into the air passages, thought by Mendelson to be due to acid irritation of material at a pH of 2·5 or below, but shown to occur with fluid of a neutral pH as well.[112] It is due to damage to the alveolar capillary membrane. Aspiration of alkali may also be harmful. The normal fasting gastric secretion has a pH of 1·5. The signs and symptoms are cyanosis, dyspnoea, tachycardia, bronchospasm and in fulminant cases either acute oedema of the lungs or acute respiratory failure. The radiograph shows a regular mottling without evidence of atelectasis. An interval of some hours may separate the initial aspiration from the development of symptoms. Most commonly seen in obstetric patients perhaps because of their acute deprivation of ACTH and corticosteroids following separation of the placenta. For treatment *see below*. (3) *Bronchopneumonia and its later complications*, e.g. lung abscess or bronchiectasis.

The Dangers of Aspiration

Aspiration of stomach contents during general anaesthesia can be made less likely by:

1. Giving only fluid and semi-solid material during labour.
2. The insertion of a No. 10 oesophageal tube before induction of anaesthesia.
3. Use of cricoid pressure (*see* Chapter 18).
4. Use of metoclopramide, 10 mg i.v., increases the lower oesophageal sphincter tone and so may reduce the incidence of regurgitation.
5. Inducing anaesthesia with the head elevated. In a reported series of 2000 cases, deliberate gastric emptying was only employed in 1% of cases and no aspirations of stomach contents were reported.[113]
6. Apomorphine to promote vomiting before induction.[114]
7. Cimetidine, 300 mg i.m. before induction—it is thought to be safe with respect to uterine activity and to the well-being of the fetus; 200 mg i.v. 60–90 min before induction results in a gastric juice of pH 5·0 on induction. It crosses the placental barrer.[115] Ranitidine is now widely employed;[116] dose 150 mg oral or 50 mg i.v.

The acid pulmonary aspiration syndrome can occur without definite vomiting or obvious regurgitation. Patients for sterilization by tubal section and ligation in the immediate post-partum days may also be at risk.

For techniques of anaesthesia in the presence of stomach contents, *see* Chapter 18.

Treatment of acid aspiration syndrome

1. Milder cases may be treated by: (*a*) The Trendelenburg position; (*b*) Lightening of anaesthesia to encourage coughing; (*c*) Pharyngeal suction.
2. Severe cases may require, in addition to careful tracheobronchial toilet, aspiration and lavage with solution of sodium bicarbonate and IPPV. Hydrocortisone in large doses reduces the inflammatory reaction and aids bronchodilatation. The same precautions are necessary to prevent aspiration during the puerperium (e.g. for sterilization) as during labour.

(*See also* Rosen M. *Anaesthesia* 1981, **36**, 145; *also* correspondence, *Anaesthesia* 1981, **36**, 910–914.)

For prevention of aspiration of stomach contents during labour, *see* The Experts Opine. *Surv. Anesthesiol.* 1985, **29**, 191–200; Nimmo W. S. *Br. J. Hosp. Med.* 1985, **34**, 176. Differing reports of the success or failure of the action of the various drugs and methods used to minimize this most serious complication, show that the problem is not yet solved.

(*See also* MacDonald A. G. in *Recent Advances in Anaesthesia and Analgesia*—15. (Atkinson R. S. and Adams A. P. ed.) Edinburgh: Churchill Livingstone, 1985; The use of antacids as a prophylaxis against Mendelson's syndrome in the United Kingdom; A survey. Sweeney B. and Wright I. *Anaesthesia* 1986, **41**, 419.)

Anaesthetic Agents

Thiopentone
A dose of 100–250 mg for induction is unlikely seriously to depress fetal respiration, but further or larger amounts are probably undesirable. Methohexitone acts similarly in doses of 60–80 mg.

Muscle Relaxants
These agents are used in labour: (1) To aid tracheal intubation; (2) To reduce reflex response to stimuli during light anaesthesia; (3) To relax the perineum and anterior abdominal wall. Clinical doses of relaxants are usually without harmful effects on the fetus, though some may cross the placenta, especially gallamine.

Hyperventilation
Oxygenation of the baby, as measured by umbilical venous P_{O_2} is maximal when maternal Pa_{O_2} is 40 kPa or $F_{I_{O_2}}$ 66%. A fall of maternal Pa_{CO_2} below 2·85 kPa causes fetal acidosis as a result of reduction in placental blood flow.[117] It is desirable to keep Pa_{CO_2} to about 4 kPa which is normal for the pregnant mother at term.

Nitrous Oxide
This analgesic with oxygen and thiopentone induction and muscle relaxants is widely used. The only complication, provided intubation can be speedily achieved to prevent aspiration of stomach contents, is awareness during operation, especially when high concentrations of oxygen are employed. The use of an $F_{I_{O_2}}$ greater than 33% results in better acid–base measurements in the fetus and $F_{I_{O_2}}$ of 66% has been recommended (reversed gas flows).[118]

Inhalation Agents
Low concentrations used as an adjuvant to nitrous oxide to prevent awareness are unlikely to affect the fetus if given for a short period and do not depress uterine retraction. Enflurane[119] 0·8% has an advantage over halothane 0·5% as uterine tone can be controlled more easily with the more insoluble agent.[120] Trichloroethylene 0·2% is safe. Isoflurane 0·7% is another alternative.

Ketamine
Ketamine increases uterine tone in the first and second, but not in the third trimester of pregnancy.[121] Has been used as the sole agent for forceps delivery,

manual removal of the placenta and similar procedures, and as an induction agent prior to Caesarean section. Should be avoided in eclampsia or hypertension. It may cause fetal respiratory depression.

Operative Obstetric Procedures

Anaesthesia for External Version
Thiopentone and a muscle relaxant will relax the abdominal wall, though not the uterus. Where uterine tone prevents version, deep anaesthesia with a volatile agent is required.

Anaesthesia for Internal Version
If the obstetrician requires a well-relaxed uterus, high into which his hand and arm must be introduced, deep anaesthesia is required, and this may be most readily obtained with ether or halothane. The technique used should avoid the risk of aspiration of stomach contents and should provide relaxation of the muscles of the pelvic floor and perineum.

Anaesthesia for Forceps Delivery
(1) Pudendal block. (2) Extradural block is satisfactory and is especially useful when an indwelling catheter is in place. (3) Low spinal analgesia has much to be said in its favour as it removes the risk of aspiration of gastric contents. Extradural sacral block is excellent, if time is available. (4) Thiopentone, suxamethonium and nitrous-oxide–oxygen, given through a cuffed tracheal tube. Severe problems may follow delayed intubation causing hypoxia (*see below*).

Anaesthesia for Breech Delivery
1. In assisted breech delivery, good oxygenation and a smooth induction at the right time are necessary. In the first and early second stages, pethidine 100–150 mg and nitrous-oxide–oxygen if necessary. When the presenting part appears, an episiotomy can be done under infiltration analgesia and pudendal block, and this gives adequate pain relief. For delivery of the aftercoming head by forceps, anaesthesia is not induced until the scapulae are delivered. If it is then necessary, it must be induced rapidly by one of the following methods: (*a*) Oxygen, thiopentone, suxamethonium, cuffed tracheal tube, nitrous-oxide–oxygen; (*b*) Thiopentone, nitrous-oxide–oxygen; (*c*) Cyclopropane and oxygen.
2. For breech extraction there is no hurry to induce anaesthesia which can follow the usually accepted techniques. Good relaxation may be required. Regional analgesia (intra- or extradural block) not contraindicated.[122]

Anaesthesia for Retained Placenta
The patient may be shocked and a retraction ring may form an obstruction. Standard techniques are satisfactory. Inhalation of one or two capsules of amyl nitrite may relax a retraction ring (but this has been denied); if it does not, deeper anaesthesia will be necessary. In the absence of facilities for general anaesthesia, trichloroethylene analgesia or intravenous opiates (e.g. morphine, 15 mg) make the manoeuvre of manual removal tolerable. Very rarely, in an

emergency and to save life in severe postpartum haemorrhage it may be justified to remove the placenta from a collapsed patient without any analgesia.

Anaesthesia for the Obstetric Flying Squad[123]
The idea of the obstetrical flying squad was suggested by Professor Farquhar Murray of Newcastle-on-Tyne in 1929, and organized in Glasgow in 1933 and in Newcastle two years later. This raises problems associated with: (1) General difficulties of all obstetric anaesthesia; and (2) Problems of the unusual location. In the absence of properly trained anaesthetists or where distances are short, it is best to transfer the patient to hospital. Equipment may include: (1) A portable anaesthetic machine; (2) Suction apparatus; (3) Case for drugs and accessories; (4) Plasma expanders for intravenous infusion and group O Rh-negative blood, and giving sets. (5) Self-inflating bag. *See also* Chapter 30.

Anaesthesia for Vaginal Termination
Thiopentone and nitrous-oxide–oxygen, with or without a narcotic analgesic or trichloroethylene. Halothane is better avoided. Ketamine affords good operative conditions with reduced blood loss.

Ergometrine
Ergometrine, although it is usually a myocardial depressant, may cause ventricular ectopic beats. There is evidence that it can stimulate α-adrenergic receptors in ordinary vessels and β-adrenergic receptors in the vessels of muscles, and if given to a patient under the influence of another α-stimulator, e.g. a pressor drug, can produce widespread vasoconstriction with hypertension, bronchoconstriction and even acute pulmonary oedema. Should be used carefully in patients with Raynaud's disease, since collapse due to intense vasoconstriction has been reported.[124] *Synthetic oxytocin*, on the other hand, may result in transient dilatation of vessels containing both α- and β-receptors and so may result in hypotension, unless the legs are in the lithotomy position or the patient in a head-down tilt. Oxytocin may be preferable if a myometrial stimulant is required in a patient who has recently been given a pressor agent.[125] Ergometrine may cause nausea and vomiting in almost half of patients.[126] It is suggested that it may contribute to the morbidity of Mendelson's syndrome.[127] Syntocinon, 10 units i.v., does not have this disadvantage.

Patients Receiving Anticoagulants
Patients on long-term anticoagulant therapy should be managed by a change to heparin at 36 weeks. Heparin does not cross the placenta. It should be reversed before extradural block and restarted 24 h after removal of the catheter.

Complications

Eclampsia and Pre-eclamptic Toxaemia
Manifestations include hypertension, reduced blood volume, increased fluid in extravascular compartment, increased risk of premature placental separation and convulsions. Death can occur from: (1) Heart failure; (2) Inhalation of saliva or vomit; (3) Cerebral haemorrhage; (4) Hepatorenal failure. May be

controlled by heavy sedation, reduction of blood pressure or special techniques. These may include: (1) Infusion of trimetaphan; (2) Lumbar extradural blockade; (3) Intravenous barbiturate and muscle relaxant with IPPV; (4) Hydralazine, 10–20 mg i.v., before induction of anaesthesia; (5) Diazepam; (6) Chlormethiazole (Heminevrin) 0·5% i.v. infusion; (7) Bromethol to produce basal narcosis. Intubation may cause harmful hypertension.

Enflurane and probably halothane are suitable agents to use during Caesarean section.[128] Extradural block is to be preferred.

Amniotic Fluid Embolism[129]

A rare and dangerous complication of delivery first recognized in 1926[130] but clinical features described in 1941.[131] Its signs and symptoms may wrongly be attributed to anaesthesia. A sudden infusion of amniotic fluid into the maternal circulation, after rupture of the membranes, gives rise to an acute shock-like state characterized by: (1) Respiratory distress; (2) Cyanosis; (3) Chest pain; (4) Peripheral vascular collapse; (5) Coma; (6) Hypofibrinogenaemia with excessive bleeding; this may occur without collapse and be the first sign of the condition; effect on blood-clotting mechanism described in 1950;[132] (7) Convulsions which must be differentiated from those of eclampsia or toxicity of local analgesics. The mortality is high. Chest X-ray reveals bilateral peri-hilar mottling. ECG shows right heart strain. Pulmonary artery and central venous pressures are raised. The pulmonary bed may be blocked by fibrin deposition. *The diagnosis* is definite when elements of amniotic fluid are found in maternal tissues. *Treatment* may include: (1) Blood transfusion to combat defibrination; (2) Administration of fibrinogen; (3) Vasopressors (ephedrine or mephenter mine are to be preferred as they do not cause pulmonary vasoconstriction); (4) Artificial ventilation with oxygen; (5) Bronchodilators; (6) Steroids; (7) Possibly digitalis; (8) Heparin has been recommended to prevent continued fibrinogen–fibrin conversion.[133]

Hypofibrinogenaemia

May follow haemorrhage, abortion, hydatidiform mole, intra-uterine fetal death, amniotic fluid embolism. May be due to: (1) Continued bleeding; (2) Destruction of fibrin and fibrinogen by plasma fibrinolysins; (3) Conversion of prothrombin to thrombin may be inactivated by release of heparin-like substance in amniotic fluid. Normal fibrinogen is 150–700 mg %. Less than 150 mg % is dangerous. *Treatment*: (1) 4 g fibrinogen rapidly and repeat in 1 h if no significant improvement; (2) If there is a circulatory fibrinolysin give epsilon aminocaproic acid, 4–5 g initial dose i.v. over 1 h, then 1 g 8-hourly; (3) When heparin-like factor diagnosed, give 20–50 mg protamine sulphate i.v. slowly. 500 ml blood contains less than 1 g of fibrinogen, 1000 ml plasma provides 3 g.

Shock

Causes of shock in the obstetric patient include: (1) Haemorrhage, e.g. antepartum or postpartum haemorrhage, lacerations of birth canal, retained placenta, uterine atony; (2) Traumatic: acute inversion of the uterus; surgical trauma; (3) Septic shock; (4) Supine hypotensive syndrome (*see below*); (5) Amniotic fluid embolism.

Awareness[137,180]

This is a problem when light anaesthesia, nitrous-oxide–oxygen with relaxants, is employed. The use of reversed gas flows, 66% oxygen and 33% nitrous oxide, makes the use of adjuvants essential, e.g. trichloroethylene 0·2%, halothane 0·5% or enflurane 0·8%. Even so, an incidence of 2·5% has been quoted as an irreducible minimum. The use of a tourniquet on one arm to prevent entry of muscle relaxant and allow the patient to use her hand on command has been advocated.[138] Following reversal of muscle relaxant at the end of operation, patient's response to command within 15 s of nitrous oxide cessation suggests that there has been a risk of awareness.

Caval Compression Syndrome

In the supine position the inferior vena cava is compressed by the gravid uterus at term. In 6% of patients this results in bradycardia, fall of cardiac output and hypotension of significant degree. Caval compression syndrome may be *latent* or *overt*. In either case placental blood flow is reduced. This may result in fall of Pao_2 and metabolic acidosis in the fetus. These ill effects are less when the fetus descends during labour and when the patient is put in the lateral position or when a tilt to the left is used on the operating table. Tilt to the left is preferred, but if this is not effective tilt to the right can be used.

Failed Intubation

Failure to intubate the patient has resulted in maternal death as a result of hypoxia. The following procedure has been recommended should tracheal intubation fail:[139] (1) Maintain cricoid pressure; (2) Patient put on left side, head down; (3) Give oxygen by IPPV; (4) If ventilation easy, ventilate with nitrous-oxide–oxygen and volatile supplement (ether or methoxyflurane) and continue by face-mask when spontaneous respiration is restored; (5) Pass wide-bore stomach tube via mouth, aspirate and instil 30 ml magnesium trisilicate before withdrawal; (6) Continue anaesthesia for operation with lateral tilt; (7) If oxygenation proves difficult ((3) *above*), allow patient to resume consciousness, and consider regional technique or general anaesthesia by face-mask with spontaneous respiration. Caval compression combined with hypoxia can precipitate cardiac arrest, so it is important to keep the patient in the lateral position until oxygenation is assured. For difficult intubation in obstetric cases, *see* Jellico J. A. and Harris N. R. *Anaesthesia* 1984, **39**, 800.

Sickle-cell Disease and Pregnancy[134]

Myasthenia Gravis in Pregnancy[135]

Disseminated Intravascular Coagulation[136]

Acute Inversion of the Uterus

Shock is out of proportion to blood loss. Immediate replacement of blood or fluid is necessary with general anaesthesia (e.g. cyclopropane).

Anaphylactoid reaction to oxytocin in pregnancy.[140]

Anaesthesia for Caesarean Section

The ideal anaesthetic or analgesic provides: (1) Good pain relief and a quiet patient; (2) Absence of respiratory depression of the fetus; (3) Good relaxation of the abdomen; (4) Absence of psychic trauma to mother and awareness during operation; (5) Absence of toxicity in mother and infant; (6) Absolute safety, especially from aspiration of stomach contents. The fetal mortality following elective section is greater than that following normal delivery.

Premedication

Many workers prohibit all sedation and allow only atropine or hyoscine. If sedation is required, diazepam, 5 mg orally, is the preferred drug.[141] Lorazepam has also been used. Mist. mag. trisil., BPC 15–30 ml or sodium citrate is given p.o.

General Anaesthesia

Proper measures to prevent aspiration of stomach contents must be taken (*see* Chapter 18). The apparatus should be checked. A standard induction technique is: preoxygenation for 3 min, thiopentone 4 mg/kg, suxamethonium 100 mg, cricoid pressure, tracheal intubation, nitrous-oxide–oxygen, non-depolarizing relaxant. The risk of awareness can be reduced if a trace of volatile agent is added (*see* p. 539). Vecuronium may be a useful relaxant in Caesarean section because of its short duration of action, rapid clearance and minimal placental transfer. The lateral position for intubation (the coma position) greatly reduces the risk of inhalation of gastric contents and might well be practised regularly in well prepared non-obstetric patients. Oxygen concentrations up to 66% have been advocated (*see above*). One disadvantage is that the mother may become aware of events during the operation.[142] Lateral tilt is employed to prevent caval compression (*see* p. 539). Full doses of relaxant are seldom necessary in Caesarean section. The abdominal muscles are stretched during pregnancy and muscle tone is seldom a problem.

Hyperventilation has been used as an aid to the production of unconsciousness. Respiratory alkalosis in the mother may, however, produce hazard to the fetus.

Extradural Lumbar Block

The method of choice in the opinion of many anaesthesists, combined with a lateral tilt and preload with 1000 ml of intravenous fluid. Extradural block for Caesarean section does not decrease the amount of placental blood flow to the fetus.[143] Previous Caesarean section is not necessarily a contraindication to extradural block in a subsequent labour, provided that careful monitoring for a ruptured scar is well maintained.[144] Injection is preferably between L.2 and L.3 of: (1) Bupivacaine 0·5%, 10 ml in the sitting position for 15 min, followed by 8–16 ml in the horizontal position, perhaps in divided doses, the aim being to produce block from T.8 to L.4;[145] (2) Bupivacaine 0·5%, 15–20 ml;[146] (3) Lignocaine 1·5%, 20–25 ml;[147] (4) Etidocaine 1% 20 ml; (5) Chloroprocaine,[148] because of its rapid onset of action, e.g. 20 ml of 3% solution;[149] cessation of action may be sudden. Insertion of a catheter is not essential.

It has been shown that patients in advanced pregnancy and labour require smaller doses of local analgesic agents than normal women. The blood pressure should be maintained at 90 mmHg or above by infusion of fluids intravenously, and if necessary by i.v. ephedrine. Hartmann's solution, 2 l given rapidly while the block is taking effect, goes some way to preventing hypotension.[150] Vomiting is not uncommon. Oxygen should be given to the mother and this can be combined with sedation or light general anaesthesia, if necessary.

One of the advantages of extradural lumbar block for Caesarean section is that the mother may remain awake with active cough reflexes. Even very nervous patients can be managed in this way if they are treated sympathetically and the surgeon is gentle. Occasionally, however, the anaesthetist must be prepared to anaesthetize the patient with a judicious mixture of thiopentone and perhaps a volatile agent with nitrous oxide and oxygen, while intubation may be necessary.

Infants born after extradural analgesia may be less acidotic and better oxygenated than those born under general anaesthesia for Caesarean section, but this is not universally accepted.[151] Lignocaine, 2% solution given extradurally for Caesarean section (elective) caused no neurobehavioural problems.[152]

The extension of extradural block given for pain relief in normal labour can be converted in those patients found to require Caesarean section by injecting 16 ml of 0·5% bupivacaine (without adrenaline), 8 ml with the patient lying on her right side followed by 8 ml on the left.[155]

It would seem that extradural analgesia reduces uterine activity; it increases the forceps delivery rate.[153] Slow controlled induction of extradural analgesia greatly reduces the risk of local analgesic toxicity.[154]

In a recent survey of 27 000 lumbar extradural blocks, exclusive of those given for elective Caesarean section operations, an extremely high rate of safety for the mother resulted when the rules of management were rigorously followed.[156]

Extradural Sacral (Caudal) Block
After a test dose of 10 ml, 20 ml bupivacaine 0·5 or 0·25% are injected, followed by 5–10 ml every 10 min until analgesia reaches the eighth dermatome. For 'one-shot' injection, 30–35 ml of 1·5% lignocaine is usually adequate. An intravenous drip and oxygen inhalation should be given before and during the operation. Not often used.

Intradural Block (Subarachnoid Block)
It is a method without bad effect on the child provided that lateral tilt is used to avoid pressure of the gravid uterus on the vena cava. It ensures good retraction of the uterus and absence of postpartum haemorrhage. The enlarged uterus, by interfering with the movements of the diaphragm, tends to produce hypoxia of the mother so 100% of oxygen should be given to the mother from the outset. The systolic blood pressure should not be allowed to fall below 90 mmHg. Following intra- or extradural block, the pressor agents to be avoided are methoxamine and phenylephrine, which may reduce the blood supply to the placenta. Ephedrine does not possess these disadvantages.

Block should reach at least to the costal margin and can be obtained with bupivacaine 0·5% plain, 3 ml injected with the patient in the right lateral position and afterwards turned on to her back on a table with a slight head-down tilt with a wedge under the right hip and shoulder to remove pressure, especially at the pelvic brim, on the vena cava from the gravid uterus.[76] Hyperbaric amethocaine hydrochloride (8 mg in 1% solution with 1 ml of 10% dextrose) can be used in the same way.

Great care is required, especially in control of the blood pressure and in adequate oxygenation of the mother and hence of the child. Hypotension can be treated by a lateral tilt, elevation of the legs, infusion of plasma-volume expander, ephedrine and oxygen administration.[156,157]

Local Infiltration
This is without serious effect on the mother or child, but is unsuitable for frightened or uncontrolled patients. The surgeon's co-operation is essential for success: he usually performs the injections himself.[158]

Intradermal and subcutaneous infiltration is carried out in the line of the incision and solution should be deposited for about 2·5 cm on each side of the midline. Extra solution is injected into the pyramidales and into the retropubic space of Retzius. Solution injected into the rectus sheath will improve relaxation. The parietal peritoneum is infiltrated, likewise the tissue overlying the lower segment if the classic operation is not to be employed. Those interested in the technique should consult the paper by A. C. Beck (*Am. J. Obstet. Gynecol.* 1942, **4**, 558 and Macintosh Marshall. *Caesarean Section; Lower Segment Operation.* Bristol: Wright, 1944). It is not very widely used today.

For some other functions of the anaesthetist in obstetric departments, *see* Crawford J. S. *Br. Med. J.* 1980, **2**, 119.

(*See also* Moir D. D. and Thorburn J. *Obstetric Anaesthesia and Analgesia*, 3rd ed. London: Baillière Saunders, 1985; Albright G. A. et al. *Anesthesia in Obstetrics*. New York: Butterworths, 1986. Schnider S. M. and Levinson G. *Anesthesia in Obstetrics*. Baltimore: Williams and Wilkins, 1979; Crawford J. S. *Principles and Practice of Obstetric Anaesthesia*, 5th ed. Oxford: Blackwell, 1986; Tunstall M. E. in: *General Anaesthesia* (Gray T. C. et al. ed.), 4th ed. London: Butterworths, 1980; Datta S. and Alper M. H. *Anesthesiology* 1980, **53**, 142.)

Resuscitation of the Newborn

One of the earliest papers on treatment was 'The Asphyxia of the Stillborn Infant and its Treatment', by Marshall Hall in 1856.[159] Intra-uterine respiration of the fetus, the rhythmical amniotic tide into and out of the air passages, was first demonstrated by J. F. Ahfelt (1843–1929), Leipzig obstetrician, in 1888 and then by the Italian, Ferroni, in 1899.[160]

The fetal blood haemoglobin is 15–20 g/100 ml and when fully saturated carries 22 vol% of oxygen. But because of the low oxygen partial pressure at which maternal blood gives up its oxygen, fetal haemoglobin is only 50% saturated. There is also a mild acidosis with P_{CO_2} of 7 kPa and a pH fall to 7·25. To compensate for this the dissociation curve of the maternal haemoglobin is shifted to the left, while the dissociation curve of fetal haemoglobin is shifted to the right, making it give up oxygen more easily. Brown fat is important in heat regulation of the newborn.

In the newborn the amount of carbonic anhydrase is half that found in adult blood so that release of carbon dioxide in lungs is handicapped.

During the process of birth, anaerobic glycolysis may aid the survival of the infant, should respiratory embarrassment occur, energy being released from glycogen.

Fluctuation in maternal carbon-dioxide tension may contribute to respiratory difficulties in the newborn, especially in premature infants. Maternal Pa_{CO_2} may fall as a result of hyperventilation towards the end of the first stage of labour, but may rise during the second stage as a result of breath-holding. The effect of hyperventilation during anaesthesia is discussed in Chapter 15.

Pneumothorax. Most infants who develop this have idiopathic respiratory distress syndrome, and it is not primarily due to artificial ventilation. With prompt diagnosis and treatment little harm to the infant results.[161]

Intrapartum Fetal Monitoring[162]

For electronic fetal heart rate monitoring *see* Pearce J. M. and Willson K. *Br. J. Hosp. Med.* 1983, **30**, 123. The signs of intrauterine hypoxia are irregularity of the fetal heart rate going on to tachycardia or bradycardia. In a cephalic presentation, the presence of meconium indicates hypoxic relaxation of the fetal anal sphincter.

Estimation of the pH of fetal blood as an index of fetal hypoxia has proved most useful. A pH of 7·15 indicates critical hypoxia.

Causes of Hypoxia in Fetus and Newborn[163]

1. Reduction of oxygen tension in maternal blood. Pa_{O_2} may be reduced at term (*see above*). Factors such as altitude, reduced F_{IO_2} or the presence of haemoglobinopathy may cause further problems. Oxygen consumption may be increased.

2. The trauma of labour.

3. Interference of passage of oxygen from mother to fetus through: (*a*) Hypotension due to caval compression, spinal or extradural analgesia; (*b*) Anaemia, e.g. haemorrhage, cardiac failure. etc; (*c*) Placental infarction or premature separation; (*d*) Prolapse or knotting of cord.

4. Fetal respiratory failure:

a. Central. Due to: (i) Immaturity of respiratory centre, perhaps associated with gross fetal abnormality; (ii) Damage to respiratory centre from trauma or from cerebral oedema due to diabetes or hydrops fetalis; (iii) Oxygen lack perhaps associated with intrapartum fetal asphyxia; (iv) Narcotics and sedatives given to mother. The threshold of maternal respiratory centre differs from that of the fetal centre, as a level of narcosis harmless to the mother may be depressing to the fetus. All general anaesthetics to mother are hazardous if the baby is premature.

b. Peripheral. Due to: (i) Immaturity of lungs; (ii) Respiratory obstruction; (iii) Muscular weakness; (iv) Fetal lungs full of liquor amnii or meconium; (v) Intranatal pneumonia.

The baby recovering from asphyxia first takes a series of gasps which give place to a series of single prolonged inspirations. Finally, rhythmic inspiration and expiration set in. Periodic breathing is not of bad prognostic significance in newborn babies and is usual in premature infants.

The diagnosis of fetal asphyxia during labour, as by measuring the pH of fetal blood,[164] indicates the need for oxygen to the mother.

All anaesthetics, except nitrous oxide and oxygen, and all analgesic agents, other than chloral in reasonable dosage, depress the fetal respiratory mechanism, an effect made worse by any hypoxia of the mother during labour. The placenta acts as no barrier to these agents. There is definite evidence that hypoxia of the fetus during labour, and of the baby at birth or shortly afterwards, may be followed by impaired cerebral function in later life. The danger is increased with premature infants.

Management of Asphyxia of the Newborn

The fetal circulation can withstand 10–15 min of anoxia but deficient cerebral blood flow may cause permanent damage. The fetus in utero is cyanosed. The normally delivered child should breathe rhythmically from the beginning, air replacing liquor amnii. Alveoli are opened up by the negative pressure exerted by normal respiratory movements ($-50\,cmH_2O$)—as in crying. In respiratory depression respiration begins differently, in gasps—the most primitive respiratory movement, involving many muscles.

Virginia Apgar[165] (1909–1975) of New York City described a system whereby the condition of a neonate can be assessed, one (or more) minutes after birth. A score of 0, 1 or 2 is given in each of five variables—heart rate, respiratory effort, muscle tone, colour and reflex irritability. The maximum score is 10. A single clinical assessment at 1 min does not distinguish beween primary apnoea (which will usually recover without treatment) and terminal apnoea (when active resuscitation is required). Important factors are: (*a*) Changes in heart rate before resuscitation; (*b*) Whether gasping precedes an improvement in colour or vice versa; (*c*) Whether or not apnoea supervenes in a baby who has initially gasped or cried. Some anaesthetists prefer to omit colour and use the A – C (Apgar minus colour) score. Subtle effects on the neonate's nervous system may be caused by drugs, local and general, used in obstetric pain relief.[166]

Table 27.1. Apgar Scoring System

	Heart rate	Respiratory effort	Muscle tone	Colour	Reflex irritability
0	Absent	Absent	Flaccid	Blue or white	No response
1	Slow, less than 100	Weak cry, hypoventilation	Some flexion of limbs	Blue hands or feet	Some movement
2	100 or over	Crying lustily	Well flexed	Healthy pink	Active movement

Indications for Oxygen and IPPV by Mask in the Newborn

(1) Central cyanosis; (2) Bradycardia; (3) Failure to cry on stimulation. Facemask resuscitation may be successful if Head's reflex[149] stimulates spontaneous respiration; if it does not, intubation will be required.[167] It requires skill and may cause damage.

Indications for Intubation of the Newborn and Short-term IPPV

The following guidelines may be considered when the baby's condition deteriorates in the minutes following birth: (1) Central cyanosis for more than 3 min; (2) Bradycardia less than 100 bpm for more than 3 min; (3) Apnoea for more than 3 min; (4) 'White asphyxia', i.e. skin vasoconstriction; (5) Cardiac arrest or depression; (6) Apgar score of 0–2.

The cyanosis will fail to respond to oxygen therapy in the presence of cyanotic heart disease, severe tracheo-oesophageal fistula, large diaphragmatic hernia and severe respiratory distress syndrome.

Blue asphyxia seldom requires more than clearing the upper air passages by suction, using a catheter (No. 6 FG), giving periods of negative pressure of 100–150 cmH$_2$O. Skin stimulation, passive limb movements, slapping, etc. are also very valuable, while oxygen given via a nasal catheter is beneficial. A useful method is to insufflate 2–3 l/min of oxygen, from a small rubber catheter into the infant's mouth, while its mouth and nares are occluded and relaxed for expiration. This is sufficient to distend the lungs, and can be continued rhythmically for some time without causing trauma. Better is the use of a neonatal inflating bag 30–40 puffs per min. (e.g. Cardiff neonatal inflating bag).[168] In feeble babies, a small stomach tube should be passed to evacuate the stomach of liquor amnii and prevent its aspiration into the lungs.

If no improvement takes place within 3–4 min the trachea should be intubated and the lungs inflated with oxygen. Incorrect insertion of tracheal tube may cause loss of the tube in the oesophagus requiring removal under general anaesthesia. Any baby born apnoeic, flaccid or with a slow heart beat should be intubated. The laryngoscope should have a straight blade.

The tracheal tube used should have an internal diameter of 2·5–3·5 mm. Various designs are available.

Oxygen is carried to the lungs by: (1) a Jackson Rees modification of Ayre's T-piece,[169] with manual compression of the reservoir bag; or (2) pressure from an oxygen supply. A small hole in the tubing is occluded by the finger to build up controlled pressure so that frequent half-second puffs of oxygen can be given. The pressure needed to expand the newborn lung is usually about 2·94 kPa (30 cmH$_2$O), but may be double this for a few inflations. Pressures greater than this may cause rupture of the lung. Excessive pressures can be avoided by use of a blow-off device, set for 30 cmH$_2$O. Should pneumothorax occur, its presence may be confirmed by X-ray and relief obtained by insertion of an i.v. cannula in the mid-axillary line which is then connected to a source of suction.

To intubate a neonate the patient should be on a flat table with no pillow. The head should not be over-extended. The straight blade of the infant laryngoscope should be inserted into the vallecula (not posterior to the epiglottis) from the right side of the mouth and then lifted vertically, but gentleness is required. Rhythmic inflation of oxygen often has beneficial results (probably because of changes in intrabronchial pressure rather than because of expansion of collapsed alveoli). There is evidence that a positive pressure of 30–50 cmH$_2$O applied through a tracheal tube for repeated short periods will cause a collapsed lung to expand. Intubation should be done by a doctor, but senior labour ward midwives may be taught how to do it also. If spontaneous breathing does not occur within 2 min, infusion of bicarbonate 1–2 mmol/kg of 8·4% solution diluted with an equal volume of water via an umbilical venous catheter slowly, and glucose into the umbilical vein should be commenced. Estimation of blood gases and electrolytes is desirable.

Closed chest massage, if required, can be carried out by pressure of two fingers over the midsternum 60 times/min. In a baby who is hypotonic and is not responding, continued resuscitation beyond 30 min is unlikely to result in a favourable outcome.[170]

Premature babies must not be given pure oxygen for any length of time. If they are cyanosed they may receive 40% oxygen for short periods only, thus reducing the danger of retrolental fibroplasia.[171]

Steps should be taken to prevent fall in temperature during resuscitation. Procedures should be carried out under a heat lamp, the infant should be wrapped up as soon as possible, and the rectal temperature taken using a low-reading thermometer.

Drugs. Injection into the umbilical vein of naloxone, 0·01 mg/kg repeated, i.v. or i.m., will counteract any respiratory depression following injection of pethidine or morphine into the mother. *Nikethamide* (0·5 ml of 5% solution) placed on the tongue has an appreciable stimulant effect on respiration. It has been suggested that respiratory stimulants have no place in perinatal asphyxia.[172]

(*See also* Davenport H. T. and Valman H. B. *General Anaesthesia* (Gray T. C. et al. ed.), 4th ed. London: Butterworths, 1980; Beard R. W. et al. *Lancet* 1979, **2**, 1117; Lissauer T. *Hosp. Update* 1981, **7**, 109.)

Respiratory Distress Syndrome[173]

The idiopathic respiratory distress syndrome of the newborn is the commonest cause of death in liveborn premature infants. The incidence is related to the degree of prematurity and is rare in infants born at term. One baby out of every 200 born alive dies of respiratory failure in the first few days of life. An equal number have respiratory distress but recover normal function. The distress may show itself from birth or may come on several hours later, and is characterized by severe retraction of the chest wall during inspiration, cyanosis, a respiratory rate above 60/min and an expiratory grunt. Recovery is usual in those babies who survive beyond the third day. The lungs are grossly atelectatic, and the radiographic appearances are those of 'ground glass'. The alveoli and terminal bronchioles are lined by a hyaline membrane, first described in 1925.[174] The material interfering with ventilation is probably formed from the lung itself and not inhaled. Lack of a surface tension-lowering substance—surfactant—in the alveolar spaces is causal.[175] Surfactant is a lipoprotein containing dipalmitoyl lecithin. Its function is to confer stability on the terminal air spaces, or to act as an anti-atelectasis factor. It increases in the amniotic fluid from the 33rd week of pregnancy. The ratio between this and another surface active phospholipid, sphingomyelin, can be determined by amniocentesis and may enable those infants who are at high risk to be diagnosed. The condition is most frequently seen in premature babies, and in babies born to mothers suffering from diabetes, toxaemia or placenta praevia. Neonatal respiratory function is related to the total lipid, phospholipid and lecithin content of amniotic fluid.

If inadequate respiration causes acid–base imbalance, hyperkalaemia may occur. It has also been suggested that routine transfusion of blood from the placenta may reduce the incidence of the condition. The infant should be nursed in an incubator in a humid atmosphere and at a temperature of 35 °C (95 °F) to minimize oxygen consumption. Careful monitoring of blood gases and pH is mandatory, and metabolic acidosis corrected by sodium bicarbonate which may be given orally or intravenously. The atmosphere should be oxygen enriched to maintain an arterial oxygen tension as near normal as possible. IPPV may be required and there is evidence that better results are obtained where a positive pressure is used in the expiratory phase whether respiration is spontaneous or not (Gregory box).[176] This can be achieved with and without tracheal intubation. Postnasal instillation of surfactant into the infant's upper respiratory tract may benefit the patient with hyaline membrane disease.[177]

The 'shake test' has been used to predict the syndrome.[178]

For drugs which can be given to nursing mothers without much harm to the infant, *see Drug Ther. Bull.* 1983, **21**, 5.

References

1. Dick-Read G. *Childbirth without Fear*, 4th ed. London: Heinemann, 1960; Brown F. J. *Antenatal and Postnatal Care.* London: Churchill, 1976.
2. Heyns O. S. *J. Obstet. Gynaecol. Br. Emp.* 1959, **66**, 220.
3. Loewe S. *Dtsch. Med. Wochenschr.* 1912, **38**, 947.
4. Vogt E. *Medsche Klin.* 1928, **24**, 24.
5. O'Sullivan J. V. and Craner W. W. *Lancet* 1932, **1**, 119; Irving F. C. et al. *Surg. Gynecol. Obstet.* 1934, **58**, 1.
6. Cleisz L. *Presse méd.* 1924, **32**, 1001.
7. Kormann E. *Monat. Gerburts. Frauenkrank.* 1860, **32**, 114.
8. Sahli L. *Münch. Med. Wochenschr.* 1909, 26.
9. Jaeger W. *Zentbl. Gynäk.* 1910, No. 46.
10. Steinbuchel R. von *Zentbl. Gynäk.* 1902, No. 48.
11. Gauss C. J. *Arch. Gynaek.* 1906, **78**, 579. (*See also* Greenwood W. O. *Scopolamine–Morphine.* London: Froude, 1918; the 5th edition of this Synopsis, 1964).
12. Korff B. *Münch. Med. Wochenschr.* 1901, **48**, 1169.
13. van Hoosen B. *Curr. Res. Anesth. Analg.* 1928, **7**, 151.
14. Duvoisin R. and Katz R. *JAMA* 1968, **206**, 1963.
15. Clark R. B. *J. Arkensas Med. Soc.* 1971, **68**, 128.
16. Akamatsu T. J. et al. *Anesth. Analg. (Cleve.)* 1974, **53**, 284; Dundee J. W. *Proc. R. Soc. Med.* 1971, **64**, 1159.
17. Pirogoff N. I. *C. R. Hebd. Séanc. Acad. Sci., Paris* 1847, **74**, 789; Secher O. *Anaesthesia* 1986, **41**, 829.
18. Gwathmey J. T. *N.Y. Med. J.* 1913, **98**, 1101.
19. Rosenfeld H. H. and Davidoff R. B. *Surg. Gynecol. Obstet.* 1935, **60**, 235.
20. Gwathmey J. T. *Am. J. Obstet. Gynecol.* 1923, **6**, 456.
21. Bepko F. et al. *Obstet. Gynecol. N.Y.* 1965, **26**, 852.
22. Kreis A. *Zentbl. Gynäk.* 1900, 747; Doleris Malartie and Dupaigne, Report to Acad. Med. Paris 22 January 1901.
23. Pitkin G. P. and McCormack F. C. *Surg. Gynecol. Obstet.* 1928, **47**, 713.
24. Adriani J. and Roma-Vega D. *Am. J. Surg.* 1946, **71**, 12.
25. Stoeckel D. *Zentbl. Gynäk.* 1909, **33**, 3; Oldham S. P. *Kenty Med. J.* 1923, **21**, 321.
26. Gellert P. *Mschr. Geburtsh. Gynäk.* 1926, 73.
27. Cleland J. G. P. *Surg. Gynecol. Obstet.* 1933, **57**, 51.
28. Bogdan E. *C. R. Soc. Biol. (Paris)* 1930, **105**, 25.
29. Bogdan E. *Bull. Soc. Obstet. Gynaecol (Paris)* 1931, **20**, 35.
30. Pickles W. and Jones S. S. *N. Engl. J. Med.* 1928, **199**, 988.
31. Graffagnino P. and Seyler L. W. *Am. J. Obstet. Gynecol.* 1938, **35**, 597.
32. Hingson R. A. and Southworth J. L. *Am. J. Surg.* 1942, **58**, 92; Edwards W. B. and Hingson R. A. *Am. J. Surg.* 1942, **57**, 459 (reprinted in 'Classical File', *Surv. Anesthesiol.* 1980, **24**, 275); Hingson R. A. and Edwards W. B. *Curr. Res. Anesth. Analg.* 1942, **21**, 301.
33. Flowers C. E. et al. *Curr. Res. Anesth. Analg.* 1949, **28**, 181.
34. Simpson J. Y. *Mon. J. Med. Sci.* (Lond. and Edin.), 1846–47, n.s., 1.
35. Simpson J. Y. *Lond. Med. Gaz.* 1847, **5**, 934.
36. Farr A. D. *Anaesthesia* 1980, **35**, 896.
37. Little D. M. *Surv. Anesthesiol.* 1980, **24**, 272.
38. Junker F. E. *Med. Times, Lond.* 1868, **1**, 171.
39. Bourne W. *JAMA* 1935, **105**, 2047.
40. Bourne W. *Lancet* 1934, **2**, 20; Griffith H. R. *Curr. Res. Anesth. Analg.* 1935, **14**, 253; Knight R. T. *Curr. Res. Anesth. Analg.* 1936, **15**, 63.
41. Hewer C. L. and Hadfield C. E. *Br. Med. J.* 1941, **1**, 924.

42. Elam J. *Lancet* 1943, **2**, 696.
43. Freedman A. *Lancet* 1943, **2**, 696.
44. Klikowitsch H. *Arch. Gynaek.* 1881, **18**, 81; Richards W. et al. *Anaesthesia* 1976, **31**, 933.
45. Webster J. C. *JAMA* 1915, **24**, 812.
46. Guedel A. E. *Indianap. Med. J.* 1911, **14**, 476; *N.Y. Med. J.* 1912, **95**, 387.
47. Minnitt R. J. *Proc. R. Soc. Med.* 1934, **27**, 1313.
48. Rivett L. C. *Br. Med. J.* 1936, **2**, 1263; Moir J. C. *Proc. R. Soc. Med.* 1936–37, **30**, 1281; Barr A. and Tindal A. *Lancet* 1937, **1**, 1271.
49. Seward E. H. *Proc. R. Soc. Med.* 1949, **42**, 745.
50. Tunstall M. E. *Lancet* 1961, **2**, 964.
51. Major V. et al. *Br. Med. J.* 1966, **2**, 1554.
52. Leboyer F. et al. *N. Engl. J. Med.* 1980, **302**, 655; Editorial, *N. Engl. J. Med.* 1980, **302**, 685.
53. Hansen R. *Klin. Wochenschr.* 1942, **21**, 301; Holmes F. J. *J. Obstet. Gynaecol. Br. Emp.* 1958, **64**, 229.
54. Mendelson C. L. *Am. J. Obstet. Gynecol.* 1946, **52**, 191 (reprinted in 'Classical File', *Surv. Anesthesiol.* 1966, **10**, 599).
55. Taylor G. and Pryse-Davies J. *Lancet* 1966, **1**, 288.
56. Scrimgeour J. B. in: *Antenatal Diagnosis of Genetic Diseases* (Emery A. E. H. ed.) Edinburgh: Churchill Livingstone, 1973.
57. Menees T. O. et al. *Am. J. Roentgenol.* 1930, **24**, 353.
58. Sweet M. de, *Br. J. Hosp. Med.* 1976, **15**, 351.
59. Bevan D. R. et al. *Br. Med. J.* 1974, **1**, 13.
60. Ang C. K. et al. *Br. Med. J.* 1969, **4**, 20.
61. Butler N. R. et al. *Br. Med. J.* 1972, **2**, 127; Cole P. V. et al. *J. Obstet. Gynaecol. Br. Commonw.* 1972, **79**, 782; Hardy J. B. and Mellitus E. D. *Lancet* 1972, **2**, 1332.
62. Hansen R. *Klin. Wochenschr.* 1942, **21**, 301; Holmes F. J. *Obstet. Gynaecol. Br. Emp.* 1958, **64**, 229.
63. Dick-Read G. *Childbirth without Fear*, 4th ed. London: Heinemann, 1960.
64. *See N. Engl. J. Med.* 1976, **294**, 1205.
65. Heyns O. S. *J. Obstet. Gynaecol. Br. Emp.* 1959, **66**, 220; Ginsburg J. *Br. J. Anaesth.* 1973, **45** (Suppl.), 790.
66. Robson J. E. *Anaesthesia* 1979, **34**, 357; Stewart P. *Anaesthesia* 1979, **34**, 361.
67. Ginsburg J. *Am. Rev. Pharmacol.* 1971, **11**, 387.
68. Weiner P. C. et al. *Br. Med. J.* 1977, **2**, 228, 229.
69. Van Hoosen B. *Anesth. Analg. Curr. Res.* 1928, **7**, 151.
70. Gauss C. J. *Zentbl. Gynäk.* 1905, 274; *Arch. für Gynek.* 1906, **78**, 579; *Münch. Med. Wochenschr.* 1907 (Jan.), **23**; von Steinbuchel N. *Zentbl. Gynäk.* 1902, No. 48.
71. Flowers C. et al. *Obstet. Gynecol. NY* 1969, **34**, 68.
72. Moir D. D. and Thorburn J. *Obstetric Anaesthesia and Analgesia*, 3rd ed. London: Baillière, Saunders, 1985.
73. *See also* Atkinson R. S. in: *Practical Regional Analgesia* (Lee J. A. and Bryce-Smith R. ed.). Amsterdam: Excerpta Medica, 1976; Moir D. D. *Obstetric Anaesthesia and Analgesia* 2nd ed. London: Baillière, Tindall, 1980; Lee J. A., Atkinson R. S. and Watt M. J. *Lumbar Puncture and Spinal Analgesia*, 5th ed. Edinburgh: Churchill Livingstone, 1985.
74. Abural E. *Bull. Soc. Obstet. Gynaec. de Paris*, 1930, **19**, 165; Cleland J. G. P. *Surg. Gynecol. Obstet.* 1933, **57**, 51.
75. Moore D. C. *Anaesthetic Techniques for Obstetrical Anaesthesia.* Springfield, Ill.: Thomas, 1964.
76. Sprague D. H. and Russell I. F. *Anaesthesia* 1983, **37**, 346.
77. Steel G. C. *Br. J. Hosp. Med.* 1972, **8**, 595; Moir D. D. and Thorburn J. *Obstetric Anaesthesia and Analgesia*, 3rd ed. London: Baillière, Saunders, 1985; Lee J. A.; Atkinson R. S. and Watt M. J. *Lumbar Puncture and Spinal Analgesia.* 5th ed. Edinburgh: Churchill Livingstone, 1985.
78. Lee J. A. *Anaesthesia* 1960, **15**, 186; 1962, **17**, 248; Doughty A. *Anaesthesia* 1974, **29**, 63.
79. Reynolds F. and Taylor G. *Anaesthesia* 1970, **25**, 14.
80. Reynolds F. and Taylor G. *Br. J. Anaesth.* 1971, **43**, 436.
81. Evans K. R. L. et al. *Anaesthesia* 1979, **34**, 310.
82. Nickel P. M., Bromage P. R. et al. *Regional Anaesthesia.* in press; Cole C. P., McMorland G. H. et al. *Anesthesiology*, 1985, **62**, 348.
83. Lund P. C. et al. *Br. J. Anaesth.* 1977, **49**, 457.

84. Abouleish F. et al. *Anesthesiology* 1977, **46**, 351.
85. Scanlon J. et al. *Anesthesiology* 1974, **40**, 121; Corke B. C. *Anaesthesia* 1977, **32**, 539.
86. Scanlon J. et al. *Anesthesiology* 1976, **45**, 400.
87. Walton P. and Reynolds F. *Anaesthesia* 1984, **39**, 218.
88. Evans J. M. et al. *Anaesthesia* 1975, **30**, 774.
89. Marinacci A. A. and Courville C. B. *JAMA* 1958, **168**, 1337.
90. Edwards W. B. and Hingson R. A. *Am. J. Surg.* 1942, **57**, 459 (reprinted in 'Classical File' *Surv. Anesthesiol.* 1980, **24**, 275); *JAMA* 1943, **121**, 225; Hingson R. A. et al. *Anesth. Analg. Curr. Res.* 1961, **40**, 119.
91. Curran J. et al. *Anaesthesia* 1975, **30**, 765.
92. Macdonald R. and Bickford Smith P. J. *Br. J. Anaesth.* 1982, **56**, 1202.
93. *See also* Rosen M. *Br. J. Anaesth.* 1971, **43**, 837.
94. Baden J. M. et al. *Br. J. Anaesth.* 1984, **56**, 523.
95. Minnitt R. J. *Proc. R. Soc. Med.* 1934, **27**, 1313; *Lancet* 1934, **1**, 1278.
96. Moir D. D. and Bissett W. I. K. *J. Obstet. Gynaecol. Br. Commonw.* 1965, **72**, 265.
97. Tunstall M. E. *Lancet* 1961, **2**, 964; *Br. Med. J.* 1963, **2**, 915; Gale C. W. et al. *Br. Med. J.* 1964, **1**, 732; MacGregor W. G. et al. *Anaesthesia* 1972, **27**, 14; Dolan P. F. and Rosen M. *Lancet* 1975, **2**, 1030.
98. Davies J. M. et al. *Br. J. Anaesth.* 1975, **47**, 370.
99. Epstein H. G. and Macintosh R. R. *Br. Med. J.* 1949, **2**, 1092.
100. Morgan B. M. *Anaesthesia* 1980, **35**, 334.
101. *See also* Tomkinson J. S. *Br. J. Hosp. Med.* 1976, **15**, 383; Moir D. D. *Br. J. Anaesth.* 1980, **52**, 1; Annotation *Br. Med. J.* 1983, **286**, 83; Morgan M. *Anaesthesia* 1986, **41**, 689.
102. A maternal death is one occurring during pregnancy or labour or as a consequence of pregnancy, within 1 year of delivery or abortion.
103. Lunn J. N. and Mushin W. W. *Mortality associated with Anaesthesia*, London: Nuffield Provincial Hospitals Trust, 1982.
104. Vella L. et al. *Br. Med. J.* 1985, **290**, 1173.
105. Crawford J. S. *Principles and Practice of Obstetric Anaesthesia*. 5th ed. Oxford: Blackwell, 1986.
106. Nimmo W. S. et al. *Lancet* 1975, **1**, 890.
107. Crawford J. S. *Lancet* 1983, **1**, 271.
108. Lord P. W. *Anaesthesia* 1984, **39**, 1144.
109. Wheatley R. G. et al. *Anesthesiology* 1979, **50**, 519.
110. Johnston J. R. et al. *Anaesthesia* 1982, **37**, 33.
111. Andrews A. D. et al. *Anaesthesia* 1982, **37**, 22.
112. Alexander I. G. S. *Br. J. Anaesth.* 1968, **40**, 408; Bannister W. K. and Sattilaro A. J. *Anesthesiology* 1962, **23**, 251; Vandam L. D. *N. Engl. J. Med.* 1965, **273**, 1206; Heaney G. A. M. and Jones H. D. *Br. J. Anaesth.* 1979, **51**, 266; Whittington R. M. et al. *Lancet* 1979, **2**, 228; Bond Y. K. et al. *Anesthesiology* 1979, **51**, 452.
113. Hodges R. J. H. and Tunstall M. E. *Br. J. Anaesth.* 1961, **33**, 572.
114. Holdsworth J. D. et al. *Br. J. Anaesth.* 1974, **46**, 375.
115. McCaughey W. et al. *Anaesthesia* 1981, **36**, 167.
116. McAuley D. M. et al. *Anaesthesia* 1983, **38**, 108.
117. Levinson G. et al. *Anesthesiology* 1974, **40**, 340.
118. *See* Rorke M. J. et al. *Anaesthesia* 1965, **23**, 585; Marx G. F. and Matter C. V. *Can. Anaesth. Soc. J.* 1971, **18**, 587; Crawford J. S. et al. *Br. J. Anaesth.* 1976, **48**, 661; Palahniuk R. J. et al. *Can. Anaesth. Soc. J.* 1977, **24**, 586.
119. Coleman A. J. and Downing J. W. *Anesthesiology* 1975, **43**, 354; Dick W. et al. *Anaesthesist*, 1977, **26**, 381.
120. Marx G. F. et al. *Obstet. Gynecol.* 1978, **56**, 695.
121. Galloon S. *Can. Anaesth. Soc. J.* 1971, **18**, 600.
122. Crawford J. S. *Br. J. Anaesth.* 1977, **49**, 19.
123. Dallas S. H. *Br. J. Anaesth.* 1967, **39**, 969; Whitford J. H. et al. *Br. J. Anaesth.* 1973, **55**, 1153.
124. Valentine B. H. et al. *Br. J. Anaesth.* 1977, **49**, 81.
125. Johnstone M. *Br. J. Anaesth.* 1972, **44**, 826.
126. Moodie J. E. and Moir D. D. *Br. J. Anaesth.* 1976, **48**, 571; Moir D. D. and Amoa A. B. *Br. J. Anaesth.* 1979, **51**, 113.
127. Crawford J. S. *Anaesthesia* 1985, **40**, 498.
128. Crowhurst J. A. and Rosen M. *Br. J. Anaesth.* 1984, **56**, 587.
129. Morgan M. *Anaesthesia* 1979, **34**, 20; Annotation, *Lancet* 1979, **2**, 398; Moore P. G. et al. *Anaesth. Intensive Care*, 1982, **10**, 40.

130. Steiner P. E. and Lushbaugh C. C. *JAMA* 1941, **117**, 1245.
131. *Brazil-Medico* 1926, **2**, 301.
132. Weiner A. E. et al. *N. Engl. J. Med.* 1950, **243**, 597.
133. *See also* Scott J. S. *Br. J. Hosp. Med.* 1969, **2**, 1847.
134. Tuck S. M. *Br. J. Hosp. Med.* 1982, **28**, 125.
135. Coaldrake I. A. and Livingstone P. *Anaesth. Intensive Care* 1983, **11**, 254.
136. Preston F. E. *Br. J. Hosp. Med.* 1982, **28**, 129.
137. *See also* Annotation *Br. Med. J.* 1980, **1**, 811.
138. Tunstall M. E. *Br. Med. J.* 1977, **1**, 1321; Tunstall M. E. *Anaesthesia* 1979, **34**, 316; Wilson M. E. *Br. Med. J.* 1980, **1**, 1270.
139. Tunstall M. E. in: *General Anaesthesia* (Gray T. C. et al. ed.), 4th ed. London: Butterworths, 1980.
140. Slater R. M. et al. *Anaesthesia* 1985, **40**, 655.
141. Crawford J. S. *Anaesthesia* 1979, **34**, 892.
142. Hutchinson R. *Br. J. Anaesth.* 1961, **33**, 463; Waters D. J. *Br. J. Anaesth.* 1968, **40**, 259.
143. Lindblad A. and Marsal K. *Br. Med. J.* 1984, **288**, 132.
144. Uppington J. *Anaesthesia* 1983, **38**, 336.
145. Moir D. D. *Br. J. Anaesth.* 1979, **51**, 79; Thorburn J. and Moir D. D. *Anaesthesia* 1980, **35**, 3.
146. Grundy E. M. et al. *Anesth. Analg. (Cleve.)* 1978, **57**, 544; Datta S. et al. *Anesthesiology* 1980, **52**, 48; Milne M. K. et al. *Anaesthesia* 1979, **34**, 992.
147. Jouppila R. et al. *Br. J. Anaesth.* 1978, **50**, 275.
148. James F. M. et al. *Anesthesiology* 1980, **52**, 488.
149. Head Hy. (1861–1940) *J. Physiol. (Lond.)* 1889, **10**, 1 and 279.
150. Hallworth D. et al. *Anaesthesia* 1982, **37**, 53.
151. Brownridge P. *Anaesth. Intensive Care* 1979, **7**, 33.
152. Kileff M. E. et al. *Anesth. Analg. (Cleve.)* 1984, **63**, 413.
153. Bates R. G. and Helm C. W. *J. R. Soc. Med.* 1985, **78**, 890.
154. Thompson E. M. et al. *Anaesthesia* 1985, **40**, 427.
155. Milne M. K. et al. *Anaesthesia* 1979, **34**, 992.
156. Crawford J. S. *Anaesthesia* 1985, **40**, 1219.
157. Russell I. F. *Anaesthesia* 1983, **37**, 346; Brownridge P. *Anaesth. Intensive Care* 1984, **12**, 334.
158. Ranney B. and Strange W. F. *Obstet. Gynecol. NY* 1975, **45**, 163.
159. Marshall Hall (1790–1857), *Lancet* 1856, **2**, 601 (reprinted in 'Classical File', *Surv. Anesthesiol.* 1977, **21**, 398).
160. Boddy K. and Robinson J. S. *Lancet* 1971, **2**, 1231; Boddy K. and Mantell C. D. *Lancet* 1972, **2**, 1219.
161. Jones R. M. et al. *Anaesthesia* 1983, **38**, 949.
162. Pipe N. G. J. *Br. J. Clin. Equip.* 1979, **4**, 216; Ostheimer G. W. *Br. J. Anaesth.* 1979, **51**, (*Suppl.* 1) 538; Weiner P. et al. *Anesthesiol.* 1979, **34**, 996.
163. See also Brownridge P. *Anaesth. Intensive Care* 1978, **6**, 5; Beard R. W. et al. *Br. J. Clin. Equip.* 1979, **2**, 1117.
164. Saling E. *Arch. Gynäk.* 1962, **197**, 108.
165. Apgar V. *Curr. Res. Anesth. Analg.* 1953, **32**, 260 (reprinted in 'Classical File', *Surv. Anesthesiol.* 1975, **19**, 401); Calmes S. H. in: *Anaesthesia: Essays on its History.* (Rupreht J. et al. ed.) Berlin: Springer-Verlag, 1985, p. 45.
166. Dubowitz V. *Br. J. Anaesth.* 1975, **47**, 1005; Brazelton T. B. *Clinics in Developmental Medicine*, No. 50, 1973, London: SIMR-Heinemann.
167. Milner A. D. et al. *Br. Med. J.* 1984, **289**, 1563.
168. Mushin W. W. and Hillard E. K. *Br. Med. J.* 1967, **1**, 416.
169. Rees G. J. in: *General Anaesthesia* (Evans F. T. and Gray T. C. ed.). London: Butterworths, 1959, Vol. 2, p. 191.
170. Addy D. P. *Br. Med. J.* 1982, **284**, 1288.
171. Terry T. L. (1899–1946), *Am. J. Ophthalmol.* 1942, **25**, 203.
172. Godfrey S. et al. *Br. Med. J.* 1970, **1**, 475.
173. Greenhough A. and Roberton N. R. C. *Br. Med. J.* 1985, **290**, 597.
174. Johnson W. C. and Meyer J. R. *Am. J. Obstet. Gynecol.* 1925, **9**, 151; Strang L. B. *Br. Med. Bull.* 1963, **19**, 45.
175. Avery M. E. and Mead J. *Am. J. Dis. Child.* 1959, **97**, 515; Hutchinson J. H. et al. *Lancet* 1963, **2**, 1019.
176. Gregory G. A. et al. *N. Engl. J. Med.* 1971, **284**, 1333.
177. Fujiwara T. et al. *Lancet* 1980, **1**, 56.

178. Evans J. J. *N. Engl. J. Med.* 1975, **292**, 1113.
179. Crawford J. S. and Lewis M. *Anaesthesia* 1986, **41**, 900.

Chapter 28   **PAEDIATRIC ANAESTHESIA**

The Neonate

Defined as an infant during the first 28 days of life. The mature 3-kg infant is normally one-third the length, has one-ninth the body surface and one-twentieth the weight of the average adult. The head is large compared with the body, and the neck muscles are inadequately developed to maintain it in position without support. The physiology of the neonate differs from that of the adult in many ways, among which are:

Respiration

In comparison with adults, neonates have a larger proportion of dead space in their lungs. Their ribs are nearly horizontal in the position of deep inspiration, while the diaphragm is pushed up by the large liver, hence respiration is rapid (30 breaths/min), diaphragmatic, and may easily become deficient. The lungs are much less efficient ventilating organs than they eventually become, with a respiratory surface per unit weight one-third that of adults. To compensate for this, the respiratory rate is increased in infants. Bucking does not occur in the first 3 months of life, although the laryngeal reflexes are very active as the child is living on fluids. In infants, the tongue is often pushed against the palate, causing respiratory obstruction under anaesthesia.

The respiratory pattern of the neonate may be one of three types: (1) *Regular*: Inspiration and expiration taking equal time in the cycle with no expiratory pause; (2) *Cogwheel*: A definite and extended respiratory pause following a lengthened expiratory phase; (3) *Periodic*: Bouts of regular pattern, interrupted by apnoeic intervals or groups of shallow respirations. Periodic respiration may be seen in premature infants, or as a result of birth injury or hypoxia of the respiratory centre. Because of the varations seen in respiratory patterns it is difficult to measure a 'normal' rate in the neonate, though average figures of 30–40/min have been found. Average tidal volumes for the neonate $V_T = 7\,\text{ml/kg}$ or 20 ml. The trachea bifurcates at the level of T.2. The airway is narrow and this causes a high airway resistance with low compliance.

In infants, a negative pressure is sometimes created in the stomach during inspiration and gas may be sucked in. To relieve this a catheter should be used as a stomach tube if the abdomen is distended or if breathing is laboured.

Intubation may be difficult because of the relatively large head, unless the anaesthetist is constantly doing this type of work. A small amount of mucus secretion may cause considerable obstruction to respiration. With inhalation induction, anaesthesia comes on more rapidly and awakening is more rapid than in adults.

The Cardiovascular System

In the fetus the left ventricle drives blood through the aorta to the body tissues and to the placenta in the proportion of one-third to two-thirds. Oxygenated blood from the placenta mixes with venous blood in its return to the heart. About half of this mixed blood passes through the foramen ovale to the left heart. The other half flows to the right heart for the pulmonary circulation, though a variable part of this passes through the ductus arteriosus to the aorta.

At birth, when the umbilical cord is tied, systemic arterial resistance rises because blood passing formerly to the placenta now has to pass through the arterial system to the body tissues. At the same time, as regular respiration is established, there is a profound reflex fall in pulmonary vascular resistance, and an increase in blood flow to the lungs. Pressure in the pulmonary artery falls and a reversal of flow occurs in the ductus arteriosus. The lumen of this vessel decreases in size over the next 7–10 days and is usually finally obliterated. The foramen ovale also closes. At birth the BP averages 80/50 mmHg.

The blood volume of the neonate is about 70–90 ml/kg, while haemoglobin is 17–21 g/dl, and this doubles by 1 year of age. Normal pulse rate 120–140/min. Cyanosis may reflect the high haemoglobin content of the neonate.

Metabolism[1]

Brown fat is an important source of energy in the newborn and its metabolic rate is nearly twice that of the adult. It contains β-adrenergic receptors. Asphyxia at birth can result in exhaustion of carbohydrate reserves in muscles, liver and myocardium, leading to hypoglycaemia and acidosis. The normal neonate has a mild metabolic acidosis and respiratory alkalosis. Exposure to cold can also give rise to the same changes. Administration of glucose is indicated, particularly if infants are starved prior to surgery. Hypoglycaemia may be present if the patient is starved for undue periods preoperatively, especially below the age of 4 years and below a weight of 15·5 kg. Hyperventilation during anaesthesia will compensate for metabolic acidosis but the calculated dose of bicarbonate should be given at the end of operation when spontaneous respiration is resumed. Blood-sugar estimations should be done in these circumstances. Figures below 1·5 mmol/l may be found. It may be necessary to infuse strong glucose solutions, 20% or 25%, into central veins. To prevent hypoglycaemia, children should, if possible, be operated on early in the day.

Heat loss is of the order of 50% by radiation to cold walls of rooms or incubators. It has recently been appreciated that it may be unwise to nurse babies naked in an air temperature of 35 °C, and it is more logical to use 'double-glazing' of the incubator or use a radiant heat shield. Draughts are to be avoided. Space blankets retain heat at first but are ineffective later when wet.

During the first year of life renal function has not developed its maximal efficiency, so that electrolytic or fluid imbalance may not be well compensated.

Premedication

Some anaesthetists aim to give heavy premedication so that children arrive in the theatre suite asleep; they can then be anaesthetized by gravity nitrous oxide or cyclopropane without the patient regaining consciousness. Other anaesthetists prefer to establish rapport with the child and to provide an environment without fear; light premedication is given and the child 'talked' to sleep, anaesthesia being induced by inhalation or intravenous routes. Sedative premedication is not necessary when the weight is less than 10 kg. Trauma, anxiety and pain may all delay emptying of the stomach. Metoclopramide 0·1 mg may aid emptying.

Prolonged fasting may result in hypoglycaemia in small infants, so many workers allow a small milk feed up to 4 h preoperatively, or bland fluids up to 3 h before.

Routes of Sedative Premedication

1. *Oral*: Some anaesthetists do not like this method because of the danger of vomiting and because absorption of drugs from the alimentary tract is uneven. Others find it a satisfactory method, acceptable to the child.

   Barbiturates. Pentobarbitone (Nembutal): This is well tolerated by children. By mouth the dosage can be 6 mg/kg, with 100 mg as the maximum. Quinalbarbitone (Seconal) has a similar dosage. Both drugs may be associated with postoperative restlessness.

   Triclofos (trichloroethyl phosphate) is rapidly metabolized in the body to form trichloroethanol. Dose 70 mg/kg by mouth.

   Diazepam. By mouth, 0·2 mg/kg satisfactory for children weighing less than 25 kg. Lorazepam: 0·05 mg/kg (long acting, 8–24 h). Temazepam: 0·3 mg/kg (short acting, 2–4 h). Midazolam by mouth is also satisfactory, accompanied by an anticholinergic drug.[2]

   Trimeprazine tartrate. This is a phenothiazine derivative and has a central sedative, antihistaminic, anti-emetic and spasmolytic action. It has none of chlorpromazine's anti-adrenaline properties. Its side-effects may include dryness of the mouth, vertigo, depression and fainting. Put up in a palatable syrup as Vallergan Forte (6 mg/ml), dose 3–5 mg/kg 1½ h before anaesthesia. Also given in a dose of 2 mg/kg 2 h preoperatively followed by intramuscular morphine 0·2 mg/kg 1 h later. Another regimen is a combination of trimeprazine 3 mg/kg (maximum 100 mg) and droperidol 0·2 mg/kg (maximum 5 mg) orally 2 h before the start of an operating session. Can be given by intramuscular injection 1 mg/kg in children under 12, and slightly less in older children and in adults, 1½ h before operation.

2. *Rectal barbiturate*. Methohexitone: 20 mg/kg or thiopentone: 40 mg/kg. A very reliable way to ensure that a child is asleep when brought to the anaesthetic room. Nursing care must be good.

3. *Intramuscular*. Papaveretum and hyoscine, premixed given on a dose-for-weight basis as compared to 20 mg papaveretum and 0·4 mg hyoscine for a 60-kg adult (although the combination is associated with a relatively high incidence of nausea and vomiting[3]). Pethidine: 1·5 mg/kg. Morphine: 0·2 mg/kg.

Atropine and Hyoscine

These drugs are well tolerated by children and are necessary as salivation is often profuse. Dose 0·015 mg/kg atropine to maximum 0·3 mg. Otherwise hyoscine may be used to prevent salivation in similar dosage. The drugs may also be given by mouth. In mongols (Down's syndrome) smaller than normal doses of atropine should be given because of its increased effect on vagal nerve endings in the heart.[4] Some workers prefer hyoscine to atropine for routine premedication by intramuscular injection because of its anti-emetic action with quietening of central nervous activity.[5] Glycopyrronium 5 µg/kg (max. 400 µg) is satisfactory.[6]

The classic method of anaesthesia in infants and children has been spontaneous respiration of various mixtures of anaesthetic gases and vapours. This has been giving place to intravenous induction of anaesthesia with a sleep dose of thiopentone, followed by a relaxant, intubation and IPPV with a nitrous-oxide–oxygen mixture.[7] In the authors' opinion, the older techniques may well be safer when applied by the occasional paediatric anaesthetist.

Intravenous Anaesthesia
A 27 SWG needle is recommended[8] but the wrist veins are to be avoided since the skin here is sensitive and extravascular injection may be dangerous. More than one venepuncture should not be allowed in the conscious child. The Butterfly needle size 23 or 25 can be used. (*See also* Whitelaw A. and Valman B. *Br. Med. J.* 1980, **2**, 602.) To facilitate intravenous puncture, a light shining from the side, casting a shadow is helpful. Suitable veins include those on the back of the hand, the dorsum of the foot, the internal saphenous vein, in front of the medial malleolus, and scalp veins in babies. Infusion sets should include a burette, so that small and measured volumes of fluid can be given. Infusion pumps and heaters may be required. Topical analgesia of the skin may help.

1. Intravenous Agents
Thiopentone 4–5 mg/kg combined with nitrous-oxide–oxygen, muscle relaxants and IPPV. *See also* Chapter 13. The dose of methohexitone is 1·1 mg/kg between 2 and 10 years and 1·2 mg/kg from 10 to 16 years.[9] This may cause discomfort on injection and restlessness; it is better avoided in patients with a history of epilepsy.

2. Ketamine
Dosage 2 mg/kg i.v. or 10 mg/kg i.m. Recommended for diagnostic procedures and minor operations in small children and infants and to control restlessness before induction of general anaesthesia. Particular examples are pneumoencephalograms, orthopaedic manipulations, burns dressing, radiology and radiotherapy,[10] examinations under anaesthesia of eye, rectum, etc. Recommended when scarring of the neck as a result of burns produces an airway problem during induction of anaesthesia for plastic surgery. The agent may produce hallucinations even in children but this can be reduced if recovery is allowed to be quiet and if diazepam is given beforehand.

Volatile Anaesthetics
Uptake rates of halothane, enflurane and methoxyflurane are more rapid in children than in adults and in younger children than in older. Age has no effect on the uptake of isoflurane.[11] These rapid rates of uptake may result in unduly high myocardial concentrations. Halothane is well tolerated in children in whom the risk of halothane-associated hepatitis on repeated administration is very small.[12] Enflurane is not as easy to use, and should be avoided in children with a history of epilepsy.

Cyclopropane gives a rapid induction, but laryngeal spasm can occur.

Open Drop Technique
Can be used for diethyl ether anaesthesia. The tidal exchange in a newborn baby may be as little as 20 ml, so even with a tiny mask, dead space must be greatly increased unless oxygen (1 litre/min) is run under it to carry away excess carbon dioxide.

Bag and Mask Anaesthesia
A suitable method of induction is to allow nitrous oxide and oxygen to flow from a mask held 5 cm above the patient's face. About 10 litre/min are required for this. When consciousness is lost, the mask is applied to the face and the gas flow reduced, a volatile agent added if necessary. Cyclopropane can be used for induction in a similar manner. Care must be taken that dead space is not too high when small children and infants are anaesthetized by these methods. Suxamethonium, syringes, needles and tracheal tubes should be at hand.

The closed system should not be used unless specially designed apparatus is available to minimize dead space such as the absorber of Cope.

Breathing Systems for Children
Dead-space and resistance to respiration must be minimal; weight and size of the equipment, with its tubing, must be suitable for small children; valves must not cause undue obstruction; inhaled gases should be humidified; the reservoir bag should be smaller than in adults so that its movements with respiration can be seen easily; for spontaneous respiration, a 'one-way' valve may be satisfactory; the face-mask must fit well to the contours of the face (e.g. the Rendall Baker mask); the Magill attachment (Mapleson-A) or Bain coaxial circuit is suitable in older children, if the fresh gas flow exceeds the alveolar ventilation, during spontaneous respiration.

Ayre's T-Piece[13]
This has a minimal resistance to respiration. *See* Chapter 9. Rees[14] has modified the system by fitting a 500-ml bag with an open tail to the expiratory limb. This makes controlled ventilation and easy monitoring of respiration possible. During spontaneous respiration the fresh gas flow should be at least twice the minute volume to eliminate rebreathing. During controlled ventilation the input need only be 200 ml/kg body weight with a minimum flow of 3 litre/min. This is likely to produce a Pa_{CO_2} of about 4 kPa. Rebreathing does not occur unless fresh gas flow falls below twice the minute volume. A flow of 3 litre/min is recommended during neonatal anaesthesia. A scavenging device is available.[15] (For detailed analysis of the T-piece, *see* Froese A. B. and Rose D. K. in: *Some Aspects of Paediatric Anaesthesia* (Steward D. J. ed.) Amsterdam: Elsevier, 1982.)

Tracheal Intubation in Small Babies
This may prove difficult in those not constantly doing it. Many workers use a straight blade, the tip of which is placed posterior to the epiglottis. A tube with internal diameter of 2·5–3 mm is suitable for neonates. During the first 4 weeks of life, awake intubation may be practised. An assistant, skilled in holding the baby, is of the greatest value.

Non-rebreathing Valves
The simplest variety is a plastic or metallic cylinder containing two unidirectional valves attached to a small reservoir bag. *See also* Chapter 9.

IPPV
Controlled respiration has the advantage that it relieves the respiratory muscles

of work and ensures adequate gas exchange. The Ayre T-piece modified by Rees,[14] is better than a closed system with absorption of carbon dioxide. Anaesthesia can be maintained at light levels with nitrous-oxide–oxygen and a muscle relaxant, and recovery is rapid. Small babies have a reduced FRC and airways closure may cause problems during spontaneous respiration.

Muscular Relaxation

In babies, muscular relaxation requires neither deep anaesthesia nor large doses of relaxants. Protrusion of the intestines from the belly is due to diaphragmatic breathing and distension due to gas in the bowel, not to the muscular tone of the abdominal wall.

Relaxants in Children

The neonate is more sensitive to tubocurarine than the adult, though this sensitivity gradually decreases over the first 2 months of life.[16] This characteristic depends on the neuromuscular junction and is not related to protein binding. Less acetylcholine is released in infants. Postoperative difficulties may be experienced if anticholinesterase drugs are not used, if hypothermia is allowed to occur, or when there is potentiation by ether or antibiotics.

Suxamethonium is probably the preferred relaxant in neonates for short operations and they require at least twice the dose (dose for weight) to produce comparable results as in adults. A dose of 5 mg can be given and repeated many times if necessary. It sometimes causes bradycardia in infants. Single doses of suxamethonium in children cause more abnormalities of cardiac rate and rhythm than in adults. Muscular fasciculation is not seen in infancy and there is no rise in intragastric pressure under 4 years of age while the rise in older children is less than in adults.[17] Cricoid pressure is effective should regurgitation be feared. Dual block may occur with large doses. Suxamethonium should be preceded by atropine, 0·05 mg/kg to reduce the greater muscarinic effects seen in children.

Doses recommended. For neonates: Tubocurarine: 250 µg/kg 0–1 week; 400 µg/kg 1–2 weeks; 500 µg/kg 2–4 weeks; supplementary doses are one-fifth the initial dose. Smaller amounts are required in premature babies, and in the presence of hypothermia, or acidosis. Smaller doses are required in babies being treated by those antibiotics which affect the neuromuscular junction.[18] Pancuronium: 30 µg/kg 0–1 week; 60 µg/kg 1–2 weeks; 90 µg/kg 2–4 weeks; supplementary doses one-quarter the initial dose.[18] Gallamine: 1·0 mg/kg initial dose and 0·25 mg/kg supplementary doses. Alcuronium: 0·1–0·2 mg/kg initial dose with incremental doses 0·05 mg/kg. Vecuronium: 0·1 mg/kg. Atracurium: 0·5 mg/kg. Suxamethonium: 1 mg/kg i.v., 2 mg/kg i.m.

For older children: Tubocurarine 0·75 mg/kg. Pancuronium 0·13 mg/kg. Gallamine 2–2·5 mg/kg.

Dose of neostigmine: 0·1 mg/kg with atropine at least 0·3 mg, 0·6 mg if over 1 year.

In children, cimetidine 10 mg/kg by mouth, 2–3 h before induction of anaesthesia reduces the volume of gastric juice and increases the pH above 2·5.[19]

For a nomogram to estimate drug dosage in children *see* Wilson M. E. and McCleod K. R. *Anaesthesia* 1982, **37**, 951.

Table 28.1. Some suggested doses

Drug	Neonate Initial dose (mg/kg)	Neonate Repeat dose (mg/kg)	Child Initial dose (mg/kg)	Child Repeat dose (mg/kg)
Atracurium	0·5	0·25	0·5	0·25
Vecuronium	0·1	0·05	0·1	0·05
Tubocurarine	0·25	0·1	0·75	0·25
Pancuronium	0·03	0·01	0·13	0·02
Alcuronium	0·2	0·05	0·5	0·1
Gallamine	1·0	0·25	2·0	0·5
Suxamethonium	1·0	1·0	1·0	1·0
Pethidine*	—	—	1·0	0·2
Morphine*	—	—	0·25	0·05
Methohexitone*	—	—	2–4	1–2
Thiopentone, i.v.*	—	—	4–8	2–4
Atropine	0·01	—	0·02	—
Hyoscine	—	—	0·01	—
Trimeprazine	—	—	3 (oral)	—
Rectal thiopentone	—	—	40	—
Ketamine	—	—	i.m. 5–10	5–10
			i.v. 1–2	1–2

*Seldom required in neonates.

Regional Analgesia
This is receiving more attention now that it has been shown that lignocaine 4 mg/kg or bupivacaine 2–3 mg/kg introduced into the body are safe doses. Extradural sacral, penile, ilio-inguinal and sciatic nerve block,[20] for pain relief in the perioperative period give good results.[21]

Anaesthesia in the Neonate[22]
The neonate may suffer from respiratory distress syndrome, haemorrhagic disease of the newborn, birth trauma, hypoglycaemia, or infection. Venepuncture may be difficult unless the skill is employed constantly. There is sensitivity to non-depolarizing relaxants but resistance to suxamethonium. Hypothermia must be avoided. No routine postoperative analgesic is necessary in neonates.

In premature infants, perioperative apnoea may be a danger so that for the first postoperative 18–24 h, respiratory monitoring, with facilities for IPPV should be considered. It has been advised that, where possible, operation before the 44th week of conceptual age, should be postponed.[23]

Causes of postoperative apnoea in the neonate are: (1) Hypothermia, 34 °C or below; (2) Overdosage of relaxant; (3) Overdosage with inhalation agent; (4) Potentiation of non-depolarizing relaxant with ether; (5) Concurrent aminoglycoside antibiotics; (6) Overdosage of narcotic analgesics (7) A combination of the above.

For anaesthetic equipment for neonates and infants *see* Hatch.[24]

See also Hatch D. J. and Sumner E. *Current Topics in Anaesthesia Series—5, Neonatal Anaesthesia.* London: Arnold, 1986.

Monitoring
It may be difficult to obtain access to the radial pulse or to see the small infant's respirations under the towels, especially when a T-piece technique is used. A

stethoscope strapped over the precordium, acts as a useful monitor of heart sounds, rate and rhythm. An oesophageal stethoscope can be used where a precordial stethoscope is impracticable. A stethoscope attached to the side-arm of a T-piece provides audible monitoring of respiration. Otherwise pulse monitors can be attached to a digit or the electrocardiogram used as a monitor. An ingenious oesophageal probe has been described which combines a stethoscope, thermistor and ECG lead.[25] For blood-pressure measurements, it is important that cuffs are of the correct size (*see* Chapter 41). Too narrow a cuff gives a reading which is too high and vice-versa; the bag should almost encircle the upper arm. Percutaneous oxygen tension monitoring makes continuous observation of the Pa_{O_2} a realistic proposition. Oxygen saturation can also be measured easily by oximetry. A temperature probe is useful, while careful observation of the condition of the patient throughout the operation is always necessary.

Blood Loss and Replacement[26]
The blood volume of an infant is small, 85 ml/kg (about 300 ml in the newborn), and so blood replacement must be accurate. This can be done with the help of calibrated small suction bottles, swab weighing or colorimetric methods to estimate blood loss. Blood transfusion can be undertaken from small reservoirs, or a three-way tap and 20-ml syringe can be used to transfuse an accurate volume in replacement. Replacement should be commenced when 10% of the estimated blood volume has been lost. Blood should be warmed to prevent hypothermia.[27] For autotransfusion *see* Church J. J. and Davidson A. M. *Anaesth. Intensive Care* 1979, **7**, 178.

Fluid Balance
It is rare for preoperative fluid and electrolyte balance to require correction during the first 12 h of life but 0·25% normal saline with 5% dextrose is suitable in small babies. Estimations of haemoglobin, haematocrit and blood sugar should be made before major surgery. In infants over 12 h of age correction of fluid and electrolyte abnormalities is of major importance. During operation Ringer lactate 2 ml/kg/h is recommended.[28]

Monitoring in major surgery may include, heart rate, arterial pressure, CVP, ECG, temperature, urinary output, respiratory rate and depth, blood gases and electrolytes.

For the accurate measurement of infused fluid, a burette should be part of the giving set or an infusion pump used. In the perioperative period, glucose-containing fluids are recommended until normal oral ingestion can be resumed.[29]

Caloric Requirements[26]
The neonate requires energy in excess of 0·45 MJ/kg/day in order to grow. Glucose and fat can provide most of the energy requirements, should parenteral nutrition be required, while amino acids are needed for protein synthesis. Peripheral veins can often be used to avoid the technical problems of central venous cannulation. Aseptic technique must be scrupulous.

Temperature
The newborn rapidly loses heat if placed in a cold environment. The heat-regulating mechanisms are unstable in the premature infant and in the mature newborn baby for some weeks. The newborn maintains its body heat through the

metabolic activity of brown fat, which is to be found mainly around the kidneys and back. This fat has a rich blood and β-adrenergic nerve supply and the cells are profusely equipped with mitochondria. It may be deficient in small or premature babies. Care must be taken that undue heat loss does not occur on the operating table. Since the baby's head has a large surface area in relation to the rest of the body, it is useful to cover it with a stockinet cap to retain warmth. Though primarily used to prevent bacterial contamination of the wound, drapes provide an efficient insulation of the exposed surface of the infant. Transfusion of cold fluids intravenously may also produce hypothermia. Blood should be warmed. Heat is also lost to provide latent heat of evaporation when dry gases are inhaled and moisture is lost via the respiratory tract. This can be avoided if warm humidified gases are supplied.[30] Cold stress and hypoxia both lead to hypoglycaemia. For major operations on small babies a mattress with circulating water coils is useful so that rewarming can be applied if necessary. Monitoring of temperature helps to give warning of accidental hypothermia.

Older children may develop (non-malignant) hyperpyrexia on the operating table. This is likely to occur: (1) When the child is pyrexial; (2) In hot climatic conditions; (3) When there are too many coverings over the child, particularly if these include macintosh sheets; (4) Inhibition of sweating following atropine premedication may interfere with heat loss. Hyperpyrexia is an aetiological factor in ether convulsions. A mattress with circulating water coils placed under the patient may be useful for cooling.

Abdominal Surgery
In neonates, muscular relaxation does not require deep anaesthesia or relaxants, except in special cases such as when a large volume of viscera has to be returned to the peritoneal cavity. Older children may be satisfactorily anaesthetized with nitrous oxide and relaxants, cyclopropane, ether or halothane. The Jackson–Rees modification of Ayre's T-piece is very convenient for both spontaneous breathing and IPPV.

Diaphragmatic Hernia[34]
Diagnosis. Shortly after birth, the child may have cyanosis resistant to oxygen; dullness of the chest, absent breath sounds, and later bowel sounds on the affected side of the chest (usually left). Chest X-ray confirms the diagnosis. There are areas of pulmonary hypoplasia on the affected side, mediastinal shift and compression of the opposite lung.
Initial Management. (1) Intubation of the trachea and gentle IPPV. The chest should not be inflated with a face-mask, as this merely fills the stomach and intestines and worsens the degree of compression; (2) Insertion of a gastric tube to prevent aeration of the gut; (3) Measurement and correction of acidosis; (4) Prevention of hypothermia, dehydration and hypoglycaemia.
Perioperative Management. The physiological problem is that some of these neonates revert to transitional circulation, with decreased pulmonary vascular bed, high pulmonary vascular resistance, and reopening of the ductus arteriosus and foramen ovale. Tolazoline, 2 mg/kg bolus, followed by the same dose infused over each hour, has been used to control these problems. Profound muscular relaxation may be required for short periods. Rapid infusion of colloids, e.g. plasma, may be required to counteract cardiovascular collapse during surgery. Postoperative elective IPPV with nasotracheal tube in severely ill cases.

To cope with possible pneumothorax, a chest drain may be inserted into each side. (*See also* Marshall A. and Sumner E. *J. R. Soc. Med.* 1982, **75**, 607.)

Omphalocele

This requires emergency operation since rupture of the thin sac covering the intestines will result in peritonitis. May be associated with the Beckwith–Wiedemann syndrome. Anaesthetic management is similar to that for diaphragmatic hernia. The intact sac can be treated conservatively by repeated painting with a suitable antiseptic solution and a synthetic sac of Silastic has been advocated.[35] Prolonged ileus is a common complication and problems of fluid and electrolyte balance and artificial nutrition may have to be solved. Peritonitis is a common cause of death and intestinal obstruction due to adhesions may occur. The overall mortality is high.

Pyloric Stenosis

The commonest disease requiring surgery in the first 6 months of life. Commoner in males and after the age of 2 weeks. The operation of pyloromyotomy was performed by Dufour[36] in 1908 and by Conrad Ramstedt (1868–1963) in 1911.[37]

This operation is not an emergency procedure.

Preoperative preparation.

1. Fluid and electrolyte replacement is the major consideration.

2. Loss of gastric acid results in metabolic alkalosis and low serum chloride.

3. There is marked loss of sodium and potassium in the urine in an effort to conserve hydrogen ions.

4. Classic signs of dehydration occur: (*a*) Weight loss (½–1 kg); (*b*) Oliguria; (*c*) Dry mouth; (*d*) Sunken eyes; (*e*) Depressed fontanelles; (*f*) Loss of skin elasticity.

5. The result is an ill, dehydrated, alkalotic, hypochloraemic, hyponatraemic, hypokalaemic infant.

6. Treatment is by intravenous drip infusion, initially normal saline with potassium chloride 20–40 mmol/l, until urine flow restarts, then 0·45% saline in 2·5% glucose with potassium chloride 20–40 mmol/l until urine flow is normal, then 0·18% saline in 4·3% glucose. A suitable drip flow-rate is 2–3 ml/kg/h. The glucose is important to prevent hypoglycaemia. Surgery should not be undertaken until the chloride is at least 90 mmol/l and the bicarbonate 24–30 mmol/l. Rarely, intravenous feeding is required.

7. Via a gastric tube, hourly gastric washouts continue until the washout fluid is returned clear and odourless. The serum standard bicarbonate should ideally be below 30 mmol/l before anaesthesia.

Premedication. Atropine: 0·1–0·2 mg i.m.

General anaesthetic technique

1. Intraoperative body warming, precordial stethoscope for monitoring, and suction on the gastric tube.

2. Either awake intubation, or inhalation or intravenous induction and cricoid pressure. Intubation with 3-mm (or smaller) tracheal tube, perhaps facilitated by suxamethonium 1–2 mg/kg i.v., or 5 mg/kg i.m. (which will last up to 20 min).

3. Maintenance with inhalational agents, supplemented if desired by relaxants and IPPV, e.g. tubocurarine 0·4 mg/kg or intermittent suxamethonium up to a maximum of 25 mg.

4. Extubation with the child awake.

5. Postoperative 0·18% saline in 4·3% glucose until the child is back on partial or full feeds.

Postoperative analgesia is usually neither necessary nor desirable.

Local analgesic technique. The maximum dose is 8 mg/kg of 0·25% lignocaine with adrenaline 1–400 000. A useful technique in the absence of a competent anaesthetist but results no better than after general anaesthesia.[38] Ketamine as sole anaesthetic is not recommended (*see* Bush G. H. *Anaesthesia* 1984, **39**, 381; Battersby E. F. et al. *Anaesthesia* 1984, **39**, 381).

Tracheo-oesophageal Fistula with Oesophageal Atresia

Aspiration of food and secretions usually results in pneumonia within a few days of birth. Operation is a hazardous procedure and successful operations were not carried out before 1939 when Leven and Ladd (independently) in the USA performed multistage operations. Primary oesophageal anastomosis was introduced by Haight in 1941.

There are various anatomical variations. Much the commonest finding is the blind upper oesophageal pouch, with a fistula between the posterior trachea and lower oesophagus.

Anaesthetic management may be difficult. Preoperative care includes safe transfer to a special unit with avoidance of hypothermia. A tube should be passed into the blind upper end of the oesophagus for suction. Controlled respiration via a tracheal tube is generally advocated. It is imperative that the anaesthetist be able to use effective suction in the airway at all times and a suitable fine catheter must be available. IPPV can result in gastric distension. Fortunately this is only a serious problem in a minority of cases, when gastrostomy may be necessary for its relief. Good relaxation enables ventilation to be carried out at minimal pressures. Accurate replacement of blood is essential.

Recommended techniques. Premedication: atropine 0·15 mg. An intravenous infusion can be set up before induction of anaesthesia. Intubation is performed while the infant is awake. Anaesthetic agents: nitrous-oxide–oxygen, and muscle relaxants, if necessary, supplemented by minimal halothane. The upper oesophageal pouch should be intubated to remove secretions. Care must be taken to avoid intubation of the fistula and inflation of the stomach.

Cleft Palate and Hare-lip in Infants

Many surgeons prefer to operate when the child is about 10–16 weeks old for hare-lip and about 1 year old for the palate. The child should be fit and healthy.

Atropine alone is suitable as premedication. Anaesthesia can be induced by any suitable method. An orotracheal tube is essential and may be used in conjunction with a Dott mouth gag. An Oxford or other non-kinking tube is recommended. Introduction may be hindered by an anteriorly displaced premaxilla obstructing the field of vision. To prevent the blade of the laryngoscope from sinking deeply into the wide cleft, gauze packing or adhesive tape can be used or the gap can be bridged by a spatula. Following removal of the tube and a careful oropharyngeal toilet, a patent airway can be ensured by a suture through the tongue. May be associated with the Pierre–Robin syndrome (*see* below) and/or congenital heart disease.

Tumours about the Face and Neck
Cystic hygromas and other tumours may occur in these regions and may make tracheal intubation difficult.

The following method of guided blind tracheal intubation for cases of cancrum oris has been described.[39] A Tuohy needle is introduced through the cricothyroid membrane and sterile vinyl plastic tubing threaded through the cords from below to coil up in the pharynx. A length of polythene tubing with a blunt hook is pushed through the nose to engage the vinyl catheter which is brought out through the nose. A Magill cuffed tracheal tube is then passed round the catheter and afterwards withdrawn. Ketamine may have a place.

Anaesthesia in Asthma
Common sense dictates that anaesthesia during an attack is undesirable. For patients on longstanding steroid therapy, preoperative injection of hydrocortisone will be required. Bronchospasm during the operation may be due to problems with a tracheal tube, e.g. irritation of the carina.

Anaesthesia for Removal of Inhaled Foreign Body
Should never be undertaken unless the services of an experienced bronchoscopist and anaesthetist are available (*see* Baraka A. *Br. J. Anaesth.* 1974, **46**, 124; Moussali H. *Br. J. Hosp. Med.* 1981, **25**, 300; Bush G. H. and Vivon E. *Br. J. Hosp. Med.* 1981, **26**, 102.) *See also* p. 573.

Anaesthetic Management of Major Spinal Surgery in Children
The surgical approach to the spine is via vascular tissues and blood loss can be large. Good intravenous lines and monitoring are essential.
Scoliosis[40] which is progressive is likely to result in long-term cardiorespiratory deterioration. Total lung capacity and vital capacity are both reduced. FEV may be diminished as a result of mechanical inefficiency of the respiratory muscles. Airways closure encroaches on the FRC earlier than in normal subjects. Abnormal ventilation/perfusion ratios may result in relative arterial hypoxaemia. During operation, full cardiovascular and respiratory monitoring is usual. General anaesthesia with muscle relaxation and IPPV is the rule. Some surgeons require the patient to wake up so that the integrity of the cord, after distraction of the spine, can be tested;[41] others use evoked potentials.[42] The wake-up technique must be explained to the patient beforehand and the timing of supplementary doses of muscle relaxant and fentanyl must be carefully gauged. Blood loss at operation may be considerable[43] and deliberate hypotension is often used. Elective IPPV may be employed postoperatively.

Neurosurgical Operations
These require light general anaesthesia via an orotracheal tube. Halothane is a useful agent in children, since respiration is usually quiet, but hypoventilation is to be avoided. Tachypnoea is usually a drawback to trichloroethylene anaesthesia in small children. Ketamine is useful for diagnostic procedures.
Operations for hydrocephalus. Intubation may be difficult due to the large forehead which makes visualization of the larynx awkward.
Meningocele. Careful anaesthetic technique is required. The operation is performed in the face-down position. Tracheal intubation is mandatory. Controlled ventilation is likely to be required as spontaneous respiration, mainly

diaphragmatic, is embarrassed in this position.

Posterior fossa exploration.[44] In infants IPPV is recommended with close attention to replacement of blood loss, avoidance of heat loss, with wrapping of abdomen and legs in bandages and elevation of the legs. Central venous pressure measurement is helpful.

Circumcision
Standard techniques of general anaesthesia are suitable. Tracheal intubation is seldom necessary but laryngeal spasm may occur; this requires temporary cessation of the surgical stimulus, then deepening of anaesthesia. Caudal block (0·25% of bupivacaine, 0·5 ml/kg[45]), performed while the child is anaesthetized, gives good postoperative analgesia[46] as does penile block[54] and dressings incorporating lignocaine spray or ointment.[47] *See* Chapter 32.

Conjoined Twins[48]
These babies may require several anaesthetics, depending on how they are joined. *Radiological investigations* require quiet babies. Each twin must be anaesthetized separately. Two anaesthetists should therefore be available. Narcosis of the first twin may be difficult. If there is a significant common circulation the anaesthetic agent will be drained away to the other twin so that the speed of induction is slowed. Conversely, the second twin is anaesthetized more readily since it has already received some anaesthesia from the first. Depending on the site of union, intubation may be technically difficult. Ketamine has a place in the management of these sometimes difficult cases.

Operations for separation of conjoined twins are likely to be long and to be associated with blood loss. (*See also* Harrison V. L. et al. *Anaesth. Intensive Care* 1985, **13**, 82; and Roy M. *Anaesthesia* 1984, **39**, 1225.)

Fibrocystic Disease
Extreme care is necessary if patients with fibrocystic disease require surgery and anaesthestics. This should be aimed at preventing accumulation of lung secretions postoperatively. Humidification and postural drainage are important. Bronchodilators and antibiotic cover can be given from the preoperative period. It is usually wise to intubate the trachea to facilitate bronchial suction and to set up an intravenous drip to prevent dehydration. There may be liver dysfunction. Hypoxia and hypotension are not well tolerated.

Burns Dressings
Problems arise when small children require frequent anaesthesia for burns dressings. Excessive starvation is to be avoided. Multiple halothane administrations are undesirable. Possible techniques include neurolept analgesia, ketamine and inhalation analgesia (e.g. nitrous oxide). (*See also* p. 447.)

Diabetic Patients
The juvenile type of diabetes is very labile and demands particular care at the time of surgery. In the severely ill, frequent estimations of electrolytes and acid–base balance are required. The anaesthetist should aim for a rapid return of consciousness at the end of the operation without vomiting. It is usually wise to seek the advice of a paediatrician regarding the insulin regimen.

Familial Dysautonomia (Riley–Day syndrome)
This was first described in 1949.[49] It is an inherited disease showing abnormally active parasympathetic system with sporadic storms of sympathetic activity. It is mainly confined to Ashkenazi Jews. The child cries without tears, is highly emotional with bouts of sweating and unexplained fluctuations of blood pressure. All volatile anaesthetic agents cause bradycardia and hypotension and thus must be used carefully. Nitrous oxide and oxygen are usually sufficient. (For anaesthetic details *see* McCaughey T. J. *Can. Anaesth. Soc. J.* 1965, **12**, 558; Inkster J. S. *Br. J. Anaesth.* 1971, **43**, 509.)

The Prader–Willi Syndrome[50]
Patients have dental caries, congenital hypotonia, mental retardation, obesity, hypogonadism and sometimes cardiovascular abnormalities. For anaesthetic problems *see* Milliken R. A. and Weintraub D. M. *Anesthesiology* 1975, **43**, 590; Palmer S. K. and Atlel J. L. *Anesthesiology* 1976, **44**, 161.

Postoperative Care
Intensive care is necessary in the neonate. Attention must be paid to: (1) Environmental temperature; (2) Feeding: a weight loss of 44 g/day/kg birth weight may occur in the first 2 days of life; it is possible for the blood sugar (normal level 3 mmol % at birth) to fall to very low levels if early feeding is not commenced—oral feeding is preferable if possible; (3) Acidaemia: if present must be corrected; (4) Oxygen therapy: respiratory failure is a not uncommon complication and assisted respiration may be necessary—rates of 60–80/min may be required using air enriched with oxygen; Po_2 estimation can be obtained using umbilical artery catheters; (5) Cross-infection is a potential hazard; (6) Jaundice: this may occur in any sick newborn baby; after surgery, blood clot provides an additional source of bile pigments.
Postoperative pain. Regional analgesia can be used when appropriate (*see* Chapters 31, 32). No routine analgesia is necessary in the neonate.[31] For infants over 5 kg in weight, codeine phosphate, 1 mg/kg is satisfactory but should not be given i.v. as it causes a severe fall in cardiac output. For children on ventilators pethidine 1 mg/kg or morphine 0·2 mg/kg is satisfactory. Older children may be given narcotic analgesics on a weight basis. Morphine has been used as a continuous infusion by syringe pump[32] in a dose of 1 mg/kg in 50 ml of saline at 1 ml/h following major surgery.
Vomiting in children after operations. Below the age of 3 there is a low incidence. There is a relatively high incidence after papaveretum and hyoscine given as premedication, as compared with those receiving other agents, or none.[33] Vomiting is high after operations for hernia, tonsils and adenoids, squint and after cardiac catheterization.

Respiratory Difficulties in Infants
1. *Asphyxia of the newborn. See* Chapter 27.
2. *Choanal atresia.*[51] Nearly always posterior. If bilateral, the infant will breathe through the mouth. The airway must be kept patent by opening the mouth, keeping the child crying, or insertion of an oropharyngeal airway until surgical correction can be performed.
3. *The Pierre Robin syndrome.*[52] Micrognathia, posterior displacement of the

tongue, a hypoplastic mandible with glossoptosis and a small epiglottis. There may also be a cleft soft palate. This produces respiratory obstruction, which tends to disappear after the age of 2 years. It may be necessary to suture the tongue to the alveolar ridge of the mandible to relieve respiratory obstruction. Such cases may be very difficult to intubate. The child should be nursed in the prone position both before and after the operation.

4. *Laryngomalacia.*[53] The commonest congenital cause of stridor. This is caused by incomplete development of the laryngeal cartilages. Inspiratory obstruction to respiration occurs as the flaccid structures are drawn in. Usually improves after the age of 18 months.

Common causes of stridor in children are (in order): laryngotracheitis, laryngotracheobronchitis, congenital stridor, acute epiglottitis and spasmodic laryngitis.

For drugs which can be given to nursing mothers, without causing great harm to the infant, *see Drug Ther. Bull.* 1983, **21**, 5).

See also Hatch D. J. in: *Recent Advances in Anaesthesia and Analgesia*—15. (Atkinson R. S. and Adams A. P. ed.) Edinburgh: Churchill Livingstone, 1985.

Cardiac Arrest in Children (*See* Wark H. and Overton J. H. *Br. J. Anaesth.* 1984, **56**, 1271; and Bray R. J. *Br. J. Hosp. Med.* 1985, **34**, 72.)

(*See also* Symposium on Pediatric Anesthesiology, *Anesthesiology* 1975, **43** (August); Inkster J. S. in: *Recent Advances in Anaesthesia and Analgesia*—12 (Hewer C. L. and Atkinson R. S. ed.). Edinburgh: Churchill Livingstone, 1976; Vivori E. and Bush G. H. *Br. J. Anaesth.* 1977, **49**, 51; Lister J. *Br. J. Anaesth.* 1977, **49**, 43; Steward D. J. *Management of Paediatric Anaesthesia* 2nd edn. London: Churchill Livingstone, 1985; Brown T. C. K. and Fisk G. C. *Anaesthesia for Children.* Oxford: Blackwell, 1979; Beasley J. M. and Jones S. E. F. *Guide to Paediatric Anaesthesia.* Oxford: Blackwell, 1980; Davenport H. T. *Paediatric Anaesthesia*, 3rd ed. London: Heinemann, 1980; Hatch D. J. and Sumner E. *Neonatal Anaesthesia* 2nd edn 1986, Arnold: London; Rees G. J. and Gray T. C. (ed.), *Paediatric Anaesthesia: Trends in Current Practice.* London: Butterworths, 1981; Sumner E. and Hatch D. J. (ed.), *Clinics in Anaesthesiology, Pediatric Anaesthesia.* London: Saunders, 1985.)

References

1. *See also* Rees G. J. in: *General Anaesthesia* (Gray T. C. et al. ed.), 4th ed. London: Butterworths, 1979.
2. Sjovall J. et al. *Anaesthesia* 1984, **39**, 224.
3. Rowley M. P. and Brown T. C. K. *Anaesth. Intensive Care* 1982, **10**, 309.
4. Harris W. S. and Goodman R. M. *N. Engl. J. Med.* 1968, **279**, 307.
5. Davenport H. T. *Paediatric Anaesthesia* 3rd ed. London: Heinemann, 1980.
6. Mirakhur R. K. *Anaesthesia* 1982, **37**, 1032.
7. Bush G. H. in: *General Anaesthesia* (Gray T. C. et al. ed.), 4th ed. London: Butterworths, 1979.
8. Inkster J. S. in: *Recent Advances in Anaesthesia and Analgesia*—12 (Hewer C. L. and Atkinson R. S. ed.). Edinburgh: Churchill Livingstone, 1976.
9. Keep P. J. and Manford M. L. M. *Br. J. Anaesth.* 1974, **46**, 685.
10. Edge W. G. and Morgan M. *Anaesth. Intensive Care* 1977, **5**, 15.
11. Gallagher T. M. and Black G. W. *Anaesthesia* 1985, **40**, 1073.
12. Wark H. J. *Anaesthesia* 1983, **38**, 237.
13. Ayre T. P. *Lancet* 1937, **1**, 561; Inkster J. S. *Br. J. Anaesth.* 1956, **28**, 512; Ayre T. P. *Br. J. Surg.* 1937, **25**, 131 (reprinted in 'Classical File,' *Surv. Anaesthesiol.* 1967, **11**, 400).

14. Rees G. J. *Br. Med. J.* 1950, **2**, 1419; *Br. J. Anaesth.* 1960, **32**, 132.
15. Flowerdew R. M. M. *Can. Anaesth. Soc. J.* 1979, **26**, 367.
16. Goudsouzian N. G. *Br. J. Anaesth.* 1980, **52**, 205.
17. Salem M. R. et al. *Br. J. Anaesth.* 1972, **44**, 401.
18. Thompson M. A. *Br. J. Hosp. Med.* 1980, **23**, 153.
19. Yildiz F. et al. *Anaesthesia* 1984, **39**, 314.
20. McNichol L. R. *Anaesthesia* 1985, **40**, 410; Arthur D. S. and McNicol *Br. J. Anaesth.* 1986, **58**, 760.
21. Brown T. C. K. et al. *Reg. Anaesth.* 1982, **7**, 64; Editorial *Anaesthesia* 1985, **40**, 407.
22. Waugh R. and Johnson G. G. *Can. Anaesth. Soc. J.* 1984, **31**, 700.
23. Liu L. M. P. et al. *Anesthesiology* 1983, **59**, 506.
24. Hatch D. J. *Br. J. Hosp. Med.* 1981, **26**, 84.
25. Inkster J. S. *Anaesthesia* 1966, **21**, 111.
26. Kay B. in: *Paediatric Anaesthesia: Trends in Current Practice* (Rees G. J. and Gray T. C. ed.) London: Butterworth, 1981.
27. Harris. F. *Paediatric Fluid Therapy.* Oxford: Blackwell, 1972.
28. Bush G. H. in: *General Anaesthesia* (Gray T. C. and Nunn J. F. ed.), 3rd ed. London: Butterworths, 1971, Vol. 2. Chap. 31.
29. Payne K. and Ireland P. *Anaesthesia* 1984, **39**, 868.
30. Inkster J. S. in: *Paediatric Anaesthesia: Trends in Current Practice* (Rees G. J. and Gray T. C. ed.). London: Butterworth, 1981.
31. Hatch D. J. and Sumner E. *Current Topics in Anaesthesia—5. Neonatal Anaesthesia.* London: Arnold, 1981.
32. Bray R. J. *Anaesthesia* 1983, **38**, 1075.
33. Rowley M. P. and Brown T. C. K. *Anaesth. Intensive Care* 1982, **10**, 309.
34. Bray R. J. *Anaesthesia* 1979, **34**, 567.
35. Schuster S. R. *Surg. Gynecol. Obstet.* 1967, **125**, 837.
36. Dufour H. and Fredet P. *Revue Chir.* 1908, **37**, 208.
37. Ramstedt W. C. *Med. Klin.* 1912, **8**, 1702.
38. Gray D. W. et al. *Ann. R. Coll. Surg. Engl.* 1984, **66**, 280.
39. Waters D. J. *Anaesthesia* 1963, **18**, 158.
40. Loach A. *Current Topics in Anaesthesia—6. Anaesthesia in Orthopaedics.* London: Arnold, 1983.
41. Vauxelle J. et al. *Clin. Orthop.* 1973, **93**, 173; Abbott T. R. and Bentley G. *Anaesthesia* 1980, **35**, 298.
42. Brown R. H. and Nash C. L. *Spine* 1979, **4**, 466.
43. Abbott T. R. and Bentley G. *Anaesthesia* 1980, **35**, 298.
44. Allan D. et al. *Can. Anaesth. Soc. J.* 1970, **17**, 227.
45. May A. E. et al. *Acta Anaesth. Scand.* 1982, **26**, 331.
46. Lunn J. N. *Anaesthesia* 1979, **34**, 552.
47. Bacon A. L. C. *Anaesth. Intensive Care* 1977, **5**, 63; White J. et al. *Br. Med. J.* 1983, **286**, 1934.
48. Ballantine R. I. W. and Jackson I. *Br. Med. J.* 1964, **1**, 1339; Furman E. B. *Anesthesiology* 1971, **34**, 95; Tovey R. M. et al. *Anaesthesia* 1979, **34**, 178; Chi-Ching Cho et al. *Can. Anaesth. Soc. J.* 1980, **27**, 565.
49. Riley C. M. et al. *Pediatrics* 1949, **3**, 648; *see also* Riley C. M. and Moore C. H. *Pediatrics* 1966, **37**, 435.
50. Prader A. et al. *Schweiz. Med. Wochenschr.* 1956, **86**, 1260.
51. Hall B. D. *J. Pediatr.* 1979, **95**, 395.
52. Robin P. *J. Med. Paris* 1923, **43**, 235; Freeman M. K. and Manners J. N. *Anaesthesia* 1980, **35**, 282; Heaf D. P. et al. *J. Pediatr.* 1982, **100**, 698.
53. Holinger P. H. and Brown W. T. *Ann. Otol. Rhinol. Laryngol.* 1967, **76**, 744.
54. Soliman M. G. and Tremblay N. A. *Anesth. Analg.* 1978, **57**, 495; Yeoman P. M. et al. *Anaesthesia* 1983, **38**, 862.

Chapter 29   # THORACIC ANAESTHESIA

History and Development

Surgery inside the thorax is complicated by the risk of pulmonary collapse unless special means to prevent it are taken. In the solution of this problem the following landmarks stand out.

The Fell–O'Dwyer apparatus for artificial respiration using a bellows and tracheal tube[1] was used in a thoracotomy by Rudolph Matas (1860–1957) of New Orleans,[2] and by Theodore Tuffier (1857–1929) and Hallion of Paris.[3]

Ferdinand Sauerbruch (1875–1951) of Breslau, assistant to Von Mickulicz (1853–1905), suggested operating in an airtight chamber with pressure reduced by 7 mmHg, while the head of the patient and the anaesthetist were outside (negative pressure breathing).[4] Leopold Brauer (1865–1951) used positive pressure enclosing the head of his patient in a positive-pressure chamber.[5]

Apnoea was produced by deep ether anaesthesia by Brat and Schmieden.[6]

M. Tiegel developed a positive-pressure apparatus which was adopted by the pioneer thoracic surgeon in Germany, Ferdinand Sauerbruch (1875–1951).[7]

An apparatus for mechanical artificial respiration was devised by Janeway and Green.[8]

Franz Volhard (1872–1950) showed that the positive-pressure technique caused hypercapnia. This led to the introduction of the insufflation technique by C. A. Elsberg (1871–1948),[9] who adapted the ideas of S. J. Meltzer (1851–1920) and Leopold Auer (1875–1948) which were employed in animals.[10] Elsberg also advocated direct vision intubation,[11] instead of blind oral intubation as practised by Franz Kuhn (1866–1929),[12] while he also showed the necessity of periodical deflation of the lungs during operation. The double-lumen tube designed for differential bronchospirometry[13] was soon employed in thoracic operations.

(*See also* Mushin W. W. and Rendell-Baker L. *The Principles of Thoracic Anaesthesia, Past and Present.* Oxford: Blackwell, 1953; Sellors T. H. *J. Ir. Coll. Phys. Surg.* 1975, **5**, 26.)

The first use of endobronchial (one lung) anaesthesia was described by Gale and Waters,[14] while a bronchus blocker was described by Archibald, at the suggestion of Harold R. Griffith, in 1935,[15] Clarence Crafoord (1899–1984) of Stockholm reported his method of artificial respiration by means of Frenckner's mechanical spiro-pulsator,[16] developed at the suggestion of the Swedish surgeon K. H. Giertz, a former assistant to Sauerbruch, in 1938,[17] and this was developed and simplified by Guedel[18] and Nosworthy (1941)[19] who advocated controlled breathing by intermittent pressure on the reservoir bag of a closed system, using cyclopropane. This technique had previously been introduced by Guedel and Treweek in 1934, using ether.[20] Cyclopropane had great popularity during the decade following 1935, but is now seldom used. The muscle relaxants have made it relatively easy to control respiration.

Early ventilating machines were those of Pinson,[21] Trier Morch (then of Denmark)[22] and Blease.[23] (For history of endobronchial anaesthesia, *see* White G. M. J. *Br. J. Anaesth.* 1960, **32**, 235; for history of various types of tube used in thoracic anaesthesia, *see* Pappin J. C. *Anaesthesia* 1979, **34**, 57.) To Ferdinand Sauerbruch is credited the first paravertebral thoracoplasty for chronic pulmonary tuberculosis. The first such operation in the UK was performed by Morriston Davies in 1912. The first pneumonectomy in the UK was performed by Tudor Edwards and Roberts in 1935 at the Brompton Hospital. For the development of cardiothoracic anaesthesia *see also* McLellan I. in: *Anaesthesia; Essays on its History* (Rupreht J. et al. ed.) Berlin: Springer-Verlag, 1985, 126.

Lateral thoracotomy is used for: (1) Operations on the lungs, pleura, oesophagus, and great vessels; (2) Access to sympathetic chain and vertebral bodies; (3) For thoracic injuries; (4) Mediastinal tumours; (5) Closed heart operations; (6) Operations on the ribs.

Midline sternotomy is used for: (1) Anterior mediastinal tumours (e.g. thymoma and thymectomy in myasthenia gravis); (2) Open heart operations; (3) For large retrosternal goitres.

The Problem of Open Pneumothorax

The lack of a solution to this problem delayed the development of surgery within the thoracic cage for many years. Normally, the lungs are kept inflated by:
1. The atmospheric pressure acting on the alveoli.
2. The adhesion of the two layers of the pleura due to the surface tension of the thin layer of fluid separating them. When the chest is opened, atmospheric pressure becomes equal on the alveolar and pleural surfaces and the elastic recoil causes collapse of the lung.

When one side of the chest is opened, negative pressure is lost. The larger the hole, the more pronounced the effect. The lung on the affected side collapses, due to recoil of its elastic tissues. The mediastinum, unless fixed by adhesions, is deviated to the sound side and presses on the sound lung. If the lung is adherent to the chest wall, these effects may not be marked. If the condition is not soon checked, death from cardiorespiratory depression follows with gross hypoxia and hypercapnia.

The management requires intermittent positive-pressure ventilation which prevents: (1) Collapse of the lungs; (2) Paradoxical breathing, i.e. as one lung is expanded in spontaneous inspiration, it sucks air partly from the other lung; in expiration the opposite occurs—the result is severe dead-space problems; (3) Mediastinal flap, i.e. movement of the mediastinum, including the heart, from side to side with spontaneous ventilation of one lung. IPPV has become standard practice in modern anaesthesia since important papers by Guedel[24], Crafoord[17] and Nosworthy[25] in the early 1940s.

Prevention of spontaneous efforts of respiration may result from one or more of the following: (1) Peripheral muscular paralysis by a relaxant; (2) Hypo-capnia; (3) Central depression from drugs; (4) Reflex inhibition of the respiratory centre due to distension of the lungs; (5) A mixture of the above.

The advantages of controlled breathing are: (1) Paradoxical breathing and hypoventilation are corrected; (2) Mediastinal flap is abolished; (3) Control of the operative field is facilitated and movement can be made to suit the surgeon; (4) Work done by the patient is reduced.

Problems which may arise include: (1) Reduction of the venous return while the chest is still closed, due to rise in intrathoracic pressure. This may reduce cardiac output temporarily; (2) In one-lung anaesthesia a low Pao_2 may occur; (3) Risk of rupture of emphysematous bullae.

Ventilatory Capacity

The functional reserve of the lungs may be limited by lung disease. This may be obvious clinically or may be found by application of lung function tests (*see* Chapter 2). These factors play a considerable part in the preoperative evaluation of the patient and help to determine the advisability and extent of surgical removal of lung tissue. They are also important in the postoperative period because a superadded lung collapse or infection may prove very serious.

Pulmonary Secretions

The patient with excessive secretion is uncommon, but wet cases occur in bronchiectasis, lung abscess, bronchopleural fistula and associated with new growths when obstruction to a bronchus may cause a pool of infected secretions to lie peripherally. Methods for controlling the spread of secretions include: (1) Preoperative preparation: postural drainage and antibiotic therapy and measures to improve the general health of the patient and dry up secretions; (2) Regional analgesia during which the cough reflex is not lost—in empyema, etc; (3) Posture during operation. When the patient is tilted head-down 35° for left thoracotomy, 55° for right thoracotomy, and is on his side, secretions from the upper—diseased—lung will flow by gravity into the trachea and can be sucked out, thus preventing contamination of the healthy lung. Similarly if the patient is prone, necessitating a posterolateral incision, secretions can be aspirated (Overholt[26] (requiring a special table); Parry Brown[27]). Useful position in children too small for the use of blockers, who are undergoing lobectomy; and in upper lobectomies in adults. When the patient is in the prone position, the table should be tilted head down by 10°. Alternatively, secretions can be retained in the diseased lobe by suitable posture, e.g. the sitting position for lower lobectomy in bronchiectasis. An empyema is also often drained with the patient sitting, especially if there is any chance of bronchopleural fistula with its risk of the patient drowning in his own secretions; (4) Tracheal suction. In wet cases routine suction every 10 min may be advisable. Secretions are likely to move into the main bronchi after changes in position and after manipulation of the lung; (5) The surgeon may be asked to apply the bronchial clamp as soon as possible when the chest is open; (6) Endobronchial intubation and blocking with inflatable cuffs.

Endobronchial Instrumentation
Isolation of one lung or major lobe has the following advantages: (1) Secretions and blood can be confined to the diseased lung or lobe; (2) The lung to be operated upon can be made quiet and collapsed; (3) A bronchopleural fistula can be isolated.

Methods include: (1) Use of a double-lumen tube (the Carlens catheter (1949) and its modifications; Bryce-Smith, 1959; Bryce-Smith and Salt, 1960; White, 1960; Robertshaw, 1962); (2) Intubation of the sound bronchus (Gale and Waters, 1931; Magill, 1936; Vellacott, 1954; Gordon and Green, 1955; Macintosh and Leatherdale, 1955; Green, 1958; Machray, 1958); (3) Use of bronchial blocker (Magill, 1934, 1936; Vernon Thompson, 1943); (4) Selective bronchial block in children.[28]

Endobronchial Tubes[29]

1. The Robertshaw Low-resistance Double-lumen Tubes[30]
Basically, two tubes fixed together, one longer, which enters the bronchus, and one shorter, which terminates just above the carina. Left and right versions exist, in three sizes—small, medium and large. For a right pneumonectomy, a

left-sided Robertshaw is used, and vice versa. The two tubes separate proximally for connection to two catheter mounts. The longer bronchial tube has a cuff which seals it in the main bronchus; a second cuff seals the instrument in the trachea. Both cuffs have pilot balloons on the inflation pipe, blue for bronchial and red for tracheal cuff. The right-sided tube has a slotted bronchial cuff to allow inflation of the right upper lobe. The tube is passed into the trachea through an ordinary laryngoscope, and then advanced blindly until the fork, where the tubes separate, is opposite the lips. The bronchial cuff is then inflated, testing for leaks by blowing down the bronchial tube and auscultating the lung to ensure correct positioning. The tracheal cuff is next inflated, using similar tests. Now either lung can be ventilated, isolated or collapsed at will. Accurate placement may be difficult owing to alterations in anatomy or as a result of pathology. A special catheter mount and precision rotary valve may be used.[31]

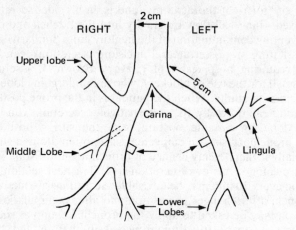

Fig. 29.1. Diagram of tracheobronchial tree.

2. Carlens Double-lumen Catheter
This was originally used for differential bronchospirometry.[32] It has a left-sided bronchial tube and a right-sided tracheal tube. There is a carinal hook to aid positioning (which may be easier than when the Robertshaw tube is used).

3. Macintosh and Leatherdale Tubes[33]
Two types exist: (*a*) A left-sided endobronchial tube with bronchial and tracheal cuffs. A small right-sided channel is used to aspirate secretions or distend the right lung. It is used for right-lung surgery; (*b*) A combined endobronchial cuffed suction blocker with inflatable cuff; for left-lung surgery.

4. The Green–Gordon Tube[34]
This has a slotted right bronchial cuff (to allow inflation of the right upper lobe), a tracheal cuff and a carinal hook. It is used for left-lung surgery.

Magill endobronchial tubes are very long Magill tracheal tubes.[35] The Machray modification has a short cuff.[36] The Pallister left endobronchial tube has a tracheal cuff and two bronchial cuffs, in case of rupture of one of them.[37] These last three are threaded over a rigid or fibreoptic[38] bronchoscope for insertion.

5. Endobronchial Tube with Movable Blocker (Univent)[116]

Endobronchial Blockers
(1) The Vernon Thompson bronchus blocker.[39] The rubber balloon is covered with nylon mesh to provide a rough surface to prevent dislodgement; (2) Magill blocker, small in size; (3) Fogarty catheters have been used in children. These bronchial blockers are passed through a rigid bronchoscope.

Problems of Endobronchial Tubes
(1) Dislodgement during positioning of patient; (2) Difficulty of insertion if the anatomy is distorted congenitally or by tumours, etc.; (3) Trauma of tracheal mucous membrane.

It may be more economical to use disposable polyvinyl chloride double-lumen tubes instead of red rubber tubes if their use is likely to be infrequent.[40] Should a double-lumen tube fail to function, a urinary catheter (Foley) with balloon can be inserted down the lumen of each side, so enabling one-lung anaesthesia to be continued.[41]

Arterial Hypoxaemia in One-lung Anaesthesia
It has been shown that shunting of blood through the collapsed lung can be as high as 65% of the cardiac output[42] and that ventilation with pure oxygen does not completely correct the hypoxaemia in such cases.[43] Unnecessary rise in intra-alveolar pressure in the ventilated lung should be avoided as this contributes to shunt of blood to the collapsed side.[44] Insufflation of oxygen to the collapsed lung may increase oxygenation of the blood if preceded by a period of inflation.[45] It is recommended that the gases used for ventilation of the sound lung should in any case contain 33% or even 50% oxygen.

Elimination of carbon dioxide may be hindered during one-lung anaesthesia, with improvement occurring on resuming two-lung ventilation.[46]

Choice of Anaesthetic Technique for a Typical Thoracotomy
Some anaesthetists prefer to use endobronchial techniques almost routinely. But *the majority of lung resections can be carried out very satisfactorily with ordinary tracheal tubes, controlled respiration and intermittent suction.* The decision to use an endobronchial instrument will depend on the nature of the operative procedure, the pathological processes present in the lungs, the equipment available, and the anaesthetist's experience.

1. Premedication
Standard premedication, including a vagolytic drug, may be used, bearing in mind the general condition of the patient. A narcotic analgesic may help to facilitate controlled respiration, provided undue depression is avoided.

2. Anaesthetic Agents
The thiopentone–relaxant–nitrous-oxide–oxygen technique, with or without narcotic analgesic, is popular and works well. Smaller doses of relaxant are often required for thoracotomy than for upper abdominal relaxation. Almost every other anaesthetic sequence has been used in thoracic surgery with good results.

3. Intermittent Positive-pressure Ventilation

Obligatory in intrathoracic surgery. High-frequency jet ventilation (HFJV) for thoracic operations offers some practical advantages over IPPV using endo-bronchial tubes.[47]

4. Blood Transfusion

Often required and it is essential to set up an intravenous drip before any thoracotomy.

Some Technical Points

1. Bronchial suture. This is usually performed with a bronchial clamp in place and presents no problem. Some surgeons sew without a clamp in an attempt to lessen the risk of bronchopleural fistula. Use of a double-lumen tube gives complete control of the opposite lung.

2. After suture of the bronchial stump is completed the anaesthetist may be asked to test for leaks. The double-lumen tube makes this easy.

3. Closure of the chest. The lungs should be fully expanded before closure. It is wise to stop ventilation at the moment of insertion of the suture needle into the chest wall; it can then be resumed.

Residual air in the pleural cavity can be removed if an intrapleural drainage tube is used and connected to an underwater seal or a Heimlich disposable flutter valve.[48]

Tracheal Resection[49]

This may present problems when performed for tracheal stenosis though preoperative dilatation of the stricture may allow passage of a tracheal tube with inflation of the cuff beyond the operation site. Difficulties are more likely to occur in children and ventilation has been maintained by use of a modification of the Sanders injector method.[50] For resection of the carina there are added problems.[51] HFPPV may also be employed (*see* Chapter 15).

Pneumonectomy

It can be performed in either the lateral or the prone position. Double-lumen tubes are popular as the diseased lung is isolated and quiescent while ventilation is maintained via the sound lung. Arterial hypoxaemia may occur (*see above*).

Most pneumonectomies can be performed under ordinary endotracheal anaesthesia, but it should be remembered that a collection of pus can be squeezed from behind a carcinoma obstructing the bronchus.

Upper Lobectomy with Sleeve Resection

Upper lobectomy is sometimes carried out for carcinoma along with a segment of the main bronchus. This means that the main bronchus will be open for some time and the large air leak may make inflation of the lungs impossible. Endobronchial anaesthesia to the sound lung, using a double-lumen tube, overcomes these difficulties.

Lower Lobectomy

This operation may be performed for bronchiectasis, and the volume of sputum may be large. Many of these operations are performed in children. In older children a Magill blocker may be useful. In young children with copious sputum the sitting position should be considered.

Segmental Resection
Resection of part of a lobe, usually for isolated tuberculous disease. A tracheal tube is satisfactory. There may be considerable alveolar air leak afterwards. Occasionally negative pressure must be applied to the drain to keep the lungs expanded postoperatively.

Thoracoplasty
First suggested by the German physician, L. Brauer (1865–1951). Usually carried out in the treatment of advanced tuberculosis with cavitation. Sometimes to reduce the residual space after pneumonectomy.

Removal of an Inhaled Foreign Body
This is most common in children and in the right lung. Removal is via a rigid bronchoscope under inhalation anaesthesia. Preoperative respiratory obstruction may be present and can act as a valve so that a segment of lung becomes hyperextended. An experienced anaesthetist should undertake such cases *See also* p. 562.

Bronchopleural Fistula
This produces two complications: (1) A leak allowing gases to escape during thoracotomy and which may make inflation of the lungs impossible; (2) A collection of fluid in the pleural cavity or post-pneumonectomy space may escape through it to flood the bronchial tree. The best solution is by use of a double-lumen tube to isolate the opposite lung. There is some danger in the use of a bronchial blocker in the bronchial stump, as it may easily be pushed through the weakened suture line, converting a small fistula into a large one. Awake intubation under local analgesia in the sitting position may be advantageous with a large fistula or empyema. For the radiological characteristics of bronchopleural fistula following pneumonectomy, *see* Lauckner M. E. et al. *Anaesthesia* 1983, **38**, 452.

Drainage of Empyema or Pneumonectomy Space Infection
An empyema is usually drained under local analgesia in the sitting position. General anaesthesia may be dangerous in the presence of unsuspected bronchopleural fistula and so should not be undertaken lightly. Rib resection may be necessary. General anaesthesia is, however, necessary for operations more extensive than simple drainage and in children and which need the lateral position. Then the technique to be used should be carefully considered in the light of a possible bronchopleural fistula. This will usually require a double-lumen tube. Anaesthesia for colobronchial fistula, *see* Swerdlow B. and Jenkins J. G. *Anaesthesia* 1985, **40**, 42.

Lung Abscess
May be caused by a breaking-down carcinoma or inhalation of infected material. A tuberculous cavity with a fluid level presents similar anaesthetic problems. Preoperative postural drainage, physiotherapy and antibiotics may reduce the amount of infected material and change its character. Endobronchial instrumentation may be used to prevent accidental flooding of the bronchial tree during surgery.

Lung Cysts

Large lung cysts cause compression of surrounding lung tissue. They may have a communication with the main bronchus which allows gases to pass in much more easily than out. Intermittent positive pressure may therefore cause a rise in tension in the cyst and may cause further collapse of surrounding tissue with deterioration in the patient's condition. Induction must be carefully carried out in such cases. The tracheobronchial reflexes are often hypersensitive. If coughing is allowed to occur it may result in further rise of tension in the cyst. Spontaneous respiration should be maintained until the cyst has been isolated via a double-lumen tube or a bronchial clamp. It may be wise to carry out full topical analgesia of the tracheobronchial tree before induction of general anaesthesia. Halothane is a useful agent since smooth quiet respiration can usually be obtained.

Pulmonary hydatid cysts are common in Middle East countries. They may be bilateral and multiple and may require surgical removal if they become large. They may erode into the bronchial wall and become infected. Accidental rupture of cyst contents into the bronchial tree may occur during surgery with the risk of flooding of the airway and dissemination of the disease. Endobronchial instrumentation is often indicated.

Surgery of the Pleura

For anaesthesia in patients with cystic fibrosis complicated by pneumothorax, requiring pleurectomy or abrasion pleurodesis, *see* Robinson D. A. and Branthwaite M. A. *Anaesthesia* 1984, **39**, 655.

Postoperative Pain

The treatment of post-thoracotomy pain. Application of the cryoprobe to the intercostal nerves adjacent to the incision from inside the chest; indomethacin by rectum, 100 mg, 8-hourly[52] may give good results.

Accidental Pneumothorax

This may occur during operations close to the pleura (e.g. cervical sympathectomy, thoracoplasty, nephrectomy, thyroidectomy), as well as a complication of local blocks (e.g. brachial plexus block, intercostal block). Accidental pneumothorax on the contralateral side can occur during thoracotomy with mediastinal dissection. When this happens during general anaesthesia the lungs should be ventilated to blow off all possible air while the hole is closed. Puncture of the lung itself will usually close spontaneously but chest drains may be required as a safety precaution. Accidental pneumothorax may be suspected by reason of altered pattern of spontaneous respiration and confirmed by absence of breath sounds on auscultation and by radiography. The air must then be aspirated.

Tension Pneumothorax

This may occur when a bulla bursts forming a one-way valve, or as a complication of fractured rib. It causes an increase in intrathoracic pressure, with shift of the mediastinum and cardiorespiratory handicap. A large 16G needle inserted into the chest in the second intercostal space anteriorly, followed by a drain. Nitrous oxide should be avoided because of its differential solubility.

Acute Massive Pulmonary Embolus
This has been successfully treated using cardiopulmonary bypass.[53]

Bronchoscopy[54]
Early history. A cylindrical metal tube, illuminated by candle-light to examine body cavities, was invented in 1807 by Bozzini (1773–1809).[55] In 1895 Gustav Killian (1860–1921) of Freiburg used a laryngoscope to peer below the cords.[56] The technique of modern bronchoscopy was developed by Chevalier Jackson (1865–1958) in the USA and by Victor Negus (1887–1974) in the UK in the early years of this century. Diffusion respiration first described (in dogs) by Draper and Whitehead in 1944[57] and apnoeic oxygenation in man in 1947 by Draper[58] and later by Holmdahl.[59] The fibreoptic bronchoscope was introduced in 1968 by Ikeda.[60]

Oesophagoscopy was pioneered by Kussmaul (1822–1902) in 1869 and by Von Mikulicz (1829–1905) in 1881.[61]

1. Topical analgesia. See section in chapter on 'Regional Analgesia' (Chapter 31). Topical analgesia, though less popular today than formerly, is safer than general anaesthesia if the patient has respiratory obstruction or is expectorating large amounts of blood or pus. It also enables the surgeon to assess the movements of the vocal cords. This cannot be accurately done if the patient is anaesthetized.

2. General anaesthesia. Patient is premedicated according to general condition. Suitable premedication is important as awareness may be a problem when using the intermittent intravenous anaesthetic and relaxant technique. The following agents may be used where appropriate: opioids, diazepam, lorazepam, tema zepam, droperidol. Whatever method of general anaesthesia is used, many authorities believe that it is best combined with topical analgesia of the larynx and trachea to prevent laryngospasm and undue straining under light anaesthesia. Intermittent intravenous agent is given whenever the previous dose is seen to be wearing off by such signs as movement of the feet, swallowing, perspiration, active dilated pupil, plus intermittent suxamethonium in small doses to prevent coughing and relax the larynx for insertion of the bronchoscope. Respiration is maintained by:

a. The Sanders Injector[62] Intermittent flow of oxygen via a small tube in the mouth of the bronchoscope entrains air and produces inflation of the lungs despite the open proximal end. Blood gases can be kept normal by this method. Apparatus can be permanently fixed to the bronchoscope, and a design has been made for use with piped oxygen supplies (410 kPa) using three different injector sizes (SWG 16, for adults and small adult, 18 for adolescent and 19 for child, infant and suckling). In the authors' opinion, this technique is the most satisfactory method of maintaining gas exchange during bronchoscopy, with full muscle paralysis. Modifications include: (1) Transtracheal ventilation, (2) Use of the oxygen side-arm of the bronchoscope which results in increased FIo_2; (3) Use of premixed N_2O and O_2 as the driving gas. Depending on the degree of air entrainment the patient is less likely to be aware during the procedure. *See also* 'Anaesthesia for Microlaryngoscopy', p. 474.

b. The ventilating bronchoscope is of special construction to allow IPPV at the same time as the operator visualizes the bronchial tree through a window.

c. The apnoeic oxygenation technique. Thiopentone and suxamethonium combined with topical spray. Suxamethonium is given to maintain apnoea during bronchoscopy. The patient can be kept oxygenated according to the principles of *aventilatory mass flow*. Oxygen is taken up from alveolar gases at a slightly faster rate than carbon dioxide is eliminated. Oxygen from a catheter in the trachea therefore moves down the bronchial tree to occupy the space. Oxygenation can be maintained; hypercapnia occurs ($Paco_2$ rising at a rate of approximately $0.4\,kPa/min$)[63] and the method should not be used for longer than periods of 15–20 min, monitoring the ECG, pulse, oxygen saturation, skin colour, etc.

d. Intermittent ventilation, using a tracheal tube pushed into the mouth of the bronchoscope.

e. Deep inhalation anaesthesia, performing bronchoscopy as anaesthesia lightens. Ether in air can be used in children. Also nitrous-oxide–oxygen–halothane.

Any method should be used so as to allow rapid return of reflexes at the end of the procedure. The patient should be placed in the lateral position afterwards to allow drainage of blood, etc. on the left side after left bronchus biopsy and vice versa, to prevent blood soiling the normal lung.

If massive haemorrhage occurs from the pulmonary artery during biopsy, a bronchus blocker or an endobronchial tube should be passed at once. These instruments should always be available during bronchoscopy.

Contraindications to general anaesthesia for bronchoscopy may include: (1) Respiratory obstruction, e.g. due to growth; (2) dyspnoea; (3) Poor general condition of patient, e.g. cyanosis at rest; (4) Large amounts of sputum.

(For bronchoscopy in children, *see* Ryan D. W. *Ann. R. Coll. Surg. Engl.* 1980, **62**, 223; for removal of foreign bodies from the trachea or bronchi, *see* Moussalli H. *Br. J. Hosp. Med.* 1981, **25**, 300.)

Fibreoptic Bronchoscopy

This instrument allows most extensive visualization of the larynx and bronchial tree, and is more comfortable to use with local analgesia than the rigid instrument. Anaesthetic techniques include:

1. Topical analgesia. The instrument can be passed through the lumen of a nasopharyngeal tube or directly through a naris, after topical application to the nose, pharynx and tracheobronchial tree. The segmental divisions can be inspected but the effect of the local analgesic may not have reached so far. Can be done in the supine or sitting position. Additional sedation is helpful, e.g. with diazepam.

2. General anaesthesia: (*a*) As for traditional bronchoscopy (*above*), though when passed down a rigid bronchoscope it may occupy a significant part of the lumen. (*b*) Use of the fibreoptic endoscope via the lumen of a standard orotracheal tube. IPPV can be maintained if a suitable airtight fit is made in the seal of a Cobb's suction connector. (The diameter of the fibreoptic bronchoscope is between 3 and 6.5 mm.)

The fibreoptic bronchoscope can also be used as an aid to tracheal intubation in difficult circumstances. Anaesthesia for transbronchial lung biopsy *see* Marshall Barr A. and Kurer F. L. *Anaesthesia* 1984, **39**, 822.

Bronchography

General anaesthesia seldom required nowadays.

For details see eighth edition of this Synopsis.

Oesophagoscopy (using a rigid oesophagoscope)

A tracheal tube should be passed. It is necessary to provide relaxation of the postcricoid sphincter and this may be achieved using muscle relaxants or deep anaesthesia. In obstructive lesions, e.g. carcinoma, it is possible for a dilated oesophagus above the lesion to contain food, etc., which may be regurgitated. Suction should therefore always be available. Oesophagoscopy may produce trauma and perforation, and bleeding may occur after biopsy or in the presence of oesophageal varices. The anaesthetic technique should allow rapid return of reflexes. At the end of the procedure the pharynx must be sucked clear of blood, etc. and the patient turned on the side.

Suggested techniques:

1. Thiopentone–suxamethonium–nitrous-oxide–oxygen and IPPV. Intermittent doses of suxamethonium as required.

2. Thiopentone → inhalation technique, nitrous-oxide–oxygen–trichloro-ethylene or nitrous-oxide–oxygen–halothane, supplemented by small doses of gallamine as required. Spontaneous or assisted respiration.

3. Oxygen–halothane.

This examination can also be performed under topical analgesia (*see* Chapter 31).

The flexible fibreoptic instrument usually requires intravenous sedation, e.g. diazepam or midazolam.[64] (*See also* Chapter 31.)

Oesophagectomy

The patient's general condition is often poor due to lack of nutrition. Preoperative assessment and treatment to correct nutritional and electrolyte deficiencies are therefore important. The problem is mainly one of starvation and responds well to 2 or more weeks of intravenous parenteral nutrition with maximum quantities of carbohydrates, e.g. 25% glucose, fats and amino acids (10–15 g of nitrogen daily) via a central venous catheter (*see* Chapter 40). The operation may be long and blood transfusion is usually required. The abdomen may be opened as well as the thorax.

Thymectomy

Pioneers in the operation of thymectomy for myasthenia gravis have been Sauerbruch (in 1912–1913), Blalock,[65] and Keynes.[66] The connection between thymus enlargement and myasthenia was noticed by Carl Weigert in 1845. The operation involves splitting of the sternum. One or both pleural cavities may be opened.

Cases should be carefully assessed preoperatively with particular reference to muscular weakness and treatment with neostigmine. For details of preoperative and anaesthetic management, *see* p. 399.

Mediastinoscopy

This is usually performed for biopsy of nodes and inspection of lesions. IPPV with tracheal intubation is usually employed and the mediastinoscope inserted through an incision above the sternum. *See* Vaughan R. S. *Anaesthesia* 1978, **33**, 195.

Crush Injuries of the Chest

See Chapter 39.

(*See also* Mansfield R. and Jenkins R. *Practical Anaesthesia for Lung Surgery*. London: Baillière, Tindall and Cassell, 1967; Mushin W. W. et al. *Automatic Ventilation of the Lungs*. Oxford: Blackwell, 1980; Gothard J. W. W. and Branthwaite M. A. *Anaesthesia for Thoracic Surgery*. Oxford: Blackwell, 1982.)

Anaesthesia for Cardiac Operations

History of Cardiac Surgery

First drainage of pericardium for suppurative pericarditis by Hilsman in 1875.[67] First successful suture of heart wound by Rehn (1849–1930) in 1896.[68] First operation for relief of valvular disease by Tuffier (1857–1929) in 1914.[69] First pericardectomy for pericarditis by Delorme (1847–1929) in 1898,[70] and Hallopeau (1876–1924) in 1921. Valvulotomy for valvular disease by Elliott Cutler (1888–1947) and Levine in 1923.[71] Digital dilatation of mitral valve through atrium by Souttar (1875–1964) in 1925.[72] Cardiac catheterization by Bleichroder in 1912 (on himself)[73] (*see* Sanders S. *Br. Med. J.* 1982, **284**, 1563), Forssmann (1904–1979) in 1929[74] and Cournand in 1941.[75] Angiocardiography by Robb and Steinberg in 1938.[76] Ligation of patent ductus by Gross and Hubbard in 1939.[77] Surgical treatment of tetralogy of Fallot by Blalock (1899–1964) and Taussig.[78] Removal of foreign body from heart by Harken in 1946. Surgical treatment of coarctation of the aorta by Clarence Crafoord and Nylin[79] in Stockholm. Pulmonary valvulotomy for the relief of pulmonary stenosis by Brock.[80] Valvuloplasty for the treatment of mitral stenosis by Harken and colleagues.[81] Pump oxygenator used in a human by Gibbon.[82] Selective coronary angiography by Sones in 1958.[83] Resection of aortic aneurysm by De Bakey in 1958.[84] Deep hypothermia, to 20 °C or below, by Drew.[85] Starr replaced the aortic valve in 1963.[86] Saphenous vein bypass grafting by Garrett in 1964.[87] Pioneering work on suture of small blood vessels by Carrel (1873–1944) in 1907.[88] First cardiac transplant carried out in man by Barnard in 1967[89] and Shumway in 1964.[90]

(*See also* History of the heart and great vessels, McKeown K. K. *Can. Anaesth. Soc. J.* 1982, **29**, 325.)

Anaesthetic Problems

Surgery of the heart raises a number of problems for the anaesthetist:

1. Open pneumothorax. *See above.*
2. Diminished cardiac reserve. Cardiac output may be reduced to the point where compensation for a sudden fall in peripheral resistance cannot take place. Anaesthetic drugs must therefore be administered with particular care. Full oxygenation must always be maintained.
3. Blood loss and replacement. Care must be taken not to overload the circulation with saline or blood. Blood loss may occur suddenly and rapidly during operation. Blood for transfusion must be instantly available with the means for rapid administration.
4. Surgical manipulations of the heart. These may cause ectopic beats or other dysrhythmias. The force of ventricular contraction may diminish with hypotension and even asystole can occur. During such manipulations it is essential to watch carefully, so that they may be interrupted if necessary to allow the heart a period of rest and recovery.

5. Open heart surgery. If the heart is to be isolated from the circulation provision must be made to prevent irreversible brain damage. Protection is provided by cardiopulmonary bypass, perhaps in association with hypothermia.

Anaesthetic Technique (without bypass)

The need is for a perfect technique providing quiet, smooth, light anaesthesia without hypoxia. (1) Premedication with morphine and atropine or hyoscine—reduced dosage in the poor risks. Some anaesthetists fear the tachycardia produced by atropine and omit it; (2) Pre-oxygenation; (3) Minimal intravenous anaesthetic to provide a smooth induction without undue depression. A slow circulation time may result in delayed response. Both thiopentone and methohexitone cause cardiac depression. Diazepam can cause fall in cardiac output in hypertensive patients; (4) Intubation using a muscle relaxant and cuffed tracheal tube. Controlled ventilation with nitrous-oxide–oxygen–relaxant and a supplement if necessary.

Many prefer suxamethonium (30–50 mg) for intubation which can then be carried out atraumatically in a light plane of anaesthesia, followed by a non-depolarizing relaxant once the effect of suxamethonium has worn off.

A slow intravenous drip is set up before surgery commences and blood must be ready in the theatre and for immediate transfusion at a rapid rate. Arterial pressure, ECG, central venous pressure, heart rate, oxygen saturation, body temperature and urine output should be monitored.

During manipulations of the heart, the heart function should be observed closely to look for evidence of the effect of such manipulations: (1) The heart watched directly; (2) The radial pulse is palpated; it may become weak or disappear for a time; (3) Blood pressure; (4) Dysrhythmias. Bradycardia with an inefficient ventricular beat is a serious sign requiring a short period of rest (unless massage is indicated) and full oxygenation. Cardiac asystole or ventricular fibrillation should be treated on the usual lines (*see* Chapter 37).

The lungs must be fully expanded before the chest is closed. At the end of operation any residual effects of relaxant drugs should be reversed with atropine and neostigmine. Full tracheobronchial toilet is advisable prior to extubation, but this has its disadvantages. The patient should be returned from theatre breathing oxygen from a portable apparatus or be attached to a ventilator.

Mitral Valvotomy,[91] Aortic Valvotomy

Anaesthesia along the lines indicated above is satisfactory for cardiac surgery that does not require the special techniques of hypothermia or cardiopulmonary bypass.

Patent Ductus Arteriosus

The ductus is a wide channel between the distal part of the aortic arch and the pulmonary artery in fetal life. If closure does not occur, blood flows from the high-pressure aorta to the low-pressure pulmonary artery, a reversal of the direction from intra-uterine life. The results are: (1) Increased intrapulmonary pressure; (2) Right ventricular hypertrophy to deal with it; (3) Small volume of blood passing down aorta, with low diastolic blood pressure and high pulse pressure—these pressures become normal when the ductus is tied; (4) Hypertrophy of left ventricle.

Cyanosis is not marked unless other congenital abnormalities exist also. There is a loud systolic and diastolic murmur, the former being more pronounced. Endocarditis frequently coexists and greatly adds to the risks of operation.

A drip should be set up as grave haemorrhage may take place while the ductus is being cleared. Tying the ductus results in increase in the peripheral blood volume, so drip must otherwise be slow.

Coarctation of Aorta
Induced hypotension, e.g. with trimetaphan or nitroprusside, has a useful place in anaesthesia for this condition. It reduces blood loss from the enlarged vessels in the chest wall and makes the actual suturing of the aorta easier. Satisfactory hypotension may be difficult to achieve, and the use of propranolol 1–2 mg to prevent tachycardia has been advocated.[92] The blood pressure should be rising again when the clamps are taken of the aorta, otherwise at this stage circulatory collapse may occur. The technique of general anaesthesia should present few special problems.

Pericardectomy
Constrictive pericarditis limits diastolic expansion of the heart. A rise in atrial pressure follows which in turn leads to venous congestion and peripheral oedema. Advanced cases present as poor risks for anaesthesia and surgery. Cardiac output may be reduced to the point where compensation for a sudden fall in peripheral resistance cannot take place. The surgical procedure involves considerable manipulation of the heart. Dysrhythmias and fall of blood pressure are likely to occur, and it may be necessary to pause from time to time to allow the heart to recover. Intravenous transfusion may be dangerous because of the risk of overloading the circulation. At the same time haemorrhage may occur and blood should be accurately replaced.

Thiopentone may be undesirable in the presence of constrictive pericarditis.[93] Many anaesthetists are, however, prepared to use the drug carefully. Otherwise induction can be by an inhalation method, providing hypoxia or excitement is not allowed to occur.

Percutaneous Lung Biopsy
(*See* Rocke D. A. *Anaesthesia* 1984, **98**, 888.)

Cardiac Tamponade
IPPV may cause severe cardiovascular depression before the pericardium is opened. Preliminary pericardiocentesis may be helpful.[94]

Anaesthesia for Cardiac Transplants[95]
The main indications for the operation are coronary artery disease and cardiomyopathy. The presence of active infection or malignant disease are absolute contraindications. The use of the immunosuppressive drug, Cyclosporin A, since 1982 has increased the survival rate which is over 75%. (For details of anaesthetic and postanaesthetic management, *see* Grebenik C. and Robinson P. N. *Anaesthesia* 1985, **40**, 131.) The anaesthetic problems do not differ from those of any open heart operation in a seriously ill patient.

Open Heart Surgery using Cardiopulmonary Bypass[95]
This is indicated when the surgical procedure needs circulatory arrest for a

period longer than the 7 min which is normally considered safe under conventional hypothermia. Operations include surgical correction of atrial and ventricular septal defects, Fallot's tetralogy, pulmonary stenosis, aortic stenosis, mitral incompetence and prosthetic operations on the heart valve. Coronary artery bypass grafts now account for the majority of open heart operations.

The use of an extracorporeal circulation allows circulation of the vital organs (the brain) while the heart is isolated from the circulation. It has been made possible by the use of heparin in preventing clotting of the blood and by the role of protamine in restoring the coagulation mechanism.

The extracorporeal circulation must incorporate a pump or pumps to provide circulation and an oxygenator for gaseous exchange. At the same time it is important that the blood is not damaged, and the apparatus must be capable of sterilization or be disposable.

The perfusion flow rate is usually calculated as 2400 ml/min/m^2 body surface[96] or as 70–80 ml/min/kg bodyweight (100–120 ml/kg in children to allow for higher oxygen consumption). The oxygenator must be capable of providing efficient gas exchange at the required flow rate and the venous and arterial cannulae must be capable of carrying this blood flow. The arterial cannula is usually inserted into the aorta or femoral artery and venous blood taken from the right atrium or superior and inferior venae cavae.

Heparin is given in a dosage of 2–3 mg/kg bodyweight or 90 mg/m^2 surface area and, in addition, the pump must be primed with 5% dextrose, Hartmann's solution or low molecular weight or other dextran mixture. Haemodilution down to 20–25% haematocrit economizes on the use of blood and is associated with less lung damage, and significantly improved perfusion of the capillaries of the body. Before bypass 500–1000 ml of blood may be taken from the patient into anticoagulated bags and the patient given dextran 70 or other plasma expander to replace it. The freshly taken blood is then reinfused after bypass to raise the haematocrit back up to 30%. Dextran may cause a fall in the level of Factor VIII in the plasma. The dosage of protamine at the end of perfusion should be 3–4 mg/kg. Hexadimethrine (Polybrene) is also used to neutralize heparin in a 1:1 ratio. Both drugs require to be given intravenously over a period of minutes. Otherwise hypotension may occur as a result of intense pulmonary artery constriction.

Pump Oxygenators

High flows of oxygen must be delivered to the oxygenators. This would normally displace too much carbon dioxide. A mixture of 2·5% carbon dioxide in oxygen (more in the presence of hypothermia) is therefore used to keep the arterial carbon dioxide tension within normal limits.

During bypass the venous return to the heart is occluded. There is, however, loss of blood which is returned to the heart; (1) From the coronary circulation; (2) From the bronchial arteries via the pulmonary veins (may be considerable in conditions such as Fallot's tetralogy); (3) From incompetent aortic valves. Such heparinized blood is removed by suction from the chest and retransfused via the bypass. Hypothermia is frequently employed down to 28 °C, using an integral heat exchanger in the bypass.

Methods designed to reduce the loss of blood from the open heart include: (1) Arrest of coronary circulation by a clamp across the root of the aorta combined with elective cardiac arrest (25% ice-cold potassium solution injected into the coronary circulation); (2) Hypothermia to 15 °C when cell metabolism is so low that cerebral circulation can be safely arrested.

Anaesthetic technique. This does not differ substantially from anaesthesia for cardiac operations without extracorporeal circulation. For elective surgery a heavy premedication has advantages, while for emergency open heart surgery, only a drying agent is required. For the anaesthetic, thiopentone–nitrous-oxide–oxygen–relaxant anaesthesia is satisfactory. Intravenous or inhalation agents may be given as a supplement if required. Coughing and straining, if allowed to occur, can impair ventilation, reduce cardiac output and even cause cardiac arrest.

A different approach is the use of large doses of morphine, 1–5 mg/kg i.v. together with muscle relaxants and IPPV.[97] High-dose fentanyl can also be used. Studies indicate that such doses have no effect on cardiac output, systemic vascular resistance, arterial pressure, pulse rate and central venous pressure in healthy subjects, but cause decreased systemic vascular resistance and increased cardiac output in patients with severe aortic valvular disease. This may be associated with liberation of catecholamines. Peripheral vasoconstriction may occur during bypass due to adrenaline release resulting from low baroreceptor stimulation, because of the non-pulsatile flow. Some workers use thymoxamine to prevent this. (N.B. thymoxamine also raises the voltage on the cerebral function monitor display.)

At least three intravenous lines may be used: (1) Right atrial pressure monitoring; (2) Drug infusion line; (3) Blood transfusion line.

Monitoring

Monitoring during cardiac surgery may include:

1. Central venous pressure. A rise in pressure suggests obstruction or malposition of the venous lines. A fall, with inadequate flow to the machine, suggests concealed blood loss. At the end of operation high pressure may be caused by over-transfusion or myocardial insufficiency; low pressure by inadequate transfusion. Right and left atrial pressures using transducers are also usually required.

2. Arterial pressure. Usually measured by cannulation of the radial artery, since during bypass the flow is not pulsatile and very rapid changes may occur.

3. Pulmonary wedge pressure and cardiac output using a balloon-tipped, flow-directed, flexible pulmonary artery catheter (Swan–Ganz).[98]

4. EEG. Gives an indication of the adequacy of cerebral perfusion. It may give warning before irreversible damage is done.

5. ECG. Gives warning of inadequate coronary flow, of injury to conducting mechanism of heart, and treatable dysrhythmias. A pacemaker lead may be inserted by the surgeon in anticipation of heart block or asystole.[99] It may be epicardial or endocardial.

6. Blood loss. Swab weighing and measurement of suction bottles should be charted at regular intervals. Blood can be transfused via the arterial line of the pump or through a separate intravenous drip. Other guides to blood loss include the reservoir of the pump, the venous pressure and the arterial pressure.

7. Arterial pH, P_{CO_2} and the standard bicarbonate. Metabolic acidosis may occur due to tissue hypoxia with low perfusion rates. Carbon dioxide is an important factor in the control of cerebral blood flow. Respiratory alkalosis may therefore be harmful if the cerebral perfusion is only just adequate during the extracorporeal circulation or the post-perfusion period. Some authorities believe

that controlled respiration should be maintained by large doses of muscle relaxants rather than by hyperventilation.

8. Arteriovenous oxygen difference. Determines the adequacy of tissue perfusion. Pao_2 should remain above 100 mmHg during perfusion. Low cardiac output contributes significantly to arterial hypoxaemia when there is venous admixture. Oxygen saturation may also be monitored.

9. Temperature recording. A nasopharyngeal probe is most frequently used as it may approximate to brain temperature. Probes at other sites reflect temperature gradients within the body. A probe in the external auditory meatus has been recommended.

10. Urine flow. A simple index of adequate renal perfusion. Output should be recorded every half-hour. The minimal acceptable volume is 0·5 ml/kg body weight per hour or 30 ml/h in the average adult.[100] Failure to achieve frusemide diuresis postoperatively may be associated with renal hypoxia due to low cardiac output or poor perfusion.

11. Serum potassium may be monitored throughout operation. There may be a shift of potassium from inside the cell, and this may cause cardiac irritability and affect the action of muscle relaxants.

12. Haematocrit. This is important when Hartmann's solution or dextrose has been used to prime the extracorporeal circuit.

13. Blood coagulability during and after reversal of heparin.

14. Blood glucose level.

See also Chapter 41.

Blood replacement. (1) *Pre-perfusion period.* It is important to keep pace with measured blood loss, and desirable to transfuse an excess of some 50–250 ml, depending on the size of the patient; (2) *Perfusion period.* The proportion of blood in the patient and in the extracorporeal system varies somewhat with vascular tone. The central venous pressure is the most reliable indication that the correct amount of blood is in the patient's circulatory system at the end of perfusion. A suitable solution for prevention of hypoglycaemia in infants and children is 10% dextrose in Hartmann's solution; 5 ml/kg/h will maintain the blood-glucose level; (3) *Post perfusion period.* Blood should be transfused according to blood loss and central venous pressure; a reading of 5–10 cmH$_2$O may be considered satisfactory; (4) *Postoperative period.* Blood may need to be given if bleeding occurs. (For maximal conservation and minimal usage of blood products, *see* Newland P. E. et al. *Anaesth. Intensive Care*, 1980, **8**, 178.)

Excessive bleeding. This may occur after perfusion and may be due to: (1) Inadequate neutralization of heparin; (2) Fibrinogen depletion (less than 100 g %); fibrinogen 4–6 mg may need to be given; (3) Reduction in platelets; (4) Failure of surgical haemostasis.

Lung changes. These may arise due to: (1) Overloading of the pulmonary vessels during surgery; (2) The post perfusion lung syndrome: perivascular oedema and haemorrhage, congestion and thickening of inter-alveolar walls, patchy collapse, intra-alveolar haemorrhage, venous admixture disturbance of ventilation perfusion relationships, presence of cells resembling immature plasma cells. Reduction in surfactant causing atelectasis in the immediate postoperative period has been reported.

Postoperative care.[101] Patients may be nursed in an intensive-care area with continued monitoring of ECG, arterial blood pressure, venous pressure, urine flow, blood pH and bicarbonate, $Paco_2$ and arteriovenous oxygen gradient. In some centres, the whole process has been computerized, with feedback of commands for the attendants, with good results. Postoperative pain can be well treated by intercostal nerve block from inside the chest using 0·5% bupivacaine in dextran 40, or a cryoprobe applied to the nerves.

Complications[102] include:

1. Cardiac arrest. Most likely to occur during induction or on termination of bypass.

2. Hypotension. Blood transfusion, pharmacological support and use of artificial pacemaker may be required. Right atrial pressure may average 12–15 cmH$_2$O. Calcium, digoxin, isoprenaline, dopamine, adrenaline, glucose/insulin mixture, and salbutamol and even noradrenaline may be required.

3. Ventilation–perfusion abnormalities.

4. Metabolic acidosis. Corrected by cautious administration of bicarbonate.

5. Cardiac dysrhythmias. Abolition includes correction of hypoxia, acid–base abnormalities, electrolyte disturbance and low $Pa\text{CO}_2$. Pharmacological agents and cardiac pacing may be indicated.

6. Oliguria. Mannitol or frusemide may be required. Haematuria from haemolysis usually clears spontaneously.

7. Pulmonary oedema. Positive end expiratory pressure may be helpful during artificial ventilation.

8. Brain damage due to preoperative ischaemia, embolism of gas bubbles, blood clot, calcific fragments from a stenosed aortic valve or fat droplets. The damage may be global or localized. Damage may be made worse by excessively low $Pa\text{CO}_2$ on bypass, acute alkalosis, CNS hydration due to haemodilution or a raised serum magnesium level. Brain damage may contraindicate PEEP following cardiac surgery. Dexamethasone may be useful, dose 10 mg i.v. immediately, followed by 4 mg 6-hourly. In skilled hands the EEG has prognostic value. Personality changes may follow.

9. Haemorrhage. The cause may be obvious or obscure. It can cause death. Treatment includes fresh blood or plasma, fibrinogen, epsilon aminocaproic acid, vitamin K and topical thrombin.

10. Artificial ventilation can be maintained postoperatively as a planned measure. Indications for weaning include the ability to maintain $Pa\text{CO}_2$ at less than 7 kPa, $Pa\text{O}_2$ over 13 kPa on 40% inspired oxygen, and a respiratory rate less than 30/min.[103]

11. Hypoglycaemia, especially in infants and children, as the glycogen stores become depleted.

12. Cardiac tamponade.

13. Hypertension after coronary artery bypass grafting (CABG) is controlled by vasodilators.

Open Heart Surgery with Profound Hypothermia[104]

As the body temperature falls below 28 °C there is a period of ventricular fibrillation which quietens into cardiac standstill as the temperature falls further.

A technique has been developed[105] using cardiopulmonary bypass with cooling. When the brain temperature is estimated to have reached 15 °C, circulation and ventilation are discontinued. The surgeon has then a period of about 1 h to operate on a dry still heart. Warming then takes place until oesophageal temperature reaches 30–32 °C when the heart is electrically defibrillated. During rewarming, serial pH, $Pa\text{CO}_2$ and $Pa\text{O}_2$ measurements are valuable.

Advantages claimed for this technique are absence of problems of 'pump-lung' postoperatively, the heart is dry and still during surgery with cardiac arrest, and coronary perfusion is not required during operations on the aortic valves. The method is especially suitable in children.[105]

Coronary Artery Grafts

The saphenous vein was used for coronary artery bypass graft in 1967 and the internal mammary artery in 1970. The anaesthetic techniques used are as described above for cardiopulmonary bypass operations.[106] For induction of anaesthesia in coronary bypass surgery, midazolam 0·3 mg/kg gives reasonable cardiovascular stability.[107] For details of anaesthesia in emergency coronary artery surgery, *see* Viljoen J. F. et al. *Br. J. Anaesth.* 1974, **46**, 953. There may be no need to withdraw β-blockers before these operations.[108]

Cardiac Catheterization[109]

This is now performed under local analgesia and sedation. (*See also* Chapter 41.)

Angiocardiography

It was common to paralyse the patient with suxamethonium or other relaxant and to ventilate with nitrous oxide and oxygen via a tracheal tube, but now sedation is employed.

Insertion of Indwelling Pacemakers

The sternal pacemaker was used in 1954,[110] the first transvenous endocardial pacing in 1958,[111] and the first totally implanted system, a few years later.[112] Advances in pacemaker design and technique have meant that patients should seldom present for anaesthesia without adequate pacing. The apparatus itself is now usually implanted in the chest wall under local analgesia. (*See also* Gothard J. W. W. and Branthwaite M. *Anaesthesia* 1979, **34**, 269.)

Patients who are paced and require surgery are dealt with on p. 409.

Anaesthesia for Cardioversion

First described in 1962.[113] Anaesthesia is necessary as the shock is painful. It can be achieved readily by administration of a sleep dose of thiopentone or methohexitone.[114] Diazepam and flunitrazepam[115] have also been used.

(*See also* Branthwaite M. A. *Anaesthesia for Cardiac Surgery and Allied Procedures.* Oxford: Blackwell, 1977; Gilston A. *Recent Advances in Anaesthesia*—13 (Hewer C. L. and Atkinson R. S. ed.). Edinburgh: Churchill Livingstone, 1979; Abbott T. R. in *Paediatric Anaesthesia. Trends in Current Practice* (Rees G. J. and Gray T. C. ed.) London: Butterworths, 1981.)

References

1. Fell G. *Buffalo Med. J.* 1887, Nov.; O'Dwyer J. P. *NY Med. J*, 1885, **42**, 145.
2. Matas R. *Ann. Surg.* 1899, **29**, 951.
3. Tuffier T. and Hallion J. *C. R. Biol. (Paris)*, 1896, **48**, 951.
4. Sauerbruch F. *Zbl. Chir.* 1904, **31**, 146; *Mitt. Grenzgeb. Med. Chir.* 1904, **13**, 399.
5. Brauer L. *Mitt. Grenzgeb. Med. Chir.* 1904, **13**, 483.
6. Brat H. and Schmieden V. *Münch. Med. Wochenschr.* 1908, **55**, 2421.
7. Tiegel M. *Zentbl. Chir*, 1908, **22**, 369; *Beitr. Klin. Chir.* 1909, **64**, 358.
8. Janeway H. H. and Green N. W. *JAMA* 1909, **53**, 1975; *Ann. Surg.* 1910, **52**, 58.

9. Elsberg C. A. *Ann. Surg.* 1910, **52**. 23.
10. Meltzer S. J. and Auer L. *J. Exp. Med.* 1909, **11**, 622.
11. Killian G. *Münch. Med. Wochenschr.* 1898, **45**, 844.
12. Kuhn F. *Dt. Z. Chir.* 1905, **76**, 148.
13. Bjork V. C. and Carlens E. *J. Thorac. Surg.* 1950, **20**, 151.
14. Gale J. N. and Waters R. M. *J. Thorac. Surg.* 1932, **1**, 432.
15. Archibald E. *J. Thorac. Surg.* 1935, **4**, 335.
16. Frenckner P. *Acta Otolaryngol.* 1934, Suppl. 20, 100.
17. Crafoord C. *Acta Chir. Scand.* 1938, Suppl. 54.
18. Guedel A. E. *Anesthesiology* 1940, **1**, 13.
19. Nosworthy M. D. *Proc. R. Soc. Med.* 1941, **34**, 479.
20. Guedel A. E. and Treweek D. N. *Curr. Res. Anesth. Analg.* 1934, **13**, 263.
21. Pinson K. B. and Bryce A. G. *Br. J. Anaesth.* 1944, **19**, 53.
22. Morch T. *Proc. R. Soc. Med.* 1947, **40**, 603.
23. Musgrove A. H. *Anaesthesia* 1952, **7**, 77.
24. Guedel A. E. *Anesthesiology* 1940, **1**, 13.
25. Nosworthy M. D. *Proc. R. Soc. Med.* 1941, **34**, 479.
26. Overholt R. H. *J. Thorac. Surg.* 1946, **15**, 384.
27. Parry Brown A. I. *Thorax* 1948, **3**, 161; *Proc. R. Soc. Med.* 1973, **66**, 339.
28. Cay D. L. et al. *Anaesth. Intensive Care* 1973, **3**, 127.
29. *See* Pappin J. C. *Anaesthesia* 1979, **34**, 57.
30. Robertshaw F. L. *Br. J. Anaesth.* 1962, **34**, 576; Black A. M. S. and Harrison G. A. *Anaesth. Intensive Care*, 1975, **3**, 334.
31. Annotation, *Br. J. Clin. Equip.* 1977, **2**, 309.
32. Carlens E. *J. Thorac. Surg.* 1949, **18**, 742; Bjork V. O. and Carlens E. *J. Thorac. Surg.* 1950, **20**, 151; Bjork V. O. et al. *Anesthesiology* 1953, **14**, 60.
33. Macintosh R. R. and Leatherdale R. A. *Br. J. Anaesth.* 1955, **27**, 556.
34. Green R. and Gordon W. *Anaesthesia* 1957, **12**, 86.
35. Magill I. W. *Proc. R. Soc. Med.* 1935, **29**, 649.
36. Machray R. *Tuberc. Index* 1958, **13**, 172.
37. Pallister W. K. *Thorax* 1959, **14**, 55.
38. Aps C. and Towney J. *Anaesthesia* 1981, **36**, 415.
39. Rusby L. N. and Thompson V. C. *Postgrad. Med. J.* 1943, **19**, 44.
40. Linter S. P. K. *Anaesthesia* 1985, **40**, 191.
41. Conacher I. D. *Anaesthesia* 1983, **38**, 475.
42. Torda T. A. et al. *Anaesthesia* 1974, **29**, 272; Kerr J. H. et al. *Br. J. Anaesth.* 1974, **46**, 84.
43. Tarhan S. and Lundborg R. O. *Can. Anaesth. Soc. J.* 1971, **18**, 594.
44. Khanam T. and Branthwaite M. A. *Anaesthesia* 1973, **28**, 132, 280.
45. O'Shea P. J. et al. *Proc. R. Soc. Med.* 1975, **68**, 772.
46. Kerr J. H. et al. *Br. J. Anaesth.* 1973, **45**, 159.
47. Hildebrand P. J. et al. *Anaesthesia* 1984, **39**, 1091.
48. Heimlich H. J. *Hosp. Topics* 1965, **43**, 122.
49. Ismail A. B. *Can. Anesth. Soc. J.* 1979, **26**, 134; Baraka A. *Anesth. Analg. (Cleve.)* 1977, **56**, 429; Lupprian M. and Mok M. S. *Br. J. Anaesth.* 1977, **49**, 383; Ellis R. H. et al. *Anaesth.* 1976, **31**, 1076; Machell E. S. *Br. J. Anaesth.* 1977, **49**, 951.
50. Lee P. and English I. C. W. *Anaesthesia* 1974, **29**, 305.
51. Clarkson W. B. and Davies J. R. *Anaesthesia* 1978, **33**, 815; Klaschik E. et al. *Anaesthesist* 1978, **27**, 430.
52. Keenan D. J. M. et al. *Br. Med. J.* 1983, **287**, 1335.
53. Akyon M. G. and Arslan G. *Br. J. Anaesth.* 1981, **53**, 903.
54. *See also* Atkinson R. S. in: *Recent Advances in Anaesthesia and Analgesia*—12 (Hewer C. L. and Atkinson R. S. ed.). Edinburgh: Churchill Livingstone, 1976.
55. Bozzini P. *Der Lichleiter.* Weimar, 1807.
56. Killian G. *Münch. Med. Wochenschr.* 1898, **45**, 844.
57. Draper W. B. and Whitehead R. W. *Anesthesiology* 1944, **5**, 262, 524.
58. Draper W. B. et al. *Anesthesiology* 1947, **8**, 524.
59. Holmdahl M.-H. *Acta Chir. Scand.* 1956, Suppl. 212, 1.
60. Ikeda S. et al. *Keio Med. J.* 1968, **17**, 1.
61. Kussmaul A. *Dtsch. Arch. Klin. Med.* 1869, **6**, 456; von Mikulicz-Radecki J. *Wien. Med. Presse* 1881, **22**, 1405.

62. Sanders R. D. *Delaware St. Med. J.* 1967, **39**, 170; Spoerel W. E. *Can. Anaesth. Soc. J.* 1969, **16**, 61.
63. Zeitlin G. L. et al. *Br. J. Anaesth.* 1965, **37**, 117.
64. Bardham K. D. et al. *Br. Med. J.* 1984, **288**, 1046.
65. Blalock A. et al. *JAMA* 1945, **128**, 189.
66. Keynes G. *Lancet* 1954, **1**, 1197; *Ann. R. Coll. Surg.* 1953, **12**, 88.
67. Hilsman F. A. *Schrift. Univ. Kiel* 1875, **2**, 20.
68. Rehn L. *Zentbl. Chir.* 1896, **23**, 1048.
69. Tuffier T. *Bull. Acad. Méd. Paris* 3rd series, 1914, **71**, 293.
70. Delorme E. *Gaz. d'Hopit.* 1898, p. 1150; Hallopeau P. *Bull. Mém. Soc. Chir. Paris* 1921, **47**, 1120.
71. Cutler E. and Levine S. A. *Boston Med. Surg. J.* 1923, **188**, 1023.
72. Souttar H. S. *Br. Med. J.* 1925, **2**, 903; Ellis R. H. *Anaesthesia* 1975, **30**, 374.
73. Bleichroder F. *Berlin Klin. Wochenschr.* 1912, **49**, 1563.
74. Forssmann W. *Klin. Wochenschr.* 1929, **8**, 2085.
75. Cournand A. and Ranges H. A. *Proc. Soc. Exp. Med. Biol.* 1941, **46**, 462.
76. Robb G. and Steinberg I. J. *J. Clin. Invest.* 1938, **17**, 507.
77. Gross R. E. and Hubbard J. P. *JAMA* 1939, **112**, 729.
78. Blalock A. and Taussig H. B. *JAMA* 1945, **128**, 189.
79. Crafoord C. and Nylin K. G. *J. Thorac. Surg.* 1945, **14**, 347.
80. Brock R. C. *Br. Med. J.* 1948, **1**, 1121.
81. Harken D. E. et al. *N. Engl. Med. J.* 1948, **238**, 804.
82. Miller B. J. et al. *Med. Clin. North Am.* 1953, **37**, 1609; Gibbon J. H. *Minn. Med.* 1954, **37**, 171; Kirklin J. W. et al. *Ann. Surg.* 1956, **144**. 2.
83. Sones F. M. and Shirley E. K. *Mod. Concepts Cardiovasc. Dis.* 1962, **31**, 735.
84. De Bakey M. E. et al. *J. Thorac. Cardiovasc. Dis.* 1958, **36**, 369.
85. Drew C. E. et al. *Lancet* 1959, **1**, 745.
86. Starr A. et al. *Circulation* 1963, **27**, 779.
87. Garrett H. E. et al. *Cardiovasc. Cent. Bull.* 1964, **3**, 15.
88. Carrel A. *Johns Hopkins Hosp. Bull.* 1907, **18**, 18.
89. Barnard C. N. *S. Afr. Med. J.* 1967, **41**, 1271.
90. Shumway N. and Lower R. R. *Ann. N.Y. Acad. Sci.* 1964, **120**, 773 (*see also* Cooley D. *Surg. Clin. North Am.* 1978, **58**, 895).
91. Bailey C. P. *Dis. Chest* 1949, **15**, 377.
92. Feldman S. A. in: *Recent Advances in Anaesthesia and Analgesia*—11 (Hewer C. L. ed.). Edinburgh: Churchill Livingstone, 1972, Chap. 5.
93. Parry-Brown A. L. and Sellick B. A. *Anaesthesia* 1953, **8**, 4; *Br. Med. Bull.* 1955, **11**, 174.
94. Möller C. T. et al. *Br. J. Anaesth.* 1979, **51**, 409.
95. *See* Farman J. V. in: *Recent Advances in Anaesthesia and Analgesia*—12 (Hewer C. L. and Atkinson R. S. ed.). Edinburgh: Churchill Livingstone, 1976.
96. Clement A. J. *Br. J. Anaesth.* 1971, **43**, 233.
97. Lowenstein E. et al. *N. Engl. J. Med.* 1969, **281**, 1389; Hasbrouck J. D. *Ann. Thorac. Surg.* 1970, **10**, 364; Lowenstein E. *Anesthesiology* 1971, **35**, 563; Stoelting R. K. and Gibbs P. S. *Anesthesiology* 1973, **38**, 45; Moffitt E. A. *Anesth. Analg. (Cleve.)* 1976, **55**, 47.
98. Swan H. J. C. et al. *N. Engl. J. Med.* 1970, **283**, 447; Shaw T. J. I. *Anaesthesia* 1979, **34**, 651.
99. Gothard J. W. W. and Branthwaite M. *Anaesthesia* 1979, **34**, 269.
100. Gilston A. *Br. J. Anaesth.* 1971, **43**, 217.
101. Hinds C. J. *Anaesthesia* 1982, **37**, 170.
102. Gilston A. *Br. J. Anaesth.* 1971, **43**, 217.
103. Sykes M. K. et al. *Anaesthesia* 1970, **25**, 525.
104. *See also* Feldman S. A. *Br. J. Anaesth.* 1971, **43**, 244.
105. Drew C. E. et al. *Lancet* 1959, **1**, 745; Drew C. E. and Anderson I. M. *Lancet* 1959, **1**, 748; Drew C. E. *Br. Med. Bull.* 1961, **17**, 37.
106. Moffatt E. A. *Can. Anaesth. Soc. J.* 1978, **25**, 462.
107. Al-Khudairi D. et al. *Br. J. Anaesth.* 1982, **54**, 831.
108. Manners J. M. and Walters F. J. M. *Anaesthesia* 1979, **34**, 3.
109. *See also* Boulton T. B. in: *Recent Advances in Anaesthesia and Analgesia*—9 (Hewer C. L. ed.). London: Churchill, 1963; Manners J. M. *Br. J. Anaesth.* 1971, **43**, 276.
110. Zoll P. M. *N. Engl. J. Med.* 1954, **247**, 768; Weinrich W. L. et al. *Surg. Forum* 1957, **8**, 360.
111. Forman S. and Schwedel J. B. *N. Engl. J. Med.* 1959, **261**, 943.

112. Chardick W. M. et al. *J. Thorac. Cardiovasc. Surg.* 1961, **42**, 816.
113. Lown R. et al. *JAMA* 1962, **182**, 548.
114. Orko R. *Br. J. Anaesth.* 1974, **46**, 947; 1976, **48**, 257.
115. Vatashsky E. *Anaesthesia* 1981, **36**, 536.
116. Hultgren B. L. et al. *Anesthesiology* 1986, **65**, A.481.

Chapter 30	ANAESTHESIA IN ABNORMAL ENVIRONMENTS

Abnormal Ambient Pressure

Altitude

In a pressurized jet plane flying at 11 000 m (35 000 ft), passengers are in effect exposed to an atmosphere equivalent to an altitude of about 2000 m (5000–7000 ft).

The anaesthetist working at high altitudes should consider:

1. The low alveolar and arterial oxygen tension which is normally present. High concentrations of oxygen should always be given in anaesthetic mixtures for inhalation.

Table 30.1. Barometric pressure related to altitude and alveolar tensions

Altitude (ft)	Barometric pressure (mmHg)	Alveolar oxygen tension (mmHg)	Alveolar carbon-dioxide tension (mmHg)	Alveolar water-vapour tension (mmHg)
0	760	103	40·0	47
5 000	632	81	37·5	47
10 000	523	61	35·5	47
15 000	429	45	32·5	47
18 000	380	38	31·0	47
20 000	349	35	30·0	47

2. Nitrous oxide has a MAC over 100%. The absolute tension and not the percentage in a mixture with oxygen is, however, important. In places at high altitude, at least 40% oxygen is required in inhaled gas mixtures. This means that nitrous oxide must be limited to 60%, so that the tension in arterial blood may be insufficient to prevent awareness. Adjuvants are then recommended.

3. Vaporizers and flow-meters are not pressure compensated and so do not read true when barometric pressure is low (*see below*).

4. Altitude is often associated with low temperatures (*see below*).

5. The pathophysiology of both the unacclimatized and acclimatized resident at high altitude. Changes include pulmonary hyperventilation, polycythaemia, hypervolaemia, rise in pulmonary blood volume, pulmonary hypertension and increase in diffusion capacity. Acute pulmonary oedema requires IPPV with 100% oxygen and descent to lower levels.

Anaesthesia at Depth[1]

This may be required as a result of illness or accident in divers who may work for several days under hyperbaric conditions as high as 26 atmospheres absolute (ATA). Surgical teams would require training to work under these conditions. Amongst other factors, the following should be considered: (1) At very high pressures, nitrogen narcosis can affect function, 15% loss of cognitive skills and 5% loss of manual dexterity at 6 ATA. This is overcome by the use of oxygen–helium mixtures; (2) Oxygen toxicity is important under hyperbaric conditions. F_{IO_2} should be less than 2% at 26 ATA; (3) High-pressure nervous syndrome (tremor, loss of fine movement control, disorientation) occurs in some individuals exposed to high pressure; (4) With rapid compression high temperatures can develop in the gases; fall of temperature with decompression; (5) Solutions in glass containers may implode at high pressures and should be opened beforehand. This raises problems of sterility, e.g. with local analgesic solutions; (6) Pressure effects on anaesthetic drugs. There is a reversal of anaesthetic action at high pressures. This affects both inhalation and intravenous drugs. (7) The skin of divers used to working at depth shows an increase in Gram-negative organisms, such as *Proteus* and *Pseudomonas spp.*, which may present a hazard when injections are made through the skin; (8) The voice requires electrical unscrambling to become intelligible; this is due to the increased density of oxygen–helium mixtures under pressure; (9) Blood-gas monitoring in impossible, though other blood samples can be decompressed before estimation at normal pressure; (10) Cuffs on tracheal tubes and Foley catheters should be filled with water, not air.

Possible suitable techniques include: (1) Ketamine—probably the anaesthetic agent least affected by pressure reversal; (2) Intravenous regional analgesia; (3) For major procedures, morphine 2–3 mg/kg with muscle relaxants and IPPV with air. The Oxford Penlon ventilator may be suitable.

Abnormal Ambient Temperature

Low Temperatures

These may be encountered at altitude or in polar regions, particularly when surgery has to be carried out under field conditions. The patient must be kept warm, and techniques of local analgesia are often unsatisfactory. Stability of Entonox may be altered.

Tropical Conditions

Care must be taken to keep certain drugs cool to prevent deterioration (e.g. suxamethonium). Gas cylinders are filled to specific standards (filling ratio) to prevent the danger of increased pressure within cylinders should the temperature rise. Tropical conditions do not prevent the use of open ether. Rubber articles are liable to perish.

Field Situations

Anaesthesia may have to be administered without the facilities of the modern general hospital: (1) In industrial accidents (e.g. mine-workings); (2) Following major disasters (earthquake, nuclear explosions, road traffic accidents); (3) On board ships at sea; (4) During exploration of remote regions; (5) In under developed countries; (6) In military surgery.

Apparatus
Medical gases are likely to be in short supply. Volatile agents may be vaporized in air, or perhaps oxygen-enriched air. Draw-over apparatus is useful, and should be light and portable. A Venturi system for oxygen enrichment is economical.

Apparatus for intravenous anaesthesia is easily carried. Tracheal tubes, laryngoscopes and connections make anaesthesia safer. Where laryngoscopes are not available, simple equipment can be improvised[2] or intubation achieved during transillumination[3] or a tube passed blindly through mouth[4] or nose.

Inhalation Methods
1. Open masks. In the first 80 years of general anaesthesia, many millions of administrations were satisfactorily accomplished using this method, which should not be totally discarded today. For induction halothane can be used with ether for maintenance, providing atropine has been given beforehand.

2. The Epstein Macintosh Oxford vaporizer for ether.[5] (EMO)The apparatus has a water jacket as a heat reservoir and an automatic thermocompensator and delivers known concentrations of ether in air. Capacity 450 ml of the volatile agent. *See* p. 161.

3. The Oxford Miniature Vaporizer.[6] Delivers 0–3·5% halothane and was designed to smooth induction with ether using the Oxford vaporizer for ether (*above*). Has a sealed water jacket but is not thermocompensated. Interchangeable scales for trichloroethylene and chloroform are available, approximate conversion factors being × 3 and × 2/3 respectively. Capacity 20 ml. Has also been used for trichloroethylene in air together with intravenous agents during major surgery (in developing countries).[7]

4. The Bryce-Smith induction unit.[8]

5. The Penlon draw-over vaporizer.[9]

6. Hewer's emergency apparatus.[10] Consists of an Ambu bag, a Goldman vaporizer and a Ruben valve. Provides halothane and air, with IPPV.

7. The Flagg can.[11] Devised during World War I. The patient breathes to and fro through a can containing ether. Modern modifications facilitate some variation of vapour strength by admitting air as a diluent via a suction union.[12]

8. Improvised vaporizers can be made out of materials which are readily available.[12] Flagg cans can be easily constructed using empty coffee tins. Inhalers can also be made from two suitable food tins with a layer of gauze between if the Schimmelbusch mask is not available.

9. Simple apparatus for administration of a non-explosive mixture of cyclopropane has been described, e.g. the CON apparatus (cyclopropane, 40%; oxygen 30%; nitrogen, 30%).[13] For short operations, nitrous oxide and air can be given (e.g. incision of abscess) and requires only a gas cylinder, a face-mask, rubber tubing and reservoir bag, and three-way stopcock.

10. The Triservice anaesthetic apparatus (Penlon), as used with success in the Falkland Islands war in 1982, consists of a Laedal self-inflating bag-valve-mask resuscitator connected to two Oxford Miniature Vaporizers (for trichloroethylene and halothane) and an oxygen supplementation attachment. For disaster medicine and flying squads.[14] For anaesthesia in battle injuries, *see* Simon E. et al. *Anaesthesia* 1984, **39**, 379.

Major Accident Procedures

Most hospitals now operate major accident procedures and emergency boxes are kept which contain resuscitation equipment, lights, distinctive protective clothing, etc. Anaesthetic equipment may include a self-inflating bag (e.g. Ambu) with valve and face-mask, tracheal tubes and connections, laryngoscopes and batteries, drugs, etc. Transfusion sets with infusion fluids in plastic containers are also required and should include a manual pressure pump.

All boxes should be lightweight and able to be carried by one person. Clear labelling and provision of an inventory are essential.

(*See also* Nancekievill D. G. *Br. J. Hosp. Med.* 1972, **7**, 593; Caro D. and Irving M. *Lancet* 1973, **1**, 1433; Finch P. and Nancekievill D. G. *Br. J. Hosp. Med.* 1975, **13**, 601; Finch P. and Nancekievill D. G. *Anaesthesia* 1975, **30**, 667; Gabriel R. W. *Anaesthesia* 1977, **32**, 252.)

Field Techniques

Intravenous apparatus, induction agents, muscle relaxants and self-inflating bags are easily carried and may be used in conjunction with tracheal tubes and a portable apparatus as described above. Ether and halothane are the two most promising agents for inhalation. There may, however, be some restrictions preventing the carriage of flammable agents in aircraft. Examples:

1. Thiopentone and muscle relaxant, combined with ether in air from the EMO vaporizer with IPPV using the Oxford inflating bellows. Another method combines thiopentone, suxamethonium, tracheal intubation and IPPV with air.[15]

2. Halothane and air, with IPPV, thiopentone and muscle relaxants, if indicated.

3. Ketamine.[16] This may be useful in the rare accident case where access to the airway is difficult, and when the patient may be shocked. A suitable agent where evacuation to hospital is not available.

4. Entonox is valuable for treatment of trapped casualties.[17] Properly administered it produces good analgesia without reduction of blood pressure or loss of consciousness.

5. Mechanical ventilation in the field.[18]

(*See also* Boulton T. B. and Cole P. V. *Anaesthesia* 1966, **21**, 268, 379, 513; 1967, **22**, 101, 435; Farman J. V. *Anaesthesia and the E.M.O. System*. London: English Universities Press, 1973; Prior F. N. *A Manual of Anaesthesia for the Small Hospital*. New Delhi: Emmanuel Hospital Association, 1974; Freyer M. E. and Boulton T. B. *Anaesthesia* 1977, **32**, 189.)

For anaesthesia in developing countries see Oduro K. A. *Anaesthesia* 1969, **24**, 307; Magbagbeola, J. A. *Br. J. Anaesth.* 1973, **45**, 1217; Simionescu R. *Anaesthesia* 1974, **29**, 318; Phillips L. A. *Anaesthesia* 1974, **29**, 230; Mimpriss T. J. *Anaesthesia* 1974, **29**, 370; Adams A. P. et al. *Anaesthesia* 1975, **30**, 73; *Internat. Forum of Anaesthesia* 1976, **3**, 1108; Hawker D. G. B. *Anaesthesia*, 1977, **32**, 654; Oduntan S. A. and Oduro K. A. *A Handbook of Anaesthesia*. Ibadan: Heinemann Educational Books, 1979; Sankaran B. in: *Regional Anesthesia 1884–1984*. Sweden: Production ICM AB, p. 176; Anaesthetics in the Third World, Prior F. N. *Br. Med. J.* 1984, **288**, 1750; Inhalation anaesthesia in developing countries, Ezi-Ashi T. I. et al. *Anaesthesia* 1983, **38**, 729 and 736;

Operating theatres and equipment for less affluent societies, Bewes P. *Br. Med. J.* 1984, **288**, 1284; *Portable ventilators under field conditions*, Harries M. G. *Anaesthesia* 1983, **38**, 279.

The greatest challenge to practitioners of Western anaesthesia is to see that the most useful parts of the knowledge we already have, is brought to all those who need it.

Anaesthesia in the Dark

Diminution of room lighting, or near-total darkness, may be requested during some endoscopy and radiological procedures. The patient is then exposed to the hazards of unrecognized cyanosis, respiratory obstruction, exhaustion of gas cylinders, etc. Adequate though subdued lighting should always be provided. When lights *have* to be extinguished, the anaesthetist should pay particular attention to the following points: (1) That gas cylinders, particularly oxygen, contain adequate reserves; (2) Tracheal anaesthesia reduces the danger of airway obstruction; (3) Monitoring of vital parameters by auditory and tactile signs; (4) Dimmed lighting must be available for inspection of the fingers, etc; (5) In some anaesthetic machines, vital parts may be fluorescent.

(*See also* Boulton T. B. in: *Recent Advances in Anaesthesia and Analgesia*—11 (Hewer C. L. ed.). Edinburgh: Churchill Livingstone, 1972, Chap. 6; Williams T. N. *Anaesthesia* 1974, **29**, 603.)

References

1. Cox J. and Robinson D. J. *Br. J. Hosp. Med.* 1980, **23**, 144.
2. Gillett G. B. and Patkin M. *Anaesthesia* 1964, **19**, 595.
3. Tate N. *Lancet* 1955, **2**, 980.
4. Siddall W. J. W. *Anaesthesia* 1966, **21**, 221.
5. Epstein H. B. and Macintosh R. R. *Anaesthesia* 1956, **11**, 83.
6. Parkhouse J. *Anaesthesia*, 1966, **21**, 498.
7. Prior F. N. *Anaesthesia* 1972, **27**, 66.
8. Bryce-Smith R. *Anaesthesia* 1964, **19**, 393.
9. Merrifield A. J. et al. *Br. J. Anaesth.* 1967, **39**, 50.
10. Hewer C. L. *Lancet* 1961, **2**, 1290.
11. Flagg P. J. *The Art of Anaesthesia* 7th ed. Philadelphia: Lippincott, 1954.
12. Boulton T. B. *Anaesthesia* 1966, **21**, 513.
13. Stephens K. F. and Bourne J. G. *Lancet* 1960, **2**, 481.
14. Houghton I. T. *Anaesthesia* 1982, **37**, 1094; Knight R. J. *Anaesthesia* 1982, **37**, 1040; Jowett M. D. and Knight R. J. *Anaesthesia* 1983, **38**, 776.
15. Boulton T. B. *Anaesthesia* 1978, **33**, 769.
16. Finch P. and Nancekievill D. G. *Anaesthesia* 1975, **30**, 667; Dobson M. B. *Anaesthesia* 1978, **33**, 868. Fiel M. S. El. *J. Irish Coll. Phys. Surg.* 1981, **11**, 69.
17. Finch P. and Nancekievill D. G. *Anaesthesia* 1975, **30**, 667.
18. Harries M. G. *Anaesthesia* 1983, **38**, 279.

5

Chapter 31   ## REGIONAL ANALGESIA

Optimism and enthusiasm on the part of the anaesthetist or surgeon are no excuse for the infliction of discomfort on the patient.

History

Modern local analgesia began with the introduction of cocaine into medical practice in 1884 by Koller.[1]

The ether spray was used by B. W. Richardson in 1866,[2] 'freezing', and the ethyl chloride spray in 1880 by Rothenstein and in 1890 by P. Redard.[3]

Karl Ludwig Schleich (1859–1922) in Berlin (1892)[4] and Reclus (1847–1914) in Paris (1890)[5] popularized infiltration analgesia, while nerve block, the mandibular, was employed by Halsted and Hall in New York in 1884.[6] As a result of acting as their own guinea-pigs during their researches on the new drug, they became cocaine addicts. First textbook on the subject by J. L. Corning, *Local Anaesthesia in General Medicine and Surgery*. New York: Appleton, 1886, Arthur E. Barker, in 1899, with β-eucaine[7] was using infiltration analgesia at University College Hospital.[8] Braun (1856–1917) introduced adrenaline in 1903 in local analgesia,[9] which was first isolated in pure form in 1897.[10]. The term 'block' first used by G. W. Crile of Cleveland.[11]

Substitutes for the toxic cocaine soon came. Giesel's tropococaine appeared in 1891; Fourneau's stovaine in 1904,[12] and Einhorn's novocaine (procaine), described in 1899,[13] in 1904, popularized by Heinrich Braun in 1905.[14]

Amethocaine described in 1931.[15]

Miescher and Uhlmann introduced Nupercaine in 1929.[16]

Lofgren and Lundqvist synthesized lignocaine in 1943, and Gordh was the first to use it in 1948.[17]

Oil of cloves (eugenol) first used as a local analgesic in dentistry in 1890.[18]

The hypodermic trocar and cannula was described by Rynd (1801–1861) of Meath Hospital and County Infirmary, Dublin in 1845,[19] and by Alexander Wood, a general practitioner, of Edinburgh who used a modified Ferguson syringe in 1855.[20] The latter also popularized hypodermic therapy for the treatment of neuralgia by injecting morphine near to the seat of the pain. Luer all-glass syringes appeared in Paris about 1896; Luer–Lok syringes in the US in 1925. (*See also* Schwidetsky O. *Anesth. Analg. Curr. Res.* 1944, **23**, 34; Jones N. H. *J. Hist. Med.* 1947, **2**, 201.) Until the 1920s, regional analgesia was almost exclusively in the hands of surgeons. For early history of regional analgesia *see* Matas R. *Am. J. Surg.* 1934, **189**, 362.

'Regional anaesthesia' was a term first used by Harvey Cushing (1869–1939) in 1901 to describe pain relief by nerve block.[21]

For history of limb blocks, *see* Bryce-Smith R. in: *Practical Regional Analgesia* (Lee J. A. and Bryce-Smith R. ed.). Amsterdam: Excerpta Medica, 1973, Chap. 3.

In the UK, R. R. Macintosh and R. J. Massey Dawkins have been pioneers and practitioners of regional techniques. Prominent and pioneering workers in regional analgesia in the USA have included R. A. Hingson, J. S. Lundy, G. P. Pitkin, G. Labat, Lincoln Sise, R. D. Dripps, L. Vandam, J. J. Bonica, D. C. Moore, P. C. Lund, P. R. Bromage and Alon Winnie. The American Society of Regional Anesthesia was founded in 1920 by G. Labat and resuscitated in 1976 with A. P. Winnie as president. The journal *Regional Anaesthesia* first published in 1976. For the history of regional block in the USA *see* Moore D. C. in: *Anaesthesia; Essays on its History* (Rupreht J. et al. ed.) Berlin: Springer-Verlag, 1985, p. 128.

General Considerations

Advantages of Regional Analgesia
Effects of drug limited to part of body to be operated on; after-effects usually less than after general anaesthesia; in long operations such as tendon transfers.

Relative Contraindications to Regional Analgesia, when used alone
(1) In children under 10; (2) In the stuporose; (3) In psychotics.

Regional analgesia is used less frequently than it might be because of: (1) Time taken to induce; (2) The fear of failure; (3) The fear of neurological complications; (4) The unpopularity of the awake patient.

Local analgesic drugs are water-soluble salts of lipid-soluble alkaloids. Each molecule is composed of an aromatic portion, intermediate chain and an amide portion. Procaine, chloroprocaine and amethocaine have ester linking the aromatic end of the molecule and the intermediate chain; lignocaine, prilocaine, mepivacaine, bupivacaine and etidocaine have an amide group between the aromatic part of the molecule and the intermediate chain. Ester-linked drugs are degraded by hydrolysis and amides by oxidative dealkylation in the liver. Overall clearance rate is fastest with prilocaine, then lignocaine, mepivacaine and finally bupivacaine. Anaphylactoid reactions are well documented in the case of ester-linked agents, but extremely rare when amide-linked drugs are administered.

With the exception of cocaine (a vasoconstrictor) and lignocaine (no effect on vessels), local analgesic drugs are vasodilators. Vasoconstricting agents such as adrenaline may be added to local analgesic solutions to delay absorption and also to prolong their action.

Adrenaline and noradrenaline do not prolong the action of local analgesic solution applied topically.

Most of the local analgesic drugs are available as hydrochlorides in modified Ringer's solution. Those containing adrenaline are often acid with a pH of 4 or 5, and contain a reducing agent sodium metabisulphite to prevent oxidation of the adrenaline. In addition, a small amount of preservative and fungicide may be added.

Theories of Impulse Conduction along Nerve Fibres

The nerve membrane consists of a bimolecular framework of phospholipid molecules associated with a globular protein mosaic. Non-specific channels, one permeant to sodium and the other to potassium, are thought to be controlled by gates which are voltage-dependent. Myelinated nerves are protected by the myelin sheath which acts as an insulator. The impulse propagation has been studied in the squid axon because of its great size compared with the mammalian fibre. There is a resting potential of $-70\,mV$ on the outside of the membrane, which rises to about $-55\,mV$, the firing threshold, before it jumps up to $+40\,mV$ to form an action potential which constitutes a change of over 100 mV. This is associated with movement of sodium ions inwards and potassium ions outwards, through their respective channels. The membrane becomes depolarized. During recovery, the ions reverse the direction of their movement across the cell membrane. Local analgesic agents may prevent depolarization and so may prevent conduction of impulses.

Impulse blockade.[22] The local analgesic solution prevents depolarization of the nerve membrane. As the concentration increases, the height of the action potential is reduced, the firing threshold is elevated, the spread of impulse conduction is slowed and the refractory period lengthened. Finally, nerve conduction is completely blocked.

It is thought that local analgesic drugs exert their effect by bonding to the internal mouth of the sodium channel.[23] It is likely that specific receptors exist to which molecules of local analgesic drug become attached. Expansion of the membrane also occurs during impulse blockade; this may be the cause of conduction block or may just be an associated phenomenon.

Site of Action

The site of action of local analgesic drugs (and of general anaesthetics too) is at the surface membrane of cells of excitable tissues. In a myelinated nerve the site of action is the node of Ranvier (1835–1909). Two or three adjacent nodes must be affected to prevent conduction; at least 6 mm and perhaps 10 mm of nerve fibre must be exposed to the local analgesic agent or else a blocked segment may be jumped.

The minimum concentration of local drug necessary to cause block of a nerve fibre of given diameter is known as the Cm. The thicker the diameter of a nerve fibre the greater the Cm required. The A delta fibres have a Cm about half that of A alpha fibres; it is therefore possible to block pain sensation while leaving sensation to pressure or position intact. The Cm of preganglionic autonomic B fibres is similar to that of small A so that sympathetic blockade is equivalent to analgesia in spinal analgesia. In practice, the sequence of block is autonomic, sensory, and finally motor block according to fibre diameter. Local analgesics affect not only nerve fibres but all types of excitable tissue, including smooth and striated muscle, e.g. in the myocardium, vessels, etc., probably by interfering with the cation fluxes across the muscle-cell membranes (as in nerve tissue). In moderate doses there is inhibition of activity of ventricular ectopic foci in the heart. The membrane stabilizing effect is shared by other drugs such as phenothiazines, antihistamines, many β-blockers, barbiturates, some antihypertensive agents, e.g. guanethidine.

Uptake

Local analgesic drugs are lipoid-soluble bases which act by penetrating lipoprotein cell membranes in the non-ionized state. In order to make a suitable solution for injection, the non-ionized base has to be converted to the ionized state.

The blocking quality of a local analgesic drug depends on its (1) Potency; (2) Latency (time between its injection and maximum effect)—this in turn depends on nerve diameter, local pH, diffusion rate and concentration of the local drug; (3) Duration of action; (4) Regression time (time between commencement and completion of pain appreciation).

Dissociation constants (pKa). The pKa is the pH at which a local analgesic drug is 50% ionized and 50% non-ionized (base). So local analgesic drugs with pKa values close to physiological pH tend to have a rapid time of onset. The degree of ionization of a molecule is important and the pKa is a measure of this. It may be calculated from the Henderson-Hasselbalch equation, pH = pKa + log base/cation. Most local analgesic agents are weak bases with pKa between 7 and 9, and are relatively insoluble in water. Examples of pKa are: lignocaine, 7·87; amethocaine, 8·50; bupivacaine, 7·74; procaine, 8·92. They are usually prepared for clinical use as the acid salt. The un-ionized form is lipid soluble and can spread through tissues and penetrate membranes; the cation is the active agent to produce the pharmacological effect. pH of local analgesic solution may be lowered by addition of adrenaline, sodium metabisulphite (antioxidant) and glucose. When the buffering effect of the tissue is low, local analgesic drugs may be less effective. This occurs in inflamed tissues. Mucous membranes also have minimal buffer reserve and this is one reason why higher concentrations of drugs are needed for topical analgesia.

Carbonated local analgesic solutions. The manufacture is difficult and expensive, so that carbonated drugs are commercially available only in Canada and West Germany. Carbonated lignocaine and prilocaine produce a shorter latent period and more intense blockade than the hydrochloride salts,[24] but trials of carbonated bupivacaine have proved disappointing.[25]

For further information about impulse conduction and impulse blockade by local analgesic drugs, *see* Corvino B. G. and Vassallo H. G. *Local Anesthetics: Mechanisms of Action and Clinical Use*. New York: Grune and Stratton, 1976; de Jong, R. H. *Local Anesthetics* 2nd ed. Springfield, Ill.: Thomas, 1977; Bromage P. R. *Epidural Analgesia*. Philadelphia: Saunders, 1978; *Lumbar Puncture and Spinal Analgesia; Intradural and Extradural* 5th ed. (Lee, J. Alfred et al. ed.) Edinburgh & London: Churchill Livingstone, 1985.

Biotransformation
Ester-linked drugs are hydrolysed in the plasma by plasma cholinesterase, the rate depending on substitution in the aromatic ring of the molecule. Half-life in plasma varies from less than 1 minute (chloroprocaine) to 8 min (amethocaine) and is prolonged in the presence of atypical cholinesterase.

Amide-linked drugs undergo biotransformation in the liver, the rate of clearance being dependent on hepatic blood flow and drug extraction by the liver.[26] Hepatic blood flow may be altered in general anaesthesia and as a result of administering vasoactive drugs. Extraction by the liver may be diminished in conditions such as cirrhosis, congestive cardiac failure, hypothermia and the administration of cimetidine. Half-life is likely to vary between 1·5 and 3 hours.

Toxicity
The following factors influence toxicity: (1) Quantity of solution; (2) Concentra-

tion of drug; (3) Presence or absence of adrenaline; (4) Vascularity of site of injection; (5) Rate of absorption of drug, e.g. rate is rapid from bronchial mucosa; (6) Rate of destruction of drug; (7) Hypersensitivity of patient; (8) Age, physical status and weight of patient. Toxic signs not always related to dosage.

A study of plasma concentration of local analgesic drugs suggests that higher levels are reached after lignocaine than after prilocaine in equal dosage. Addition of adrenaline to the local infiltration reduces the plasma concentration of lignocaine but not of prilocaine. Higher plasma levels are found after intercostal block than after extradural injection.[27] Plasma concentrations of local analgesic drugs correspond very poorly with the patient's body weight. The site of injection is far more important.[28] There is no maximum safe dose for all procedures. Skeletal injuries, including dislocation of the shoulder joint, have been caused by convulsions due to the toxicity of local analgesic agents.[251]

1. Central Nervous System
Central stimulation followed by depression, restlessness, hysterical behaviour, vertigo, tremor, convulsions and respiratory failure. Treatment consists in: (1) Artificial ventilation with oxygen or air; (2) Intravenous or intramuscular injection of suxamethonium or just sufficient thiopentone to control convulsions (100–150 mg). Diazepam may be useful. A rise in Pa_{CO_2} increases tendency to convulsions, so treatment should include hyperventilation with oxygen.

2. Cardiovascular System
Hypotension. Acute collapse—primary cardiac failure. This has followed moderate amounts given intravenously of etidocaine and bupivacaine.[29] Feeble pulse and cardiovascular collapse, bradycardia, pallor, sweating, and hypotension. This type of intoxication may be due to a rapid absorption of the drug.
Treatment. Elevate legs; give oxygen by IPPV; rapid intravenous infusion; raise blood pressure; cardiac massage if necessary. Resuscitation after the longer acting drugs, bupivacaine and etidocaine, may be difficult and lengthy.[30] High-energy shock electrical defibrillation may be required.[31]

3. Respiratory Depression
This may progress to apnoea from medullary depression or respiratory muscle paralysis. It may have delayed onset.

4. Allergic Phenomena
Allergy, a term introduced by C. P. von Pirquet (1874–1929) in 1906. Rare: may take form of bronchospasm, urticaria or angioneurotic oedema.[32] Well documented in association with the use of ester-linked agents, including contact dermatitis in personnel handling procaine.[33] Cross-sensitivity can occur. Allergy to amide-linked agents is extremely rare but has been reported.[34] In many thousands of administrations the authors have never seen this. Injections of adrenaline, hydrocortisone and oxygen therapy by IPPV and i.v. colloid solutions may be necessary.

Reactions to vasoconstrictor drugs may include pallor, anxiety, palpitations, tachycardia, hypertension and tachypnoea and may respond to a β-blocker. Care should be taken in patients receiving mono-amine oxidase inhibitors or tricyclic antidepressants.

Toxicity may occur as a result of simple overdosage, by inadvertent intravenous injection, or because of susceptibility of the patient to normal dosage. Injection with a moving needle, together with frequent aspiration testing, minimizes risk of intravenous injection. No preservatives such as phenol, chlorocresol or sodium sulphite should be used when any large volume of local analgesic solution is to be injected. Allergic reactions may be due to methylparaben, sometimes used in commercial preparations of local analgesic solutions as a stabilizing agent.[35]

Toxic signs are often due to intravenous injection.

There is evidence that local analgesic drugs may have cytotoxic effects, although harmful clinical consequences are difficult to find.[36]

(*See also* Scott D. B. *Br. J. Anaesth.* 1981, **53**, 553.)

Improving Duration and Quality of Local Analgesia
1. Addition of adrenaline, e.g. 1–200 000 to 1–500 000 solution.
2. Free base is liberated quickly due to rapid buffering and liberation of CO_2 which diffuses across cell membranes. Thus the analgesic base is brought closer to nerve tissue more rapidly and in higher concentration, resulting in a more widespread and more intensive block. The amount of free base available determines the rate of diffusion of the local analgesic solution. Adjusting the pH to about 7 (alkalinization) reduces the time of onset and the duration of analgesia. Substitution of the carbonated salts of local analgesic drugs for the hydrochloride, the pH of carbonated salts (6·5) is relatively higher than other acid salts so that speedy buffering occurs with liberation of free base and CO_2 which diffuses to lower the pH inside the nerve sheath (diffusion trapping).[37,62]

Premedication
Adequate premedication is essential for successful local analgesia in major surgery. The subject is set out in the chapter on Spinal Analgesia (*see* Chapter 32).

Methods of Local Analgesia
(1) Infiltration analgesia, to abolish the pain due to surgical intervention and to ease pain associated with trauma and the injection of irritant drugs. The direct injection of drugs into the area to be incised and between bone ends in fractures; (2) Field block. The injection of a local analgesic so as to create a zone of analgesia around the operative field; (3) Nerve block (conduction anaesthesia). The injection of a solution of local analgesic drug near the nerve or nerves supplying the area to be operated on. The use of a peripheral nerve stimulator increases the accuracy of needle placement and the success of the block;[38] (4) Refrigeration analgesia (*see* Chapter 17); (5) Intravenous local analgesia; (6) Topical or surface analgesia; (7) Central neural blockade (Chapter 32).

Pharmacodynamics and Pharmacokinetics of Drugs used in Local Analgesia

A molecule of local analgesic drug possesses an aromatic or lipophilic group and a hydrophilic group with a linking chain between them which may be an ester (COO—) or an amide (NH·CO—).

A. Ester-linked Drugs

1. Cocaine (Benzoyl methylecgonine hydrochloride)[39]

A derivative of the nitrogenous base ecgonine and an ester of benzoic acid. Cocaine is extracted from the leaves of *Erythroxylon coca*, a shrub indigenous to Bolivia and Peru, which the natives have chewed for centuries for their stimulant effect; 100 g of leaves yield 200 mg of cocaine. Easily decomposed by heat sterilization. Cocaine is soluble in water and alcohol and is now used solely for topical analgesia. It is an excellent surface analgesic and has a vasoconstrictor effect, 4% being a suitable strength. It is often toxic when injected.[40] A dangerous drug of addiction. Duration of effect, 20–30 min. Solutions should be protected from the light. pKa 8·7. (For history of coca plant, *see* Christensen E. M. *Anaesthesia*, 1947, **2**, 4; *Time Magazine* 1981, 6th July, p. 42; Images of cocaine *Lancet* (Leader) 1983, **2**, 1231.)

History. Specimens of the leaves and bark of the plant containing cocaine were brought to Europe in the middle of the 19th century by Dr Scherzer, scientific officer in an Austro-Hungarian round-the-world voyage in the naval frigate *Novara*. Several sacks of the leaves were made available to Viennese investigators and an alkaloid was isolated in 1855 by Gaedcke. Niemann (1840–1921), a pupil of Wohler (1800–1882), purified erythroxylon and described its numbing effects and named the alkaloid in 1860[41]; its local analgesic effects were noticed in 1868 by Moreno y Maiz, surgeon-in-chief to the Peruvian Army,[42] and also by von Anrep (1852–1902) of Würzburg in 1878.[43] Was prescribed by Freud (and used by Sherlock Holmes!) for its stimulating effects and as a cure for morphine addiction.[44] Carl Koller (1858–1944) introduced to cocaine by Sigmund Freud (1856–1939) proved its use in surgery (of the cornea) in 1884[45] using 2% solution in water; this was reported on 15 September 1884, at the Congress of Ophthalmology at Heidelberg.[46] The drug was originally prepared by Merck of Darmstadt. Used by W. C. Burke of South Norwalk, Connecticut, for removal of a revolver bullet from a hand (5 minims of 2% solution) in November 1884, in urology by F. N. Otis (1825–1900) in 1884 in New York, and also by R. J. Hall (1856–1897) and William Stewart Halsted (1852–1922)[47] at the Roosevelt Hospital in New York, each of whom injected it into his own arms[48] and each becoming an addict. First synthesized in 1924.[49]

Pharmacodynamics

Central Nervous System. This is stimulated from above downwards:

On the cortex, excitement and restlessness are caused and mental powers increased. There is euphoria and a decreased sense of fatigue, hence its tendency to cause addiction. In higher dosage convulsions are followed by apnoea and death.

The sympathetic nervous system is stimulated. As cocaine is a powerful vasoconstrictor, adrenaline added to it is not only unnecessary but also increases the risks of cardiac dysrhythmia and ventricular fibrillation. The two drugs should not be used together.[50]

It inhibits mono-amine oxidase. It is not destroyed by cholinesterase.

Cardiovascular system. Small doses increase the pulse rate, raise the blood pressure and potentiate the effects of adrenaline on capillaries (dilatation or constriction). Dysrhythmias may occur, but can be reversed by beta blockade.

Eye. Mydriasis, perhaps due to sympathetic stimulation; there is blanching of the conjunctiva from vasoconstriction, clouding of the corneal epithelium and, rarely, ulceration, together with excellent analgesia. Used as 1% solution for analgesia. Eserine counteracts the mydriatic effect of cocaine and atropine increases it. Now seldom employed in ophthalmology.

Pharmacokinetics

Absorption. From all mucous membranes, including the urethra and bladder. There is some evidence that stronger solutions are absorbed less readily than weaker solutions, owing to the increased vasoconstriction they produce. In nose and throat surgery used in 1% to 20% solution. Can be employed usefully as a spray to produce ischaemia of the nose, e.g. before nasal intubation.

Excretion. Cocaine is detoxicated in the liver, one metabolite being ecognine, a CNS stimulant. About 10% is excreted by the kidneys, unchanged.

A safe dose of cocaine for surface analgesia is 2 ml of 4% solution. It was for years used to overcome drowsiness due to chronic morphine addiction in the treatment of severe pain in terminal disease (e.g. in the Brompton cocktail).[51] *See also* Gay G. R. *Anesth. Analg. (Cleve.)* 1976, **55**, 582.

2. Procaine Hydrochloride, BP (Novocain, Planocaine, Ethocaine, Neocaine) *p*-amino-benzoyl-diethyl amino-ethanol hydrochloride.

pKa 8·9. The standard local analgesic agent until the advent of lignocaine. Synthesized by Alfred Einhorn (1856–1917) of Munich in 1899.[13] Like amethocaine, it inhibits the bacteriostatic action of *p*-aminosalicylic acid and the sulphonamides. Should be stored in a cool place to retard hydrolysis.

For infiltration the strength used is 0·25–1%; for nerve block, 1–2%. Procaine 5·05% in water is iso-osmotic, with pH of 6·4. Hydrolysed by serum cholinesterase, diethyl amino-ethanol and *p*-aminobenzoic acid being formed. Biotransformation requires absorption into the bloodstream as neural tissue and cerebrospinal fluid lack esterases.

Analgesia lasts from 45 to 90 min when adrenaline is added. Relatively non-toxic.

Procaine has been recommended as the agent of choice in patients with a history of malignant hyperpyrexia.[52] A concentration of 5% may be necessary for successful extradural block.[53]

Procaine intravenously has been recommended for the treatment of malignant hyperpyrexia, in almost toxic doses. (*See* Chapter 18.)

3. Chloroprocaine Hydrochloride

An ester of para-aminobenzoic acid. has been in use in the USA since 1952. Quick onset of effect, but analgesia may disappear suddenly. Rapid hydrolysis makes it relatively non-toxic and it is not easily transferred across the placenta. Effect lasts about 45 min. Used as a 2 or 3% solution, pKa 8·7. Initial dose for obstetrical extradural block 8–10 ml, which can be followed by bupivacaine.[54,55] The most acid of local analgesic agents commonly used (3% solution has pH of 3·3). Paraplegia has been reported following its use, particularly after intradural injection for which it is not recommended. This may be due to sodium metabisulphite in the commercial solution.[56] *See also* Chapter 32.

4. Amethocaine   Hydrochloride,   BP (Pantocaine,   Pontocaine,   Decicain,

Butethanol, Anethaine, tetracine (USP)
Synthesized by O. Eisleb in Germany in 1928. pKa 8·2. Solutions prepared under sterile conditions remain sterile and bactericidal. Like cocaine, it may cause cardiac asystole or ventricular fibrillation. Used for topical and corneal analgesia in 0·5% solution. The solution can be boiled once or twice without deterioration, but is rendered inactive by alkalis. It should be protected from light. For infiltration the usual strength is 1–2000 to 1–4000, preferably with adrenaline. Up to 200 ml of 1–2000 solution with adrenaline can safely be used for infiltration analgesia. It is hydrolysed completely by serum cholinesterase but four times more slowly than is procaine. None is found in bile or urine. Used for intradural block (*see* Chapter 32).

The maximum dose is 100 mg or 1·5 mg/kg of body weight. Large doses are unwise and maximum for surface analgesia should be 8 ml of 0·5% solution in two or three divided doses with an interval of 5 min between each dose. A lozenge containing 60 mg amethocaine is available. Absorption from the bronchial tree—when analgesia for bronchoscopy is being induced—is almost as rapid as that following intravenous injection.

Its effect lasts longer than that of procaine and lignocaine, roughly 1½–3 h. Onset of analgesia slow. For intradural block, 0·5–1% solution may be used; for extradural block 0·25–0·5% with adrenaline. The addition of adrenaline greatly reduces its toxicity, toxic signs being similar in appearance and treatment to those of cocaine.

B. Amide-linked Drugs

1. *Lignocaine Hydrochloride, BP* (Xylocaine, Duncaine, lidocaine)
The most commonly used local analgesic agent in the UK today. A tertiary amide, synthesized by Nils Lofgren (1922–1953) and Lundqvist in 1943 in Sweden.[57] First used by Gordh (1907–)of the Karolinska Hospital, Stockholm in 1948.[58] Very stable, not decomposed by boiling, acids or alkalis. The pKa is 7·86. Solutions of 0·25–0·5% for infiltration, with adrenaline 1–250 000; 4% for topical analgesia, in surgery of throat, larynx, pharynx, etc. For nerve block 1·5–2% with adrenaline, and for extradural block 1·2–2% with adrenaline. For corneal analgesia 4%; this causes no mydriasis, vasoconstriction or cycloplegia. For urethral analgesia 1–2% in jelly and for tracheal tubes 5% as an ointment. Toxicity not great, but cardiovascular and central nervous symptoms of poisoning may occur. Can be toxic when ingested orally. The clearance of lignocaine is reduced in the presence of propranolol, with increased risk of toxicity. As in the case of prilocaine, the metabolism of lignocaine can give rise to the formation of methaemoglobin. It is not a vasodilator nor does it interfere with the vasoconstrictive action of adrenaline. It has a cerebral effect, causing drowsiness and amnesia. It is metabolized by oxidases and amidases from microsomes in the liver, but this is retarded in chronic liver disease.[59] It is excreted renally, hastened when the urine is acid. Duration of effect of 1% solution, 1 h; with adrenaline, 1½–2 h. Has rapid onset. Has been given intravenously in 40-mg doses at 5-min intervals, to potentiate the analgesia of thiopentone–gas–oxygen–relaxant combination, and also intramuscularly in 250-mg doses in 2% solution. Has been used in the treatment of status epilepticus, and due to its cell membrane-stabilizing effect on cardiac tissue for ventricular dysrhythmias, by intravenous injection. As lignocaine may facilitate the release of calcium from

sarcoplasmic reticulum, it should not be used in patients susceptible to malignant hyperpyrexia.[60] Its use in the treatment of cardiac infarction is not proven. While it controls the non-dangerous unifocal ectopics, it is far less successful in cases of multifocal ectopics. Suggested maximum safe dose of lignocaine for a 70-kg man—with adrenaline, 500 mg, i.e. 7 mg/kg; without adrenaline, 200 mg, i.e. 3 mg/kg body weight.

The carbonate of lignocaine (and prilocaine) has been investigated[61] and found to give greater speed of onset and intensity of both sensory and motor block, in comparison with the hydrochloride salt, especially in the L.5 and S.1 segments. On injection the CO_2 diffuses out of the drug, so raising the tissue pH and increasing the concentration of the un-ionized base.[62]

Toxic effects are twitching, convulsions, apnoea and acute cardiac failure.

2. Mepivacaine (Carbocaine, Meaverin)

This is a tertiary amine synthesized in 1956 by Ekenstam and Egner[63] and used first by Dhuner in 1956.[64] It is clinically comparable with lignocaine. It is resistant to acid and alkaline hydrolysis. The pKa is 7·8. Seventy per cent of the drug becomes protein bound (greater than in the case of lignocaine but less than with bupivacaine). Most of the drug is metabolized in the liver and some has been recovered from the urine (increased by acidification). Unlike lignocaine, it is not metabolized by neonates; eliminated via the kidneys. It is claimed to be a little less toxic than lignocaine while its local analgesic effects last rather longer. The subconvulsive dose in man is 5 mg/kg.[65] When injected into the extradural space of patients in labour it passes rather rapidly into the fetal circulation where it may cause harm. It would appear to have few advantages over lignocaine. A dose of 400 mg should not be exceeded (about 5 mg/kg body weight). For extradural analgesia 15 ml of 2% or 20 ml of 1·5% solution; for intradural block 1–2 ml of heavy 4% solution. Has anti-dysrhythmic properties.

3. Bupivacaine (Marcain, Marcaine, Sensorcaine, Carbosterin)

This amide-type local analgesic drug was synthesized in Sweden by Ekenstam and his colleagues in 1957,[66] and used clinically by L. J. Telivuo (1923–1970) in 1963.[67] The base is not very soluble but the hydrochloride readily dissolves in water. The pKa is 8·2. It is very stable both to repeated autoclaving and to acids and alkalis, but solutions containing adrenaline should not be autoclaved more than twice. It is reputed to be four times as potent as both mepivacaine and lignocaine, so that a 0·5% solution is roughly equivalent to 2% lignocaine. More cardiotoxic than lignocaine and this is made worse by hypoxia, hypercapnia and by pregnancy.[68] It causes more sensory than motor block. It is not recommended for intravenous regional analgesia as leakage past the tourniquet into the bloodstream may cause toxic or even fatal complications. Duration of effect is between 5 and 16 h, one of the longest acting local analgesic known. This may be more related to binding to nerve tissue than to its overall retention in the body. Duration of action of a local analgesic drug correlates with binding to plasma lipoproteins. At the same concentration bupivacaine is longer acting than etidocaine. A small percentage of a given dose of bupivacaine is excreted unchanged in the urine. The remainder is metabolized in the liver. The N-dealkylated metabolite, pipecolyloxylidine, is found in the urine.[69] Maximal dose is 2 mg/kg body weight (25–30 ml of 0·5% solution) and the strength used is 0·125–0·75% with or without adrenaline 1–200 000 or 1–400 000;

adrenaline does not greatly prolong its effect but reduces its toxicity. The carbonated form probably has few advantages over the hydrochloride salt. A plain solution of 0·5% has been much used for intradural block, either alone or made hyperbaric with dextrose (*see* Chapter 34) and for extradural analgesia. The pH of the 0·5% solution with adrenaline is 3·5 and its density 0·997 g/ml at 37 °C.

4. *Etidocaine Hydrochloride* (Duranest, W-19053)

This long-acting local analgesic drug is related chemically to lignocaine and was described in 1972.[70] It is a stable compound and can be autoclaved up to five times without deterioration. The onset of action is rapid and the duration of action is long (comparable to bupivacaine). It is very lipid-soluble and almost completely protein-bound; metabolic pathways not yet determined. Probably retained in the body longer than other local analgesic drugs. It is probably less toxic than bupivacaine but certainly more toxic than lignocaine.[71] Gives good motor block. pKa 7·7.

The drug has been used in extradural block but in obstetric analgesia has the disadvantage that motor block is readily produced. It has been used in 0·25 and 0·5% concentration. The former may give inadequate analgesia, the latter inappropriate motor block.

Concentrations of up to 1·5% have been used with success in extradural block for surgical operations. Maximal dose: 4 mg/kg.

It is a useful topical analgesic, similar to bupivacaine and stronger than lignocaine.

5. *Prilocaine Hydrochloride* (Citanest, Xylonest, Distanest)

A close relation of lignocaine to which it is clinically comparable. A secondary amide. Described by Lofgren and Tegner,[72] tested pharmacologically by Wiedling,[73] and used clinically by Gordh in 1959.[74] A very stable compound, pharmacologically resembling lignocaine but less toxic, pKa 7·9. Whereas lignocaine is metabolized in the liver, prilocaine is metabolized also in the kidneys and lungs and more rapidly, partly by amidase. Little drug reaches the urine. This rapid metabolism may account for the methaemoglobinaemia sometimes seen after its use, if more than 600 mg are injected. A maximal safe dose without adrenaline is 400 mg; with adrenaline 600 mg.

Methaemoglobin is continuously formed during red-cell metabolism but normally does not exceed 1% of the haemoglobin at any one time. The cause of this oxidation of haemoglobin to methaemoglobin is not prilocaine itself but one of its degradation products. The degree of cyanosis due to methaemoglobin following prilocaine varies in different individuals and usually disappears spontaneously in 24 h. It is of little clinical importance unless there is severe anaemia or circulatory impairment. The presence of cyanosis indicates that 1·5% or more of the haemoglobin is circulating as methaemoglobin. There is an associated shift of the oxygen dissociation curve of the remaining haemoglobin which hinders oxygen liberation at tissue level. Methaemoglobin crosses the placenta. A dose of 16 mg/kg or more is necessary to cause symptoms of hypoxia and is only likely to be seen after extradural block with repeated injections through a catheter. Congenital or acquired methaemoglobinaemia are probably contraindications to the use of the agent. Treatment is by intravenous injection of 1% methylene blue, 1–2 mg/kg.

In extradural block the drug has been shown to give a slower onset and spread with a longer duration of effect and greater intensity than lignocaine, with less toxicity. The addition of adrenaline prolongs the duration of effect less with prilocaine than with lignocaine. Can be used for intradural block (*see* Chapter 32).

It is most useful when high dosage and strong concentration are required of a local analgesic drug as when injection is into vascular areas, e.g. pudendal block and blocks about the face and neck, and for Bier's intravenous local analgesia in 0·5% solution, for which it is most suitable.[75] For topical analgesia 10 ml of 4% solution is reasonable. A rough guide to dosage is to regard 4 mg/kg as reasonably safe.

See review 'Citanest' (Wielding S. ed.), *Acta Anaesth. Scand.* 1965, Suppl. 16.

6. *Cinchocaine Hydrochloride* (Nupercaine, dibucaine, Percain, Sovcaine, Dulzit) Synthesized by Karl Miescher in 1925[76] and used for many years for spinal analgesia (intradural) with great satisfaction, and also for infiltration and surface analgesia. No longer commercially available in the UK.

For chemistry of local analgesic agents, *see* Geddes I. C. *Br. J. Anaesth.* 1967, **34**, 229; Cousins M. and Maher L. E. *Anaesth. Intensive Care* 1980, **8**, 257.

Lecithin-coated microdroplets of methoxyflurane produce long-lasting local analgesia which is stable and localized.[77]

Autoclaving of Local Analgesic Drugs
The commonly used agents are very stable chemical compounds. Ampoules of the hydrochloride salts of lignocaine, prilocaine, mepivacaine, bupivacaine, etidocaine and procaine can all be autoclaved and thereafter show no chemical change on chromatographic analysis. They are not inactivated by gamma radiation (25 Mrad).

Drugs Used for Vasoconstriction

For history of sympathomimetic amines, *see* Runciman W. B. et al. *Anaesth. Intensive Care* 1980, **8**, 289.

Vasoconstrictor drugs have been used in local analgesia since Braun introduced adrenaline in 1902.[78]

The adrenaline-induced contraction of the smooth muscle of vessel walls is modified to different degrees by the same molar concentrations of different local analgesic agents and by different concentrations of the same agent.[79] The vascularity of the tissues receiving the injection is also a factor to be considered in estimating the optimal concentration in a given case. Vasoconstrictors are employed: (1) To retard absorption and reduce toxicity; (2) To prolong analgesic activity; (3) To produce ischaemia.

Adrenaline BP (Epinephrine USP)
The tartrate, which is synthetic, is used for injection and contains a stabilizer, potassium metabitartrite, 0·1% which increases the acidity of the solution. Many workers add their own adrenaline to local analgesic solutions, preferring this to the commercially available mixtures, in extradural block. It is used less

frequently in intradural block. The hydrochloride, which is of animal origin, is for topical application. For infiltration it is probably unnecessary to use a strength greater than 1–200 000, although dentists employ 1–80 000. Discoloration indicates decomposition; it can be autoclaved once but not repeatedly. For infiltration to produce ischaemia before incision the usual amount added is 1 mg to 250–500 ml of saline, giving a 1–250 000 to 1–500 000 solution. It is probably unwise to inject more than 0·5 mg at one time. The addition of adrenaline reduces the uptake of lignocaine by the circulation more than that of the other amide-linked agents.

It is an α-adrenergic stimulant and may produce pallor, tachycardia and syncope. It should be used with the greatest care if chloroform, cyclopropane or halothane is to be given, lest the combination should cause ventricular fibrillation. It has been suggested that, providing there is no hypercapnia or hypoxia, 10 ml of 1–100 000 adrenaline solution can be injected with safety in any 10-min period and not more than 30 ml/h.[80] Vasoconstrictors help to produce a dry operative field. Adverse reactions to adrenaline and noradrenaline are most likely to occur following intravascular injection, especially in patients with diabetes, heart disease, thyrotoxicosis, epilepsy and those receiving some halogenated anaesthetics or drug therapy involving tricyclic antidepressants or adrenergic neuron-blocking drugs. (*See also* Chapter 19.)

Phenylephrine (Neosynephrine)
Used for vasoconstriction during local analgesia, 0·25–0·5 ml of 1% solution added to each 100 ml of local analgesic solution. Causes no cerebral stimulation or tachycardia.

Noradrenaline
This can be used to produce local vasoconstriction but is less effective than adrenaline as it is a weaker α-receptor stimulant. Does not stimulate the β-receptors in muscle so causes no ischaemia there. It is oxidized in the body more rapidly by amine oxidase than is adrenaline. Tricyclic antidepressants increase its pressor effects. (*See also* Chapter 19.)

Felypressin (PVL-2, Octopressin)
This is 2-phenylalanine-8-lysine vasopressin and may prove to be a good local vasoconstrictor for use along with halothane, cyclopropane, trichloroethylene, etc. It is a synthetic derivative of the octapeptide hormone, vasopressin, from the posterior pituitary. It causes constriction of all smooth muscle but has little oxytocic or antidiuretic effect. May result in coronary arterial constriction, but has little influence on cardiac rhythm. Unlike adrenaline it does not alter cardiac rate or rhythm in dental surgery. Available with 3% prilocaine for dental use.

Techniques of Regional Analgesia

Before any large volume of local analgesic solution is injected, the following should be available: (1) An open vein; (2) A tilting table or trolley; (3) Facilities for IPPV with oxygen; (4) Suction equipment and catheters; (5) Syringes, needles and ampoules of thiopentone, suxamethonium, diazepam and pressor drugs; (6) Fluid for infusion.

Uses of Vasoconstrictors in Patients on Other Drugs

Vasoconstrictors are unlikely to cause special dangers in patients taking mono-amine oxidase inhibitors, the common tranquillizers or hypotensive agents, as catecholamines are not destroyed by metabolic processes. If volatile anaesthetic agents are being given at the same time, suitable β-blocking agents should be available and of course both hypoxia and hypercapnia avoided. Some dental cartridges contain adrenaline 1–80000 solution, but felypressin can be substituted. With tricyclic antidepressants, the cardiovascular effects of catecholamines may be increased. They should not be used together.

Identification of Nerves

Facilitated in many nerve blocks by an electric current (6–8 V, 2 Hz) via a needle, insulated apart from its tip. Muscular contraction shows proximity to nerve.[81] Nerves can be located using voltages high enough to stimulate motor fibres without causing sensory discomfort as sensory stimulation requires a higher voltage than motor stimulation.[82]

Topical Analgesia[83] (Greek *topos*, 'a place')

Can be applied: (1) On gauze swabs; (2) As a liquid in a spray; (3) As a paste or ointment; (4) As an aerosol; (5) By direct instillation, e.g. conjunctival sac, nose and trachea.

Sites

(1) The upper air passages, e.g. 4% lignocaine, 5 ml. A 10% aerosol of lignocaine, two squirts is safe;[84] (2) The nasal cavities, e.g. 4% cocaine is potentiated by sodium bicarbonate; (3) The external ear, e.g. 10% lignocaine aerosol for paracentesis; (4) The conjunctival sac, e.g. 4% lignocaine or 2–4% cocaine or 0·5% amethocaine. Stinging pain on instillation can be eased if the drug is dissolved in methyl cellulose; (5) Perineum and vagina in obstetrics, e.g. 10% lignocaine aerosol for spontaneous delivery or for suture of simple lacerations; (6) Urethra, e.g. 1% lignocaine gel; (7) Before open wound closure.[263]

Infiltration Analgesia

Popularized by C. L. Schleich (1853–1922) of Berlin in 1892. A weal is raised with a fine needle and through this weal a larger needle is used to inject the main bulk of solution. Procaine or lignocaine 0·5–1% solution, each with adrenaline, is ideal for this procedure. *For painless skin incisions, infiltration should be intradermal as well as subcutaneous.* For maximal intradermal analgesia the adrenaline should be omitted.[85] A slow, gentle technique is important, and the solution should be injected while the needle is moving to reduce the chances of intravenous injection.

A patient taking debrisoquine (Declinax) for hypertension may develop total ischaemia in areas infiltrated with lignocaine–adrenaline solutions.[86]

As with all forms of local analgesia, the effect is not instantaneous and a proper interval must elapse between injection and incision. Patience!

Transverse Injection Anaesthesia

A name given by Russian surgeons to a method (Vishnevsky technique) in which a transverse disk of tissue of a limb is infiltrated from skin to bone with a dilute solution of an analgesic drug such as 0·5% procaine in large volume. In the vernacular 'the squirt-and-cut' technique.

Field Block of Scalp and Cranium

Anatomy
The trigeminal nerve supplies the anterior two-thirds, the posterior divisions of cervical nerves the posterior third. (*Fig.* 31.1.)

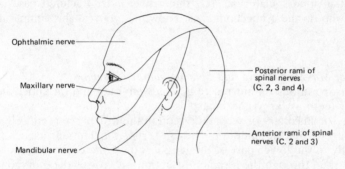

Fig. 31.1. Showing the cutaneous nerve areas of the face and scalp. (*From 'Gray's Anatomy', by kind permission of the Editor.*)

There are five sensory nerves in front of the ear and four behind it.

These nerves all converge towards the vertex of the scalp, so that a band of infiltration passing just above the ear through the glabella and the occiput will block them all.

Technique
Injections of 0·5% lignocaine with adrenaline solution must be made in three layers: (1) The skin, intradermal; (2) The subcutaneous tissues superficial to the epicranial aponeurosis in which the nerves and vessels lie, and also below the aponeurosis; (3) The periosteum.

In addition, solution should be injected into the substance of the temporalis muscle. The dura is insensitive except at the base of the skull.

For removal of sebaceous cysts or suturing of small wounds, the area is surrounded by a zone of infiltration. Periosteal injection is only necessary if bone is to be removed.

Useful in some cases of acute head injury and also to reduce haemorrhage in intracranial operations under general anaesthesia.

Nerve Block for Nose Operations

Anatomy
The nerve supply is from the first or ophthalmic division and from the second or

maxillary division of the trigeminal nerve.

In more detail: *The skin of the nose* is supplied by the supratrochlear branch of frontal nerve of the ophthalmic; the anterior ethmoidal branch of the nasociliary (ophthalmic); the infraorbital branch of the maxillary. *The maxillary antrum of Highmore*: its lining is supplied by the maxillary nerve via the sphenopalatine ganglion. *The frontal sinus*: frontal nerve; branch of ophthalmic. *The ethmoid region*: the anterior and posterior ethmoidal branches of the nasociliary.

The sensory supply of the nasal cavities—fifth nerve—is as follows: The anterior one-third of the septum and lateral walls by the anterior ethmoidal branch of the nasociliary nerve (division 1). The posterior two-thirds of the septum and lateral walls by the long sphenopalatine nerves from the sphenopalatine ganglion (division 2).

Injections into the nose or orbit (ethmoid region, septum, middle turbinates, etc. may result in total spinal block (cf. rhinorrhoea after fractured base of skull). Surgeons who do these injections must know how to treat this complication.[87]

Techniques

1. Block of Maxillary Nerve and Sphenopalatine Ganglion
Useful for operations on antrum (e.g. Caldwell–Luc) and on upper lip, palate and upper teeth as far as the bicuspids.

Anatomy. The maxillary or second division of the fifth nerve is entirely sensory. It is given off from the middle of the Gasserian ganglion and passes forwards horizontally in the lower part of the lateral wall of the cavernous sinus until it leaves the skull through the foramen rotundum. It crosses the pterygomaxillary fissure to enter the orbit through the inferior orbital fissure and ends as the infra-orbital nerve after emerging on to the face through the infraorbital foramen. The sphenopalatine ganglion of Meckel is situated in the pterygopalatine fossa in the upper part of the pterygomaxillary fissure, lateral to the sphenopalatine foramen. Blocking of the nerve causes analgesia in the lateral nasal, inferior palpebral and superior labial nerves, the posterior, middle and anterior superior alveolar nerves, and the palatal nerves which supply the skin of the upper lip, side of nose, lower eyelid and malar region, the teeth of the upper jaw and the underlying periosteum, the mucosa of the maxillary antrum and of the hard and soft palate, and the posterior part of the nasal cavity.

A weal is raised 0·5 cm below the midpoint of the zygoma, which is over the anterior border of the coronoid process, and through it a needle is introduced at right angles to the median plane of the head until it strikes the lateral plate of the pterygoid process at a depth of about 4 cm. Set marker 1 cm from skin surface and reinsert needle slightly anteriorly so that its point glances past the anterior margin of the external pterygoid plate and advances as far as the marker. The needle point should be in the pterygomaxillary fissure. The needle has been known to enter the pharynx or the orbit. If aspiration test is negative, 3–4 ml of 1·5% solution of lignocaine is injected and a similar amount as the needle is slowly withdrawn.

Transient paralysis of the sixth cranial nerve may result; it soon passes off.

2. Block of Anterior Ethmoidal Nerve (Median Orbital Block)
This is a branch of the nasociliary nerve and is blocked in the medial wall of the orbit as the nerve passes through the anterior ethmoidal foramen. A weal is

raised 1 cm above the caruncle at the inner canthus of the eye. A small needle is introduced along the upper medial angle of the orbit for 3·5 cm keeping near the bone. Injection is made of 2 ml of 1·5% lignocaine.

3. Block of Frontal Nerve
From the same weal as in anterior ethmoid block, the needle is introduced more laterally towards the central part of the roof of the orbit where the frontal nerve lies between the periosteum and the levator palpebrae superioris. Lignocaine, 1 ml of 2% solution, is injected in close contact with the bone.

4. Block of Infraorbital Nerve
The infraorbital nerve, the terminal portion of the maxillary nerve, divides at the infraorbital foramen into inferior palpebral, external nasal and superior labial branches. These supply the side of the nose, the lower eyelid, the upper lip and its mucosa. The infraorbital foramen is in line with the supraorbital notch and canine fossa—both of which are palpable—or the second upper premolar tooth; it is 1 cm below the margin of the orbit, below the pupil when the eyes look forwards. The mental foramen is in the same straight line, as is also the second bicuspid tooth.

A needle is inserted through a weal 1 cm below the middle of the lower orbital margin, a finger-breadth lateral to the ala of the nose. Lignocaine, 2 ml of 2% solution, is deposited near the nerve as it issues from the foramen, not while it is in the foramen. By this injection the upper lip and tip of the nose are made insensitive.

For radical operation on the antrum, a maxillary block is indicated, together with local infiltration inside the upper lip, over the canine fossa.

For radical operation on the frontal sinus, anterior ethmoidal and frontal blocks are necessary.

For operations for dacryocystitis, anterior ethmoidal and infraorbital blocks are required.

Intraoral Nerve Block for Extraoral Lesions[88]
Useful for repair of lacerations of face and removal of skin lesions. No tissue distortion; injections less painful than through the skin.

Infraorbital nerve. Injection in mucobuccal fold, just medial to canine tooth; 1–2 ml of solution injected, advancing needle 1 cm. The entire upper lip is anaesthetized. Can be done bilaterally.

Mental nerve. Injection between apices of premolar teeth of lower jaw of 1–2 ml of solution; lower lip anaesthetized. (*See* Smith J. S. et al. *Anaesth. Intensive Care* 1985, **13**, 407.)

Long buccal nerve. Can be blocked as it crosses the anterior border of mandible. Injection immediately in front of the ramus, in the mucobuccal fold opposite the first molar tooth. Needle is inserted just anterior to the margin of the mandible and 2–3 ml of solution injected while needle is withdrawn. Useful for blocking 'cross-over' fibres.

Topical Analgesia of the Nasal Cavities

Sometimes managed by the surgeon. Useful in co-operative patients with reasonably patent nares.

1. Packing

The nasal cavities are first sprayed with 4–10% cocaine, all excess solution being rejected and not swallowed. With a good light and a speculum, the cavity is now packed with gauze soaked in 4–5% cocaine. Cocaine is a powerful vasoconstrictor and so adrenaline, although beloved of rhinologists, is not necessary. Trauma must be avoided.

After 10 min the packing is removed and the mucosa will be found to be avascular.

2. Sluder's Method[89]

3. Use of Cocaine Paste[90]

Cocaine is toxic! (*See* Pearman T. *J. Laryngol. Otol.* 1979, **93**, 1191.)

4. Moffett's Method[91]

The solution is a mixture of 2 ml of 8% cocaine hydrochlor, 2 ml of 1% sodium bicarbonate, 1 ml of 1–1000 adrenaline solution. A 2-ml syringe with bent cannula is required.

Position 1: Patient lies on left side with pillow under left shoulder and head in lateral position at angle of 45° with vertical. One-third of solution is drawn up, half being squirted into each naris along the floor of the nose.

Position 2: After 10 min second third of solution is drawn up and is similarly divided between the two sides of the nose; patient pinches nose, turns prone, lies on face for 10 min.

Position 3: With the remainder instilled the patient rolls on to right side as in position 1 and remains 10 min. If the septum is to be operated on, 2 ml of 1% lignocaine-adrenaline should be injected into the columella and base of septum in addition, as this area is covered by squamous epithelium which will not absorb the topical agent.

The method gives good analgesia, free from the unpleasantness of gauze packing and its resulting mild trauma.

5. Curtiss' Method[92]

6. Macintosh and Ostlere's Method[93]

7. Bodman's Method.[94]

(*See also* Oldham K. W. *Br. J. Anaesth.* 1968, **40**, 979.)

These methods of local analgesia are useful for the surgery of nasal septal defects, removal of polypi, turbinectomy, cauterization, etc.

For puncture of the antrum cotton-wool swabs on applicators soaked in 4% cocaine solution are inserted under the middle and inferior turbinates for 10 min. The nasal cavity is then sprayed with two or three squirts of 10% lignocaine aerosol spray.

Local Infiltration for Dental Extraction

This can be done for all teeth with the possible exception of the lower molars. Lignocaine 2% with 1–80 000 adrenaline solution is commonly used, and 3%

prilocaine with felypressin is now also used. A 26-gauge needle is inserted at the junction of the adherent mucoperiosteum of the gum with the free mucous membrane of the cheek and directed parallel to the long axis of the tooth; 0·5–1 ml of solution is injected superficial to the periosteum on the buccal and either the lingual or palatal side. Analgesia is tested for after 5 min by pushing the needle down the periodontal membrane on each side of the tooth to be extracted. If required more solution can be injected. Where there is infection involving teeth in the lower jaw, a 5% solution may give better analgesia than the usual 2%. It has a shorter latency but a similar duration of activity.[95]

(For details of technique *see* Wahlin A. and Nordenram A. in: *Anaesthesia and Sedation in Dentistry* (Coplans M. P. and Green R. A. ed.) Amsterdam: Elsevier, 1983, p. 175.)

Mandibular (Inferior Dental) Block
This may be required for extraction of several teeth of the lower jaw or for removal of the second or third molars. Infiltration cannot always be relied on to make these teeth insensitive. A single well-placed injection makes one-half of the lower jaw and tongue analgesic, except for the central incisor which gets some nerve supply from the other side, and the lateral buccal fold and molar buccal alveolar margin and gum supplied from the buccinator nerve. Both of these areas can be infiltrated with a small volume of solution to make them painless.

With the mouth open palpate the anterior border of the ramus of the mandible, the retromolar fossa and the internal oblique ridge. The needle is inserted just medial to this ridge lateral to the pterygomandibular ligament for a distance of 1·5 cm, keeping the syringe parallel to the occlusal plane of the lower teeth with its barrel over the premolar teeth of the opposite side; 2 or 3 ml of solution are now injected.

Transient amaurosis after mandibular nerve block has been reported[96] and may be due to intra-arterial injection of adrenaline with the local analgesic solution in patients whose orbital blood supply is derived from the middle meningeal artery—a rare anomaly. Unusual reactions to lignocaine in dental surgery (fixed drug eruption) may occur.[261]

Paracentesis of the Eardrum

Two or three metered (10-mg) doses of lignocaine aerosol spray are applied to the superior wall of the external auditory canal and allowed to trickle down onto the eardrum. This is repeated in 2 min and the incision can be made 3 min later. Useful in cooperative children. In adults, in the absence of acute inflammation, no form of pain relief is necessary.

Lingual Nerve Block

The lingual nerve block is the only sensory nerve supplying the floor of the mouth between the alveolar margin and the midline.

A finger in the retromolar fossa of the mandible will palpate the internal oblique line. The lingual nerve can be injected, just medial to this line, with 2 ml of 2% lignocaine. A useful method of analgesia for removing calculi from the submaxillary duct.

Facial Nerve Block

For hemifacial spasm.[97] The nerve is blocked as it crosses the neck of the mandible (*see also* Chapter 24).

Vagus Nerve Block

This was described[98] as a method of analgesia for broncho-oesophagoscopy and in the diagnosis of pain arising in the thorax, but is now seldom used. (For details *see* sixth edition of this Synopsis, p. 329.)

Superior Laryngeal Nerve Block

The internal laryngeal nerve passes forwards and downwards and pierces the thyrohyoid membrane to reach the space between the epiglottis and the pharyngeal mucosa posteriorly and the membrane in front. Its terminal twigs convey sensation from the larynx above the cords, the epiglottis, vallecula and the base of the tongue. This nerve is blocked at its point of division into the internal and external laryngeal nerve, slightly below and anterior to the greater cornu of the hyoid bone. Block of the internal branch causes analgesia of the lower pharynx, the laryngeal aspect of the epiglottis, the vallecula, the vestibule of the larynx, the aryepiglottic fold and the posterior part of the rima glottidis. There is no motor block.

1. A weal is raised over the thyroid notch in the midline, the hyoid grasped between the thumb and index finger of the left hand and displaced laterally towards the side to be injected. Through the weal, an 8-cm needle is introduced laterally and 2% procaine solution is injected as the needle is advanced to the greater cornu—but not beyond it for fear of injuring the great vessels of the neck. A further few millilitres of solution are injected as the needle is withdrawn. A similar procedure is carried out on the other side, through the same weal.[99]

2. A 22-gauge, 4-cm needle is passed through the skin, just above the thyroid cartilage, at a point one-third of the distance between the midline and the tip of the superior cornu; it is advanced upwards and medially for 1–2 cm until a 'give' is felt as it pierces the thyrohyoid membrane, and enters the space containing the internal laryngeal nerve. With the needle moving slightly in and out, 2–3 ml of solution are injected. If the needle advances too far it may enter the pharynx and air can be aspirated.

This block causes analgesia of the posterior surface of the epiglottis and of the larynx above the cords, so that food and drink must be prohibited for an adequate period depending on the drug and strength used.

It is useful, in conjunction with topical analgesia of the nose and pharynx, to enable blind nasotracheal intubation to be performed for tracheobronchial toilet; the coughing which results from irritation of the larynx below the cords soon passes off.

Topical analgesia, coupled with superior laryngeal and glossopharyngeal nerve block, gives good results for awake intubation, tonsillectomy and bronchoscopy.[100] (*See also* p. 207.)

Transtracheal Block

(*See* pp. 217 and 655.)

For technique for awake intubation, *see* Pedersen B. *Acta Anaesth. Scand.* 1971 **15**, 107; Anand J. S. *Br. J. Anaesth.* 1974, **46**, 413; Bromage P. R. *Epidural Analgesia*. Philadelphia: Saunders, 1978, p. 476.

Accessory Nerve Block
The nerve has both cranial and spinal roots. it leaves the skull through the jugular foramen, enters the deep surface of the sternomastoid, pierces it and emerges just above the midpoint of its posterior margin. It crosses the posterior triangle of the neck and enters the anterior border of the trapezius, giving motor fibres to it and to the sternomastoid.

Technique: Needle inserted 2 cm below the tip of the mastoid and 5–10 ml of solution injected into muscle.

Indications: To relax sternomastoid and trapezius muscles during physio-therapy for pain in the shoulder and neck, e.g. torticollis.[101]

Stellate Ganglion Block[102] (Cervicothoracic sympathetic block)

Sympathetic block is most commonly carried out: (1) In the neck (stellate ganglion block); (2) In the abdomen (splanchnic or coeliac plexus block); (3) In the lumbar region (L.1–L.4).

The stellate ganglion is formed by the fusion of the lowest of the three cervical ganglia with the first thoracic ganglion. It is irregular in size and position, being usually 1–3 cm long, and differs in the same individual on the two sides. Stellate ganglion block was first used for cerebral vascular accidents by Leriche and Fontaine in 1934.[103] This should be named cervicothoracic sympathetic block, as when 10–15 ml of analgesic solution are injected into the correct plane at the base of the neck, the middle cervical, stellate and the second, third and usually the fourth thoracic ganglia and their rami are blocked. This results in interruption of all sympathetic fibres to most of the thorax, head, neck and arm (except possibly the nerve of Kuntz[104]). Certain visceral afferent fibres are also blocked, e.g. the cervical cardiac nerves.

The stellate ganglion is often blocked by spill-over following supraclavicular brachial plexus block.

Anatomy
The cervical sympathetic chain and its three ganglia lie in front of the head of the first rib and the seventh cervical and first thoracic transverse process, just behind the subclavian artery and origin of the vertebral artery. It lies posterior to the carotid sheath on the longus colli and longus cervicis muscles. It is anterior to the eighth cervical and first thoracic nerves, so paraesthesia involving these nerves shows, if stellate ganglion block is done from the front, that the needle is too deeply placed. On the right side, the apex of the lung and the dome of the pleura are anterior relations; on the left side these structures are 2·5 cm lower and so are not in such close relationship to the ganglion. Vasoconstrictor fibres pass from the stellate and the other cervical sympathetic ganglia to a plexus around the internal carotid artery. Twigs from the second and sometimes also from the third thoracic sympathetic ganglion often go directly to the upper extremity via the first thoracic nerve, thus bypassing the stellate ganglion (the nerve of

Kuntz[104]). But this nerve is usually blocked by spread of the analgesic solution down to the region of the fourth thoracic ganglion.

It sends grey rami to the seventh and eighth cervical nerves, gives origin to the inferior cervical cardiac nerve, and supplies twigs to the vessels in its vicinity. It may communicate with the vagus.

Its most frequent indication is to release vascular tone, and it may need to be repeated several times.

As pointed out by Winnie[105] postganglionic sympathetic fibres are also distributed to the arm with the somatic nerves of the brachial plexus and are distributed from them to the vessels, supplying vasoconstrictor impulses to the whole limb.

Indications

There are few indications for stellate ganglion block today, although in the recent past it was widely practised (*see* the seventh edition of this Synopsis, 1973, p. 356). The control of the tone of intracranial vessels is now known to be more humoral than nervous. It has been used to treat quinine blindness[106] and acute deafness.[107] Its use in the treatment of blindness due to quinine poisoning is doubtful.[108] Has been used for relief of the acute pain due to herpes zoster ophthalmicus.[252]

Technique

Stellate ganglion block performed on a patient with an increased bleeding time or a decreased clotting time may result in a large haematoma in the deep planes of the neck. Long-acting drugs, e.g. 6% phenol or absolute alcohol, are used chiefly to control cardiac pain. Bilateral block should not be carried out at the same time.

1. Paratracheal approach.[109] The patient lies supine, chin forwards, neck extended without a pillow. Weal raised two finger-breadths lateral to the suprasternal notch and a similar distance above the clavicle, which is on the medial border of the sternomastoid overlying the transverse process of the seventh cervical vertebra. The position can be checked by palpating the tubercle of Chassaignac and the cricoid cartilage, both of which are at the level of the sixth cervical transverse process, i.e. a little higher than the weal. A fine 5–8-cm needle is inserted directly backwards through the weal, while downward and backward pressure is exerted on the sternomastoid to draw the muscle and the carotid sheath laterally. When contact is made with bone (C.7) the needle is withdrawn 0·5–1 cm so that its point lies in front of the longus colli muscle and, after careful aspiration for blood (the vertebral artery is very near) and for cerebrospinal fluid, 15–20 ml of 0·5% lignocaine or similar solution are injected. This will, if correctly placed, diffuse up and down in the fascial plane and will block the ganglia and rami from C.2 to T.4 inclusive. Thirty minutes may elapse before Horner's syndrome and vasodilatation of the arm appear. This technique is, in the authors' opinion, the safest and easiest.

2. Anterior approach (Apgar).[110]

3. Lateral approach (Goinard).[111]

4. Posterior approach (Kappis et al. 1947; Labat, 1930; White, 1940).

5. Tissue displacement method.[112]

Signs of Successful Block
(1) Horner's syndrome[113]—miosis, enophthalmos and ptosis. This does not guarantee sympathetic paralysis of the vessels of the arm; (2) Flushing of the cheek, face and neck and arm. Engorged veins of arm. Increase in skin temperature; (3) Flushing of the conjunctiva and sclera; (4) Anhidrosis of the face and neck; (5) Lacrimation; (6) Stuffiness of the nostril (Guttmann's sign); (7) Mueller's syndrome: injection of tympanic membrane and warmth of face; (8) Sympathetic block can be assessed by the cobalt blue and ninhydrin sweat tests which are more informative than the sympatho-galvanic response.[114]

Complications and Dangers of the Block
(1) Pleural shock; (2) Perforation of the oesophagus, with infection; (3) Intrathecal injection causing a total spinal block;[115] (4) Intravascular injection, e.g. sending volume of solution via the vertebral artery straight up to the medulla; (5) Pneumothorax; (6) Cardiac arrest—very rare, although it has resulted from surgical cervicothoracic sympathectomy (a permanent stellate block);[116] (7) Alteration of voice from recurrent laryngeal nerve block; (8) Phrenic nerve block; (9) Brachial plexus block; (10) Extradural or intradural block; (11) Mediastinitis; (12) Intercostal neuralgia.[253]

Death has been reported after stellate ganglion block, so that it should not be lightly undertaken.

Field Block for Tonsillectomy

Anatomy
The tonsil and its immediate surroundings are supplied by the lesser palatine (from maxillary), the lingual (from mandibular) nerves, and the glossopharyngeal nerve, via the pharyngeal plexus, which gives off filaments which form a plexus called the circulus tonsillaris.

Technique
Half an hour before the analgesia is commenced, an amethocaine lozenge 60 mg is given, after which the mouth and pharynx should be sprayed with 4–10% cocaine solution; some operators object to this, preferring to the keep the cough reflex active throughout.

Injections of 3–5 ml of 1·5% lignocaine and adrenaline are now made: (1) Into the upper part of the posterior pillar; (2) Into the upper part of the anterior pillar—both pillars must be made oedematous throughout their whole extent; (3) Into the triangular fold, near the lower pole; (4) Into the supratonsillar fossa, after drawing the tonsil towards the middle line.

The patient is sitting, well supported, in a chair. Adequate time must be given for the analgesic to act. Fainting is sometimes seen, while the depression of the tongue by the spatula may cause discomfort.

The technique finds little favour in the UK.

Glossopharyngeal Nerve Block[117]

Head fully rotated to opposite side with patient lying supine. At midpoint of a line joining the tip of the mastoid process to the angle of the jaw a needle inserted vertical to the skin makes contact with the styloid process 2–4 cm deep. Needle partially withdrawn and reinserted 0·5 cm deep to and posterior to styloid process. Injection of 6 ml of solution at this point will produce analgesia of posterior one-third of tongue.

Another technique for block of the glossopharyngeal nerve is to deposit solution near the jugular foramen. A 5-cm needle is introduced through a weal just below the external auditory meatus, anterior to the mastoid process. It is advanced perpendicularly to the skin until it meets the styloid process 1·5–2 cm deep and passes it posteriorly for a further 2 cm. Analgesia involves the 9th to 12th nerves inclusive and has been maintained with a long-acting drug in cases of malignant disease in the posterior third of the tongue, and in severe cases of neuralgia. Successful block results in analgesia of the posterior one-third of the tongue, uvula, soft palate and pharynx. There is no motor block. The gag reflex is suppressed. Also used in differential diagnosis between glossopharyngeal and atypical trigeminal neuralgias. An intraoral approach has been described.[118] (*See also* Mackintosh R. R. and Ostlere M. *Local Analgesia. Head and Neck*, 2nd ed. Edinburgh: Churchill Livingstone, 1967.)

Suprascapular Nerve Block[119] (C.5–6)

The nerve is the sole pathway of somatic pain from the shoulder and acromioclavicular joints and structures surrounding them. The block does not result in any skin analgesia, but when successful, relieves pain in the shoulder-joint.

Technique
Patient should be sitting with arms to the sides and head and shoulders slightly flexed. With a skin pencil the spine of the scapula is lined in: the inferior scapular angle is located and bisected by a line which crosses the first line. A weal is raised one finger-breadth from the crossing, in the upper outer angle, and a needle inserted downwards and medially to make contact with the bone of the surpaspinatus fossa, just lateral to the notch. Needle then withdrawn and reintroduced more medially until its point lies in the notch. Paraesthesiae take the form of pain at the tip of the shoulder, and after aspiration 10 ml of analgesic solution are injected. The block must be at the suprascapular notch as there the nerve is accessible to a needle and no afferent branches leave it before it passes through the notch. Types of shoulder pain relieved by this block include subacromial bursitis, painful abduction of the arm; calcified deposits about the capsule of the shoulder-joint. Used for pain relief, not surgery.

Cervical Plexus Block (C.1–4)

This is paravertebral cervical analgesia. It is not commonly used but is convenient for the removal of superficial tumours and cysts from the neck.

Anatomy
Formed by the anterior primary divisions of the upper four cervical nerves, each one of which, after leaving the intervertebral foramen, passes behind the vertebral artery and comes to lie in the sulcus between the anterior and posterior

tubercles of the transverse process of the appropriate cervical vertebra. Each nerve lies between the scalenus medius deeply and the levator anguli scapulae, under cover of the sternomastoid. Each of these four nerves, except the first, divides into upper and lower branches, which form three loops lateral to the transverse processes. The loops are between C.1 and C.2; C.2 and C.3; C.3 and C.4. The lower branch of C.4 joins C.5 in the formation of the brachial plexus. The upper loop is directed forwards, the lower two, backwards.

Branches are superficial (cutaneous), deep (muscular) and communicating. *Superficial branches* emerge posterior to the lateral border of the sternomastoid, near its midpoint. They are:

1. *Ascending Branches*. Lesser occipital (C.2) and great auricular (C.2 and C.3). They supply skin of the occipitomastoid region, auricle, and parotid.

2. *Transverse Branch*. The anterior cutaneous nerve of the neck (C.2 and C.3) supplying skin of anterior part of neck between the lower jaw and the sternum.

3. *Descending Branches*. The lateral, intermediate and medial supraclavicular nerves (C.3 and C.4) supplying skin of shoulder and upper pectoral region. C.1 has no cutaneous branch.

Deep branches of the plexus are: (1) Phrenic nerve—C.3, C.4 and C.5; (2) Anterior (deep) muscular branches; (3) Posterior muscular branches to sterno-mastoid, levator scapulae, trapezius and scalenus medius.

Communicating branches are: (1) Sympathetic—each cervical nerve receives a grey ramus from the cervical sympathetic chain—the upper four nerves from the superior cervical ganglion; (2) To vagus; (3) Branch to hypoglossal nerve from C.1 and C.2, the descendens hypoglossi which joins the descendens cervicalis (C.2–C.3) to form the ansa hypoglossi.

The posterior primary divisions of the cervical nerves supply skin and muscles of the back of the neck. Their cutaneous distribution spreads like a cape over the upper thorax and shoulders, and this area is made insensitive in cervical plexus block.

Nerve supply of thyroid is from middle and inferior cervical sympathetic ganglion; of the oesophagus, the vagus (and sympathetic); of the trachea, recurrent laryngeal (and sympathetic); of the sternomastoid, the 11th cranial, and 2nd and 3rd cervical nerves.

Technique

The patient lies supine with shoulders slightly elevated and neck and head extended—as for thyroidectomy, but with his head turned away from the side to be injected. Solution used is 0·5–1% lignocaine, or one of its congeners, with adrenaline.

Deep cervical block requires the deposition of analgesic solution just lateral to the transverse processes of the 2nd, 3rd and 4th cervical vertebrae (the 6th, 7th and 8th nerves having no sensory branches in the neck, and the first is purely motor). A needle is inserted to a depth of 1·5–2 cm perpendicular to all planes of the skin so that the transverse processes are contacted. (For details, *see* the eighth edition of this Synopsis.)

Superficial cervical block is carried out by injecting 20 ml of analgesic solution between skin and muscle along the posterior border of the sternomas-toid near its midpoint, usually just below the position where it is crossed by the external jugular vein, so as to cut off impulses from the ascending, transverse and descending superficial branches of the plexus.

Cervical plexus block gives analgesia of the front and back of the neck, the occipital region, and a cape-like area over the shoulders to below the clavicle, the skin above the third rib anteriorly and above the upper border of the scapula posteriorly. Its chief indication is in thyroidectomy.

Complications may include: (1) Phrenic block; (2) Intrathecal or intravascular injection; (3) Vagus and/or recurrent laryngeal nerve block causing aphonia; (4) Cervical sympathetic block and Horner's syndrome.

For single-injection interscalene cervical plexus block, *see* Winnie A. P. et al. *Anesth. Anal.* 1975, **54**, 370.

Brachial Plexus Block (C.5–T.1)

History

Halsted (1852–1922) of New York in 1884, Matas of New Orleans[120] (1860–1957) and Crile[121] (1864–1943) of Cleveland in 1897, injected the plexus under direct vision following exposure under local infiltration (intraneural block). Hirschel injected the plexus blindly through the skin.[122] Kulenkampff, assistant to Heinrich Braun at Zwickau, after experimenting on himself, used the supraclavicular technique in 1912.[123] Patrick[124] in Sheffield published his modification of the Kulenkampff technique in 1940. Macintosh and Mushin[125] in Oxford describe this method in their excellently illustrated book. The method involves blocking the plexus as it lies on the first rib, lateral to the subclavian artery. (*See Plexus Anesthesia*, Vol. 1. Winnie A. P. Edinburgh: Churchill Livingstone, 1983.)

Anatomy

The brachial plexus is formed from the anterior primary divisions of C.5, C.6, C.7, C.8 and T.1. It forms the entire motor and almost the entire sensory nerve supply to the arm. It receives communicating twigs from C.4 and T.2. These nerves unite to form three trunks, which lie in the neck above the clavicle. Its roots pass through the fascia-enclosed space between the scalenus anterior and the scalenus medius accompanied by the subclavian artery, invaginate the scalene fascia to form a neurovascular space; this fascia then becomes the axillary sheath or axillary perivascular space which surrounds the plexus. This space may be entered at the supraclavicular, interscalene, axillary or infraclavicular level; a single injection into it will produce analgesia, the extent of which will depend on the volume of solution injected and the level of injection. Each trunk divides, behind the clavicle, into anterior and posterior divisions, which unite in the axilla to form cords.

The plexus is broad above and converges to the first rib. Its anterior relations are the skin, superficial fascia, platysma and supraclavicular branches of the cervical plexus, the deep fascia and external jugular vein; the clavicle is in front of its lower part, the scalenus anterior is in front of its upper part. Its posterior relations are the scalenus medius and the long thoracic nerve. Its inferior relations are the first rib, where the plexus lies between the subclavian artery anteriorly and the scalenus medius behind.

The plexus emerges from the intervertebral foramina and passes between the scalenus anterior and the scalenus medius. Close to their emergence the 5th and 6th nerves each receive a grey ramus from the middle cervical sympathetic ganglion. The 7th and 8th nerves each receive a grey ramus from the inferior cervical ganglion. The thoracic nerve receives a grey ramus from and sends a white ramus to the first thoracic sympathetic ganglion. As the plexus converges on the first rib it is enclosed in a fibrous sheath contributed by the scalenus anterior and medius muscles. It lies first above, and then to the outer side of, the subclavian vessels and just above the clavicle lies between the skin and the first rib, immediately behind the deep fascia.

The upper trunk is formed by the anterior rami of C.5 and C.6.

The middle trunk is formed by the anterior ramus of C.7.

The lower trunk is formed by the anterior rami of C.8 and T.1. Behind the clavicle the trunks each divide into anterior and posterior divisions, i.e. in relationship to the axillary artery.

The posterior cord is formed by the three posterior divisions.

The medial cord is formed by the lowest anterior division.

The lateral cord is formed by the upper two anterior divisions.

Branches are given off from: (1) Roots; (2) Trunks; (3) Cords.

1. *Branches from roots*: The nerve to the serratus anterior (of Bell) from C.5, C.6 and C.7. Dorsalis scapulae nerve from C.5. Muscular branches to the longus cervicis (C.5–C.8) and the three scaleni (C.5–C.8), the rhomboids (C.5) and a twig to the phrenic (C.5).

2. *Branches from trunks*: Suprascapular nerve (C.5 and C.6). Nerve to subclavius (C.5 and C.6).

3. *Branches from cords*: From lateral cord (three): Lateral pectoral (C.5–C.7); lateral head of the median (C.5–C.7); musculocutaneous (C.5, C.6, C.7). From the posterior cord (five): Radial (C.5, C.6, C.7, C.8 and T.1); axillary (C.5 and C.6); thoracodorsal nerve to the latissimus dorsi (C.6, C.7, C.8); upper and lower subscapular nerves (C.5 and C.6). From the medial cord (five): Medial head of the median; medial pectoral; ulnar; medial cutaneous of the forearm (all from C.8 and T.1); medial cutaneous of the arm (T.1).

The scalenus anterior arises from the anterior tubercles of the transverse processes of the 3rd, 4th, 5th and 6th cervical vertebrae. It is inserted into the scalene tubercle on the inner border of the first rib. The muscle lies anterior to the plexus, being separated from it below by the subclavian artery. Its lateral border, if it is palpable, is a guide to the position of the plexus.

The scalenus medius arises from the posterior tubercles of the six lowest cervical vertebrae and is inserted into the upper surface of the first rib behind the groove made by the plexus and the subclavian artery. The plexus thus lies in front of the muscle.

The first rib lies in an almost horizontal plane, being inclined slightly downwards and forwards. It passes below the clavicle at about the junction of its inner and middle thirds. Its surfaces look upwards and downwards and its borders inwards and outwards.

The head has a single articular facet which articulates with the body of the first thoracic vertebra. The tubercle articulates with the transverse process of the same vertebra.

The upper surface has two transverse grooves: an anterior for the subclavian vein and a posterior for the subclavian artery and the lowest trunk of the brachial plexus. On the inner border, between the grooves, is the scalene tubercle. The subclavius muscle originates in front of the anterior groove and the scalenus medius is inserted behind the posterior groove. The lower surface has no costal groove; the inner border embraces the dome of the pleura; while the outer border gives origin to the first slip of the serratus anterior.

The subclavian artery extends from its origin to the outer border of the first rib. The right subclavian comes from the innominate artery, the left from the aortic arch. At its highest point, each artery is about 2 cm above the clavicle. Three parts of the artery are described: one medial, one behind and one lateral to the scalenus anterior.

The relations of the third part, i.e. the part lateral to the scalenus anterior, are: anteriorly, the skin, superficial fascia, platysma, deep fascia, descending branches of the cervical plexus, a plexus formed by the external and anterior jugular veins, and the transverse cervical and transverse scapular veins, the transverse cervical and transverse scapular arteries. Above and laterally is the plexus, while below is the first rib.

The subclavian vein is separated from the plexus by the scalenus anterior. As it is well protected by the clavicle, it is unlikely to be punctured.

It has been pointed out[126,127] that a continuous fascia-enclosed perineural and perivascular compartment exists, extending from the origins of the brachial plexus at the intervertebral foramina to the upper arm. This compartment can be entered at various levels and different volumes of local analgesic solution can be injected into it, as is the case with the extradural space, producing different effects. Thus the need for the elicitation of paraesthesiae with the needle is diminished.[127] The importance of this anatomical concept to anaesthetists should be recognized by its being known as 'Winnie's fascial compartment'. The connective tissue forming the neurovascular sheath of the plexus is denser proximally than distally. Connective tissue septa between the components of the plexus make the sheath multicompartmental and the compartments do not always intercommunicate. Thus, using any technique of block, certain nerves may remain unblocked.[128]

Technique (Patrick's Method)[124]

Not easy for the tyro. Patrick's aim was to infiltrate a sector of tissue lying between the midclavicular point on the skin and the first rib. He advocated starting the injections lateral to the plexus and slowly working medially, until the subclavian artery pulsations transmitted along the needle indicated that the lower trunk of the plexus had been reached. Macintosh and Mushin[125] modified this by starting the injections into the lower trunk close to the subclavian artery and working laterally. This modification is described below.

The patient should be sitting or lying supine. The head is rotated to the other side and the arm and shoulder depressed. A weal is raised 1 cm above the midpoint of the clavicle, a position: (1) Midway between the sternoclavicular and acromioclavicular joints; (2) Crossed by a line produced downwards from the external jugular vein, made prominent by blowing out the cheeks; (3) Just lateral to the pulsating subclavian artery, often palpable; (4) Lateral to the outer border of the scalenus anterior, sometimes palpable under cover of the sternomastoid.

A needle is inserted through the weal downwards, inwards and backwards, so that it is pointing to the spine of the second to fourth thoracic vertebra, a finger meanwhile guarding the subclavian artery and drawing it slightly medially. A cough from the patient is a warning that the pleura is being irritated by the needle. If paraesthesia is felt, the needle is steadied and 30 ml of the solution are injected. The following nerves are blocked: the median, the musculocutaneous, the radial, the axillary, the ulnar, the medial cutaneous nerve of the arm and the medial cutaneous nerve of the forearm.

If paraesthesiae are not felt in the arm and hand after one or two needle thrusts, the upper surface of the first rib is contacted and the needle inserted on to it so that the pulsations of the subclavian artery are transmitted to the needle. This is at a depth of 1·2–2·5 cm. Doppler ultrasound will aid localization.[129] After a negative aspiration test, 10 ml of solution are injected between the first rib and the skin. The needle is reintroduced on to the first rib, 1 cm laterally to the first position, and 10 ml similarly deposited. Third and fourth injections are made, each 1 cm lateral to the last, and at each point 10 ml are deposited beween skin and rib. Efficiency is improved if a nerve stimulator and an insulated needle are used. If stimulation is felt in the second, third or fourth fingers, a successful block results in over 90% of cases. It may be incomplete if only the first and fifth fingers react to stimulation.[130]

Analgesia is rapid in onset if paraesthesiae are present; if not, an interval of 20 min may be necessary. A feeling of warmth and 'pins and needles' precedes analgesia, while motor paralysis, when it occurs, follows analgesia.

An area of skin over the point of the shoulder and another on the inner aspect of the upper arm from the axilla to its midpoint (intercostohumeral T.2) are not made insensitive. A subcutaneous band of injection downwards from the acromioclavicular joint and surrounding the shoulder will render these areas analgesic. Occasionally, median nerve block at the wrist is necessary, as the palm of the hand, supplied by the middle trunk (C.7) of the plexus via the median nerve, is the most resistant area to successful block.

Lignocaine 2% solution with adrenaline, or longer-acting drugs, will produce sensory and motor paralysis. Solution of 1% will give sensory loss alone for about 1 h. Nerve suturing or trimming requires the use of the stronger solutions. Toxic and ill or feeble patients should have the strength of solution and not the volume reduced. For prolonged block *see* Hempel V. *Anesth. Analg. (Cleve.)* 1981, **60**, 352.

Horner's syndrome may or may not follow injection. It is due to paralysis of the cervical sympathetic chain. For details *see* above.

Complications

1. Paralysis of phrenic nerve often occurs.[131] At the level of the first rib, the phrenic nerve is separated from the brachial plexus by the scalenus anterior muscle. Higher in the neck it is the same fascial compartment as the upper components of the plexus. Analgesic solution injected into the tissue surrounding the plexus can thus ascend to block the phrenic nerve. Such a block is harmless and causes no symptoms, even if bilateral, but if the patient has a respiratory difficulty, e.g. emphysema or kyphosis, or if a general anaesthetic is to be administered, the possibility of diaphragmatic paralysis must be borne in mind. There is a high hemidiaphragm on X-ray examination.

2. Puncture of vessels, including subclavian artery. Haematomata may form but cause no trouble. Intravascular injection must be avoided.

3. Pneumothorax. Due to piercing Sibsons fascia.[132] Trouble seldom occurs. The axillary approach avoids this complication. Silent pneumothorax is unlikely as air in the chest is usually accompanied by pain. Surgical emphysema may be seen, probably due to wounding of the lung by the needle. If a radiograph shows a large area of lung collapse, air should be withdrawn from the chest. Bilateral pneumothorax may be a dangerous condition.

Pain in the chest during needling may also be due to irritation of the nerve to the serratus anterior.

4. Toxic effect of drug injected. Slow injection lessens chance of this.

5. Postoperative disability following brachial plexus block is rare, although the paralysing effects of bupivacaine may last many hours.[133]

Interscalene Approach[134]

Described by Labat in 1927[135] but modern use is due to Alon Winnie.[136] The sheath of the plexus can be entered via the interscalene space between the anterior and middle scalene muscles at the level of C.6. The patient lies supine, arms by the sides and head turned away from the side to be injected. The level of C.6 may be obtained by palpation of the cricoid cartilage or of the sixth transverse process (Chassaignac's tubercle). At the edge of the sternomastoid muscle the palpating finger lies on the scalenus anterior muscle and more laterally the groove between the anterior and middle scalene muscles can be felt. A needle is inserted perpendicular to the skin and passing the external jugular vein advanced until the point is felt to enter the perivascular space by a click. After the injection of a small volume of fluid, there should be a 'flow-back' on aspiration.[137] After careful aspiration tests the desired volume of analgesic solution is injected (e.g. 25–40 ml). When this is completed the patient may be sat up and gentle massage used to aid downward spread of solution. For complete analgesia of the inner aspect of the upper arm, block of the intercostohumeral nerve (T.1–2) may be required (*see* p. 624). Permanent neurological damage has been reported.[138] Though the dangers of pneumothorax are avoided, there is risk of injection into the extradural space, into CSF or the vertebral artery and bilateral block of the cervical and brachial plexuses.[139] The needle should not be inserted more than 3 cm.[140] Successful injection blocks both the cervical and brachial plexuses. Suitable for operations on the shoulder joint[141] and for the reduction of Colles' fracture. The complications are the same as may arise from the supraclavicular approach. 30 ml of 0·375% bupivacaine with adrenaline may be used. Complete onset of block may take 30 min. An acute exacerbation of asthma has been reported in an asthmatic patient.[142]

The Subclavian Perivascular Technique

(*See* Winnie A. P. and Collins J. J. *Anesthesiology* 1964, **25**, 353; Winnie A. P. *Plexus Anesthesia* Vol. 1. Edinburgh: Churchill Livingstone, 1983, p. 145.) The recumbent patient is told to turn his head to the opposite side and to touch his knee. The tip of the anaesthetist's index finger is placed posterior to the lateral border of the relaxed sternomastoid at the level of C.6 (cricoid cartilage). The tip of the finger moves medially behind the belly of the sternomastoid and enters the interscalene groove and edged inferiorly. A 5-cm 22-g short bevelled needle is then inserted just above the finger and pushed downwards (caudally) until it enters the perivascular space, shown by paraesthesia in the arm (not the shoulder as this may be due to irritation of the suprascapular nerve) or by a click as the needle pierces the fascia. After aspiration, 20–40 ml of solution is injected slowly. The intercostobrachial and the medial brachial cutaneous nerve (C.8–T.1 must in addition be blocked by a few ml of solution injected subcutaneously over the axillary artery if a tourniquet is to be applied.

Infraclavicular Brachial Plexus Block
(*See* Winnie A. P. *Anesthesiology* 1964, **25**, 353; Raj P. P. et al. *Anesth. Anal. Curr. Res.* 1973, **52**, 897; Sims J. K. *Anesth. Analg. (Cleve.)* 1977, **56**, 554; Whiffler K. *Br. J. Anaesth.* 1981, **53**, 845.)

Parascalene Technique
(*See* Vongveses P. et al. *Anesth. Analg. (Cleve.)* 1979, **58**, 267.)

Axillary Approach to Brachial Plexus
Used by Labat in 1922,[143] by Burnham[144] a surgeon, who revived the idea of Reding,[127] concerning a fascial compartment, and Eather[145] in 1958. Hirschel injected it 'blind', through the axilla, in 1911.[146] In the axilla the nerves from the brachial plexus, together with the main artery, are enclosed in a fibrous neuromuscular fascial sheath. The median and musculocutaneous nerves together with their sensory branches are anterior or anterolateral, i.e. above and beyond the artery; the ulnar nerve is inferior; the radial nerve is posterolateral or below and behind the vessel. The musculocutaneous and axillary nerves are given off high in the axilla.

Block follows if analgesic solution is injected periarterially into the fibrous neurovascular sheath.

Technique. The patient lies supine with the arm abducted to a right angle, the humerus externally rotated and the elbow flexed. The skin of the axilla is not shaved but is well cleaned and a weal is raised at the highest part of the axilla at which arterial pulsation is felt, proximal to the lower border of the pectoralis major. The pulsating vessel is identified and through the weal a 2·5–5 cm short bevelled needle is inserted until a click shows that the neurovascular sheath has been entered; a paraesthesia shows that the point has entered the sheath. It is easy to push the needle too deeply and to thus avoid the sheath. Local analgesic solution, e.g. 20 ml of 1–2% lignocaine with adrenaline, is placed in each quadrant surrounding the vessel. Alternatively, bupivacaine may be employed to a total dose of 1·5 mg/kg. The addition of potassium chloride to 0·25% solution of bupivacaine (but not to prilocaine) causes a more rapid onset of sensory block.[254] To prevent dissipation of the solution downwards in the neurovascular space firm finger pressure is applied below the needle during and after the injection or the arm elevated. Occasionally the musculocutaneous nerve (C.6), which is a continuation of the lateral cord of the plexus, is given off higher than usual and consequently escapes the effects of local analgesic solution deposited in the neurovascular space. In such cases it can be dealt with by the injection of 10–15 ml of solution from a point 2·5 cm distal to the crease of the elbow joint in the cleft between the tendon of the biceps and the brachioradialis where it becomes the lateral antebrachial cutaneous nerve, or the original needle can be inserted superior to the vascular bundle and 5 ml of solution injected into the substance of the coracobrachialis muscle. Similarly, a few drops of solution may be deposited just superficial to the neurovascular bundle, to block the intercostobrachial nerve which supplies the inner and outer aspects of the upper arm. An area of skin over the point of the shoulder supplied by the intercostohumeral nerve (T.1 and T.2) is not blocked by this approach. Onset of analgesia takes up to 30 min. If necessary, reinforcement of the ulnar distribution will follow ulnar nerve block just proximal to the ulnar nerve sulcus above the 'funny' bone. The use of a nerve stimulator before injection increases the efficiency of brachial plexus block by the axillary route.[255]

Extent of block by axillary approach. Complete analgesia below the elbow joint. Good sympathetic block of arm. Shoulder joint, supplied by the suprascapular nerve (C.5 and C.6), not made insensitive, so reductions of dislocation of this joint cannot be performed under axillary block as they can under the supraclavicular block. A subcutaneous ring injection at the level of the initial weal may be required for the painless application of a tourniquet. Pain from ischaemia due to an arterial tourniquet may not be completely obtunded unless a 2% solution of lignocaine, mepivacaine or prilocaine is used.

Advantages. Only one landmark, the axillary artery. No paraesthesiae so less chance of nerve damage. No possibility of pneumothorax, stellate ganglion, recurrent laryngeal nerve block or phrenic nerve block. Less pain during injection. Difficult in obesity or when the arm cannot be abducted. (*See also* Bosomworth P. P. et al. *Ann. Surg.* 1961, **154**, 911; Moir D. D. *Anaesthesia* 1962, **17**, 274; Lofström B. in: *Local and Conduction Anaesthesia* (Crul J. F. ed.). Nijmegen: Drukkerij/Uitgeverij, 1970). Continuous block, using a catheter, eases pain following trauma to the arm.[147]

Brachial plexus block is a most satisfactory method of analgesia though less popular since the reintroduction of intravenous regional analgesia. For dislocations of the shoulder joint or elbow joint, for tendon suture, for manipulation of fractures under the X-ray screen, for suturing of lacerations, etc., the method is excellent. A tourniquet may be applied to the upper arm even in the absence of analgesia of the inner aspect of the upper arm. It is more successful in cases with a previously painless limb than in those with an existing painful lesion, e.g. a fracture or abscess.

Injury to the brachial plexus following brachial plexus block may be due to lack of support for the anaesthetized limb after operation.[148]

Major operations on the breast are not satisfactory under regional analgesia, but biopsies can be obtained without pain using lignocaine and adrenaline.[256]

Intravenous Regional Analgesia

History

This was first described by Bier in 1908 who used procaine[149] but it never became popular. Its use today follows the work of Holmes in 1963, then of Oxford, who substituted the more powerful lignocaine for procaine.[150] It was also described by Riha in 1962.[151]

(*See also* Holmes C. McK. *Acta Anaesth. Scand.* 1969, Suppl. **36**, 11.)

Intravenous injection of local analgesic agents has been used for: (1) General anaesthesia; (2) In the treatment of cardiac dysrhythmias; (3) To produce local analgesia.

Local analgesia involves the injection of a local analgesic solution into a vein of a limb which has been made ischaemic by a tourniquet. Most useful for operations on arms but can also be used in the leg.

Technique

A Butterfly needle is inserted into a vein on the dorsum of the hand (preferably not in the forearm) and very firmly secured; another should be in a vein in the other limb in case of toxic signs. Veins in the forearm or antecubital fossa are better avoided. The limb is drained of blood by elevation for 5 min, with or without compression of the brachial artery. An Esmarch bandage,[152] the Rhys-Davies exsanguinator (an inflatable pneumatic cylinder which is easier to apply and less uncomfortable[153]) or an orthopaedic pneumatic splint[154] can also be used for this purpose. Two narrow sphygmomanometer cuffs are securely placed on the upper arm, one proximal to the other, and the upper one inflated to a pressure a little above the systolic blood pressure, before removal of the compression or pneumatic bandage (if used). Injection of the local analgesic solution now follows, and after 5–10 min, the lower cuff is inflated and the upper one released, to minimize discomfort. A tourniquet that does not occlude the brachial artery throughout the operation may result in congestion of the limb, absorption of the drug and imperfect analgesia. Close attention to detail and to the efficiency of the apparatus is most important.[155] The patient is ready for operation after an interval of 10 minutes. Analgesia and motor weakness continue while the tourniquet remains inflated. The block has been used successfully in children,[161] and also on the lower extremity, in which case the cuff should be placed on the mid-calf.[162]

Intravenous analgesia below the knee, using prilocaine has been used, but for perfect results requires near-toxic doses.[162]

Local Analgesic Solutions

While 0·5% lignocaine or prilocaine are effective and popular, 0·2% bupivacaine is efficient but potentially toxic and should not be used. Volumes: lignocaine or prilocaine[157] 0·5%, 3–4 mg/kg, e.g. 30–40 ml. Solutions should be free of preservative.

The information derived from angiography of the upper limb may be increased if guanethidine is used to produce sympathetic block, using the Bier technique.[159]

Cuff Deflation

This is better done in stages although interosseous leak may occur.[158] Analgesic drug is released into the circulation in a biphasic manner. There is an initial fast release of 30%, but 50% may still be present in the limb 30 min later.[160] Toxic signs may be drowsiness, twitches, jactitations or convulsions, bradycardia proceeding to asystole, hypotension and ECG abnormalities. The patient should be carefully observed during the 10 min following release of the cuff. Reinflation may be considered if signs of toxicity arise.

Contraindications

These may include Raynaud's disease, sickle-cell anaemia and scleroderma.

Reactionary oedema may follow release of the cuff, so that in plaster work a back splint should be applied and splintage completed in a few days' time.

The site of action of the drug is on the peripheral nerve endings,[156] and also on nerve trunks when stronger solutions are used. (*See also* Evans C. J. et al. *Br. J. Anaesth.* 1974, **46**, 668.)

Intravenous regional analgesia of one finger has been reported.[164]

Because of its toxicity, bupivacaine should not be used.

Intravenous Sympathetic Block

Guanethidine 10–20 mg with 500 units of heparin in 25 ml of saline has been used to reduce pain; a form of regional blockade.[163]

(For a full review of this subject *see Acta Anaesth. Scand.* 1969, Suppl. 336; Thorne-Alquist A.-M. *Acta Anaesth. Scand.* 1971, **15**, 23; Suppl. 40; Goold J. E. *Br. J. Hosp. Med.* 1985, **33**, 335.)

Intra-arterial Local Analgesia

Introduced by Goyanes, a Spaniard, in 1912.[165]

A pneumatic cuff is applied to the upper arm, and a fine, short-bevel needle, attached to a 20-ml syringe containing 0·5% lignocaine solution, is introduced into the brachial artery near the elbow. The cuff is then inflated until arterial pulsations are occluded and the solution injected intra-arterially 5 ml at a time until the desired analgesic effect is obtained. The average dose in adults is 14–15 ml, considerably less than would be required in intravenous regional analgesia. Unsuccessful attempts at intra-arterial injection may cause temporary vascular spasm, but no other complications were seen in van Niekerk and Coetzee's series of 300 cases.[166]

Distal Nerve Blocks

Elbow Block

Intradermal and subcutaneous circles of infiltration are made just proximal to the internal epicondyle.

Median block is obtained by injecting through a weal placed midway between the outer side of the tendon of the biceps and the medial epicondyle or from a weal 1 cm medial to the brachial artery at the bend of the elbow. The needle should be inserted in an upward direction. If paraesthesiae are felt, success is likely: 5 ml of 2% lignocaine are used. The median nerve supplies the lateral part of the palm of the hand and fingers.

Radial block together with block of the lateral cutaneous nerve of the forearm, the sensory continuation of the musculocutaneous nerve, is performed through a weal 1 cm lateral to the tendon of the biceps at the line of the bend of the elbow. The needle is directed upwards to reach the front of the outer surface of the lateral epicondyle and solution deposited between the bone and the skin

Alternatively, a weal is raised four finger-breadths proximal to the lateral epicondyle of the humerus which overlies the point at which the nerve pierces the intermuscular septum and is close to the bone. The needle is advanced perpendicularly to the skin towards the bone and 20 ml of analgesic solution are deposited above and below the point of injection.

Ulnar block is performed 2 or 3 cm proximal to the point where the nerve can be palpated behind the medial epicondyle, using 2–4 ml of 2% lignocaine. The ulnar nerve supplies skin on the medial side of the palmar and dorsal aspects of the hand and 5th and medial part of 4th fingers.

Wrist Block

Circular lines of intradermal and subcutaneous infiltration are carried out just above the wrist-joint.

Median nerve (C.5–T.1). The median nerve at the wrist lies deeply between the flexor carpi radialis laterally and the palmaris longus and flexor digitorum sublimis medially. It is injected with 5 ml of 1% lignocaine immediately lateral to the tendon of the palmaris longus with the hand dorsiflexed. Attempts to elicit paraesthesiae are made, but if unsuccessful the solution is injected nevertheless. The median nerve supplies the skin of the thenar eminence and of the anterior aspects of the lateral three and a half fingers together with the skin over the dorsal aspects of their terminal phalanges. Median nerve block at the wrist or elbow may be followed by neuritis.

Ulnar nerve (C.7–T.1) divides (5 cm) above the wrist joint into superficial terminal or palmar mixed, and dorsal sensory branches.

The superficial terminal branch lies between the flexor carpi ulnaris tendon and the ulnar artery. It supplies the medial part of the palm of the hand and the palmar aspect of the fifth and medial side of the ring finger. The pisiform bone is immediately medial to it. Its sensory branch is blocked from a weal immediately lateral to the flexor carpi ulnaris.

The dorsal branch is anaesthetized by intradermal and subcutaneous injection along a line at the level of the ulnar styloid from the medial side of the tendon of the flexor carpi ulnaris to the middle of the back of the wrist. It supplies the ulnar border of the dorsum of the hand.

Radial or musculospiral nerve (C.5–T.1) is the sensory nerve of the back of the lateral part of the hand. After accompanying the radial artery along the medial border of the brachioradialis, it passes 6–7 cm above the wrist joint beneath the tendon of that muscle and comes to lie beneath the skin on the extensor aspect of the lower forearm and wrist. It can be blocked by infiltrating between the skin and the bone on the posterolateral aspect of the wrist joint near the base of the thumb lateral to the radial artery.

Wrist block, with a finger tourniquet, is useful for surgery of the hand, especially if motor function is required during the operation. It does not remove the discomfort of an Esmarch bandage on the forearm.

Elbow and wrist block are often unwise in the presence of neuritis or carpal tunnel syndrome, but intravenous regional analgesia is not contraindicated.

Nerve supply of the palm of the hand is from the ulnar and median nerves, with the radial supplying part of the thumb. (The sole of the foot is supplied by the sural and the lateral and medial branches of the tibial nerve.) The palm can be blocked at the wrist and the sole at the ankle.

Field Block for Operation on the Digits

Two palmar and two dorsal nerves supply each digit. With a fine (25 gauge) needle an intradermal weal is raised on the dorsum of the finger near its base.

2 ml of 1 or 2% lignocaine (or one of its congeners) solution are injected into the substance of the finger through this weal between the bone and the skin and repeated on the other side of the digit. The weals should be connected by 1 ml of solution between skin and bone on the dorsal aspect. Analgesia may take 15 min to become established. The palmar skin is not pierced. *Adrenaline should not be used*. Another method of blocking the finger is to deposit 5–7 ml of 1% lignocaine solution in the interosseous spaces at each side of the metacarpal bone, entering from the dorsal aspect and carrying the needle almost to the palmar skin. Spread of infection due to this technique is very rare, providing that solution is not injected into infected tissue.

If a tourniquet is used, no more than 3 ml of solution should be injected; a tourniquet must not remain on the finger for more than 15 min and not used at all in patients with Raynaud's disease.[167]

A similar technique—using less solution—can be employed on the toe. Intravenous regional analgesia of one finger has been reported.[164]

Paravertebral Somatic Block
This method was introduced by Hugo Sellheim of Leipzig (1871–1936) in 1906[168] and developed by Läwen in 1911, who called it 'paravertebral conduction anaesthesia',[169] and by Kappis (1881–1938).[170] It involves injecting a local analgesic close to the vertebral column where the nerve trunks emerge from the intervertebral foramina.

Macintosh and Bryce-Smith, in a well-illustrated book,[171] describe the paravertebral space as a wedge-shaped compartment, bounded above and below by the heads and necks of adjoining ribs; posteriorly by the superior costotransverse ligament; medially it communicates with the extradural space through the intervertebral foramen; laterally its apex leads into the intercostal space. The base is formed by the posterolateral aspect of the body of the vertebra and the intervertebral foramen and its contents.

There is no direct communication between one paravertebral space and another, but an indirect communication exists medially through the intervertebral foramen with the extradural space. Spread from one paravertebral space to another, across the extradural space, is frequent and may involve nerves on the same or on the opposite side of the body.

When the first thoracic to second lumbar nerve roots are blocked, their rami communicantes are blocked too.

Paravertebral Cervical Block
Described under Cervical Plexus Block.

Paravertebral Thoracic Block
It is indicated for operations on the chest or abdominal wall, for relief of postoperative, post-herpetic pain and the pain of fractured ribs.[172]
Technique. Skin weals are raised 4 cm from the midline, opposite the lower borders of the vertebral spines. Through each weal, a needle is inserted perpendicularly to strike bone near the lateral extremity of the transverse process. It is then redirected to pass upwards and slightly medially over the upper border of the transverse process and at this point local analgesic solution is injected. Aspiration tests should be made to ensure that the needle point has not

entered a vessel or the dura. Puncture of the pleura is also possible. (*See also* Cleland J. G. P. *Surg. Gynecol. Obstet.* 1933, **57**, 51.)

Lumbar Sympathetic Block

Surgical lumbar sympathectomy was described at the Mayo Clinic in 1929[173] and by Leriche (1879–1955) and Fontaine in 1934.[174] Phenol injected by Mandl in 1947.[175] A technique using phenol dissolved in a radio-opaque medium and an image intensifier has been used.[176] (*See also* Cleland J. G. P. *Surg. Gynecol. Obstet.* 1933, **57**, 51; reprinted in 'Classical File' *Surv. Anesthesiol.* 1981, **25**, 341.)

Anatomy

The sympathetic trunk in the lumbar region consists of four ganglia and their interconnecting fibres. It lies on the anterolateral aspect of the bodies of the lumbar vertebrae, immediately medial to the psoas muscle, which fills the triangular space between the vertebral bodies and the transverse processes. A tendinous arch, which gives part origin to the psoas muscle, connects the upper and lower borders of each lumbar vertebra and forms a tunnel around the side of the bone in which the lumbar vessels and the grey ramus communicans run. The lumbar arteries are posterior but the veins may be anterior. The fatty tissue occupying this tunnel is an extension of that in the extradural space and it passes through the intervertebral foramina as far forward as the sympathetic chain. The chain lies in a fascial plane bounded by the vertebral column, the psoas sheath and the parietal peritoneum. L.1 is on a level with the intersection of the last rib and the outer border of the erector spinae. The L.4–L.5 interspace corresponds to the highest point of the iliac crests in many patients.

In the sacral region, each chain consists of four ganglia with intervening fibres lying medial to the anterior sacral foramina. Preganglionic fibres (white rami) are derived from the anterior primary rami from T.4 to T.12 and each ganglion gives off a grey ramus to the corresponding sacral nerve, to supply sympathetic innervation to the lower limbs. On the coccyx, the two chains unite to form the ganglion impar.

Disturbances of function of the sympathetic nervous system can produce: (1) Vasospasm: (2) Pain; (3) Visceral dysfunction. Sympathetic block can remedy all of these, either temporarily, for diagnosis, or permanently, by interrupting a vicious circle.

Indications

See Chapter 33.

Technique

Posterior approach.[177] The patient is placed in the prone position, with two pillows flexing the lumbar spine, or in lateral spinal position with the affected side uppermost and the spine flexed. He should be premedicated with a sedative. The procedure can be carried out in the patient's bed if necessary.

1. Skin weals are raised at points 5 cm lateral to the upper borders of the spinous processes of the 2nd, 3rd and 4th lumbar vertebrae. Successful injection at these points blocks all the vasoconstrictor impulses to the lower limb. These points lie immediately above the transverse processes of the corresponding vertebrae. A 12–16-cm needle is introduced through each weal at right angles to

the skin for 4–5 cm and should encounter the transverse process; it is slightly withdrawn and directed upwards so that it passes between the transverse processes; it is also directed slightly inwards. After travelling 3–4 cm from the transverse process, the needle should make contact with the anterolateral aspect of the body of the vertebra. After careful aspiration to exclude both blood and cerebrospinal fluid, 10 ml of 1% lignocaine are injected at each site. (If force is required, needle tip is in anterior vertebral ligament or the psoas muscle and should be slightly withdrawn.) It spreads out in the retroperitoneal tissue. The spinal lumbar nerves run midway between the spinous processes, so if the needle point is kept in relation to the upper border of the transverse process, pain from hitting a nerve should be avoided. The lumbar arteries—branches of the aorta—with their veins must also be avoided. After 5–20 min the leg becomes less painful, its temperature increases and it becomes dry, its superficial veins dilate, and there is hyposensitivity to pin-prick.

2. A 12-cm needle is inserted at an angle of 70° through a weal three finger-breadths lateral to the superior point of the spinous process of L.3. It should miss the transverse process and come into contact with the body of the vertebra in the psoas tunnel: 15–20 ml of analgesic fluid are now injected.[178]

Use of X-ray control with an image intensifier greatly adds to the accuracy of needle placement.[176] Results of chemical lumbar sympathectomy can be assessed by taking infrared thermograms before and after the injections.[179]

For chemical sympathectomy three needles are placed against the bodies of L.2, L.3 and L.4 and their position verified radiologically; 3 ml of either 6% phenol in water or absolute alcohol, preceded by local analgesia, are injected through each correctly placed needle.[180]

Lateral approach. See Wallace C. *Anesthesiology* 1955, **16**, 254.

For assessment and monitoring of sympathetic block, *see* Cronin K. D. and Kirsner R. L. G. *Anaesth. Intensive Care* 1979, **7**, 353.

(*See also* Klopper G. T. *Anaesth. Intensive Care* 1983, **11**, 43.)

Complications
   1. Intradural injection and spinal analgesia.
   2. Intravascular injection.
   3. Hypotension.
   4. Haemorrhage into the sheath of the psoas muscle with pain referred to the groin and upper and inner part of the thigh.
   5. Neuritis of the genitofemoral nerve.

Caudal block gives the same results but is not unilateral: it produces, in addition to sympathetic paralysis, motor paresis and analgesia which may be useful objective signs of successful sympathetic block.

(*See also* Cherr D. A. et al. *Anaesth. Intensive Care* 1978, **6**, 164; Walker P. M. et al. *Surg. Gynecol. Obstet.* 1978, **146**, 741; Goldring J. R. et al. *J. R. Coll. Surg. Edinb.* 1979, **24**, 83; Cousins M. J. et al. *Anaesth. Intensive Care* 1979, **7**, 121.)

Intercostal Nerve Blocks
The cutaneous distribution of spinal nerves was worked out by O. Foerster (1873–1941) of Breslau and by Henry Head (1866–1940) of London.

The Cutaneous Nerves of the Trunk (*Figs*. 31.2–31.4)
Anteriorly

1. The lateral, intermediate and medial supraclavicular branches of the superficial division of the cervical plexus (C.3–C.4) to the second interspace.

2. The anterior rami of the thoracic nerves, excluding T.1.

3. The iliohypogastric and ilio-inguinal nerves (L.1).

Posteriorly. The posterior rami of C.2–C.5; T.1–T.12; L.1–L.3; the five sacral and the coccygeal nerves.

Anatomy of Spinal Nerves

Typical intercostal nerves are the 3rd to 6th inclusive. Each nerve is formed by the union of the anterior (motor) and the posterior (sensory) root: the latter has a ganglion on it. The mixed spinal nerve soon divides into anterior and posterior primary divisions (rami). The thoracic or dorsal nerves then are distributed as follows:

The posterior rami are smaller than the anterior. They turn backwards and divide into medial and lateral branches (except C.1, S.4 and S.5, coccygeal) which supply the muscles and skin of the back.

The anterior rami in the thoracic region of the 2nd to 6th nerves are each connected to the lateral sympathetic chain by a grey and a white ramus communicans. Each crosses the paravertebral space between the necks of contiguous ribs and then enters the subcostal groove where it lies below the vein

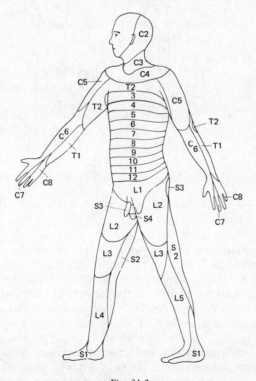

Fig. 31.2

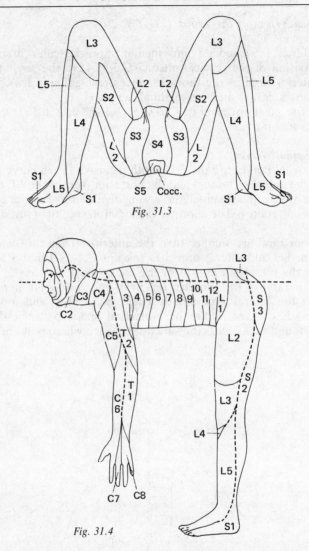

Fig. 31.3

Fig. 31.4

Figs. 31.2–31.4. Distribution of cutaneous nerves. (*After* Foerster O. *Brain* 1933, **56**, 1.)

and artery in a triangular space, bounded above by the rib, the posterior intercostal membrane and the internal intercostal muscle (intercostal intima)[181] until it reaches the anterior axillary line, at which point the nerves come into direct relationship with the pleura, as the innermost intercostal muscle terminates. There is a communication between each space and those contiguous to it, while analgesic solution spreads medially to surround the sympathetic chain in the paravertebral space.[181] Each intercostal nerve supplies muscular branches to the intercostal muscles and lateral and anterior cutaneous branches to supply the skin of the chest and abdomen. The 7th to 11th nerves pass below and behind the costal cartilages, between the slips of the diaphragm running between the internal oblique and transversus muscles (again between the second and third layers) to enter the posterior layer of the rectus sheath. They run deep into the rectus, pierce and supply it, and end as anterior cutaneous nerves.

The lateral cutaneous branch emerges in the midaxillary line, and divides into anterior and posterior branches which supply the skin on the lateral wall of the chest as far forward as the nipple line.

The anterior cutaneous branch is the termination of the intercostal nerve; it supplies the skin on the front of the chest, internal to the nipple line.

Exceptions. The 1st nerve parts with most of its fibres to the brachial plexus and gives neither lateral nor anterior cutaneous branches, the skin over the first intercostal space being supplied by the descending branches of the cervical plexus (C.3–C.4). The lateral cutaneous branch of the second intercostal nerve crosses the axilla and becomes the intercostobrachial nerve supplying the skin on the medial aspect of the arm. The lateral cutaneous branch of the 12th thoracic nerve, which does not divide into anterior and posterior branches, crosses the iliac crest to supply the skin of the upper part of the buttock as far as the greater trochanter. The 12th thoracic and 1st lumbar nerves supply sensory branches to the anterior chest and anterior abdominal wall, the parietal pleura and the parietal peritoneum.

The 10th nerve—lateral and anterior cutaneous branches—supplies the area of the umbilicus.

The 9th, 8th and 7th nerves supply the skin between the umbilicus and the xiphisternum.

The 11th, 12th and 1st lumbar nerves supply the skin between the umbilicus and the pubis.

Technique of Intercostal Nerve Block

1. At the angle of the ribs (Sellheim (1871–1936), 1906,[182] James, 1943[183]). At this point the nerve becomes relatively superficial, lateral to the erector spinae muscle. In this technique the rami communicantes conveying afferent impulses may be blocked by the local analgesic solution tracking medially but splanchnic analgesia will be necessary in addition for intra-abdominal surgery. The patient is arranged in the lateral spinal position with his back well arched over the edge of the table. After swabbing with antiseptic and fixing sterile towels, two lines are drawn, one on each side four finger-breadths from the middle line, the lines should extend from the spines of the scapulae to the iliac crests. At a point where the lower border of the 11th rib on the patient's upper side crosses the line, a needle is introduced (through an intradermal weal if necessary) until it makes contact with the rib. It is then partially withdrawn and advanced until it slips past the lower border of the rib for 3 mm; 2–3 ml of local analgesic solution with adrenaline are then injected, while the needle point is slightly advanced and withdrawn so as to surround the nerve with analgesic solution. The intercostal nerve is thus surrounded by a zone of solution as it lies in the subcostal groove between the intercostalis internus and the internal intercostal muscles. The needle should be mounted on a syringe, so that should the pleura be punctured no air will enter the pleural cavity. The needle is then withdrawn until its point is just beneath the skin, so that it can act as a marker. The 10th to the 6th nerves are now injected on the upper side, followed, after turning, by the lower seven nerves on the patient's other side. The 12th nerves are deeper and require special care. Before the 6th and 7th nerves can be injected the patient's scapulae must be drawn laterally by crossing his arms over his chest. The needle pierces the trapezius, the latissimus dorsi and the two intercostal muscles. Good analgesia for up to 12 h results if the abdominal incision is subcostal. For paramedian or midline incisions, bilateral block is necessary.[181] A possible complication is pneumothorax.[182] Another is intradural injection.[257]

Posterior splanchnic block can be performed with the patient in the same position if the abdomen is to be opened.

2. *In the posterior axillary line.* First reported in 1915.[183] Similar injections can be carried out with the patient supine and with his arms abducted to a right angle. In this position the ribs, and so the intercostal nerves, are not so deeply placed. A block in the midaxillary line misses the lateral cutaneous nerve. Local analgesic solution injected via an extradural catheter often spreads to several spaces above and below the point of injection, external to the pleura.[168] This spread was not seen in Moore's cases.[185] Massive haematoma formation has been reported.[181,184]

3. *In the midaxillary line.* It has been shown that the intercostal nerves can be blocked at the level of the midaxillary line in supine patients as effectively as at the posterior angle of the ribs.[186]

Indications

Blocking of the lower seven intercostal nerves on each side results in analgesia of the anterior abdominal wall from just below the nipple line to a level just above the pubic bone. In addition, it produces analgesia of the parietal peritoneum and relaxation of the muscles of the anterior abdominal wall. It is especially useful when scars from previous operations disturb the relations of the abdominal wall making abdominal field block difficult. For analgesia of the viscera, splanchnic analgesia is required in addition.

To give a longer period of analgesia, 0·25 or 0·5% bupivacaine or amethocaine hydrochloride 1–2000 to 1–4000 solution may be used, 3 ml being injected at 12-hourly intervals for up to 36 hours.[184] Care must be taken to avoid a toxic dose of these and other agents and adrenaline should be added. Absorption is rapid.

Intercostal block is also useful to enable deep breathing and coughing to take place in a patient with severe postoperative abdominal pain or with fractured ribs but does not always produce good results.[262]

Blood levels of local analgesic solutions injected near the intercostal nerves rise rapidly.

A cryoprobe applied to intercostal nerves within the thorax has been used to reduce postthoracotomy pain.[187] There is evidence that more complications follow attack on the intercostal nerves from inside the thorax than when it is injected percutaneously.[188]

Intercostal Block for Rib Resection and Insertion of a Drain

The surgeon is asked to mark out the position of the incision he wishes to make, and it is infiltrated intradermally and subcutaneously with 0·5–1% lignocaine solution. An intradermal and subcutaneous line of infiltration is carried out one rib above and one below the length of rib to be removed. Their lines extend 2·5 cm in front and 2·5 cm behind the proposed incision, and the extremities are joined by intradermal and subcutaneous infiltrations, so that a rectangle is marked out. The intercostal nerves within this rectangle are blocked at their posterior extremities with 2% lignocaine solution. There may be slight discomfort during the stripping of the periosteum from the rib by the surgeon.

Local block is usually the preferred method of anaesthesia in these operations. If the patient is well enough, he should sit sideways across the table, to prevent him drowning in his own pus if the abscess ruptures into a bronchus. Otherwise he is placed in the lateral position with the head and shoulders elevated. This position is also suitable for general anaesthesia.[189]

Splanchnic Analgesia; Coeliac Plexus Block

Anatomy[190]
Semilunar or coeliac plexus. Two in number, one on each side of the midline, lying on the aorta and the crura of the diaphragm just above the pancreas, at the level of the 1st lumbar vertebra between the adrenal glands and behind the stomach and lesser sac. The renal vessels are inferior to the plexus while the vessels to the adrenals often pass through it. They are connected with each other and with their associated ganglia (superior mesenteric and inferior mesenteric, etc.) by a network of nerve fibres around the coeliac artery. These fibres are postganglionic fibres of the greater and lesser splanchnic nerves. From this mass of retroperitoneal nerve tissue fibres pass with the arteries to the abdominal viscera. These plexuses also receive twigs from the right vagus and the phrenic nerves. The semilunar or coeliac ganglia with the aorticorenal and superior mesenteric ganglia together make up the solar or epigastric plexus.

Afferent fibres from the abdominal viscera, both sympathetic and parasympathetic (vagus), pass through the coeliac ganglia. Afferent fibres from the pelvic viscera, travelling through the nervi erigentes (S.2–S.4) do not.
Greater splanchnic nerve (the superior thoracic splanchnic nerve), like the lesser and the lowest splanchnic, is composed of pre-ganglionic fibres which are, in effect, elongated white rami. The majority of its fibres are myelinated. It rises from the union of four or five roots coming from the thoracic sympathetic ganglia which receive white rami from the 5th to the 10th thoracic nerves, sometimes higher. The nerve enters the abdomen through the crus of the diaphragm on each side, with the lesser and lowest splanchnic nerves, and enters the corresponding semilunar ganglion. It mainly contains visceral afferent fibres. Within the abdomen the nerve lies between the diaphragm and the adrenal gland on each side.
Lesser splanchnic nerve (the middle thoracic splanchnic nerve). This arises from the lower thoracic ganglia of the sympathetic cord, connected with the 10th and 11th thoracic nerves. It enters the corresponding aorticorenal ganglion.
Lowest splanchnic nerve (the inferior thoracic splanchnic nerve). This arises from the last thoracic ganglion and enters the renal plexus and the posterior renal ganglion.
The lumbar splanchnic nerves. Are presumably blocked when the coeliac plexus is blocked, by spreading of solution. The 1st lumbar splanchnic nerve arises from the 1st lumbar ganglion; the 2nd from the 2nd and 3rd ganglia (they join the coeliac plexus): the 3rd from the 2nd, 3rd and 4th ganglia; the 4th from the 4th and 5th ganglia. The last two join the superior hypogastric plexus.
The hypogastric nerve (presacral nerves). Extends from the 3rd lumbar vertebra to the 1st sacral where it ends by dividing into the right and left hypogastric

nerves or plexuses. It lies in front of the lower part of the abdominal aorta, behind the peritoneum.

The Superior Hypogastric Plexus

Formerly known as the presacral nerve. It is retroperitoneal, lying on the body of the fifth lumbar vertebra. It receives fibres from the sympathetic trunk via lumbar ganglia 3 and 4; fibres known as the intermesenteric plexus coming from the coeliac, mesenteric and pararenal plexuses; and parasympathetic fibres. From it are derived fibres supplying, via the inferior mesenteric artery the transverse, descending and sigmoid colon; the inferior hypogastric nerves to the rectum and ureters which contain both sympathetic and parasympathetic elements.

The Inferior Hypogastric Plexus

A collection of ganglia and nerve fibres where preganglionic sympathetic fibres synapse. It receives fibres from the inferior hypogastric nerves, together with parasympathetic fibres and supplies the viscera of the female pelvis (except the ovaries). Its sympathetic element provides sensory and motor fibres to the urinary and anal sphincters; the parasympathetic fibres are motor to the bladder and rectum. These fibres travel with blood vessels.

Many of these structures are damaged in pelvic operations. Division of the superior hypogastric plexus (presacral neurectomy) is used in the treatment of dysmenorrhoea.[191]

Afferent Pathways from Upper Abdominal Viscera

These visceral afferents travel from sensory nerve endings in the walls of the viscera, mesentery, etc. via the splanchnic nerves and enter the cord with the white rami of the lower seven thoracic nerves (and sometimes higher), having their cell stations in the posterior root ganglia of these nerves. Afferent impulses also travel up in the vagi and the phrenics.

Visceral afferent fibres, travelling with the sympathetic, enter the cord at the following levels: stomach, T.6–10; small gut, T.9–10; large gut to middle of transverse colon T.11–L.1; distal colon, L.1–2; liver and biliary tract T.7–9; pancreas T.6–10; kidney and ureter T.10–L.2; bladder and prostate T.11–12; testis and ovary T.10–11; uterus T.10–11.

Nerve Supply to Adrenal Glands

Preganglionic fibres do not synapse in coeliac or other pre-aortic plexuses, but pass directly to end around chromaffin cells of the medulla. In addition to the lesser splanchnic, fibres go to the adrenals from the 10th thoracic to 2nd lumbar nerves.

Technique of Splanchnic Block

Splanchnic block can be performed before laparotomy (Wendling) or during laparotomy from the front (Braun), or before laparotomy from behind (Kappis). The Braun technique is usually performed by the surgeon.

1. *Braun's method.*[192] With the abdomen opened, the liver is gently retracted upwards and the stomach is drawn to the left. The anterior aspect of the body of the 1st lumbar vertebra is located medial to the lesser curvature of the stomach; the aorta is retracted laterally and the long Braun needle is inserted down to the bone and 50 ml of solution injected (e.g. 0·5% lignocaine).

2. Kappis's method. Described by Max Kappis (1881–1938) in 1914.[193] The patient is in the spinal position, sitting or lying prone. The 4th interspace is located, lying on or before the intercristal line; by counting upward, the spine of the 1st lumbar vertebra is identified. Weals are raised four finger-breadths from this spine, one in each side of the midline. The weals must be below the 12th rib.

A long needle is inserted at an angle of 45° to the median plane through this weal with its bevel facing inwards. It is directed slightly upwards and thrust in until it makes contact with the body of the 1st lumbar vertebra. It is then partly withdrawn and its point directed more laterally until its bevel is felt to glance past the lateral aspect of the body of the vertebra. The needle is then advanced a further 1 cm and, after a most careful aspiration test, 20–40 ml of solution are injected. The average distance between the skin and the plexus is 7–10 cm. If blood is aspirated into the syringe, the needle point may be in the vena cava or the aorta and must be moved until it is free of these vessels. Bilateral block is probably unnecessary. The technique has been modified.[194] Fluoroscopy aids accurate placement of the needle. Computerized aided tomography guided coeliac plexus block has been described,[195] while insertion of the needle at the level of L.2 has been advocated.[196]

The usual strengths of solution employed are prilocaine, 0·5%; lignocaine, 0·5%; amethocaine, 1–2000 to 1–4000. Adrenaline should be added.

Splanchnic block causes a profound fall in blood pressure which can be partially controlled by an intravenous infusion of fluid or by ephedrine or one of its congeners, should it be considered necessary. It produces analgesia of the abdominal viscera, with the exception of the pelvic viscera, i.e. the sigmoid colon, rectum, bladder and reproductive organs. The bowel becomes contracted and ribbon-like. The patient must be particularly well premedicated, intravenous narcotic analgesic being given until his mental state is calm. The surgeon must be light-handed, especially when the peritoneal cavity is being explored, as its lateral walls are not rendered insensitive either by the splanchnic block or the abdominal field block (but by posterior intercostal block).

Therapeutically, splanchnic block is useful in the treatment of carcinoma of the pancreas and acute pancreatitis (perhaps because it relaxes the sphincter of Oddi). It causes a greater blood supply to be diverted to the pancreas. If these conditions are found at laparotomy, splanchnic block with phenol has much to recommend it.[197] The block may be repeated if desirable. It has also been used in the terminal stages of upper abdominal cancer to relieve pain. Alcohol in saline, 50%, preceded by local analgesic solution, has been employed.[198] Paraplegia has followed this block.[199]

Abdominal Field Block

Described in 1905.[201]

Anatomy

The superficial fascia in the upper abdomen is a single fatty layer, but from a point midway between the umbilicus and the pubis two layers are described, the deep layer (fascia of Antonius Scarpa; 1747–1832) and the superficial layer (fascia of Petrus Camper; 1722–1789).

Camper's fascia passes over the inguinal ligament and is continuous with the superficial fascia of the thigh. It is continued over the penis, spermatic cord and scrotum where it helps to form the dartos muscle. In the female it is continued into the labia majora.

Scarpa's fascia is tougher. It blends with the deep fascia of the thigh and, like Camper's fascia, is continued over the penis and helps to form the dartos. From the scrotum it becomes continuous with Colles's fascia (1811) over the perineum. There is no deep fascia covering the abdomen.

External oblique. The largest and most superficial of the muscles of the anterior abdominal wall. The aponeurosis is attached below to the anterior superior spine and to the pubic crest and tubercle; it thus forms the inguinal ligament. In the midline it forms the linea alba which runs from the symphysis pubis to the xiphisternum. The subcutaneous or external inguinal ring is an opening in the aponeurosis.

The fibres of the external oblique pass downwards and inwards, like those of the external intercostal muscles.

Internal oblique. This is a thinner layer than the above.

The fibres of this muscle run upwards and inwards.

Transversus abdominis. The fibres of the muscle run transversely. Between it and the external oblique run the lower intercostal, iliohypogastric and ilio-inguinal nerves. Below the level of the iliac crest the fibres of these three muscles are aponeurotic and run downwards and medially.

Rectus abdominis. Each muscle *arises* from the crest of the pubis and from the ligaments in front of the symphysis. *Inserted* into the anterior aspects of the 5th, 6th and 7th costal cartilages and into the xiphisternum.

Three tendinous intersections cross the muscle and are firmly attached to the anterior layer of its sheath, but not to the posterior layer. One is at the level of the xiphisternum, one at the umbilicus and the third one midway between.

The rectus sheath contains, in addition to the rectus and pyramidalis muscles, the superior and inferior epigastric vessels and the terminations of the lower six intercostal nerves and vessels. The nerves pierce the lateral margin of the sheath and run in relation to its posterior wall, before they enter the substance of the muscle.

Pyramidalis. A small muscle on each side, within the rectus sheath. It is well developed in marsupial mammals and serves to strengthen the linea alba.

The abdominal muscles are supplied by the anterior rami of the lower six thoracic nerves and by the iliohypogastric and ilio-inguinal nerves.

They are accessory muscles of expiration and help to compress the abdominal viscera, as in defaecation, straining, coughing, etc. They are not muscles of normal inspiration.

Transversalis fascia. A thin membrane, continuous with the iliac and pelvic fascia. In the inguinal region it is stronger and thicker than elsewhere and through it, at the abdominal inguinal (internal inguinal); ring, passes the spermatic cord or the round ligament.

Sensory nerve supply of abdominal wall. The anterior primary rami of the lower six thoracic nerves, via the intercostal nerves. The skin in the region of the nipple is supplied by the 5th thoracic nerve. Skin in the epigastrium is supplied by the 7th nerve. Skin in the region of the umbilicus is supplied by the 10th nerve. Skin midway between the umbilicus and the pubis is supplied by the 12th nerve. Skin of the groin is supplied by the iliohypogastric nerve (L.1).

Intercostal nerves and the last thoracic nerve pass under the costal margin between the slips of the diaphragm and run forwards between the internal oblique and the transversus abdominis before they pierce the lateral margin of the rectus sheath. After lying behind the rectus muscle, they pierce its substance and supply it, and end as anterior cutaneous nerves.

Vessels of the abdominal wall. The only vessels likely to be injured by the anaesthetist are the superior and inferior epigastric arteries and veins. The superior artery is the termination of the internal mammary and enters the rectus sheath posterior to the 7th costal cartilage. The inferior epigastric artery arises from the external iliac artery and enters the rectus sheath behind the arcuate line of Douglas.

Surface markings. The xiphoid is on a level with the body of T.9. The subcostal plane is at L.3. The highest part of the iliac crest is on a level with L.4 or the L.4–L.5. interspace.

Technique of Abdominal Field Block

In all operations performed under field block analgesia it is necessary to infiltrate the line of incision both subcutaneously and intradermally. The injections should be commenced 15–20 min before the incision is to be made.

Weals are raised: (1) At the tip of the xiphisternum opposite the body of T.9; (2) One on each side at the 9th costal cartilage, where the rectus muscle crosses it; (3) One on each side at the lateral margin of the rectus, just above the umbilicus; (4) One on each side at the lateral margin of the rectus, below the umbilicus—if the incision is to be prolonged.

Through weals 2, 3 and 4 a needle is inserted perpendicularly until it meets the resistance of the rectus sheath. If the patient is conscious he will experience pain when the anterior layer of the rectus sheath is pierced. The needle is advanced a further 0·5 cm and 5 ml of solution are injected into the sheath. After withdrawal into the subcutaneous tissue, the needle is inclined upwards and downwards so that more solution is deposited into the rectus sheath. It is important to remember the positions of the tendinous intersection so that solution is deposited between each pair to ensure even distribution of the analgesic drug. Posterior to the muscle, these intersections do not impede the spread of solution. After completion of the deep injections the weals are joined together along the lateral margin of the rectus by lines of subcutaneous injection. Similarly weal 1 is joined to each weal 2 along the costal margin. A total of 50–100 ml of solution is used (e.g. 0·5% lignocaine).

A costo-iliac block gives a wider zone of analgesia and relaxation than the rectus-sheath block outlined below, but is more difficult to carry out successfully. Weals are raised on each side along the costal margin and vertically downward to the iliac crest. Solution is deposited, from needles passed through these weals, into the subcutaneous and muscular layers of the abdominal wall, remembering that laterally the intercostal nerves lie between the transversalis and internal oblique. The weals are joined together by subcutaneous infiltration, as described for rectus-sheath block. In muscular subjects, in addition, solution can be injected into the rectus sheath. The volume of solution required is 150–200 ml.

Rectus-sheath block (Carl Ludwig Schleich, 1859–1922)[202] is an excellent method of producing muscular relaxation when combined with a light general anaesthetic, and if the incision is to be midline or paramedian it is usual to do both sides. Perforation of the peritoneum should be avoided, but in the absence of peritonitis or adhesions no serious harm is likely to result. The anterior layer of the rectus sheath is detected by the needle throughout its whole extent, but the posterior layer only for about 7·5 cm above and below the umbilicus. Solution is placed posterior to the muscle so that the intercostal nerves supplying it, together with the zone of skin medial to its outer border, are blocked. If the abdomen shows the scar of a previous operation, abdominal field block may be difficult and undesirable, and intercostal block or paravertebral block may be indicated if the operation is to be performed under local analgesia.

Intermittent injection through a small plastic catheter can be used to produce good postoperative analgesia.

Abdominal field block renders the abdominal wall and its underlying parietal peritoneum insensitive. To block pain impulses from the viscera, and postero-lateral parietal peritoneum, either light general anaesthesia or a splanchnic block and posterior intercostal block is required.

Regional analgesia for intra-abdominal surgery, requiring multiple punctures and near-toxic doses of local analgesic drugs, finds little favour today although Hans Finsterer (1876–1954), leading surgeon from Vienna, considered it to be the best method of pain relief for gastric surgery in his time (1923).[200]

Field Block for Repair of Inguinal Hernia

Anatomy
The inguinal canal is 4 cm long and extends from the internal inguinal ring laterally to the external inguinal ring medially. It lies above the inner half of the inguinal ligament.

The internal or abdominal ring is just above the midpoint of the inguinal ligament; it is an opening in the transversalis fascia and just medial to it is the inferior epigastric artery.

The subcutaneous or external ring lies above and lateral to the pubic crest. It is an opening in the external oblique, and through it passes the spermatic cord in the male and the round ligament in the female. They lie lateral to the pubic spine.

The walls of the inguinal canal are:
1. Anteriorly: external oblique; internal oblique in its lateral third.
2. Posteriorly: fascia transversalis in its whole length; conjoint tendon or falx inguinalis in its inner two-thirds; reflected part of the inguinal ligament in its inner third; the femoral vessels.
3. The floor: inguinal ligament.
4. The roof: arching fibres of the conjoint tendon of the transversus abdominis and the internal oblique.

The contents of the inguinal canal are the ilio-inguinal nerve and the spermatic cord (or the round ligament of the uterus). The spermatic cord comprises the internal and external spermatic arteries and the artery to the vas deferens, the pampiniform plexus of veins, the lymphatic vessels, the autonomic nerve-fibres and the vas deferens in the male.

Indirect inguinal hernia. All inguinal hernias are protrusions through the fascia transversalis. An indirect hernia protrudes through the deep inguinal ring, descends into the cord and receives a covering from the external spermatic fascia, cremesteric muscle and internal spermatic fascia (from the fascia transversalis).

Direct inguinal hernia. This protrudes through the fascia transversalis in the more medial part of the posterior wall of the canal through the triangle of Hesselbach (1759–1816),[203] the boundaries of which are: lateral, the inferior or deep epigastric artery; medial, the outer border of the rectus; inferior, the inguinal ligament.

Nerve supply. The nerve supply of the inguinal region is from the last two thoracic and the first two lumbar nerves via the iliohypogastric, the ilio-inguinal and the genitofemoral.

The last two thoracic nerves run downwards and inwards, just above the anterior superior iliac spine, between the internal oblique and transversus muscles. They end by piercing the rectus sheath.

The iliohypogastric and ilio-inguinal nerves come from the first lumbar root. They are inferior to the last two thoracic nerves and curve round the body just above the iliac crest, gradually piercing the muscles and ending superficially; the ilio-inguinal nerve traverses the inguinal canal, lying anterior to the spermatic cord, and becomes superficial through the external ring and supplies the skin of the scrotum. The iliohypogastric nerve, after running between the internal oblique and the transversus abdominis, pierces the internal oblique just above the anterior superior iliac spine and supplies the skin over the pubis.

The genitofemoral nerve comes from the 1st and 2nd lumbar nerves and divides into a genital and a femoral branch. The former enters the inguinal canal from behind through the internal ring.

Indications

1. In slim, elderly, poor-risk patients, to avoid the risks of general anaesthesia or the possible risks of hypotension associated with intra- or extradural analgesia. Used routinely by some surgeons.[204]

2. To reduce the risks of aspiration of intestinal contents in cases of strangulation. Bowel resection usually requires other methods of pain relief.

3. For day-stay surgery.[205]

4. Ilio-inguinal and ilio-hypogastric block eases postoperative pain.

Contraindications

Obesity, lack of cooperation by the surgeon and nervousness of the patient.

Technique

Three weals are made as follows: (1) A finger-breadth internal to the anterior superior iliac spine; (2) Over the spine of the pubis; (3) 1·5 cm above the midpoint of the inguinal ligament.

Through weal 1 a larger needle is introduced vertically backwards until it is felt to pierce the aponeurosis of the external oblique with a slight click.[206] After aspiration, 30 ml of solution (+ or −) are injected so that both the ilio-inguinal and iliohypogastric nerves are surrounded. At this point a needle introduced perpendicularly to the skin will not pierce the peritoneum. Solution is deposited in all layers including that small area of tissue between the weal and the anterior superior spine. (*See* p. 643.)

Through weal 2 a larger needle deposits solution in the intradermal and subcutaneous layers in the direction of the umbilicus. This blocks nerve twigs overlapping from the opposite side.

Through weal 3 a needle is inserted perpendicularly to the skin until it pierces the aponeurosis of the external oblique. At this level 20 ml of solution (+ or −) are injected so that the genital branch of the genitofemoral nerve is blocked.[207]

Intradermal and subcutaneous infiltration along the line of the incision may be necessary to get perfect analgesia; in addition, infiltration of the periosteum near the pubic tubercle and Astley Cooper's ligament, the conjoint tendon and the lateral border of the rectus abdominis muscle should be performed in cases of direct inguinal hernia.[208]

The use of 0·5% solution of prilocaine with adrenaline allows a generous volume of relatively non-toxic local analgesic solution to be employed. Otherwise 0·25% bupivacaine or 0·5% lignocaine, both with adrenaline, are suitable. Dose of bupivacaine should not exceed 2 mg/kg. There is no advantage in the use of dextran to prolong local analgesic effect.[258]

If the hernia is strangulated or irreducible, deeper layers should be injected by the surgeon, under vision, as he goes along.

The patient may complain of temporary discomfort when the neck of the sac is under tension; this can often be relieved by infiltration of local analgesic solution around the neck. Infiltration analgesia is a perfectly acceptable method of pain relief in elective inguinal and femoral hernias and patients require less postoperative analgesia and vomit less than after general anaesthesia.[204,205]

In these operations, the surgeon often gives his own injections.[209] Following his experience with 100 000 operations under local analgesia, using the Shouldice surgical technique, Glasgow[210] advises first weight reduction. Then premedication sodium pentobarbitone, 200–250 mg by mouth, 1½ h before operation, then pethidine 50–75 mg i.m. Procaine 2% solution (for those over 70, 1–1·5%) without adrenaline; total volume 150 ml (a big dose!); 80–100 ml subcutaneously with a further 10–20 ml beneath the external oblique aponeurosis, with a similar volume round the internal ring, avoiding the inferior epigastric vessels. Advantages of regional analgesia: avoids the risks of general anaesthesia; makes the surgeon gentle; patient can cough during the operation if required; surgeon uses less tension in his sutures; patient can walk off the table and be treated as a day-stay case; catheterization is eliminated; and a quicker turn-round of cases.

Field Block for Repair of Femoral Hernia

Anatomy
A femoral hernia passes through the femoral canal and the saphenous opening or fossa ovalis, an opening in the deep fascia of the thigh, 3·8 cm (1½ in) below and 3·8 cm (1½ in) lateral to the pubic tubercle.

The femoral canal is the most medial of three compartments, the most lateral containing the femoral artery and the intermediate one the femoral vein. The femoral canal is 1·2 cm long, and at its mouth is the femoral ring.

The femoral ring is bounded in front by the inguinal ligament and behind by the pectineus, laterally by the femoral vein, and medially by the lacunar ligament of Gimbernat (1734–1790). Astley Cooper's (1768–1841) ligament is a backward extension of the lacunar ligament, along the pelvic brim (iliopectineal line) for 1·5 cm. The ring contains the femoral septum or fatty pad.

The coverings of a femoral hernia are, from within outwards: the fat from the femoral septum, the prolongation of the fascia transversalis forming the anterior wall of the femoral sheath, and the cribriform fascia of the fossa ovalis.

Technique

The technique is similar to that for repair of inguinal hernia, with the addition that the lump in the thigh is surrounded by subcutaneous and intradermal weals.

Paravertebral block from T.10 to L.3 may also be carried out; it is a suitable procedure for operation on strangulated herniae, both inguinal and femoral. The authors have no experience of it.

Iliac Crest Block

A weal is raised 4 cm from the anterior superior iliac spine on a line joining this spine to the xiphisternum. A needle is inserted laterally, first just beneath the skin and then deeper until the ilium is touched. Solution is injected so that it anaesthetizes the 12th thoracic, iliohypogastric and ilio-inguinal nerves as they lie between the internal oblique and the transversus abdominis muscles. (*See* p. 645.)

Field Block for Appendicectomy

This can be useful in interval cases, but is seldom successful in operation for acute appendicitis.

Two weals are raised, one just above and behind the anterior superior iliac spine, the second below the costal margin at the tip of the 10th rib on the right side. The tissues between the skin and peritoneum in this line are infiltrated, and subcutaneous infiltration is made between the two weals and downwards between the lower weal and the iliac bone. Thus the 10th, 11th and 12th thoracic nerves are blocked, together with the ilio-inguinal and iliohypogastric.

Splanchnic block and bilateral somatic block are usually necessary, except in the very simplest operations on thin subjects.

Field Block for Operations on the Anal Canal

A weal is made on each side of the anus and 2·5 cm away from it. From these weals a subcutaneous rhomboidal zone of infiltration is made, using 20 ml of 0·5% bupivacaine and adrenaline. Deep injections are now made from the infiltrated zone into each quadrant, 5 ml into each with a finger in the rectum preventing perforation of the mucous membrane. The nerve to the external anal sphincter is the perineal branch of the 4th sacral nerve. The operation can be done satisfactorily with the patient in the prone position with the pelvis raised, and heavy premedication should be employed, e.g. pethidine and promethazine 50 mg of each i.m. with diazepam i.v.[211]

Penile Block; Field Block for Circumcision

Anatomy

The sensory nerves of the penis are derived from the terminal twigs of the internal pudendal nerves. The dorsal nerves of the penis travel beneath the pubic bone, one on each side of the midline, lying against the dorsal surface of the corpus cavernosum. The skin at the base of the organ is supplied by the ilio-inguinal and perhaps the genitofemoral nerves. In addition, the posterior scrotal branches of the perineal nerves run para-urethrally to the ventral surface and fraenum, so four nerves have to be blocked.

Technique

An intradermal and subcutaneous ring weal is raised around the base of the penis; the subcutaneous infiltration should precede the intradermal. The dorsal nerve is next blocked on each side by injected 5 ml of solution into the dorsum of the organ just below but not deep to the symphysis so that the needle point lies against the corpus cavernosum. If the needle pierces the corpus cavernosum, pain is experienced. For the ventral injection of the para-urethral branches, the penis should be pulled upwards and 2 ml of solution injected near the base of the organ into the groove formed by the corpora cavernosa and the corpus spongiosum. Infiltration of 5 ml of 1% lignocaine or 0·5% bupivacaine into each dorsal nerve provides good postoperative analgesia.[212] In infants, smaller volumes are used. Postoperative pain can be relieved by repeated penile block in awake patients, even in children, without undue discomfort.[213]

Adrenaline must not be used lest necrosis of tissue results, as the arteries of the penis are end-arteries.

Care must be taken not to cause haematoma formation as this may contribute to gangrene of skin; subpubic injection must be avoided.[214]

Pain following circumcision under general anaesthesia can be relieved by sacral extradural analgesia (*see* Chapter 32) or by infiltrating each dorsal nerve at the root of the penis[215] with 1–3 ml of local analgesic solution, e.g. 0·5% bupivacaine, without adrenaline. This is a satisfactory alternative to extradural sacral block, with fewer complications.[216] Lignocaine spray or gel, applied topically gives useful relief.

Nerve Block at the Upper Part of the Thigh (*Figs.* 31.5–31.8)

Anatomy of Lumbar Plexus

The ventral rami of the lumbar nerves each receive a grey ramus communicans from a lumbar ganglion, while the 1st and 2nd lumbar nerves are also connected with the trunk by a white ramus.

They form the lumbar plexus lying in the psoas major, anterior to the transverse process of the lumbar vertebrae. A branch from the 4th unites with the 5th nerve to form the lumbosacral trunk which joins the sacral plexus.

The branches of the lumbar plexus are:

The iliohypogastric nerve from L.1. It leaves the psoas major, crosses the quadratus lumborum, perforates the transversus abdominis and then divides into lateral and anterior cutaneous branches. Its lateral cutaneous branch supplies the skin on the anterior part of the gluteal region after piercing the internal and external oblique muscles 5 cm behind the anterior superior iliac spine and just above the iliac crest, while the terminal part of the nerve supplies the skin over the pubic bone after piercing the aponeurosis of the external oblique, 2 cm medial to the anterior superior iliac spine. It does not divide into anterior and posterior branches. Block after operation reduces pain.

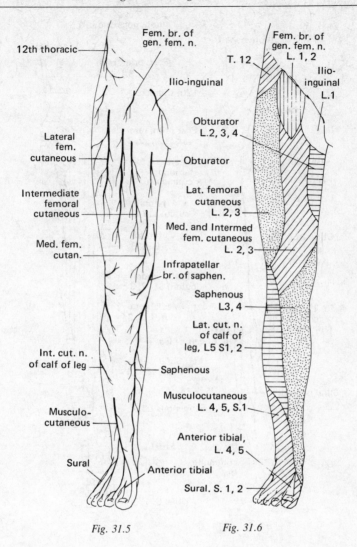

Fig. 31.5   Fig. 31.6

Fig. 31.5. The cutaneous nerves of the right lower extremity. Anterior aspect.

Fig. 31.6. The segmental distribution of the cutaneous nerves of the right lower extremity. Anterior aspect.

The ilio-inguinal nerve from L.1. This accompanies the iliohypogastric nerve, in its early course, lying just inferior to it in close relationship to the iliac crest. About 2 cm anterior and just below the anterior superior spine, it pierces the internal oblique and runs medially behind the aponeurosis of the external oblique. It then passes with the spermatic cord through the inguinal canal and supplies the skin of the upper and medial part of the thigh and the adjacent skin

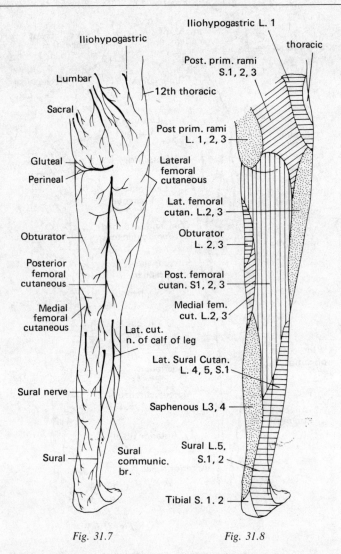

Fig. 31.7.   *Fig. 31.8.*

Fig. 31.7. The cutaneous nerves of the right lower extremity. Posterior
aspect.

Fig. 31.8. The segmental distribution of the cutaneous nerves of the right
lower extremity. Posterior aspect. (*Figs. 31.5–31.8 after 'Gray's Anatomy'
by kind permission.*)

covering the external genitals. It has no lateral cutaneous branch, unlike the
iliohypogastric nerve, and in the inguinal canal is sensory.(*See also* p. 643.)
The genitofemoral nerve from L.1 and L.2. Its genital branch supplies the skin
of the scrotum or labium majus, and the cremaster muscle. Its femoral branch
supplies an area of skin on the middle of the anterior surface of the upper part of
the thigh.

The lateral cutaneous nerve of the thigh (lateral femoral cutaneous) from L.2 and L.3 (posterior divisions). It supplies the skin of the anterolateral aspect of the thigh as far as the knee anteriorly, but laterally not quite so low after passing behind the inguinal ligament and the sartorius muscle, just medial and slightly inferior to the anterior superior iliac spine. (*See* p. 649.)

The femoral nerve from L.2, L.3 and L.4 (posterior divisions). It emerges from the psoas major, passes between it and the iliacus and enters the thigh behind the inguinal ligament and just lateral to the femoral artery, from which it is here separated by a slip of the psoas major. It has anterior and posterior divisions, the latter giving rise to the saphenous nerve and the medial and intermediate cutaneous nerves of the thigh. The femoral nerve supplies the hip joint and knee joint, the skin of the anterior part of the thigh and the anteromedial part of the leg. It is motor to the quadriceps femoris, the sartorius and the pectineus.

The obturator nerve from L.2, L.3 and L.4 (anterior divisions). It emerges from the medial border of the psoas muscle where it is a posterior relation of the external iliac vessels. After running forwards on the lateral wall of the pelvis it pierces the obturator canal, the nerve divides into anterior and posterior branches; the former supplies the adductor longus and brevis and the gracilis, with a twig going to the hip joint; the posterior branch supplies the adductor magnus and the hip joint. It supplies an area of skin on the medial aspect of the thigh and sends a small branch to the knee joint. An *accessory obturator nerve* is present in about 25% of people and runs a variable course across the superior pubic ramus and not via the obturator foramen; it comes from L.3 and L.4 (anterior divisions). (*See* p. 649.)

Anatomy of Sacral Plexus

The anterior primary rami of the five sacral and the coccygeal nerves receive each a grey ramus from the sympathetic trunk. From the 2nd, 3rd and 4th sacral nerves white rami (visceral afferent) join the pelvic plexuses, the sacral outflow of the autonomic nervous system or pelvic splanchnic nerves.

The sacral and pudendal plexuses are composed of the lumbosacral trunk (L.4 and L.5) and the ventral rami of the upper four sacral nerves. They lie on the posterior wall of the pelvic cavity between the piriformis and the pelvic fascia and have in front the ureter, internal iliac vessels, and the sigmoid colon on the left.

The following branches are given off:

The posterior cutaneous nerve of the thigh (S.1–S.3) supplies the skin of the lower part of the gluteal region, the perineum and the back of the thigh and leg.

The great sciatic nerve (L.4 and L.5; S.1–S.3) supplies the skin at the back of the leg and sole of the foot, after dividing into tibial and common peroneal nerves usually at the upper extremity of the popliteal fossa. It leaves the pelvis through the greater sciatic foramen, lying between the piriformis and the superior gemellus muscles, and occupies the space between the ischial tuberosity and the greater trochanter. After splitting into: (1) the tibial nerve, which gives origin to the sural and divides near the ankle into the medial and lateral branches, and (2) the common peroneal, from which originate the deep and superficial peroneal nerves. (The tibial is synonymous with the medial popliteal and posterior tibial, while the common peroneal is synonymous with the lateral popliteal, and from it arise the deep peroneal or anterior tibial and the superficial peroneal or musculocutaneous nerves.)

The perforating cutaneous nerve (S.2 and S.3) supplies the skin over the medial and lower parts of the gluteus maximus.

The pudendal nerve leaves the pelvis through the greater sciatic foramen, crosses the ischial spine medial to the pudendal vessels and goes through the lesser sciatic foramen. With the pudendal vessels it passes upwards and forwards along the lateral wall of the ischiorectal fossa, in Alcock's canal, a sheath of the obturator fascia. It gives off: (1) The inferior rectal nerve supplying the external anal sphincter and the skin around the anus. (2) The perineal nerve supplying the skin of the scrotum or labium majus and small twigs to muscles. (3) The dorsal nerve of the penis or clitoris. (4) The medial and lateral posterior scrotal (or labial) nerves. (5) Visceral branches supplying the rectum and bladder. From the 2nd, 3rd and 4th sacral nerves. They communicate with the sympathetic pelvic plexuses. (Sometimes called the pelvic splanchnic nerves of Gaskell, homologous with the white rami communicantes of the thoracic and upper lumbar nerves.) The levator ani and the coccygeus, and also the external anal sphincter, are supplied by the 4th sacral nerve.

Technique of Femoral Nerve Block

A weal is raised a finger-breadth to the outer side of the femoral artery, just below the inguinal ligament. A needle is inserted for 3–4 cm so that the pulsations of the artery are transferred to the needle and 20 ml of 2% lignocaine are injected. The nerve lies beneath the deep fascia. Femoral nerve block, following injection of solution lateral and deep to the femoral artery, greatly reduces pain, following fractured neck of the femur during movement in adults and children.[217]

Sciatic and femoral nerve blocks in combination are useful in operations on the leg and foot from a point 5 cm below the patella.[218] Operations on or above the knee require, in addition, lateral femoral cutaneous and obturator block, the latter being difficult. Manipulations of the lower half of the femur can, however, be carried out under sciatic and femoral block.

Nerve to quadratus femoris. This branch of the femoral nerve supplies the hip-joint. To block it the patient is placed in the prone position with leg externally rotated. A line is drawn with a skin pencil joining the posterior superior iliac spine and the sacrococcygeal joint. The junction of the middle and lower thirds is marked. A weal is raised 5 cm posterior to the greater trochanter on a level with the lower end of the sacrum and a 14-cm 16-gauge needle inserted at 45° to the horizontal towards the point previously marked until it hits bone. The needle point is worked medially 1–2 cm while 20 ml of solution are deposited along the flat surface of the body of the ischium. Useful for relief of pain in the hip joint and to allow gentle physiotherapy in patients with osteoarthritis.

Regional Hip Blockade

Regional hip blockade involves injection into the region of the nerve to the quadratus femoris and the obturator nerve, with the aim of ameliorating the severe pain due to osteoarthritis of the hip-joint.[219] Some workers have found the block of doubtful utility.[220] Some pain relief follows the injection into the hip joint of 10 ml of 0·5% bupivacaine.[221]

Inguinal Perivascular Block[222]
Injection of 25–40 ml of solution into the region of the femoral nerve, after eliciting paraesthesia, from just below the inguinal ligament, will block the femoral, obturator and external femoral cutaneous nerves (the 'three-in-one block'). Useful together with sciatic block for analgesia of the leg.

Saphenous Nerve Block
This is the terminal branch of the femoral nerve and becomes subcutaneous immediately below the sartorius muscle at the medial side of the knee joint; it accompanies the long saphenous vein to the medial malleolus. It can be blocked by a subcutaneous injection of 10–15 ml of local analgesic solution in the close vicinity of the vein just below the knee joint, taking care to avoid intravenous injection. For long saphenous vein stripping under regional analgesia *see* Bromage et al.[223]

Technique of Block of Lateral Cutaneous Nerve of Thigh[259]
A weal is raised one finger-breadth below and medial to the anterior superior spine of the ilium. A needle is inserted perpendicularly to the skin and 1% lignocaine is deposited between the skin and the iliac bone and along the pelvic brim for two finger-breadths internally to the anterior superior spine; 10–15 ml of solution are used. The nerve lies deep to the fascia lata of the thigh.

When associated with femoral block, adequate analgesia is produced for taking skin grafts from the front of the thigh. Alternatively, infiltration analgesia of the skin of the front of the thigh can be performed, using intradermal and subcutaneous injections to cover the desired area.

Technique of Obturator Block (*See also* p. 647.)
The obturator nerves arise from the 2nd, 3rd and 4th lumbar nerves. Block is required for operations involving the knee joint, the medial aspect of the thigh, and may be necessary to make application of an arterial tourniquet above the knee tolerable.

The anterior and posterior divisions of the nerve are blocked as they lie in the obturator canal below the superior ramus of the pubis, between the pectineus and the obturator externus. The following techniques can be used:

1. The patient lies supine with leg slightly abducted. A skin mark is made halfway between the pubic tubercle and femoral artery, 2–3 cm below the inguinal ligament. The pubic ramus is palpated here and a disposable 18-gauge spinal needle inserted to strike the bone. The needle is then slightly withdrawn and turned through 90° to a point about 2 cm below the superior ramus and parallel to the shaft of the femur. The needle is now advanced into the obturator foramen by a forward movement of 4–5 cm. After aspiration tests, and provided there is no resistance to injection, 10 ml of solution are deposited.

2. A skin weal is raised just below the midpoint of the superior pubic ramus and a 5-cm needle introduced perpendicular to the plane of the obturator foramen and advanced just below the ramus for 1·5 cm. Paraesthesiae should be elicited after the injection of 5 ml of 1·5% lignocaine solution.

3. A weal is raised 1 cm below and lateral to the pubic tubercle and through it a 5-cm needle is thrust backwards until it strikes bones; as it is withdrawn, 10 ml

of solution are injected. An 8-cm needle is now inserted in the track of the first one and moved gently laterally until its point enters the obturator foramen where 10 ml of solution are injected. An additional similar volume is finally injected as the needle is withdrawn.[224] Successful block is shown by weakness when the patient attempts to adduct the leg.

Block of the above nerves (other than the saphenous, included in femoral block), together with the sciatic, will produce analgesia of the lower extremity below the level of the symphysis pubis. It can also be used for the treatment of pain in the region of the hip joint or of adductor spasm. The position of the needle point can be checked radiographically or by electrical stimulation (0·5 mA rheobase) using a Teflon-covered needle.[225] Eases the pain during transport.

For nailing, etc. a fractured neck of fractured femur, the line of incision is infiltrated down to the bone with 0·5% lignocaine or 1–2000 amethocaine. Solution is injected between the ends of the fractured neck from above the great trochanter and from a point just external to the pulsating femoral artery.

For *arthroscopy of the knee*, femoral and lateral femoral cutaneous nerve block has been recommended.[226] Intradural spinal analgesia also gives good results and is used in day-stay surgery.[260]

Doppler localization of the popliteal artery combined with nerve localization with a peripheral nerve stimulator facilitates knee-block by reducing discomfort and increasing efficacy.[227]

Lumbar Plexus Block[228] (Psoas Compartment Block)

A single injection of solution or serial injections through a catheter introduced via a needle from a weal 5 cm lateral to the upper border of the 4th lumbar vertebra. A 15-cm needle is inserted perpendicularly to the skin until contact with the transverse process is made. It is then partially withdrawn and glided over the transverse process. The injection is made until loss of resistance is felt, and thereafter 40 ml of 0·25% bupivacaine solution with adrenaline 1–200 000 are placed within the psoas compartment. This is said to be safe and is recommended for surgery of the hip, including arthroplasty together with light general anaesthesia.[229] This is a useful block in the management of fractured femur before, during and after operation and during transport.

Technique of Sciatic Nerve Block (See p. 647.)

Patient lies on sound side with hip slightly flexed. *Methods*: (1) A line connecting the sacral hiatus with the most prominent part of the greater trochanter is drawn and a weal raised at its midpoint. A 21-gauge spinal needle is inserted at right angles to the skin and through it 10–15 ml of 2% lignocaine with adrenaline are injected after eliciting paraesthesia;[230] (2) A line is traced between the upper extremity of the great trochanter and the posterior superior iliac spine. From the midpoint of this line a perpendicular is dropped 3–5 cm long, and at its end a weal is raised and a needle introduced at right angles to the skin plane until it reaches the ischial spine, 5–7·5 cm from the skin surface. The nerve lies on this area of bone so that paraesthesiae must be elicited before the needle strikes bone; 10–15 ml of 2% lignocaine are then injected. Intraneural injection is undesirable; (3) A surface marking is the junction of the medial third with the lateral two-thirds of a line joining the ischial tuberosity to the greater femoral trochanter—the needle being inserted at right angles to the skin surface until paraesthesiae are felt by the patient; (4) A guide to the position of the nerve is the midpoint of a line joining the posterior superior iliac spine to the ischial tuberosity.

The block is useful for reduction of fractures around the ankle, combined if necessary with a saphenous nerve block just below the knee joint as it accompanies the long saphenous vein. It can be used together with femoral block for ligation of varicose veins on the front of the leg. An alternative for operations below the knee is injection into the region of the tibial and common peroneal nerves in the popliteal fossa, and the saphenous nerve adjacent to the knee. Efficacy is enhanced by the use of a peripheral nerve stimulator.[231]

It also causes almost complete vasoconstrictor paralysis of the foot and is better, safer and less painful than lumbar sympathetic block for this purpose. A rise in skin temperature starts in 10 min and is maximal in 20–30 min. Sciatic nerve block gives analgesia of the whole foot with the exception of an area of skin over the medial malleolus supplied by the saphenous branch of the femoral nerve. The pain caused by gangrene of the foot can be relieved by continuous sciatic nerve block in which a catheter is inserted into the neurovascular sheath by the posterior approach.[232]

Anterior Approach.[233] This may be useful when the patient cannot be easily moved from the supine position and when intervention on the foot or lower leg is required. Other nerve blocks in the leg may be combined with it. The needle passes between the sartorius laterally and the rectus femoris medially and reaches the sciatic nerve below the lesser trochanter.

For technique of lateral approach with the patient supine *see* Ichiyanagi K. *Anesthesiology* 1959, **20**, 601.

Dorsal Superior Approach. See Raj A. A. et al. *Anesth. Analg. (Cleve.)* 1975, **54**, 489.

Pudendal Nerve Block
See Chapter 27.

Ankle Block

A subcutaneous and intradermal weal is raised circumferentially around the ankle just above the medial malleolus.
The deep peroneal (anterior tibial; S.1 and S.2) is blocked by inserting a needle midway between the most prominent points of the medial and lateral malleoli, on the circular line of infiltration in front of the ankle joint. It is directed medially towards the anterior border of the medial malleolus and solution is injected between the bone and the skin; paraesthesia should be elicited if possible. Instead of blocking this nerve at the ankle, its parent trunk, the common peroneal nerve, can be blocked at the neck of the fibula where it can be rolled under the finger—the only palpable nerve in the leg. It supplies the skin on adjacent sides of the first and second toes, dorsal aspect. The amount of solution used should be 10–15 ml.

The superficial peroneal (musculocutaneous, S.1 and S.2), also a branch from the common peroneal nerve, can be blocked immediately above the ankle joint by a subcutaneous weal extending from the front of the tibia to the lateral malleolus. It supplies the dorsum of the foot (with the exception of the small area innervated by the tibial nerve).

The sural nerve (L.5; S.1 and S.2). formed with twigs from the tibial and common peroneal nerves and descends with the short saphenous vein below and posterior to the lateral malleolus to supply the outer part of the foot and heel. It is blocked by subcutaneous infiltration between the tendo Achillis and the prominence of the lateral malleolus, using 5–10 ml of solution.

The saphenous nerve (L.3 and L.4). This is the terminal branch of the femoral nerve and accompanies the long saphenous vein anterior to the medial malleolus where it can be blocked by the injection of 10 ml of local analgesic solution. It supplies an area of skin just below and above the medial malleolus.

The tibial nerve (S.1 and S.2) passes behind the medial malleolus to divide into medial and lateral plantar nerves after giving off the medial calcaneal branch. With the patient in the prone position it is blocked by 10 ml of solution introduced through a point on the circular weal just internal to the tendo Achillis, deep to the flexor retinaculum near the palpable posterior tibial artery. It is easiest with the patient lying prone. The needle is inserted forwards and slightly outwards towards the posterior aspect of the tibia, near which the solution is deposited.

After waiting 10 min, ankle block is suitable for operation on the foot. Tibial block is useful for testing vasodilatation of the foot.

Following infiltration of any peripheral nerve there results a vasomotor paralysis over the area of anaesthetized skin.

Block for Hallux Valgus

A weal is raised near the proximal end of the first intermetatarsal space, superior surface, and, from this, solution is deposited between the two layers of skin, dorsal and plantar, as far forwards as the web between the toes. More solution is injected between the dorsal skin and the first metatarsal bone. A second weal medial to the first one, on the internal aspect of the metatarsal, is raised, and injection made between it and the bone between the plantar skin and the bone. A 10–15 min pause is made before the operation is commenced. From 30 to 50 ml of solution are used (e.g. 1 to 1·5% lignocaine).

Local Analgesia of Foot[234]

Sole of Foot

Supplied by the medial (L.4 and L.5) and lateral (S.1 and S.2) branches of the tibial nerve (plantar from sciatic), supplying the medial and lateral anterior part of the sole; the sural nerve supplying the posterior and lateral part of the sole and heel; and the tibial nerve (S.1 and S.2) supplying the medial part of the heel. The plantar surface of the heel is supplied by calcaneal branches of the tibial nerve, but not by the sural nerve.[235]

Tibial Nerve Block. See above under Ankle Block.

Dorsum of Foot

Supplied by medial terminal branch of deep peroneal nerve (the adjacent sides of the first and second toes). The sural innervates the lateral side of the fifth toe, the superficial peroneal supplies the remainder. Midtarsal block for surgery of the forefoot (*see* Sharrock N. E. et al. *Br. J. Anaesth.* 1986, **58**, 37.)

Medial Side of Foot

Supplied by saphenous nerve from the femoral nerve. Also from the medial plantar branch of the tibial nerve.

Lateral Side of Foot

Supplied by sural nerve from the tibial and common peroneal, which goes to fifth toe and lateral side of foot.

Ring Block of Toe

Lignocaine plain, 1·5 ml of 2% solution, to be injected into each side of the proximal phalanx near its base. Injection from dorsal aspect with small amount of solution across from side to side. After an interval of 7–10 min, the operation, e.g. removal of toe nail, can commence.[236]

(*See also* Schuman D. J. *Anesthesiology* 1976, **44**, 348; Edmonds-Seal J. et al. *J. R. Soc. Med.* 1980, **73**, 111; Robertson J. F. R. and Muckart D. J. *J. R. Coll. Surg. Edinb.* 1985, **30**, 237.)

Local Analgesia for Reduction of Closed Fractures

After localizing the exact site of fracture by means of X-rays, a weal is raised near the fracture and a needle introduced into the haematoma between the broken bone ends. Aspiration of old blood confirms the position and must be obtained: injection is then made of 1·5 or 2% lignocaine without adrenaline. For Colles' fracture[237] the amount required is 15–20 ml; injection should be made from the extensor aspect of the wrist and, in addition, a few millilitres should infiltrate the ulnar styloid. The method is easier, quicker and does not carry the possible risks of intravenous local analgesia; though pain relief is superior with the latter.[238] For Pott's fracture, 10–20 ml of solution with hyaluronidase can be used; for fractured femur, 20–30 ml. These are high doses so the possibility of toxic signs must be borne in mind. Cases of recent fracture are the most suitable for this method of reduction, especially fractures of the metatarsal or metacarpal bones. Good results are claimed for the addition of 1000 units of hyaluronidase to each 20 ml of solution. With lignocaine, analgesia lasts 2–3 h and comes on after 10 min. This technique does not produce complete pain relief but may be employed when dealing with mass casualities or when anaesthetists are not available.

Topical Analgesia for Gastroscopy, Fibreoptic Endoscopy and Oesophagoscopy

Cocaine was first used for oesophagoscopy by Stoerk and Von Hacker in 1887. Fibreoptic endoscopes employ very fine bundles of glass fibres which carry images around corners, an invention patented by J. L. Baird of the UK in 1927; developed by H. H. Hopkins of Reading University.[239] Gastrointestinal endoscopy developed following pioneering work by Hirschowitz in 1958.[240]

Sedation

Personality traits as measured by e.g. the Eysenck personality inventory, influence the tolerance and future compliance with gastrointestinal endoscopy. Drugs producing amnesia make repeat examinations more acceptable.[241] The following drugs have been suggested: lorazepam, 2·5–5 mg, 90 min before pharyngeal analgesia, then Diazemuls 10–60 mg before endoscopy.[242] Flunitrazepam,[243] midazolam 0·1 mg/kg i.v.,[244] pentazocine and Buscopan may also have their indications.

After administration of the sedative of choice the patient is given a tablet of amethocaine (60 mg) or lignocaine to suck. Too much atropine may make this difficult. Additional intravenous diazepam may be necessary, 5 mg i.v. each minute until ptosis or dysarthria occurs. In cirrhotic patients, diazepam may result in hepatic coma. Chlormethiazole (Heminevrin) may be used instead in hypotensive patients.[245] The gums, tongue, palate and pharynx are now sprayed with 4% lignocaine, 4% cocaine, 1% amethocaine or some other suitable analgesic solution. He can be given amethocaine hydrochloride 2% to gargle, or Xylocaine Viscous to swallow, a 2% solution in a mucilage base, very pleasantly flavoured. In active bleeding, topical analgesia increases the risk of aspiration.[246]

Gargling with 4% lignocaine makes the passage of the small fibreoptic endoscope tolerable in over 90% of patients, without premedication or intravenous sedatives.[247]

Many operators have now discarded the use of local analgesia prior to fibreoptic gastroscopy, relying on the use of intravenous sedative and/or analgesic drugs alone.

Topical Analgesia for Bronchoscopy

Since the introduction of the Sanders injector technique with general anaesthesia,[248] topical analgesia has lost much of its popularity. Flexible fibreoptic bronchoscope introduced in 1968.[249]

The gums, tongue, palate and pharynx are sprayed as for oesophagoscopy on two occasions, à few minutes apart. After a short interval, the piriform fossae and the terminal twigs of the internal laryngeal nerve beneath its mucosa are made analgesic by application of swabs soaked in the solution (with excess of it removed), applied on a curved applicator or with Krause's laryngeal forceps. After this has been done, and after spraying the epiglottis and the cords, a swab is gently introduced into the glottis and held there for a short while, so that its analgesic solution completes the block of the superior laryngeal nerve endings.

In addition, the trachea must be anaesthetized by:

1. The transtracheal method of Canuyt (1920),[250] which consists in inserting a No. 1 hypodermic needle through the middle line of the neck into the trachea. The needle should be 3–4 cm long so that if breakage occurs, which is usually near the hub, the remains of the shaft can be easily removed. Aspiration of air proves its presence in the trachea. An injection of 2–3 ml of 4% lignocaine or cocaine is now made after a deep expiration and the patient told not to cough until the solution has trickled down the trachea into the bronchi. Insertion of the

needle can be preceded by 100–150 mg of thiopentone. Complications are: (1) Infection; (2) A broken needle; (3) Surgical emphysema; (4) Haemorrhage.

2. By instillation from a laryngeal syringe, holding the tongue forward, using an indirect laryngeal mirror if thought necessary. For doses of local analgesic solution *see* pp. 599–602.

A 10% lignocaine aerosol spray is available and enables a measured (10-mg) dose of drug to be given with each 'squirt'. Deep penetration into the bronchial tree can be achieved.

Such topical solutions should not be used on inflamed or traumatized surfaces.

Regional analgesia is probably safer than general anaesthesia for those examinations where there is copious sputum, airway obstruction or when the general condition of the patient is poor. It enables the movements of the vocal cords to be seen also.

As an aid to comfortable endoscopy under local analgesia, the concurrent use of divided doses of a narcotic analgesic, neurolept agent or diazepam given intravenously is beneficial.

After topical laryngeal analgesia, instruction must be given to the patient not to eat or drink for at least 3 h, i.e. until the sentinel of the larynx has returned to duty.

Even without the administration of extra oxygen, oxygen saturation of the blood increases during bronchoscopy performed under local analgesia.

(*See also* Magill I. W. *J. Laryngol. Otol.* 1939, **54**, 425; Bonica J. J. *Anesthesiology* 1949, **10**, 736; Bromage P. R. *Epidural Analgesia*. Philadelphia: Saunders, 1978, p. 476.)

Topical Analgesia of the Urethra

Technique
A useful preparation is Xylocaine Gel, a 1–2% preparation put up in 30-ml tubes with carboxymethylcellulose. The maximum dose should probably not exceed 10 ml, i.e. 100–200 mg of lignocaine. The plastic nozzle supplied by the makers of the preparation is used to squeeze the jelly into the urethra. A clamp is applied to the penis and the paste gently massaged into the posterior urethra. After an interval of 10–15 min instrumentation can begin. It is sometimes helpful to pass a small catheter into the urethra connected to the plastic nozzle, so as to deposit gel in the posterior urethra. The gel is also useful for postoperative comfort after general anaesthesia.

Alternatively, 30 ml of a mixture of 0·5% cocaine and 0·5% sodium bicarbonate is instilled into the urethra with a urethral syringe. Sufficient volume is injected to distend the anterior urethra and allow some to be massaged back to the posterior urethra. The syringe is removed and a penile clamp applied to keep the solution in contact with the urethral mucosa. This is removed after 5 min and an applicator with cotton-wool soaked in 10% cocaine is placed inside the meatus and allowed to remain for a further 5 min.

For patients who react abnormally to ordinary analgesics, 2% solution of pyribenzamine, the antihistamine, gives reasonable analgesia without toxic reactions, other than occasional drowsiness.

Analgesia of the Peritoneal Cavity by Lavage

Lignocaine, 0·5%, prilocaine, 0·5%, or procaine, 0·5–1%, is used. Volume 200 ml. This is poured into the peritoneal cavity and the peritoneal edges are drawn together. After 5–8 min the solution is sucked out. Results: slackening of the peritoneum, contraction of the bowel, absence of reflex response from visceral trauma. Toxic reactions are said to be rare. Good results are not seen in cases of peritonitis or where the bowel is grossly distended.

(For good illustrations showing some of the techniques described in this and the next chapter the reader is referred to the following books: Moore D. C. *Regional Block*, 4th ed. Springfield, Ill., 1965; Macintosh R. R. and Ostlere M. *Local Analgesia: Head and Neck*, 2nd ed. Edinburgh: Livingstone, 1967; *Practical Regional Analgesia* (Lee J. A. and Bryce-Smith R. ed.). Amsterdam: Excerpta Medica, 1976; *Illustrated Handbook of Local Anaesthesia* (Ericksson E. ed.), 2nd ed. London: Lloyd-Luke, 1980; Cousins M. J. and Bridenbaugh P. O. *Neural Blockade in Clinical Anaesthesia and the Management of Pain*. Philadelphia: Lippincott, 1980; Lee J. A., Atkinson R. S. and Watt M. J. *Macintosh's Lumbar Puncture and Spinal Analgesia*, 5th ed. Edinburgh: Churchill Livingstone, 1985; Scott D. B. et al. (ed.) Regional Anaesthesia: 1884–1984, Sondertalje, Production ICM AB. 1984.

References

1. Koller C. *Klin. Mbl. Augen.* 1884, **22**, 60; *Wien. Med. Wochenschr.* 1884, **34**, 1276, 1309 (translated and reprinted in 'Classical File', *Surv. Anesthesiol.* 1963, **7**, 74); *Lancet* 1884, **2**, 990.
2. Richardson B. W. *Med. Times. Gaz.* 1866, **1**, 115.
3. Redard P. Vera. *Xth. Int. Med. Cong.* 1890, **5**, 14, Abstract 71.
4. Schleich K. L. *Verh. Dtsch. Ges. Chir.* 1892, **21**, 121; *Gesellsch. f. Chir.* 1892, **21**, 121; *Therap. Monats.* 1894, **8**, 429; *Schmerzlöse Operationen.* Berlin: Springer, 1894.
5. Reclus P. *Gaz. Hebd. Med. (Paris)*, 1890, p. 106; *La Cocaine en Chirurgie.* Paris, Masson, 1895.
6. Halsted W. S. *NY Med. J.* 1885, **42**, 294; Hall R. J. *NY Med. J.* 1884, **40**, 463.
7. Vinci G. *Berlin Klin. Wochenschr.* 1896, 27.
8. Barker A. E. *Lancet* 1899, **1**, 282.
9. Braun H. *Arch. Klin. Chir.* 1902, **69**, 541.
10. Abel J. J. *Johns Hopkins Hosp. Bull.* 1897, **8**, 151.
11. Crile G. W. *Cleveland Med. J.* 1897, **11**, 355.
12. Fourneau E. (1872–1949), *Bull. Soc. Pharmacol.* 1904, **10**, 141.
13. Einhorn A. *Münch. Med. Wochenschr.* 1899, **46**, 1218.
14. Braun H. *Dtsch. Med. Wochenschr.* 1905, **31**, 1667.
15. Eisleb O. et al. *Arch. Exp. Path. u. Phar.* 1931, **160**, 53.
16. Uhlmann T. *Narkose und Anaes.* 1929, **6**, 168.
17. Gordh T. *Anaesthesia* 1949, **4**, 4.
18. Redman A. in: *Hollander-Schneidermühl's 'Handbuch des Zahnartzl'.* Heilmittellehre, 1890, p. 149.
19. Rynd F. *Dublin Med. Press* 1845, **13**, 167; *Dublin J. Med. Sci.* 1861, **32**, 13.
20. Wood A. *Edin. Med. Surg. J.* 1855, **82**, 265.
21. Cushing H. W. *Ann. Surg.* 1902, **36**, 321.
22. *See also* Ritchie J. M. *Br. J. Anaesth.* 1975, **47**, 191; de Jong R. *Local Anesthetics.* 2nd ed. Springfield, Ill.: Thomas, 1977.
23. *See also* Hiele B. *J. Gen. Physiol.* 1977, **69**, 497.
24. Bromage P. R. et al. *Br. J. Anaesth.* 1967, **39**, 197.

25. Appleyard J. N. et al. *Br. J. Anaesth.* 1974, **46**, 530.
26. Branch R. A. et al. *J. Pharmacol. Exp. Ther.* 1973, **184**, 515; Munson E. S. et al. *Anesthesiology* 1975, **42**, 471; Burney R. G. and Di Fazio C. A. *Anesth. Analg. (Cleve.)* 1976, **55**, 322.
27. Braid D. P. *Br. J. Anaesth.* 1964, **36**, 742.
28. Braid D. P. and Scott D. B. *Br. J. Anaesth.* 1965, **37**, 394; Tucker G. T. et al. *Anesthesiology* 1965, **37**, 277.
29. Editorial, *Anesthesiology* 1979, **51**, 285.
30. Albright G. A. *Anesthesiology* 1979, **51**, 285.
31. Scott D. B. *Br. J. Anaesth.* 1984, **56**, 437.
32. Noble D. S. and Pierce G. F. M. *Lancet* 1961, **2**, 1436.
33. Moore D. C. *Regional Block*, 4th ed. Springfield, Ill.: Thomas, 1965.
34. Brown D. T. et al. *Br. J. Anaesth.* 1981, **53**, 435; Fisher M. McD. and Pennington J. C. *Br. J. Anaesth.* 1982, **54**, 893; Reynolds F. *Br. J. Anaesth.* 1982, **54**, 901.
35. Nagel J. F. and Fuscaldo J. T. *JAMA* 1977, **237**, 1594.
36. Sturrock J. E. and Nunn J. F. *Br. J. Anaesth.* 1979, **51**, 273.
37. Bromage P. R. et al. *Br. J. Anaesth.* 1967, **39**, 197; Catchlove R. F. H. *Br. J. Anaesth.* 1973, **45**, 471.
38. Chapman G. M. *Anaesthesia* 1972, **27**, 185.
39. Pearman T. *J. Laryngol. Otol.* 1979, **93**, 1191.
40. Van Essen E. J. and Ploeger E. J. *Anaesthesia* 1981, **36**, 713.
41. Niemann A. *Justus Liebig's Annals of Chemistry* 1860, **114**, 213.
42. Von Ottingen W. F. *Ann. Med. Hist.* 1933, n.s., **5**, 275; Moréno y Maiz T. *Thèse de Paris*, 1868, 91.
43. von Anrep B. *Arch. Physiol.* 1880, **21**, 38.
44. Musto D. F. *JAMA* 1968, **204**, 27.
45. Koller C. *Wiener Med. Blatt.* 1884, **7**, 1352.
46. Koller C. *JAMA* 1928, **90**, 1742; 1941, **117**, 1284; Koller-Becker H. *Psychoanal. Q.* 1963, **32**, 309; Gay G. B. et al. *Anesth. Analg. (Cleve.)* 1976, **55**, 582, Sigmund Freud, *Cocain Papers.* (Byck R. ed.). New York: Stonehill, 1974; Gay G. B. et al. *Anesth. Analg. (Cleve.)* 1976, **55**, 582.
47. Halsted W. S. *NY Med. J.* 1885, **42**, 294.
48. von Oettingen W. F. *Ann. Med. Hist.* 1933, n.s., **5**, 275; Olch P. D. *Anesthesiology* 1975, **42**, 479.
49. Willstatter R. *Münch. Med. Wochenschr.* 1924, **71**, 849.
50. Delikan A. E. et al. *Anaesth. Intensive Care* 1978, **6**, 328.
51. Martindale J. J. *The Extra Pharmacopoeia* (Wade A. ed.), 27th ed. London: Pharmaceutical Press, 1977, pp. 960, 974; Annotation, *Br. Med. J.* 1979, **1**, 971.
52. Cousins M. J. and Mather L. E. *Anaesth. Intensive Care* 1980, **6**, 270.
53. Ansbro F. P. et al. *Anesth. Analg. Curr. Res.* 1953, **32**, 73.
54. Allen P. R. and Johnson R. W. *Anaesthesia* 1979, **34**, 874.
55. Reisner L. S. et al. *Anesth. Analg. (Cleve.)* 1980, **59**, 452.
56. Wang B. C. and Hillman D. E. *Anesth. Analg. (Cleve.)* 1984, **63**, 445.
57. Lofgren N. *Xylocaine.* Stockholm: Haeggstroms, 1948; *Archiv. Kemi Mineral Geol.* 1946, **18**, 22A.
58. Gordh T. *Anaesthesia* 1949, **4**, 4 (reprinted in 'Classical File', *Surv. Anesthesiol.* 1977, **21**, 314).
59. Forrest J. A. et al. *Br. Med. J.* 1977, **1**, 1384.
60. Katz J. D. and Krich L. B. *Can. Anaesth. Soc. J.* 1976, **23**, 285.
61. Bromage P. R. *Acta Anaesth. Scand.* 1965, **16**, Suppl. 55; Cousins M. J. and Bromage P. R. *Br. J. Anaesth.* 1971, **43**, 1149; Cole C. P. et al. *Anesthesiology* 1985, **62**, 348; Sukhani R. et al. *Anesthesiology* 1985, **63**, A209.
62. Soderman M. and Duke P. C. *Can. Anaesth. Soc. J.* 1983, **30**, S.71; Bokesch P. M. et al. *Anesth. Analg. (Cleve.)* 1987, **66**, 9.
63. Af Ekenstam B. et al. *Br. J. Anaesth.* 1956, **28**, 503.
64. Dhuner K. G. et al. *Acta Chir. Scand.* 1956, **112**, 350.
65. Jorfeldt L. et al. *Acta Anaesth. Scand.* 1968, **12**, 153.
66. Af Ekenstam B. et al. *Acta Chem. Scand.* 1957, **11**, 1183.
67. Telivuo L. *Ann. Chir. Gynaecol. Fenn.* 1963, **52**, 513. *See also* Watt M. J. et al. *Anaesthesia* 1968, **23**, 2, 331; 1970, **25**, 24.
68. Marx G. *Anesthesiology* 1984, **60**, 3; Rosen M. A. et al. *Anesth. Analg. (Cleve.)* 1985, **64**, 1039.
69. Reynolds F. *Br. J. Anaesth.* 1971, **43**, 33.

70. Adams H. J. et al. *J. Pharm. Sci.* 1972, **61**, 1829.
71. Scott D. B. et al. *Br. J. Anaesth.* 1975, **47**, 56; Lund P. C. et al. *Br. J. Anaesth.* 1975, **47**, 313.
72. Lofgren N. and Tegner C. *Acta Chem. Scand.* 1960, **14**, 486.
73. Wiedling S. *Acta Pharmacol. Toxicol. (Copenh.)* 1960, **17**, 233.
74. Eriksson E. and Gordh T. *Acta Anaesth. Scand.* 1959, Suppl. 2, 81.
75. Wildsmith J. A. W. et al. *Anaesthesia* 1979, **34**, 919.
76. Meischer K. *Helv. Chim. Acta* 1932, **15**, 163; Uhlmann T. *Narkose u. Anaesth.* 1929, **2**, 168.
77. Haynes D. H. and Kirkpatrick A. *Anesthesiology* 1985, **63**, 430.
78. Braun H. *Münch. Med. Wochenschr.* 1903, **50**, 352; *Lokalanaestesie*, 4, Auflage, Leipzig: Barth Verlag, p. 163.
79. Astrom A. *Acta Physiol. Scand.* 1964, **60**, 30.
80. Matteo R. S. et al. *Anesthesiology* 1962, **23**, 360, 597.
81. Montgomery M. B. et al. *Anesth. Anal.* 1973, **52**, 827; Raj P. P. et al. *Anesth. Anal.* 1973, **52**, 897; Zeh D. W. et al. 1978, **57**, 13; Ford D. J. et al. *Anesth. Analg. (Cleve.)* 1984, **63**, 925.
82. Smith D. C. and Miah H. *Anesthesiology* 1985, **60**, 569.
83. Boulton T. B. *Anaesthesia* 1967, **22**, 101.
84. Scott D. B. et al. *Br. J. Anaesth.* 1976, **48**, 899.
85. Morris R. W. and Whish D. K. M. *Anaesth. Intensive Care* 1984, **12**, 113.
86. French A. J. and Patel Y. U. *Lancet* 1980, **2**, 482.
87. Hill J. N. et al. *Anesthesiology* 1983, **59**, 144.
88. Macht S. D. et al. *Surg. Gynecol. Obstet.* 1978, **146**, 87.
89. Greenfield Sluder (1865–1928), originator of guillotine tonsillectomy in 1911.
90. Barton R. P. E. and Gray R. F. E. *J. Laryngol. Otol.* 1979, **93**, 1201.
91. Moffett A. J. *Anaesthesia* 1947, **2**, 31.
92. Curtiss E. S. *Lancet* 1952, **1**, 989.
93. Macintosh R. R. and Ostlere M. *Local Analgesia, Head and Neck*, 2nd ed. Edinburgh: Livingstone, 1967.
94. Bodman R. I. and Boyes-Korkis F. *Br. Med. J.* 1960, **2**, 1956.
95. Sowray J. H. *SAAD Digest* 1980, **4**, 128.
96. Blaxter P. L. and Britten M. J. A. *Br. Med. J.* 1967, **1**, 681.
97. Takahashi T. and Dohi S. *Br. J. Anaesth.* 1983, **55**, 333.
98. Mushin W. W. and Macintosh R. R. *Proc. R. Soc. Med.* 1945, **38**, 308.
99. Gaskill J. R. and Gillies D. R. *Arch. Otolaryngol.* 1966, **84**, 654; Gaskill J. R. *Arch. Otolaryngol.* 1967, **86**, 697; Coghlan C. J. *Anesth. Analg. Curr. Res.* 1966, **45**, 290; Young T. M. *Anaesthesia* 1976, **31**, 570.
100. Cooper M. and Watson R. L. *Anesthesiology* 1975, **43**, 377.
101. Ramamurthy S. et al. *Anesth. Analg. (Cleve.)* 1978, **57**, 591.
102. *See* Moore D. C. *Stellate Ganglion Block*. Springfield. Ill.: Thomas, 1954.
103. Leriche R. and Fontaine R. *Presse Méd.* 1934, **41**, 849 (reprinted in 'Classical File', *Surv. Anesthesiol.* 1973, **17**, 297); *Rev. Chir.* 1936, **74**, 751.
104. Kuntz A. *The Autonomic Nervous System*, 3rd ed. Philadelphia: Lea and Febiger, 1945.
105. Winnie A. P. *Plexus Anesthesia* Vol. 1, Edinburgh: Churchill Livingstone, 1983, p. 43.
106. Valman H. B. et al. *Br. Med. J.* 1977, **1**, 1065; Boscoe M. J. et al. *Anaesthesia* 1983, **38**, 669; Bateman D. N. et al. *Anaesthesia* 1984, **39**, 71; Robertson D. B. *Anaesthesia* 1984, **39**, 603.
107. Cook T. G. et al. *Anesthesiology* 1981, **54**, 421.
108. Dyson F. H. et al. *Br. Med. J.* 1985, **291**, 31.
109. Moore D. C. *Stellate Ganglion Block*, Springfield, Ill.: Thomas, 1954, p. 83.
110. Apgar, Virginia, *Anesth. Analg. Curr. Res.* 1948, **27**, 49.
111. Goinard P. *Acad. di. Chir.* 1936, 258.
112. Smith D. W. *Am. J. Surg.* 1951, **82**, 344.
113. Horner J. F. *Klin. Mbl. Augenheilk.* 1869, **7**, 193. It was described by Horner, a Swiss ophthalmologist (1831–1886), in 1869, having been previously noted by Claude Bernard in 1862 and by François Pourfois du Petit in 1727; and by Jonathan Hutchinson in 1866 (Hutchinson J. *Illustrations in Clinical Surgery*. London: Churchill, 1878, Vol. 1, p. 203).
114. Benzon H. T. et al. *Anesth. Analg. (Cleve.)* 1985, **64**, 415.
115. Whitehunt L. et al. *J. Bone Joint Surg.* 1977, **A/4**, 541.
116. Zee R. F. Y. *Anaesth. Intensive Care* 1977, **5**, 76.
117. Rovenstine E. A. and Papper E. M. *Am. J. Surg.* 1948, **75**, 713; Montgomery W. and Cousins M. J. *Br. J. Anaesth.* 1972, **44**, 383.
118. Barton S. and Williams J. D. *Arch. Otolaryngol.* 1971, **93**, 186.
119. Wertheim H. M. and Rovenstine E. A. *Anesthesiology* 1941, **2**, 541; Milougky J. and

Rovenstine E. A. *Anesthesiology* 1948, **9**, 76.
120. Matas R. *Johns Hopkins Hosp. Bull.* 1925, **2**, 8.
121. Crile G. W. *Cleveland Med. J.* 1897, **2**, 355.
122. Hirschel G. *Münch. Med. Wochenschr.* 1911, **58**, 1555.
123. Kulenkampff D. *Dtsch. Med. Wochenschr.* 1912, **38**, 1878.
124. Patrick J. *Br. J. Surg.* 1940, **27**, 734.
125. Macintosh R. R. and Mushin W. W. *Local Anaesthesia: Brachial Plexus*, 4th ed. Oxford: Blackwell, 1967. (1st ed. 1943.)
126. Winnie A. P. *Plexus Anesthesia* Vol. 1, Edinburgh: Churchill Livingstone, 1983.
127. Reding M. *Presse Med.* 1921, **29**, 294.
128. Thompson G. E. and Rorie D. K. *Anesthesiology* 1983, **59**, 117.
129. La Grange P. et al. *Br. J. Anaesth.* 1978, **50**, 965.
130. Yasuda I. et al. *Br. J. Anaesth.* 1980, **52**, 409.
131. Knoblanche G. E. *Anaesth. Intensive Care* 1979, **7**, 346.
132. Sibson F. (1814–1876), *Trans. Prov. Med. Surg. Assoc.* 1844, **12**, 307.
133. Moraitis K. *Anaesthesia* 1977, **32**, 161.
134. Mulley K. *Beitr. z. Clin. Chirurg.* 1919, **114**, 666; Etienne J. (1925), *see* Vidal-Lopez F. *Anesth. Analg. (Cleve.)* 1977, **56**, 486; Winnie A. P. *Anesth. Analg. (Cleve.)* 1970, **49**, 455; Ward M. E. *Anaesthesia* 1974, **29**, 147; Winnie A. P. *Surg. Clin. North Am.* 1975, **55**, 874; Vester-Andersen T. et al. *Acta Anaesth. Scand.* 1981, **35**, 81.
135. Labat G. *Br. J. Anaesth.* 1927, **4**, 174; Livingstone E. M. and Wertheim H. *JAMA* 1927, **88**, 1464.
136. Winnie A. P. *Anesth. Analg. (Cleve.)* 1970, **49**, 455; Mathews P. J. and Hughes T. J. *Anaesthesia* 1983, **38**, 813.
137. Miranda D. R. *Br. J. Anaesth.* 1977, **49**, 722.
138. Barutell C. et al. *Anaesthesia* 1980, **35**, 365.
139. Huang K. C. et al. *Anaesth. Intensive Care* 1986, **14**, 87.
140. Edde R. R. et al. *Anaesth. Analg. (Cleve.)* 1977, **54**, 446.
141. Lim E. K. *Anaesth. Intensive Care* 1979, **7**, 53.
142. Lim E. K. *Anaesthesia* 1979, **34**, 370.
143. Labat G. *Br. J. Anaesth.* 1926, **4**, 174.
144. Burnham R. J. *Anesthesiology* 1958, **19**, 281.
145. Eather K. F. *Anesthesiology* 1958, **19**, 683.
146. Hirschel G. *Münch. Med. Wochenschr.* 1911, **58**, 1555 (translated and reprinted in *Surv. Anesthesiol.* 1963, **7**, 281).
147. Rosenblatt R. et al. *Anesthesiology* 1979, **51**, 565; Winnie A. P. *Surg. Clin. North Am.* 1975, **55**, 861.
148. Boures J. B. *Anaesthesia* 1984, **39**, 1250.
149. Bier A. *Arch. Klin. Chir.* 1908, **86**, 1007 (translated and reprinted in 'Classical File', *Surv. Anesthesiol.* 1967, **11**, 294).
150. Holmes C. M. *Lancet* 1963, **1**, 245
151. Riha J. *Anaesthesist* 1962, **11**, 230.
152. Johann Friedrich von Esmarch (1832–1908), professor of surgery in University of Kiel (when August Bier gave his first spinal block in 1898). Esmarch became, by marriage, uncle of Kaiser Wilhelm II of Germany (*Samml. Klin. Vortr.* 1873, **58**, 373.)
153. Rhys-Davies N. and Stotter A. T. *Ann. R. Coll. Surg. Engl.* 1985, **67**, 193.
154. Finlay H. *Anaesthesia* 1977, **32**, 357.
155. Davies J. A. H. et al. *Anaesthesia* 1984, **39**, 416.
156. Fleming S. A. et al. *Can. Anaesth. Soc. J.* 1966, **12**, 21.
157. Kerr J. H. *Anaesthesia* 1967, **22**, 562; Thorne-Alquist A.-M. *Acta Anaesth. Scand.* 1971, **15**, 23; Wildsmith J. et al. *Anaesthesia* 1979, **34**, 919.
158. Davies J. A. H. et al. *Anaesthesia* 1984, **39**, 996.
159. Vaughan R. S. et al. *Ann. R. Coll. Surg. Engl.* 1985, **67**, 309.
160. Tucker G. T. and Boas R. A. *Anesthesiology* 1971, **34**, 538.
161. Fitzgerald B. *Br. J. Anaesth.* 1976, **48**, 485.
162. Wallace W. A. et al. *Hosp. Update.* 1978, **17**, 999; Davis J. A. H. and Walford A. J. *Acta Anaesth. Scand.* 1986, **30**; 145; Valli H. and Rosenberg P. H. *Anaesthesia* 1986, **41**, 1196; Nusbaum L. M. and Hamelberg W. *Anesthesiology* 1986, **64**, 91; Turner P. L. et al. *Aust. N. Z. J. Surg.* 1986, **56**, 153.
163. Hannington-Kiff J. G. *Lancet* 1984, **1**, 2019. *See also* Kepes E. R. et al. *Region. Anaesthe.* 1982, **7**, 52.

164. Ryding F. N. *Anaesthesia* 1981, **36**, 969.
165. Goyanes J. *Rev. Clin. Madr* 1912, **8**, 401.
166. Van Niekerk J. P. de V. and Coetzee T. *Lancet*, 1965, **1**, 1353.
167. Bradfield W. J. D. *Br. J. Surg.* 1963, **50**, 495.
168. Sellheim H. *Verh. Dtsch. Ges. Gynäk* 1906, 176; Crossley A. W. H. and Hosie E. E. *Br. J. Anaesth.* 1987, **59**, 149.
169. Läwen A. *Münch. Med. Wochenschr.* 1911, **58**, 1390.
170. Kappis M. *Zentbl. Chir.* 1912, **39**, 249.
171. Macintosh R. R. and Bryce-Smith R. *Local Analgesia: Abdominal Surgery*, 2nd ed. Edinburgh: Livingstone, 1962.
172. Eason M. J. and Wyatt R. *Anaesthesia* 1979, **34**, 638.
173. Adson A. W. et al. *Surg. Gynecol. Obstet.* 1929, **48**, 577.
174. Leriche R. and Fontaine R. *Presse Méd.* 1934, **2**, 1843 (translated and reprinted in 'Classical File', *Surv. Anesthesiol.* 1974, **18**, 430).
175. Mandl F. *Paravertebral Block.* New York: Grune & Stratton, 1947.
176. Sanderson C. J. *Ann. Roy. Coll. Surg. Engl.* 1981, **63**, 420; Correspondence, *Ann. R. Coll. Surg. Engl.* 1982, **64**, 135; Duncan J. A. T. *Today's Anaesthetist* 1986, **1**, No. 2, 4.
177. Mandl F. *Paravertebral Block.* London: Heinemann (Medical Books) Ltd., 1928 (translated into English, 1947) and Parke F. W. and Chalmers J. A. *J. Obstet. Gynaecol. Br. Commonw.* 1957, **64**, 420.
178. Bryce-Smith R. *Anaesthesia* 1951, **6**, 159; 1955, **10**, 173.
179. McCollum P. T. and Spence V. A. *Br. J. Anaesth.* 1985, **57**, 1146.
180. Lofström B. *Illustrated Handbook of Local Anaesthesia* (Eriksson E. ed.)., 2nd ed. London: Lloyd-Luke, 1979.
181. Nunn J. F. and Slavin G. *Br. J. Anaesth.* 1980, **52**, 253; Cronin K. D. and Davies M. J. *Anaesth. Intensive Care* 1976, **4**, 259.
182. Sellheim H. *Verh. Dtsch. Ges. Gynäk.* 1906, 176.
182. Moore D. C. *Br. J. Anaesth.* 1975, **47**, 284.
183. James N. R. *Regional Analgesia for Intra-abdominal Surgery.* London: Churchill, 1943.
183. Adams L. *Dtsch. Z. Chir.* 1915, **133**, 1.
184. Cronin K. D. et al. *Anaesth. Intensive Care* 1976, **4**, 259.
184. Baxter A. D. et al. *Br. J. Anaesth.* 1984, **56**, 665; Murphy D. F. *Br. J. Anaesth.* **56**, 627.
185. Moore D. C. *Br. J. Anaesth.* 1981, **53**, 1235. *See also* Moore D. C. *Br. J. Anaesth.* 1985, **57**, 543.
186. Mulroy M. F. *Region. Anesth.* 1985, **10**, 39.
187. Katz J. et al. *Anesthesiology* 1979, **51**, 233; Orr I. A. et al. *Ann. R. Coll. Surg. Engl.* 1983, **65**, 366.
188. Shretting P. *Br. J. Anaesth.* 1981, **53**, 527; Moore D. C. *Br. J. Anaesth.* 1981, **53**, 1235.
189. Moore D. C. and Bridenbaugh L. D. *Anesth. Analg. Curr. Res.* 1962, **41**, 1.
190. Nauss L. A. et al. *Anesthesiology* 1979, **51**, Suppl. 237; Ward E. M. et al. *Anesth. Analg. (Cleve.)* 1979, **58**, 465.
191. Lavelle J. J. *J. Irish Coll. Phys. Surg.* 1983, **12**, 101.
192. Braun H. *Beitr. Klin. Chir.* 1919, **115**, 161; Braun H. *Die Lokal-Anaesthesie.* Leipzig, 1905, p. 311; Kappis, K. M. Bruns. *Beitr. Klin. Chirg.* 1919, **115**, 161.
193. Kappis M. *Zentbl. Chir.* 1920, **47**, 98; *Dtsch. Med. Wochenschr.* 1920, **40**, 535; *Klin. Wochenschr.* 1923, **2**, 1441.
194. Reid W. et al. *Br. J. Surg.* 1970, **57**, 45.
195. Filshie J. et al. *Anaesthesia* 1983, **38**, 498.
196. Umeda S. and Hashida T. *Abs. 8th World Cong. Anaesth. Manila*, 1984, **1**, 90.
197. Gardner A. M. H. and Soloman G. *Ann. R. Coll. Surg. Engl.* 1984, **66**, 498.
198. Jones N. et al. *Ann. R. Coll. Surg. Engl.* 1977, **59**, 46.
199. Cherry D. A. and Lamberty J. *Anaesth. Intensive Care* 1984, **12**, 59.
200. Mayerhofer O. in: *Regional Anaesthesia (1884–1984)* Scott D. B. et al. ed. Production ICM AB. Sodertalje, 1984.
201. Braun H. *Die Lokal-Anaesthesie.* Leipzig. 1905, p. 311.
202. Schleich C. L. *Schmerzlöse Operationen.* Berlin: Springer, 1899, p. 240.
203. Hesselbach F. C. *Anatomisch-chirurgische Abhandlung.* Würzburg: Baumgartner, 1806.
204. Alexander-Williams J. and Keithley M. R. B. *Ann. R. Coll. Surg. Engl.* 1979, **61**, 251.
205. Glassow F. *Ann. R. Coll. Surg. Engl.* 1976, **58**, 133; Flanagan L. and Bascom J. V. *Surg. Gynecol. Obstet.* 1981, **153**, 557.

206. Bainton A. *Anaesthesia* 1982, **37**, 696.
207. Macintosh R. R. and Bryce-Smith R. *Local Analgesia: Abdominal Surgery*, 2nd ed. Edinburgh: Livingstone 1962, p. 70; Glassow F. *Ann. R. Coll. Surg. Engl.* 1976, **58**, 133.
208. Magbagbeola J. A. O. *Br. J. Anaesth.* 1970, **42**, 184.
209. Glassow F. *Ann. R. Coll. Surg. Engl.* 1976, **58**, 133.
210. Glassow F. *Ann. Surg.* 1976, **58**, 134; Glassow F. *Ann. R. Coll. Surg. Engl.* 1984, **66**, 382.
211. Feeley M. et al. *J. Irish Coll. Phys. Surg.* 1974, **3**, 83.
212. Bacon A. L. C. 1977. *Anaesth. Intensive Care* 1977, **5**, 63; White J. et al. *Br. Med. J.* 1983, **266**, 1934; Yeoman P. M. et al. *Anaesthesia* 1983, **38**, 862.
213. Muir J. G. *Anaesthesia* 1985, **40**, 1021.
214. Sara C. A. and Lowry C. J. *Anaesth. Intensive Care* 1985, **13**, 79.
215. Soliman M. G. and Trembley N. A. *Anesth. Analg. (Cleve.)* 1978, **57**, 495; Goldberg P. J. *J. Urol.* 1981, **126**, 337.
216. Yeoman P. M. et al. *Anaesthesia* 1983, **38**, 862.
217. Berry F. R. *Anaesthesia* 1977, **32**, 576; Khoo S. T. and Brown T. C. K. *Anaesth. Intensive Care* 1984, **11**, 40; Grossbard G. D. and Love B. R. T. *Aust. N.Z. J. Surg.* 1979, **49**, 592.
218. Gjessing J. and Harley N. *Anaesthesia* 1969, **24**, 213.
219. James C. D. T. and Little T. F. *Anaesthesia* 1976, **31**, 1060.
220. Coates D. P. et al. *Anaesthesia* 1983, **38**, 588.
221. Casale F. F. and Thomas T. L. *Anaesthesia* 1983, **38**, 1090.
222. Winnie A. P., Ramamurphy S. et al. *Anesth. Analg.* 1973, **52**, 989; Winnie A. P. *Surg. Clin. North. Am.* 1975, 55, 881.
223. Taylor R. W. et al. *Ann. R. Coll. Surg. Engl.* 1981, **63**, 207.
224. Loftström B. *Illustrated Handbook of Local Anaesthesia*, 2nd ed. London: Lloyd-Luke, 1979, p. 106.
225. Magora F. et al. *Br. J. Anaesth.* 1969, **41**, 695.
226. Patel N. *Region. Anesth.* 1985, **10**, 40.
227. Wedel D. J. et al. *Region. Anesth.* 1985, **10**, 48.
228. Chayen D. et al. *Anesthesiology* 1976, **45**, 95; Brands E. et al. *Anaesth. Intensive Care* 1978, **6**, 256.
229. Odoom J. A. et al. *Anaesthesia* 1986, **41**, 155.
230. Bryce-Smith R. *Postgrad. Med. J.* 1966, **42**, 367; Bryce-Smith R. in: *Practical Regional Analgesia* (Lee J. A. and Bryce-Smith R. ed.). Amsterdam: Excerpta Medica, 1976, p. 70.
231. Kempthorne P. M. and Brown T. C. K. *Anaesth. Intensive Care* 1984, **12**, 14.
232. Smith B. E. et al. *Anaesthesia* 1984, **39**, 155.
233. Beck G. P. *Anesthesiology* 1963, **24**, 222; Winnie A. P. *Surg. Clin. North Am.* 1975, **45**, 887.
234. *See also* Schurman D. J. *Anesthesiology* 1976, **44**, 348.
235. Bradshaw E. G. and Earlam C. M. *Br. Med. J.* 1982, **285**, 977.
236. Orr C. M. E. et al. *Hosp. Update* 1977, **3**, 465.
237. Dinley R. J. and Micjelinakis E. *Injury* 1972–73, **4**, 345; Cobb A. G. and Houghton G. R. *Br. Med. J.* 1985, **291**, 1683; Cobb A. G. *Br. J. Emerg. Med.* **1**, 9.
238. Cobb A. G. and Houghton G. R. *Br. Med. J.* 1985, **291**, 1683.
239. Hopkins H. H. and Kapany N. S. *Nature* 1954, **173**, 39.
240. Hirschowitz B. I. et al. *Gastroenterology* 1958, **35**, 50.
241. Webberley M. J. and Cuschieri A. *Br. Med. J.* 1982, **285**, 260.
242. Jones R. *Br. Med. J.* 1982, **285**, 512.
243. Vatashki H. et al. *J. R. Soc. Med.* 1982, **75**, 627.
244. Al-Khudhairi D. et al. *Anaesthesia* 1982, **37**, 1002; Kauar P. et al. *Ann. R. Coll. Surg. Engl.* 1984, **66**, 283; Brophy T. et al. *Anaesth. Intensive Care* 1982, **10**, 344.
245. Galizia E. J. et al. *Br. J. Anaesth.* 1975, **47**, 402.
246. Hoare A. M. *Br. J. Hosp. Med.* 1980, **23**, 347.
247. Beavis A. K. et al. *Br. Med. J.* 1979, **1**, 1387.
248. Sanders R. D. *Delaware St. Med. J.* 1967, **39**, 170.
249. Ikeda S. et al. *Keio J. Med.* 1968, **17**, 1.
250. Allen H. A. et al. *Anesth. Analg. Curr. Res.* 1956, **35**, 386.
251. Pagden D. et al. *Anesth. Analg. (Cleve.)* 1986, **65**, 1063.
252. Harding S. F. et al. *Br Med. J.* 1986, **292**, 1428.

253. McCallum M. I. and Glynn C. G. *Anaesthesia* 1986, **41**, 850.
254. Parris M. R. and Chambers W. A. Br. *Br. J. Anaesth.* 1986, **58**, 297.
255. Toumineu M. K. et al. *Anaesthesia* 1987, **42**, 20.
256. Dixon J. M. and Crofts T. J. *J. R. Coll. Surg. Edinb.* 1983, **28**, 292.
257. Surg M. R. J. and Bingham R. M. *Anaesthesia* 1986, **41**, 401.
258. Armstrong D. N. and Kingsnorth A. N. *Ann. R. Coll. Surg.* 1986, **68**, 207.
259. Brown T. C. K. and Dickens D. R. V. *Anaesth. Intensive Care* 1986, **14**, 126.
260. Atkinson R. S. and Lee J. A. *Anaesthesia* 1985, **40**, 1059.
261. Curley R. K. et al. *Br. Dent. J.* 1987, **162**, 113.
262. Ross W. N. et al. *Br. J. Surg.* 1987, **74**, 63; Baxter A. D. et al. *Br. J. Anaesth.* 1987, **59**, 162.
263. Cook J. H. *Ann. R. Coll. Surg.* 1987, **69**, 4.

Chapter 32   **SPINAL ANALGESIA: INTRADURAL; EXTRADURAL**

It is the opinion of the authors of this book, based on very considerable practical experience, that well-conducted and skilfully applied spinal analgesia, both intra-and extradural, are techniques of pain relief which, when indicated, give results just as satisfactory from the points of view of the patient, surgeon and anaesthetist as well-given general anaesthesia. These blocks provide profound muscular relaxation and analgesia while, in addition, they are usually associated with some degree of ischaemia and contraction of the bowel, which gives the abdominal surgeon more room for manoeuvre.

In recent years, intradural spinal analgesia has been increasing in popularity, partly owing to the introduction of plain 0·5% bupivacaine solution.

INTRADURAL SPINAL ANALGESIA

History
Cerebrospinal fluid discovered by Domenico Cotugno (1736–1822) in 1764;[1] its circulation described by F. Magendie in 1825, who named it.[2]

Cocaine isolated from *Erythroxylon coca* in 1860 by Niemann and Lossen; its analgesic properties described by Schroff in 1862 and von Anrep in 1880.[3] Introduced into medicine as local analgesic for ophthalmology by Carl Koller (1858–1944) encouraged by Sigmund Freud (1856–1939) in 1884.

First spinal analgesia by J. Leonard Corning (1855–1923), New York neurologist, in 1885.[4] He accidentally pierced the dura while experimenting with cocaine on the spinal nerves of a dog. Later he deliberately repeated the intradural injection, called it spinal anaesthesia and suggested it might be used in surgery. 'Be the destiny of this observation what it may, it has seemed to me, on the whole, worth recording.' This failed to influence his contemporaries. Wrote first book on local analgesia, 1886.[5]

Lumbar puncture standardized as a simple clinical procedure by Heinrich Irenaeus Quincke (1842–1922) of Kiel[6] in Germany in 1891 and by Essex Wynter (1860–1945) in England in the same year.[7]

First planned spinal analgesia for surgery in man performed by August Bier (1861–1949) on 16 August 1898, in Kiel when he injected 3 ml of 0·5% cocaine solution into a 34-year-old labourer.[8] After using it on 6 patients, he and his assistant each injected cocaine into the other's theca. Advised it for operations on legs, but gave it up owing to toxicity of cocaine. Tuffier[9] (1857–1929) and Sicard (1872–1929) in Paris soon afterwards extended its scope to include the external genitals and the abdomen. Frederick Dudley Tait (1862–1918) and Guido E. Caglieri (1871–1951)[10] of San Francisco, and also Rudolf Matas (1860–1957) of New Orleans,[11] were its first users in the US in 1899, their works being published in the following year.

Adrenaline used to increase duration and reduce toxicity of spinal analgesia in 1903.[12]

Stovaine synthesized by Fourneau (French, *fourneau*, stove) (1872–1949) in 1904,[13] used first in spinal analgesia in 1904 by Henri Chaput (1857–1904),[14] and novocaine (procaine) described by Einhorn (1956–1917) in Munich the following year.[15] It was used in spinal analgesia soon after its discovery.[16]

Alfred E. Barker (1850–1916) of London, the leading pioneer of spinal analgesia in Britain, was the first to realize (in 1906–7) the importance of the curves of the vertebral canal and the use of gravity in control of level of analgesia.[17] He introduced heavy Stovaine solutions in 1907 in Britain. Other early users of spinal analgesia in the UK were Robert Jones, the Liverpool orthopaedic surgeon,[18] Dean of the London Hospital[19] and Tyrrell Gray in children.[20] Babcock of Philadelphia first to use light solution, his formula containing Stovaine, alcohol, lactic acid, strychnine, etc.[21]

Spinal analgesia little used until Gaston Labat's work in 1921.[22] He urged use of neocaine (procaine) crystals dissolved in cerebrospinal fluid, together with barbotage and early Trendelenburg position. Then came George Pitkin, pupil of Babcock, with his light (spinocain) and heavy (duracaine) solutions and his use of the fine-bore, short-bevel needle (1927).[23]

Chen and Schmidt introduced ephedrine in 1923,[24] while Ocherblad and Dillon[25] and Rudolf and Graham[26] used it to maintain the blood pressure in spinal analgesia in 1927. The associated hypotension was first thought to be due to anterior abdominal wall paralysis causing decreased intrathoracic pressure during inspiration.[27] Later it was suggested that the cause was paralysis of the vasoconstrictor nerves supplying the splanchnic and other vessels.[28] Gaston Labat insisted that the hypotension itself was not so important as the cerebral ischaemia it might cause, unless a head down tilt was maintained.

Spinal analgesia was used for surgery of the head, neck and thorax by Jonnesco in 1909[29] and Koster, the Brooklyn surgeon, in 1928.[30]

Miescher discovered the analgesic properties of Percaine (nupercaine) in 1929; it was used in hyperbaric solution by Keyes and McLelland of New York in 1930,[31] while Howard Jones of London published his technique, using a hypobaric solution, in 1930,[32] Kirschner of Heidelberg in 1932,[33] and Sebrechts of Bruges in 1934.[34]

Etherington Wilson's work appeared in 1934,[35] and Walter Lemmon's first account of continuous spinal analgesia was published in 1940[36] (although Dean of the London Hospital had described this technique as early as 1907[37]).

Lincoln Fleetwood Sise (1874–1942) of Boston in the US popularized amethocaine (tetracaine)[38] which was synthesized by Eisleb in 1928.[39] Bupivacaine was first used for intradural block in 1966.[40]

In the UK intradural spinal analgesia was for many years under a cloud, partly because of the tendency to litigation should complications follow, such as the Woolley and Roe case in which paraplegia followed spinal analgesia in two patients operated on on the same day, and was thought to be due to contamination of the analgesic solution by phenol which had entered the ampoules through minute cracks in the glass.[41] The articles 'The Grave Spinal Cord Paralyses Caused by Spinal Analgesia' by Foster Kennedy[42] and 'Neurological Complications after Spinal Anaesthesia'[43] also had an important effect on the climate of opinion. They stimulated Dripps (1911–1974) and Vandam[44] to write their article entitled 'The Long-term Follow-up of Patients who received 10 098 Spinal Analgesics: Failure to Discover Major Neurological Sequelae' (reprinted in *Surv. Anesthesiol.* 1970, **14**, 308); later articles confirmed this good result. Anxiety is made worse as the causes of some of these complications, such as adhesive arachnoiditis, are not fully understood. The method is, however, a valuable one, and if proper care is taken in the technique, it yields, in a very large proportion of cases, admirable results and satisfaction to all concerned.[45] Extradural analgesia can be substituted for intradural (spinal) analgesia in nearly every case. The ready availability of 0·5% solution of bupivacaine which has been used for a number of years for extradural block, has led to its use for intradural analgesia[46] and over the past decade a large number of successful cases has been reported for operations on the legs and perineum. For lower abdominal operations a hyperbaric solution gives better results. The long period during the 1950s and 1960s during which intradural spinal analgesia lay under a cloud of suspicion in the UK now appears to be coming to an end as an increasing experience, both here and in other countries, with bupivacaine and lignocaine bears witness to its efficiency and relative freedom from complications.

(*See also* Lee J. A. et al. ed. *Sir Robert Macintosh's Lumbar Puncture and Spinal Analgesia*, 5th ed. Edinburgh: Churchill Livingstone, 1985, Ch. 1; The Early History of Regional Anesthesia in the United States, Winnie A. P. *Regional Anesthesia 1884–1984*. Sweden. Production ICM AB, 1984.)

Anatomy

The Vertebrae
The vertebral column consists of 7 cervical, 12 thoracic, 5 lumbar, 5 sacral and 4 or 5 coccygeal vertebrae. The sacral and coccygeal vertebrae are fused in adult life.

Vertebral Column
This has four curves, of which the thoracic and sacral are primary and are concave anteriorly; thus, when the spine is fully flexed, the cervical and lumbar

curves are obliterated. In the supine position the 3rd lumbar vertebra marks the highest point of the lumbar curve, while the 5th thoracic is the lowest point of the dorsal curve. Kyphosis, lordosis, scoliosis and hypertrophic arthritis of the spine may upset the curves and make lumbar puncture difficult.

The direction of the spinous processes determines the direction in which the spinal needle must be inserted. The spinous processes of the cervical, the first two thoracic, and the last four lumbar vertebrae are all practically horizontal and are therefore opposite the bodies of their respective vertebra. The other spinous processes are inclined downwards, their tips being opposite the bodies of the vertebrae next below; exception, the tip of the first lumbar is opposite the intervertebral disk. The 5th lumbar spine overhangs the lumbosacral interspace.

Some Useful Surface Markings

The vertebra prominens (spine of C.7) is easily palpable. The tip of the spine of T.3 is opposite the roots of the spines of the scapula, with the arms at the sides of the body.

The tip of the spine of T.7 is opposite the inferior angle of the scapula, with the arms to the sides.

The highest points of the iliac crests are usually on a line crossing the spine of L.4 or the L.4–5 interspace.

The dimples overlying the posterior superior iliac spines are on a line crossing the second, posterior sacral foramina and at this level the dural sac in the adult usually ends. The lower end of the spinal cord terminates at the level of the upper border of the body of L.2.

The Intervertebral Disks

At least one-quarter of the length of the vertebral column is made up of these disks, each of which consists of an outer cover, the annulus fibrosus, enclosing a core of gelatinous material, the nucleus pulposus. The disks give flexibility to the column and act as 'shock-absorbers'. The annulus may rupture, usually posteriorly, so causing pressure on nerve roots. Such a prolapsed disk has been described following a lumbar puncture.

The Vertebral Canal

Bounded in front by bodies of the vertebrae and intervertebral disks; posteriorly by the laminae, ligamenta flava and the arch which bears spinous processes and by ligaments between them called the interspinous; laterally by pedicles and laminae. Size and shape vary, but is larger in cervical and lumbar regions.
Contents. (1) Roots of spinal nerves; (2) Spinal membranes with their enclosed cord and cerebrospinal fluid (*see* Chapter 2); (3) Structures—vessels, fat and areolar tissue of extradural space. The narrowest part is between T.4 and T.9.

Stenosis of the vertebral canal may cause cord compression after central neural blockade.[47] This may be intensified should there be extradural haemorrhage.[48]

The Vertebral Ligaments bounding the Canal

1. *Supraspinous ligament*, passes longitudinally over tips of spinous processes from C.7 to the sacrum.
2. *Interspinous ligaments*, joining spinous processes together. Cyst formation

in the interspinous ligament may result in a false positive sign of entry into the extradural space.[49]

3. *Ligamenta flava*, running from lamina to lamina, composed of yellow elastic fibres. Half of the substance of the posterior wall of the vertebral canal is composed of the bony laminae, half by the ligamenta flava. They become progressively thicker from above downwards.

4. *Posterior longitudinal ligament*, within the vertebral canal on posterior surfaces of bodies of vertebrae, from which it is separated by the basivertebral veins.

5. *Anterior longitudinal ligament*, runs along the front of the vertebral bodies to which, as also to the intervertebral disks, it is adherent.

Midline spinal puncture pierces the first three of these. In lateral approach only ligamenta flava are encountered.

The Spinal Cord

The elongated part of the central nervous system which occupies upper two-thirds of vertebral canal and is 45 cm long. Extent is from upper border of atlas to upper border of 2nd lumbar vertebra, and lower still in infants. At its rostral end, continuous with medulla oblongata; below, ends in conus medullaris, from apex of which filum terminale descends as far as coccyx. In fetal life length of cord corresponds with that of vertebral canal, but the canal grows more rapidly than the cord. Thus nerve roots which pass out transversely in early fetal life come to be more and more oblique in direction, so that in adult life lumbar and sacral nerves descend almost vertically to meet their foramina, and are known as the cauda equina. They are bathed in cerebrospinal fluid and will be affected by local analgesic solution injected in the lumbar area. The point of a lumbar puncture needle may touch one or more nerve roots but is unlikely to injure them, if the injection is given below the level of the upper border of L.2 where the cord ends.

The spinal cord is ensheathed by three membranes from without inwards.

Dura mater. The spinal dura mater represents only the inner or meningeal layer of the cerebral dura mater; the outer, or endosteal layer, being represented by the periosteum lining the vertebral canal which is separated from the spinal dura by the extradural space. It is connected by fibrous slips to the posterior longitudinal ligament, especially near the lower end of the vertebral canal. The dural sheaths of the spinal nerves fuse with the connective tissue in, or slightly lateral to, the intervertebral foramina. A strong fibrous layer forms a tubular sheath attached above to margins of foramen magnum, and ending below at lower border of second sacral vertebra. This does not prevent solutions of local analgesic from passing into the cranial cavity when excessive doses are injected. Main fibres are longitudinal, so the lumbar puncture needle should be introduced with its bevel separating rather than dividing these fibres.

Arachnoid. This is a thin transparent sheath closely applied to the dura. It surrounds the cranial and spinal nerves as far as their points of exit from the skull and the vertebral canal.

Pia mater. This is separated from the arachnoid by the subarachnoid space filled with cerebrospinal fluid. Here local analgesic drugs are deposited in spinal analgesia. The pia closely invests the cord and sends delicate septa into its substance. From each lateral surface of the pia mater a fibrous band, the denticulate ligament, projects into the subarachnoid space, and is attached by a series of pointed processes to the dura as far down as the first lumbar nerve. A posterior midline septum, the septum posticum has been described.[50] This may give rise to unilateral analgesia.[51] The pia mater ends as a prolongation—the filum terminale—which pierces the distal end of the dural sac and is attached to the periosteum of the coccyx. Although in some ways the intradural space is like the glass spine modelled for Barker (1907), being filled with fluid and the spinal cord, it is also broken up by nerve roots, the denticulate ligaments and fine trabeculae which attach the arachnoid to the pia mater. These may cause obstruction to the free flow of analgesic solution by forming baffles, with uneven distribution and occasional unexpected effects.

There are two enlargements of the cord, one in the cervical, the other in the lumbar region, corresponding to the origins of the nerves of the arms and legs.

Spinal Segments
The cord is divided into segments by the pairs of spinal nerves which arise from it. These pairs are 31 in number and are as follows: (*a*) 8 cervical; (*b*) 12 thoracic; (*c*) 5 lumbar; (*d*) 5 sacral; (*e*) 1 coccygeal.

The nerve roots within the dura have no epineural sheaths and are therefore easily affected by doses of analgesic drugs brought into contact with them. The cord is not transversely blocked by spinal analgesia, but it is probable that there may be some block of the longitudinal columns by penetration of the drug.[52]

Spinal Nerves
Anterior root is efferent and motor.

Sympathetic preganglionic axons arise from cells in the intermediolateral horn of the spinal cord from T.1 to L.2 inclusive. Blockade of these fibres influences the response of some of the endocrine glands to surgical stress.

Posterior root is larger than anterior. All the afferent impulses from the whole body, including viscera, pass into the posterior roots (largely sensory).

Each posterior root has a ganglion and conveys fibres of: (1) Pain; (2) Tactile; (3) Thermal sensation; (4) Deep or muscle sensation from bones, joints, tendons, etc.; (5) Afferents from the viscera (accompanying sympathetic); (6) Vasodilator fibres.

Pain and temperature fibres enter the posterior horn where they end around cells in the grey matter; fibres then cross to the contralateral side within three segments and ascend in the lateral spinothalamic tract to the thalamus. Tactile impulses ascend in the ventral spinothalamic tract to the thalamus. Deep or muscle sensory impulses ascend in the posterior columns and spinocerebellar tracts. Vibration impulses ascend in the posterior columns.

The anterior and posterior roots each with its covering of pia–arachnoid and dura cross the extradural space and unite in the intervertebral foramina to form the main spinal nerve trunks, which soon divide into anterior and posterior primary divisions—mixed nerves. These are blocked only secondarily in spinal analgesia; it is block of the nerve roots which gives the effect. There is evidence, however, that analgesic drugs after subarachnoid injection can soak along the nerve trunk for as much as 2 cm beyond the intervertebral foramen. Analgesic drugs affect autonomic, sensory and motor fibres in that order, while fibres which block easily hold the drug longest; thus sensory block lasts longer than motor and usually ascends two segments higher up the cord than motor block. *Segmental levels (Fig. 32.1)*. Perineum, S.1–S.4; Inguinal region, L.1; Umbilicus,

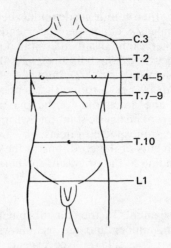

Fig. 32.1 Segmental levels

T.10; Subcostal arch. T.6–T.8; Nipple line, T.4 and T.5; Second intercostal space, T.2; Clavicle, C.3–C.4.

The skin above the nipple line has a double innervation from C.3 and C.4 and from T.2, T.3 and T.4, so even with a successful block to C.8 there will be some sensation above the nipple line. The success of a block to T.1 is proved by the inability of the patient to hold a sheet of paper between the fingers (innervation of interossei, C.8 and T.1).

Segmental Levels of Spinal Reflexes. Epigastric, T.7 and T.8; Abdominal, T.9 and T.12; Cremasteric, L.1 and L.2; Plantar, S.1 and S.2; Knee jerk, L.2–L.4; Ankle jerk, S.1 and S.2: Anal sphincter and wink reflexes, S.4–S.5.

Movement of joints. Hip flexion L.1–L.3; extension, L.5, S.1. Knee flexion L.5, S.1; extension L.2–L.3. Ankle flexion L.4–L.5; extension S.1–S.2.

Blood Supply to Spinal Cord

The posterior spinal arteries, two on each side, branch from the posterior inferior cerebellar arteries at the level of the foramen magnum. They supply the posterior columns of the cord.

The anterior spinal artery, a single vessel lying in the substance of the pia mater overlying the anterior median fissure, arises at the level of the foramen magnum from the junction of a small branch from each vertebral artery. It receives communications from the intercostal, lumbar and other small arteries. It supplies the lateral and the anterior columns, three-quarters of the substance of the cord. Thrombosis of this artery causes the anterior spinal artery syndrome in which there is paralysis sparing the posterior columns (joint, position, touch, vibration sense). Communicating branches at the level of T.1 and T.11 are larger than the others and help to supply the enlargements of the cord (the arteries of Adamkiewicz).[53] The artery at T.11 supplies the cord both upwards and downwards; that at T.1 only downwards from this level. There are thus three vascular areas in the cord with no anastomosis between them.[54] Normal intra-arterial capillary pressure is 30–35 mmHg. Deprivation of blood supply for 2–3 min may result in infarction of the cord.[55] (*See also* Dommisse G. F.

Arteries and Veins of the Human Spinal Cord from Birth. Edinburgh: Churchill Livingstone, 1976.)

The Extradural Veins
These largely form a plexus, most dense in the anterolateral part of the extradural space. They receive blood from the cord and the vertebral canal with its contents and communicate with both the intracranial sinuses and the tributaries of the inferior vena cava and the azygos system. The main longitudinal channels are without valves,[56] thus there is a continuous vascular connection between the cranium and the pelvis bypassing the vena cava. They dilate when either the thoracic or the intra-abdominal pressure is increased as by coughing, straining or due to swellings, such as a cyst or uterus at term. These veins have an important influence on both the spread of local analgesic solutions and on their absorption.

Nerve Supply of Meninges
The posterior aspect of the dura and arachnoid contains no nerve fibres and so no pain is felt on dural puncture. The anterior aspect is supplied by sinovertebral nerves; each of these enters an intervertebral foramen and passes up for one segment and down for two segments.[57]

The Subdural Space
This is a potential space between the dura and the pia–arachnoid into which a catheter, contrast medium or local analgesic solution may track.[58] Injection into it of local analgesic solution may cause inadequate block, abnormally high block or even total central neural blockade[94]. It does not communicate with the subarachnoid space but is in free communication with the lymph spaces of the nerves.

The Extradural Space (*see* p. 694)

The Subarachnoid Space
This is between the arachnoid and the pia mater and in the lumbar region it occupies more than half the anterior-posterior diameter of the vertebral canal. Communicates with the ventricular system at the base of the brain.

The contents of the space are the spinal nerve roots, the denticulate ligaments, a spongy reticulum of fibres connecting the pia to the arachnoid the cerebro-spinal fluid and the larger vessels.

The Cerebrospinal Fluid (*see* Chapter 2)
Its specific gravity averages 1004·5.[59]

Physiology of Central Neural Blockade

Zone of Differential Block
Sensory
In intradural block sympathetic fibres are blocked two to three segments higher than sensory fibres. In extradural block the relationship is complex. Some sympathetic afferent fibres escape the block, and when reflex response is high,

as in the young anxious patient, considerable sympathetic function may persist.[60] Sympathetic block will be greater when more concentrated solutions are used or when adrenaline is added, as this has a similar effect.[61]

Motor
In intradural block, the difference between sensory and motor block is slight (two segments). In extradural block, the difference in levels is greater,[62] depending very much on the nature of the local analgesic solution.[63]

Spinal analgesia will control hyper-reflexia in patients with chronic spinal cord injury.[64]

Nervous System
Order of blocking nerve fibres. (1) Autonomic preganglionic B fibres; (2) Temperature fibres—cold before warm; (3) Pin-prick fibres; (4) Fibres conveying pain greater than pin-prick; (5) Touch fibres; (6) Deep pressure fibres; (7) Somatic motor-fibres; (8) Fibres conveying vibratory sense and proprioceptive impulses.

During recovery, return of sensibility in the reverse order was assumed, but it has been suggested that sympathetic activity returns before sensation.[65] It has been asserted[66] and denied[67] that the cells of the posterior horn of the spinal cord are anaesthetized during both intra- and extradural block.

For work on the susceptibility of nerve fibres to analgesic solution, *see* Nathan P. W. and Sears T. A. *Anaesthesia* 1963, **18**, 467.

Spinal analgesia may also exacerbate pain in patients who have severe pain in a limb, e.g. sciatica.[68] In spinal analgesia, entirely adequate for surgery of a lower limb, a patient may complain of pain due to the tourniquet. A concentration of a solution of local analgesic drug may give excellent analgesia for ordinary sensation, conveyed by small nerve fibres, but may not be adequate to block transmission in larger fibres transmitting pressure-pain sensation. An increased concentration will avoid this. Another explanation of bizarre pains occurring during otherwise adequate low spinal analgesia may be that some pain fibres pass with sympathetic nerves to reach the cord at a higher level.[69]

Local analgesic drugs act mainly on the nerve roots leaving the cord, though some drug molecules reach its substance.[70] This depends on: (1) Accessibility; diffusion across the pia; the spaces of Virchow–Robin; the arachnoid villi;[71] (2) Lipid solubility; (3) Tissue blood flow. Drug molecules are removed from the intradural space[72] by absorption into blood vessels in the pia mater and by movement into the cord substance.

Drugs are removed from the extradural space via the extradural veins; their molecules can also pass through the dura in both directions. Such movement depends on: (1) Molecular weight; (2) Molecular shape; (3) Liposolubility; (4) The degree of ionization of the molecule. This movement is more important than may be obvious as the dura, although 0·3 mm in thickness in the lumbar area presents a total surface area up to the T.10 level of the order of $70 \, cm^2$.[73]

Cardiovascular System
There are six different ways in which intra- and extradural spinal block can influence the cardiovascular system: (1) Vasodilatation of resistance and capacitance vessels; (2) Block of cardiac efferent sympathetic fibres from T.1 and T.4 resulting in loss of chronotropic and inotropic drive and fall in cardiac

output; (3) The atrial or Bainbridge reflex causing bradycardia; (4) The operation of Marey's law causing tachycardia; (5) Depression of vascular smooth muscle and β-adrenergic blockade of myocardium with fall in cardiac output, following systemic absorption of the local analgesic drug (in some circumstances moderate levels of plasma lignocaine may be associated with increased cardiac output, arterial pressure and heart rate, but this is probably a central mechanism dependent upon an intact autonomic system);[74] (6) Adrenaline effect (if used) following absorption, resulting in β-stimulation and associated rise in cardiac output and reduction in peripheral resistance. The overall effect is likely to be a greater fall in mean arterial pressure than if adrenaline had not been used.[75]

Block not extending above T.4 is not always associated with fall of blood pressure in fit young adults[76] though the elderly may suffer significant hypotension when moderate volumes are injected into the extradural space.[77] Hypotension is also likely in the debilitated or hypovolaemic subject, and very rarely this may lead to cardiac arrest. When there is cardiac decompensation removal of sympathetic tone may be dangerous.

Blood pressure fall is usually seen in the first 20 min after injection. Hypotension is seldom a cause for anxiety if the peripheral pulses are easily palpable. Administration of inotropic and chronotropic drugs may cause an increase in the oxygen requirements of cardiac muscle as well as in the oxygen supply. Corrective measures may be considered if arterial pressure falls more than one-third below its preoperative level.[78]

Slowing of the heart rate is caused if any of the anterior roots carrying sympathetic cardiac-accelerator fibres are blocked, as may happen in high spinals above T.4–T.5. A further cause of slow pulse rate is the lowering of blood pressure in the right auricle consequent on diminished venous return (Bainbridge (1874–1921) effect).[79] On the other hand, *tachycardia* during spinal analgesia may result from the operation of Marey's (1830–1904) law[80] (a pulse of low tension is fast). Bradycardia is the more frequent effect.

Theories of Causation of Fall in Blood Pressure

1. Diminished cardiac output consequent on reduction of venous return to heart, and lack of muscular propulsive force on veins.

2. Dilatation of post-arteriolar capillaries and small venules due to paralysis of vasoconstrictors. It is seen in entire vascular area, somatic and visceral, where anterior roots are paralysed, together with their sympathetic vasoconstrictor fibres. Compensatory vasoconstriction takes place in areas not anaesthetized, via carotid sinus reflexes. In high spinal blocks, majority of vasoconstrictor fibres—including those to arm (T.2–T.10)—are paralysed, hence low blood pressure. As a concentration of solution less than that required to cause muscular relaxation or analgesia will produce sympathetic block, vasoconstrictor paralysis is often complete even if sensory block is only up as high, say, as T.8. The warm, dry arm with dilated veins is often seen in cases of high spinal analgesia. Total peripheral resistance decreases by only 18% following complete sympathetic block in healthy young adults.[81]

3. Paralysis of sympathetic nerve supply to the heart (T.1–T.4).

4. Paralysis of sympathetic nerve supply to adrenal glands (splanchnic nerves), with consequent catecholamine depletion.

5. Absorption of drug into circulation. This is much more likely to be a cause

of hypotension after extradural than after intradural analgesia because of the larger amount of analgesic drug injected.

6. Ischaemia and hypoxia of vital centres.

7. Hypovolaemia, if present, may give rise to severe falls in blood pressure if central neural blockade is employed.

8. Compression of the great vessels within the abdomen by the pregnant uterus, abdominal tumours or abdominal packs may cause severe hypotension in the presence of central neural blockade.

Spinal analgesia may not cause much fall in blood pressure in the absence of surgical stimuli or bodily movement. Blood pressure drop below 80 mmHg systolic and 60 diastolic should be taken notice of while systolic blood pressure below 50 is unsatisfactory. Blood pressure and pulse rate often fall together. A palpable superficial temporal artery is a reassuring sign, while a palpable carotid pulse accompanied by adequate tidal exchange indicates that the patient is not gravely collapsed.

Treatment of Lowered Blood Pressure (if thought to be necessary)

Intravenous fluid; oxygen inhalation; injection of pressor drug, e.g. ephedrine or ergotamine tartrate 0·25 mg;[82] elevation of the legs. When there is brady-cardia, atropine 0·2 mg alone will often elevate blood pressure.[83] When hypotension is accompanied by bradycardia, phenylephrine and methoxamine are probably better avoided, unless accompanied by atropine. Some anaesthetists use vasopressors prophylactically in high blocks and other cases judged to be doubtful risks. It has been suggested that ephedrine, to increase the cardiac output and venous return, is a more satisfactory drug than methoxamine, etc.

Electrolyte solutions used to treat hypotension are successful in a large proportion of cases in amounts up to 2 litres.

The vasoconstrictor reflex produced by haemorrhage is abolished by spinal block, in proportion to the height of the block, so that the patient is unable to protect himself against this stress. Infusion is necessary.

Respiratory System

The phrenic nerve supplying the diaphragm rises from the anterior roots of C.3, C.4 and C.5, and should not be encroached on in spinal analgesia, but phrenic paralysis can occur. Apnoea may be due to medullary ischaemia or to a toxic effect of the drug—in extradural blocks. During spinal analgesia, breathing becomes quiet and tranquil. This is due not only to motor blockade, but also to deafferentation with reduction of sensory input to the respiratory centre. Lowered arterial and venous tone also lessens the work of the heart and tends to relieve any pre-existing pulmonary congestion. The ventilation–perfusion relationship during extradural block is not greatly altered and the effect on respiratory function is relatively small with no evidence of change in FRC or V/Q ratio. The pulmonary gas exchange is preserved. The effect of block is largely on the cardiovascular system.[84] Vital capacity and forced expiratory volume may be reduced, especially in cigarette smokers.[85] Intercostal paralysis is compensated for by increased descent of the diaphragm which is made easier by the lax abdominal walls. This is not accompanied by hypoxia and hypercapnia[86] though the ability to cough forcibly to expel secretions is impaired.[87] Although resulting respiratory function is little affected by spinal analgesia there is less reserve.[88] Obesity is associated with reduced inspiratory capacity.[89] If there is any effect on the phrenic roots, patient cannot talk, but can whisper. Such a condition requires oxygen immediately. Oxygen therapy is beneficial in high block as it decreases heart rate and cardiac output and increases total peripheral resistance, and when a block is accompanied by general anaesthesia.[90] Breathing is quiet and in obstructive airways disease there is some reflex bronchodilatation from stimulation of pressor receptors in the aorticocarotid sinuses by hypotension.[91] There is decreased pulmonary blood volume and pulmonary arterial blood pressure from reduced venous return to the right heart.

After upper abdominal surgery[92] but not following lower abdominal procedures,[93] respiratory function is better if the pain of the operation is relieved by extradural block, rather than by centrally acting analgesics. There is less reduction of FRC and consequent physiological shunting which may arise from airways closure.

The patient may stop breathing so that respiratory support by IPPV and, if necessary, tracheal intubation may be required. Causes may be: (1) Inadequate medullary blood flow due to inadequate cardiac output: a serious situation demanding immediate cardiorespiratory support; (2) Total spinal analgesia with denervation of all the respiratory muscles. True phrenic paralysis is uncommon as the motor roots are large while the analgesic solution is likely to be weak when it reaches the cervical region; (3) Massive extradural spread; (4) Accidental subdural injection.[94] A small volume of solution may travel to an unexpectedly high level in this potential space; (5) Toxic effects of the local analgesic drug; (6) Injection of narcotic analgesic drug (*see* p. 711).

Gastrointestinal System

Preganglionic sympathetic fibres from T.5 to L.1 are inhibitory to gut. No effect on the oesophagus, the innervation of which is vagal. The small gut is contracted as the sympathetic inhibitory impulses are removed, the vagus being all-powerful. Sphincters are relaxed and peristalsis is active although not more frequent. Pressure within the bowel lumen is increased.[95] Handling of the small bowel by the surgeon may cause it to dilate, as may the injection of atropine before operation. Nausea and vomiting due to the hypotension may occur and usually come on in waves lasting a minute or so and then passing away spontaneously. The spleen enlarges two or three times in high block, when its sympathetic efferent fibres (splanchnic nerves) are paralysed. Stimuli arising in the upper abdomen may ascend along the unblocked vagi and perhaps the phrenics, and cause discomfort if the patient is conscious. Para-oesophageal infiltration of local analgesic solution may prevent this by blocking vagal afferents. Colonic blood supply and oxygen availability are increased in animals following spinal analgesia[96] perhaps an important factor in the prevention of anastomotic breakdown following gut resection. (*See* p. 690.)

Theories of Causation of Nausea and Vomiting

(1) Hypotension; (2) Increased peristalsis; (3) Traction on nerve endings and plexuses, especially via vagus; (4) Presence of bile in stomach due to relaxation of pyloric and bile-duct sphincters; (5) Narcotic analgesics (premedication); (6) Psychological factors; (7) Hypoxia. Gastric emptying time is quicker when extradural block is employed for postoperative pain relief than when narcotic analgesics are used.[97]

Treatment

This consists in attending to the hypotension and hypoxia, if present; intravenous atropine; deep breathing through the mouth; reassurance and attention to general comfort; anti-emetics; supplementary intravenous anaesthesia with thiopentone and nitrous-oxide–oxygen, or a volatile agent, etc., if the condition persists or if the surgeon's work is being interfered with. Full general anaesthesia may be required.

The Liver[98]

There are no specific effects of significance. The degree of hypotension which compromises liver function is not known. Liver disease may interfere with the metabolism of local analgesic drugs.

Electrolytes

Following surgery and trauma there is water and salt retention. Continuous extradural block abolishes sodium retention but not water retention in patients undergoing upper abdominal operations.[99]

Endocrine System

The release of antidiuretic hormone is suppressed during surgery.[100] Spinal block delays adrenal response to trauma, whereas operations under general anaesthesia cause a rise in the blood steroids.[101] (*See also* Kehlet H. et al. *Br. J. Surg.* 1979, **66**, 543.) The rise in blood cortisol levels associated with surgery performed under general anaesthesia may be less marked if afferent impulses are blocked by spinal analgesia. There is, however, no difference when the surgery is major and involving the abdomen or thorax,[102] and in any case there is no difference in the postoperative period once the effects of the block are discontinued.

Spinal block suppresses the hyperglycaemic response to surgery[103] and stress and so is useful in diabetic patients but this does not extend into the postoperative period.[104,105] The response to insulin is augmented and the anaesthetist should be aware of the possibility of hypoglycaemia. Infused glucose is well utilized.[106] Extradural block prevents lymphopaenia and granulocytosis after operation, thus inhibiting the metabolic endocrine response to surgery and preventing immuno-depression.[107]

Stress Response

Regional analgesia which blocks afferent impulses plays an important part in avoiding stress responses to surgery. With single-dose blocks the effect is likely to be transitory so that the most effective method is probably continuous extradural block, though even this is not very effective following upper abdominal operations, being better in lower laparotomies. This may be because some afferent pathways remain unblocked (*see also* p. 670).[108] Stress responses to intubation may be obtunded by i.v. fentanyl.[109] Intra- or extradural block may modify stress responses, whether hormonal, cardiovascular or metabolic, but are more likely to do so in lower than in upper abdominal operations.[109]

Genito-urinary System

Sympathetic supply to kidneys from T.11 to L.1, via the lowest splanchnic nerves.

Any effects on renal function are due to hypotension. Autoregulation of renal blood flow is impaired if mean arterial pressure falls below about 50 mmHg. These changes are transient and disappear when blood pressure rises again.

Sphincters of bladder not relaxed, so soiling of table by urine is not seen, and tone of ureters not greatly altered. The penis is often engorged and flaccid due to paralysis of the nervi erigentes (S.2 and S.3); this is a useful positive sign of successful block. Post-spinal retention of urine may be moderately prolonged as S.2 and S.3 contain small autonomic fibres and their paralysis lasts longer than that of the larger sensory and motor fibres. During prolonged blockade of the lumbar and sacral segments, the bladder must be palpated so that catheterization can be employed when necessary. Spermatorrhoea is sometimes seen. Block of the nerves from T.11 downwards results in painless labour.

The tone of the uterus is not greatly altered after spinal analgesia in pregnancy so that block is not contraindicated then. In late pregnancy smaller doses of analgesic solution are required.[110] Tone of uterus increased in third stage of labour. (*See* Chapter 27.)

Body Temperature[111]

Vasodilatation favours heat loss; absence of sweating favours hyperpyrexia in hot environments. Catecholamine secretion is depressed, hence less heat is produced by metabolism. There is evidence that the extradural space is a temperature sensitive zone, whereas the intradural space is not. Cold solutions injected into the former may induce shivering:[412] (1) because the large veins act as heat exchangers; (2) as a result of the sensory input; (3) possibly because of the existence of thermal sensors. Extradural pethidine 25 mg may induce control.[420]

(*See also* Greene N. M. *Physiology of Spinal Anesthesia* 3rd ed. Baltimore: Williams and Wilkins, 1981.)

Factors Influencing Height of Analgesia in Intradural Block

1. Dose of Drug Injected
Probably the most important single factor. Nerve tissue absorbs local analgesic drugs as blotting-paper absorbs ink; a limited amount of nerve tissue can only absorb so much drug, the surplus being available for convection or absorption into the bloodstream. The greater the dosage and concentration, the higher is the block likely to spread, the longer will its effect last.

2. Volume of Fluid Injected
Recent work suggests that this is much less important than was once thought. Increasing the volume of a fixed concentration of analgesic solution is synonymous with increase in the dose of drug injected. If a fixed amount is given in varying volumes, the spread may be identical.[112]

3. Barbotage
A method of mixing the dose in an increasing volume of CSF and so increasing dispersion; it thus increases the volume injected. Some workers of experience advocate barbotage.[113] Others find it less valuable.[114]

4. Force and Rate of Injection
Forceful injection has only a marginal effect on the height of block obtained. Slow injection, especially of a viscid hyperbaric solution, is likely to limit spread (*see* p. 682).

5. Specific Gravity of Solution

Baricity. This is the weight of one substance compared with the weight of another substance at the same temperature. Analgesic solutions for intradural injection may be hypo-, iso- or hyperbaric in relation to cerebrospinal fluid.

Plain solutions of local analgesic drugs are likely to be iso- or slightly hypobaric. Addition of glucose between 5 and 8% makes the solution hyperbaric. Recent work confirms that when the patient is tilted head-down the resulting height of segmental block is likely to extend a few segments higher when hyperbaric solution is used in place of plain solution in the same dosage and volume.[115] This may make all the difference between success and failure in spinal analgesia for abdominal surgery.

6. Position of Patient during Injection

If the patient sits during the injection and for a short time afterwards, heavy solutions tend to fall, especially if injected slowly, and hypobaric solutions to rise. After injection in the lateral position with the patient turned supine immediately afterwards, the bolus of analgesic solution, if it is hyperbaric, will tend to move either cephalad or caudad, the direction being controlled by the cephalad or caudad inclination of the vertebral canal which can be influenced by the tilt of the table. The lowest point of the thoracic curve is at the level of T.5 and spread above this level is limited unless a very steep head-down tilt is adopted. Further cephalad spread can be inhibited by elevating the head and shoulders of the patient on pillows. A so-called 'brake action' occurs because an analgesic drug becomes fixed to nerve tissue and the concentration in solution becomes less as distance increases from the site of injection.[116]

7. Interspace Chosen

The higher the interspace chosen for injection the higher will be the resulting analgesia, leaving other factors out of account. A good rule is to choose the L.2–L.3 interspace for upper abdominal cases; the L.3–L.4 interspace for lower abdominal and leg operations; and the L.4–L.5 interspace for perineal procedures. In the very tall a space higher is sometimes advantageous, while in the very short, one space lower may be chosen (except for perineal operations).

8. Posture of Patient after Injection

If patient remains on the side, curves of spine are without effect, and specific gravity of solution partially controls side of analgesia although a predominantly unilateral block soon becomes bilateral.

If patient is supine:

a. Hyperbaric solutions pass to the bottom of sacral and dorsal curves; some of it to both, if injection is made at apex of lumbar curve. Lowest point of dorsal curve coincides with the 5th thoracic vertebra, so upward spread of a reasonable volume of a heavy solution will not occur unless a steep Trendelenburg position is assumed. Similarly, hyperbaric analgesic fluid placed in the sacral curve cannot spread upwards over the hollow of the back, without a head-down tilt. *Thus, for blocks above the perineum with these solutions, the back of the patient, who is in the lateral position, should be slightly inclined head downwards during injection and slightly head up for sacral blocks, ensured by tilting the table appropriately.*

b. Hypobaric solutions gravitate to the top of the lumbar curve, but few solutions are truly hypobaric in practice.

c. Isobaric solutions are uninfluenced by gravity, and their maximum effect is at point of injection.

In the lithotomy position lumbar curve is obliterated. In the Trendelenburg position hypobaric solutions travel caudad, while hyperbaric solutions move cephalad. The normal spinal curvature limits this movement. Raising the head and shoulders accentuates the dorsal curve and tends to prevent spread of hyperbaric solutions to the cervical area with its phrenic roots.

In a most comprehensive review of factors which influence the distribution of solutions of local analgesic within the subarachnoid space, Greene[117] regards the following as having clinical importance: age; height; anatomy, and abnormalities of anatomy of the vertebral canal and spinal column; site of the injection; direction of the needle (at right angles or pointing upwards); effective volume of CSF in the lumbar region; density of CSF; density and baricity of local analgesic solution; position of the patient (unless an isobaric solution such as 0·5% plain bupivacaine is used); the amount or mass of the drug injected; the volume of solution injected.

The following factors are probably not important in influencing the spread of local analgesic solutions: sex of patient; weight; direction of needle bevel during injection; composition, pressure and circulation of CSF; addition of vasoconstrictors; turbulence or its lack, during injection; varying with speed and force of injection; barbotage.

We await a clear pathway through this jungle of uncertainties because of many mutually contradictory statements which perplex all experienced anaesthetists.

Duration of Analgesia
Depends on the drug used and the dose administered. The upper end of an abdominal incision regains sensation before the lower end. Cinchocaine, bupivacaine,[118] etidocaine and amethocaine last longer than lignocaine and procaine.

Fixation Time
For lignocaine, about 5 min. For procaine, 5–10 min. Amethocaine, etidocaine, bupivacaine and cinchocaine take longer. These drugs are removed from the intradural space by blood vessels in the pia mater and cord, a process related to lipid solubility. The extradural space has greater vascularity and transfer of analgesic drug to the bloodstream is likely to result in significant plasma levels.

Drugs Used to Produce Intradural Spinal Analgesia

(For Pharmacology, *see* Chapter 31.)

Bupivacaine
Plain bupivacaine 0·5% is satisfactory. Higher concentrations result in greater variability of spread[120] and are seldom necessary. In 1% solution, the drug precipitates when mixed with CSF.[121] Hyperbaric solutions are likely to result in block a few segments higher than when plain solutions are used. Dose up to 4 ml of 0·5% solution; this should be reduced in the elderly. (*See also* Chambers W. A. Editorial, *Br. J. Anaesth.* 1982, **54**, 799.)

Lignocaine Hydrochloride, BP
For spinal analgesia has been used in a strength of 5% with dextrose 3·0 and 7·5%; 1·5 ml of this solution gives about 2 h of good analgesia up to the umbilicus.[119]

Prilocaine
A 5% solution in 5% dextrose (sp. gr. 1022) is a clinically acceptable solution with a duration of action similar to that of lignocaine. Can be autoclaved. As the onset of analgesia is rapid there should be minimal delay in commencing the operation.

Amethocaine Hydrochloride, BP
Put up in ampoules containing 20 mg of dried powder, also in solution 1%, each ml containing 10 mg. Can be combined with dextrose solution to make it hyperbaric or with distilled water to make it hypobaric.[122] The maximal intrathecal dose is 20 mg. A long-acting drug for *extradural block* (1–1000 to 1–2000) which can be added to lignocaine 1·5%.

Etidocaine
This precipitates in CSF.[123] It produces more motor than sensory block, but may not be unique in this respect.[124]

Procaine Hydrochloride, BP
Can be autoclaved. The crystals are dissolved in cerebrospinal fluid and injected. In 5% strength or less, procaine is not irritating to nervous tissue and meninges. Analgesia lasts from 40 to 80 min.

Chloroprocaine
Not recommended for intradural injection as the commercial preparation contains sodium metabisulphite in an acid solution which may cause neurological irritation.[125]

Cinchocaine Hydrochloride, BP
It has a slow onset but lasting effect, and may give analgesia for 1½–3 h. Like amethocaine, it is easily destroyed by traces of alkali, so that needles, syringes, etc. should be washed through with cinchocaine solution which is subsequently discarded. Weight for weight it is highly toxic, but not dose for dose. A well-tried and very useful agent for intradural block; no longer manufactured.

Mepivacaine Hydrochloride[126]
Satisfactory for surgical operations not exceeding 1 h. The spinal preparation is 4% and contains 10% glucose and is hyperbaric.

Vasoconstrictors
Adrenaline (0·2 ml of 1–1000 solution) or phenylephrine (0·5 ml of 1% solution), added to amethocaine prolongs both sensory and motor blockade.[127] Adrenaline added to hyperbaric solutions of bupivacaine[128] or lignocaine[129] does not have this prolongation effect. Vasoconstrictors are seldom used in the intradural space in the UK for fear of compromising the blood supply of the cord, while in addition, the development of extradural catheter technique has made the

indications for prolonged intradural block uncommon. Spinal cord blood flow can be reduced in the region of an injection of lignocaine with phenylephrine into the intradural space, not by lignocaine alone.[130]

Preliminary Medication

Inadequate premedication during spinal analgesia shows callous unconcern for the patient. It may also wreck the smoothness of an otherwise correct technical procedure. Patients who come to the theatre in an anxious state of mind should be helped by further intravenous doses of a suitable sedative or narcotic analgesic.

Many anaesthetists prefer to give premedication such as morphine, 10 mg, with hyoscine, 0·4 mg, while agents such as diazepam, midazolam and the neuroleptics are alternatives. (*See also* Chapter 8.)

Armamentarium

Sterilization is most important and the whole pack should be sterilized by gamma radiation or autoclaved. Ampoules should not be stored in spirit or other antiseptic solution, as minute faults in the glass may result in contamination of the contents with untoward results.[131] Disposable sets are available. It has been suggested that plastic containers for analgesic solution should not be used as they may be contaminated with particles of plastic which may be injected and cause trouble.[132]

The lumbar puncture needle should be of fine gauge (20–25 gauge) and have a short bevel. Size 22 gauge is easy to use but a 25 gauge is preferable. To facilitate insertion of a fine (e.g. 25-gauge) needle, it can be inserted into the extradural space through a Sise introducer or shorter 20-gauge needle and then advanced through the dura.[133] A 2-ml and 5-ml all-glass syringe and a needle for aspirating the local analgesic solution, with an intradermal needle, swabs, swab-holder, antiseptic solution and container, complete the set.

Technique of Lumbar Puncture for Intradural Block[134]

The technique consists, in the words of the pioneer Barker,[135] 'To enter the lumbar dural sac effectually with the point of the needle, and to discharge through this all the contemplated dose of the drug, directly and freely into the cerebrospinal fluid, below the termination of the cord.'

The lumbar puncture must be done in a good light on a table which can be tilted. Pain can be minimized by the infiltration of local analgesic solution into the subcutaneous and deeper tissues, especially, during the paramedian approach, near the lamina.[136]

Lumbar puncture is contraindicated in patients with papilloedema or cerebral oedema, especially as the result of tumours in the posterior fossa, for fear of producing a cerebellar pressure cone. Unilateral space-occupying lesions may result in herniation through the tentorial hiatus. It is contraindicated in suspected spontaneous subarachnoid haemorrhage, unless a CT scan has been performed.[137] Relative contraindications include blood dyscrasias and those patients on full *anticoagulant therapy*. Skin sepsis and marked spinal deformity are also contraindications.

Puncture in Lateral Position
The patient should be supported by a nurse and positioned with back at edge of table and parallel to it, knees flexed on to abdomen, head brought down to knees, and hips and shoulders *vertical to the table* to avoid rotation of the vertebral column. Sudden movement is to be avoided. In the obese the median crease sags downwards sometimes as much as 2·5 cm, so the point of the needle should be inserted above the crease in these cases.

The line joining the highest points of the iliac crests crosses either the spine of the 4th lumbar vertebra or the interspace between L.4 and L.5. Precise identification of the lumbar spines may be impossible, but this does not matter so long as the first lumbar interspace (and those above this level) are avoided. When the chosen interspace is located the intradermal needle is inserted after careful palpation, midway between the two spines, and a small weal of analgesic solution is raised. The hands of the anaesthetist have been scrubbed up and he has donned a sterile gown and gloves. The back has been painted over a large area with antiseptic and towels arranged suitably. While the skin weal is taking effect, a syringe is filled with analgesic solution. A small incision is made in the skin with a large skin needle to prevent a tough skin from grasping the spinal needle tightly and to prevent a core of skin being carried into the intra- or extradural space with the lumbar puncture needle.[138] Some prefer to use a Sise or a Rowbotham introducer as a cannula through which to introduce the spinal needle. A 19-gauge Butterfly needle can also be used as an introducer for a 25-gauge spinal needle.[139] The needle is then slowly pushed forwards through the skin and tough superficial tissues *parallel to the floor* and at right angles to the back, with its bevel in the plane to separate and not to divide the longitudinal fibres of the dura. If bone is met, it is necessary to withdraw and slightly alter direction either upwards or downwards. The extradural space can be identified in many cases if a drop of analgesic solution is left on the hub of the needle after withdrawal of the stylet as it is pushed inwards; the negative pressure of the space causes the drop to be indrawn.[140] From this point, the dura is only a few millimetres away. When the dura is pierced a click can often be felt. A successful puncture is followed by a free flow of CSF on withdrawal of the stylet. Flow must be free, not an occasional drop. Rotation of needle and pushing it in an extra millimetre will often ensure a free flow. If CSF does not drip from a needle the point of which the anaesthetist is fairly certain is correctly placed, it may be made to do so by applying a bilateral Queckenstedt test, which increases CSF pressure.[141] Bloodstained CSF is of no importance and usually becomes clear after a millilitre has leaked away. Withdrawal of pure blood shows that needle point is probably in a vein, and another puncture must be made.

Paramedian Approach. A needle is inserted 1·5 cm from the midline directly opposite the centre of the interspace, and the needle is inserted at an angle of 25° to the midline. With this approach, flexion of the back is not so important. It is said to cause minimal pain as tough ligaments are avoided and the sense of touch and needle control are more accurate. Sometimes it is successful when attempts using median approach have failed. (*See also* Armitage E.N. *Anaesthesia* 1977, **32**, 672; Chapman G. M. *Anaesthesia* 1977, **32**, 671.)

Some advantages of the paramedian approach: (1) The inter- and supraspinous ligaments, sometimes bony hard, are not penetrated, so possibly less backache; (2) The lamina, if touched by the needle, indicates the depth of the extradural space if a marked needle is used; (3) Flexion of the back is not as important as with the median approach: this may be beneficial in late pregnancy; (4) The more oblique insertion of the needle into the extradural space makes the passage of the catheter from the needle into the extradural space easier.

Puncture in Prone Position—Lumbosacral Approach. A weal is raised 1 cm medial and 1 cm inferior to the lowermost prominence of the posterior superior iliac spine. The patient lies prone with a pillow under the hips. A 12-cm needle is inserted at an angle of 55° aiming for the midline at the L.5–S.1 junction. The ligamentum flavum and the dura are punctured in the usual way. A useful approach in arthritic and obese patients.[142] This approach may also be used for lumbar extradural blocks.

Should positioning cause pain, as in fractured hip, ketamine 0·5 mg/kg i.v. may be beneficial.

Puncture in the Sitting Position

Many workers find this easier than the lateral. Patient is placed across the table with his feet resting comfortably on a stool; spine should be flexed with chin pressed on to sternum. Flexion of the spine rather than flexion of the hips is the aim. It is convenient when block of the sacral roots by hyperbaric solutions is to be done, although this latter block can be done equally well if the puncture is made with the patient in the lateral position, provided that the caudal end of the patient is tipped downwards and the patient placed supine after withdrawal of the needle.

Puncture in the lumbar region requires no after-treatment other than a dab with antiseptic to the skin. Infection seldom occurs in the skin and subcutaneous tissues.

If the needle touches a root of the cauda equina the patient will complain of pain, probably in the leg; usually no harm results from this, but if injection of the drug causes pain the position of the needle should be slightly altered. Such events should be documented. It shows that the needle point is within the vertebral canal and has pierced the ligamentum flavum. If failure results from puncture in one interspace, it can often be made successfully if an adjacent interspace is used.

Injection of the Analgesic Drug

The prepared solution is drawn up in correct amount into a suitably graduated syringe. It is beneficial to rinse out the syringe first with some of the solution, which is later discarded. To prevent particulate matter from being injected and causing neurological complications, injection into both the intra- and extradural spaces can be made from a syringe fitted with an appropriate filter, pore size 0·22 μm.[143] During injection, occasional aspiration of a small quantity of CSF confirms that all of the solution reaches the subarachnoid space. The needle should remain in situ for a few seconds after injection to prevent leak of analgesic solution through the dural puncture hole.

The patient must then be placed in the required position without delay so that fixation of the drug does not occur before the desired spread has taken place. When head-down tilt has been employed, levelling off should take place when sensory loss reaches two spinal segments below the desired level. This allows for a little spread with advancing time. For almost any work inside the abdominal cavity analgesia should reach to the subcostal arch (T.6–T.8), so that the table can be levelled when analgesia reaches the umbilicus (T.10). Upper abdominal procedures require block to T.4–T.5. The cough test is useful in estimating height of block. The patient is asked to cough: the relaxed part of the abdomen bulges out, and any segment not relaxed remains firm and rigid. Disappearance of the knee-jerks shows block at least up to L.2, of the ankle-jerk, block of the sacral segments.

Specimen Techniques

Doses quoted in the following section are for guidance only. All experienced workers in this field have found the spread of solutions within the intradural space capricious, so that exact levels of analgesia following injection of a given dose cannot always be forecast.

a. Low spinal

Block of S.2–S.5 (piles, anal fissure, etc.): Lumbar puncture in L.4–L.5 interspace; patient sitting or lying lateral with definite caudad tilt; injection of 1 ml of a heavy solution slowly, so that it trickles into the bottom of the subarachnoid space. After 1 min patient can lie supine, as lumbar curve prevents spread upwards.

Block of S.1–S.5 (urethra, bladder-neck, prostate, etc.): Lumbar puncture, L.3–L.4 interspace; patient sitting or lying on side, with caudad tilt; injection of 2 ml of a heavy solution slowly, and patient lies level after 1 min.

Block of L.1–S.5, i.e. of lumbar and sacral plexuses: For unilateral analgesia, sound side upwards; puncture in L.3–L.4 interspace; patient in lateral position with spine level. Inject 2–3 ml of a heavy solution and maintain lateral position for 5–15 min. Unilateral analgesia gradually spreads to the other side unless patient is maintained in lateral position throughout operation. Suitable for operations on leg.

For bilateral blocks make injection with *spine* tilted 5°, head down, to prevent solution from accumulating in sacral curve. Immediately after injection turn patient on to back and level table.

b. Mid-spinal: For lower abdominal analgesia (T.7–T.8 to L.4). Puncture, L.3–L.4 interspace; patient in lateral position with spine showing 5° head-down tilt. Inject 3 ml of a heavy solution and maintain position for 5 min for unilateral cases. For bilateral and intra-abdominal cases patient turned supine after injection and tilt maintained.

c. High spinal: For upper abdominal analgesia (T.2–T.5 to L.4). Puncture, L.2–L.3 interspace; patient in lateral position with 5° head-down tilt of spine. Inject up to 4 ml of a heavy solution using a little barbotage. After injection, patient turned supine and tilt maintained. No steep tilt allowed for 15 min after injection. Any excess solution pools at bottom of thoracic curve opposite roots of T.5.

Bupivacaine

Plain bupivacaine 0·5% solution; 1–4 ml injected in the lumbar region is satisfactory for operations on the lower limbs or perineum (L.1–S.5), the exact volume depending on the age and physical status of the patient. Even in expert hands, plain bupivacaine solution is an unpredictable agent (concerning extent of block).[144] For lower abdominal surgery (T.8) the hyperbaric solution with added glucose is recommended in a dosage up to 4 ml. For transurethral prostatectomy 2·5 ml of heavy solution[145] or 2–3 ml of plain solution is satisfactory. (*See also* Nolte H. et al. *Anaesthesist* 1977, **26**, 33; Moore D. C. *Anesthesiology* 1979, **51**, Suppl. 211; Ryan D. W. et al. *Ann. R. Coll. Surg.* 1983, **65**, 40; Tattersall M. P. *Anaesthesia* 1983, **38**, 115; Cummings G. C. et al. *Br. J. Anaesth.* 1984, **56**, 573; Lee J. A. et al. ed. *Sir Robert Macintosh's Lumbar Puncture and Spinal Analgesia*, 5th ed. Edinburgh: Churchill Livingstone, 1985.)

Amethocaine Hydrochloride

This is used as crystals dissolved in CSF; as 1% solution either alone or mixed with 10% glucose; as 1% solution in 5 or 6% glucose. When 1% solution is mixed with one and a half parts of 10% glucose, sp. gr. of mixture is 1013. Popular in the USA.

Plain amethocaine solution. (*a*) A 0·1% solution in water is slightly hypobaric. It has been used for procedures performed in the prone or jack-knife positions and for operations on the lower limb. The injection can be made with the patient in the prone position if the paramedian approach is used (*see* p. 681). The dose in mg is similar to that used for hyperbaric amethocaine, though the volume is greater. The block produced has a shorter duration of action; (*b*) A 1·0% solution has been used in the belief that it is isobaric and so is unlikely to spread with changes in the position of the patient. (*See also* Carron H. et al. *Regional Anesthesia*. Orlando: Grune & Stratton, 1984.)

Sise's technique.[146] The dose of 1% solution is drawn into a 5-ml syringe (1 ml = 10 mg) and 3 ml 10% glucose solution added. Puncture in L.3–L.4 interspace and injection made in 30 s. Table put into 10° Trendelenburg and patient turned supine; 1 min from time injection was started, lessen tilt to 5°. In a further minute, table levelled off and height of analgesia tested. Patient's head and neck raised on sandbag throughout proceedings. For blocks of lumbar and sacral nerves alone, after patient is turned on to back, table is put into reverse Trendelenburg tilt of 3–4°, and there maintained. Dosage is based on size and condition of patient. Small dose for frail, old, small patient; large dose for tough, tall, young patient; medium dose for average patient.

For operations of anus: amethocaine, 8, 7, 6 mg (according to type). For operations on perineum, bladder, legs, vagina: 14, 12, 10 mg. For hernia and appendix operations: 16, 14, 12 mg. For lower abdominal operations: 18, 16, 14 mg. For upper abdominal operations: 20, 17, 14 mg.

Lignocaine

Has been recommended for transurethral prostatectomy, given with the patient sitting, in a dose of 1·5 ml, hyperbaric, when analgesia should extend to about T.10.

Prilocaine

Five per cent in 5% glucose (sp. gr. 1022). Dosage: 1–2 ml. Not satisfactory for operations lasting more than 1 h.

Mepivacaine

Four per cent in 10% glucose.[147] (*See* p. 678.)

Heavy Cinchocaine

No longer manufactured. Previously popular as the heavy solution (1–200) with

No longer manufactured. Previously popular as the heavy solution (1–200) with 6% glucose.[148] Also used formerly as a hypobaric solution (1–1500). For details *see* 7th edition of this Synopsis (1973) and Lee J. A. and Bryce-Smith R. ed. *Practical Regional Analgesia.* Amsterdam: Excerpta Medica, 1976.
Etherington–Wilson's technique.[149]
Lake technique.[150]

Total Spinal Analgesia
This was used by Le Filliatre in 1921[151] and by Koster in 1928[152] (whose paper should be read by all anaesthetists interested in producing ischaemia by spinal block) and was reintroduced by Griffiths and Gillies of Edinburgh[153] as a method of providing the surgeon with an almost bloodless operation field. The technique causes block of all the vasoconstrictors (T.1–L.2) together with analgesia and relaxation. Posture is employed to ensure adequate blood supply to the brain with head-down tilt.

While this technique was an important advance in its day it is seldom employed now, although it has been recently revived.[154]

Serial or Continuous Spinal (Intradural) Analgesia

First described by Dean of the London Hospital in 1907.[155] Reintroduced by Lemmon, a Philadelphia surgeon, in 1940.[156] The method was very useful when either the scope or the duration of the operation was uncertain. It enabled minimal dosage to be given without fear of inadequate analgesia, and so was desirable in the aged, the very young and the physically handicapped. In ill patients, a short-acting agent such as procaine hydrochloride 5%, dissolved either in CSF or 5% glucose solution, is useful.[157] Tuohy[158] used a special lumbar puncture needle, very slightly angulated at its point (Huber point). Through it he put in a plastic catheter and directed it either caudad or cephalad by means of the direction of the angulation of the needle. This technique, suitably modified, is nowadays popular for continuous *extradural* block. When used for intradural block, top-up doses equal to half the original dose may be injected, due allowance being made for the dead-space of the catheter which averages about 0·25 ml.

Conduct of the Analgesia

Nausea, fairly common, and vomiting may sometimes be controlled by deep mouth-breathing. If analgesia ascends high up the body, consciousness may be lost, as afferent impulses reaching the cortex become fewer and fewer. Apparatus for general anaesthesia and for oxygen therapy should be at hand, as also should suitable intravenous fluids and pressor drugs. *There must always be an open vein.* It is the duty of the anaesthetist to exercise constant vigilance—of the circulation and of the respiration. The patient should usually be asleep, if not he should be made comfortable on the table. We favour either small intermittent doses of a narcotic analgesic with or without intermittent doses of thiopentone or nitrous oxide and oxygen. For major operations, e.g. resection of the colon, we prefer to intubate and allow spontaneous respiration with light general anaesthesia. Diazepam and ketamine,[159] and midazolam,[160] also chlormethiazole[161] have also been given via an i.v. drip. Blood pressure should be monitored. (*See also* Bromage P. R. *Epidural Analgesia*. Philadelphia: Saunders, 1978, p. 475.)

Difficulties and Complications during the Operation

The following troublesome symptoms and signs may occur: (1) Nausea; (2) Vomiting; (3) Headache; (4) Precordial discomfort; (5) Paraesthesiae in the limbs; (6) Difficulty in phonation; (7) Hypotension; (8) Restlessness; (9) Inability to cough effectively; (10) Hiccups.

Broken Needles
If a needle breaks, the proximal part and the stylet should, if possible, be left in place to serve as a guide to the distal part. If the proximal part has already been removed, another needle is thrust along the track of the first one for purposes of localization. Removal should be attempted at once. With patient prone, a portable X-ray with image intensifier may be helpful.[162]

Poor Flow of CSF
This may be due to a component of the cauda equina or of the pia–arachnoid obstructing the needle point. Slight movement or rotation usually overcomes this difficulty. A free flow of CSF is desirable at all times.

The Intradural Spinal that does not take
Usual cause is failure to deposit all of the analgesic solution in the proper part of the subarachnoid space. May be due to difficulty with lumbar puncture; displacement of needle point, after successful puncture, by syringe, movement, etc.; use of a long-bevelled needle which allows part of the solution to be injected inside, part outside, the intradural space; faults in the use of gravity, tilts, dosage, etc. to control level of block; faults in the solution, alkalinization, etc.; idiosyncrasy, or the so-called rachi-resistance. This last is a definite entity. It may be impossible to aspirate CSF from a needle, the point of which is truly in the subarachnoid space, the patient being in the lateral position.

(If an *extradural block* does not come on after the injection of a reasonable amount of local analgesic solution, the injection has gone astray. A congenital midline diffusion barrier in either the intra- or extradural space may result in inadvertent dural puncture[163] or unilateral block.)

Retching and Vomiting
See Chapter 18. Hiccups may interfere with the operation and if simple sedation fails to control them, general anaesthesia may be required.

Treatment of Collapse during Spinal Analgesia (Intradural and Extradural)
Turn patient on to back (except in patients in advanced pregnancy or with large abdominal tumours which may cause pressure on the vena cava and interfere with venous return to the heart—in these cases a bolster placed under the right flank may relieve pressure on the vessel). Tilt the patient head-down. The lungs must be inflated with oxygen, the legs elevated, intravenous fluids infused, and cardiac massage instituted if there is no evidence of cardiac action. A pressor drug (e.g. ephedrine) will be required.

The causes of collapse in spinal analgesia are: (1) Lowering of blood pressure to point where coronary arteries are not adequately perfused; (2) Hypoxia of vital centres; (3) Progressive upward paralysis of respiratory mechanism— should not cause hypoxia as IPPV will carry the patient on until the paralysis wears off; (4) Occasional toxic reaction to drugs injected in extradural block.

Sequelae

Headache

Most frequently seen following an inadvertent dural puncture with a Tuohy needle in an attempt to locate the extradural space. A patient with a postlumbar puncture headache should not be discharged from hospital. Only seen after intradural block, never after extradural. This occurs in up to 20% of patients[163] and up to 75% of patients when a large size (e.g. a Tuohy) needle is used.[164] Onset in first three postoperative days. Usually worse when the patient sits or stands and frequent after small operations such as haemorrhoidectomy. Often occipital and associated with pain and stiffness in neck; may be vertical or frontal, can cause pain in the orbit.[413] Headaches are not rare after simple lumbar puncture. The incidence of postlumbar puncture headache in medical wards was estimated at 30%.[165] Sicard first suggested in 1902 that cause might be leakage of CSF into extradural space.[166] The average loss is about 10 ml/h[167] and healing, according to radio-isotope myelography, may take 3 weeks.[168] Jet air travel, soon after dural puncture, may cause a recurrence of headache.[169] Headache may last days, weeks or months, but usually 1–2 weeks. Loss of up to 10 ml of fluid during lumbar puncture probably has no effect on subsequent headaches. Dural tap has brought to light unsuspected arteriovenous malformations, with delayed neurological signs.[170]

Puncture with an unflexed back may reduce the incidence of headaches as the dural hole is not stretched open.

Theories of causation

1. Low CSF pressure. The rate of leakage of CSF exceeds its rate of formation, and this results in changes in the hydrodynamics of the fluid, with loss of cushioning of the brain and pressure or traction on vessels and sensitive brain structures, basal dura, tentorium, etc. In cases of traumatic leakage of CSF, the choroid plexus can form 500 ml/day.

2. High CSF pressure—a response to meningeal irritation. This is the mechanism of headache caused by chemical or bacterial invasion. Queckenstedt's test eases pain if applied to patients with low-pressure headache, makes it worse in those with high-pressure headache.[171]

Diagnosis. A postspinal headache is probably caused by the method of analgesia if: (1) It is different from any headache previously experienced by the patient; (2) It is initiated or made worse by adoption of the sitting or erect posture; (3) It has occipital and nuchal components; (4) It is relieved by abdominal compression—which raises the venous pressure.

Treatment. This is prophylactic and combative. *Prophylactic*: (1) The elimination of neurotic and unsuitable patients before operation, including those with a history[172] of frequent severe headaches; (2) The use of a small needle; incidence has been reduced to 3·5% with a 25-gauge needle,[173] and 1·4% with a 32-gauge needle.[174] The fine-bore needle can be inserted inside a larger needle previously placed in the extradural space, or through a No. 19 Butterfly needle;[175] (3) Intravenous infusion of excess fluid containing electrolytes (e.g. 15 ml/kg of bodyweight/h), in addition to blood replacement if required; (4) Separation rather than cutting of longitudinal fibres of dura, by situation of needle bevel; (5) Surgical and chemical cleanliness.

Low pressure headache is ameliorated by analgesics. Straining and coughing are predisposing factors. (*See* Handler C. E. et al. *J. R. Soc. Med.* 1981, **75**, 404.)

Treatment of established headache depends on CSF pressure; if this is thought to be low the following measures may help: (1) Frequent long drinks; (2) A tight abdominal binder;[176] (3) A continuous drip of Hartmann's solution, via a catheter in the lumbar extradural space, for 24 h;[177] injection of normal saline, 25–50 ml, into either the sacral or lumbar extradural space (injection of saline into the sacral canal has recently been found not to raise the CSF pressure significantly);[178] (4) Injection of 10–20 ml of autologous blood into the extradural space, to form a blood patch for sealing the dural puncture;[179] Blood patch, using 20 ml had a 92% success rate in 244 cases of postspinal headache.[180] This is occasionally followed by minor neurological changes.[181] Failure of a blood patch to ease headache may be due to incorrect position of the injection or to too small a volume of blood; (5) Oxygen inhalations may do good while carbon dioxide increases the cerebral blood flow;[182] (6) Simple analgesics, e.g. aspirin (introduced into medicine by Dreser (1860–1924) in 1899[183])—apart from alcohol, the most popular drug in the world!—may also be helpful. (Dreser also introduced the use of diamorphine.)

Backache
Probably not much more common after spinal than after general anaesthesia. A small pillow under the lumbar region reduces incidence of postoperative backache irrespective of method of anaesthesia. Damage to intervertebral disk by the needle has been reported.

Retention of Urine
No more common after spinal than after general anaesthesia. Usually yields to carbachol, 0·5–1 mg i.m., repeated if necessary, or neostigmine, 0·5 mg i.m. Very occasionally prolonged retention due to spasm of vesical sphincter consequent on spinal analgesia is seen.

Meningitis[184]
Usually due to faulty asepsis, but can occur with a seemingly flawless technique. Aseptic meningitis has been reported.[185] Contamination with chemical antiseptics, starch powder from gloves,[186] detergents, concentration of the drug and variations in pH have all been blamed. Autoclaving of the whole pack is the ideal to be aimed at. The authors have never seen a case of meningitis following intra- or extradural block in many thousands of cases.

Paralysis of 6th Cranial Nerve
Palsy of external rectus causing diplopia. First reported in 1907.[187] Onset commonly between 5th and 11th postoperative days and associated with headache. May be delayed for three weeks, while simple lumbar puncture without injection of analgesic solution can cause it. Has been said to occur in about 1 in 300 cases of spinal analgesia. Paralysis is never complete and is a different entity from the total paralysis associated with such conditions as skull fracture.

Causes. (1) Mechanical, due to upset of hydrodynamics of CSF pressure causing stretching of the abducens nerve. As the 6th nerve runs forwards from the posterior margin of the pons it is crossed by either the anterior inferior cerebellar or the internal auditory artery, or by both, so that if slight displacement of the cerebellum occurs, these arteries are stretched and, being fixed below to the basilar artery, may cut into the nerve like a tight band; (2) Inflammatory, low-grade meningitis; (3) Toxic, due to specific action of drug used acting on an unstable binocular vision mechanism, phylogenetically a recently acquired one; a similar condition is seen in acute alcoholic intoxication.

When severe headache occurs, steps must at once be taken to prevent diplopia. The patient must be sent back to bed and rehydrated both orally and parenterally. The antidiuretic hormone in posterior pituitary extract may be useful.

While the condition persists, dark glasses should be worn, with the outer one-third of glass of affected eye made opaque. About 50% of cases recover within a month. If after 2 years spontaneous recovery of function has not occurred, operative cure may be considered. About 25% of the cases show bilateral nerve involvement.

Paralysis of every cranial nerve except the 1st, 9th and 10th has been reported after spinal analgesia, and transient deafness or tinnitus is not uncommon. Diplopia has been reported following general anaesthesia and after the use of relaxants and may then persist for some time.[188]

Other Neurological Lesions[189]

Permanent neurological sequelae first reported by Koenig in 1906. Transient lesions of cauda equina causing abnormalities of leg reflexes, incontinence of faeces, retention of urine, loss of sexual function, sensory loss in lumbosacral distribution and temporary paralysis of peroneal nerve. Most of these clear up spontaneously.[190]   Radiculitis, ascending myelitis, transient transverse myelitis,[191] adhesive arachnoiditis paraplegia,[42] meningo-encephalitis and bulbar involvement have all been reported. Their cause is not fully understood nor is it always due to the method of pain relief.[192] It may well be the result of the drug injected. Distinguished neurologists have blamed the local analgesic drug,[193] while the low pH of a large volume of injected solution has also been blamed. Haematoma formation may cause trouble due to pressure on the cord.[194] Severe back pain with paraplegia requires emergency neurological examination and, if necessary, surgical exploration. Ischaemia of the cord due to severe hypotension, or the use of local vasoconstrictors, may be causal. Electromyographic studies enable lesions of the lower motor neuron type due to spinal analgesia to be differentiated from other neurological and myopathic conditions.[195] In the dog, severe hypotension and/or the intravenous infusion of large volumes of non-colloid solutions, poor in electrolytes (e.g. 5% dextrose solution), tend to increase the incidence of neurological signs.[196] An extradural abscess following several spinal blocks, without causing either sensory or motor impairment, only localized pain, in a diabetic patient with an infected leg, has been reported.[197] Spinal stenosis may be responsible for neurological sequelae.[198]

Anterior spinal artery syndrome (*see* Lancet 1958, **2**, 515; Wells C. E. C. *Proc. R. Soc. Med.* 1966, **59**, 790) is a lower motor neuron paralysis (paraplegia) without involvement of the posterior columns of the spinal cord, subserving joint position sense, touch and vibration sensibility. It has followed spinal analgesia. (*See* Annotation, *Lancet* 1967, **2**, 143; Bryce-Smith R. in: *Recent Advances in*

Anaesthesia and Analgesia—11 (Hewer C. L. ed.), Edinburgh: Churchill Livingstone, 1972, Ch. 7, p. 260.)

A constricting pachymeningitis may develop some time after intradural block. Horner's syndrome has been reported following extradural sacral block in obstetric patients.[199] Phantom limb pain after amputation may be caused by intradural block and may be so severe as to require general anaesthesia for its relief.[200] Intracerebral haematoma formation causing hemiparesis, coincident with a lumbar puncture with a 19-gauge needle, in a previously fit patient, has been reported.[201] Pruritus following intradural block, in patients with peripheral neuropathy has been seen.[202] The addition of sodium metabisulphite as an anti-oxidant, to solutions for intradural injection (e.g. chloroprocaine) may cause neurological damage.[203] Spinal stroke can occur independently of central neural blockade. An infarcted cord does not recover.[204]

Conditions which may cause signs and symptoms referable to the central nervous system in any postoperative patient may include: vascular, neoplastic, infective or viral disease, myopathies, neuropathies, operative trauma, e.g. due to the position of the patient on the table, retractors, etc. Careful clinical and electromyographic investigation is always necessary. Prolonged block following extradural injection of 1% etidocaine has been reported.[205] Subdural haematoma with delayed neurological signs, ending in death, has also occurred.[206]

There was formerly some emphasis on the serious neurological sequelae of intradural spinal analgesia but the pendulum of popularity is swinging back towards the method, although complications other than headache are no more frequent after intradural than after extradural block.[207] On the other hand, the technique is not without its strong supporters, who, after most careful postoperative assessment, are not able to blame it for the production of significant neurological sequelae. Among these may be mentioned Vandam L. D. and Dripps R. D. *Surgery* 1955, **38**, 463 (reprinted in 'Classical File', *Surv. Anesthesiol.* 1970, **14**, 308); *JAMA* 1956, **161**, 586; Moore D. C. and Bridenbaugh L. D. *JAMA* 1966, **195**, 907; Gordh T. *Illustrated Handbook of Local Anaesthesia*. London: Lloyd-Luke, 2nd ed., 1979; Noble A. B. and Murry J. C. *Can. Anaesth. Soc. J.* 1971, **18**, 5.

Neurological complications following spinal analgesia are not necessarily due to the method,[192,208] while such complications following surgical operations may be seen in patients who have had general anaesthesia.[209] Epidermoid spinal tumours have been reported.[210] Lumbar canal stenosis can result in compression of nervous structures.[211] (For neurotoxicity of drugs used for intra- and extradural block, *see* Steen P. A. and Michenfelder J. D. *Anesthesiology* 1979, **50**, 437.)

The Choice Between Spinal Intra- and Extradural Analgesia and General Anaesthesia

Advantages of Spinal Analgesia
Prevents the tough, strong patient from being soaked with muscle relaxant and preserves spontaneous respiration; cheap; ideal for fit patients who object to being put to sleep; lessens risk of vomiting causing pulmonary aspiration in patients with full stomach; quiet relaxed abdomen together with small

contracted intestines and spontaneous breathing helps surgeon; as intubation is unnecessary the cough of extubation is avoided; upset of body chemistry minimal; intestinal function returns early; risk of explosion absent; wound bleeding reduced; return to normo-tension is gradual. Since the advent of muscle relaxants, the need for spinal analgesia has decreased, but it is still a useful method which has stood the test of time. Can be employed deliberately to produce hypotension and so less bleeding during operation.

Intradural block can be said to have the following advantages over extradural: (1) It is easier; (2) It is quicker; (3) It requires less skill and experience; (4) It provides slightly better relaxation of the abdomen; (5) It gives better control over the height of the block; (6) The danger of toxic signs due to the drug are negligible. Very rarely, unilateral spinal block occurs, probably due to a posterior midline septum of the pia mater.[212]

Disadvantages of Spinal Analgesia
Spinal analgesia affects the cardiovascular system more than general anaesthesia by tending to cause hypotension in some patients; the incidence of postoperative headache (in intradural block). It does not reduce the incidence of postoperative chest complications. May take some time to induce.

Indications for Spinal Analgesia (Intradural and Extradural)
These vary greatly with different surgeons and anaesthetists. Specially indicated in strong muscular patients. Useful when muscle relaxants are contraindicated, or when it is thought advantageous to preserve spontaneous respiration. Patients with chronic respiratory disease often do well with central neural blockade as tracheal intubation may be avoided. Following the insertion of a catheter into the extradural space, postoperative pain can be relieved by repeated injections of either opioids or local analgesics, without interfering too much with respiratory function. Some patients fear loss of consciousness and prefer to remain awake. Acute cases, including obstetric patients, with a full stomach may be at less risk under spinal than general anaesthesia (the stomach cannot always be emptied by a stomach tube). Some patients with compromised hepatorenal function may do well with central neural blockade.[213] Skilled workers may meet fewer difficulties with central neural blockade than with general anaesthesia in the morbidly obese patient, using a thoracic approach.[214] For prolonged distension of the bladder, e.g. with a Helmstein balloon.[215]

Examples of procedures particularly suited to spinal methods are: amputations; hip surgery,[216] when blood loss and postoperative thrombophlebitis are reduced;[217] transurethral manipulations and in some cases of prostatectomy, especially if done per urethram; abdominoperineal resection of the rectum; colectomy;[218] hysterectomy and vaginal repair; haemorrhoids when the surgeon requires an atonic sphincter; in operative obstetrics.[219] Useful whenever a bloodless field is desirable, or when a contracted bowel (not seen with muscle relaxants) is advantageous. In surgery of the colon, central neural blockade may improve vascularity at the site of anastomosis; reversal of relaxants which could be harmful, is unnecessary.[220] For vascular surgery, the use of central neural blockade is controversial. Combined intra- and extradural injection may be performed using a 25 or 26-g needle inserted through a Tuohy needle (than which it must be 1 cm longer). This may give rapid onset of analgesia followed by an extradural catheter. In hip surgery, extradural block is associated with a smaller incidence of deep vein thrombosis than general anaesthesia.[221] The changes produced in the cardiovascular system under low block are usually small, unlike those caused by a block to a higher level. Low spinal analgesia may often be indicated in poor-risk cases instead of general anaesthesia.

Contraindications to Intra- and Extradural Block

Should not, without a good reason, be used on unwilling or uncooperative patients, including young children. Often unwise in the following groups without careful consideration:

1. Cardiovascular. Severe shock; hypovolaemia; dehydration; hypotension below 80–90 mmHg systolic; gross hypertension; patients unable to do reasonable physical work because of obesity; senility; myocardial degeneration, toxaemia; severe ischaemic heart disease, especially with history of recent infarction, because of the dangers of hypotension; cerebral atheroma. In any patient with a fixed cardiac output (severe valvular stenosis, heart block, medication with β-blocking drugs, etc.) and therefore unable to respond to dilatation of the vascular bed, sudden blood loss, etc. Hypertensive patients whose hypertension is uncontrolled medically are more at risk than those whose blood pressure is controlled when given extradural block. They need careful monitoring and are doubtful anaesthetic risks.[222]

2. Mechanical. Spinal analgesia, properly performed, is safe for obese patients and for those with obstructive lung disease.[223] Patients with a splinted diaphragm which interferes with breathing, such as hydramnios, large ovarian and uterine tumours, e.g. pregnancy; ascites, omental obesity. Dangers to be considered include hypoxia due to respiratory inadequacy and aortocaval compression by the tumour mass. Lateral tilt, oxygen and IPPV should be used when indicated. Dosage should be reduced in such patients.

3. Respiratory. Patients who are breathless from any cause; these may become hypoxic, especially if level of analgesia is high. On the other hand, patients with emphysema or bronchospasm often do surprisingly well after spinal blocks.

4. Abnormalities of the central nervous system. Spinal analgesia should not be given to a patient with an abnormality of the central nervous system, whether it be congenital or acquired, infective or degenerative, active or inactive or healed unless the indications are compelling, although this view has been contested by experienced workers.[224] Any subsequent symptoms may be blamed on the spinal. Patients who are chronic sufferers from headaches will in all probability get a headache of moderate severity after operation following intradural block. If it is suspected on the history (headache, vomiting, blurred vision) or the physical signs (papilloedema, bradycardia, drowsiness) that the patient has an expanding cerebral lesion, a tumour, cyst or abscess, which may, if the intracranial pressure is suddenly altered, cause obstruction to the cerebrospinal fluid or blood circulation (the pressure cone), intradural block is absolutely contraindicated.

5. Gastrointestinal perforations. Contraction of the gut adds to the soiling of the peritoneum in these cases.

6. Genito-urinary. Patients who may have an enlarged prostate (which is not the reason for the surgical procedure). Bladder difficulty may be complained of after operation and blamed on the method of pain relief. Ephedrine is perhaps not the best pressor agent to use in this type of patient. In renal failure, the low blood pressure associated with spinal analgesia may result in temporary oliguria which may upset the subnormal renal function.

7. *Cases with deformed backs*. Because of difficulty in the performance of lumbar puncture.

8. *Skin sepsis* in lumbar region.

9. *Neurological operations*. In operations for lesions of the spinal cord or cauda equina, on medicolegal grounds. Many anaesthetists, however, favour the use of extradural block for laminectomy for prolapsed disk with the patient on his side during operation. (Thorne T. C. and Watt M. J. personal communication.)

10. *Patients with disorder of blood clotting and those on anticoagulants*. The precise risk in undertaking lumbar puncture in these patients is unknown. In patients receiving small doses of heparin for the prophylaxis of venous thrombosis, the risk is unknown. Lumbar puncture may be dangerous if the thrombotest value is less than 10% at the time of the procedure.[225]

11. *In cases of dehydration*. These are bad risks and a much smaller dose of drug than usual is required.

Spinal Intradural Analgesia in Children

Advocated by Tyrrell Gray in 1909,[226] but seldom used today. Risk of circulatory depression minimal because of elasticity of their cardiovascular systems. Puncture should be in the L.4–L.5 interspace because cord extends lower in children than in adults.

(*See also* Slater H. M. and Stephen C. R. *Anesthesiology* 1950, **11**, 709; Berkawitz S. and Greene B. A. *Anesthesiology* 1951, **12**, 376; Leigh M. D. *Int. Anesthesiol. Clin.* 1963, **1**, 3; Harnik E. V. et al. *Anesthesiology* 1986, **64**, 95 and Correspondence, *Anesthesiology* 1986, **65**, 559.)

Spinal Intradural Analgesia in Pregnancy

Spinal and extradural block for surgery in pregnancy do not materially increase the uterine tone and do not harm the fetus. (*See* Chapter 27.)

Spinal Intradural Analgesia in Urology

Very useful in cystoscopies and transurethral procedures. If retrograde pyelography is to be done soon after cystoscopy, block must not ascend higher than the roots of L.2, otherwise overfilling of the renal pelves will not be prevented by the patient feeling pain. For transurethral resection of the prostate 1·5 ml of lignocaine (5% with glucose), or 0·5% bupivacaine plain, 2–3 ml has been used successfully. In suprapubic prostatectomy some surgeons appreciate the relaxation and freedom from toxic effects obtained with spinal analgesia. Block must ascend to T.8–T.9 and then hyperbaric solutions may be advantageous in obtaining a higher level. For nephrectomy or nephrolithotomy, done with the patient in the lateral position, hypobaric or hyperbaric solutions may be used; fat, heavy patients may suffer respiratory difficulty in this position and so may do better with general anaesthesia.

Spinal Intradural Analgesia in Acute Injury

Acute war injuries of the lower limbs and perineum have been successfully managed by 0·5% plain solution of bupivacaine, intradurally, controlling the resulting hypotension with large infusions and metaraminol. The head-down position can be adopted early, there is prolonged postoperative analgesia and little risk of aspiration of gastric contents.[227]

Spinal Analgesia in Thoracic Surgery

This is seldom, if ever, used today for thoracic surgery, although thoracic extradural block is sometimes used for abdominal surgery and for pain relief.

Supplementary Anaesthesia (for Intradural and Extradural Analgesia)

No patient should receive a spinal injection without having an open vein or a drip. This is to enable acute hypotension or convulsions to be rapidly reversed.

Supplementary anaesthesia may be: (1) Planned from the beginning, and may be given either before or after the spinal injection; (2) Given during the course of the operation because of the partial failure or wearing off of the analgesia or extension of scope of the operation; because of the emotional discomfort and anxiety of the patient; because of persistent vomiting or restlessness.

The authors prefer to use minimal thiopentone in 2·5% solution, injected as necessary into an indwelling needle; to this is sometimes added nitrous oxide and oxygen. An intravenous infusion of either methohexitone or propofol provides satisfactory and controllable sedation.[228] Intravenous diazepam[229] can usefully be given too. Midazolam i.v. (12 mg) is a satisfactory sedative.[230] Chlormethiazole (Heminevrin, Hemineurin), e.g. 4 g in 500 ml of glucose solution as an intravenous infusion at an initial rate of 20 ml/min has also been advocated.[231] Chlormethiazole may result in nasal irritation with sneezing and restlessness.[232] A tracheal tube may be desirable: (1) If the airway is difficult to maintain without it; (2) If the operation is likely to last a long time, especially if it takes place in the upper abdomen. It can be passed, using a relaxant, or following transtracheal injection of 3 ml of 4% lignocaine, using thiopentone to relax the jaw, after an interval of 2–3 min.[233] If the tube is used, nitrous oxide and oxygen, a volatile anaesthetic or a narcotic analgesic are suitable supplements.

Intravenous diamorphine, 1–4 mg, may be sufficient to settle a nervous patient if there is a little return of sensation towards the end of an operation. Intraperitoneal swabbing with 100 ml of 0·5% procaine will also have a beneficial effect if mild pain stimuli are causing discomfort. Infiltration of the peri-oesophageal branches of the vagus, at the cardiac end of the stomach, will do much to prevent sensations of nausea and faintness from worrying the patient in upper abdominal operations, if he is conscious, and to prevent hiccup if he is not.

For intradural narcotic analgesics, *see* p. 711.

(There are few aspects of intradural block which are not fully and clearly discussed by Peere C. Lund in *Principles and Practice of Spinal Anesthesia* 1971, Springfield, Ill.: Thomas. *See also* Lee J. A. et al. ed. *Sir Robert Macintosh's Lumbar Puncture and Spinal Analgesia,* 5th ed. Edinburgh: Churchill Livingstone ed.), 1985.

Injections of Contrast Medium for Radiological Diagnosis

A meticulous technique of lumbar puncture and thecal tap is essential. The medium used may be iophendylate (Myodil) but this has caused spinal arachnoiditis, so that metrizamide (Amipaque) or lopamidol which are water-soluble and do not dissociate in solution, may be substituted. Usual dose of iophendylate is 5–10 ml, and before the injection the CSF pressure should be measured with a manometer, and one or more specimens of the fluid taken for examination. Injection is made in either the lateral or the sitting position. The viscous solution should be warmed to blood heat and a needle no narrower than 20-gauge used. Epidurography is sometimes preferred to myelography using metrizamide as the contrast medium.[234]

EXTRADURAL BLOCK

Definition
Blockage of nerve roots outside the dura. A method giving reflex flaccidity of muscles, analgesia, a degree of hypotension and consequent ischaemia secondary to sympathetic blockade while allowing spontaneous respiration to continue relatively unimpaired. May be used for: (1) The relief of pain during and/or following surgical operations; (2) The relief of pain during labour; (3) The reduction of bleeding by producing hypotension during surgery; (4) To supplement light general anaesthesia and so suppressing the transmission of afferent impulses and hormonal and autonomic responses to surgery.[235] It will provide relaxation of the abdomen without the use of myoneural blocking agents.

History
Introduced by Corning, and used in dogs by Cathelin[236] and Sicard (1872–1929)[237] in 1901, and in man, tentatively, by Kappis[238] and by Bleeck and Strauss,[239] and applied in clinical surgery by Pages[240] in 1921 and by Dogliotti[241] and Aburel[242] in 1931. Popularized in Britain by Massey Dawkins.[243] The publications and researches of Bromage and of the Seattle school have led to a reappraisal of many opinions formerly held concerning the physiology and pharmacology of the method.[244] Curbelo of Cuba was the first worker to insert a catheter into the extradural space in 1949.[245] *See also* Little D. M. *Surv. Anesthesiol.* 1981, **25**, 340.

Anatomy of the Extradural Space
The spinal dura mater represents the meningeal layer of the dura mater of the brain; the periosteum lining the vertebral canal represents the outer layer of the cerebral dura. Between the spinal dura and the vertebral canal is the extradural (epidural, peridural) space. Its average diameter is 0·5 cm and it is widest in the midline posteriorly in the lumbar region.

Its boundaries are: superiorly the foramen magnum and inferiorly the sacrococcygeal membrane; posteriorly the anterior surfaces of the laminae and their connecting ligaments, the roots of the vertebral spines and the ligamenta flava; anteriorly the posterior longitudinal ligament covering the vertebral bodies and the disks; laterally the pedicles and intervertebral foramina. The interspinous ligaments and the ligamenta flava, dense gristly tissue, are important in locating the extradural space.

The contents include the dural sac and the spinal nerve roots, the extradural plexus of veins and the spinal arteries, lymphatics and fat. The veins become distended when the patient strains or coughs, i.e. during bouts of increased intrathoracic or intra-abdominal pressure. The veins form a network which runs in four main trunks along the space. They communicate with venous rings at each vertebral level, with the basivertebral veins on the posterior aspect of each vertebral body, and with the ascending and deep cervical, intercostal, iliolumbar and lateral sacral veins. These veins have no valves and constitute the valveless vertebral venous plexus of Batson.[246] They connect the pelvic veins below with the intracranial veins above, so that air or local analgesic solution injected into one of them may ascend straight to the brain. They drain into the inferior vena cava via the azygos vein, so that when there is obstruction to vena caval flow, as with large abdominal tumours, advanced pregnancy, etc., they become distended. They form an alternative venous pathway to the caval system. There are 58 intervertebral foramina and the degree of their patency is an important factor in controlling the height of analgesic a given volume of analgesic solution will produce. They tend to be more permeable in the young than in the old, so that a given volume of solution tends to cause a higher block in the old than in the young. The shape of the space is triangular with the apex dorsomedial. A dorsomedial fold of dura mater occasionally divides the space into a ventral and two dorsomedial compartments which do not always communicate freely with each other. Such abnormalities may explain patchy analgesia or inadvertent dural puncture when the midline approach is used.[247] Reports of two cases of unilateral extradural block support the existence of a dorsomedial septum.[414]

The dura mater is attached to the margins of the foramen magnum, but this does not prevent the passage of analgesic drug into the cranial cavity. It is also attached to the 2nd and 3rd cervical vertebrae and to the posterior longitudinal ligament. It ends at the lower border of the 2nd sacral vertebra, a point corresponding in level with the posterior superior iliac spines. Prolongations of the dura surround the spinal nerve roots and fuse with the epineurium of the complete spinal nerves, as they traverse the intervertebral foramina. Extradural block includes blocking of the sympathetic fibres travelling with the anterior or ventral roots, which soon become the white rami. Usual distance between skin and extradural space 4–5 cm.[248] For topography of the lumbar extradural space, *see* Husemeyer R. P. and White D. C. *Anaesthesia* 1980, **35**, 7.

Causes of Negative Pressure in Extradural Space

There is a negative pressure in the extradural space in about 80% of patients.[249]

Possible causes: (1) Dimpling of dura by needle;[250] (2) Transfer of negative pressure from thorax via paravertebral spaces (especially in the thoracic region);[251] (3) Full flexion of the back;[252] (4) The initial bulge forwards of the yellow ligament in front of the advancing needle, followed by its rapid return to the resting position once the needle has perforated the ligament;[253] (5) One cause of the negative pressure is the redistribution of CSF in the intradural space which creates a negative pressure between the dura and the walls of the vertebral canal. This is greater in the recumbent than in the vertical position.[254]

Negative pressure in extradural space is not the same at all levels and in the sacral canal it is absent. It may be less in the thoracic region than in the lumbar part of the space.

This negative extradural pressure may account for the leakage of CSF into the extradural space after lumbar puncture, contributing to headache.

Caval compression from large intra-abdominal tumours can cause extradural venous distension. A rise in pressure may favour spread of local analgesic solution.[255] The pressure may be positive in labour.[256] Injection of a small volume of fluid is likely to increase both the extradural and the CSF pressure.[257]

Site of Action

When a solution of a local analgesic is injected into the extradural space it may exert its effect: (1) On the nerve roots in the extradural space; (2) On the nerve roots in the paravertebral spaces after they have shed their dural sheaths;[258] (3) On the nerve roots in the intradural or subarachnoid space after inward diffusion of the drug across the dura;[259] (4) Diffusion into the subperineural and subpial spaces from the so-called 'ink-cuff' zone[260] where the anterior and posterior nerve roots fuse. Analgesic drug may eventually pass centripetally and reach the substance of the cord and diffuse out from this into the CSF, where its concentration is significant.[261] Injected solution can thus spread up and down the space, especially in the elderly; laterally into the paravertebral space, especially in the young, although this has been questioned, and centripetally into the neuraxis along the subepineural (subperineural) spaces.[262]

The following fibres are blocked: (1) Anterior nerve roots; (2) Posterior nerve roots and their ganglia; (3) Mixed spinal nerves; (4) White and grey rami communicantes; (5) Visceral afferents accompanying sympathetic fibres; (6) Certain descending pathways in the spinal cord.[244]

Factors influencing spread of solution: (1) The volume of solution injected; (2) The age of the patient, the old requiring less than the young—the largest dose is required at about the age of 19; (3) The force of injection—fast injection spreads the solution thinly over a wide area and may give an incomplete but extensive zone of analgesia; (4) The amount of drug used; (5) The level at which an injection is given;[263] (6) Gravity—a head-down tilt aids cephalad diffusion of the solution and vice versa; an injection given in the sitting position will spread higher than if given in the lateral position due to the hydrostatic bulging of the dural sac and its encroachment on the extradural space[264]—the side on which the patient is lying influences spread;[265] (7) The length of the vertebral column; (8) Full-term pregnancy or abdominal tumours—one-third to one-half normal doses required; (9) Concentration of local analgesic solution—a given volume of a high concentration will spread further than an equal volume of a lower concentration; (10) In diabetes and in occlusive arterial disease less solution is required, although in the latter condition, this has been questioned.[266] *The height of analgesia produced by a given volume of solution is one of the great uncertainties of anaesthesia.* Four segments on each side of the point of injection are said to be affected by the extradural injections of 10–15 ml of analgesic solution.

Combined intra- and extradural block in the same patient has been described, using either two needles one intra- and the other extradural[267] or inserting a long needle into the intradural space through a wider needle in the extradural space.[268]

Local Analgesic Solutions Used

Lignocaine 1–2% which has a rapid onset in about 10 min and gives good relaxation. Duration of effect 1½–2 h—depending on strength of solution employed; 0·8% solution gives good sensory without motor block. The writers have had very considerable experience of the use of 1·5% solution for surgical work and find it most satisfactory. In very muscular patients, 2% solution may produce more intense muscular relaxation. Lignocaine and bupivacaine have been given in a mixture.[269]

Bupivacaine (Marcain) is a long-acting drug which has been used in 0·5% concentration, with or without adrenaline, giving analgesia for up to 8 h.[270] Volumes in excess of 20 ml need to be given with care. Motor block is not quite so intense as that produced by 1·5% lignocaine. In obstetrics, 0·25–0·375% solutions are popular. For surgical operations, 0·75% has been advocated.[271]

Amethocaine hydrochloride can be added to lignocaine solution, e.g. 50 mg added to 50 ml giving a 0·1% strength. It increases the duration of analgesia by about 50% and gives good motor block.

Prilocaine is excellent for extradural blockade and lasts longer than lignocaine in the same concentrations. Strengths of 1·5, 2 and 3%, with adrenaline 1–200 000, have been recommended. It is a little less toxic than lignocaine. Doses in excess of 600 mg may cause cyanosis from methaemoglobinaemia.

Etidocaine[272] has been used for extradural block in 1 or 1·5% solution.

Chloroprocaine hydrochloride.[273] A drug current in the USA has been employed in the UK, in 2–3% solution.[274] Short latency and duration of activity (about 45 min), its effects ceasing suddenly. Gives more intense motor block than bupivacaine. Hydrolysed by serum cholinesterase and so is relatively non-toxic. The commercial solution has a low pH and contains sodium metabisulphite as an anti-oxidant. Its use is being reassessed. *See also* Chapter 31. May cause more hypotension in Caesarean section than bupivacaine.

Adrenaline. This may be added in the usual strength, i.e. 0·2 ml of the 1:1000 solution in 20 ml of local analgesic solution (making 1–200 000). It causes positive inotropic and chronotropic effects on the heart,[275] while the peripheral resistance and mean blood pressure are decreased. This causes a rise in cardiac output.[275] Locally, by preventing absorption of the analgesic drug it may cause more intense blockade of nerve fibres and hence greater sympathetic blockade.[244] Some workers omit adrenaline as they fear the combined effect of hypotension and vasoconstriction on the nerve tissue. It may also be omitted in the presence of thyrotoxicosis, in those receiving tricyclic antidepressant drugs and in labour. The acidity of local analgesic solutions is increased when adrenaline is contained in commercial solutions from about pH 6 to 3. If used, adrenaline is better added freshly.

Potentiation of Local Analgesic Solutions

By raising the alkalinity of solution. Combination of local analgesic bases with CO_2 to form bicarbonate salts, which have a pH of about 6·5. The free base is rapidly liberated in the tissues due to buffering and the liberated CO_2 diffuses, causing a fall in the intracellular pH in the vicinity, so that the local analgesic base is brought close to the nerve membrane in higher concentration, for combination with the receptors.[276] These salts are said to combine low toxicity, rapid onset and sensory and motor block of intense degree.[277] Carbonated salts of lignocaine, prilocaine and bupivacaine have been prepared, but are not commercially available in the UK.

Methods of Location of the Extradural Space

Before any block is attempted, an open vein must be guaranteed (by indwelling needle, drip, etc.). No block must be attempted without this supremely important precaution. During the insertion of the spinal needle, we prefer usually to have the patient conscious but lightly sedated. The extradural space may be entered from the midline or laterally, with the patient either on the side or sitting. For *midline approach* great care must be taken to insert the needle in the sagittal plane to minimize injury to extradural veins. The back should be painted with antiseptic solution and not completely covered by sterile towels. The type of lumbar puncture needle selected depends on the anaesthetist, some workers preferring a standard needle of 20-gauge, others favour a larger bore, e.g. 16 or 18 SWG, or the Tuohy,[278] the use of which reduces the incidence of dural puncture to a minimum.[279] A thin-wall 18-SWG needle serves well. The needle should be suitably marked to enable the depth of the point to be instantly recognized[280] (*Fig. 32.2*). Full flexion of the spine should be employed for the insertion of the needle into the ligamentum flavum, but this position stretches the dura and makes it more liable to be punctured. The back should therefore be slightly deflexed as the needle is advanced towards the space from the ligamentum flavum. The level from which the block is made is not very important and any easily palpable interspace below L.1/L.2 should be chosen. The depth of the extradural space has been measured by ultrasound.[281]

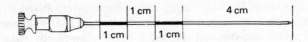

1 cm   1 cm   1 cm   4 cm

Fig. 32.2 The Lee marked needle (Medical & Industrial Equipment Ltd)

For the *lateral* or *paramedian approach* a weal is raised 1 cm from the midline opposite the lower edge of the spinous process.[282] The needle is then inserted at right angles to the back until the body lamina is touched and the depth of this noted. The needle is next withdrawn as far as the muscle sheath and reinserted at an angle of 10° upwards and 10° medially. When the needle lies at the depth of the laminae, the stylet is withdrawn and the loss of resistance test applied. Useful for mid-thoracic approach.

Both the midline and the lateral entry into the space may be performed with the patient in the sitting position, and this may be the easier way in obese and in some arthritic cases, and also for thoracic puncture, using a negative-pressure method. For discussion on choice of lateral or paramedian approach *see* Armitage E. N. *Anaesthesia* 1976, **31**, 1287; **32**, 672; Carrie L. E. S. *Anaesthesia* 1977, **32**, 620; Chapman G. M. *Anaesthesia* 1977, **32**, 671.

An easily palpable interspace should be selected, if possible a high one above L.3 for a high block and a lower space for a low block.

Injection in the *thoracic region* is more difficult and is best avoided between T.4 and T.9. The patient should either be sitting up and a negative pressure test employed or the loss of resistance test used. Injection between T.10 and L.1 causes little difficulty and is similar to injection between L.2 and L.5, although the extradural space is shallower. In the midthoracic region, the needle should be inserted at an angle of 40°.[249] Care must be taken not to damage the cord. The angulation, however, renders accidental dural puncture unlikely, since the Tuohy needle tends to 'toboggan' along the dura. The paramedian approach is useful in the thoracic region (*see above*). The prone position, with lumbar elevation by an inflatable rubber pillow beneath the lower abdomen, has been successfully used for gaining access to the extradural space.[283] The tyro can be taught the 'feel' of the extradural puncture in the post-mortem room.[284]

The following points suggest that the needle is in the extradural space:

1. Sudden lack of resistance to advancing needle as it leaves the dense ligamentum flavum.

2. Sudden ease of injection of a little air or liquid from a freely running syringe attached to a needle. If point is in ligamentum flavum, plunger rebounds: if it is in the space, plunger can be pushed in easily (Sicard and Forestier, 1921;[285] Dogliotti, 1931[241]). In the authors' opinion this is by far the best method in the lumbar region. It is the 'loss of resistance to injection' test, the medium being injected can be air (preferably), local analgesic solution or saline. A false-positive test may result if the needle point enters a small cyst in the yellow ligament.[286] The presence of much blood is a contraindication to injection.

3. Withdrawal of hanging drop of saline on hub of needle.[287] Gutiérrez's sign;[288] useful in the thoracic region but unreliable in the lumbar. Negative pressure in the extradural space described in 1926.[289]

4. Movement of bubble on Odom's indicator[252] (a glass tube with fine bore containing saline and an air bubble) which can be attached to hub of spinal needle.

5. Macintosh's extradural space indicator—a small rubber balloon attached to an adaptor which is connected to the needle when it lies in the interspinous ligament. With a fine hypodermic needle, air is injected into the thick rubber of the neck of the balloon, and when the extradural space is entered, the small balloon diminishes in size.[290]

6. The Macintosh spring-loaded needle,[291] devised by R. H. Salt.[292]

7. Ultrasonic localization.[293]

8. The Oxford epidural space indicator.[294]

In the unconscious patient the rapid injection of liquid into the extradural space is accompanied by an increase in the rate and depth of respiration (Durrans' sign[295]). This test is not always positive in conscious patients, if injection is made slowly, or if injection is made into subarachnoid space. The injection of 5 ml of distilled water will cause some discomfort to the patient if it is placed in the extradural space—an additional help in localization (Lund). All of the solution injected by even experienced anaesthetists, after a positive loss of resistance test, does not always enter the extradural space.[296] In very difficult cases, or where accuracy is imperative (e.g. in pain therapy), X-ray control may be advisable.

Injection must only commence when position of needle point is certain.

Test dose. An initial injection (following aspiration test) of either 1 ml of hyperbaric lignocaine with adrenaline[297] or 2 ml of 0·5% bupivacaine with adrenaline[298] is made and if in 5 min there is no evidence of intradural block, e.g. inability to move the feet, or tachycardia from possible intravenous injection of adrenaline, the main injection can be made.[415] A volume of 1·5 ml has also been recommended.[299] It has been suggested that 5% lignocaine is more satisfactory than 0·5% plain bupivacaine (which may spread too high and take too long).[416] Many workers of experience omit this test dose. It is more logical when used under stable conditions following insertion and secure fixation of an extradural catheter. There are advantages in injecting the total dose in four aliquots to reduce toxic effects; such a procedure does not influence the eventual height of the block, at least in Caesarean section.[300]

Rate of injection has no effect on the extent of the block.[301]

The patient is then turned on the back with slight head-down tilt.

Procedure if dura is pierced. In the hands of skilled workers, the incidence of dural puncture should not exceed 1%.[302] Although dural puncture is usually due to lack of delicacy in technique, it may result from congenital narrowing of the vertebral canal.[303] (This spinal stenosis has caused intermittent claudication of the cauda equina.) The choice is as follows: (1) Leave needle in theca so that it occludes the dural puncture and attempt to locate the extradural space from a higher or lower level. Withdraw first needle after injection of local analgesic solution through the second needle into the extradural space; (2) Convert the block into an intradural (subarachnoid) one; (3) Abandon the method and use general anaesthesia.

Cerebrospinal fluid dripping from the needle can be differentiated from local analgesic solution by: (1) Difference in temperature; (2) Testing for glucose and protein on urine-testing paper strips; (3) Allowing a few drops to fall onto thiopentone solution, when local analgesic solution causes turbidity (pH of thiopentone is 10; of analgesic solution, about 5).[304]

Thoracic Extradural Block

Used mainly for the relief of postoperative pain as it is possible to block thoracic roots selectively while sparing the lumbar and sacral roots. The ideal puncture site for thoracic operations is T.2–T.6; for the upper abdomen, T.6–T.8; the paramedian approach is recommended. A skin weal is placed just lateral to the spinous process at the inferior aspect of the interspace and the needle directed 10° medially and 45° cephalad. After identification of the space and the usual aspiration test, a test dose may be injected, followed by the insertion of an extradural catheter. Puncture of the theca is less likely than in the lumbar region because of the angulation of the needle and the tendency of the Huber point to 'toboggan' over the dura mater. The dose of solution may vary from 3 to 5 ml of 1·5% lignocaine or 0·5% bupivacaine for a block of 2–4 segments, or up to 10–15 ml when a greater zone of analgesia is required as in abdominal surgery. A constant infusion of 0·125% bupivacaine at 10–15 ml/h has been used for postoperative analgesia. (*See also* Bromage P. R. *Epidural Analgesia*. Philadelphia: Saunders, 1978; Carron H. et al. *Regional Anesthesia*. Orlando, Florida: Grune & Stratton, 1984.)

The technical difficulties of cervical and thoracic block are greater than those associated with the lumbar approach.

Cervical Extradural Block

Used for the management of intractable pain and by some enthusiasts, for thyroidectomy and for carotid endarterectomy. The concentration of solution should be such as to provide sensory block without motor block of the phrenic nerves, e.g. lignocaine 1% or bupivacaine 0·25%. For the injection the patient sits with the head and neck flexed forward. The C.7–T.1 interspace (vertebra prominens) is identified and a skin weal made over it in the midline. By the median approach the extradural needle is advanced slowly, inclined at an angle of

30° cephalad. The hanging drop method of localizing the space has been recommended as the negative pressure in the extradural space is likely to be greatest in this situation. Variations with respiration may be noticed if a second drop is placed in the correctly placed needle, while a deep inspiration will usually pull this drop into the needle. Usual dose is 6–8 ml of solution for neck analgesia. Technically, it is easy, although potentially very harmful, should the cord be pithed. Nonetheless, experienced workers advocate it. The extradural space is relatively superficial and the yellow ligament thin.

Assessment of Successful Blockade

Onset of complete analgesia may require 10–20 min and can be checked by: (1) Disappearance of anal tone (S.4–S.5); (2) Disappearance of knee-jerks (L.2–L.4), Westphal's sign 1875;[305] (3) Disappearance of tone of abdominal muscles (T.8–L.1); (4) Disappearance of ankle-jerk (S.1–S.2); (5) The existence and extent of skin analgesia, tested with an ether swab, needle, or ice cube; (6) Absence of muscle tone is shown by weakness or abolition of movement of the hips, knees and ankles.

The maximal concentration of lignocaine in the bloodstream after extradural block occurs, on average, 18 min after injection, and after a shorter period if adrenaline is not used.[306]

Delayed extension of the block (and even delayed apnoea) may be due to medial spread of the local analgesic solution in nerve trunks from the extradural space into the spinal cord itself (intraneural spread). Delay may be as long as 40 min.

Absorption into the intraneural spaces and centripetal spread is said to occur from the region of the junction of the anterior and posterior nerve roots.[307]

Injection of local analgesic solution into the extradural space may cause temporary headache and vertigo. Absorption of drug from this situation or its direct intravascular injection may result in disorientation, psychic abnormalities and twitching or convulsions. The last should be treated by intravenous barbiturate, suxamethonium or diazepam and hyperventilation with oxygen.

Continuous Extradural Analgesia

Greater control over duration and extent of analgesia can be gained if instead of a single injection of solution, repeated injections are made through a plastic catheter introduced into the extradural space. The plastic catheter, made of nylon or polyvinyl chloride, with markings at 5-cm intervals from the tip,[308] is passed through a larger needle (e.g. Tuohy),[309] the slightly angulated tip of which is accurately placed in the extradural space. The angle at the tip carries the catheter either up or down within the space according to the direction of its opening. This special needle, though rather large in bore (16–18 gauge), is relatively easy to insert and many workers use it routinely,[310] even for 'one-shot' injections. The catheter, however, does not always travel in the desired direction. Many workers give the first dose through the needle before the catheter is introduced. Kinking of the catheter within the hub of the spinal needle can be avoided by partly filling the lumen of the hub by the sawn-off nozzle of a plastic syringe.[311]

The insertion of a catheter into the extradural space is especially useful: (1) When the extent of the operation is uncertain; (2) When the duration is uncertain; (3) When the time of commencement is uncertain—the catheter can be put in at leisure and the injection given when necessary; (4) In handicapped patients, to enable small doses to be given and later increased; (5) For postoperative pain relief, especially in patients with chronic bronchitis. Supplemental doses should be one-half to two-thirds of the original dose and great care taken to prevent the introduction of infection by various methods including the Millipore bacterial filter. The catheter should not be inserted more than 5 cm into the extradural space. The catheter should be firmly fixed to the back so as to avoid kinking and its proximal end taken to the pillow from which serial injections can be given. (6) In obstetrics.

For management of the knotted catheter *see* Browne R. A. and Politi V. L. *Can. Anaesth. Soc. J*. 1979, **26**, 142.

Volumes of solution of 1·5% lignocaine required (for extradural block). For suprapubic prostatectomy, 10–20 ml; for vaginal and perineal repair, 20–35 ml; for herniae, appendicectomies, etc. 20–30 ml of solution are required; for hysterectomies, etc. 25–35 ml; for upper abdominal operations, 35–40 ml. For *Caesarean section*, 15–25 ml, taking care to control the blood pressure. In infants 5–6 ml of 1% lignocaine has been reported to give good results (or 1 ml/2 lb bodyweight).[312]

Those workers who regard the mass of solute as more important than the volume of solution in judging dosage suggest that 35 mg per spinal segment to be blocked at age 20, decreasing to 15 mg per segment at age 80, when using solutions between 2 and 5%, is a suitable guide. Adrenaline is added (1–200 000) to the lignocaine solution.

Prilocaine 1·5–2% in dosage a little less than that for lignocaine.

Volumes of bupivacaine for extradural block. Onset of analgesia and duration of block is longer than when lignocaine is used. The addition of adrenaline increases the duration only marginally. Maximum safe dose 2 mg/kg (25–30 ml 0·5% solution in the average adult); 0·75% solution gives a slightly more profound effect and 0·25% solution is useful for postoperative pain relief. Average dose for lower laparotomy 15–25 ml of 0·5% solution, for upper laparotomy, 30 ml.

Indications for Extradural Block

1. In upper abdominal operations. A block to T.4 or T.5 is required and this obtunds all afferent impulses from upper abdominal viscera. It does not block those conveyed up the vagus or phrenic nerves and so reflex disturbances, hiccups, nausea and retching, and laryngeal spasm (Brewer–Luckhardt reflex) may cause trouble. The method is suitable in fit young patients. By introducing the catheter from the thoracic region through a Tuohy needle at an angle of 40°, much smaller volumes of solution are required, e.g. 16–22 ml. Greater control is obtained if a tracheal tube is passed before or after the extradural injection, and this allows unimpeded spontaneous respiration of inhalation agents.

2. In lower abdominal operations. The method is seen at its best advantage in these cases. Muscular relaxation, contracted bowels, wound ischaemia with adequate spontaneous respiration combine to give excellent conditions for surgery.

3. In hernia repairs. An excellent method unless the patient is grossly obese, arthritic or unfit.

4. In operations on the lower limbs. Extradural block gives excellent results in relatively fit patients and has been recommended (as has intradural block)[313] for total hip replacement, fractured neck of femur, and for arthroplasty of the hip in elderly patients.[314] For operations below the knee, a low level of injection with a relatively concentrated solution has been recommended.[315]

5. *Operations on the vertebral column.* In laminectomies the injection of a full dose of solution produces wound ischaemia which many surgeons find most welcome. Experienced workers employ volumes up to 40 ml of 1·5% lignocaine with adrenaline in fit patients.[316]

6. *Obstetric analgesia* (*see* Chapter 27). If a catheter is inserted analgesia can be limited to the lower thoracic and upper lumbar segments for the first stage of labour and extended by tilting the vertebral column to the sacral segments for the second stage. It may also be useful to relieve the distress of delayed dilatation of the cervix. Initial dose 6–7 ml of bupivacaine (0·25–0·5%).

7. *For postoperative pain relief. See* Utting J. E. and Smith J. M. *Anaesthesia* 1979, **34**, 320. (*See* Chapter 8.)

8. Has been used in infants and young children.[419]

Management of the Patient during Extradural Block

The general effects are similar to those described in the section on spinal analgesia. Management of the patient on the operating table is the same as in intradural block (*see* pp. 684 and 693).

The blood pressure is likely to be higher in a conscious than in an unconscious patient. Most anaesthetists have their patients drowsy, under the influence of, e.g. an intravenous thiobarbiturate, diazepam, droperidol, a continuous drip of chlormethiazole[317] or under full general anaesthesia. The blood pressure can be controlled as outlined below, the actual degree of hypotension depending on the amount of ischaemia thought desirable and the general condition of the patient. The proponents of high spinal analgesia believe that, given adequate ventilation and oxygenation, a systolic blood pressure of 35 mmHg is adequate as it is greater than the sum of the venous pressure and the osmotic pressure of the plasma, always provided that peripheral resistance is abolished by the vasodilatation consequent on sympathetic block.[318] The blood pressure of the authors begins to rise if that of their patients descends very much below 60 mmHg. During periods of hypotension a head-down tilt should, if possible, be adopted and maintained into the postoperative period until the blood pressure rises satisfactorily. There is evidence that elevation of the legs is preferable to the Trendelenburg position as the latter may interfere with cerebral perfusion.[319] Intravenous infusions must be given. Breathing pure oxygen causes a decrease in heart rate and cardiac output and an increase in total peripheral resistance, i.e. a decreased myocardial work load without decrease in oxygen transport to the tissues; it is beneficial for patients with a high block.

Breathing during extradural block is generally quieter and easier than under general anaesthesia, probably consequent upon deafferentiation.[60] Controlled ventilation is relatively easily superimposed if desired. There may be a reflex bronchodilatation initiated by baroreceptors stimulated by low blood pressure, in the aorticocarotid sinuses, or it may be due to relative ischaemia of the mucosae of the bronchi consequent on the low blood pressure in their supplying vessels, the bronchial arteries. During high extradural block the respiratory minute volume, the tidal volume, blood-gas estimations and the vital capacity are not greatly altered.

Complications

1. Inadequate block: this must be covered by some convenient form of general anaesthesia. Unilateral block can occur; its cause is unknown. Occasionally, one or more nerve roots (e.g. L.5, S.1 or 2) remain unblocked.[320]

2. Hypotension and cardiovascular depression: this should be dealt with *secundum artem*—posture, pressor drugs, intravenous infusions, atropine in the presence of severe bradycardia, oxygen.

3. Hypopnoea: this will need careful attention to the airway and may call for assisted respiration. It may progress to frank apnoea,[321] and this need not be due to either total spinal or to total extradural block, but to medullary depression from the local analgesic drug. It may take up to 45 min to become established. It may well be a sign of toxicity of the analgesic drug. It usually lasts about 1 h and need not interrupt the operation providing respiration is controlled or assisted.

4. Nausea and vomiting: this can be managed by additional intravenous or inhalation anaesthesia by intravenous atropine, or antiemetic.

5. Spasmodic muscular movements of the arms and shoulders: these may be seen in patients kept lightly asleep with thiopentone or other i.v. agents. Intravenous narcotic analgesic, diazepam, more barbiturate or light general anaesthesia may be required.

6. Total central neurological blockade (total spinal analgesia): the possibility of this must always be present in the mind of the anaesthetist performing an extradural block. While it usually comes on soon after the injection, it may be delayed for 30–45 min.[322] If this has occurred the patient is likely to show, within 3 min of injection of the analgesic drug: (*a*) marked hypotension; (*b*) apnoea; (*c*) dilated pupils; (*d*) loss of consciousness. He is in grave danger of death from asphyxia. *Management*: turn patient into the supine position (but not in labour) ventilate the lungs, elevate legs, inject a pressor drug into the open vein, give intravenous fluid. This will in most cases rescue the patient. Later, a tube can be passed and ventilation can be controlled with equal volumes of oxygen and nitrous oxide. The operation can in most cases proceed and breathing will probably recommence within the hour. Unpleasant sequelae are unlikely.

7. Toxicity due to the injected drug: this may occur after rather small amounts of drug, but is not common. It can follow intravascular (usually) or extradural injection, that is the subsequent block may be absent or good. The signs are disorientation, going on to twitching, convulsions and perhaps apnoea.[323] They usually come on soon after injection but may be delayed. Management consists of injecting a barbiturate (e.g. thiopentone, 150 mg) into the open vein (to find a vein of a violently convulsing patient may be impossible); diazepam may also have a place; the administration of oxygen by IPPV; protection of the patient's teeth and tongue from the trauma of the fits; injection of 50 mg of suxamethonium. In the authors' experience the last has never been necessary.

8. Unblocked segments,[324] e.g. S.1 or L.5, supplying sensation to the outer border of the foot and ankle. The incidence of this is decreased if carbonated salts of the analgesics are substituted for the hydrochlorides.[325]

9. Prolonged analgesia; 60 h of analgesia have been reported, following the extradural injection of 18 ml of 0·5% bupivacaine (without adrenaline).[326]

10. Unilateral block.[327]

11. Horner's syndrome.[328] Recovery may be delayed.[329]

12. High block possibly due to subdural injection.[330] Subdural migration of an extradural catheter, verified by X-rays, has been described.[417]

13. Epiduro-cutaneous fistula (successfully treated by a blood patch).[331]
14. Unexplained pain during injection.[332]
15. Trigeminal nerve palsy following lumbar extradural analgesia.[418]

Advantages claimed for the method as against intradural analgesia are: (1) Less danger of meningitis and neurological sequelae; (2) Absence of postoperative headache; (3) Prolonged postoperative analgesia—up to 48 h after bupivacaine, cinchocaine or amethocaine, especially if a catheter is inserted. Neurological sequelae much the same in the two methods, fortunately rare in both.[333]

Advantages, as compared with general anaesthesia: (1) Protection of the patient from stress responses of the operation—the benefits of this are not proved; (2) Maintenance of spontaneous respiration; (3) Provision, by one injection, of analgesia, of relaxation, ischaemia and contracted bowels; (4) Very suitable in certain patients with asthma, bronchitis or emphysema; (5) Can be employed in patients who are not suitable for muscle relaxants, e.g. in myasthenia; (6) Neostigmine not required (e.g. in colon surgery).

Disadvantages are: (1) Difficulty of being sure of position of needle point, with risk of subarachnoid injection of a large volume of solution; (2) Time taken over the block; (3) Time taken before onset of analgesia.

Contraindications

These are similar to those set out above for intradural block. Patients who are over 65, and those with large abdominal tumours, arteriosclerosis and diabetes need special care. Hypovolaemia is a relative contraindication.

Sequelae

1. Paraplegia[334]—a rare occurrence. May be due to infarction of the cord or stenosis of the vertebral canal or extradural spinal cord tumour.[335] Intracranial complication e.g. subdural haematoma.[336] In a reported series of 50 000 blocks, 2 patients developed paraplegia, 1 of whom had metastatic carcinoma.[337] Sometimes the cause remains obscure.

2. Anterior spinal artery syndrome.[338] Paraplegia not involving the posterior column of the cord, so that joint, position sense, touch and vibration sense are spared. This was first described in 1909 by Miller.[339] An extremely uncommon occurrence.

3. Intraocular haemorrhage has been reported after the rapid injection of 30 ml.[340] This may raise the CSF pressure with resulting subhyaloid bleeding.

4. Occasional backache caused by the needle.

5. Extradural abscess,[341] which may take up to 16 days to develop, may be metastatic. Extradural haematoma has been reported in a patient, 3 days after delivery who received neither extradural block nor anticoagulants.[342] Extradural abscess or haematoma must be drained immediately after diagnosis, otherwise paraplegia may result.[343]

It is interesting that up to 20 ml of thiopentone[344] and 160 ml of parenteral nutritional solution[345] have been accidentally injected into the extradural space, both without harm.

Neurological sequelae following extradural block are not necessarily due to the method of analgesia. *See* Lee. J. A. et al. ed. *Sir Robert Macintosh's Lumbar Puncture and Spinal Analgesia*, 5th ed. Edinburgh: Churchill Livingstone, 1985, p. 180; Neumark J. et al. *Anesthesiology* 1980, **52**, 518.

(*See also* Dawkins C. J. M. *Anaesthesia* 1969, **24**, 554.)

Therapeutic Use of Extradural Injections

(1) Postoperative pain relief and for prevention of postoperative chest complications.[346] Insertion of an extradural catheter into the upper thoracic region, either by the midline or by the lateral route, between T.1 and T.4 or between T.7 and T.8 will enable local analgesic solution (e.g. 0·5–1·5% lignocaine 8–10 ml or 0·25% bupivacaine 5–7 ml), or narcotic analgesic (*see* p. 711) to be deposited in the region where afferent fibres from the abdominal wall enter the posterior roots. Puncture in the upper thoracic region, using a hanging drop test in the sitting position, is easier than in a mid-thoracic approach, owing to the obliquity of the spinous processes. In this way analgesia of the wound and anterior abdominal wall is produced so that the patient can be encouraged to cough and breathe deeply without the severe pain usually caused by such activity. Improvement in postoperative ventilatory capacity results from continuous block. This may be due to factors other than pain relief. Fresh injections can be given as frequently as necessary. If the patient is kept flat for 20 to 30 min thereafter he can then get up and walk about without much fall in blood pressure. Respiratory function is restored much more efficiently by afferent blockade than by systemic narcotic analgesics, although it confers no marked advantage in blood-gas status.[347] The usual fall in functional residual capacity (FRC) following abdominal surgery is less in the presence of extradural block; (2) In the management of closed chest injuries, e.g. fractured ribs;[348] (3) To control the severe pain of acute pancreatitis and dissecting aneurysm; (4) To relieve status asthmaticus; (5) In eclampsia as a method of deliberate hypotension; (6) To control chronic pain due to ischaemia or to cancer; (7) In acute occlusive vascular conditions; (8) In obstetrics for pain relief; (9) To aid the passage of renal calculi; (10) In the treatment of post-spinal headache;[349] (11) In the treatment of the lumbar-sciatic syndrome,[350] with the addition of steroids (which may cause systemic side-effects even after one dose).[351] (*See also* Doughty A. *Anaesthesia* 1975, **30**, 741.)

The whole subject of extradural block is fully discussed by Lund P. C. *Peridural Analgesia and Anesthesia*. Springfield, Ill.: Thomas, 1966; Bromage P. R. *Epidural Analgesia*. Philadelphia: Saunders, 1978.

Extradural Sacral Block (Caudal Block)

This method of analgesia was introduced by Cathelin[352] and Sicard[353] (1872–1929) of Paris in 1901 but neither employed it for operations. It was used by Schlimpert in 1910, [354] and in obstetrics by Stoeckel[355] in 1909, who was the first to report painless vaginal delivery following injection of the recently discovered agent procaine into the extradural space, and by Läwen,[356] who potentiated his solution by the addition of sodium bicarbonate. Arthur Läwen placed extradural block via the sacral route on a firm foundation when he made use of the observation of Gros[357] that procaine acts more effectively in an alkaline medium.[358] Hingson in the US has been a pioneer and proponent of the method.[359] Has been used in animals, especially in cattle, since 1925. Very suitable for block of the sacral and lumbar nerves. For higher block the lumbar approach to the extradural space is preferable as less solution will thereby be used.

Anatomy of Sacrum

A large triangular bone formed by the fusion of the five sacral vertebrae, articulating above with the 5th lumbar vertebra and below with the coccyx.

Posterior surface is convex and down its middle line runs the median sacral crest with its three or four rudimentary spinous processes. The laminae of the 5th and sometimes of the 4th sacral vertebrae fail to fuse in the midline; the deficiency thus formed is known as the sacral hiatus. The tubercles representing the inferior articular processes of the 5th sacral vertebra are prolonged downwards as the sacral cornua. These cornua, with the rudimentary spine of the 4th vertebra above, bound the sacral hiatus. Four posterior sacral foramina correspond with the anterior foramina. Each transmits a sacral nerve posterior ramus and communicates with the sacral canal.

Apex is directed downwards and articulates with the coccyx.

Coccyx represents four rudimentary vertebrae—sometimes three or five.

Sacral canal is a prismatic cavity running through the length of the bone and following its curves. Superiorly it is triangular on section and is continuous with the lumbar vertebral canal. Its lower extremity is the sacral hiatus, closed by the posterior sacrococcygeal membrane. Fibrous strands sometimes occur in the canal and divide the extradural space into compartments. These may account for some cases of failure to produce uniform analgesia. Its anterior wall is formed by fusion of the bodies of the sacral vertebrae; its posterior wall, by fusion of the laminae. On each lateral wall of the canal, four foramina are present, which divide in the form of a Y into anterior and posterior sacral foramina. The contents of the sacral canal are: (1) The dural sac which ends at the lower border of the second sacral vertebra, on a line joining the posterior superior iliac spines. The pia mater is continued as the filum terminale; (2) The sacral nerves and the coccygeal nerve, with their dorsal root ganglia; (3) A venous plexus formed by the lower end of the internal vertebral plexus. These vessels are more numerous anteriorly than posteriorly and so the needle point should be kept as far posteriorly as possible; (4) Areolar and fatty tissue—more dense in males than in females.

Each sacral nerve is provided with a thick sheath from the dura.

The *sacral hiatus* is a triangular opening, caused by failure of the 5th (and sometimes of the 4th) laminar arch to fuse, with apex upwards formed by the 4th sacral spine, and a sacral cornu on each side below and laterally. (But this is so in only 35% of sacra.[360]) It is covered over by the sacrococcygeal membrane which is pierced by the coccygeal and 5th sacral nerves. It is superior to the sacrococcygeal junction, usually about 3·8–5 cm from the tip of the coccyx and directly beneath the upper limit of the intergluteal cleft.

Anatomical abnormalities of the sacrum are not uncommon. They include: (1) Upward and downward displacement of the hiatus; (2) Pronounced narrowing or partial obliteration of the sacral canal, making needle insertion difficult; (3) Ossification of the sacrococcygeal membrane; (4) Absence of the bony posterior wall of the sacral canal, due to failure of laminae to fuse; (5) Dural extension to the level of S.3–S.4 in 2% of patients, quoted by Louis,[361] or even to the sacrococcygeal membrane itself.[362]

The average capacity of the sacral canal is 34 ml in males and 32 ml in females. Its average length is 10–15 cm.

When a local analgesic solution is injected into the sacral canal it ascends upwards in the extradural space for a distance proportional to the volume of solution, the force of injection, the amount of leakage through the eight sacral foramina and the consistency of the connective tissue in the space. While the first two are controllable, the last are not, so precise placement of the solution is impossible and sometimes leads to unexpected results.

Technique of Injection

Careful antiseptic preparation of the skin is essential. A needle (e.g. a Butterfly) is inserted into a vein. The patient is in the prone position with hips slightly flexed over two pillows. To prevent tensing of the gluteal muscles the patient should be asked to abduct his legs and turn his toes in. Other positions are the lateral, Sims position, knee–chest and knee–elbow. After cleaning and towelling, the tip of the coccyx is identified and the triangular sacral hiatus palpated about 3·5–5 cm above it. The hiatus must be clearly palpated. Its anatomy is not constant; sometimes it is larger, sometimes smaller, than normal. Relatively easier to palpate in Negroes.[363] It is difficult to feel in fat patients. If necessary, an intravenous agent can be injected into an indwelling needle just before the block is commenced.

A weal is raised over the hiatus, with a fine intradermal needle using no more than 2 drops of solution, as oedema obscures the landmarks. A 5-cm needle, No. 1, is inserted through the sacrococcygeal membrane so that it makes an angle of about 20° with the line drawn at right angles to the skin surface. Once through the membrane the needle is depressed a further 45° towards the intergluteal cleft and the needle is advanced into the sacral canal for 2–3 cm keeping in the midline. The point must not ascend higher than the line joining the posterior superior iliac spines lest the dura, which ends at this level, be pierced. Occasionally the dural sac extends lower down than the level of the second piece of the sacrum. The mean distance between the apex of the hiatus and the dural sac is 4·5 cm. In many cases the needle used for the skin weal can be used to enter the sacral canal by workers of experience.

After aspiration tests for blood and CSF have been proved negative, a test dose can be injected if thought necessary. Should *blood* flow through the needle, its position must be slightly altered. Should *cerebrospinal fluid* appear, the method of analgesia must be abandoned and intradural injection substituted for it in suitable cases, the proper amount of drug being introduced into the theca through the sacral needle.

Five minutes after the test injection, movement of the toes is called for; if this is present, a intradural block has not resulted and the needle point is not in the theca; further injection can then be proceeded with. When the needle is correctly placed, injection is easy, no great force being required to depress the plunger of the syringe. Should the needle be *posterior to the canal*, a tumour is raised over the sacrum as the injection proceeds. Injection of a few millilitres of air will produce surgical emphysema with its crepitus. If the needle point comes to lie *between periosteum and bone* the force needed for injection will be great—a sure sign of an incorrect position. Young males, because of the tough nature of their extradural fat, require larger doses, injected with greater force, than females, while 2% solution of lignocaine gives better results than 1·5% solution in these patients. Usually easily accomplished.

Drugs

Lignocaine 1–2% or bupivacaine 0·25–0·5% solution with or without adrenaline are excellent, giving a rapid onset and a profound degree of analgesia.

Dosage. Level of analgesia is governed by: (1) Quantity of solution; (2) Speed of injection; (3) Gravity; (4) Age and height of patient. Poor-risk cases require a smaller dose by at least 20%.

Low block, i.e. up to L.2–L.4, for operations on anus, rectum, perineum or urethra, circumcision, vaginal plastics, etc.: up to 30 ml. In 10 min analgesia will develop and will last 1–2 h; 15–20 ml of solution are sufficient for the average case of haemorrhoids or anal fissure.

Toxic reactions to the drugs used are sometimes seen, as dosage is fairly large. Injection of the drug into the venous plexus may also be a cause of this. An occasional twitch requires no treatment, but convulsions should be combated with intravenous suxamethonium or thiopentone, together with IPPV with oxygen. Collapse due to cardiovascular depression consequent on reduction of the blood pressure is treated on the usual lines by elevating the lower limbs, giving a plasma-volume expander, giving oxygen and injecting a pressor drug, if required. Too rapid a rate of injection may cause transient unconsciousness.[364]

The extent of analgesia is not by any means related only to the volume of solution injected, but also to the volume which leaks through the sacral foramina and the intervertebral foramina and to the degree of the lumbosacral angle. The best control of the height of analgesia is obtained by the use of the continuous technique via a plastic catheter.

Indications. (1) Haemorrhoidectomy and other perianal operations; (2) Forceps delivery in obstetrics; (3) Operations on the lower limbs and transurethral operations, e.g. lignocaine 6 mg/kg of 2% solution or bupivacaine 2·2 mg/kg of 0·75% solution, both with adrenaline.[365] The extradural injection of large volumes of procaine, e.g. 50 ml of 0·5% solution or other agents, is extensively used for the relief of skeletal pain. Extradural injection of steroid, especially if repeated, can prevent a patient mounting a normal cortisol response to stress.[366] Neurolytic solutions have been used for the relief of intractable pain. (Neurolytic *trans-sacral* injections of phenol have been used successfully for the relief of severe and intractable pain due to malignancies.[378] S.4 and S.5 are the main nerves to be treated. A trial injection of 0·5% bupivacaine 2·5 ml should precede the phenol.)

Sacral Extradural Block in Infants and Children

First described in 1933.[367] Perhaps because of their healthy cardiovascular systems, young children stand this form of analgesia well though collapse has been reported.[42] Light general anaesthesia is required for the block and for the operation. Excellent postoperative analgesia is obtained. The use of bupivacaine 0·25%, 0·5 ml/kg after operation, provides good pain relief and does not interfere with ventilation.[368]

Some recommended doses: (1) Bupivacaine plain, 0·5% solution, 0·5 ml/year of age[369] or 1·5 mg/kg;[370] 0·25%, 1 ml/year[371] or 0·5–1·25 mg/kg.[372] (2) Lignocaine with adrenaline, 1% solution, 1 ml/year of age[371] or 0·1 ml/dermatome/year of age, with upper limit of 6 mg/kg.[373] (*See also* Touloukian R. J. et al. *Anesth. Analg. Curr. Res.* 1971, **50**, 565; Hassan S. Z. *Anesth. Analg. (Cleve.)* 1977, **56**, 686; McGown R. G. *Anaesthesia* 1982, **37**, 806; Hain W. R. *Br. J. Anaesth.* 1978, **50**, 303.)

Advantages

Absence of postoperative headaches. The method is excellent for cystoscopies, haemorrhoidectomies and gynaecological plastic operations and is highly recommended by the present authors. Useful also for outpatients in whom an intravenous infusion of 500 ml of Hartmann's solution helps to prevent any hypotension produced. It is also very suitable for forceps deliveries in obstetrics, owing to the excellent relaxation of the cervix and pelvic floor and perineum. It can be used for orthopaedic operations on the foot, for ligation of varices and for the prolonged relief of postoperative pain after, for example, haemorrhoidectomy;[422] in this case a plastic cannula is left in the sacral canal and through it doses of 12 ml of local analgesic solution can be injected as required. Its therapeutic indications include low backache, sciatica (sometimes combined with a steroid),[374] vasospastic disease of the lower limbs, and intractable pelvic pain.

Disadvantages
(1) Length of time taken for development of analgesia; (2) Lack of accurate control of height of analgesia; (3) Muscular relaxation not maximal in mid and high blocks, although it is excellent in low blocks; (4) Technical difficulty; (5) Risk of inadvertent subarachnoid injection (but very slight); (6) Hypotension and possible signs of drug toxicity;[375] (7) It produces complete flaccidity of the anal sphincters, a condition unpopular with some surgeons doing operations for fistula-in-ano.

Continuous Caudal (Extradural Sacral) Block

This is chiefly used to produce painless labour. Single extradural sacral injections have been used for many years in obstetrics (Stoeckel, 1909; Schlimpert, 1913), but the continuous technique was introduced in 1942 by Edwards and Hingson,[376] who used a needle connected to rubber tubing. Manalan substituted a ureteric catheter.[377] (*See* Chapter 27.)

Trans-sacral Block

First performed by Victor Pauchet (1869–1936) (Labat's teacher), Läwen in 1909 and Danis of Brussels in 1913, this involves blocking the sacral nerves through the posterior sacral foramina; it is usually associated with extradural sacral (caudal) block, but is frequently quite unnecessary, solution deposited in the sacral canal through the sacral hiatus usually producing excellent analgesia. It is, however, useful when an extradural sacral block is required but cannot be induced because of the difficulty of introducing a needle into the sacral canal.

Technique
The posterior superior iliac spines are located, as the patient lies prone with his pelvis supported on a sandbag. In the obese, a dimple overlies the spine. The 2nd foramen is a finger-breadth caudad and a finger-breadth medial to the spine. The 3rd, 4th and 5th foramina are one finger-breadth apart on the same line, while the 1st foramen is a finger-breadth above the spine and a similar distance medial to it. The 5th foramen is usually between the sacrum and the coccyx.

The foramina underlie a line of finger-breadth lateral to the median line.

To prevent painful injections, caudal block should be induced a quarter of an hour before the needles for the trans-sacral block are inserted.

Weals are raised and needles introduced no more than halfway through each foramen. With a negative aspiration test for cerebrospinal fluid and blood, 0·5% lignocaine is injected on each side: First sacral foramen, 15 ml; second foramen, 10 ml; third foramen, 4 ml; fourth foramen, 3 ml; fifth foramen, 2 ml.

Block of the posterior divisions of the sacral nerves by long-acting agents by the trans-sacral route is said to be useful in the treatment of severe sciatica and of the hypertonic bladder in paraplegics. Block of S.3 or S.2 and S.3 on each side will not prevent a patient from micturating. (*See* p. 709.)

Extradural and Intradural Narcotic Analgesics

The identification of opiate receptors in the central nervous system[379] and the isolation of endorphins led to an interest in the production of analgesia by spinal application of narcotic analgesics. Intrathecal narcotics have been used in animals[380] and in man.[381] The first reports of clinical use of extradural narcotic analgesics came from Jerusalem[382] and it was shown[383] that pethidine was soon transferred from the extradural space to the CSF.

Extradural Narcotic Analgesics
These have been administered in the treatment of intractable pain,[382] postoperative pain,[384] trauma,[385] ischaemic pain[423] and obstetrics.[386] Poor results have generally been obtained in labour,[387] perhaps because the pain pathways involved differ from those associated with other types of pain or perhaps because of increased vascularity of the space in labour and hence quicker absorption to the systemic circulation, though this theory is not supported by measurement of blood levels. Sacral injection has been used in children.[388]

Pharmacokinetics and Pharmacodynamics
Analgesic drug injected into the extradural space has to pass through the dura into the intradural space to reach the substance of the cord, the greatest concentration of opioid receptors being in lamina 2 (substantia gelatinosa) and lamina 5 of the cord.

The dura presents a substantial barrier to drug diffusion. The concentration gradient may be several hundred fold.[383] In the lumbar region the dura is about 0·3 mm thick and it becomes thicker in the cephalad direction. Factors affecting molecular movement include molecular weight, molecular shape, solubility in fat and the concentration of the drug.[389] Fentanyl has a relatively high permeability.

Human studies are difficult[390] but animal work[391] shows that following extradural injection of morphine, the concentration in lumbar CSF can peak at high levels after 2 h. There is a considerable concentration gradient in the CSF with very low concentrations near the fourth ventricle. Activities such as coughing can, however, disturb the equilibrium, allowing much higher concentrations to reach the brain.[392] The volume in which the drug is dissolved is also probably important.[393]

Systemic absorption also takes place from the extradural space. The plasma profile resembles that following intramuscular injection,[394] although peak blood levels tend to be lower. Systemic absorption contributes to analgesia and also decreases the concentration gradient across the dura. Some of the drug also diffuses into extradural fat to form a depot.

Addition of adrenaline to the injected solution is likely to enhance both analgesia and side-effects.[395] The danger of respiratory depression is greater when a patient has recently received an intramuscular injection of a narcotic analgesic drug.[396]

Clinical use. Although it may be more logical to inject local analgesic solution directly into the intradural space and hence near to the cord itself, extradural placement allows the use of repeated doses via a catheter. The correct positioning may be validated by injection of local analgesic solution. The segmental level of injection should be as near to the cord segment where analgesia is desired as possible. This is higher than would be required when local analgesic drugs are used. Narcotic analgesic drug without preservative is used, though the shelf life of morphine is then only 1 week. A 0·1% morphine hydrochloride solution (1 mg/ml) in 10% glucose may be prepared in the pharmacy. The desired dose, 2–4 mg morphine, is then made up to 10 ml by addition of isotonic saline.

The onset of analgesia can be expected in 20–30 min and the duration of effect may vary between 4 and 36 h. Arterial pressure, heart rate and respiratory rate should be monitored, though cardiovascular stability is the rule. Posture is not important in relation to spread of analgesic effect. Other analgesics which have been used include pethidine[383] fentanyl[397] methadone,[398] buprenorphine, lofentanil[399] and sufentanil.[400] Fentanyl has been used successfully in an infusion without causing respiratory depression.[397] Ketamine 4 mg in 10 ml of 5% dextrose in water injected into the extradural space provides potent analgesia postoperatively, without side-effects.[401] Extradural opiates do not directly influence the metabolic response to surgery, but decrease the cortisol response postoperatively, secondary to improved analgesia.[402]

Advantages. (1) Reduced dosage compared to intramuscular injection; (2) Good and prolonged analgesia without depression of consciousness, skin numbness or motor block; (3) Cardiovascular stability due to lack of sympathetic block; (4) Absence of constipation.

Complications.[403] (1) Severe respiratory depression, sometimes delayed, can occur;[404] (2) Itching, particularly in the area supplied by the 5th cranial nerve; (3) Some nausea and dizziness has been reported; (4) Urinary retention may occur[405] but is difficult to assess. Urinary retention after extradural morphine may be relieved or prevented by 4 oral doses of phenoxybenzamine 10 mg given before and after surgery;[406] (5) Poor results have been obtained in obstetrics; (6) May cause temporary inability to ejaculate in males.[405]

Extradural opioid injection is now widely employed in the management of postoperative pain, though patients are best nursed in an intensive care or high dependency unit so that continuous observation is possible, with instant correction of respiratory depression, perhaps by the use of naloxone. This reverses the respiratory depression without diminishing analgesia, but its duration of action is less than that of the extradural opioid, so that continuous observation is still necessary.

Choice of drug. Some drug doses which have been recommended for extradural injection for pain relief include: morphine, 2–4 mg; diamorphine, 0·1 mg/kg; methadone, 5–6 mg (top-up dose 4 mg); fentanyl, 1·5 µg/kg (bolus), infusion, 0·5 µg/kg/h); buprenorphine, 0·3 mg; lofentanil 5 µg; pethidine 25 mg.

The dose is commonly dissolved in 10 ml, sometimes in 20 ml saline. A wide variety of narcotic analgesic drugs have been employed, as have other agents such as midazolam.[407] Morphine has been used in many studies perhaps because it is regarded as the standard for reference, but since most other narcotic analgesics are more lipophilic than morphine, it might be more logical to use another agent. If less of the drug is dissolved in cord lipid, more may remain free to diffuse rostrally to cause respiratory depression.

Intradural Narcotics

Intradural injection has been used in the management of various types of pain.[408] Morphine 1·5 mg has been used successfully in labour.[409] However, there is no doubt that intrathecal narcotics are associated with a much higher incidence of severe respiratory depression than when the drugs are given extradurally, and apnoea has been described many hours later.[410] Close observation of patients is therefore required and naloxone should be available for immediate use in case of respiratory depression.[411] It reverses respiratory depression without loss of analgesia. The danger is less if hyperbaric solutions are used and head-up tilt maintained and can probably be disregarded when elective IPPV is carried out postoperatively. Drug doses for intradural injection, morphine 0·5–1 mg.

(*See also* Bullingham R. E. S. et al. in *Recent Advances in Anaesthesia and Analgesia*—14 (Atkinson R. S. and Hewer C. L. ed.) London: Churchill Livingstone, 1982; Symposium 'Opioid Receptors'; *Br. Med. Bull.* 1983, **39**, January; Cousins M. J. and Mather L. E. *Anesthesiology* 1984, **61**, 276; Lee J. A. et al. ed. *Sir Robert Macintosh's Lumbar Puncture and Spinal Analgesia*, 5th ed. Edinburgh: Churchill Livingstone, 1985.)

References

1. Viets H. R. *Bull. Hist. Med.* 1935, **3**, 701.
2. Magendie F. *J. Physiol. Exp. Path.* 1827, **7**, 66.
3. von Anrep B. *Arch. Physiol.* 1880, **21**, 38.
4. Corning J. L. *NY Med. J.* 1885, **42**, 483 (reprinted in 'Classical File', *Surv. Anesthesiol.* 1960, **4**, 332); *Med. Rec.* (NY) 1888, **33**, 291.
5. Corning J. L. *Local Anesthesia.* New York: Appleton. 1886; *See also* Little D. M. 'Classical File', *Surv. Anesthesiol.* 1979, **23**, 271.
6. Quincke H. I. *Berl. Klin. Wochenschr.* 1891, **28**, 930; *Verh. Kongr. Inn. Med.* 1891, **10**, 321.
7. Wynter W. E. *Lancet* 1891, **1**, 981.
8. Bier A. *Dtsch. Z. Chir.* 1899, **51**, 361 (translated and reprinted in 'Classical File', *Surv. Anesthesiol.* 1962, **6**, 352).
9. Tuffier T. *C. R. Soc. Biol. (Paris)* 1899, **51**, 882.
10. Tait F. D. and Caglieri G. E. *JAMA* 1900, **35**, 6.
11. Matas R. *Phil. Med. J.* 1900, **6**, 820.
12. Donitz A. *Münch. Med. Wochenschr.* 1903, **50**, 1452; Bier A. *Verh. Dtsch. Ges. Chir.* 1905, **34**, 115.
13. Fourneau E. *Bull. Soc. Pharmacol. (Paris)* 1904, **10**, 141.
14. Chaput H. *Bull. Soc. Chir. (Paris)* 1904, n.s., **30**, 835.
15. Einhorn A. *Dtsch. Med. Wochenschr.* 1905, **31**, 1668.
16. Heineke H. and Läwen A. *Dtsch. Z. Chir.* 1905, **80**, 192; Braun H. *Dtsch. Med. Wochenschr.* 1905, **31**, 1667.
17. Barker A. E. *Lond. Clin. J.* 1906, **28**, 4; *Br. Med. J.* 1907, **1**, 665; 1908, **1**, 244; **2**, 453; Lee J. A. *Anaesthesia* 1979, **34**, 885.
18. Brownlee A. *Practitioner* 1911, February, p. 214.
19. Dean H. P. *Br. Med. J.* 1906, **1**, 1086; Akhtar M. *Anaesthesia* 1972, **27**, 330.
20. Gray H. T. *Lancet* 1909, **2**, 913.
21. Babcock W. W. *NY St. J. Med.* 1914, **50**, 637.
22. Labat G. *Ann. Surg.* 1921, **74**, 673.
23. Pitkin G. P. *J. Med. Soc. NJ.* 1927, **24**, 425; *Am. J. Surg.* 1928, **5**, 537.
24. Chen K. K. and Schmidt C. F. *J. Pharmacol. Exp. Ther.* 1924, **24**, 331; *JAMA* 1926, **87**, 836.

25. Ocherblad N. F. and Dillon T. G. *JAMA* 1927, **88**, 1135.
26. Rudolf R. D. and Graham J. D. *Am. J. Med. Sci.* 1927, **173**, 399.
27. Gray H. T. and Parsons L. *Q. J. Med.* 1912, **5**, 339.
28. Smith G. S. and Porter W. T. *Am. J. Physiol.* 1915, **38**, 108.
29. Jonnesco T. *Br. Med. J.* 1909, **2**, 1396 (reprinted in 'Classical File', *Surv. Anesthesiol.* 1978, **22**, 301).
30. Koster H. *Am. J. Surg.* 1928, **5**, 554 (reprinted in 'Classical File', *Surv. Anesthesiol.* 1968, **12**, 306).
31. Keyes E. L. and McLelland A. M. *Am. J. Surg.* 1930, **9**, 1: *JAMA* 1931, **96**, 2085.
32. Jones H. W. *Br. J. Anaesth.* 1930, **7**, 146.
33. Kirschner M. *Surg. Gynecol. Obstet.* 1932, **55**, 317.
34. Sebrechts J. *Br. J. Anaesth.* 1934, **12**, 4.
35. Wilson W. E. *Br. J. Anaesth.* 1934, **11**, 43.
36. Lemmon W. T. *Ann. Surg.* 1940, **111**, 141.
37. Dean H. P. *Br. Med. J.* 1907, **2**, 870.
38. Sise L. F. *Surg. Clin. North Am.* 1935, **15**, 1501 (reprinted in 'Classical File', *Surv. Anesthesiol.* 1957, **1**, 266).
39. Eisleb O. *Arch. Exp. Path. Pharmak.* 1931, **160**, 53.
40. Ekblom L. and Widman B. *Acta Anaesth. Scand.* 1966, Suppl. 23, 419.
41. Cope R. W. *Anaesthesia* 1954, **9**, 249; *Br. J. Anaesth.* 1954, **26**, 233.
42. Foster Kennedy G. et al. *Surg. Gynecol. Obstet.* 1950, **91**, 385 (reprinted in 'Classical File', *Surv. Anesthesiol.* 1964, **8**, 273).
43. Thorsen G. *Acta Surg. Scand.* 1947, Suppl. 95, 121.
44. Dripps R. D. and Vandam L. D. *JAMA* 1954, **156**, 1486.
45. Lee J. A. *Anaesthesia* 1967, **22**, 342; Macintosh R. R. *Anaesthesia* 1975, **30**, 476; Bryce-Smith R. *Proc. R. Soc. Med.* 1976, **69**, 75; Scott D. B. and Thorburn J. T. *Br. J. Anaesth.* 1975, **47**, 421.
46. Nolte H. et al. *Anaesthesist* 1977, **26**, 33.
47. Critchley E. M. R. *Br. Med. J.* 1982, **284**, 1588.
48. Newman B. *Anaesthesia* 1983, **38**, 350.
49. Sharrock N. E. *Br. J. Anaesth.* 1979, **51**, 253.
50. Key E. A. H. and Retzius M. G. *Studien in der Anatomie des Nervensystems.* Stockholm: Samson and Wallin, 1875.
51. Jenkins J. G. *J. R. Soc. Med.* 1986, **79**, 110.
52. Shantha T. R. and Evans J. A. *Anesthesiology* 1972, **37**, 543.
53. Adamkiewicz A. *Sber. Akad. Wiss. Wien.* Abt. **II**, 1882, **85**, 101.
54. Djindjian R. *Proc. R. Soc. Med.* 1970, **63**, 181.
55. Dommisse G. F. *Ann. R. Coll. Surg.* 1980, **62**, 369.
56. Batson O. V. *Ann. Surg.* 1940, **112**, 138; Dommisse G. F. *Arteries and Veins of the Human Spinal Cord from Birth.* Edinburgh: Churchill Livingstone, 1976.
57. Edgar M. A. and Nundy S. J. *J. Neurol. Neurosurg. Psychiatry* 1966, **29**, 530.
58. Sechzer P. H. *Anesthesiology* 1963, **24**, 869; Cohen C. A. and Kallos T. *Anesthesiology* 1972, **37**, 352; Boys J. E. and Norman P. F. *Br. J. Anaesth.* 1975, **47**, 1111.
59. Bryce-Smith R. *Proc. R. Soc. Med.* 1976, **69**, 75.
60. Bromage P. R. *Epidural Analgesia.* Philadelphia: Saunders, 1978.
61. Consino M. J. and Wright C. J. *Surg. Gynecol. Obstet.* 1971, **133**, 59.
62. Walts L. F. et al. *Anesthesiology* 1964, **25**, 634; Freund F. et al. *Anesthesiology* 1967, **28**, 834.
63. Rosenberg P. H. and Heinonen E. *Br. J. Anaesth.* 1983, **55**, 163.
64. Barker I. et al. *Anaesthesia* 1985, **40**, 533.
65. Roe C. F. and Cohn F. L. *Surg. Gynecol. Obstet.* 1973, **136**, 265.
66. Urban B. J. *Anesthesiology* 1973, **39**, 496.
67. Forbes A. R. and Roisen M. F. *Anesthesiology* 1978, **48**, 440.
68. Harrison, Gwendolen *Anaesthesia* 1951, **6**, 115; Leatherdale R. A. *Anaesthesia* 1956, **11**, 249.
69. de Jong R. H. and Cullen S. C. *Anesthesiology* 1963, **24**, 628.
70. Bromage P. R. et al. *Science* 1963, **140**, 392; Moller I. W. et al. *Acta Anaesth. Scand.* 1982, **26**, 58; Traynor C. et al. *Br. J. Anaesth.* 1982, **54**, 319.
71. Shantha T. J. and Evans J. A. *Anesthesiology* 1972, **37**, 543.
72. Greene N. M. *Anesth. Analg. (Cleve.)* 1983, **62**, 1013.
73. Moore R. A. et al. *Br. J. Anaesth.* 1982, **54**, 1117.
74. McWhirter W. R. et al. *Anesthesiology* 1973, **39**, 398.

75. Bonica J. J. et al. *Acta Anaesth. Scand.* 1966, Suppl. 23, 429.
76. Bonica J. J. and Berges P. V. *Anesthesiology* 1970, **33**, 619.
77. Dohi S. et al. *Anesthesiology* 1979, **50**, 319.
78. Greene N. M. *Region. Anesth.* 1982, **7**, 55.
79. Bainbridge F. A. *J. Physiol.* 1914, **48**, 332; 1915, **50**, 65.
80. Marey E. J. *C. R. Acad. Sci. (Paris)* 1861, **53**, 95.
81. Sansetta S. M. et al. *Circulation* 1952, **6**, 559.
82. Klingstrom P. *Acta Anaesth. Scand.* 1960, Suppl. 4.
83. Germann P. A. S. et al. *Anaesth. Intensive Care* 1979, **7**, 229.
84. Cundh R. et al. *Acta Anaesth. Scand.* 1984, **27**, 410.
85. Aldrete J. A. et al. *Anesth. Analg. (Cleve.)* 1973, **52**, 809.
86. Moir D. D. *Br. J. Anaesth.* 1963, **35**, 3; Moir D. D. and Mone J. G. *Br. J. Anaesth.* 1964, **36**, 480; Askrog V. F. et al. *Surg. Gynecol. Obstet.* 1964, **119**, 563; de Jong R. H. *JAMA* 1965, **191**, 698; Ward R. J. et al. *JAMA* 1965, **191**, 275; Wishart H. Y. *Anaesthesia* 1971, **26**, 37; James M. L. and Fisher A. *Anaesthesia* 1969, **24**, 511.
87. Egbert L. D. and Tamersoy K. *Anesthesiology* 1961, **22**, 882.
88. Takasaki M. and Takasaki T. *Br. J. Anaesth.* 1980, **52**, 1271.
89. Catenacci A. J. and Sampathacher K. R. *Anesth. (Cleve.)* 1969, **48**, 48.
90. James M. L. and Fisher A. *Anaesthesia* 1969, **24**, 511.
91. Bromage P. R. *Anaesthesia* 1956, **11**, 139.
92. Spence A. A. and Smith G. *Br. J. Anaesth.* 1971, **43**, 144.
93. Drummond G. B. and Littlewood D. G. *Br. J. Anaesth.* 1977, **49**, 999.
94. Boys J. E. and Norman P. F. *Br. J. Anaesth.* 1975, **47**, 1111; Mehta M. and Maher R. *Anaesthesia* 1977, **32**, 760.
95. Eckenhoff J. E. and Cannard T. H. *Anesthesiology* 1960, **21**, 96.
96. Aitkenhead A. R. et al. *Br. J. Anaesth.* 1980, **52**, 1071.
97. Nimmo W. S. et al. *Br. J. Anaesth.* 1978, **50**, 559.
98. Kennedy W. F. et al. *Anesth. Analg. (Cleve.)* 1971, **50**, 1069.
99. Bevan D. R. *Anaesthesia* 1971, **26**, 188.
100. Bonnet F. et al. *Br. J. Anaesth.* 1982, **54**, 29.
101. Kehlet. H. *Region. Anesth.* 1982, **7**, 538.
102. Bromage P. R. *Surg. Gynecol. Obstet.* 1971, **132**, 1051; Lines J. G. *Br. J. Anaesth.* 1971, **43**, 1136.
103. Traylor C. et al. *Br. J. Anaesth.* 1982, **54**, 319.
104. Oyoma T. and Matsuki A. *Br. J. Anaesth.* 1970, **42**, 723; Moller I. W. et al. *Acta Anaesth. Scand.* 1982, **58**; Traynor C. et al. *Br. J. Anaesth.* 1982, **54**, 319.
105. Buckley F. P. et al. *Br. J. Anaesth.* 1982, **54**, 325.
106. Houghton A. et al. *Br. J. Anaesth.* 1978, **50**, 495.
107. Rem J. et al. *Lancet* 1980, **1**, 283.
108. Kehlet H. *Clin. Anesthesiol.* 1984, **2**, 315.
109. Blunnie W. P. et al. *Br. J. Anaesth.* 1983, **55**, 611.
110. Bromage P. R. *Br. J. Anaesth.* 1962, **34**, 161.
111. *See also* Downey J. A. et al. *J. Appl. Physiol.* 1969, **27**, 209; Bromage P. R. *Epidural Analgesia.* Philadelphia: Saunders, 1978; Bazeman P. M. and Chandra P. *Anesthesiology* 1980, **52**, 356.
112. Wildsmith J. A. W. et al. *Br. J. Anaesth.* 1981, **53**, 1103.
113. Nolte H. and Farrar M. D. *Anaesthesia* 1983, **38**, 811.
114. Chambers W. A. et al. *Br. J. Anaesth.* 1982, **54**, 799.
115. Sinclair C. J. et al. *Br. J. Anaesth.* 1982, **54**, 497.
116. Bryce-Smith R. *Proc. R. Soc. Med.* 1976, **69**, 75.
117. Greene N. M. *Anesth. Analg. (Cleve.)* 1985, **64**, 715.
118. Watt M. J. et al. *Anaesthesia* 1968, **23**, 2.
119. Adams B. W. *Anaesthesia* 1956, **11**, 297.
120. Chambers W. A. et al. *Br. J. Anaesth.* 1982, **54**, 75.
121. Moore D. S. *Anesthesiology* 1982, **57**, 134.
122. Lund P. C. and Cameron J. D. *Anesthesiology* 1945, **6**, 565.
123. Messakel F. M. et al. *Br. J. Anaesth.* 1983, **55**, 169.
124. Winnie A. P. et al. *Region. Anesth.* 1984, **9**, 146.
125. Moore D. C. et al. *Anesth. Analg. (Cleve.)* 1982, **61**, 155; *see also* Gissen A. J. et al. *Region. Anesth.* 1984, **9**, 124 and 125.
126. Siker E. et al. *Anesth. Analg. Curr. Res.* 1966, **45**, 191; El-Shirbiny H. M. *Arch. Chir. Scand.* 1966, Suppl. 23, **1**, 442.

127. Armstrong I. R. et al. *Anesth. Analg. (Cleve.)* 1983, **62**, 793; Concepcion M. et al. *Anesth. Analg. (Cleve.)* 1984, **63**, 134.
128. Chambers W. A. et al. *Br. J. Anaesth.* 1982, **54**, 230P; Chambers W. A. et al. *Anesth. Analg. (Cleve.)* 1982, **61**, 49.
129. Chambers W. A. et al. *Anesth. Analg. (Cleve.)* 1981, **60**, 417.
130. Dohi S. et al. *Anesthesiology* 1984, **61**, 238.
131. Cope R. W. *Anaesthesia* 1954, **9**, 249 (description of the 'Woolley and Roe Case').
132. Seltzer J. L. et al. *Anesthesiology* 1977, **47**, 378.
133. Slattery P. J. et al. *Anaesthesia* 1980, **35**, 392.
134. *See also* Clough C. and Pearce J. M. S. *Br. Med. J.* 1980, **1**, 297.
135. Barker A. E. *Br. Med. J.* 1907, **1**, 665.
136. Griffin R. M. and Scott R. P. F. *Anaesthesia* 1984, **39**, 584.
137. Dufy G. P. *Br. Med. J.* 1982, **285**, 1163.
138. Charlebois P. A. *Can. Anaesth. Soc. J.* 1966, **13**, 585.
139. Ariaraj S. J. P. *Anaesthesia* 1981, **36**, 72.
140. Gutiérriez A. *Rev. Cirug., B. Aires* 1932, **12**, 665.
141. Dvir E. and Collins G. I. *Anaesthesia* 1985, **40**, 1018.
142. Taylor J. A. *J. Urol.* 1940, **43**, 561 (reprinted in 'Classical File', *Surv. Anesthesiol.* 1969, **13**, 325); Surks S. N. and Wood P. *Anesthesiology* 1951, **12**, 239.
143. Crawford J. S. et al. *Br. J. Anaesth.* 1975, **47**, 807.
144. Logan M. R. et al. *Br. J. Anaesth.* 1986, **58**, 292; Logan M. R. et al. *Br. J. Anaesth.* 1986, **58**, 292.
145. Shribman M. J. and Hanning C. D. *Eur. J. Anaesth.* 1986, **3**, 103.
146. Sise L. F. *Surg. Clin. North Am.* 1935, **15**, 1501 (reprinted in 'Classical File', *Surv. Anesthesiol.* 1957, **1**, 266).
147. Siker E. S. et al. *Anesth. Analg. Curr. Res.* 1966, **45**, 191.
148. Silverton R. J. *Aust. N.Z. J. Surg.* 1934, **3**, 223; Fisher A. and Bryce-Smith R. *Anaesthesia* 1971, **26**, 324.
149. Etherington-Wilson W. *Proc. R. Soc. Med.* 1934, **27**, 323; 1944, **38**, 109.
150. Lake N. C. *Lancet* 1938, **2**, 241; 1958, **1**, 387.
151. Le Filliatre G. *Précis de Rachianesthésie générale.* Paris: Libraire Le François, 1921.
152. Koster H. *Am. J. Surg.* 1928, **5**, 554 (reprinted in 'Classical File', *Surv. Anesthesiol.* 1968, **12**, 306).
153. Griffiths H. W. C. and Gillies J. *Anaesthesia* 1948, **3**, 134 (reprinted in 'Classical File', *Surv. Anesthesiol.* 1980, **24**, 342).
154. Evans T. I. *Anaesth. Intensive Care* 1974, **2**, 158.
155. Dean H. P. *Br. Med. J.* 1907, **2**, 870; Akhtar M. *Anaesthesia* 1972, **27**, 330.
156. Lemmon W. T. *Ann. Surg.* 1940, **111**, 141.
157. Lee J. A. *Lancet* 1943, **2**, 156.
158. Tuohy E. B. *Surg. Clin. North Am.* 1945, **111**, 141 (reprinted in 'Classical File', *Surv. Anesthesiol.* 1971, **15**, 310).
159. Austin T. R. *Anaesthesia* 1980, **35**, 392.
160. McClure J. H. et al. *Br. J. Anaesth.* 1983, **55**, 1089.
161. Mather L. E. and Cousins M. J. *Anaesth. Intensive Care* 1980, **8**, 421; Runciman, W. B. et al. *Anaesth. Intensive Care* 1981, **9**, 34.
162. Eng. M. and Zorotovitch R. A. *Anesthesiology* 1977, **46**, 147; Maxon L. H. *Spinal Anesthesia.* Philadelphia: Lippincott, 1938, p. 172; Lahey F. H. *JAMA* 1929, **93**, 518.
163. Phillips O. C. et al. *Anesthesiology* 1969, **30**, 284; Abouleish E. et al. *Anesth. Analg. (Cleve.)* 1975, **54**, 459; Flaatten H. et al. *Anaesthesia* 1987, **42**, 202.
164. Croft J. B. et al. *Anesth. Analg. (Cleve.)* 1973, **52**, 228.
165. Gibb W. R. G. and Wen P. *Br. Med. J.* 1984, **289**, 530.
166. Sicard A. *Le Liquide céphalo-rachidien.* Paris: Masson, 1902.
167. Franksson C. and Gordh T. *Acta Chir. Scand.* 1946, **94**, 443.
168. Liebermann L. R. et al. *Neurology* 1971, **21**, 925.
169. Vacanti J. J. *Anesthesiology* 1972, **37**, 358; Mulroy M. F. *Anesthesiology* 1979, **51**, 479.
170. Wark R. J. *Anaesthesia* 1977, **32**, 336.
171. Queckenstedt H. *Dtsch. Z. Nerv. Heilk.* 1916, **55**, 325.
172. Greene B. A. *Anesthesiology* 1950, **11**, 464.
173. Sears R. T. *Br. Med. J.* 1959, **1**, 755.
174. Frumin M. J. *Anesthesiology* 1969, **30**, 599.
175. Ariaraj S. J. P. *Anaesthesia* 1981, **36**, 72.
176. Mosavy S. H. and Shafei M. *Anaesthesia* 1975, **30**, 807.

177. Crawford J. S. *Br. J. Anaesth*. 1972, **44**, 598.
178. Usubiaga J. E. et al. *Anesth. Analg. Curr. Res*. 1967, **46**, 293.
179. Gormley J. B. *Anesthesiology* 1960, **21**, 565; Ostheimer G. W. et al. *Anesthesiology* 1974, **41**, 307; Walpole J. B. *Anaesthesia* 1975, **30**, 783; Abouleish E. *Anesthesiology* 1978, **49**, 291; Crawford J. S. *Anaesthesia* 1980, **35**, 513; Brownridge P. *Anaesth. Intensive Care*. 1983, **11**, 384.
180. Crawford J. S. *Anaesth. Intensive Care* 1983, **11**, 384.
181. Rainbird A. and Pfitzner J. *Anaesthesia* 1983, **38**, 481.
182. Sikh S. S. and Agawal G. *Anaesthesia* 1974, **29**, 297.
183. Dreser H. *Pflügers Arch. Ges. Physiol*. 1899, **76**, 306.
184. Rifaat M. et al. *J. Neurosurg*. 1973, **36**, 366.
185. Seigne T. D. *Anaesthesia* 1970, **25**, 402.
186. Dunkley B. and Lewis T. T. *Br. Med. J*. 1977, **2**, 1391.
187. Venua E. *Wien. Klin. Wochenschr*. 1907, **20**, 566.
188. Norman J. E. *Anaesthesia* 1955, **10**, 87.
189. Kane R. E. *Anesth. Analg. (Cleve.)* 1981, **60**, 150.
190. Ballin N. C. *Anaesthesia* 1981, **36**, 952; Sarate G. S. *Can. Anaesth. Soc. J*. 1981, **28**, 283.
191. Birkhahn H. J. and Rosenberg B. *Anaesthesia* 1977, **32**, 680.
192. Lee J. A. *Anaesthesia* 1967, **22**, 342; Neumark J. et al. *Anesthesiology* 1980, **52**, 518; Schremer E. et al. *Anaesthesia* 1983, **38**, 226.
193. Walsh F. M. R. *Lancet* 1956, **1**, 859.
194. Scott D. B. *Br. Med. J*. 1982, **285**, 1048.
195. Marinacci A. A. *JAMA* 1959, **168**, 1337; *Bull. Los Angeles Neurol. Soc*. 1960, **25**, 170; Marinacci A. A. and Courville C. B. *JAMA* 1958, **168**, 1337.
196. Funkquist B. *Acta Anaesth. Scand*. 1967, **11**, 237.
197. Beaudoin M. G. and Klein L. *Anaesth. Intensive Care* 1984, **12**, 163.
198. Yates D. A. H. *J. R. Soc. Med*. 1981, **74**, 334.
199. Clayton K. I. *Anaesthesia* 1983, **38**, 583.
200. MacKenzie N. *Anaesthesia* 1983, **38**, 886.
201. Wedel D. J. and Mulroy M. F. *Anesthesiology* 1983, **59**, 475.
202. Cashman J. N. *Anaesthesia* 1984, **39**, 248.
203. Wang. B. C. et al. *Region. Anesth*. 1982, **7**, 85.
204. Silver J. R. and Buxton J. H. *Brain* 1974, **97** (III) 539; Annotation *Lancet* 1974, **2**, 1299.
205. Ramachandran S. et al. *Anesth. Analg. (Cleve.)* 1978, **57**, 361.
206. Edelman J. D. and Wingard D. W. *Anesthesiology* 1980, **52**, 166.
207. Scott D. B. and Thorburn J. T. *Br. J. Anaesth*. 1975, **47**, 421.
208. Leatherdale R. A. L. *Anaesthesia* 1959, **14**, 274; Wark H. J. *Anaesthesia* 1977, **32**, 336.
209. Hewer C. L. and Lee J. A. *Recent Advances in Anaesthesia and Analgesia*, 8th ed. London: Churchill, 1957, p. 133; Lett Z. *Br. J. Anaesth*. 1964, **36**, 266; 'Current Comment', *Anesthesiology* 1948, **9**, 439; Newbery J. M. *Anaesthesia* 1977, **32**, 78.
210. Rifaat M. *J. Neurosurg*. 1973, **38**, 366; Shaywitz B. A. *J. Pediatr*. 1972, **80**, 638; Batnitzky S. et al. *Lancet* 1977, **1**, 635.
211. Hawkes C. H. and Roberts G. M. *Br. J. Hosp. Med*. 1980, **23**, 498.
212. Jenkins J. G. *J. R. Soc. Med*. 1986, **79**, 110.
213. Runciman W. B. et al. *Br. J. Anaesth*. 1984, **56**, 1247.
214. Buckley F. P. et al. *Anaesthesia* 1983, **38**, 840.
215. Helmstein K. *Br. J. Urol*. 1972, **44**, 434; Ramsden P. D. et al. *Br. J. Urol*. 1972, **48**, 623.
216. Sculco T. P. et al. *J. Bone. Joint Surg*. 1975, **57A**, 173; Loudon J. R. et al. *Br. Med. J*. 1978, **1**, 1550.
217. Thorburn J. et al. *Br. J. Anaesth*. 1980, **52**, 1117; McDonogh A. J. and Cranney B. S. *Anaesth. Intensive Care* 1984, **12**, 364.
218. Aitkenhead A. R. et al. *Br. J. Anaesth*. 1980, **52**, 1071.
219. Crawford J. S. *Br. J. Anaesth*. 1979, **51**, 531.
220. Aitkenhead A. R. et al. *Br. J. Anaesth*. 1978, **50**, 177.
221. Davis F. M. and Quince M. *Br. Med. J*. 1980, **281**, 1528; Thorburn J. et al. *Br. J. Anaesth*. 1980, **52**, 1117.
222. Dagnino J. and Prys-Robers C. *Br. J. Anaesth*. 1984, **56**, 1065.
223. Bonica J. J. *Surv. Anesthesiol*. 1970, **14**, Annotation, p. 270.
224. Crawford J. S. et al. *Anaesthesia* 1981, **36**, 821.
225. Odoom J. A. *Anaesthesia* 1984, **39**, 602.
226. Gray H. T. *Lancet* 1909, **2**, 913; 1910, **1**, 1611.
227. Bion J. F. *Anaesthesia* 1984, **39**, 534.

228. Jessop E. et al. *Br. J. Anaesth.* 1985, **57**, 1173.
229. Pearce C. *Br. J. Anaesth.* 1974, **46**, 439.
230. McClure J. H. et al. *Br. J. Anaesth.* 1983, **55**, 1089.
231. Wilson J. et al. *Br. J. Anaesth.* 1969, **41**, 840; Schweitzer S. A. *Anaesth. Intensive Care* 1978, **6**, 248; Mather L. E. and Cousins M. J. *Anaesth. Intensive Care* 1980, **8**, 421.
232. Seow L. T. et al. *Anaesth. Intensive Care* 1984, **12**, 127; Seow L. T. et al. *Br. J. Anaesth.* 1984, **56**, 666.
233. Bromage P. R. *Epidural Analgesia*. Philadelphia: Saunders, 1978, p. 476.
234. Hamilton C. J. *Irish Coll. Phys. Surg.* 1983, **76**, 126.
235. Germann P. A. S. et al. *Anaesth. Intensive Care* 1979, **7**, 229.
236. Cathelin F. *C. R. Soc. Biol. (Paris)* 1901, **53**, 452.
237. Sicard J.-A. *C. R. Soc. Biol. (Paris)* 1901, **53**, 396.
238. Kappis M. *Münch. Med. Wochenschr.* 1912.
239. Bleeck and Strauss *Zeit. Geburtsch. Gynek.* 1912, **2**, 72.
240. Pagés-Miravé F. *Revta Sanid. Milit. (Madrid)*, 1921, **11**, 351 (translated and reprinted in 'Classical File', *Surv. Anesthesiol.* 1961, **5**, 326).
241. Dogliotti A. M. *Zbl. Chir.* 1931, **58**, 3141.
242. Aburel E. *Bull. Soc. d'Obstet. Gynaecol. (Paris)* 1931, **20**, 85.
243. Dawkins C. J. M. *Proc. R. Soc. Med.* 1945, **38**, 299.
244. Bromage P. R. *Epidural Analgesia*. Philadelphia: Saunders, 1978.
245. Curbelo M. M. *Anesth. Analg. Curr. Res.* 1949, **28**, 13.
246. Batson O. V. *Ann. Surg.* 1940, **112**, 138; *Am. J. Roentgenol*, 1942, **48**, 715.
247. Husemeyer R. P. and White D. C. *Anaesthesia* 1980, **35**, 7.
248. Harrison G. R. and Clowes N. W. B. *Anaesthesia* 1985, **40**, 685.
249. Dawkins C. J. M. and Steel G. C. *Anaesthesia* 1971, **26**, 41.
250. Janzen E. J. *Dtsch. Z. NervHeilk.* 1926, **94**, 280; Aitkenhead A. R. et al. *Anaesthesia* 1979, **34**, 14.
251. Macintosh R. R. and Mushin W. W. *Anaesthesia* 1947, **2**, 100.
252. Odom C. B. *Am. J. Surg.* 1936, **34**, 547.
253. Zazur E. *Anaesthesia* 1984, **39**, 1101.
254. Andrade P. *Br. J. Anaesth.* 1983, **55**, 85.
255. Usubiaga J. E. et al. *Br. J. Anaesth.* 1967, **39**, 612.
256. Galbert M. W. and Marx G. F. *Anesthesiology* 1974, **40**, 499.
257. Shah J. L. *Anaesthesia* 1981, **36**, 627.
258. Flowers C. E. *Anaesthesia* 1954, **9**, 146.
259. Usubiaga J. E. et al. *Anesthesiology* 1964, **25**, 752.
260. Brierly J. B. *J. Neurol. Psychiatry* 1950, **13**, 203.
261. Shantha T. R. and Evans J. A. *Anesthesiology* 1972, **37**, 543.
262. Bromage P. R. *Br. J. Anaesth.* 1974, **46**, 504.
263. Sharrock N. E. et al. *Br. J. Anaesth.* 1984, **56**, 285.
264. Erdemir H. A. and Soper L. E. *Anesth. Analg. (Cleve.)* 1965, **44**, 223; Usubiaga J. E. et al. *Anesth. Analg. (Cleve.)* 1968, **47**, 440.
265. Grundy E. M. et al. *Anesth. Analg. (Cleve.)* 1977, **57**, 95.
266. Sharrock N. E. *Anesthesiology* 1977, **47**, 307; Grundy E. M., Ramamurthy S., Winnie A. P. et al. *Brit. J. Anaesth.* 1978, **50**, 805.
267. Brownridge P. *Anaesthesia* 1981, **36**, 70.
268. Forster S. J. *Anaesthesia* 1983, **38**, 72.
269. Magee D. A. et al. *Can. Anaesth. Soc. J.* 1983, **30**, 174.
270. Watt M. J. et al. *Anaesthesia* 1968, **23**, 2, 311; 1970; **25**, 24; Ekblom L. and Widman B. *Acta Anaesth. Scand.* 1966, Suppl. 21, 33.
271. Moore D. C. et al. *Anesth. Analg. (Cleve.)* 1978, **57**, 42.
272. Abdel-Salem A. R. et al. *Br. J. Anaesth.* 1975, **47**, 1081; Galindo A. et al. *Br. J. Anaesth.* 1975, **47**, 41; Stanton-Hicks M. et al. *Anesthesiology* 1975, **42**, 398; Buckley F. P. et al. *Br. J. Anaesth.* 1978, **50**, 171.
273. Ravindran R. S. et al. *Anesth. Analg. (Cleve.)* 1980, **59**, 447; Editorial. *Anesth. Analg. (Cleve.)* 1980, **59**, 401.
274. Allen P. R. and Johnson R. W. *Anaesthesia* 1979, **34**, 874; Reisner L. S. et al. *Anesth. Analg. (Cleve.)* 1980, **59**, 452.
275. Bonica J. J. et al. *Acta Anaesth. Scand.* 1966, Suppl, 23, 429.
276. Schulte-Steinberg O. et al. *Anaesthesia* 1970, **25**, 191.
277. Bromage P. R. *Acta Anaesth. Scand.* 1965, Suppl. 16, 55; Bromage P. R. et al. *Br. J. Anaesth.* 1967, **39**, 179; Bromage P. R. *Epidural Analgesia*. Philadelphia: Saunders, 1978, pp. 82, 314.

278. Tuohy E. B. *Surg. Clin. North Am.* 1945, **25**, 834.
279. Bromage P. R. *Epidural Analgesia.* Philadelphia: Saunders, 1978, pp. 179, 476.
280. Lee J. A. *Anaesthesia* 1960, **15**, 186.
281. Currie J. M. *Br. J. Anaesth.* 1984, **56**, 345.
282. Bonica J. J. *Principles and Practice of Obstetrical Anesthesia and Analgesia.* Philadelphia: Davis, 1967; Lee J. A. et al. ed. *Sir Robert Macintosh's Lumbar Puncture and Spinal Analgesia,* 5th ed. Edinburgh: Churchill Livingstone, 1985.
283. Mustafa K. et al. *Anesthesiology* 1983, **58**, 464.
284. Duffy B. *Anaesth. Intensive Care* 1982, **10**, 373.
285. Sicard J. A. and Forrestier J. *Rev. Neurol.* 1921, **28**, 1264.
286. Sharrock N. E. *Br. J. Anaesth.* 1979, **51**, 253.
287. Soresi A. L. *Med. Rec. (New York)* 1932, **35**, 165.
288. Gutiérrez A. *Rev. Cirg. B. Aires* 1932, **12**, 665; 1933, **13**, 255.
289. Jansen E. *Dtsch. Z. NervHeilk.* 1926, **94**, 280.
290. Macintosh R. R. *Anaesthesia* 1950, **5**, 98.
291. Macintosh R. R. *Br. Med. J.* 1953, **1**, 398.
292. Salt R. H. *Anaesthesia* 1963, **18**, 404.
293. Cork R. C. et al. *Anesthesiology* 1980, **52**, 513.
294. Evans J. M. *Lancet* 1982, **2**, 1432.
295. Durrans S. F. *Anaesthesia* 1947, **2**, 106.
296. Mehta M. and Salmon N. *Anaesthesia* 1985, **40**, 1009.
297. Moore D. C. and Batra M. S. *Anesthesiology* 1982, **57**, 141.
298. Peters G. C. *Anaesthesia* 1983, **38**, 72.
299. Kumar C. M. et al. *Anaesthesia* 1985, **40**, 1023.
300. Batra M. S. and Bridenbaugh L. D. *Region. Anesth.* 1985, **10**, 32.
301. Husmeyer R. P. and White D. C. *Br. J. Anaesth.* 1980, **52**, 55; Burn J. M. B. and Langdon L. *Br. J. Anaesth.* 1980, **52**, 707.
302. Macdonald R. *Anaesthesia* 1983, **38**, 71.
303. Ehni G. *Proc. Staff Meet. Mayo Clin.* 1975, **50**, 327; Verbiest H. *J. Bone Jt Surg.* 1954, **34B**, 230; *Clin. Neurol.* 1973, **20**, 204; Sullivan M. *Br. J. Hosp. Med.* 1976, **15**, 25.
304. Catterberg J. *Anesthesiology* 1977, **46**, 309.
305. Westphal A. K. O. (Berlin neurologist, 1833–1890), *Arch. Psychiatr. Nervenkr.* 1975, **5**, 803.
306. Bromage P. R. and Robson G. *Anaesthesia* 1961, **16**, 461.
307. Shantha T. R. and Evans J. A. *Anesthesiology* 1972, **37**, 543.
308. Lee J. A. *Anaesthesia* 1962, **17**, 248.
309. Tuohy E. B. *JAMA* 1945, **128**, 262.
310. Bromage P. R. *Epidural Analgesia.* Philadelphia: Saunders, 1978, p. 465.
311. Keane P. W. *Anaesthesia* 1983, **38**, 701.
312. Ruston F. G. *Can. Anaesth. Soc. J.* 1954, **1**, 37; 1964, **11**, 12.
313. Thorburn J. et al. *Br. J. Anaesth.* 1980, **52**, 1117.
314. Hole A. *Acta Anaesth. Scand.* 1980, **24**, 279; Modig J. et al. *Acta Anaesth. Scand.* 1980, **24**, 305.
315. Bromage P. R. *Epidural Analgesia.* Philadelphia: Saunders, 1978, p. 131.
316. Thorne T. C. and Watt M. J. personal communications; Scovill W. B. *Surg. Neurol.* 1977, **7**, 163.
317. Mather L. E. and Cousins M. J. *Anaesth. Intensive Care* 1980, **8**, 421.
318. Griffiths H. W. C. and Gillies J. *Anaesthesia* 1948, **3**, 134.
319. Gunteroth W. G. et al. *Surg. Gynecol. Obstet.* 1964, **119**, 245; Taylor J. and Weil M. H. *Surg. Gynecol. Obstet.* 1969, **124**, 1005.
320. Galindo A. and Hernandes J. *Br. J. Anaesth.* 1975, **47**, 41.
321. Holmboe J. et al. *Anaesthesia* 1982, **37**, 60.
322. Woerth S. D. et al. *Anesthesiology* 1977, **47**, 380.
323. Scott D. B. *Br. J. Anaesth.* 1981, **53**, 553.
324. Bryce-Smith R. *Anaesthesia* 1954, **9**, 201; Ducrow M. *Br. J. Anaesth.* 1971, **43**, 1172; Roberts R. B. *Br. J. Anaesth.* 1972, **44**, 628; Bray M. C. and Carrie L. E. S. *Anaesthesia* 1978, **33**, 232.
325. Bromage P. R. *Br. J. Anaesth.* 1972, **44**, 676; *Epidural Analgesia.* Philadelphia: Saunders, 1978, p. 559; Sorigge J. S. *Anaesth. Intensive Care* 1979, **7**, 182.
326. Pathy G. V. and Rosen M. *Br. J. Anaesth.* 1975, **47**, 520.
327. Bose H. *Br. J. Anaesth.* 1975, **47**, 806.
328. Evans J. M. et al. *Anaesthesia* 1975, **30**, 774.
329. Hertz R. et al. *Anesth. Analg. Curr. Res.* 1980, **59**, 299.

330. Brindle-Smith G. et al. *Anaesthesia* 1984, **39**, 355; Pearson R. M. G. *Anaesthesia* 1984, **39**, 262 and 460.
331. Longmire S. and Joyce T. H. *Anesthesiology* 1984, **39**, 1115.
332. Edwards G. M. and Sprigge J. *Anaesthesia* 1984, **38**, 194.
333. Scott D. B. and Thorburn J. T. *Br. J. Anaesth.* 1975, **47**, 421.
334. Urquhart-Hay D. *Anaesthesia* 1969, **24**, 461; Harrison P. D. *Anaesthesia* 1975, **30**, 778; Ballin N. C. *Anaesthesia* 1981, **36**, 952.
335. Hirlekar G. *Anaesthesia* 1980, **35**, 363.
336. Eerola M. et al. *Acta Anaesth. Scand.* 1981, **25**, 115.
337. Hillmann K. *Can. Anaesth. Soc. J.* 1965, **12**, 4.
338. Annotation, *Lancet* 1958, **2**, 515; Davies A. et al. *Br. Med. J.* 1958, **2**, 654.
339. Miller *J. Nerv. Ment. Dis.* 1909, **36**, 601.
340. Kelman H. *Am. J. Surg.* 1944, **64**, 183; Clark C. J. and Whitwell J. *Br. Med. J.* 1961, **2**, 1612.
341. Chaudhari L. S. et al. *Anaesthesia* 1978, **33**, 722; Loarie D. J. and Fairley H. B. *Anesth. Analg. Curr. Res.* 1978, **57**, 351.
342. Crawford J. S. *Br. J. Anaesth.* 1975, **47**, 412.
343. Male C. G. and Martin R. *Lancet* 1973, **1**, 609.
344. Cay D. L. *Anaesth. Intensive Care* 1984, **12**, 61.
345. Patel P. C. et al. *Anaesthesia* 1984, **39**, 383.
346. Spence A. A. and Smith G. *Br. J. Anaesth.* 1971, **43**, 144; Utting J. E. and Smith J. M. *Anaesthesia* 1979, **34**, 320.
347. Drummond G. B. and Littlewood D. G. *Br. J. Anaesth.* 1977, **49**, 999.
348. Dittman M. et al. *Intensive Care Med.* 1978, **4**, 193.
349. Crawford J. S. *Br. J. Anaesth.* 1972, **44**, 598.
350. Swerdlow M. and Sayle-Creer W. *Anaesthesia* 1970, **25**, 341; Daly P. *Anaesthesia* 1970, **25**, 346.
351. Knight C. L. and Burnell J. C. *Anaesthesia* 1980, **35**, 593.
352. Cathelin F. *C. R. Soc. Biol. (Paris)* 1901, **53**, 452.
353. Sicard J. A. *C. R. Soc. Biol. (Paris)* 1901, **53**, 396 (both Cathelin's and Sicard's papers are translated and reprinted in 'Classical File', *Surv. Anesthesiol.* 1979, **23**, 271).
354. Schlimpert H. and Schneider K. *Münch. Med. Wochenschr.* 1910, **57**, 2561.
355. Stoeckel W. *Zbl. Gynäk.* 1909, **31**, 1.
356. Läwen A. *Zbl. Chir.* 1910, **37**, 708; *Dtsch. Z. Chir.* 1910, **108**, 1; Läwen A. and von Gaza W. *Dtsch. Z. Chir.* 1911, **111**, 289.
357. Gros O. *Arch. Exp. Pathol. Pharmac.* 1910, **63**, 80.
358. Läwen A. and von Gaza A. *Dtsch. Zahnarztl. Chir.* 1911, **111**, 289.
359. Hingson R. A. and Southworth J. L. *Am. J. Surg.* 1942, **58**, 92; Hingson R. A. and Edwards W. B. *Anesth. Analg. Curr. Res.* 1942, **21**, 301; *JAMA* 1943, **121**, 252.
360. Trotter M. and Letterman G. S. *Surg. Gynecol. Obstet.* 1944, **78**, 418.
361. Nolte H. and Farrar M. D. *Anaesthesia* 1984, **39**, 1142.
362. Meyer R. J. *Anaesthesia* 1984, **39**. 610.
363. Norenberg A. J. et al. *Anesthesiology* 1979, **50**, 549.
364. Semple A. J. and Bissett W. I. K. *Anaesthesia* 1985, **40**, 380.
365. Freund F. R. et al. *Anesth. Analg. (Cleve.)* 1984, **63**, 1017.
366. Burn J. M. B. and Langdon L. *Anaesthesia* 1984, **39**, 295; Pullan P. T. *Anaesthesia* 1984, **39**, 496.
367. Campbell M. F. *Am. J. Urol.* 1933, **30**, 245.
368. Hatch D. J. et al. *Anaesthesia* 1984, **39**, 873.
369. Davenport H. T. *Paediatric Anaesthesia* 3rd ed. 1981; Kay B. *Anaesthesia* 1974, **29**, 610.
370. Lunn J. N. *Anaesthesia* 1979, **34**, 610.
371. Soliman M. G. et al. *Can. Anaesth. Soc. J.* 1978, **25**, 226.
372. Armitage E. N. *Anaesthesia* 1979, **34**, 396.
373. Schulte-Steinberg O. and Rahles V. W. *Br. J. Anaesth.* 1970, **42**, 1093.
374. Gordon J. *Anaesthesia* 1980, **35**, 515.
375. Prentiss J. E. *Anesthesiology* 1979, **50**, 51.
376. Edwards W. B. and Hingson R. A. *Am. J. Surg.* 1942, **57**, 459 (reprinted in 'Classical File', *Surv. Anesthesiol.* 1958, **2**, 424); Hingson R. A. and Edwards W. B. *Anesth. Analg. Curr. Res.* 1942, **21**, 301.
377. Manalan J. A. *J. Indiana State Med. Assoc.* 1942, **35**, 564.
378. Robertson D. H. *Br. J. Anaesth.* 1983, **55**, 873.
379. Snyder S. H. *N. Engl. J. Med.* 1977, **296**, 266; Pert C. B. and Snyder S. H. *Science* 1973, **179**, 1011.

380. Yaksh T. L. and Rudy T. A. *J. Pharmacol. Exp. Ther.* 1977, **202**, 411; Yaksh T. L. and Rudy T. A. *Pain* 1978, **4**, 299; Yaksh T. L. and Rudy T. A. *Science* 1976, **192**, 1357.
381. Wang J. K. *Ann. Anaesth. Franc.* 1978, **19**, 371; Wang J. K. et al. *Anesthesiology* 1979, **50**, 149.
382. Behar M. et al. *Lancet* 1979, **1**, 527; Howard R. P. et al. *Anaesthesia* 1981, **36**, 51.
383. Cousins M. J. et al. *Lancet* 1979, **1**, 1141.
384. Graham J. L. et al. *Anaesthesia* 1980, **35**, 158; Bromage P. R. et al. *Anesth. Analg. (Cleve.)* 1980, **59**, 473; Gjessing J. and Tomlin P. J. *Anaesthesia* 1981, **36**, 268; Boskovski N. et al. *Anaesthesia* 1981, **36**, 67; McClure J. H. et al. *Lancet* 1980, **1**, 975.
385. Johnson J. R. and McCaughey W. *Anaesthesia* 1980, **35**, 155.
386. Perriss B. W. *Lancet* 1979, **2**, 422; Perriss B. W. *Anaesthesia* 1980, **35**, 380.
387. Husemeyer R. P. et al. *Anaesthesia* 1980, **35**, 161.
388. Jensen B. H. *Acta Anaesth. Scand.* 1981, **25**, 373.
389. Moore R. A. et al. *Br. J. Anaesth.* 1982, **54**, 1117.
390. Jorgensen B. C. et al. *Anesthesiology* 1981, **55**, 714.
391. Strube P. J. et al. *Br. J. Anaesth.* 1985, **56**, 921.
392. Kafer E. R. et al. *Anesthesiology* 1983, **58**, 418.
393. Chrabasik J. et al. *Lancet* 1984, **1**, 793.
394. Wedel S. J. and Ritter R. R. *Anesthesiology* 1981, **54**, 210.
395. Bromage P. R. et al. *Anesthesiology* 1983, **58**, 510.
396. Magora F. et al. *Br. J. Anaesth.* 1980, **52**, 247.
397. Bailey P. W. and Smith B. E. *Anaesthesia* 1980, **35**, 1002; Welchew E. A. and Thornton J. A. *Anaesthesia* 1982, **37**, 309; Welchew E. A. *Anaesthesia* 1983, **38**, 1037; Lam A. M. et al. *Can. Anaesth. Soc. J.* 1983, **30**, 578; Lomessy A. et al. *Anesthesiology* 1984, **61**, 466; Ahuja B. R. and Strunin L. *Anaesthesia* 1985, **40**, 949.
398. Welch D. B. and Hrynaszkiewicz A. *Anaesthesia* 1981, **36**, 1051; Nyoka M. et al. *Br. Med. J.* 1986, **293**, 1347.
399. Bilsback P. et al. *Br. J. Anaesth.* 1985, **57**, 943.
400. Donadoni R. et al. *Anaesthesia* 1985, **40**, 634.
401. Islas J. A. et al. *Anesth. Analg. (Cleve.)* 1985, **64**, 1161.
402. Normandale J. P. et al. *Anaesthesia* 1985, **40**, 748.
403. Reiz S. and Westberg M. *Lancet* 1980, **2**, 203; Boas R. A. *Anaesth. Intensive Care* 1980, **8**, 377.
404. Glynn C. J. et al. *Lancet* 1979, **2**, 356; Liolios A. and Andersen F. H. *Lancet* 1979, **2**, 357; Scott D. B. and McClure J. *Lancet* 1979, **1**, 1410; Sidi A. et al. *Anaesthesia* 1981, **36**, 1044.
405. Torda T. A. et al. *Br. J. Anaesth.* 1980, **52**, 939.
406. Evron S. et al. *Br. Med. J.* 1984, **288**, 190.
407. Niv D. et al. *Br. J. Anaesth.* 1983, **55**, 541.
408. Samil K. et al. *Lancet* 1979, **1**, 1142; Samil K. et al. *Anesthesiology* 1979, **50**, 149.
409. Scott P. V. et al. *Br. Med. J.* 1980, **281**, 351.
410. Daines G. K. et al. *Anesthesiology* 1980, **52**, 280; Davies G. K. *Anaesthesia* 1980, **35**, 1080.
411. Jones R. D. M. and Jones J. G. *Br. Med. J.* 1980, **281**, 645; Gjessing J. and Tomlin P. J. *Anaesthesia* 1981, **36**, 268.
412. Walmsley A. J. et al. *Br. J. Anaesth.* 1986, **58**, 1130; Walmsley A. J. et al. *Anesth. Analg. (Cleve.)* 1986, **65**, S.164; Crawford J. S. *Anaesthesia* 1986, **41**, 765.
413. Kumar C. M. and Dennison B. *Anaesthesia* 1986, **41**, 556.
414. Nunn G. and Mackinnon R. P. G. *Anaesthesia* 1986, **41**, 439.
415. *See also* Prince G. and MacGregor D. *Anaesthesia* 1986, **41**, 1240; McKeown D. W. et al. *Anaesthesia* 1986, **41**, 1262.
416. Mallaiah S. *Anaesthesia* 1986, **41**, 334.
417. Abouleish E. and Goldstein M. *Br. J. Anaesth.* 1986, **58**, 1194; Lee A. and Dodd K. W. *Anaesthesia* 1986, **41**, 847.
418. Shigematsu L. et al. *Anesth. Analg. (Cleve.)* 1985, **64**, 653.
419. Dalens B. et al. *Anesth. Analg. (Cleve.)* 1986, **65**, 1060; Desparmet J. *Anaesthesia* 1986, **41**, 338.
420. Brownridge P. *Anaesth. Intensive Care* 1986, **14**, 412.
421. Matsumiya N. et al. *Anesth. Analg. (Cleve.)* 1986, **65**, 1074.
422. Bailey P. M. and Sangwan S. *Anaesthesia* 1986, **41**, 499.
423. Clemensen S. E. et al. *Br. Med. J.* 1987, **294**, 475.

Chapter 33   **THE PAIN CLINIC**

Algology is the specialty of chronic pain relief. 'Pain is an unpleasant experience which is associated with tissue damage or described in terms of tissue damage, or both.' It consists of the sensation of pain, together with the patient's psychological response to it, both of which need attention.[1] For history *see* Roll R. J. *J. R. Soc. Med.* 1982, **75**, 812; Bonica J. J. *Clin. Anaesthesiol.* 1985, **3**, 1. The patient with intractable pain requires careful evaluation, diagnosis and sympathetic understanding. The patient should know that the doctor will welcome him back for further treatment.

Organization of the Clinic[2]

A clinic requires outpatient room, an interested and dedicated consultant in charge, a secretary, operating theatre sessions, a drug cupboard, data storage, ECG, EMG, skin thermometers, nerve stimulator, cryoprobe, muscle strength assessment equipment, full resuscitation equipment, a wide range of diagnostic tools, if possible with an image intensifier (and a back door for the staff to escape, if necessary!)

Three levels of provision have been described, minimal, average and comprehensive. The multidisciplinary approach has been advocated, for example, while it is important to have primary referrals from family doctors, many of these patients will need an exact diagnosis to be made by hospital colleagues before treatment is attempted.

The patient should, if possible, see the same members of staff at each visit.

Assessment of Pain[3]

Type—e.g. central or peripheral. This may only become clear after treatment has started.

Duration—How long has it existed? Has it changed?

Location—Is it focal or diffuse? Superficial, deep, neurological, psychological? Is it false? i.e. a habit reference to some previous site of pain? (30% of cancer patients have two or more pains, about half have no pain).

Quality—Is it aching, crushing, tight, lancinating, vice-like, sharp, throbbing, burning, pressing, colicky, stabbing, pricking, constricting?

Intensity: The patient is asked to complete a linear analogue scale (0 = no pain, 10 = terrible pain) or categorical scale (no pain—just noticeable—weak—mild—moderate—strong—severe—excruciating)

Modifying factors: food, drugs, exercise, rest.

Time relations: variation from day to day, hour to hour (e.g. migraine in the early morning). Presence of a basic background with exacerbations.

Physiological effects—e.g. nausea and vomiting, dysuria, diarrhoea. Do these need treatment in their own right?

Habits—interference with work or sleep, physiological functions, tolerance of others, relationships (including doctor/patient).

Mental changes—depression, anxiety, tension, aggression, obsession, introversion, hypochondriasis, hysteria? What is the home situation like? Have there been mental changes only since the pain started or did they exist previously?

The emotional content and intensity of the patient's language are noted for future comparison (the existence of denial, anger, depression, acceptance, and the extent to which emotional conditioning is contributing to the pain).[5] Also demeanour, facial expression, posture, gait, and a full physical examination.

Has the patient got 'total pain'? i.e. pain + hopelessness + fear of impending death?

Cancer pain is often continuous, at the same location (which enlarges progressively), and is preoccupying and demoralizing.

A pain map may be drawn.

Further investigations—urine and blood analysis (untreated intractable pain from malignant disease produces a metabolic alkalosis related to the severity of the pain),[6] ESR, coagulogram, ECG, perhaps EEG, EMG, appropriate X-rays and endoscopy.

Reassessment

Reassessment is made regularly to determine whether there is good control or poor control of pain, bearing in mind that pain relief is not usually an instant cure, because old pains reappear and new pains may develop. Partial relief may enable the patient to regain control, and that pain is often not the only form of suffering for the patient. It is especially difficult to achieve relief in the depressed, anxious, and those whose pain is worsened by activity.

The patient and appropriate relatives should participate fully in decisions about timing and type of treatment. Informed consent is obtained.

Approach to Treatment of Chronic Pain[7]

Each individual aspect of treatment is used as part of a comprehensive multimodular therapeutic strategy. Enabling the patient to get a good night's sleep has high priority.

Notes on drugs used for intractable pain
Anthranilic acids—mefenamic and flufenamic (500 mg daily). Not gastric irritants, but may cause diarrhoea.
Aspirin—(max dose 3 g daily). Especially good for metastatic bone pain. Gastric irritant, faecal blood loss may occur, controlled by cimetidine 300 mg or ranitidine 150 mg, without affecting plasma salicylate levels.
Brompton Cocktail—no longer employed.
Buprenorphine—strong, long-acting agonist–antagonist. May be given sublingually, (onset in 1/2–1 h, peak effect in 2 h). Some patients are excessively sensitive or excessively resistant to this drug.
Butorphanol—strong agonist–antagonist.[8]
Carbamazepine—good for trigeminal neuralgia, glossopharyngeal neuralgia, migraine, and lightening pains of tabes. May cause aplastic anaemia, leucopenia and liver damage in prolonged use.
Chlorpromazine—25–50 mg anti-emetic, antidepressive, potentiates analgesics, reduces responsiveness of CNS. May produce subcutaneous oedema with other antidepressants. May cause Parkinsonism.
Codeine—30 mg. Slightly stronger than aspirin, antitussive, antidiarrhoeal.

Dextromoramide—5–10 mg orally or rectally. Rapid onset, good for 'breakthrough pain'.

Dextropropoxyphene—65 mg q.d.s. Equal strength to codeine; oral route only; may cause euphoria.

Diamorphine—5 mg. Euphoric, soluble in very small volumes. Advantage over morphine, is that it causes less nausea and vomiting.

Diazepam—5–10 mg. Central muscular relaxation, good with minor analgesics, may be useful at night, not as potent as phenothiazines.

Diflunisal (Dolobid)—Duration of action 10 h. Similar to aspirin.

Dihydrocodeine—30–60 mg. For moderate to severe pain, good when combined with aspirin or paracetamol.

Dipipanone—25–50 mg. Similar to methadone.

Ethoheptazine—75–150 mg/t.d.s. For moderate pain. Antispasmodic.

Indomethacin—up to 150 mg/day. Gastric irritant; can be given rectally.

Levorphanol—long acting, very strong analgesic, less sedating, less nauseating than morphine. Very lipid-soluble. Said to be ten times more effective than morphine when given by mouth.[9]

Methadone—5–10 mg orally. Long acting, very strong analgesic, less sedating, less nauseating than morphine, good for weaning morphine addicts. Should not be given i.v. Plasma half-life 15 h, increases after 2–3 days therapy. The plasma concentration plateau is reached only after 1–3 weeks. Cimetidine inhibits its metabolism. Rifampicin speeds up its metabolism.

Methyl salicylate—absorbed through the skin, for athletic strains.

Morphine (*see* Chapter 8)—best given orally, twice daily as MST, or by subcutaneous infusion in chronic pain.[10] Some pains are not morphine-sensitive, regardless of dose or route. Oral, rectal/parenteral potency ratio is 1–3.[11] Anti-emetics and laxatives likely to be required.

Nalbuphine—10–20 mg. Medium to strong analgesic, and sedative.[12]

Nefopam—15 mg. Peak effect at 2 h, ceiling effect at 20–30 mg, side-effects; insomnia, dry mouth, nausea, nervousness, light-headedness, vomiting, blurred vision, tachycardia, sweating, urinary retention, enhanced motor neurone activity, anticholinergic effects.

Oxycodone—10 mg. Less addictive and sedating than morphine. Long acting when given as the pectinate. Can be given rectally.

Papaveretum (Omnopon)—a basic opiate analgesic (*see* Chapter 8).

Pericyazine—25 mg t.d.s. (more at night). Effective phenothiazine tranquillizer.

Pentazocine—Moderate analgesic with marked dysphoria.

Pethidine—up to 100 mg. Good antispasmodic for gut and uterus. Dysphoric, may cause hypotension, tachycardia and dryness of mouth. Reacts with mono-amine oxidase inhibitors giving hypertension, or coma and hypotension.

Phenoperidine—1–2 mg. Strong analgesic and respiratory depressant, low incidence of vomiting.

Tricyclic antidepressants—antidepressive, analgesic, hypnotic, in moderate pain, potentiate other analgesics, antagonize guanethidine, potentiate adrenaline, may produce oedema with phenothiazines (*see* chlorpromazine, above).

Methods of Pain Relief[13]

1. Analgesics
Classically divided into mild and strong, the stronger ones having more

side-effects. (Doxapram, 1 mg/kg, or small doses of naloxone reverse respiratory depression without influencing analgesia.)

With any analgesic, there is a ceiling dose, above which there is no more analgesia, only more side-effects. Then progression to more powerful analgesics is needed. Some pains are untouched by morphine, but respond to other analgesics. The longer-acting analgesics e.g. diflunisal and levorphanol produce a smoother result, especially at night.

2. Co-analgesics

Antidepressives potentiate analgesics, by stimulating the descending modulating pathways, elevate mood, and may relax muscle spasm. They are not always helpful, may have unpleasant side-effects (dry mouth, blurred vision, urinary retention, constipation and diaphoresis) and their withdrawal may lead to more severe depression. *Anxiolytic drugs* e.g. benzodiazepines, have a role for controlling agitation and producing sleep at night. *Antispasmodic drugs* e.g. Baclofen and orphenadrine.

3. Hyperstimulation Analgesia[14]

This includes cupping, transcutaneous electric nerve stimulation (TENS),[15] acupuncture, needling and ice massage. A brief, intense stimulation encourages the central biasing mechanism to inhibit chronic pain which the brain or spinal cord has remembered and repeated long after the initial injury had healed.[16]

4. Occupational Therapy/Psychotherapy

Unsuitable for patients with a major language barrier, severe deafness, dementia, severe cardiac failure or cognitive deficit. This type of therapy is particularly appropriate for the 'learned pain syndrome' (*see below*), and in overcoming self-perpetuating inactivity caused by pain and the fear that activity will cause harm especially in the elderly and depressed. Such inactivity causes insomnia, muscle loss, bone decalcification, hypercalcuria, joint fibrosis, reduced lung function, altered eating habits, constipation, and obesity or cachexia.

5. Nerve Blockade (sensory, autonomic or motor)[76]

For diagnostic, prognostic, prophylactic and therapeutic purposes. For diagnosis, differential subarachnoid block is sometimes employed. Isotonic saline is injected. A short response indicates a placebo effect. A prolonged response indicates that the pain was psychogenic. A response to 0·25% procaine suggests sympathetic pain; a response to 0·5% procaine suggests a sensory problem; a response to 1% procaine suggests a motor problem. In the course of time after a phenol block, the C fibres may make new connections, producing various abnormal shunts, e.g. afferent input via anterior roots, and reappearance of the pain. For technique of various blocks *see* Chapters 31 and 32 and below. Extradural block with catheter is most suitable for short term pain relief.[17] Long-term implantation can be employed using tunnelling techniques.

6. Hypnosis

This is a state of altered consciousness characterized by heightened suggestibility, narrowed awareness, selective wakefulness, and restricted attentiveness. About 10–15% of adults are not susceptible. Children are the most susceptible and adults over 55 yr the least susceptible. A trance is usually brought about by repetitive auditory, visual or tactile stimuli. The aim is a reduction of sensory intake to one or two monotonous stimuli.[18] Sedative drugs may help. The advantage of hypnosis is that there is no danger of the toxic side-effects of drugs. However, it is difficult and time-consuming, and not suitable for every patient. The contraindications are: (1) Refusal of the patient; (2) Psychiatric illness; (3) Absence of quiet surroundings. Naloxone does not abolish analgesia produced by hypnosis (Needham, Joseph, personal communication).

(*See also* Merskey H. *Postgrad. Med. J.* 1971, **47**, 572.)

7. Deafferentation Drugs

E.g. carbamazepine, clonazepam, sodium valproate, L-tryptophan. Helpful where nerve blocks have failed to relieve pain.

8. Central Nervous Stimulation, and Destructive Procedures.[19]

Agents Used for Nerve Block
1. Local analgesics. Their effect is often prolonged, perhaps by closing the 'gate' at spinal level.
2. Phenol 5% in glycerin[20] 0·5–1 ml. Duration 1 week–3 months. Patients should be warned about the effects of motor block from this agent. This solution is hyperbaric and is used for intradural posterior root block with the patient lying semi-supine with the appropriate segment at the lowest point.
3. Chlorocresol 2% in glycerin.[21] 0·5–1 ml intradurally. Duration weeks to months.
4. Absolute alcohol.[22] 0·5–1 ml. Onset in days, duration in months or years. This is hypobaric, and for intradural block the affected segment is placed uppermost with the patient in the semi-prone position. Injection is very painful and so should be preceded by local analgesia. Arachnoiditis is a complication. Has been used via the trans-sphenoidal approach to destroy the pituitary for metastatic bone pain,[23] when X-ray control in two planes and washout check for sphenoidal sinus infection is required.
5. Intradural ice-cold saline.[24] Selectively blocks C fibres, lasting for weeks, but the injection is very painful. Spinal barbotage[25] is used in a similar way.
6. Cryoprobe block, percutaneously.[26] Duration 6–10 weeks block, including pituitary ablation.[27] Post-cryoprobe neuritis and dyaesthesia are very rare.
7. Opioids[28] *(intradural or extradural).* See also Chapter 32. Should be free of preservatives.[29] Act on the substantia gelatinosa of the posterior horn of the spinal cord.[30] Extradural opioids act partly by systemic absorption, and in the case of water-soluble agents, e.g. morphine, by cephalad spread in the CSF.
Complications—non-segmental pruritus, nausea, vomiting, retention of urine, and, uncommonly, respiratory depression (onset up to 24 h after block, especially by water-soluble opioids). Extradural opioid sedation and respiratory depression, but not analgesia, is reversible by naloxone.
8. Ammonium salts. These are reputed to have a lower incidence of neuritis.
Placebo blocks are used for weaning patients off spinal blocks, and training patients to cope with pain.
Nocebo blocks are where complaints of bodily impairments follow nerve blockade, not fitting any known pattern of anatomical or physiological effect, sometimes seen in patients with disability settlements pending.[31] One source of failure of intradural nerve blocks is the existence of afferent fibres in the anterior roots.[32] Another is 'central pain', which may be treated by deafferentation drugs (*see above*).

Notes on Various Intractable Pains

Amputation Pains
1. *Phantom limb pain (see below)*
2. *Stump pain.* Injection of trigger points or TENS therapy.
3. *Brachial plexus avulsion injury.* TENS may help. Radiofrequency cervical block has been used. The patient may request amputation, but this is of no help.

Anaesthesia Dolorosa
Pain in the desensitized face.[33] Deafferentation treatment (*see above*).

Anal Pain
Involves spinal segments S.2–S.5 (*or supratentorial*!). Proctalgia fugax may occur.

Angina
Differential diagnosis from: (1) Costal cartilage pain; (2) Oesophageal reflux spasm; (3) Left mammary pain due to anxiety; (4) Neuralgias; (5) Mediastinitis; (6) Pericarditis; (7) Gastric pain.
Management (Chronic) glyceryl trinitrate, calcium antagonists (e.g. verapamil 360 mg daily, diltiazem 360 mg daily) β-blockers, left stellate ganglion block and trigger point injection.

Atypical Facial Pain
(Typically maxillary, in a middle-aged female, unresponsive to trigeminal nerve block). Sphenopalatine block (*see* p. 608) and deafferentation (*see above*).

Backache
(15% of pain referrals in India, 70% of referrals in the USA).[34] Treat bad posture, poor muscle tone, obesity, gynaecological pathology, or pancreatitis as appropriate. Bed rest, analgesics required. In selected cases, facet nerve blocks and cryotherapy are effective. Chemical sympathectomy may help for referred buttock and leg pains.

Muscle and ligament strain backache—there is a wide spectrum of patients, from those with excellent coping skills (low pain behaviour, well-documented pathology, good prognosis) to those with poor coping skills (high pain behaviour, no clear pathology, poor prognosis). Moderate to major analgesics, diazepam, and physiotherapy and correction of obesity are a starting point in treatment.

Extradural steroid injection is indicated for acute intervertebral disk pathology, nerve root irritation, myofascial syndrome, interlaminar joint problems and sciatica. Methylprednisolone 80 mg (or 50 mg of triamcinolone) in lignocaine or bupivacaine, has an onset in some days, and may need repeating two or three times. A short general anaesthetic is often required for the injection.

Cancer pain in the back—analgesics, radiotherapy, neurolytic blocks.

Postmyodil arachnoiditis—prevention is better than cure!

Ankylosing spondylitis—posture control; radiotherapy has been used. The biggest problem in this area is postlaminectomy pain.

Bladder Pain
Involves spinal segments S.2–S.4.

Carcinomatosis Bone Pain
Analgesics, aminoglutethimide, tamoxifen, cyproterone, consider hypophysectomy. Aspirin and non-steroidal anti-inflammatory drugs (NSAIDS) are specific, and may reduce the rate of tumour growth.

Causalgia[35]
Regional sympathetic blockade; tranquillizers to control emotional crises.

Central Pain
(1) Post-stroke, thalamic in origin (self-limiting, but pituitary alcohol injection has been used); (2) Residual pain, in a patient whose peripheral source of pain has been controlled, e.g. rendered numb by nerve block, deafferentation (*see above*).

Cluster Headache
(*See* migrainous neuralgia.)

Gallbladder Pain
Pethidine, splanchnic (coeliac plexus) block if surgery is not appropriate.

Geniculate Neuralgia
Analgesia, divide nervus intermedius.

Giant-cell Arteritis
Corticosteroids.

Glossopharyngeal Neuralgia
(*See* p. 616)

Herpes Zoster Neuralgia
Early and completely adequate analgesia is important in preventing post-herpetic neuralgia. Extradural block and steroids, perhaps repeated, nerve blocks, repeated, sympathetic blocks.[36] (*See* postherpetic neuralgia.)

Ischaemic Pain
Alcoholic night-caps, α-blockers, sympathectomy, surgery.

Learned Pain Syndrome (Chronic intractable benign pain syndrome)[37]
There is:
  1. Dramatization of complaints, the descriptions of which have a high emotional content.
  2. Disuse—self-perpetuating prolonged physical inactivity.
  3. Drug misuse—need for multiple or frequently changed prescriptions.
  4. Dependency—helplessness and parasitism on others.
  5. Disability—need for social security handouts and litigation awards. Exact diagnosis is not wanted because of a desire for the reward factors of chronic illness, e.g. discharge from military service.

Treatment by behaviour modification.[38] The behaviour to be modified is first defined from as many sources as possible (to avoid bias) e.g. (1) Pavlovian or conditioned behaviour—the sight of a bottle of tablets or alcohol leads to unnecessary consumption; (2) Social modelling, where the patient reacts as he thinks others expect him to—for better or worse depending on the model chosen; (3) Helplessness, where the patients feels that he is the victim of disease, at the mercy of an inevitable fate.

The basic tenets of behaviour modification are: (1) Removal of the conditioning stimulus (e.g. a bottle), focusing the patient's attention away from the pain, and replacing it by rewards for the target behaviour; (2) Correction of unhelpful antecedents, e.g. muscle tension, overwork, bad posture, idleness; (3) Setting positive goals for progress, e.g. in the area of physical activity; (4) Reinforcement of new healthy habits and attitudes, e.g. sleep, posture, drug-taking, with emphasis on *self*-improvement, i.e. it is the patient's responsibility to get well; (5) Return to suitable work at a graded pace; (6) Sorting out unsatisfactory relationships.

Measurement of progress is necessary, e.g. using biofeedback techniques such as EMG levels in migraine and low back pain. The fully informed support of close relatives is crucial.

Migraine[39]
Treatment—possibly avoid starvation and tyramine-containing foods (chocolate, cheese, red wine). Counselling and minor tranquillizers useful. Ergotamine, 0·25 mg s.c. or i.m., or 0·5 mg orally for the acute attack, with metoclopramide 10 mg i.m. Clonidine and methysergide are used for prophylaxis. Acupuncture has been tried.[40] Simple measures like keeping the hands warm and deliberately relaxing muscle tension are encouraged.

Migrainous Neuralgia
Often unilateral in eye and cheek, occurring in the early hours of the morning, in the middle-aged. Precipitated by alcohol. Sphenopalatine and stellate ganglion blocks are used. Ergotamine is used.

Myofascial Pain (Muscular Rheumatism; Myalgia; Myositis; Fibrositis; Fibromyositis)
'Trigger points' are identified.[41] They are sometimes palpable, exquisitely sensitive, produce intense sharp pain and muscle spasm on needling or pressure, may occur anywhere (especially back and pectoral girdle), and are sometimes related to surgical scars. Histologically they show oedema and accumulation of mast cells. Infiltration with 5–10 ml of 0·25% bupivacaine often removes the original pain which sensitized the trigger point.

Neck Pain
When originating in the neck, is usually due to muscle spasms and responds to analgesics and physiotherapy. When the pain radiates outside the neck, it probably arises from meninges or spondylosis.

Nerve Entrapment
There is burning, tingling or shooting pain, tenderness, weakness, muscle wasting, or loss of sensation. Treatment is surgical, with or without repeated

local analgesic injections. Radiotherapy may help if the nerve is trapped by tumour.

Occipital Pain
Usually due to nerve root pain from the neck, responding to cervical collar wearing, nerve block, manipulation, or surgery. May also be due to a form of migraine.

Painful Scars
Classically the wound has been healed for several weeks. Local or regional blocks are required, perhaps repeated, with surgical excision of neuroma if present.

Pancreatic Pain
Involves dermatomes T.6–T.12 and may require splanchnic or coeliac ganglion block. Under general anaesthesia, needles are inserted bilaterally, preferably under image intensifier control and the effect tested with local analgesic. Absolute alcohol is then injected in divided doses. Resultant postural hypotension lasting from minutes to weeks may be controlled by elastic stockings. Extradural block is satisfactory for acute pancreatitis.[4]

Phantom Limb
(1) Local analgesic block of nerves to the phantom limb, but not spinal block, which may make the pain worse; (2) TENS; (3) Infiltration of trigger points in trunk and opposite limb (*see above*); (4) Sympathectomy; (5) Cordotomy in the worst cases.

Posthemiplegic Dystrophy/Postsympathetic Dystrophy/Post-traumatic Dystrophy
I.V. regional sympathetic blockade may relieve superficial but not deep pain.

Postherpetic Neuralgia
(Prevention—*see* herpetic neuralgia.) Onset as the scabs separate or up to 4 weeks later, with background soreness and episodic sharp stabbing pain, triggered by touching, draughts, or emotions. May last many years, but when resolved, is soon forgotten. Treatment is by analgesics, TENS, local anaesthetic creams, local analgesic subcutaneous injections, nerve and extradural blocks (occasional permanent relief). Intradural alcohol and phenol is often disappointing. Neurosurgery for head and neck neuralgia, or anterolateral cordotomy, is reserved for the worst cases. Steroids (extradural or systemic) and idoxyuridine have been recommended.[42] Sodium valproate and amitriptyline may help at night. The painful area recedes with time.

Raynaud's Disease
Treatment includes avoidance of cold, i.v. regional sympathetic blockade (*see below*) and sympathectomy.

Reflex Dystrophy
E.g. shoulder–hand syndrome in myocardial ischaemia. Regional sympathetic blockade may help.[43]

Renal Pain
Involves dermatomes T.11–L.2.

Temporomandibular Joint Pain
May be due to arthritis or masseter spasm (bruxism). The latter is usually unilateral, may radiate in any direction, or may trigger trigeminal neuralgia and migraine. It is relieved by local analgesic injection into the masseter, dental attention to occlusion, wearing better fitting new dentures.

Tennis Elbow and Various other Joint Pains
Bupivacaine and steroid injection, under anaesthesia, if necessary.

Trigeminal Neuralgia
Intermittent unilateral pain, with or without twitches, usually in an elderly patient. An infraorbital trigger zone is especially common. There is no sensory loss except in postherpetic trigeminal neuralgia. Treatment is by carbamazepine, 100 mg–1 g daily, phenytoin, clonazepam, valproate,[44] local analgesic blocks of trigger points, trigeminal ganglion block (thermocoagulation or neurolytic)[45] or surgical extirpation. Some patients develop postoperative 'anaesthesia dolorosa' which is resistant to treatment.

Percutaneous Cordotomy[46]

Technique originally introduced by Mullan (Chicago) in 1963 using a strontium needle. Later modified by Rosomoff who used radiofrequency current to create a high cervical lesion. Lin and Polakoff have developed an anterior approach for percutaneous lower cervical cordotomy. These techniques are effective and may replace open cordotomy. However, a bilateral high cervical lesion can cause damage to the respiratory outflow fibres with the risk of death when the patient goes to sleep and relies on the involuntary mechanism. Radiological control is used for accurate placement of the needle.[47] Has been reported as giving good results in 64% of patients.[48]

Dorsal Column Stimulation

By an implanted electrode attached to a subcutaneous implanted receiver. The patient operates the transmitter power and frequency; 30% success.[49] Antero-lateral tracts, thalamic and internal capsule have also been similarly stimulated.

Sympathetic Block

Sympathetic dysfunction can cause symptoms due to vasospasm, the production of pain and alteration of function, so that therapy is directed to vasodilatation, relief of pain and restoration of function. Pain due to central nervous system lesions can be treated with either sympathetic blocks or intravenous guanethidine.[50]

Vasomotor block may be performed at any of five levels; (1) Peripheral nerve block, e.g. the ulnar nerve, causing vasodilatation of the skin of the little finger; (2) The sympathetic ganglia, e.g. the stellate or the 2nd and 3rd lumbar ganglia, causing release of vasomotor tone in the upper and lower limbs; (3) The vascular smooth muscle using intravenous guanethidine[51] for reflex sympathetic dystrophies and arterial insufficiency;[52] (4) Extradural block; (5) Subarachnoid block. The last two are examples of preganglionic block and must extend in the case of the lower limb to the 10th thoracic segment so as to paralyse all the preganglionic fibres going to the limb.

Indications for Sympathetic Block[53]

Painful limbs due to vascular disease. Raynaud's (1834–1881) phenomena;[54] vasospasm associated with lesions of the spinal cord, e.g. poliomyelitis and some cases of pyramidal disease; arteriosclerosis and thrombophlebitis obliterans; chronic ulceration of the extremities; embolism of major vessels; thrombophlebitis; erythromelalgia (Weir Mitchell, 1878) and after intra-arterial thiopentone injection. Peripheral arterial disease. This may be: (1) Vasospastic; (2) Vasospastic and organic (Buerger); (3) Degenerative organic (arteriosclerosis). Increased blood supply to the limb is shown by: (1) Increased surface temperature; (2) Increased oscillations shown by an oscillometer; (3) Increased function, e.g. later onset of claudication.[55]
Conditions due to idiopathic and post-traumatic pain of limbs. Causalgia;[52] amputation stump neuralgias; Sudeck's atrophy.[56]
Unclassified conditions of the limbs. Hyperhidrosis; after embolectomy; in the posthyperaemic stage of the immersion foot syndrome.
Abdominal Disease. Pancreatitis (bilateral block of T.6–12) and splanchnic block;[57] inoperable carcinoma (coeliac plexus—splanchnic block);[58] eclampsia (*see* Chapter 27).

The pain associated with neurolytic sympathetic block can be prevented by first giving a segmental extradural block using 2–3 ml 2% lignocaine at L.2/L.3.[59]

'Escape' of sympathetic drive from stellate ganglion block may be stopped by upper thoracic paravertebral blocks.

Intravenous Regional Sympathetic Block (Arms or Legs)[52,64,65]

Advantages. Few complications, still works after excision of stellate ganglion, etc.
Disadvantages. Effects of tourniquet and risk of effects of release of the agent into the general circulation.
Precautions. The following are available: resuscitation facilities, a tilting table, a reliable tourniquet at 100 mmHg above the patient's systolic pressure, an i.v. cannula in place, in both the limb to be treated and another limb.
Procedure. Average dose is guanethidine 10–20 mg with 500 units heparin in 25 ml saline for the arm (double these for the leg). Duration of treatment 5–10 min. Tourniquet released for 30 s then reinflated for 5 min before removal. Effects assessed 30 min after release.

Other Techniques

Transnasal destruction of the pituitary with alcohol, under X-ray control, in certain forms of carcinomatosis.[60] Percutaneous vibration or electrical stimulation[61] has a 30–50% success rate in postherpetic neuralgia.[62] Portable stimulators are available. Acupuncture in the affected dermatome is under assessment.[63] (*See also* p. 733.) Rubbing counter-irritants into the overlying skin is traditional treatment. Cryoprobe application to the spinal cord at open operation has been described, and also to the painful area[65] (e.g. the perineum[66]).

These techniques give results which tend to be poor when employed by the occasional anaesthetist. However, keen, dedicated workers who are willing and able to devote time and attention to acquiring experience in their performance, tell a different tale.

(*See also* Mehta M. *Recent Advances in Anaesthesia and Analgesia*—14 (Atkinson R. S. and Hewer C. L. ed.). Edinburgh: Churchill Livingstone, 1982).

Acupuncture

Acupuncture[67] for pain relief goes back 4000 years, but its use in anaesthesia dates from 1958.[68] The idea is that the 'vital life force' (ch'i) flows in 'meridians' in the body, being disturbed in disease. The location of the disturbed meridian is found by 'pulse diagnosis' and insertion of a needle to stimulate one of over 1000 'acupuncture points' corrects the disturbance, leading to analgesia. Opinions differ widely about the right points for needle insertion.

Acupuncture may be acceptable for chronic pain not amenable to conventional forms of therapy.[69] Acupuncture points are points of low skin resistance, detected by neurometers which measure current flow at 6 V, e.g. Ta-ch'ang yü is 3·6 cm from the midline of the back at the L.4–L.5 interspace. Ch'êng-san is between the heads of the gastrocnemius and Jen Chung is in the middle of the philtrum.

Stimulation. May be electrical (12 V, 100–200 µA, 3–10 Hz for 30 min at 2–3-day intervals) or manual (twirling of needles) or thermal (burning of moxa tufts on the skin or a hot probe at 80 °C).

Naloxone inhibits the analgesic effects of acupuncture[70] (suggesting that endorphin release may be one of the mechanisms) but not the autonomic effects.[71] Controlled studies have shown acupuncture to have a marked pain relieving effect, equal to that of a placebo.[72] Stimulation is continued until Te Chi is developed, i.e. a sensation of numbness, heat, tingling and distension at the needle site. Traumatic sympathetic dystrophy has been successfully treated by electro-acupuncture.[73] Complications include haematomas, infection (including AIDS), pneumothorax and serum hepatitis.[74] Care with the sterility of acupuncture needles is most important. Perichondritis of the pinna has been reported.[75]

Enthusiasm for acupuncture for surgical operations has declined recently, even in the Republic of China. (For history of acupuncture, *see* Loh S. T. *Anaesth. Intensive Care* 1980, **8**, 373.)

References

1. Wall P. D. and Melzack R. *Textbook of Pain.* Edinburgh: Churchill Livingstone, 1984; Glynn C. J. *Br. Med. J.* 1986, **292**, 222.
2. Annotation, *Lancet* 1982, **1**, 486; Rolls R. J. R. *J. R. Soc. Med.* 1982, **75**, 151 and 818.
3. Aronoff G. N. et al. *Pain* 1983, **16**, 1; Bromm B. (ed.) *Pain Measurement in Man.* Amsterdam: Elsevier, 1984; Foley K. M. *Clin. Oncol.* 1984, **3**, 17; Smith G. and Covino B. G. *Acute Pain.* Butterworth: London, 1985.
4. Bromage P. R. *Epidural Analgesia.* Philadelphia: Saunders, 1978, p. 612.

5. Pilowsky I. *Clin. Anesthesiol.* 1985, **3**, 143.
6. Evans R. J. and MacKay I. M. *Can. J. Surg.* 1972, **15**, 50.
7. Twycross R. G. and Lack S. A. *Therapeutics in Terminal Cancer.* London: Pitman, 1983; Twycross R. G. *J. R. Coll. Phys.* 1984, **18**, 32.
8. Heel R. C. et al. *Drugs* 1978, **16**, 473.
9. Williams N. E. in: *Persistent Pain* (Lipton S. ed.) Vol. 1. London: Academic Press, 1977.
10. Oliver D. J. *Br. Med. J.* 1983, **287**, 1218.
11. Aherne G. W. et al. *Br. J. Clin. Pharmacol.* 1979, **8**, 577.
12. Lewis J. R. *JAMA* 1980, **243**, 1465.
13. Mehta M. in: *Recent Advances in Anaesthesia and Analgesia*—14 (Atkinson R. S. and Hewer C. L. ed.) Edinburgh: Churchill Livingstone, 1982.
14. Melzack R. *Clin. Anesthesiol.* 1985, **3**, 81.
15. Navarathnam R. G. et al. *Anaesth. Intensive Care* 1984, **12**, 345; *Advances in Pain Research and Therapy*, Vol. 2. New York: Raven Press, 1984, p. 509.
16. Melzack R. and Wall P. D. *The Challenge of Pain.* Harmondsworth: Penguin Books, 1982.
17. Forrest J. B. *Can. Anaesth. Soc. J.* 1978, **25**, 218; Perkins H. M. and Hanlon P. R. *Arch. Surg.* 1978, **113**, 253.
18. Pilowsky I. in: *The Therapy of Pain* (Swerdlow M. ed.). Lancaster: MTP Press, 1981.
19. Editorial *J. R. Soc. Med.* 1983, **76**, 905.
20. Maher R. M. *Lancet* 1955, **1**, 18; Nathan P. W. and Scott T. G. *Lancet* 1958, **1**, 76.
21. Maher R. M. *Lancet* 1963, **1**, 965; Swerdlow M. *Anaesthesia* 1973, **28**, 297.
22. Dogliotti A. M. *Presse méd.* 1931, **39**, 1249.
23. Moricca G. in: *Advances in Neurology* (Bonica J. J. ed.). No. 4. Liverpool: Raven Books, 1974; Corssen G. et al. *Anesth. Analg. (Cleve.)* 1977, **56**, 414; Cook P. R. et al. *Anaesthesia* 1984, **39**, 540.
24. Hitchcock E. *Lancet* 1967, **1**, 1133.
25. Lloyd J. W. et al. *Lancet* 1972, **1**, 354; Lloyd J. W. *Proc. R. Soc. Med.* 1973, **66**, 540.
26. Evans P. J. D. *Anaesthesia* 1981, **36**, 1003.
27. Duthrie A. *Anaesthesia* 1983, **38**, 448 and 495.
28. Behar M. et al. *Lancet* 1979, **1** 527.
29. Mathews E. *Lancet* 1979, **1**, 1724.
30. Snyder R. H. *Sci. Am.* 1977, **236**, 44.
31. Parris W. C. V. *Clin. Anesthesiol.* 1985, **3**, 93.
32. Coggeshall R. E. *Physiol. Rev.* 1980, **6**, 716.
33. Sweet W. H. and Wespic J. G. *J. Neurosurg.* 1974, **40**, 143.
34. Chaturvedi S. K. et al. *Pain* 1984, **19**, 87.
35. Richards R. L. *Arch. Neurol.* 1967, **16**, 339.
36. Lipton S. *Br. Med. J.* 1984, **289**, 98.
37. Brena S. F. and Chapman S. L. *Postgrad. Med.* 1981, **69**, 53; Tyrer S. P. *Br. Med. J.* 1986, **292**, 1.
38. Chapman S. L. *Clin. Anesthesiol.* 1985, **3**, 111.
39. Whitty C. W. M. et al. *Lancet* 1966, **1**, 856.
40. Marcus P. *J. R. Soc. Med.* 1983, **76**, 983.
41. Travell J. G. and Simons D. G. *Myofascial Pain and Dysfunction, the Trigger Point Manual.* Baltimore: Williams and Wilkins, 1983.
42. Lipton S. *Br. Med. J.* 1984, **298**, 98.
43. Cronin K. D. and Kirsner R. D. *Anaesthesia* 1982, **37**, 848.
44. Swerdlow M. and Cundill J. G. *Anaesthesia* 1982, **37**, 1129.
45. Jefferson A. L. *J. Neurol. Neurosurg. Psychiatry* 1963, **26**, 345.
46. Finneson B. E. *Diagnosis and Management of Pain Syndromes.* Philadelphia: Saunders, 1969. p. 325; Lipton S. in: *Recent Advances in Anaesthesia and Analgesia*—12 (Hewer C. L. and Atkinson R. S. ed.). Edinburgh: Churchill Livingstone, 1976; Otrofio B. M. *Proc. Staff Meet. Mayo Clin.* 1970, **45**, 689; Lipton S. *Anaesthesia* 1978, **33**, 953; Lipton S. in: *Textbook of Pain* (Wall P. D. and Melzack R. ed.) Edinburgh, Churchill Livingstone; 1984, Sect. 3B. No. 1.
47. Lipton S. *Clin. Oncol.* 1984, **3**, 195.
48. Lahuer J. et al. *Ann. R. Coll. Surg. Engl.* 1985, **67**, 41.
49. Nashold B. and Friedman H. *J. Neurosurg.* 1972, **36**, 590.
50. Loh L. et al. *Br. Med. J.* 1981, **1**, 1026.
51. Holland A. J. C. et al. *Can Anaesth. Soc. J.* 1977, **24**, 597.
52. Hannington-Kiff J. C. *Br. Med. J.* 1979, **2**, 367; Kepes E. R. et al. *Region. Anesth.* 1982, **7**, 52.
53. Walker P. M. et al. *Surg. Gynecol. Obstet.* 1978, **146**, 741.

54. Raynaud A. G. M. *Local Asphyxia and Symmetrical Gangrene of the Extremities*. London: The New Sydenham Soc., 1888, p. 150.
55. Feldman S. A. and Yeung M. L. *Anaesthesia* 1975, **30**, 174; Fyfe T. and Quin R. O. *Br. J. Surg.* 1975, 62, **68.**
56. Sudeck P. H. M. *Arch. f. Klin. Chir.* 1900, **62**, 147.
57. Kune G. A. et al. *Med. J. Aust.* 1975, **2**, 789; Thompson G. F. et al. *Anesth. Analg. (Cleve.)* 1977, **56**, 1
58. Jones J. and Gough D. *Ann. R. Coll. Surg.* 1977, **59**, 46; Thompson G. E. and Moore D. C. *Anesth. Analg. (Cleve.)* 1977, **56**, 1.
59. Morris R. W. and Loong E. D. *Anaesth. Intensive Care* 1984, **12**, 177.
60. Corssen G. et al. *Anesth. Analg. (Cleve.)* 1977, **56**, 414; Lipton S. *Anesthesiology* 1978, **33**, 953; Williams N. E. *Ann. R. Coll. Surg. Engl.* 1980, **62**, 263.
61. Pike P. M. H. *Anaesthesia* 1978, **33**, 165.
62. Nathan P. W. and Wall P. D. *Br. Med. J.* 1974, **3**, 645.
63. Lipton S. *Proc. R. Soc. Med.* 1974, **67**, 731.
64. Hannington-Kiff J. G. *Lancet* 1974, **1**, 1019; *Br. Med. J.* 1979, **2**, 367; Hannington-Kiff J. G. in: *Textbook of Pain* (Wall P. D. and Melzack R. ed.) Edinburgh, Churchill Livingstone; 1984, Sect. 3B, No. 1.
65. Hannington-Kiff J. G. *Lancet* 1978, **2**, 816; Barnard D. *Ann. R. Coll. Surg. Engl.* 1980, **62**, 180.
66. Evans P. J. D. et al. *J. R. Soc. Med.* 1981, **74**, 805.
67. Mehta M. in: *Recent Advances in Anaesthesia and Analgesia—14* (Atkinson R. S. and Hewer C. L. ed.) Edinburgh: Churchill Livingstone, 1982.
68. *Acupuncture Anaesthesia*. Peking: Foreign Language Press, 1973; Diamond E. G. *JAMA* 1971, **218**, 1558.
69. Yamaichi N. *Can. Anaesth. Soc. J.* 1976, **23**, 196.
70. Mayer D. J. et al. *Brain Res.* 1977, **124**, 523.
71. Lee D. C. *Can. Anaesth. Soc. J.* 1979, **26**, 410; Pomeranz B. *New Scientist* 1977, **73**, 12.
72. Edelist G. et al. *Can. Anaesth. Soc. J.* 1976, **23**, 303.
73. Chan C. S. and Chow S. P. *Br. J. Anaesth.* 1981, **53**, 899.
74. Carron H. et al. *JAMA* 1974, **228**, 1552; Bonica J. J. *JAMA* 1974, **228**, 1544.
75. Warwick-Brown N. P. and Richards A. E. S. *Br. Med. J.* 1985, **291**, 450.
76. Bonica J. J. in: *Textbook of Pain* (Wall P. D. and Melzack R. ed.) Edinburgh, Churchill Livingstone; 1984, Sect. 3B. No. 1.

Section 6 — Cardiorespiratory Intensive Therapy (Critical Care)

Chapter 34 — THE INTENSIVE THERAPY UNIT[1]

History of Intensive Care

An intensive therapy unit was opened in Copenhagen in 1953 by Björn Ibsen; the first to be run by anaesthetists. *See also* Hilberman M. *Crit. Care Med.* 1975, **3**, 159 and Symposium on Critical Care, *Anesthesiology* 1977, **47** (August).

Intensive therapy consists of the care of patients who are deemed to be recoverable[2] but who need continuous supervision and who need, or are likely to need, specialized techniques by experienced skilled personnel.[3]

Intensive therapy units provide for the management of the critically ill patient who requires facilities greater than those available in the traditional ward. They provide additional space, staff and equipment. The vital functions of the body can be continuously observed and when necessary supported promptly and efficiently.

Admission criteria should be worked out.[4] Certain broad groups may be defined: (1) Patients requiring the use of an artificial machine to support a vital system until the primary disease of the system is cured (e.g. ventilator, renal dialysis); (2) Patients requiring continuous monitoring (e.g. certain cases of cardiac infarction); (3) Certain patients with severe metabolic or electrolyte disorders; (4) Those who require heavy or specialized nursing (e.g. difficult tracheostomy, the comatose patient); (4) A place of safety for patients at risk of lethal complications.

Patients should not be admitted to an intensive therapy unit unless a definite therapeutic advantage for the patient is to be gained. The number of beds set aside for this purpose has been stated to be 1% of the acute bed complement of a hospital.[3] The anaesthetist has a major role to play in the management of patients in the unit because of (1) His special knowledge of ventilatory and resuscitation problems; (2) Wide knowledge of medical and surgical conditions; (3) Commitment to continuous communication with colleagues, nurses, patients and relatives, i.e. liaison.

Prediction of survival is possible and is a major aspect of the intensivist's work. The Apache system is gaining international recognition.[5] (*See* Chapter 39.)

Care of the dying patient is also an important intensive care skill.[6]

Design of the Unit[7]

A unit of 6–8 beds is an economic size (a 4-bed area and 2 side wards). Wall-mounted monitoring boxes are useful.[8] The plan should be as flexible as possible to allow for future changes. Mobile partitions are useful. About 18–28 m² floor space should be allowed for each bed. Piped oxygen, suction, adequate light, a wash-basin, fresh-air inlet pipe, exhaust pipe, sealable waste-disposal facilities and 8 electric sockets[9] per bed should be provided. The danger of cross-infection is a particular hazard.[10] Division into cubicles and the wearing of gowns and masks by the staff help to reduce this. Adequate storage space for equipment must be provided, and a small laboratory is advantageous. Staff facilities will occupy a space equal to the patient space. So will the storage area. A high staff/patient ratio is important.[11]

Stress in the Intensive Care Unit

Psychological aspects also require consideration.[12] Outside window views, radio, television and occupational therapy are vital factors for some patients. Diurnal rhythm of patients is maintained by modifying the regime at night: (1) Reduction of light to minimal adequate intensity; (2) Reduction of disturbance due to recording, to the safe minimum; (3) Silence as far as possible; (4) Sedation[13] is increased at night if possible; (5) Artificial feeding is 'cyclical' when possible.

Effects of stress include psychosis, exacerbated by cimetidine,[13] hallucinations, acute peptic ulceration (largely prevented by early enteral nutrition)[14] and reduced immunocompetence.[32] Prophylactic measures include sedation, antacids, cimetidine 200 mg i.v. t.d.s., clomipramine 25 mg t.d.s. and prevention of awareness in paralysed patients. (For importance of environmental conditions, especially temperature, *see* Lord Brock, *Br. J. Surg.* 1975, **62**, 253.) The critical environmental temperature for adults is 21 °C and for infants, 24 °C.

Cross-infection

Any organism may be involved, bacteria[15] (especially pseudomonas aeruginosa),[16] fungi,[17] viruses, e.g. AIDS.[18] Reduced by careful hygiene, handling of fomites, and hand cleansing of staff when moving between patients.

Computers in Intensive Care[19]

Development of the Computer
The first calculating machine was the abacus; then the 'pascaline' devised by Blaise Pascall (1623–1662) in 1644; the analytical engine of Babbage, 1832; the 'punch-card' (Hollerith) 1890; first electronic computer designed by Eckert and Mauchley in the US to calculate artillery firing tables (the ENIAC) in 1943.

Computer Terminology
Data = information. *File* = a stored quantity of data, with a name. *Terminal* = a typewriter keyboard with TV screen. *Network* = a computer with a group of terminals. *Address* = to ask or consult. *Intelligent* = having computing capability. *Slave* = under the control of a computer. *Core memory* = the data and programs within a computer (2 types, *ROM* = read only memory, this cannot be changed by the ordinary user, and *RAM* = random access memory, which can be added to, and erased by the user. *Dump* = to move data from memory to printer,

cassette or disc. *Disc* = a type of permanent data storage. *Call-up* = to move data from storage to memory. *Dedicated* = a device with just one function. *Basket* = a group of ideas. *VDU* = a TV screen. *BASIC* = a language (very similar to English) for making programs. *Program* = a set of instructions. *Software* = programs. *Hardware* = computers and similar equipment. *Password* = a code which allows access to confidential information.

The fields that are most useful at the present time include:
1. Data storage and retrieval.
2. Signal analysis—monitoring, diagnosis and prognosis making.
3. Medical education.
4. Word processing.
5. Trend analysis in results.[20]

A computer is only as accurate as the data entered and the person who operates it. (*See also* Computer Symposium, *Anaesth. Intensive Care* 1982, **10**, August; Hunter A. R. *Anaesthesia* 1984, **39**, 487; Prakash C. et al. *Computing in Anaesthesia and Intensive Care*, Boston: Martinus Nijhoff, 1984.)

Intensive Care of the Neonate[21] *and Infants*[22]

1. Temperature. The neonate is liable to heat loss and care should be taken not to expose the baby unnecessarily. A mattress with coils for circulation of warm water or an incubator is useful. Note that a stockinet cap is valuable since the head has a larger proportion of body-surface area than in the case of the adult. The normal neonate makes use of the metabolic activity of the brown fat to maintain body temperature. Small or premature babies or babies who have suffered from intrauterine malnutrition may have a lack of brown fat and so are at a disadvantage in the heat losing environment. Hyperthermia is also a risk.[23]
2. Feeding. This must be considered under the heading of water, electrolytes and calories. Dehydration can lead to fever, acidaemia, shock and brain damage. The normal weight loss in the first two days of life may be taken as 44 g/day/kg birth weight—about half as urine and faeces, and about half as insensible fluid loss. The small or premature baby is liable to severe hypoglycaemia if unfed, and this may be severe enough to produce brain damage or death. Hypernatraemia is also a risk and 1/5 normal saline is usually the strongest salt solution which should be given for maintenance infusion.
3. Acidaemia. If present this should be corrected before surgery. Arterial sampling is avoided if possible. If it is essential, the greatest care is taken with the arteries.
4. Oxygen. This is important in that while hypoxaemia may be dangerous, administration of high concentrations of oxygen may result in retrolental fibroplasia. Arterial oxygen tension can be measured, sampling being undertaken from umbilical artery catheters. Hypoxaemia results in inhibition of the brown-fat metabolism (*see above*). Assisted respiration may be necessary.
5. Cross-infection. One hazard particular to the neonate is that the cord stump can act as a culture medium for pathogenic organisms. This can be reduced by the use of a Polybactrin spray to the cord stump daily. *Pseudomonas pyocyanea* is a hazard and polymyxin methane sulphonate may be given as a protection. In babies on respirators it can be instilled into the trachea.
6. IPPV, e.g. in respiratory distress syndrome.[24] The small size of the patient calls for specially designed small tracheal tubes (e.g. Jackson Rees), small

ventilators, light weight small connections, fine suction catheters, all difficult in an incubator. Measurement of tidal volume is equally difficult, as is arterial sampling for blood-gas estimation. To prevent damage to the lungs from attempted spontaneous respiration during IPPV muscle relaxation with pancuronium has been recommended.[25] Special ventilators have been designed.[26]

7. *The Haemorrhagic shock and encephalopathy syndrome* has recently appeared.[27]

The Geriatric Patient in Intensive Care

An increasing number of elderly patients are to be seen in intensive care units. They present the following particular problems: (1) They frequently have low total body potassium;[28] (2) Many of them receive long-term digoxin therapy; (3) The serum albumin is frequently below 30 g/l with reduced colloid osmotic pressure and plasma drug binding; (4) Poor respiratory function is common; (5) Circulatory support is often needed; (6) The skin is more fragile; (7) Orientation may be poor; (8) There is a higher risk of the hyperosmolar syndrome, which presents as flushed facies with falling cardiac and renal output; (9) Significant disease is often not revealed by careful physical examination.[29]

Mobile Intensive Care[30]

For history of mobile medical emergency units (*see* Drouet N. *Br. Med. J.* 1982, **284**, 1924; Park G. R. and Johnson S. *Anaesthesia* 1982, **37**, 1204.)

Specially designed and equipped ambulances and helicopters have been used[31] to provide a resuscitation and ambulance service outside the hospital. They are equipped to a high level for intubation of the trachea, IPPV, monitoring and ventricular defibrillation. Foot-operated aspirators are carried. In some areas a mobile coronary care service has been provided, in conjunction with education of the public in first-aid resuscitation. Radiocommunication and facilities for ECG telemetry may be available. An anaesthetist may go with the team. For portable lung ventilators *see* Gray A. J. G. *Br. J. Hosp. Med.* 1981, **25**, 173; Marsh R. H. K. and Ledingham I. McA. *Br. J. Hosp. Med.* 1981, **25**, 377.

Transport of sick and injured children (*see* Owen H. and Duncan A. W. *Anaesth. Intensive Care* 1983, **11**, 113). Airway management in transfer of the unconscious patient (*see* Robinson N. and Macleod K. G. H. *Ann. R. Coll. Surg. Engl.* 1983, **63**, 372). Ambulance equipment (*see* Woollam H. M. *Br. J. Hosp. Med.* 1982, **27**, 538).

References

1. Hinds C. J. *Intensive Care.* Baillière Tindall, 1987; Rippe J. M. et al. *Intensive Care Medicine.* Boston: Little Brown, 1985: Oh T. E. *Intensive Care Manual.* Australia: Butterworth, 1985.
2. Champion H. R. *Crit. Care Med.* 1982, **10**, 552.
3. BMA Planning Unit Report No. 1, *Intensive Care*, November 1967.
4. Telpick R. et al. *Anesth. Analg. (Cleve.)* 1983, **62**, 572.
5. Le Gall J. R. et al. *Crit. Care Med.* 1982, **10**, 575; Keene A. R. and Cullen D. J. *Crit. Care Med.* 1983, **11**, 1.
6. Cohen C. B. *Crit. Care Med.* 1982, **10**, 776; Micetich K. C. *Arch. Intern. Med.* 1983, **143**, 975.

7. Robinson J. S. *Br. J. Anaesth*. 1966, **38**, 132; Sherwood Jones E. *Postgrad. Med. J*. 1967, **43**, 339; BMA Planning Unit Report No. 1 *Intensive Care*, November 1967.
8. Ryan D. W. et al. *Br. Med. J*. 1982, **285**, 1634.
9. *Hospital Building Note, Intensive Therapy Unit*, No. 27, 1970, London: HMSO.
10. Seal D. V. and Strangeways J. M. *Anaesth. Intensive Care* 1981, **19**, 260.
11. Gribbens R. E. and Marshall R. E. *Crit. Care Med*. 1982, **10**, 865; Phillips G. D. et al. *Anaesth. Intensive Care* 1983, **11**, 118.
12. Fuller B. F. and Foster G. M. *Heart Lung* 1982, **11**, 457.
13. Cerra F. B. *Ann. Surg*. 1982, **196**, 565.
14. Pringleton S. and Hadzima S. K. *Crit. Care Med*. 1983, **11**, 13.
15. Muder R. R. et al. *JAMA* 1983, **249**, 3184.
16. Freeman R. and McPeake P. K. *Thorax* 1982, **37**, 732.
17. Craven P. C. et al. *Ann. Intern. Med*. 1983, **98**, 160.
18. Davis K. C. et al. *Ann. Intern. Med*. 1983, **98**, 284.
19. Blackburn J. P. *Br. J. Clin. Equip*. 1976, **1**, 122; Franklin C. B. in: *Recent Advances in Anaesthesia and Analgesia—13* (Hewer C. L. and Atkinson R. S. ed.). Edinburgh: Churchill Livingstone, 1979; Paull J. D. *Anaesth. Intensive Care* 1980, **8**, 336; Phillips G. D. et al. *Anaesth. Intensive Care* 1982, **10**, 223; Prakash O. et al. *Crit. Care Med*. 1982, **10**, 811.
20. Kendall R. I. *Am. J. Clin. Pathol*. 1983, **79**, 217.
21. Tizard J. P. M. *Proc. R. Soc. Med*. 1967, **60**, 935; Inkster J. S. in: *Recent Advances in Anaesthesia and Analgesia—12* (Hewer C. L. and Atkinson R. S. ed.). Edinburgh: Churchill Livingstone, 1976; Boyle M. H. et al. *N. Eng. J. Med*. 1983, **308**, 1330.
22. Boyle M. H. *N. Engl. J. Med*. 1983, **308**, 1330.
23. David P. and Mughal R. *J. R. Soc. Med*. 1985, **77**, 721.
24. Valman H. B. *Br. Med. J*. 1979, **2**, 1483.
25. Pollitzer M. J. et al. *Lancet* 1981, **1**, 346.
26. Hall M. W. and Peevy K. J. *Crit. Care Med*. 1983, **11**, 26.
27. Levin M. et al. *Lancet* 1983, **2**, 64.
28. Morgan D. B. et al. *Postgrad Med. J*. 1978, **54**, 72.
29. Del Guerico L. R. M. and Cohn J. D. *JAMA* 1980, **243**, 1350.
30. Harries M. G. *Br. Med. J*. 1979, **2**, 426; Ledingham I. Mc. A. and Banks J. G. *Hospital Update* 1980, **6**, 43; Simpson D. S. and Thys D. M. *Anaesthesia* 1978, **33**, 965; Harber T. W. and Lucas B. G. B. *Ann. R. Coll. Surg. Engl*. 1980, **62**, 291; Park G. R. et al. *Br. J. Anaesth*. 1982, **54**, 1081.
31. Cruikshank A. D. N. *Anaesthesia* 1981, **36**, 427.
32. Watkins J. and Salo M. *Trauma, Stress and Immunity in Surgery and Anaesthesia*. London: Butterworth, 1982.

Chapter 35   # FAILURE OF THE CARDIOVASCULAR SYSTEM, INCLUDING SHOCK

Acute Myocardial Infarction[1]

Patients with recent infarction are liable to develop cardiac asystole or ventricular fibrillation. This is thought to be due to an electrical imbalance in the myocardium and is not necessarily related to the size of the infarct. If resuscitation can be carried out promptly and cerebral hypoxia is prevented, there is a good chance of restoration of cardiac function and the prognosis is hopeful.

Such patients require intensive monitoring. The electrocardiogram is usually recorded continuously, and alarm systems are activated if the heart rate rises above or falls below preset limits. Apparatus for cardiac resuscitation is kept immediately at hand so that defibrillation or cardiac pacing can be carried out at once if required. Blood pressure must be recorded frequently and some workers prefer a direct arterial line for continuous recording. Other parameters to be monitored may include central venous pressure and blood-gas analysis, pulmonary artery wedge pressure, cardiac output, lactate levels, urinary output.

Indications for Admission of Infarction Patients to Intensive Care Units
(1) Infarction with pump failure requiring balloon pumping[2] or emergency or planned coronary artery bypass grafting;[3] (2) Infarction plus other organ failure, e.g. cerebral hypoxia, respiratory failure requiring IPPV, severe hypovolaemia, etc.; (3) Severe dysrhythmias.

Cardiopulmonary Resuscitation[4]
See Chapter 37.

Treatment
1. *Relief of pain.* Opioids in full dose i.v. with anti-emetics, buprenorphine, Entonox. Diamorphine is often used.
2. *Oxygen.* May be given by mask, nasal catheter or tent. Hyperbaric oxygen has been used.
3. *Dysrhythmias.* About 80% of patients show some form of dysrhythmia in the first few days following infarction. Occasional atrial or ventricular ectopic beats may be ignored, but R upon T ectopics may lead to ventricular fibrillation. Slow intravenous injection of lignocaine up to 100 mg (or 1–2 mg/kg) is suitable for ventricular ectopic beats. Supraventricular bradycardia may be treated by atropine in doses of 0·3 mg up to a total of 2 mg. Heart block, when complete and associated with a failing circulation, must be treated by electrical pacing.[5] β-blockers, especially those with intrinsic sympathomimetic activity, e.g. practolol, in doses up to 20 mg i.v. are useful for supraventricular ectopic beats. Verapamil, lignocaine, flecainamide and quinidine may also be required. Indications for and complications of temporary cardiac pacing by the transvenous method.[6]
4. *Cardiac shock (pump failure).* Profound hypotension (systolic blood pressure below 60 mmHg) further reduces coronary perfusion. Treatment may include: (a) Catecholamines, e.g. dopamine 5–20 µg/kg/min, isoprenaline or ephedrine; the calcium channel blockers nifedipine and diltiazem; and the vasodilators nitroprusside and nitroglycerin; (b) Careful increase of preload with CVP monitoring; (c) Reduction of after-load by α-blockade and nifedipine; (d) Frusemide diuresis for congestive failure. Balloon pumping in the aorta is an effective method of prolonging life when the patient is *in extremis*[7] and may allow time for coronary bypass graft to be carried out. Extracorporeal membrane oxygenation and urgent coronary artery bypass graft may be needed in the extreme case.
5. *Digitalis.*[8] Digoxin, 0·25–0·5 mg, may be given for uncontrolled atrial fibrillation.
6. *Corticosteroids.*
7. *Anticoagulants.*
8. *Measurement of acid–base state.* This may show the presence of metabolic acidosis. Correction with intravenous sodium bicarbonate may result in a rise in systolic blood pressure.

Shock[9]

Shock may be described as any haemodynamic disturbance causing such a degree of reduced capillary flow that tissue hypoxia leading to functional and/or morphological changes is produced. In the past the main emphasis has been on indirect blood pressure and pulse rate measurement. Account must also be taken of venous return and venous pressure, cardiac output, peripheral resistance, velocity of blood flow, tissue perfusion, and maintenance of organ function.

History

The term 'shock' was coined in the sense in which it is now employed by Thomas A. Latta, of Leith, Scotland, in 1832,[10] who used an intravenous infusion of salt solution in the treatment of cholera in 1831–2. Sir Christopher Wren (1632–1723) more than 150 years before this gave an intravenous infusion, using a quill and bladder, the first intravenous syringe, into a dog.[11]

Theories of causation have included the following: (1) Vasomotor collapse or vasodilatation (G. W. Crile (1865–1943), 1899); (2) Vasoconstriction (Malcolm, 1905); (3) Carbon-dioxide depletion—acapnic theory of shock (Yandell Henderson (1873–1944), Yale physiologist, 1909);[12] (4) Increased capillary permeability leading to hypovolaemia, the cause being toxic substances liberated in the injured area (W. B. Cannon (1871–1945), Boston physiologist, and Sir W. M. Bayliss (1860–1924), London physiologist, 1919); (5) Fluid loss at site of injury (Alfred Blalock (1899–1964), 1930); (6) Vasoconstriction due to hypovolaemia (Freeman, 1933); (7) Left ventricular failure as a contributing factor (C. J. Wiggers (1893–1963), of Cleveland, 1947); (8) Bacteraemia.

First scientific investigation into the causes of shock took place during the First World War. Haemorrhage is the commonest cause of shock.
(*See also* The pathophysiology of haemorrhagic shock. Runciman W. B. and Skowronski G. A. *Anaesth. Intensive Care* 1984, **12**, 193.)

Signs and Symptoms of Blood Loss

Loss of up to 15% blood volume; BP normal, tachycardia, postural hypotension. Loss of up to 30% BP begins to fall, heart to beat faster, complaint of thirst, patient feels ill and weak. Up to 40% progressive fall in BP, restlessness, oliguria, air hunger, confusion, coma and death.

The chief factor in shock is relative or absolute depletion of blood flow and replacement of that flow is the major therapeutic exercise. In severe shock congestion and haemorrhagic necrosis of mucosa of the small intestine may occur. Bacterial endotoxins play a part in the production of the syndrome.

What was formerly known as primary shock is now termed 'vasovagal collapse', which is characterized by a slow pulse, unlike the tachycardia associated with true (secondary) shock. The elderly and dysautonomic often lack the protective responses to shock.

Assessment of Shock

The clinical examination is still of primary importance: (1) Peripheral skin perfusion; (2) Pulse volume; (3) Arterial blood pressure; (4) Level of consciousness; (5) Skin/core temperature gradient; (6) Urine output; (7) Central venous pressure; (8) ECG (S–T segment depression); (9) Acid–base status (including blood lactate); (10) Cardiac output measurement; (11) Diuretic test. For prognosis *see* Ledingham.[13]

Assessment of Response to Treatment

(1) Ability to think and converse shows reasonable brain perfusion; (2) Urine flow shows reasonable renal perfusion; (3) Acidosis may worsen temporarily from washing out of lactate from previously ischaemic extremities.

Causes

1. Hypovolaemia. A loss of up to 1000 ml of blood is usually well compensated by splanchnic and cutaneous vasoconstriction. The body reacts by an increase in sympathetic activity with increased heart and respiratory rates, cold, pale, clammy skin, thirst and oliguria. If bleeding continues, true oligaemic shock is seen. Heart rate may rise. In early stages, haemoglobin percentage is no index of blood lost. The decreased blood volume causes a decreased venous pressure, a decreased venous return and so a decreased cardiac output. Arterial pressure is well maintained at first, but falls later. Pulse pressure is increased early.

Should the patient with haemorrhagic or wound shock not receive intravenous fluid he may:

a. Become rehydrated from his own tissue fluids, his cardiac output returning to normal, but he remains anaemic. This is the hyperkinetic phase and in it rapid blood or fluid transfusion may overload the circulation and cause heart failure. A slow drip of packed red-cell suspension is required, or—

b. He fails to rehydrate himself and passes into peripheral circulatory failure. A normal man has a blood volume of 5 litres.

Shock may also be due to fluid depletion, e.g. (*a*) plasma, electrolyte fluid, due to burns or trauma; (*b*) dehydration; (*c*) losses into the gut.

2. Central circulatory collapse

Causes of Cardiogenic Shock. (1) Myocardial ischaemia; (2) Dysrhythmias; (3) Acidosis, toxins and drugs; (4) Respiratory failure hypoxia; (5) Damage during bypass; (6) Cardiac trauma and tamponade; (7) Disruption of cardiac structure (e.g. valves); (8) Pulmonary embolism.

Management of Acute Central Circulatory Failure (Cardiogenic Shock). (1) Correction of hypovolaemia if present, using CVP if possible; (2) Loop diuretics, e.g. frusemide 20–100 mg; (3) Catecholamines, e.g. (*a*) dopamine 5–20 µg/kg/min i.v. (also specifically raises renal blood flow); (*b*) dobutamine 5–10 µg/kg/min; (*c*) salbutamol 100 µg and isoprenaline 1 µg/kg/min—may cause dysrhythmias; (*d*) noradrenaline and adrenaline; (4) Balloon pumping (*see* p. 765); (5) Cardiopulmonary bypass with membrane oxygenator (*see* Chapter 29); (6) Diuretics and vasodilators—*see below*; (7) Digoxin has undergone a revival of interest in recent years.[14]

(*See also* Fisher M. McD. *Anaesth. Intensive Care* 1986, **14**, 17.)

3. Peripheral circulatory collapse.

a. Hormone Deficiency, e.g. adrenal cortical deficiency.

b. Anaphylaxis.[15] (Anaphylaxis is the opposite of prophylaxis meaning 'to be on guard', a neologism coined by Richet C. R. (Nobel prizewinner, 1913), *Anaphylaxis*, Eng. transl. Liverpool University Press, 1913, p. 2). Classically, a reaction to foreign protein. Onset usually within a few minutes of exposure and is characterized by pruritus, urticaria, dyspnoea, wheezing, syncope, nausea and vomiting, rhonchi and râles in the chest, hypotension, cyanosis and flushing or pallor. Treatment may include: oxygen, attention to pulmonary ventilation and removal of secretions, an intravenous drip with colloid fluids (500–1000 ml) and vasopressors, massive corticosteroids. Antihistamines must be used with care as they increase vasodilatation. Cimetidine prophylaxis may be considered.

c. Tissue Trauma. Circulating toxins, the results of tissue autolysis or infection, are absorbed into the circulation from damaged tissue. They injure the endothelial lining of the capillaries, causing leakage of fluid into tissue spaces and producing a reduced blood volume, hypotension and oliguric renal failure (reduced glomerular filtration rate). If condition is progressive, venous return to heart and cardiac output are reduced and blood pressure falls. But this fall is not a sign of incipient shock; rather it is a sign that the circulatory system is not able to cope with the emergency. Renal failure may be due to the effect of these same toxins on the renal epithelium.

4. Bacteraemic; septicaemic; endotoxic shock.[16] Prevention is better than cure! Mortality is up to 30%.[17] Septic infection, with Gram-negative organisms (e.g. *Escherichia coli*), but also *Strep. pneumoniae* and other organisms, can cause a state of acidosis, acute hypotension, oliguria and reduced peripheral blood flow and reduced liver function.[18] Jaundice is common and is an indication to search for undrained pus or other nidus of infection. Plasma thromboxane A_2 is raised in non-survivors but not in survivors.[19] There is intrapulmonary shunting and perhaps mental confusion. The condition may come on acutely over a period of a few hours. Treatment includes intravenous fluids, especially colloids and blood, antibiotics, metronidazole, corticosteroids,[20] naloxone,[21] and adjustment of acid–base balance. The pulmonary complications (adult respiratory distress syndrome) also require intensive care. *See* Chapter 38.

5. Neurogenic

a. Operative Trauma or Injuries may cause shock due to sudden afferent stimulation, e.g. disarticulation of the hip joint; rapid dilatation of a pregnant cervix uteri; traction on the spermatic cord; perineal injuries; acute inversion of the uterus; traction on the gallbladder or cardiac end of the stomach. Signs often disappear with the cessation of the stimulus.

b. Subjection to Massive G Forces. Sudden deceleration in aerospace and motor-racing accidents, or sudden acceleration, e.g. in bomb blasts, without other injury may lead to cessation of circulation and respiration. This resolves spontaneously after a few minutes of cardiac massage and mouth-to-mouth respiration.

c. Head Injuries. Subarachnoid haemorrhage, quadriplegia.

Shock may be made worse by: cold; pain; rough movement of the patient; hypoxia.

6. Haemorrhagic shock and encephalopathy. A fulminant fatal disease of infants.[22]

Effects of Shock

1. Decreased oxygen consumption and carbon dioxide production.

2. Fall in body temperature.

3. Secretion of adrenaline with all its effects. Hyperglycaemia in the initial period, followed by hypoglycaemia in late shock as glycogen stores are depleted.

4. Rise of blood lactate[23] and pyruvate. The concept of excess lactate production as an indication of tissue hypoxia was introduced by W. E. Huckabee.[24] In severe and prolonged shock a greater rise in blood lactate is

observed. The lactate/pyruvate or L/P ratio may be valuable if an early estimation is available for comparison.

5. Metabolic acidosis[25] commonly occurs.

6. Depletion of body protein, with increase of urinary nitrogen (catabolism).

7. Secretion of ADH and aldosterone. Fall in serum sodium and chloride and rise in potassium. Reduced excretion of sodium, chloride and water.

8. Fall in serum levels of ascorbic acid and decreased excretion of ascorbic acid, riboflavin, thiamine and nicotinamide.

9. Increase of hypothalamic–pituitary–adrenal activity. Increase of ACTH secretion.

10. Impairment of liver function—tests may be abnormal.

11. The kidneys ('shock kidney'). During shock the rate of urine flow indicates parallel changes in glomerular filtration rate. The urine may contain protein casts. The relationship of shock to the development of acute renal insufficiency is not clear. Patients particularly at risk include those who have shock in association with septic abortion, Gram-negative septicaemia, haemoglobinuria, myoglobinuria, intra-abdominal trauma, aortic surgery, acute liver failure and burns. Renal function often recovers in up to 2 weeks. Dialysis may be needed in the meantime.

12. The lungs. Shock lung may occur.[26] Adult respiratory distress syndrome, *see* 'Respiratory failure'.

13. Reduced coronary perfusion. Myocardial infarction may occur.

14. Hypoxic brain damage.

15. Stagnant hypoxia and disseminated intravascular coagulation.

16. Blood thyroxine levels are reduced.[27]

17. Reflex tachycardia and vasoconstriction.

The following conditions may be confused with shock:

Fat embolism. See Chapter 39.

Air embolism. See Chapter 18.

Amniotic fluid embolism. See Chapter 27.

Differential Diagnosis of Hypovolaemic Shock

The following conditions may also give rise to a shock-like state: (1) Perforation of viscera; (2) Acute high intestinal obstruction; (3) Severe burns; (4) Certain drugs used in anaesthesia, e.g. opiates, phenothiazines, halothane; (5) Interference with venous return to heart due to position or to pressure on the vena cava from abdominal tumours, e.g. the pregnant uterus near term; (6) Following intradural or extradural analgesia; (7) Anaphylaxis; (8) Disseminated intravascular coagulopathy.[28]

Methods of Estimating Blood Loss

See Chapter 41.

Management of Hypovolaemic Shock[29]

The aim is maintenance of organ function (especially brain). Try to arrest haemorrhage. Elevate legs 15–20°. Lowering of the head is not now recommended; 10° head-down tilt has been shown to cause fall in arterial blood pressure.[30] Prolonged head-down position may also be disadvantageous as there is a risk of cerebral oedema, retinal detachment, brachial plexus damage, and nursing care is made more difficult. Antishock trousers—(pneumatic)[31] and simple raising of the legs are effective and do not affect lung function. Thirst may be more distressing than pain, but is better relieved by mouthwashes and intravenous fluid than by drinks, if operation is pending.

Opioids should be injected intravenously to ensure rapid controlled absorption. Only about one-quarter of seriously injured and shocked patients require opioids for pain relief and rarely should 10 mg of morphine be exceeded. They should not be given if there is severe brain injury, respiratory depression or an acute abdomen. Naloxone prevents respiratory depression.

Transfusion of whole blood is of paramount importance, especially if haemorrhage has been marked, and it should be given at a rapid rate, controlled, if necessary, by central venous pressure monitoring. *See* Chapter 41.

Oxygen inhalation helpful as intrapulmonary shunting occurs. Very useful in cases where oxygenation is deficient, e.g. wounds of chest, patients who are cyanosed. Should be given if there is severe haemorrhage, tachycardia or respiratory depression and may need to be combined with IPPV.

Infusion of colloids and crystalloids. If blood is not immediately available any isotonic fluid should be infused as a temporary measure.[32] Blood acid–base balance and Pao_2 levels are very useful estimations and are a guide to treatment. Venous blood oxygen tension is a measure of the adequacy of oxygen flow to the tissues. 4 kPa or more is a normal value. If the intravenous route is not available, oral, rectal and subcutaneous routes may be employed. PAWP and CVP are invaluable diagnostic aids.

Drugs in Shock

Pressor drugs.[29] Pressor agents reduce blood flow to the renal cortex and medulla. These drugs have little place, except in the operating theatre to buy time.

Isoprenaline. A β-stimulator. When given by intravenous infusion (1–450 000) this causes peripheral vasodilatation and has achieved success, especially in cases of endotoxic shock and in heart failure and in open heart surgery. Salbutamol i.v. can be used.

Dopamine. Said to have the advantages of isoprenaline without its disadvantages. It acts on dopaminergic β_1- and α-receptors; the biological precursor of noradrenaline. It dilates renal and mesenteric vascular beds. Available in a 4% solution. A naturally occurring catecholamine. Dobutamine is also a selective inotropic drug. (*See* Chapter 19.)

Vasodilators. Only used after full volume replacement.

1. Phenoxybenzamine, 0·1 mg/kg, repeated. Duration 24 h. Also has a sedative effect. Recommended for endotoxic shock.

2. Thymoxamine 0·1 mg/kg, repeated. α-blocker. Onset in 15 min, duration 2–4 h.

3. Phentolamine 10 mg, repeated. α-blocker. (Also recommended for hypertensive crises and phaeochromocytoma.)

4. Nitroprusside.

5. Nitroglycerin.

Sodium bicarbonate. For the correction of any metabolic acidosis which may be present. A reasonable first dose would be 50 mmol. Further dosage would depend on laboratory findings.

Hydrocortisone. This has, as well as anti-inflammatory, positive inotropic and α-blocking effects. Dose: 25–50 mg/kg i.e. up to 2 g intravenously in a short period. The plasma volume must be maintained as vasodilatation results. Dexamethasone and methylprednisolone are alternatives.

Antibiotics, if septic shock is suspected.

More can be achieved in the treatment of shock by promoting tissue perfusion than by simply raising the blood pressure. The administration of vasodilator agents must always be accompanied by infusion of adequate amounts of plasma-volume expanders. Central venous pressure measurement is a valuable guide to intravenous infusion. Oxygen should be administered to prevent hypoxia and to improve the oxygen supply to the brain.

Salt and Water Balance

Definitions
A mole (mol) is the molecular weight expressed in grams. A millimole (mmol) is a thousandth of a mole. Molality is the number of moles of solute in 1000 grams of solvent. Molarity is the number of moles of solute in 1 litre of solution (a molar solution) and so depends partly on temperature.

Fluid Balance
The healthy adult may have a daily water intake of 2600 ml (1100 ml in food and 1500 ml as drink). An output of 2600 ml may consist of 1500 ml as urine, 100 ml in faeces, 400 ml from the lungs and 600 ml via the skin. The healthy kidney can concentrate the 24-h excretory products into 500 ml with a specific gravity as high as 1032. Fluid control in the postoperative patient is a delicate balance between dehydration and waterlogging. Balance is easily achieved in the younger patient but is difficult in the elderly. The young are often run too dry and the old, too wet.

Deficit
Fluid losses may be increased in many circumstances. In hot climates the insensible loss may be as high as 2000 ml in 24 h. Losses are also increased with diarrhoea, vomiting, paralytic ileus, intestinal fistulae and cholera. Clinical signs of dehydration occur when 6% of body water has been lost, and in severe dehydration 10% may have been lost.

Diagnosis. On clinical and laboratory evidence.

Clinical. Thirst, dryness of mouth (because of scantiness of saliva) and oliguria. Thirst is more characteristic of fluid than of salt depletion. Loss of skin elasticity, sunken eyes.

Laboratory. Raised blood urea, haemoglobin, haematocrit and plasma proteins. High specific gravity of urine with decreased output. Raised plasma osmolality above 300 mosmol/kg.

Treatment. Abnormal loss of fluid should be replaced by an equal volume of fluid of the same electrolyte composition to that lost, in addition to the normal fluid requirements of the body. In exceptional cases, as much as 6 litres a day may be necessary, e.g. intestinal fistulae.

Prophylactic. Use of an intravenous drip during operation.

Curative. Water by mouth, rectum, vein or hypodermocylsis. Isotonic fluids infused i.v. include physiological saline, Hartmann's solution and 5% glucose. It is common practice to administer 500 ml 4-hourly, 1 unit of physiological saline to 2 units of isotonic glucose.

Table 35.1 Composition of some fluids used for intravenous infusion

Constituents		g %	Na	K	Cl	Lactate
					mmol/l	
Isotonic saline	NaCl	0·9	153	—	153	—
Ringer lactate	NaCl	0·6	102	—	102	—
(Hartmann's solution)	Na lactate	0·31	28	—	—	29
	KCl	0·03	—	4	4	—
	CaCl$_2$	0·02	—	—	4	—
			130	4	110	29
Extracellular fluid			140	5	103	—
(for comparison)						

Table 35.2 Average figures for electrolyte losses in secretions from various sites

	Na	K	Cl	vol/day (ml)
		mmol/l		
Stomach	60·4	9·2	84·0	1500
Small intestine	111·3	4·6	104·2	3000
Bile	148·9	4·98	100·6	1500
Pancreatic juice	141·1	4·6	76·6	1000
Recent ileostomy	129·4	11·2	116·2	1000
Established ileostomy	46	3·0	21·4	700
Caecostomy	52·5	7·9	42·5	700

Electrolyte Balance. *See* Chapter 3.

The Metabolic Response to Injury

This occurs after operation and is characterized by: (1) Impairment of water excretion. Lasts 24–36 h. Independent of salt and water intake; (2) Impairment of sodium excretion. Lasts 4–6 days. Independent of sodium intake; (3) Increased potassium excretion. Maximal in 24 h. Usually lasts only 48 h; (4) Hyperglycaemia.

This response is associated with an increased secretion of adrenocortical hormones, an impairment of their breakdown and an increased production of antidiuretic hormone. The essential stimulus is probably via a nervous reflex, relaying in the hypothalamus.

Problems from Infusion Fluid Containers

1. Sepsis. Growth of organisms within an intravenous pack can reach 10^6 or 10^7 organisms/ml without turbidity being detected and this concentration infused can cause severe and fatal septicaemia. Infection also occurs at the point where the intravenous line penetrates the skin; Giving sets should be changed every 24–48 h and always after blood has been used. Infusion teams to supervise intravenous drips have been employed.

2. Pulmonary microembolism. The particles may be plastic, rubber, bacterial, air or dust.

In-line filtration is available, which removes these particles during infusion without seriously impeding flow. The mesh size within a filter diminishes progressively in the direction of flow from about 10 µm down to around 0·1–0·5 µm. These filters are not satisfactory for using with blood transfusion!

References

1. *See also* Chamberlain D. in: *Intensive Care* (Gerson G. ed.). 2nd ed. London: Heinemann, 1981.
2. Tobias M. A. et al. *Anaesthesia* 1979, **34**, 844.
3. Gilston A. in: *Recent Advances in Anaesthesia and Analgesia*—13 (Hewer C. L. and Atkinson R. S. ed.). Edinburgh: Churchill Livingstone, 1979.
4. Donovan K. D. *Anaesth. Intensive Care* 1985, **13**, 41 and 63.
5. Donovan K. D. *Anaesth. Intensive Care* 1985, **13**, 41.
6. Donovan K. D. and Lee K. Y. *Anaesth. Intensive Care* 1985, **13**, 63.
7. Dunkman W. B. et al. *Circulation* 1972, **46**, 465; Mundth E. D. et al. *Circulation* 1972, **45**, 1279; *Ann. Surg.* 1973, **178**, 379; Curtis J. J. et al. *Mayo Clin. Proc.* 1977, **52**, 723.
8. Withering W. M. (1741–1799) *An Account of the Foxglove and some of its Medical Uses,* Birmingham, 1785.
9. Wilson R. F. *Int. Care Med.* 1980, **6**, 89.
10. Latta J. A. *Lancet* 1832, **1**, 274 (reprinted in 'Classical File'. *Surv. Anesthesiol.* 1970, **14**, 563).
11. Wren C. *Phil. Trans. R. Soc.* 1665, **1**, 128.
12. Hendeson Y. *Am. J. Physiol.* 1908, **21**, 126.
13. Ledingham I. McA. *Br. Med. J.* 1982, **284**, 643.
14. Berman W. et al. *N. Engl. J. Med.* 1983, **308**, 363.
15. Portier P. and Richet C. R. *C. R. Séanc. Soc. Biol.* 1902, **54**, 170; Thornton J. A. *Br. J. Anaesth.* 1982, **51**, 1; Levy J. H. *Anaphylactic Reactions in Anaesthesia and Intensive Care.* London: Butterworth, 1986.
16. Wardle M. *Br. J. Hosp. Med.* 1979, **21**, 223; Thomas D. and Withington P. S. *Ann. R. Coll. Surg. Engl.* 1985, **67**, 156.
17. Hook E. W. *JAMA* 1983, **249**, 1055.
18. Banks J. G. *J. Clin. Pathol.* 1982, **35**, 1249.
19. Reines H. D. et al. *Lancet* 1982, **2**, 174.
20. Lansing A. M. *Can. Anaesth. Soc. J.* 1963, **89**, 583; Annotation, *Lancet* 1963, **2**, 1265.
21. Weissglas I. S. *J. Surg. Res.* 1982, **33**, 131.
22. Levin M. et al. *Lancet* 1983, **2**, 64.
23. Vincent J. L. *Crit. Care Med.* 1983, **11**, 449.
24. Huckabee W. E. *J. Clin. Invest.* 1958, **37**, 264.
25. Root W. S. et al. *Am. J. Physiol.* 1947, **149**, 52.
26. Beyer A. *Br. J. Hosp. Med.* 1979, **21**, 248.
27. Vitek V. *Surgery* 1983, **93**, 768.
28. Preston F. E. *Br. J. Hosp. Med.* 1982, **28**, 129.
29. Tinker J. *Br. J. Hosp. Med.* 1979, **21**, 261.
30. Taylor J. and Weil M. H. *Surg. Gynecol. Obstet.* 1967, **124**, 1005; Gunteroth W. G. et al. *Surg. Gynecol. Obstet.* 1964, **119**, 245.
31. Abraham E. *Crit. Care Med.* 1982, **10**, 754.
32. Alexiv O. et al. *Anaesthesia* 1975, **30**, 609; McGowan R. G. *Anaesthesia* 1975, **30**, 623.

Chapter 36   *OXYGEN THERAPY*[1]

Modern oxygen therapy initiated in 1917 by J. S. Haldane (1860–1936).[2] The first satisfactory measurement of blood oxygen content performed in 1924.[3]

The fundamental aim of oxygen therapy is to restore the tissue oxygen tension towards normal. A partial pressure of at least 1·3 kPa is required at the cellular mitochondria.[4] An increase in the percentage of oxygen in the inhaled gases results in a rise in alveolar oxygen concentration and a rise in oxygen tension in the blood leaving the lungs. Oxygen therapy is most valuable when the blood oxygen tension is low (hypoxic hypoxia). In anaemic and stagnant hypoxia it does not greatly increase the amount of oxygen carried by haemoglobin, though the rise in dissolved oxygen in the plasma is significant. It is doubtful whether histotoxic hypoxia is benefited by oxygen therapy.

Some Relevant Physiological Data

Oxygen content of air 20·93%. Oxygen content of expired air 16·3%. Oxygen content of alveolar air 14·2%. Partial pressure of oxygen in air 21 kPa (160 mmHg). Partial pressure of oxygen in alveolar air 13·3 kPa (104 mmHg). Partial pressure of oxygen in venous blood 5·3 kPa (40 mmHg). Solubility of oxygen in plasma 0·3 ml/100 ml. Oxygen capacity of haemoglobin 1·34 ml/g Hb. Oxygen capacity of arterial blood 19·8 vol%. Oxygen saturation of arterial blood 97%. Oxygen tension of arterial blood 13 kPa (100 mmHg).

Oxygen Flux

The amount of oxygen available in the body can be calculated as follows: 100 ml of blood contains 19·8 ml of oxygen when fully oxygenated. If the cardiac output is 5 l/min, then the oxygen available (oxygen flux) to the body is 19·8 × 50 = 990 ml/min. Normal oxygen consumption is 250 ml/min. There is thus a large reserve. In severe exercise, cardiac output increases to 20 l/min, quadrupling the oxygen flux. Demands in excess of this build up a temporary oxygen debt, by anaerobic metabolism. Oxygen monitoring (*see* Chapter 41):[5] pulse oximetry.[6]

Oxygen flux to individual organs (e.g. brain) also merits consideration.

Types of Oxygen Lack

'Oxygen lack not only stops the machine, but wrecks the machinery' (J. S. Haldane).

Cyanosis may be detected by trained observers when the reduced Hb is only 1·5 g/dl, though for many people, detection is only possible at 5 g/dl (Pa_{O_2}=8 kPa, 55 mmHg).[7]

Reduced utilization of oxygen by tissues may be of the following types—the first three were described by Joseph Barcroft[8] (1872–1947) (1920), the fourth by Peters and van Slyke[9] (1883–1971) (1931).

1. Hypoxic hypoxia. The arterial Po_2 is low. It occurs whenever oxygen is prevented from reaching the pulmonary capillaries.

Diffusion hypoxia may occur during recovery from nitrous oxide anaesthesia. Air containing nitrogen enters the alveoli. This results in a reduction of concentration of oxygen since there is also a large concentration of nitrous oxide present. The remedy is to give oxygen in high concentration towards the end of the anaesthesia and for some time after its termination.[46]

Alveolar oxygen tension is also reduced when the concentration of carbon dioxide in alveolar gas is increased. Pa_{O_2} and Pa_{CO_2} are linked by the *alveolar air equation:*

$$PAO_2 = PIO_2 - \frac{PACO_2}{R}$$

R is the respiratory exchange ratio (usually 0·8). The equation can also be written:

$$PAO_2 = PIO_2 - 1·25 \times PACO_2.$$

The relationship between PAO_2 and $PACO_2$ is linear, and the line will be shifted if PIO_2 is changed.
2. *Anaemic hypoxia.* Oxygen-carrying capacity of blood is reduced in proportion to degree of anaemia although the oxygen tension is normal.
3. *Stagnant hypoxia.*[10] Two types: (*a*) Low cardiac output; (*b*) Local, due to partial or complete vascular occlusion.
4. *Histotoxic or cytotoxic hypoxia.* Occurs when tissues are unable to utilize the normal supply of oxygen brought to them; seen in cyanide poisoning and overdosage of narcotics and anaesthetics due to interference with dehydrogenase systems.

The Effects of Oxygen Want
For physiological effects of oxygen lack at altitude *see* Mills F. J. and Harding R. M. *Br. Med. J.* 1983, **286**, 1269. Commercial aircraft are pressurized to between 5000 and 7000 ft (1524–2134 m).
1. *The respiratory system.* Hyperpnoea is due to reflex stimulation of respiratory centre by chemoreceptors in aortic and carotid bodies which react to the lowered oxygen tension. The glomus cells normally have a high oxygen uptake; when tension falls, anaerobic metabolism causes the release of substances which stimulate pericellular chemosensory nerve endings. The respiratory centre becomes less sensitive to carbon dioxide with increasing hypoxia. Dyspnoea and hyperpnoea are not necessarily indications for oxygen therapy, as both may be seen without hypoxia, just as hypoxia can occur without these symptoms.
2. *The cardiovascular system.* Coronary systemic and cerebral vasodilatation, with large decreases in afterload, increased cardiac output, stroke volume and tachycardia. Arterial pressure falls in simple hypoxia, but rises if hypercapnia coexists. Effects similar in the anaesthetized and conscious subject. In severe hypoxia, cardiovascular collapse occurs. The ECG: T wave becomes inverted or decreased and there is slowing of conduction and a lengthening of the P–R interval. Capillaries lose their tone and their walls allow the leakage of fluid and cells into the tissues. Pulmonary vasoconstriction occurs.
3. *The central nervous system.* In healthy young men, the oxygen utilization of the brain is 3·3 ml/100 g of brain/min or about one-fifth of the body's total oxygen consumption. The nervous tissue is more susceptible to oxygen want than any tissue in the body. The blood flow to the brain is increased, an effect also produced by the raised carbon dioxide tension which is often concurrent. Later oedema of the brain results from capillary damage. The CSF pressure is increased. Hypotension greatly magnifies the brain-damaging effect of hypoxia.

The Effects of Inhalation of 100 per cent Oxygen
Using a well fitting mask and breathing pure oxygen, 96% of nitrogen is eliminated from the lungs, with a Magill (Mapleson-A) system.[11]
Oxygen carriage in the blood (*see* Chapter 2).

Nitrogen is eliminated from the lungs in 2 min, from the blood in 5 min, from the brain in 20 min and from the body in about 2 h.[11]

Carbon dioxide. As reduced haemoglobin aids in the transport of carbon dioxide, inhalation of 100% oxygen, by lessening the amount of reduced haemoglobin, interferes with the transport of carbon dioxide, especially if the gas is given at a raised pressure.

Table 36.1 Results of inhalation of pure oxygen

	Breathing air O_2 21 kPa (159 mmHg)	Breathing 100 per cent oxygen O_2 104 kPa (760 mmHg)
Alveolar air		
Oxygen tension	13·3 kPa (104 mmHg)	90 kPa (675 mmHg)
Arterial blood		
Oxygen tension	13 kPa (100 mmHg)	85 kPa (637 mmHg)
Oxygen saturation	97%	100%
Oxygen combined with haemoglobin	19·5 ml %	20·1 ml %
Oxygen in solution in plasma	0·3 ml %	1·9 ml %
Total oxygen content	19·8 ml %	22·0 ml %
Mixed venous blood		
Oxygen tension	5·3 kPa (40 mmHg)	7 kPa (52 mmHg)
Oxygen saturation	75%	85%
Oxygen combined with haemoglobin	15·07 ml %	17·19 ml %
Oxygen in solution in plasma	0·12 ml %	0·16 ml %
Total oxygen content	15·19 ml %	17·35 ml %

Arterial blood contains an additional 2·2 vol %, a rise of more than 10%, after inhalation of pure oxygen. This represents about 50 ml O_2 transported to the tissues per min or about one-fifth of requirements. Fluorocarbon (Fluosol DA 20%) carries 0·75 ml/100 ml 10 kPa[47] (i.e. 7·5 ml/100 ml at FIo_2 100%).

Respiration. This is often slightly depressed at first, owing to the removal of the stimulating effect through chemoreceptors.

Circulation. There is decrease in the pulse rate, from chemoreceptor effect. Slight increase in diastolic blood pressure. Blood vessels directly constricted (reflexly, via chemoreceptors, dilated), former effect predominating. Cerebral vessels constrict, coronary vessels also constrict, but pulmonary artery dilates, constricting in hypoxia. Very prolonged administration of oxygen may interfere with red-cell formation.

Adverse Effects of High Oxygen Concentrations

Chronic bronchitis and emphysema. In patients who develop respiratory failure, oxygen is needed to correct hypoxia, but it must be given in a controlled manner otherwise a dangerous rise in arterial Pco_2 may occur as the hypoxic drive is removed. The danger is that a state of CO_2 narcosis may develop with loss of consciousness and ultimately death. The risk of this chain of events is said to be greater when arterial Pco_2 is already above 10 kPa.

Controlled oxygen therapy is required. The aim is to give enough oxygen to relieve hypoxia, but not enough to remove the respiratory drive. The characteristics of the dissociation curve for haemoglobin are such that a relatively small rise in oxygen tension will result in a relatively large increase in saturation in the middle part of the curve. Pao_2 estimations aid therapy. 'Pink puffers' may be benefited by oxygen.[12]

Intermittent oxygen therapy is particularly dangerous since the increased alveolar CO_2 concentration which may then occur results in an even lower O_2 concentration when the patient breathes air. (*See* the alveolar air equation, *see* p. 752).

Should oxygen administration, carefully regulated, fail to correct hypoxia without depressing respiration, then IPPV becomes necessary.

Following hypoxia. The oxygen paradox was first described by Ruff and Strughold in 1939. Has subsequently been re-examined by Latham.[13] It is a temporary blackout due to the sudden administration of a high oxygen atmosphere, seen in airmen. If the gas is first inhaled at normal tensions, and later gradually increased, ill effects are not seen.

Retrolental fibroplasia. The formation of a fibrovascular membrane, posterior to the lens, may occur in premature babies who have been exposed to high concentrations of oxygen. (There are other causes of this condition.) Pao_2 should be kept between 6·5 and 13 kPa by adjusting inspired concentration. Danger exists when Pao_2 remains high for a significant period of time and inspired oxygen concentration should not normally exceed 40%. Higher oxygen concentrations may carry a risk with regard to lung toxicity even for short periods during active resuscitation. Doubt has been cast on the relationship of the administration of a high oxygen atmosphere to neonates and retrolental fibroplasia.[14]

Oxygen toxicity. *Acute* oxygen poisoning is manifest as convulsions, the Paul Bert effect.[15] These are similar in nature to idiopathic epilepsy, and do not occur except under hyperbaric conditions (3 atmospheres). The causes have not been fully elucidated, though the incidence appears to be related to an increased cerebral Pco_2. *Chronic* poisoning may occur when concentrations over 60% are inhaled for prolonged periods at atmospheric pressure. Perhaps due to inactivation of surfactant and damage to pulmonary epithelium. Untoward effects reported[16] include substernal distress, reduction in vital capacity, paraesthesiae, joint pains, anorexia, nausea, contracted visual fields, vomiting, bronchitis and atelectasis, and mental changes.

This is a problem in the intensive care unit when IPPV is carried out with high inspired oxygen concentrations over a long period.[17] X-ray changes may then occur due to oxygen toxicity. These take the form of bilateral patchy opacities spreading to the whole of the lung fields.[18] There is then increase of alveolar–arterial Po_2 difference, so that despite high inspired oxygen, Pao_2 may be low. The mechanism of such lung damage by oxygen in uncertain. Suggested effects are: (1) Airways closure leading to atelectasis in the absence of nitrogen; (2) Loss of surfactant; (3) Lesions may be due to the primary condition requiring IPPV. It may nevertheless be justified to administer high concentrations of oxygen when Pao_2 cannot be raised to acceptable levels by any other means.

While in a healthy person inspiration of 100% oxygen may be harmful if continued for more than a few hours, 40% can be inhaled indefinitely, with impunity. The crucial level may be the arterial Po_2. Free oxygen radicals are proposed as the causative factor in alveolar damage in these circumstances, by inactivating the antiprotease α_1-antitrypsin of alveolar cells. Leucocytes activated by complement then flood the area giving the typical picture of leucoaggregates and intra-alveolar haemorrhage and exudation.[19]

(*See also* Karsner H. T. *J. Exp. Med.* 1916, **23**, 149 (reprinted in 'Classical File', *Surv. Anesthesiol.* 1972, **16**, 495); Poulton E. C. *Aerospace Med.* 1974, **45**, 482.)

Indications for Oxygen Therapy

The relief of all forms of hypoxia other than histotoxic. Cardiac output is important as well as arterial oxygen tension.

1. Cyanosis of recent origin. Cardiopulmonary disease. Venous to arterial shunts, intracardiac or intrapulmonary, are the only types of hypoxaemia not completely corrected by the inhalation of 100% oxygen.[20]

2. Following major operations, chest wounds or rib fractures. The 35% Ventimask is satisfactory as is the nasal catheter or cannula.[21] After major surgery under general anaesthesia many patients suffer from periodic episodes of apnoea if pain is controlled by morphine. Oxygen therapy increases oxygen saturation without influencing the number of such attacks.[22] If pain is controlled by some form of regional analgesia, such attacks do not occur.[23]

3. In shock and severe haemorrhage and coronary occlusion. The central feature of shock is diminished cardiac output leading to reduction in cellular oxygenation. In shock there is an increase in physiological dead space and a compensatory hyperventilation. Reduction of this hyperventilation by airway obstruction, chest injuries, drugs, etc. may be dangerous. Oxygen administration may prevent the vicious circles which end in death.

4. To decompress distended bowels, reduce surgical emphysema, pneumothorax and air embolism. The gas imprisoned in these cases is 70% nitrogen. Prolonged inhalation of 100% oxygen reduces the nitrogen tension in the blood, so that the molecules of gas in the tissues diffuse into the blood and are carried away.

5. When metabolic rate is raised, e.g. in postoperative thyrotoxicosis and hyperthermia, because in these conditions the demand for oxygen is increased.

6. In carbon monoxide poisoning.

7. In the treatment of pneumatosis coli.[24]

8. In cases of severe headache due to retained intracranial air following encephalography. In migraine to produce vasoconstriction of cerebral vessels.

9. Preoxygenation before induction of anaesthesia.

Commercial oxygen is pure enough for inhalation and is much cheaper than medicinal oxygen. Oxygen therapy presents a definite fire hazard. In all cases a patent airway must be ensured.

Inspired oxygen concentration and Pa_{O_2} should be considered together. It is sometimes possible to predict the change in Pa_{O_2} which will occur with changes in $F_{I_{O_2}}$. In theory, measurement of cardiac output would also be valuable in conjunction with Pa_{O_2}. Or Pv_{O_2} might be measured directly.[25]

Technique of Administration

The first method of oxygen administration was from a glass funnel held some distance from the face. The first to advocate a closely fitting face-mask was Leonard Hill.[26] Modern oxygen therapy requires separate devices for administering oxygen in high and low concentration.

Oxygen-administration devices can be classified into:[27] (1) Fixed-performance system—patient independent; (*a*) high air flow oxygen enrichment

(HAFOE)—Ventimasks;[28] (*b*) lower flow—anaesthetic circuits; (2) Variable performance system—patient dependent; (*a*) without rebreathing—catheters and cannulae; (*b*) with rebreathing—MC, Polymask. The former group supply the predetermined oxygen concentration irrespective of the patient's ventilatory parameters. The latter group vary in their performance according to the patient's inspiratory flow-rate and duration of the expiratory pause.

Reservoirs. Use of a reservoir prevents wastage of oxygen but may allow rebreathing with low flows. The T-piece system can be used, the degree of air dilution or rebreathing being determined by flow-rates, tidal volumes and the volume of the expiratory limb. The majority of commercial face-masks may be considered as modifications of the T-piece system, the mask dead space being equivalent to the expiratory limb of the T.

1. *The MC (Mary Catterall) oronasal masks.*[29] A plastic cone mask with padded foam to encourage a good fit to the face. A flow of 6 l/min oxygen provides an F_{IO_2} of about 60%, but there is significant dead space at low flows.[30]

2. *Harris mask.* Made from stiff semi-translucent plastic with small dead-space volume. F_{IO_2} approaches 60% with a flow of 6 l/min.

3. *Ventimask.* A HAFOE device (*see above*). Oxygen is entrained in air on the Venturi principle to provide a concentration of 24, 28 and 35%. The oxygen flow-rates are written on the mask. There is no apparatus dead space. The Venturi[31] method is useful for providing controlled oxygen concentration, such as is required in the treatment of chronic lung disease.[32] It has been shown that the oxygen concentration in the trachea may be up to 5% less than that delivered from the Ventimask,[33] probably due to the addition of water vapour, also when peak flow exceeds the 32 l/min supplied by the 35% mask (*see also* Bethune D. W. and Collis J. M. *Br. J. Clin. Equip.* 1977, **2**, 305).

4. *Edinburgh mask.*[34] This is a semi-rigid mask designed to give controlled oxygen at low concentrations. At 1 l/min the F_{IO_2} is 25–29%; at 2 l/min 31–35%; at 3 l/min 33–39%.

5. *A nasal catheter.* First used by Arbuthnot Lane in 1907. Size 9 (Jaques) is suitable, and its terminal 7–10 cm should be smeared with analgesic cream. The distal end lies in the nasopharynx. When a pharyngeal airway is in place, the catheter should be inserted into it.[35] With it an oxygen flow of 3 l/min raises inspired oxygen concentration to 30–60%. Accidental rupture of the stomach has been reported following oxygen therapy by nasopharyngeal catheter.[36] A T-piece dipping into 5 cm of water in a vessel is a safety factor and acts as a blow-off if the tip of the catheter slips into the oesophagus. A humidifier should be used.

6. *Plastic nasal cannulae.* These are now available.

7. *BLB mask* (Boothby, Lovelace and Bulbulian, 1938).[37] The oronasal and the nasal types.

8. *The portable oxygen apparatus*, e.g. the B.O.C. Portogen.

9. *An oxygen chamber or tent.* This is best for babies and young children, and when prolonged administration is necessary. To enable real benefit to be obtained from a tent, it must be flushed with 10 l/min of oxygen and maintained with a flow of 8 l/min. It gives lower levels of oxygen concentration than the various masks and spectacles.

The Head Tent[38] (Vickers) is an alternative form. A Venturi system is used to provide oxygen concentrations up to 34%.

The Croupette Type D apparatus is useful for paediatric use. It can yield concentrations of 27–49% with oxygen flow-rates between 2 and 20 l/min.[39] With the Intensive-care Isolette Incubator and oxygen flow between 1 and 4·5 l/min, the oxygen concentration at the baby's lips may be between 58 and 71%.[39] For adults, an uncooled low-volume tent (HiCon Tent) has been described, which gives a rapid rise in oxygen concentration and a high equilibrium level.

10. *IPPV* can be carried out in ill patients or following major surgery. It can be maintained for 12–24 h and allows administration of analgesic drugs, e.g. narcotic analgesics, without depression of ventilation. The F_{IO_2} can be controlled by dilution of oxygen with air, using flow-metres or a blending device.

Choice of Method

1. When high F_{IO_2} required: MC mask; anaesthetic circuit.

2. When controlled F_{IO_2} required: Ventimask or Edinburgh mask.

3. When small rise in F_{IO_2} required but dose not critical: above masks or nasal catheter.

4. When the patient is uncooperative: oxygen tents. IPPV after sedation and tracheal intubation may be considered.

A study of different methods of oxygen administration[40] showed that patients found nasal cannulae more comfortable than face-masks. The latter are likely to be hot and sweaty and patients cannot eat or spit. Oxygen tents hold little advantage and the patient is less accessible and less easy to observe. Cannulae, the Edinburgh mask and the Ventimask are without significant rebreathing. Oxygen given by cannulae requires humidification. *See also* a study of dead space in various types of mask.[41]

Oxygen therapy should be controlled by serial estimations of F_{IO_2} and Pa_{O_2} when carried out over a period of days, to prevent use of unnecessarily high concentrations with risk of lung damage. Positive end-expiratory pressure may be advantageous when high inspired concentrations fail to correct arterial hypoxaemia (*see* Chapter 15). (*See also* Symposium on Oxygen Therapy and Physiology, *Anaesth. Intensive Care* 1979, **7**, 77; Benson M. K. *Prescriber's Journal* 1979, **19**, 9.) Pulse oximetry may be useful.[6]

Oxygen Concentrators

These produce oxygen (94% pure) from room air by the absorption of atmospheric nitrogen on Zeolite (Gk—to seethe) crystals (an aluminosilicate). Two or more absorption tanks are used alternately in each machine, one producing oxygen and the other being purged of nitrogen ready for its next cycle. The smallest machines produce 3 l/min, at a cost of about 3·7 pence/l, slightly more than liquid oxygen and ⅔ of the price of cylinder oxygen.[42]

Hyperbaric Oxygen

Breathing air, 100 ml of plasma will dissolve 0·3 ml of oxygen. For each 13 kPa (100 mmHg) of oxygen tension 0·3 vol% oxygen is dissolved in the plasma. Breathing 100% oxygen, 100 ml of plasma will thus dissolve 2·1 ml of oxygen. Breathing 100% oxygen at 2 atmospheres, 100 ml of plasma will dissolve 4·2 ml of oxygen. Breathing 100% oxygen at 3 atmospheres, 100 ml of plasma will dissolve 6·5 ml of oxygen.

An efficient and rapid method of restoring cellular oxygenation is to give the gas under pressure. At 2 atmospheres pressure, although the oxygen carried as oxyhaemoglobin will only increase by 1 vol %, the gas carried in solution in the plasma rises from 0·3 to 4·2 vol %. The pressure gradient is greatly increased between the arterial and the hypoxic tissue tension and this allows an increased rate of oxygen transport from blood to cells.

Vascular resistance is increased during hyperbaric oxygenation, especially in the brain and pulmonary circulation.

Oxygen at high pressure can be given from a pressure chamber into which patient and attendants enter. The patient then receives oxygen from an ordinary mask and cylinder. A pressure of 2 atmospheres is generally employed. Decompression is accompanied by a sharp fall in temperature with mist formation due to condensation. This may be uncomfortable for patients and staff. Otherwise the hyperbaric oxygen bed can be used. This consists of a steel chamber with perspex dome in which the patient lies at an oxygen pressure of 2·5 atmospheres. Rate of compression and decompression is controlled from an adjacent console.

High-pressure Oxygen in Medical Conditions[43]
(1) In treatment of carbon-monoxide poisoning; (2) In the treatment of infections by anaerobic organisms, e.g. gas gangrene. The growth of aerobic organisms may also be inhibited; (3) In incipient gangrene and frostbite; (4) For topical application in the treatment of pressure-sores and skin ulcers; (5) In purpura fulminans; (6) In burns; (7) Acute trauma;[44] (8) In acute ischaemic vasculitis; (9) Acute and chronic sepsis, resistant to orthodox treatment.

Elimination of Carbon Dioxide
During hyperbaric oxygenation, haemoglobin remains fully saturated, even in the venous blood. The buffering capacity of the blood is not increased by the presence of desaturated haemoglobin. Carbon dioxide is therefore transported in venous blood at a higher cost in terms of P_{CO_2}. Arteriovenous difference in P_{CO_2} may double. The rise in venous and tissue P_{CO_2} occurs also at the respiratory centre to give an increase in ventilation. The fall in arterial P_{CO_2} which results compensates in part for the raised tissue P_{CO_2} and is probably partly responsible for the cerebral vasoconstriction which occurs with hyperbaric oxygen.

The finding of a significant rise in P_{CO_2} of the blood during exercise in the hyperbaric chamber has little to do with the above. It is due rather to the increased density of the inhaled gas mixture, and occurs with both air and oxygen under pressure. The resistance to gas flow is such that there is an increase in the work of breathing. The body adapts by lowering alveolar ventilation and allowing a higher P_{CO_2}.

High-pressure Oxygen during Radiotherapy[45]
There is evidence that this has a definite advantage during treatment of tumours of the head and neck, cervix and bronchus.

Dangers of Hyperbaric Oxygenations
These include: (1) Risk of fires and explosions; (2) 'Bends', unless nitrogen has been eliminated; (3) Acute oxygen toxicity and convulsions; (4) Avascular necrosis of bone; (5) Barotrauma—ear discomfort; (6) Inflammation of the lungs (Lorraine-Smith effect).

(*See also* Leigh J. M. in: *General Anaesthesia* (Gray T. C. et al. ed.), 4th ed. London: Butterworth, 1980, Vol. 1. Ch. 27.)

References

1. *See also Uses and Dangers of Oxygen Therapy*. Edinburgh: HMSO, 1969; Leigh J. M. in: *Scientific Foundations of Anaesthesia* (Scurr C. and Feldman S. A. ed.), 2nd ed. London: Heinemann, 1974, p. 253; Sykes M. K. et al. *Respiratory Failure*, 2nd ed. Oxford: Blackwell, 1976, Chap. 7; Leigh J. M. in: *General Anaesthesia* (Gray T. C. et al. ed.), 4th ed. London: Butterworth 1980, vol. 1. Chap. 27.
2. Haldane J. S. *Br. Med. J.* 1917, **1**, 181.
3. Van Slyke D. D. and Neill J. M. *J. Biolog. Chem.* 1924, **61**, 523.
4. Flenley D. C. *Lancet* 1967, **1**, 270.
5. Hanning C. D. *Br. J. Anaesth.* 1985, **57**, 359.
6. Byrick R. J. *Can. Anaesth. Soc. J.* 1984, **31**, 397; Nunn J. F. *Anaesthesia* 1987, **42**, iv.
7. Kelman G. R. and Nunn J. F. *Lancet* 1966, **1**, 1400.
8. Barcroft J. *Lancet* 1920, **2**, 485.
9. Peters J. P. and van Slyke D. D. *Quantitative Clinical Chemistry*. Baltimore: Williams and Wilkins, 1932, Vol. 2, p. 579.
10. Barcroft J. *Nature* 1920, **106**, 125.
11. Berthoud T. M. et al. *Anaesthesia* 1983, **38**, 96.
12. Woodcock A. A. et al. *Lancet* 1981, **1**, 907.
13. Latham F. *Lancet* 1951, **1**, 77.
14. Flynn J. T. *Anesthesiology* 1984, **60**, 485.
15. Bert, Paul, *La Pression Barométrique*. Paris, 1878.
16. Barach A. L. *Ann. Intern. Med.* 1938, **12**, 454.
17. Leading Article, *Lancet* 1970, **4**, 1292; Winter P. M. and Smith G. *Anesthesiology* 1972, **37**, 210; Sevitt S. *J. Clin. Pathol.* 1974, **27**, 21; Deneke S. M. and Fanburg B. L. *Br. J. Anaesth.* 1982, **54**, 737.
18. Joffe M. and Simon M. *Radiology* 1969, **92**, 460.
19. Till G. O. *J. Trauma* 1983, **23**, 269.
20. Drummond G. B. *Br. J. Anaesth.* 1975, **47**, 491; Drummond G. B. and Wright D. J. *Br. J. Anaesth.* 1977, **49**, 789; Drummond G. B. and Milne A. C. *Br. J. Anaesth.* 1977, **49**, 1093; Leigh J. M. *Br. J. Anaesth.* 1969, **41**, 376.
21. Tantum K. R. *Anesthesiology* 1969, **31**, 376.
22. Jones J. G. et al. *J. R. Soc. Med.* 1985, **78**, 1019.
23. Catley D. M. et al. *Anesthesiology* 1985, **63**, 20.
24. Watson R. D. S. *Br. Med. J.* 1976, **1**, 199.
25. Flenley D. C. et al. *Br. Med. J.* 1973, **1**, 78.
26. Hill L. *Br. Med. J.* 1912, **1**, 71.
27. Leigh J. M. *Anaesthesia* 1971, **25**, 210.
28. Campbell E. J. M. *Lancet* 1982, **2**, 1206.
29. Catterall M. et al. *Lancet* 1967, **1**, 415.
30. Bethune D. W. and Collis J. M. *Thorax* 1967, **22**, 221.
31. 'Venturi and Bernoulli' *Lancet* 1983, **1**, 183.
32. Cox D. and Gillbe C. *Anaesthesia* 1981, **36**, 958; Campbell E. J. M. *Lancet* 1982, **2**, 1206.
33. Gibson R. L. et al. *Anesthesiology* 1976, **44**, 71.
34. Flenley D. C. et al. *Br. Med. J.* 1963, **2**, 1081.
35. Komesaroff D. *Anaesth. Intensive Care* 1974, **2**, 182.
36. Fenton E. N. S. *Br. J. Anaesth.* 1956, **28**, 220; Walstad P. M. and Conklin W. S. *N. Engl. J. Med.* 1961, **264**, 1201.
37. Series of papers, *Proc. Staff Meet. Mayo Clin.* 1938, **13**, 641 et seq.
38. Campbell E. J. M. and Gebbie T. *Lancet* 1966, **1**, 468.
39. Simpson H. and Russell D. J. *Br. Med. J.* 1967, **4**, 201.
40. Green I. D. *Br. Med. J.* 1967, **2**, 593.
41. Bethune D. W. and Collis J. M. *Anaesthesia* 1967, **22**, 43.
42. *Drug Ther. Bull.* 1982, **20**, 65; Harris C. E. and Simpson P. J. *Anaesthesia* 1985, **40**, 1206; Carter J. A. et al. *Anaesthesia* 1985, **40**, 560.
43. Loder R. E. *Anaesthesia* 1980, **35**, 761.

44. Loder R. E. *Ann. R. Coll. Surg. Engl.* 1979, **61**, 472.
45. Henk J. M. et al. *Lancet* 1977, **2**, 101 and 104, Report of MRC, Working Party, *Lancet* 1978, **2**. 881.
46. Fink B. R. *Anesthesiology* 1955, **16**, 511.
47. Faithfull N. S. *Anaesthesia* 1987, **42**, 234.

Chapter 37   **RESUSCITATION**

Historical[1]

It is now well known that a patient is not necessarily dead because his heart has stopped beating but this was not always so. Attempts at cardiopulmonary resuscitation are of comparatively recent date.

Expired air ventilation has been used throughout history in an effort to revive the apparently dead.[2] Tracheostomy was performed in the twelfth and thirteenth centuries in the treatment of drowned persons. Paracelsus (1493–1541) is usually credited with the introduction of the bellows to ventilate the lungs.

Modern history of resuscitation begins in the middle of the eighteenth century. This was a period when a wave of humanitarianism spread through Europe. A Society for the Recovery of Drowned Persons was founded in Amsterdam in 1767. In Britain the Humane Society, later the Royal Humane Society, was established by William Hawes in 1771. Classic early contributions to the literature include those of John Hunter (1718–1783)[3] in 1776, Kite[4] in 1788 and Herholdt and Rafn.[5]

Artificial ventilation of the lungs was advocated by Marshall Hall (1790–1857)[6] in 1856, the discoverer of reflex action, who described a method of rotating the patient's body combined with pressure on the back to aid expiration. Silvester (1818–1902)[7] described his method in 1858, and Holger Nielsen[8] published details of a new technique in 1932. In the same year Eve (1871–1952) introduced the tilting board method.[9] Artificial respiration by direct laryngeal intubation with a modified O'Dwyer's tube was performed by Rudolph Matas of New Orleans in 1902.[10] In the past four decades positive-pressure ventilation applied to the upper airways has displaced these methods.[11] First use of IPPV in respiratory paralysis by Lassen of Copenhagen in 1952.[12]

Reports of deaths during anaesthesia, in the years following 1846, led to interest in the study of cardiac arrest. The first successful internal cardiac massage was probably performed in Norway in 1901[13] and by Beck in 1947.[20] The first in Britain was reported by Starling (1866–1927)[14] in 1902. Beck[15] successfully defibrillated the human heart in 1937. First external defibrillation of the human heart in 1956.[16] External cardiac compression became popular following the work of Kouwenhoven and others in 1960.[17] Teaching aids in resuscitation are valuable.[18] First successful cardiopulmonary resuscitation outside the operating theatre by Beck in 1956.[19] Cardiopulmonary resuscitation should form part of the curriculum of every young doctor.[21] In some hospitals cardiopulmonary resuscitation officers are now being appointed.

(For history of resuscitation in the nineteenth century, *see* McLellan I. *Anaesthesia* 1981, **36**, 307.)

Cardiac Arrest

Coronary artery disease is the commonest cause.[22]

Cessation of the heart beat occurs in two entirely different forms: (1) Cardiac asystole; (2) Ventricular fibrillation. The two cannot be differentiated by clinical observation, but only by electrocardiography or direct inspection of the heart.

Asystole and ventricular fibrillation can change one to the other, either spontaneously or as a result of treatment.

Asystole. No complex on the ECG.

Ventricular fibrillation. First described by MacWilliam (1857–1937),[23] of Aberdeen. There is a fine or coarse irregular uncoordinated twitching of the heart-muscle fibres. Metabolism continues at about the normal rate. During fibrillation blood pressures of 20–30 mmHg have been observed, but this is due to residual vascular tone and there is no flow of blood.

Causes of Cardiac Arrest

1. Cardiac disease. Certain forms of cardiac disease are particularly prone to sudden arrest; (*a*) Where there is a danger of acute circulatory obstruction (atrial myxoma or ball-valve thrombus with change of posture); (*b*) In fixed output states (tight valvular stenosis, constrictive pericarditis, severe pulmonary hypertension, cardiac tamponade); (*c*) Cardiac myopathies; (*d*) Myocardial ischaemia; (*e*) Acute myocarditis.

2. Haemorrhage. Massive haemorrhage may cause cardiac arrest due to a fall in coronary perfusion pressure. There is also the danger of hyperkalaemia in massive transfusions of stored blood.

3. Hypoxia. Hypoxia results in: (*a*) Tachycardia and rise of blood pressure (sympathetic stimulation) leading to bradycardia, heart block and asystole; (*b*) Serum potassium may rise by 50% in 5 min; (*c*) Potentiation of the depressant effects of drugs. The end-result is usually cardiac asystole.

4. Fainting. This may be fatal if the patient is prevented from assuming the horizontal position. There is a danger of this during anaesthesia (e.g. in the dental chair) and in the postoperative period if the patient is sat up in bed.

5. Electrocution. See Chapter 5.

6. Drowning. See p. 767.

7. Electrolyte changes. Administration of *potassium* ions leads to loss of conductivity, contractility and a decreased theshold to vagal stimulation. Eventually, if given slowly, the heart action ceases in diastole. If given quickly, causes ventricular fibrillation. *Calcium* administration leads to increased contractility, prolongation of systole, shortening of diastole and eventual cardiac arrest in systole. The ratio of potassium to calcium in the blood is important. Rise of serum potassium occurs in anuria, dehydration, diabetic acidosis, drowning in fresh water, extensive tissue breakdown, in transfusion of stored blood, and in hypoxia. Intravenous iron and mercurial diuretics have caused cardiac arrest.

8. Effect of drugs. Has occurred during administration of all the anaesthetic agents in common use (especially halothane when increasing the inspired tension too rapidly during induction, in an effort to save time), cyclopropane, chloroform, intravenous agents, local and spinal techniques. Anaesthetic drugs may exert an effect on the heart in a variety of ways: (*a*) Direct myocardial depression (specific impairment of contraction of the muscle fibres); (*b*) Vagotonic effect; (*c*) Sympathetic stimulation; (*d*) Increased excitability of ventricular muscle; (*e*) Hypotension, especially in patients with inability to increase cardiac output (severe valvular stenosis, heart block, constrictive pericarditis); (*f*) Hypoxia as a result of respiratory depression; (*g*) Hypercapnia associated with respiratory depression.

9. *Hypercapnia.* Results in: (*a*) Increase of circulating catecholamines; (*b*) Increase of serum potassium level; (*c*) Prolongation of the period of asystole induced by vagal stimulation.

In a healthy patient, moderate hypercapnia is well tolerated in the absence of hypoxia.

Sudden hypocapnia after a period of hypercapnia is associated with severe dysrhythmias and even ventricular fibrillation in dogs, the Brown and Miller effect.[24]

In asphyxia there is both hypoxia and hypercapnia.

10. *Hypothermia. See* Chapter 17.

11. *Acute hypotension.* For example, after central neural blockade.

12. *Cardiac catheterization and angio-cardiography.* Ventricular fibrillation may occur, most likely when the tip of the catheter is in the right ventricle.

13. *Vagal reflex mechanisms.* Sources of stimuli which may provoke bradycardia or asystole include the rectum, uterus and cervix, glottis, bronchial tree, bladder and urethra, mesentery, the carotid sinus, heart, biliary tract, traction on extraocular muscles (especially the medial rectus) and testis. Atropine may prevent them.

14. *Circulating catecholamines.* The heart is more sensitive to adrenaline in the presence of anaesthetic drugs, especially chloroform, cyclopropane, halothane, trichloroethylene and in the presence of myocardial hypoxia. A rise in the blood catecholamine level occurs with injection of adrenaline, anxiety, adrenal tumours and after haemorrhage. Fenfluramine (a common obesity treatment) acts as a catecholamine. Discontinuation for 1 week before anaesthesia, has been recommended.[25]

15. *Air embolism and pulmonary embolism. See* Chapter 18.

Diagnosis of Cardiac Arrest

1. *The pulse.* Inability to palpate any arterial pulsation. It is sometimes impossible to feel a peripheral pulse in the obese, vasoconstricted or shocked patient, even though a circulation to the brain is obviously maintained, since other vital functions are present. Continuous monitoring of the pulse is valuable in rapid diagnosis. The electrocardiogram is useful if it has been giving a continuous record and in the differential diagnosis between asystole and ventricular fibrillation. But normal tracings do not necessarily imply that the circulation is effective. Femoral and carotid pulses are the easiest to feel.

2. *Auscultation of the heart.* Absence of heart sounds.

3. *The pupils.* The pupils dilate, but they may be dilated due to hypoxia, drugs, etc. The intensely constricted pupil (e.g. after morphine) may not dilate at once in cases of arrest. During resuscitation the pupils should be examined frequently. Diminution in size is a most valuable and sensitive sign of effective treatment. If the pupils become smaller within 3 min of the arrest the prognosis is good.

4. *Absence of bleeding.* Venous bleeding may occur and should not be confused with arterial bleeding which is absent.

5. *Respiration*. Blood flow to the respiratory centres ceases and respiratory arrest occurs, which may be preceded by some irregular gasps, 1–3 min after the cardiac arrest.

6. *On ophthalmoscopy* the veins of the fundus show segmentation of the blood column.

7. *General appearance of the patient*. Cyanosis occurs and there are no signs of a circulation. In other cases pallor is present.

The Effects of Cardiac Arrest on the Brain

1. Unconsciousness supervenes in about 15 s.

2. EEG changes occur in 4 s and the tracing is flat within 20–30 s.

3. The Po_2 of cerebral blood falls to 2·5 kPa at the time consciousness is lost. Tissue Po_2 falls to zero within 1 min.

4. Histological changes.[26] Diffuse neuronal damage is not restricted to any particular vascular territory of the brain. Petechial haemorrhages also occur. Brain damage may be diffuse or focal. The mildest structural damage is selective neuronal necrosis, but with more severe hypoxia neuroglial cells are affected also and areas of infarction may arise.

(*See also* Brain ischaemia, its prevention and treatment, Editorial, McDowall D. G. *Br. J. Anaesth.* 1985, **57**, 1.) Resuscitation of the brain (*see* Thurlow A. C. in: *Anaesthesia Review*—(Kaufman L. ed.) Edinburgh: Churchill Livingstone, 1982, Ch. 13.)

Barbiturates were formerly thought to aid brain resuscitation after hypoxia[27] but this has been questioned.[28]

Treatment of Cardiac Arrest[29]

The person who should treat cardiac arrest is the person immediately available. There are two vital factors which must be accomplished quickly if adequate cerebral circulation is to be restored: *Pulmonary ventilation* and *cardiac compression or massage*. Time must not be wasted giving intracardiac injections (first described by Velden in 1919),[30] intravenous infusions or waiting for asepsis. It is, however, permissible that when arrest has been instantly recognized, elevation of all four limbs to 90° may be tried for a maximum of 15 sec. This simple manoeuvre may be successful in restoring heart beat without resort to cardiac massage.

Procedure recommended.[31] (1) Continue external cardiac massage; (2) Maintain ventilation of the lungs; (3) Immediate diagnosis of cardiac rhythm by ECG with defibrillation if indicated; (4) Immediate infusion of sodium bicarbonate, 100 mmol in the adult; (5) If possible, remove cause of arrest. (Sometimes taught as 'A' for airway, 'B' for breathing, and 'C' for cardiac output).[32]

Expired air ventilation. This is the method described by Sibson (1814–1876)[33] and Safar of Pittsburgh. The patient lies in the supine position and the airway must be maintained by extending the neck and holding the jaw forwards. The nares are occluded, and the operator expires directly into the mouth of the patient. Alternatively, the mouth-to-nose method may be used. In either case, movements of the chest should be observed to check that adequate expansion of the lungs has occurred. A simple pharyngeal airway is a valuable aid, and two airways may be cemented by their flanged ends to provide a mouthpiece for the donor. The Brook airway is a more elaborate apparatus, which has a valve permitting exhaled gases from the patient to escape directly to the atmosphere.

IPPV with *oxygen* is of course always to be preferred, if available.

Cardiac compression

1. *External Cardiac Compression*. First performed by Janos Balassa (1814–1865) of Budapest in 1858 (who introduced ether anaesthesia into Hungary).[34] Developed by Kouwenhoven and others of the Johns Hopkins Hospital.[35] The heart is compressed against the vertebral bodies sixty times a minute. The patient should be on a rigid surface such as the operating table or the floor. Pressure is applied to the lower sternum about sixty times a minute. Head-down position is of doubtful benefit as it is not helpful in shock, but the legs should be elevated 30–40° to facilitate venous return to the heart. This does not provide adequate ventilation of the lungs which must be inflated independently. Advantages lie in the simplicity of the technique and its ready applicability both inside and outside the operating theatre. It has also been applied to the newborn infant.

External cardiac compression should be abandoned when it becomes clear that sinus rhythm cannot be obtained, when cardiac output is not maintained despite resuscitative measures (e.g. if femoral or carotid pulses cannot be felt or if the pupils remain fixed and dilated) or when the general condition of the patient including existence of pre-existing pathology does not justify its continuance. External cardiac compression may cause visceral injuries. This possibility should be considered if a patient does not do well after the restoration of the heart beat.[32]

2. *Direct Cardiac Compression*. This was first done in animals by Schiff of Florence in 1874 and in man by Igelsrud in 1901.[36] Electrical defibrillation came later, followed by the work of Zoll.[37] The first successful cardiac massage in England was by Arbuthnot Lane (1856–1943) of Guy's Hospital in 1902, at the suggestion of Ernest Starling (1866–1927).[38]

Indicated: (*a*) When the chest or upper abdomen is already open; (*b*) In the presence of multiple rib fractures; (*c*) In cardiac tamponade.

Technique of internal cardiac massage

1. *Transthoracic route*. An incision is made in the left fifth intercostal space from the midaxillary line to one inch from the sternum (avoiding the internal mammary artery). A small hole is made in the pleura before incising it (to avoid cutting the lung). The left arm is abducted. The heart is compressed 60 times per min against the sternum by the flat of one hand. Later, the pericardium can be incised and both hands used.

2. *Transabdominal route*. If the abdomen is already open, the heart can be compressed against the sternum by one hand via the intact diaphragm. The other hand is held over the sternum.

Further treatment of asystole. The following measures have been suggested: (*a*) Continue cardiac compression until a normal beat returns; (*b*) If the returning beat is weak, stimulate the myocardium by injection into a large vein as near to the heart as possible, or even into the atrium—adrenaline, 0·5–1·0 mg every 3–4 min. It has, however, been argued that catecholamine administration is illogical, since there is already a high endogenous level.[39] Coronary perfusion is increased.[40] The dose in neonates is 0·1–0·2 mg. The positive inotropic effect of adrenaline is opposed by metabolic acidosis and enhanced by alkalosis. Isoprenaline may also be given 0·1–0·2 mg every 3–4 min. This is also affected by acidosis and alkalosis; (*c*) If the response is still unsatisfactory, 10 ml of 1% calcium chloride should be similarly injected to restore the cardiac tone. The dose in neonates is 1–2 ml. These injections may initiate ventricular fibrillation which must be appropriately treated. Cardiac compression may be necessary for a long period and bicarbonate infusion given (*see below*).

Further treatment of fibrillation. Adrenaline 0·05–0·2 mg may be administered to convert a slow fibrillation to a rapid fibrillation before defibrillation. The average adult can safely be given 100 mmol $NaHCO_3$ in 10–15 min and repeated over 20–30 min if necessary. Calcium salts can also be used to convert slow to rapid fibrillation. Calcium gluconate is less irritating to the tissues, when extravascular.[41] The passage of an electrical current through the heart causes all its muscular fibres to have their refractory period simultaneously; a normal beat is then stimulated by manual compression.

D.C. defibrillation. 100–400 watt-seconds or joules (J) externally. Most patients respond satisfactorily to 100 J and only rarely is 300–400 J required. The D.C. shock is produced by the discharge from a condenser and is of brief duration. D.C. defibrillation is more effective and causes less myocardial damage than A.C. defibrillation. D.C. defibrillators can also be used for synchronous discharge in the treatment of atrial fibrillation or ventricular tachycardia. Low-energy D.C. shock from a relatively cheap, miniaturized defibrillator may have a place.

The operating team should wear rubber gloves to protect themselves from electric shock. Repeated shocks of more than 150 J may cause myocardial (especially epicardial) damage, especially in the newborn.

To raise the blood pressure and stimulate the coronary circulation once the beat has been restored, isoprenaline sulphate may be useful. Acting almost exclusively on the β-receptors it is a potent cardiac stimulant; 2 mg may be added to 540 ml of isotonic saline and infused at a rate just sufficient to maintain adequate blood pressure. Dopamine infusion, 5 mg in 500 ml (5–20 µg/kg/min), or ephedrine, 10 mg i.v., are also highly effective. β-adrenergic blocking agents may sometimes be of value in preventing a recurrence of ventricular fibrillation, but facilities for emergency artificial pacemaking should be available. The blood pressure may need support for some hours from intravenous infusions. Hydrocortisone, 1 g i.v., may also have a pressor effect. Verapamil, i.v. slowly, has been recommended for ventricular fibrillation refractory to all treatment.[42]

Balloon pumping.[43] This is a temporary resuscitative measure for reversible myocardial dysfunction. Indications are based on clinical judgement, about half being after cardiopulmonary bypass, a quarter having had severe myocardial ischaemia, e.g. unstable angina, severe rest pain and evolving infarcts, and a further quarter having had cardiogenic shock due to various mechanical causes, such as ventricular septal rupture, acute ventricular aneurysm and severe mitral regurgitation. Such cases will naturally proceed to cardiac surgery. The main benefit is a reduction of after-load, and it reduces the highly energy consumptive phase of isometric ventricular contraction.

When indicated, balloon pumping is started early, within 2 h of the onset of severe cardiogenic shock and before organ death develops. It can be continued for up to 2 weeks. Balloon inflation coincides with aortic valve closure, being triggered by the ECG QRS complex. Monitoring includes right radial intra-arterial pressure recording or pulse tracing to give the correct time delay for balloon inflation. The main use for balloon pumping is to maintain circulation until emergency cardiac surgery can be carried out. A percutaneous model balloon is available, in which the balloon is wrapped round a Seldinger wire, for insertion into the femoral artery.

Resuscitation of the Brain
(*See* Thurlow A. C. in: *Anaesthesia Reviews*—(Kaufman L. ed.), Edinburgh: Churchill Livingstone, 1982. *See also* pp. 763 and 786) Therapeutic intervention to protect the brain after hypoxia remains controversial.[44]

Biochemical Changes during Cardiac Arrest
These occur as a result of tissue hypoxia, and inadequate removal of the products of metabolism. Even with external cardiac compression, the flow of blood (up to 1500 ml/min) is not sufficient to perfuse tissues normally. There is thus a maximum arteriovenous-oxygen and carbon-dioxide difference with resultant tissue acidosis. As a result of tissue hypoxia, there is movement of water and sodium into the cells and a movement of potassium ions out of cells into extracellular fluid. This results in a rise in packed cell volume and in plasma proteins, while plasma potassium concentration can reach levels as high as 7 mmol/l in a few minutes. There is a rise in lactic acid in the blood, together with a fall of bicarbonate, pH may fall to levels as low as 6·8 or 6·9. Blood sugar also rises as a result of hypoxia and levels up to 20 mmol/l (360 mg %) are commonly observed.

Drugs for cardiac resuscitation service in hospital.[45] The following drugs have been recommended: adrenaline, calcium chloride, atropine, dextrose, heparin, isoprenaline, dopamine, ephedrine, lignocaine, methohexitone, flecainamide, calcium blockers (especially verapamil and diltiazam),[46] diazepam, noradrenaline, pancuronium, practolol, normal saline, sodium bicarbonate 8·4% solution and suxamethonium. Also equipment for IPPV.

Correction of acidaemia. Bicarbonate infusion is given to correct the metabolic acidosis (2·74% is twice isotonic; 8·4% contains 1 mmol/ml). About 500–1000 ml of 2·74% solution may be required in an adult, with further doses on subsequent days as indicated by biochemical measurement of the deficit. It has been suggested that the initial dose may be related to the estimated duration of arrest:

Dose of bicarbonate in mmol =

$$\frac{\text{Wt of patient in kg}}{5} \times \frac{\text{Duration of arrest in minutes}}{2}$$

After treatment. The main cause of hypoxic brain damage is cerebral oedema from damage to the cerebral capillaries.

Clinical Signs of Cerebral Hypoxia. These may follow either an acute hypoxic episode after cardiac standstill or a prolonged period of suboxygenation. Recovery may occur after the episode and the patient may regain consciousness after the resuscitation, but may relapse into coma later. Respiration is gasping and stertorous and may be accompanied by a tracheal tug. There may be sweating, hyperpyrexia, dilated pupils and a coarse nystagmus. There may be restlessness, rigidity, choreo-athetosis or fits and twitching. These may progress to deepening coma, periodic breathing, tachycardia and death.

Treatment. The following measures may be required. Dehydration with use of hypertonic intravenous fluids to reduce cerebral oedema. Dexamethasone.

Reduction of body temperature by surface cooling, if raised; there is doubt whether hypothermia is useful in the absence of hyperpyrexia. Elevation of the head. Support of the circulation, physiotherapy, antibiotics, tracheostomy and IPPV to maintain $Paco_2$ of 3·5 kPa (25 mmHg).

(*See also* Tinker J. *Br. J. Hosp. Med.* 1981, **25**, 83.)

Prediction of Awakening After Cardiac Arrest

A reasonably accurate prognosis can be made,[47] based on the following variables: the arrest was witnessed; resuscitation was started immediately; the first observed ECG was asystole; spontaneous eye movements were present; pupil light reflex was present; corneal reflex was present; the heart responded in less than 2·5 min by reasonable pulse and arterial pressure; normothermia; arterial blood gases rapidly returned to normal.

Prognosis after Cardiac Arrest

In one series[48] of 108 patients, 21% left the hospital with 0·9% of these showing cerebral impairment; 53% died immediately, and 25% died later. (*See also* Annotation, *Br. Med. J.* 1984, **288**, 1324.)

(*See also* National Conference on Cardiopulmonary Resuscitation and Emergency Cardiac Care. *JAMA* 1980, **244**, 453. These have been adopted by the British Heart Foundation and appear in the First Aid Manual of the British Red Cross & St John Ambulance Brigade.)

Training for Cardiopulmonary Resuscitation

(*See* Stross J. K. *JAMA*, 1983, **249**, 3339 and *JAMA* 1980, **244**, 453.)

Management of Cardiac Arrest in Infants and Children

(*See* Bray R. J. *Br. J. Hosp. Med.* 1985, **34**, 72.)

For a discussion on the usefulness of a resuscitation trolley and its contents, *see* Hilton P. J. *Anaesthesia* 1985, **40**, 486; and Conroy P. J. and Wilson A. M. *Anaesthesia* 1985, **40**, 1142.

Drowning (the Immersion Incident)[49]

About 700 fatalities from drowning occur in the UK every year, about a quarter in the sea. There are pathophysiological differences between fresh and salt water drowning though these are largely of academic interest since survivors who reach hospital need similar therapeutic measures in both situations.

Fresh Water

Due to the difference in osmotic pressure, water passes rapidly from the lungs to the general circulation. There may be a 50% increase in circulatory volume within 3 min. This results in haemolysis, and ventricular fibrillation, resistant to treatment, occurs at an early stage. The heart is submitted to hypoxia, overfilling, potassium excess and sodium deficit. The clinical features can be demonstrated readily in animals, but there is evidence that the haemodilution is much less in man, and it is possible that some other factor may be operative. The prognosis is poor.

Salt Water

The osmotic effect is exerted in the opposite direction. Fluid passes out from the circulation into the alveoli to produce pulmonary oedema. In practice, fresh and salt water drowning are clinically very similar.

Vagal Inhibition

Death from vagal inhibition can occur without entrance of fluid into the lungs. Or vagal inhibition may prevent fluid entering the lungs for several minutes. Prompt resuscitation is likely to be successful in this type of case.

Other Effects

Drowning is likely to be complicated by: (1) Hypothermia (*see also* Chapter 17); (2) Acute pulmonary oedema; (3) Respiratory distress syndrome; (4) Pulmonary infection; (5) Cerebral oedema (not a common complication).[50]

Monitoring

Temperature, blood pressure, pulse, blood-gases, chest auscultation, venous filling, CVP, even intracranial pressure and cerebral perfusion pressure.[51]

Treatment

Speed is vital. Experiments in Denmark on cadavers suggest that the lungs cannot be emptied by posture, and that regurgitation from the stomach does not occur except with inflation pressures greater than $25\,cmH_2O$. Treatment should consist of: (1) Very quick efforts to clear the mouth and pharynx of debris and efforts to drain the lungs in salt water drowning. (2) Artificial ventilation, mouth-to-mouth, mouth-to-nose or by means of an apparatus, if possible while the subject is still in the water; (3) External cardiac compression; (4) Administration of pure oxygen as soon as practicable and transfer to hospital; (5) Treatment of hypothermia, if present, by rapid rewarming in water at $37\,°C$ and intravenous glucose and steroid administration. (6) Tracheal intubation and IPPV if indicated; (7) Chest X-ray, blood and urine analysis, blood-gas estimation and intensive therapy as indicated; (8) 1 litre of quadruple strength human albumin solution infused rapidly i.v.; (9) Don't give up easily.

Prognosis

Better after immersion in salt water than in fresh water. Recovery unlikely if the lungs have been flooded with fresh water for a period of over 2 min owing to the rapid circulatory changes with irreversible ventricular fibrillation. Hypothermia may, however, exert a protective effect, and when a cold subject is rescued from the water, resuscitation should always be attempted, even when no sign of life is apparent. Survival can occur after 18 min cardiac arrest.[52] Severe near-drowning is defined as requiring cardiopulmonary resuscitation in hospital. Survival of this is around 14%.[50]

References

1. *See also* Hawkins L. H. *Br. J. Hosp. Med.* 1970, **4**, 495; *History of Resuscitation*, Little D. M. 'Classical File', *Surv. Anesthesiol.* 1981, **25**, 415; ABC of resuscitation, *Br. Med. J.* 1986, **292**, 1002, 1123, 1257 and 1316.
2. Holy Bible, 2 Kings iv. 34–35.

3. Hunter J. *Phil. Trans.* 1776, **66**, 412.
4. Kite C. *An Essay on the Recovery of the Apparently Dead.* London: Dilly, 1788.
5. Herholdt J. D. and Rafn C. G. *Life Saving Measures for Drowning Persons.* Copenhagen, 1796 (Reprinted by Scandinavian Society of Anaesthesiologists, 1960, Aarhus).
6. Marshal Hall M. *Lancet* 1856, **1**, 229; Ellis R. *Lancet* 1868, **2**, 538.
7. Silvester H. R. *Br. Med. J.* 1858, **2**, 576.
8. Nielsen H. *Ugeskr. Laeg.* 1932, **94**, 1201.
9. Eve F. C. *Lancet* 1932, **2**, 995.
10. Matas R. *Am. Med.* 1902, **3**, 97 (reprinted in 'Classical File', *Surv. Anesthesiol.* 1978, **22**, 401).
11. Safar P. *JAMA* 1958, **167**, 335.
12. Lassen H. C. A. *Lancet* 1953, **1**, 37.
13. Keen W. W. *Ther. Gaz.* 1904, **28**, 217.
14. Starling E. A. *Lancet* 1902, **2**, 1397 (reprinted in 'Classical File', *Surv. Anesthesiol.* 1975, **19**, 497).
15. Beck C. S. and Mautz F. R. *Ann. Surg.* 1937, **106**, 525.
16. Zoll P. M. and Paul M. H. *Circulation* 1956, **14**, 745.
17. Kouwenhoven W. B. et al. *JAMA* 1960, **173**, 1064.
18. Woolam C. H. M. *Br. J. Clin. Equip.* 1979, **4**, 182; Eaton J. M. *Br. J. Hosp. Med.* 1984, **31**, 67.
19. Beck C. S. et al. *JAMA* 1956, **161**, 434.
20. Beck C. S. et al. *JAMA* 1947, **135**, 985.
21. Correspondence, *Br. Med. J.* 1985, **290**, 1985 et seq.
22. Bedell S. E. *N. Engl. J. Med.* 1983, **309**, 569.
23. MacWilliam J. A. *J. Physiol., Lond.* 1887, **8**, 291; *Br. Med. J.* 1889, **1**, 6.
24. Brown F. B. and Miller F. *Am. J. Physiol.* 1952, **169**, 56.
25. Bennett J. A. and Eltringham R. J. *Anaesthesia* 1977, **32**, 8.
26. Adams J. H. *Br. J. Anaesth.* 1975, **47**, 121.
27. Rockoff M. A. and Shapiro H. M. *Anesthesiology* 1978, **49**, 385.
28. Gisvold S. E. et al. *Anesthesiology* 1984, **60**, 88.
29. *See also* Report of Joint Cardiology Committee. *Br. J. Hosp. Med.* 1985, **53**, 477.
30. Velden R. *Münch. Med. Wochenschr.* 1919, **66**, 274.
31. Clifton V. *Anaesth. Intensive Care* 1979, **7**, 396; Taylor G. J. et al. *N. Engl. J. Med.* 1977, **296**, 1515.
32. Barrowcliffe M. P. *Anaesthesia* 1984, **39**, 347.
33. Maltby J. R. *Anaesthesia* 1977, **32**, 53.
34. Balassa J. *Orv. Hétil.* 1858, **2**, 653, quoted by Husveti J. and Ellis H. *Anaesthesia* 1969, **24**, 113.
35. Kouwenhoven W. B. et al. *JAMA* 1960, **173**, 1064; *Br. Med. J.* 1960, **2**, 1582; Jude J. R. et al. *JAMA* 1961, **178**, 1062 (reprinted in 'Classical File'; *Surv. Anesthesiol.* 1981, **25**, 418).
36. Keen W. W. *Therap. Gaz.* 1904, **28**, 217.
37. Zoll P. M. *N. Engl. J. Med.* 1952, **247**, 768.
38. Starling E. A. and Lane W. A. *Lancet* 1902, **2**, 1397.
39. Frayn K. N. and Maycock P. F. *Clin. Chem.* 1983, **27**, 1426; Laing G. S. and Redmond A. D. *J. R. Soc. Med.* 1982, **75**, 567.
40. Otto C. W. *Anesthesiology* 1979, **51**, 152.
41. Heining M. P. D. et al. *Anaesthesia* 1984, **39**, 1079.
42. Kapur P. A. and Norel P. *Anesth. Analg. (Cleve.)* 1984, **63**, 460.
43. Clauss R. H. et al. *J. Thorac. Cardiovasc. Surg.* 1961, **41**, 447; Curtis J. J. et al. *Mayo Clinic Proc.* 1977, **52**, 723; Tobias M. A. et al. *Anaesthesia* 1979, **34**, 844; Bregman D. *Curr. Prob. Surg.* 1976 **13**, 12.
44. Michenfelder J. D. *J. Irish Coll. Phys. Surg.* 1983, **12**, 154.
45. Gilston A. *Br. J. Clin. Equip.* 1979, **4**, 236.
46. Garcia J. H. *Arch. Pathol. Lab. Med.* 1983, **107**, 157; Shiu G. K. et al. *Crit. Care Med.* 1983, **11**, 452.
47. Longstreth W. T. et al. *N. Engl. J. Med.* 1983, **308**, 1378.
48. Sowden G. R. et al. *Anaesthesia* 1984, **39**, 39; *Br. Med. J.* 1984, **288**, 1324.
49. Orlowski P. *Crit. Care Med.* 1978, **6**, 94; Conn A. W. et al. *Can. Anaesth. Soc. J.* 1978, **25**, 259; Golden F. S. *Br. J. Hosp. Med.* 1980, **23**, 371.
50. Oakes D. D. *J. Trauma* 1982, **22**, 544.
51. Nussbaum E. and Galant S. P. *J. Pediatr.* 1983, **102**, 215.
52. Singh S. V. *J. R. Soc. Med.* 1980, **73**, 292.

Chapter 38   **RESPIRATORY FAILURE**

Respiratory failure is a common indication for admission to an intensive therapy unit. Defined by Campbell[1] as a state present in a patient at rest, breathing air at sea level if, because of impaired respiratory function, the arterial Po_2 is below 60 mmHg or the Pco_2 is above 49 mmHg. (*See also* MacNee W. *J. R. Soc. Med.* 1985, **78**, 61.) (Artificial ventilation of the lungs is dealt with in Chapter 15; Intubation of the trachea in Chapter 12.)

Causes of Failure to Maintain Normal Blood-gas Homeostasis[69]
(1) Respiratory depression, either central or neuromuscular; (2) Respiratory obstruction; (3) Pulmonary failure, including chronic bronchitis, acute bronchiolitis, emphysema, fibrosis, asthma, adult respiratory distress syndrome (shock lung), pneumothorax, pneumonia and pulmonary oedema; (4) Cardiac failure; (5) Acidosis; (6) Hypermetabolism, e.g. hyperpyrexia, thyroid crisis.

Signs of Respiratory Failure
Restlessness, fatigue, sweating, cyanosis, tachycardia, ectopic beats, dyspnoea, tachypnoea, use of accessory muscles of respiration, facial anxiety patterns and tracheal tug. Reduction of number of words per breath.

Assessment of Respiratory Failure
(1) Respiratory rate, depth, paradox, pattern; auscultation of chest; (2) Cough and sputum; (3) Respiratory volumes. Patient's FVC (below 2 litres surgery is a problem: below 1·5 litres they cannot cough; below 1 litre/min they need respiratory assistance; below 0·8 litre cannot sleep; below 150 ml/min need continuous IPPV); (4) Blood-gas analysis and pulmonary diffusion gradient; (5) Pulse and pulsus paradoxus, blood pressure, CVP and ECG; (6) Chest X-ray; (7) Pulmonary shunt estimation.

IPPV
Common indications
   1. Chronic respiratory failure, either for an acute exacerbation, or nocturnal ventilation at home in the very long term, e.g. using a cuirass ventilator. This may reverse the hypersomnolence, polycythaemia, and pulmonary hypertension seen in chronic severe respiratory failure. Some permanent ventilation units exist.
   2. Oncology. Immunosuppressed patients with opportunistic infections may be referred for IPPV and antibiotic therapy, with reverse barrier nursing. Their thrombocytopenia is often such that they require platelet transfusion even for insertion of central venous lines. The pulmonary problem may be a very fast-growing tumour, infection, superinfection, cardiac failure, or due to toxic effects of drugs. Early lung biopsy is frequently very helpful.
   3. Post cardiopulmonary bypass patients (*see* Chapter 29).
   4. Neurosurgery, a 48-h period of elective ventilation in the patient with raised intracranial pressure (ICP). ICP monitoring is standard and is reduced as necessary by lowering $Paco_2$, infusing a diuretic such as mannitol or frusemide. Patients with poor cranial pressure compliance, while responding well at first,

sometimes show a decreasing response to these therapeutic measures. Sedation is maintained with fentanyl and midazolam.

Management of Respiratory Failure[2]
This depends on the severity of the failure. It includes: (1) General respiratory care, education of the patient, nursing expertise, physiotherapy, monitoring of signs, blood gases, X-rays, bacteriology, hydration of the patient, humidification of inspired air. Specific drug administration, including antibiotics, bronchodilators, diuretics and cardiac stimulants; (2) Oxygen therapy (*see* Chapter 36) plus IPPB; (3) Mechanical ventilation of the lungs (IPPV). The time for intervention may be judged on clinical grounds, e.g. fatigue, pulmonary measurements (e.g. inadequate tidal volume or blood-gas estimation as when the Pa_{O_2} is lower than the Pa_{CO_2} even when breathing oxygen-enriched mixtures. The wave-forms, pressures and frequencies of the machine must be tailored to the particular needs of the patient. F_{IO_2} is set to maintain Pa_{O_2} at 14 kPa (100 mmHg) and is normally 21–40%. If IPPV with 50% oxygen fails to correct hypoxaemia, PEEP may be tried or even reduction of oxygen consumption by induced hypothermia to 34 °C.[3] When on IPPV the inspired gases should be humidified (*see* p. 775) and the patient sedated (whether relaxants are required or not). Tracheostomy may be performed after 5 days of oral or nasal intubation. Facilities may exist for this operation to be performed in the intensive therapy unit; (3) Diaphragmatic pacing.[4]

Long-term Ventilation (Days or Weeks)

Nursing Care of Patient on Artificial Ventilation
In addition to care of the tracheostomy (*see below*): (1) The patient should never be left unattended; (2) In case of mechanical failure, alternative means of ventilation must be available and understood by the nursing attendants.

The Control of Long-term Ventilation
1. *Clinical.* The underventilated patient may show discomfort, restlessness, rise in pulse rate, rise in blood pressure, sweating, cyanosis. The overventilated patient may show increased muscular irritability leading to tetany.
2. *Analysis of blood gases.* See Chapter 41.

Positive End-expiratory Pressure (PEEP)
See Chapter 15.

Management of the Patient
1. *Fluid balance and calorie intake.* Generally speaking, the intake (via gastric tube) should be above 2 litres of fluid and 2000 calories/day. For information about parenteral and tube feeding, *see* Chapter 40.
2. *Infection.* The relapse may have been precipitated by an infection. Chest infections may occur unless prophylactic measures are taken. Suction catheters should be sterile and used on one occasion only before resterilization. Antibiotic cover is advisable.[5] Patients should be turned at regular intervals (2-hourly) and physiotherapy three or four times daily helps to prevent atelectasis. Visitors may be required to wear gowns and masks.

3. Pressure areas. These require careful nursing attention.

4. Sedation. This may be required: (*a*) To help the patient to become accommodated to artificial ventilation, particularly in the early stages; (*b*) To ensure adequate rest at night.

5. Communication. The conscious patient must be given bell, mirror, pencil and paper.

6. Eyes. If the muscles of the eyelids are paralysed corneal abrasions may occur unless protective measures are taken.

7. Bladder and bowels. Function may become automatic in the unconscious or immobilized patient. Manual removal of faeces sometimes requiring sacral extradural blocks and manual compression or catheterization of the bladder may be necessary.

8. Monitoring. Charts must be kept of blood pressure, pulse, tidal volume, respiratory rate, etc. Special record charts are useful. Blood-gas estimation, chest radiographs and examination of sputum for organisms and sensitivity may be helpful, especially in the early stages. Blood-gas analysis may be required hourly at first, daily after the first day, weekly after the first week, unless fresh problems arise, when they are performed more frequently. Blood-sugar level is also monitored. Pulse oximeters are useful.

Transcutaneous oxygen monitoring. Although not yet free of electrode damage to the skin, this is of the greatest value in monitoring IPPV in the intensive therapy unit.

9. Psychological aspects.[6] These are important in long-term cases on ventilator treatment. Special arrangements must be made to enable patients to read newspapers and books, and watch television, etc. Windows, calendars and clocks help to keep the patient orientated as do visits by close relatives.

10. Artificial ventilation in neurological disease.[7]

Advantages of IPPV

(1) Gas exchange is improved; (2) It takes over the work of breathing; (3) It permits heavy sedation and analgesia without danger; (4) It re-expands collapsed lung tissue; (5) It reverses pulmonary oedema (although this has been questioned[7,38]); (6) It maintains gas exchange when relaxants must be used or when muscles are otherwise inadequate, or when there is a flail segment.

Complications of Long-term IPPV

(1) Tracheal tube enters right main bronchus; (2) Tracheal tube becomes blocked by kink, sputum, occlusion of tracheal end by wall of trachea; (3) Failure or disconnection of mechanical ventilator; (4) Pressure ulceration of mouth or nose or vocal cords or trachea; (5) Sputum retention and chest infection from inadequate humidification and bacterial contamination. The difference should be noted between bacterial colonization of the airways and lung infection, where there may be all the usual signs of infection, including pyrexia, leucocytosis, purulent sputum, bacteraemia and rising blood-sugar level. Lung abscess. Absorption collapse of lung tissue in a patient on IPPV is an emergency; (6) Hypotension due to CO_2 wash-out and raised intrathoracic pressure; (7) Difficulties in communication; (8) Psychological disturbances, including hallucinations; (9) Surgical emphysema and pneumothorax; (10) Water and sodium retention with oedema (not reduced by PEEP); (11) Rarely, tracheal stenosis;[8] (12) Subpleural air cysts;[9] (13) Bronchiolectasis.

Long-term nasotracheal is preferable to long-term orotracheal intubation,[10] although neither is free from complications.[11] To change a nasotracheal tube, a long suction catheter may be passed down it and the tube withdrawn, leaving the catheter as a guide for the new tube.[12]

Permanent IPPV
A tracheostomy tube, if used, is uncuffed. Such intubation may of course be unnecessary if an 'iron lung' or rocking bed is used. Tunnicliffe jackets or cuirasses may also be employed.

For complications of PEEP *see* Chapter 15.
For HFPPV *see* Chapter 15.

Weaning from a Ventilator

It is usually easier to put a patient on a ventilator than to take him off it. Weaning may take anything from minutes to weeks. It is indicated when the original disease process has been cured to a stage where: (1) The patient can cough; (2) The chest compliance is good; (3) Oxygen exchange is good, the Pa_{O_2} being normal while the patient is ventilated with 25% oxygen; (4) Chest infection has been substantially cleared; (5) The chest X-ray shows absence of atelectasis, consolidation, oedema or pneumothorax; (6) Muscle power, especially respiratory muscles, and nutrition are as normal as possible (i.e. there is no abdominal paradox within spontaneous respiration and the vital capacity is one litre or more). Allowing the patient to breathe against the ventilator, within limits, during prolonged IPPV, will tend to keep the respiratory muscles in reasonable condition.

1. *IMV* (*see* Chapter 15). First, analgesics, muscle relaxants and sedatives are stopped. The Pa_{CO_2} is allowed to rise to normal or above. The patient is instructed and encouraged to breathe; then the ventilator is switched to IMV; this should preferably take place in the morning. The patient is watched carefully for signs of respiratory distress, sweating, struggling, cyanosis (extra oxygen may be given by mask) or exhaustion. If these appear the ventilator is returned to complete IPPV. A trial period of up to an hour, repeated later, or prolonged as necessary is a good start. If PEEP was required during IPPV, then CPAP is likely to be required during weaning.

2. *Traditional methods.* With similar preparation to that for IMV weaning, the patient is allowed spontaneous ventilation for a short period. If the respiration is satisfactory, the period may be doubled, and so on, up to several hours. The following day, the process is repeated, either with longer periods of spontaneous ventilation, or progressively shorter periods of IPPV in between. Arterial blood-gas monitoring and $A\text{-}aD_{O_2}$ measurements are useful. Various ventilators can add safety and comfort to this process by employing triggered ventilation (which is varied progressively) or mandatory minute volume (MMV)—facilities (*see* Chapter 15) especially valuable where experienced nursing is in short supply. *Extubation* of the trachea may follow 24 h adequate spontaneous ventilation, provided there is reasonable brainstem function, or earlier if the patient is intolerant of the tube.

Tracheostomy[13]

History[14]

Performed by Pedro Virgili (1699–1776) of Cadiz for the relief of quinsy. George Martine (1702–1741)[15] was the first to employ it in a case of diphtheria in Britain. Heister (1683–1758) introduced the term 'tracheotomy' in place of 'bronchotomy' in 1718 and this gave place to 'tracheostomy' at the suggestion of Negus (1887–1974) of London in 1938 (*see* Wath J. M. *Br. J. Surg.* 1963, **50**, 954). Employed to relieve laryngeal diphtheria by Brettonneau (1778–1862) in 1818 (which was its chief use for the next 120 years),[16] and in the treatment of poliomyelitis in 1943.[17]

Tracheostomy reduces the anatomical dead space by 30–50%.

Indications for Tracheostomy

1. In obstruction of the upper airway. Sudden death from choking when a food bolus sticks in the laryngeal aperture occurs in about 300 people each year in Britain. First-aid treatment may include the 'Heimlich manoeuvre', sudden pressure on the epigastrium in an inward and upward direction to produce a sudden sharp rise in intrathoracic pressure which may eject the bolus.[18]

2. To permit artificial ventilation if an ordinary tracheal tube will not suffice.

3. For aspiration of the trachea and bronchial tree.

4. To prevent inhalation of foreign material, usually in the unconscious patient or when pharyngeal reflexes are depressed.

Except in the rare case of sudden complete obstruction to the upper airway, tracheostomy is not an operation of extreme urgency and is perhaps too often performed.[19]

Types of Tube

1. The King's College Hospital pattern silver tube. Size 32 or 34 for men. Size 28 for women. Later a valved tube can be inserted which enables the patient to speak.

2. Cuffed plastic tracheostomy tube. Low-pressure cuffs are preferable to high-pressure cuffs as they cause less damage. Other types which have been advocated include double cuffs, solid cuffs and automatic inflating cuffs.

Laryngostomy

Easier to perform than tracheostomy and need not result in postoperative laryngeal obstruction.[20]

Minitracheostomy

Can be rapidly performed using a set designed for the purpose. Useful in a life-saving situation. Has also been used for short-term tracheobronchial toilet.

Needle Tracheostomy

In extremis, e.g. after failed intubation, the insertion of a plastic intravenous cannula No. 12 (internal diameter 2·3 mm, length 7 cm) into the trachea, above or below the cricoid, will provide oxygenation if connected to a source of oxygen or even air from a reservoir bag or Ambu bag. A minute volume of 3–4 litres can be provided while over-inflation can be prevented by a vent controlled by a finger, on the rubber tubing. Such cannulae and connectors should be readily available in all operating suites. As a 'last ditch' airway, the spike which enters an infusion bottle can be thrust into the trachea, following a small incision and connected to an oxygen supply line[21] (*see also* The Penlon tracheotome).[22]

Complications of Tracheostomy

1. Early complications include: Haemorrhage; displacement or obstruction of the tube; difficult insertion or reinsertion of the tube; injury to the trachea, tracheitis, crust formation; respiratory complications; surgical emphysema and pneumothorax.

2. Infection. May arise from: (*a*) Contamination during tracheal suction. Aseptic 'no-touch' methods, with the use of disposable gloves, help to minimize this; (*b*) The wound itself is liable to become infected. Hourly spraying with polybactrin aerosol is helpful, and so is application of nystatin; (*c*) The humidifier: can be prevented by raising the temperature of the water to 60 °C (140 °F) so that pasteurization occurs. Despite all measures, tracheostomy wounds may become infected.

3. Tracheal ulceration. Erosions of the tracheal mucous membrane are not uncommon. In some cases, ulceration has produced exposure of the tracheal rings, secondary haemorrhage from erosion of a major vessel, and even ulceration into the oesophagus.

4. Tracheal dilatation.[23] Mechanism not fully understood.

5. Tracheal stenosis. The Björn flap[24] is unlikely to be associated with stenosis.[25] Many surgeons make a circular opening in the trachea at the level of the third tracheal ring the size of the proposed tube, the edges being sutured to the skin. Symptoms do not occur unless the tracheal diameter is 60% reduced. Respiratory distress indicates a diameter of 6 mm or less. It may occur: (1) In the subglottic region; (2) At stoma level; (3) At the level of the cuff; (4) Below the tube. Commonest sites are at cuff and stoma sites. Symptoms may not arise until late, usually after the patient has left hospital. In severe cases, definitive treatment by resection of the stenosed area with primary suture is required. Dilatation usually affords temporary benefit only.

Soft-cuff or floppy-cuff tracheal tubes overcome the problem of pressure ulceration of the trachea to a large extent. The position of the curve of a tracheostomy tube should be checked by lateral soft-tissue X-ray of the neck.

6. Cardiovascular collapse.[26]

Humidification

When the normal humidifying mechanisms of the upper respiratory tract are bypassed by a tracheal tube or tracheostomy, there is a tendency for fibrinous exudation with crusting to occur in the trachea and larger bronchi. In 1 h, 20 ml of water are lost from the lungs.

During artificial ventilation a humidifier should be incorporated between the ventilator and the patient. During spontaneous respiration through a tracheostomy, crusting can be discouraged by blowing humidified air into a plastic mask fitting loosely over the tracheostomy.

Methods of Humidification[27]

1. The classic humidifier is a can of warm water over which the gases are

blown. Tubing between humidifier and patient should be lagged to prevent condensation. A water trap placed between expired gases and a volume meter helps to prevent false readings caused by condensation. Colonization by bacteria has proved to be a major disadvantage, but it can be prevented if chlorhexidine is added to the water and the temperature of the water is maintained at 60 °C (140 °F) so that a process of pasteurization occurs. This type of humidifier is surprisingly efficient and is particularly useful when incorporated in the ventilator circuit.

2. Nebulizers are used to produce a supersaturated mist. (*a*) Gas-driven nebulizers. Droplets from 5 to 20 μm; (*b*) Spinning-disc humidifiers. Water is drawn from a reservoir by an Archimedean screw to impinge on the surface of a rapidly rotating disc which flings water to produce a wide range of droplet sizes.

3. Ultrasonic humidifiers. Water drops on to a vibrating plate and is broken up into particles of 1–2 μm size.

4. Condenser humidifiers ('artificial nose'). Layers of wire gauze may be interposed between the tracheostomy tube and the external air. Dead space can be as low as 17 ml. May offer some resistance to respiration. Not suitable for use in small children. Can also act as reservoirs of infection. To prevent this they should be changed 3-hourly.

5. A simple method, requiring no sophisticated apparatus, is to insufflate oxygen via a catheter placed in the mouth of the tracheostomy tube at 2 litres/min. A fine needle is inserted through the wall of the catheter and water allowed to pass through at a rate of 4 drops/min using a standard transfusion set.

Whatever method of humidification is used it is important to make sure that the patient is adequately hydrated.

Nursing Care of Patient with Tracheostomy[28]
The following points are important:

1. All conscious patients should have a bell, pencil and paper, and mirror at hand.

2. The inner tube of a silver tracheostomy tube should be cleaned at regular (4-hourly) intervals.

3. The cuff of a cuffed tube may be deflated at regular intervals and reinflated with just enough air to make an airtight seal. The pharynx should be sucked out before, and the trachea after, carrying out such a manoeuvre. Many workers now prefer to inflate the cuff carefully and then leave it with pressure unchanged until it is time to remove the tube.

4. Use a humidifier to prevent crusting. Maintain hydration.

5. The trachea should be sucked out as indicated. All catheters should be sterile and used only once.

6. Sterile dressing to tracheostomy wound daily, using no-touch technique.

Artificial Ventilation of the Lungs. *See* Chapter 15.

Oxygen Therapy. *See* Chapter 36.

Acute Exacerbations of Chronic Bronchitis and Emphysema

An acute infection may precipitate acute respiratory failure. Arterial oxygen tension falls and arterial carbon dioxide tension rises. Respiration is maintained by the hypoxic drive via the aortic and carotid body reflexes in the very severe case. Where there is a danger that oxygen administration may remove this drive, further depression of respiration occurs and a state of carbon dioxide narcosis results. In other circumstances, long-term oxygen therapy has been given in the home.[29] Oxygen must, however, be administered to relieve hypoxia and respiration maintained. This may be achieved by:

1. The use of controlled concentrations of oxygen.[30] Hypoxic hypoxia is always very responsive to the Po_2 of the inspired air. Raising this from normal 20 to 26 kPa (28% O_2) has a very significant effect. Intermittent oxygen therapy may be dangerous (*see* Chapter 36).

2. Sedatives and hypnotics should be avoided.

3. Full humidification of inspired gases is important, perhaps with nebulized medication (antibiotics, sputum solvents, etc.).

4. Regular and vigorous chest physiotherapy although a session of therapy may temporarily increase the hypoxia.

5. Respiratory stimulants (e.g. Doxapram) may be useful in marginal cases as may intermittent positive-pressure breathing (IPPB). This has been disputed.

6. IPPV via tracheal tube. First used in the treament of respiratory failure in 1952.[31] This is indicated if: (*a*) Tidal volume is inadequate; (*b*) $Paco_2$ exceeds Pao_2; (*c*) Patient is becoming exhausted and cannot effectively cough or clear his secretions.

The tracheal tube may be oral or nasal. If treatment is prolonged beyond 1 week, tracheostomy may be indicated. (*See above.*) It is unwise to provide mechanical ventilation for patients with emphysema in the absence of a clearly remediable pathology. Bronchoscopy can be useful in identifying the causative organism.[32]

Status Asthmaticus

Status asthmaticus can be defined as a severe and prolonged episode of broncho-spasm, causing distress to the patient, and not relieved by conventional therapy. Reports of deaths show an incidence of between 1·6 and 7·07/100 000 population per annum in various series.[33]

Treatment[34]

1. Oxygen. Arterial oxygen tensions as low as 6 kPa (35–40 mmHg) are common in severe cases. The aim should be to maintain it above 7·5 kPa (50 mmHg). As hypercapnia may be present in late stages and the chemoreceptor drive lost, oxygen must be given with care, in controlled concentrations. Sedatives are not given unless the patient is on IPPV.

2. Drugs. Aminophylline and theophylline (first used in the treatment of bronchial constriction in 1937)[36] may be given intravenously or per rectum. They improve the contractile properties of the diaphragm, cause bronchodilatation and stimulate respiration.[37] Isoprenaline or salbutamol is useful as an aerosol inhalation. Salbutamol may be given intravenously and orally (100–300 mg). Terbutaline has a longer duration of action. Dose: 0·25 mg s.c. or slowly i.v.; 0·25 mg by inhalation; oral, 5 mg 8-hourly.

3. Fluid replacement to correct dehydration. The deficit may be great and should be corrected with normal saline using CVP monitoring.[32]

4. *Lignocaine* spray to laryngeal mucosa; deep anaesthesia with halothane[35] or ether and oxygen.

5. *Indications for IPPV in status asthmaticus.* (1) Exhaustion apnoea; (2) Pneumothorax (after insertion of chest drain), pneumomediastinum; (3) Deteriorating general condition, reduced consciousness, oliguria, acidosis, peripheral circulatory failure, rising pulse, dysrhythmias; (4) Pulsus paradoxus greater than 40; (5) Pao_2 less than 9 kPa (60 mmHg); $Paco_2$ more than 9 kPa (60 mmHg); (6) Night. Many deaths from asthma occur soon after midnight. The serum potassium should be above 3 mmol/l and a pneumothorax, if present, should be drained. Sodium bicarbonate is rarely needed. The trachea is sprayed with lignocaine prior to insertion of the tracheal tube. The ventilator is timed to start inspiration when the expiratory wheeze (auscultated) ceases. Inspiration is usually short; expiration, long; (7) Antacids and a nasogastric tube are frequently required; (8) Membrane oxygenators have been used.[39]

6. *Corticosteroids.*[40] The effect may not be seen for 12 h.[41] These should be given, often in massive dosage, especially when the patient is already on long-term steroid therapy.

7. *Antibiotics.* Unless the precipitating factor is obviously allergic or psychological, it is wise to give a bactericidal antibiotic.

Legionnaires Disease[42]

Caused by a virulent mycobacterium, *Legionella pneumophila*; causes severe pneumonia often requiring oxygen therapy and IPPV. The organism multiplies in warm water and has airborne spread, especially via air-conditioning systems. Cross-infection is common and severe epidemics occur. The organism is frequently sensitive to erythromycin.[43]

Adult Respiratory Distress Syndrome (ARDS)[45]

A term first used by Ashbaugh.[44] This is a form of pulmonary failure once thought to be due to depletion of surfactant. It is frequently caused *by* diseases which are remote from the lung itself. These include massive (especially unfiltered) blood transfusion, Gram-negative septicaemia, fat embolism, pulmonary micro-embolism, cardiopulmonary bypass, pancreatitis, ulcerative colitis, peritonitis, barbiturate overdose and prolonged severe hypotension. Some authorities also include drowning, prolonged pulmonary oedema (including neurogenic), crushed chest, radiation, burns, explosions, smoke, gas or acid inhalation, immunosuppression, pulmonary oxygen toxicity, anaphylactic reactions and prolonged IPPV. The commonest cause is sepsis. Two types have been described: Type A—wet lung, responds to diuretics. Type B—obstructed lung, the one described here. It should be noted that ARDS also occurs in children.[46]

Symptoms
Progressive respiratory distress with decreased lung compliance and increased work of breathing; acute hypoxaemia, not relieved by inhalations of oxygen.[47] In addition, there is often multiple organ failure.

Diagnosis

Early stage, dyspnoea and tachypnoea existing with or following the above conditions. Later, diffuse patchy clouding in chest X-ray, increasing dyspnoea and hypoxia. Later still, circulatory instability, hypotension, deepening cyanosis, loss of consciousness, moribundity and finally cardiac arrest. Swan–Ganz catheterization is useful. Lung biopsy has a place.

Pathophysiology[69]

Multiple pulmonary microthromboses, pulmonary interstitial oedema, cellular infiltration,[48] alveolar oedema and hyaline membrane.[49] Pulmonary thromboxane-A_2 production may cause pulmonary vasoconstriction, resulting in right ventricular failure and high CVP and PAP. The lung does not exchange gases very well, but it can recover function.

Treatment

1. Correction of the primary cause if possible, e.g. removal of pus.
2. Humidified oxygen therapy up to F_{IO_2} 40% to maintain Pa_{O_2}.
3. Massive dose of steroids, e.g. 40–120 mg methylprednisolone, 6-hourly, given early. The value of this is disputed.
4. Fluid restriction and possibly diuretic therapy.
5. IPPV, if necessary; the indications being: A respiratory rate greater than 35/min, vital capacity less than 10 ml/kg, Aa_{PO_2} gradient of 7 kPa on air or 40 kPa on pure oxygen, Pa_{CO_2} greater than 7 kPa, Vd/Vt greater than 60%, right to left shunt greater than 15%. PEEP[50] is likely to be of value and is adjusted to keep Pa_{O_2} greater than 5 kPa with F_{IO_2} less than 50% if possible. Any resulting reduction of cardiac output can be reversed by dopamine. However, raising the cardiac output may also raise the shunt fraction. *Prophylactic* IPPV has been advocated.[51]
6. The patient is turned every half hour.
7. Plasma colloid osmotic pressure is maintained by giving plasma to keep the serum albumin above 30 g/l.
8. Anticoagulation with heparin.
9. Streptokinase therapy sometimes.
10. Sedation, paralysis and hypothermia to reduce oxygen demand.
11. Reduction of pulmonary vascular resistance by: (*a*) Pulmonary vasodilators, nitroprusside and α-blockade; (*b*) Ibuprofen 400 mg to antagonize thromboxane-A_2; (*c*) Prostacyclin treatment may have a place.
12. Possibly fibrosis inhibitors, e.g. *d*-hydroxyproline.
13. Extracorporeal membrane oxygenation will buy time but not cure. The carbon dioxide membrane lung (CDML) has been used in this condition in an effort to rest the lung, with a little success.
14. Prevention of failure of other organs, e.g. kidney.
15. Extracorporeal removal of CO_2 by the Gattinoni method[52] appears to be a promising technique.[53]

Prognosis

The mortality of established ARDS is about 90% without special treatment; about 40% with treatment. Additional failure of other organs in the body, e.g. kidney, increases mortality considerably. The survivors show reduced pulmonary function for a long time.

Other Conditions which may require IPPV

AIDS (Acquired Immune Deficiency Syndrome)[70]
The indications for intensive therapy in AIDS include life support of a promptly reversible complication, and to allow time for affairs to be settled, family visits, etc. The average survival may be extendible to 6 months in the case of *Pneumocystis carinii* pneumonia (PCP) or about 18 months in the case of Kaposi sarcoma. PCP is by far the commonest complication and may respond to trimethoprim, sulphamethoxazole or pentamidine, giving a survival rate of 30–50% from the first attack and about half this from the second attack. Sputum for bacteriological analysis is obtained by hypertonic saline sputum induction and has a high yield for *P. carinii*, but bronchoscopy and even lung biopsy may be required. PCP shows a dry, granular appearance on chest X-ray. Many AIDS patients also have oral candidiasis. A few have open TB. Those AIDS patients with CNS complications are not usually presented for intensive therapy. The H/V is usually killed by 1% glutaraldehyde for 30 min or 5% hypochlorite for 5 min (good for cleaning surfaces). (*See also Guidance for Staff treating Patients with AIDS*, London: DHSS 1986.)

Poliomyelitis
This may be spinal, bulbar or bulbospinal. Patients with bulbar poliomyelitis can breathe but cannot maintain the integrity of their upper air passages. The semi-prone head-down position together with suction will prevent soiling of the bronchial tree. Bulbospinal poliomyelitis is the dangerous type as it is a combination of the first two above.

The tracheostomy and cuffed tube technique provide for suction of the airways, protection of the airways from soiling and an easy route for IPPV.

(*See also* Permanent IPPV, p. 773.)

Tetanus[54]
Tetanus presents some problems very similar to those seen in poliomyelitis. There may be pharyngeal and laryngeal insufficiency due to spastic, not flaccid, muscles. Mild cases have been treated with sedatives (e.g. diazepam). When reasonable doses fail to control convulsions, muscle relaxants and IPPV must be considered, often through a tracheostomy, although tracheal narrowing may occur later.[55] Tetanus may be accompanied by overactivity of the sympathetic nervous system, shown by rise in heart rate and arterial pressure. These changes may be aggravated by tracheal suction. For these *autonomic storms* β-blockade and calcium antagonists are used to protect the heart; atropine controls salivation and α-blockade controls the blood pressure.

The Autonomic System in Tetanus
Overactivity of the sympathetic system, which may occur in the early stages of severe tetanus, is evidenced by rises in arterial pressure and pulse rate (Domenighetti G. M., Savary G. et al. *Br. Med. J.* 1984, **288**, 1483). Tracheal suction in curarized patients on artificial ventilation may result in marked rises in arterial and central venous pressure.

Autonomic depression may be seen in neuropathies, e.g. diabetic, Guillain–Barré syndrome, cervical cord injuries and familial dysautonomia.

Myasthenia Gravis
Cases may require IPPV and careful supervision over a long period of time. (For details of management, *see* Chapter 22.)

Status Epilepticus
Muscle paralysis and IPPV are sometimes required and diazepam or a thiopentone[56] drip has been used.[57]

Management of Rabies Encephalitis
In the present state of knowledge, the aim should be to provide full supportive therapy in the hope that immunoglobulins and immunization at the time of diagnosis might allow recovery to occur. This will include IPPV, and cardiovascular support with appropriate sedation. Muscle spasms are controlled by muscle relaxant drugs; intubation will prevent pulmonary soiling; loss of vasomotor tone may result in the need for vasopressors (e.g. dopamine). Brainstem death is likely to supervene. Monitoring may include direct arterial pressure, arterial oxygen tension, Swan–Ganz catheterization, and use of the cerebral function monitor.

Barrier nursing should be carried out and the number of medical and nursing attendants kept to a minimum. Those in direct contact with the patient or the patient's ventilator, should receive active immunization. (*See also* DHSS Memorandum on Rabies. London: HMSO, 1977; Editorial, *Br. Med. J.* 1975, **3**, 721; Cohen S. L. et al. *Br. Med. J.* 1976, **1**, 1041; Cundy J. M. *Anaesthesia* 1980, **35**, 35.)

Respiratory Problems in Children[58]

Respiratory Problems in Infants
Special factors to be considered include: (1) Restricted vital capacity; (2) Increased right-to-left shunt; (3) Increased closing volume; (4) Narrow airways; (5) Pulmonary and neurological developmental immaturity; (6) Susceptibility to infection; (7) Specific abnormalities, e.g. pulmonary dysplasia with high pulmonary vascular resistance, congenital cardiac lesions, respiratory distress syndrome; (8) Diazepam increases pulmonary vascular resistance in infants; tolazoline, 1–2 mg/kg, reduces it; (9) Considerable adrenergic activity leading to early severe hyperglycaemia, exhaustion of glycogen followed by severe hypoglycaemia; (10) Inspiratory stridor suggests obstruction above larynx, expiratory stridor, below.

Indications for IPPV in Infants
(1) Clinical (in the words of Sir William Osler (1849–1919): 'Don't touch the patient; note first what you see'): Tachypnoea, tachycardia, facial distress, indrawing of the ribs, tracheal tug, use of accessory muscles of respiration, irregular gasping and exhaustion. (2) Pao_2 less than 9 kPa (60 mmHg). (3) Prophylaxis, i.e. strong likelihood of failure. (4) Post-cardiac surgery.

Acute Epiglottitis
This is an acute inflammatory condition which may cause respiratory obstruction and is a danger to life. The history is short, usually a matter of hours. There is

stridor, sore throat, irritability, fever, dysphagia and the child looks toxic; he often prefers to sit up with the neck extended. If viewed with a spatula or laryngoscope the epiglottis is seen to be red and oedematous. The causal agent is often *Haemophilus influenzae* and this organism can be grown from the pharynx and sometimes the bloodstream. There are general signs of fever and toxicity. Suspicion of this condition demands urgent admission to hospital. The tongue frequently protrudes, the stridor is often inspiratory. Age range mostly 2–6 years. The leucocyte count is usually less than 10 000.

As soon as the condition is diagnosed, steps must be taken to ensure the adequacy of the airway. The child is not left alone, nor laid flat, nor sent to the X-ray department. The mouth and tongue are not manipulated. Crying can precipitate laryngeal obstruction in acute epiglottitis.[59] Where the necessary facilities are to hand, tracheal intubation by a skilled anaesthetist can be performed.[60] This should be accomplished in the operating-theatre environment with facilities for immediate tracheostomy available (in other circumstances, tracheostomy may be preferred). The child is given an oxygen/halothane induction, which, though slow, is safe. The tracheal tube should be small enough to allow a slight leak. An i.v. cannula may be inserted after the child is asleep. A nasogastric tube may be passed. Humidified oxygen-enriched air is breathed, usually spontaneously. Diazepam, 0·1 mg/kg, or morphine, 0·1 mg/kg, or chloral hydrate, 30 mg/kg, may be used for sedation following intubation.

Once the airway is secured, the child will usually sleep, but sedatives can be given if necessary. The tube should stay in position for 24–36 h after the commencement of antibiotic treatment[61] to allow resolution of the condition. Antibiotics (e.g. ampicillin or chloramphenicol[62]) are given, and hydrocortisone may help to reduce oedema.[67] Hydrocortisone cream may be smeared on the tracheal tube. Oxygen–helium mixtures have been used.[63]

Pulmonary oedema may follow relief of acute infective upper airway obstruction and may require IPPV and PEEP.[64]

Spasmodic croup may occur in adults.[65]

Supraglottitis has been described.[66]

Suggested protocol for management of children suspected of suffering from acute epiglottitis *see* Baines D. B. et al. *Anaesth. Intensive Care* 1985, **13**, 25. Fulminating acute epiglottitis and supra-epiglottitis is becoming more frequent in adults and may progress rapidly.[66] Parenteral chloramphenicol, with or without tracheostomy, is the treatment, pending definitive microbiological diagnosis.

Acute Laryngotracheitis

Acute infection is often viral in origin, with superimposed bacterial infection. Obstruction occurs due to oedema and exudate, and is most likely in the immediate subglottic region in the 1–2 year age group. Tracheal intubation and gentle suction may be necessary. Tracheostomy is to be avoided if possible. The child may develop acute pulmonary oedema.

Reye's Syndrome

Acute non-inflammatory encephalopathy with microvesicular fatty infiltration of the liver confirmed by biopsy or suggested by liver function test results (aspartate transaminase, alanine transaminase, blood ammonia) greater than three times normal. Incidence 80 cases/year in UK. Average age 15 months.

Prognosis—4% outcome unknown. Aspirin is under suspicion as a cause. 43% survived intact, 41% died, 12% neurologically damaged.[68]

(*See also* Brown T. C. K. in: *Paediatric Anaesthesia. Trends in Current Practice* (Rees G. J. and Gray T. C. ed.) London: Butterworth, 1981; Hatch D. J. in: *Recent Advances in Anaesthesia and Analgesia*—15. (Atkinson R. S. and Adams A. P. ed.) Edinburgh: Churchill Livingstone, 1985.

Septicaemia

See Chapter 35.

Poisoning

Buy time for recovery by life support of respiratory and other organ function. For self-poisoning, psychiatric advice is an important part of the follow-up.

References

1. Campbell E. M. J. *Br. Med. J.* 1965, **1**, 1451.
2. Petheram I. S. and Branthwaite M. A. *Anaesthesia* 1980, **35**, 467.
3. Sherwood Jones E. *Essential Intensive Care*. Lancaster: MTP Press, 1978.
4. Lozewicz S. et al. *Br. Med. J.* 1981, **282**, 1015.
5. Darrell J. H. and Uttley A. H. C. *Br. J. Anaesth.* 1976, **48**, 13.
6. *See also* Tomlin P. *Br. Med. J.* 1977, **2**, 441; Atkinson R. S., Hamblin J. J. and Wright J. E. C. *Handbook of Intensive Care*. London: Chapman & Hall, 1981, Ch. 22.
7. Douglas J. G. et al. *Br. Med. J.* 1983, **286**, 1943.
8. Flowers M. W. and Edmondson R. S. *Br. Med. J.* 1980, **1**, 303.
9. Albelda S. M. *Am. Rev. Respir. Dis.* 1983, **127**, 360.
10. Slavin G. et al. *Br. Med. J.* 1982, **285**, 931.
11. Dubick M. N. and Wright B. D. *Anesth. Analg. (Cleve.)* 1978, **57**, 663; Pippin L. K. and Bowes J. B. *Anaesthesia* 1983, **38**, 791.
12. Moller C. T. *Anaesth. Intensive Care* 1979, **7**, 192.
13. *See also* Atkinson R. S. et al. *Handbook of Intensive Care*. London: Chapman & Hall, 1981, p. 58.
14. McCelland R. M. A. *Progress in Anaesthesiology*. Amsterdam: Excerpta Medica, 1970, p. 195.
15. Martine G. *Phil. Trans. R. Soc.* 1730, **36**, 448.
16. Brettonneau P. F. *New Sydenham Soc. (Lond.)* 1859.
17. Galloway T. *JAMA* 1943, **128**, 1096.
18. Heimlich H. *JAMA* 1975, **234**, 398; Editorial, *N. Engl. J. Med.* 1979, **300**, 990; *Emerg. Med.* 1974, **6**, 154; *Paediatrics* 1982, **70**, 120.
19. Gilston A. *Anaesthesia* 1979, **34**, 912.
20. Hardy R. H. *Accidents and Emergencies*. 2nd ed. Oxford: Oxford University Press, 1978.
21. Fisher J. A. *Can. Anaesth. Soc. J.* 1979, **26**, 225.
22. Hayes B. *Br. Med. J.* 1978, **1**, 854.
23. Fryer M. E. and Marshall R. D. *Anaesthesia* 1976, **31**, 470.
24. Björk V. O. *J. Thorac. Cardiovasc. Surg.* 1960, **39**, 179.
25. Magregor I. A. and Neill R. S. *Anaesthesia* 1984, **39**, 718.
26. Didier E. P. *Anesth. Analg. (Cleve.)* 1962, **41**, 154.
27. Hayes B. and Robinson J. S. *Br. J. Anaesth.* 1970, **42**, 94; Boyes J. E. and Howells T. H. *Br. lJ. Anaesth.* 1972, **44**, 879.
28. Robbie D. S. and Feldman S. A. *Br. J. Anaesth.* 1963, **35**, 771; Matheson M. A. et al. *Lancet* 1963, **2**, 31; Gregory I. C. *Br. J. Hosp. Med.* 1970, **3**, 611.
29. Annotation *Lancet* 1981, **1**, 681, 701.
30. Campbell E. J. M. *Lancet* 1960, **2**, 10; *The Uses and Dangers of Oxygen Therapy*. Edinburgh: HMSO, 1969, Ch. 12.
31. Lassen R. C. A. *Lancet* 1953, **1**, 37.
32. Hedemark L. L. et al. *Am. Rev. Respir. Dis.* 1982, **126**, 981.
33. Rees H. A. *Postgrad. Med. J.* 1967, **43**, 225.

34. James O. F. et al. *Anaesth. Intensive Care* 1977, **5**, 11.
35. Raine J. M. *Br. Med. J.* 1981, **1**, 520.
36. Hermann G. and Aynesworth M. *J. Lab. Clin. Med.* 1937, 23, 1244.
37. Aubier M. et al. *Am. Rev. Respir. Dis.* 1983, **127**, 148.
38. Stoddart J. S. in: *Recent Advances in Anaesthesia and Analgesia*—13 (Hewer C. L. and Atkinson R. S. ed.) Edinburgh: Churchill Livingstone, 1979.
39. Goujon M. and Raphael P. H. *Intensive Care Med.* 1978, **4**, 173.
40. Haskell R. J. *Arch. Intern. Med.* 1983, **143**, 1324.
41. Fanta C. H. et al. *Am. J. Med.* 1983, **74**, 845.
42. Muder R. R. *JAMA* 1983, **249**, 3184.
43. Popp A. J. *J. Neurosurg.* 1982, **57**, 784.
44. Ashbaugh D. G. and Bigelow D. B. *Lancet* 1967, **2**, 319.
45. Boggis C. R. M. and Greene R. *Br. J. Hosp. Med.* 1983, **29**, 167.
46. Pfenninger et al. *J. Paediatr.* 1982, **101**, 352.
47. Boggis C. R. M. and Greene R. *Br. J. Hosp. Med.* 1983, **29**, 167; Wallace P. M. G. and Spence A. A. *Br. Med. J.* 1983, **286**, 1167.
48. Zimmerman G. A. *Am. Rev. Respir. Dis.* 1983, **127**, 290.
49. Last J. A. *Thorax* 1983, **38**, 364.
50. Viquerat C. E. *Chest* 1983, **83**, 509.
51. Goris R. J. A. *J. Trauma* 1982, **22**, 895.
52. Gattinoni L. et al. *Lancet* 1980, **2**, 292.
53. Hickling K. G. *Anaesth. Intensive Care* 1986, **14**, 46.
54. Edmondson R. S. and Flowers M. W. *Br. Med. J.* 1979, **1**, 1401; Edmondson R. S. *Br. J. Hosp. Med.* 1980, **23**, 596.
55. Flowers M. W. and Edmondson R. S. *Br. Med. J.* 1980, **1**, 303.
56. Partinen M. et al. *Br. Med. J.* 1981, **1**, 520.
57. Chin L. S. et al. *Anaesth. Intensive Care* 1979, **7**, 50.
58. Hatch D. J. in: *Recent Advances in Anaesthesia and Analgesia*—15 (Atkinson R. S. and Adams A. P. ed.) Edinburgh: Churchill Livingstone, 1985.
59. Tarnow-Mordi W. O. and Berill A. M. *Br. Med. J.* 1985, **290**, 629.
60. Hannallah R. and Rosales J. K. *Can. Anaesth. Soc. J.* 1978, **25**, 270.
61. Phelan P. D. *Anaesth. Intensive Care* 1980, **8**, 402.
62. Love J. B. et al. *Anesth. Intensive Care* 1984, **12**, 264; Warner J. A. and Findley W. E. I. *Anaesthesia* 1985, **40**, 348.
63. Duncan P. G. *Can. Anaesth. Soc. J.* 1979, **26**, 206.
64. Donnelly J. et al. *Anaesth. Intensive Care* 1981, **9**, 29; Kamal R. S. and Agha S. *Anaesthesia* 1984, **39**, 464; Barin E. S. et al. *Anaesth. Intensive Care* 1986, **14**, 54.
65. Collett P. W. et al. *Am. Rev. Resp. Dis.* 1983, **127**, 500.
66. Yardley T. H. *Br. Med. J.* 1985, **290**, 861.
67. Warner J. A. and Finlay W. E. I. *Anaesthesia* 1985, **40**, 348.
68. Report, *Br. Med. J.* 1985, **291**, 329.
69. Nunn J. F. *Applied Respiratory Physiology* 3rd ed London: Butterworth, 1987.
70. Kunkel S. E. and Warner M. A. *Anesthesiology* 1987, **66**, 195.

Chapter 39   **MULTIPLE INJURIES**

First-aid treatment of multiple trauma is very important;[1] 25% of those mortally injured in accidents die from respiratory obstruction, so that it is essential that a clear airway is established as a first priority in the unconscious subject. This includes placing these patients on their side in anticipation of the first vomit. The services of an experienced anaesthetist may be invaluable, as urgent tracheal intubation may be required, also pain relief and experienced triage. Post-traumatic pulmonary insufficiency may develop within hours or days.

An aggressive ventilation and fracture fixation regime has been advocated.[2]

Chest Injuries[3]

Respiration is embarrassed should bleeding occur into the airway or into the pleural cavity. Blood clot, saliva, stomach content and other debris may be inhaled to produce suffocation. The flail chest embarrasses physiological ventilatory exchange as some degree of paradoxical respiration occurs.[4] Pain from fractured ribs may also prevent proper excursion of the diaphragm and thoracic cage. Pain relief without respiratory depression is thus important. Up to a quarter of these patients require IPPV, one-fifth are severely shocked and about a third will have other (especially head) injuries. In major thoracic injury the first priority is to treat hypoxia and hypovolaemia. In some cases, IPPV will be required[3] and chest infection is common in these patients. Correct treatment results in fixation of a flail segment in the normal position and prevents a thoracoplasty-like deformity.

Other thoracic injuries which may require treatment include haemothorax (which requires drainage), pneumothorax (requiring intercostal tube to water-seal), chylothorax, direct lung trauma, diaphragmatic rupture, or injury to heart and great vessels. Bronchial tears may give rise to large leaks requiring negative pressure to intercostal drains. They usually heal in time. If air enters the mediastinum the whole body may become bloated with surgical emphysema. Stabbing is a difficult problem, often requiring emergency surgery. Early CVP measurement is helpful in detecting concealed haemorrhage and cardiac tamponade.

Crush Injury of the Chest

This may cause painful breathing or subsequent hypoxia and cardiorespiratory embarrassment. Injury (and operation) to the chest wall is likely to interfere with the patient's ability to rid the tracheobronchial tree of secretions. Pulmonary contusion is common.

To help the patient to breathe and cough, extradural block via an indwelling catheter in the thoracic region is invaluable. Intercostal block may also be helpful. A patent airway must be maintained using suction, endotracheal intubation or tracheostomy. The control of paradoxical movements of the chest wall may be managed by IPPV. Surgical fixation using Rush nails has also been advocated in suitable cases as the patient becomes mobile in a shorter time.

Chest injury can be treated by extradural bupivacaine with morphine.[5]

For outcome of chest injury, *see* Moore P. C. et al. *Anaesth. Intensive Care* 1985, **13**, 362.

Head Injuries[6]

It is vital that proper oxygenation of the brain is maintained. Primary efforts should therefore be directed to maintenance of the airway and adequate pulmonary ventilation, arrest of any serious haemorrhage and maintenance of an adequate blood circulation. The brain may be damaged by contusion, haemorrhage, local or global ischaemia, with diffuse axonal injury,[7] hypoxia (low Pa_{O_2}), very low Pa_{CO_2} or very low BP, hyperthermia, alkalosis, oedema due to fluid overload or embolism. Blood loss from scalp wounds can be significant, so that transfusion is required. Uncomplicated head injury should not prevent the treatment of abdominal injuries, compound limb fractures or haemothorax, though faciomaxillary fractures can usually be left to a later date. Astrocytes and endothelial cells appear to protect against cerebral oedema, and these cells may be spared, even when ischaemia has damaged neurons. Hyperglycaemia (and hypoglycaemia) increases the infarction associated with ischaemia, especially with brain lactate levels above 16 mmol/kg.[8]

Middle Meningeal Haemorrhage

This is the most frequent serious remediable head injury and requires urgent operation.

The most important physical signs are: (1) Progressive deterioration of consciousness; (2) Progressive dilatation of a previously normal pupil; (3) Progressive bradycardia, perhaps with a rising systolic blood pressure; (4) Progressive weakness of the face, arm and even leg on the side opposite to the injury; (5) Apnoea: This sign carries the gravest prognosis, even when instantly remedied by IPPV.

Management of Head Injuries[9]

1. First aid—airway management. Lateral position in anticipation of vomiting, control of haemorrhage, speedy hospitalization.

2. Clinical diagnosis of injuries (*see above*)—Is the head injury localized or diffuse? Glasgow coma scale[39] recording is established and an agreed flow chart commenced. Skull, cervical spine and chest X-rays may be taken.[10] Other injuries are treated.

3. Reduction of raised intracranial pressure by IPPV, etc. Mannitol may be needed later. The value of steroids is in doubt.

4. Evaluation of extent of injury, by CT scan,[11] NMR, isotope scans, etc.

5. Control of clinical or subclinical fits, as shown on the EEG, by barbiturates or benzodiazepines.

6. Monitoring of cerebral function within the controlled neurosurgical environment, by intracranial pressure and compliance (and ICP waveform analysis), EEG and cerebral function monitoring, brainstem auditory evoked potentials (BSAEP), spinal evoked potentials, cerebral blood flow, cerebral oxygen consumption ($CMRO_2$)—normally 3–4 ml/100 g/min, cerebral arterio-venous oxygen difference ($A-JDO_2$)—normally 6–7 vol%, phosphorus spectroscopy, positron emission tomography, etc.

7. Brain protection.[12]

8. General intensive care—early enteral feeding, H_2 blockers, and antacids prevent gastric ulceration.[13] Cholecystitis may complicate head injuries,[14] as may pulmonary damage, due to increased alveolar cholesterol.[15]

Calcium channel blockers may improve cerebral blood flow in the head-injured patient.[16]

Procedure for Transfer of a Patient to a Neurosurgical Unit[17]

(1) The airway is secured by tracheal intubation, or facilities are carried for this if the patient is conscious. Oxygen and a self-inflating bag should be alongside the patient;[18] (2) One or two intravenous cannulae are in place before leaving. A pressure infusor will be required because of the limited head-room for elevation of the fluid container; (3) Recording blood pressure and pulse rate is very difficult. Occasional stops may be necessary. The ECG is monitored continuously; (4) The

doctor and nurse are advised to take travel sickness pills! (5) Suction equipment must be available; (6) The following drugs should be carried: atropine, barbiturate, e.g. thiopentone, suxamethonium, ephedrine, dexamethasone and diuretics. Cardiac arrest equipment must be to hand.

Hyperventilation is advocated in the management of head injuries. The cerebral vasoconstriction which results in normal brain tissue from hypocapnia may result in increased blood supply to the damaged areas.[19]

The long-term effects of head injury can seldom be assessed at the time of admission to the intensive therapy unit. In general the younger the patient the better is the prognosis. Recovery may be complete or partial. Social and personality problems may arise subsequently.

Prognosis
Prognosis after head injury is related to CSF enzyme levels. A CPK level > 150 units/l and LDHi > 150 units/l both carry a bad prognosis.[20] Of those patients in coma for 6 h or more, mortality is up to 40%. In patients more than 40 yr old, mortality is up to 70%.[21]

Brainstem Death[28]

First described clinically in 1959.[32]
For this diagnosis *all* the following signs must be present, in addition to a clear diagnosis of the underlying condition, for at least 12 h: Pupils have no response to light. Oculovestibular reflex absent.[29] (There should be no wax in the ear.) The 'doll's-eye reflex' does not mean that there is brain death. Corneal reflex absent. Gag reflex absent. Carinal reflex absent. No response to pain inflicted on head. No spontaneous respiration for 4 min[30] in the absence of hypothermia, and anoxia, with a normal ($> 6 \cdot 6$ kPa) Pa_{CO_2} provided that no drugs which affect these reflexes persist in the body. PEEP is useful here.[31] EEG confirmation is useful but opinions vary concerning its necessity. Such a diagnosis is made by two doctors independently and is confirmed by re-examination at least 24 h later. It should be noted that spinal reflexes may persist after brain death.

(*See also* Annotation, *Br. Med. J.* 1982, **285**, 1487; Pallis C. *Br. Med. J.* 1983, **286**, 123; Editorial, Jennett B. *Br. J. Anaesth.* 1981, **53**, 111; *ABC of Brain Stem Death.* (Pallis C. ed.) London: BMA, 1985.)

Spinal Column Injuries

The utmost care is necessary during transport and movement.[33]

Early Management
Should tracheal intubation be necessary to procure a patent airway, the production of muscle relaxation with suxamethonium may remove the protective splinting provided by the support muscles to allow subluxation and cord damage. After 72 h, a non-depolarizing relaxant should be used, to avoid the occurrence of hyperkalaemic cardiac standstill from massive potassium efflux from denervated muscle.[34]
(*See also* Swain A et al. *Br. Med. J.* 1985, **291**, 1558.)

Abdominal Injuries

All penetrating wounds of the abdomen require laparotomy. The signs of intra-abdominal trauma may be misleading in the presence of other injuries, but an accurate diagnosis should not be necessary in making the decision to perform laparotomy.

Blood Transfusion

This will often be required where there are multiple injuries. An estimate of blood loss from fractures can be made as follows: Humerus 500–1000 ml; radius and ulna, 500 ml; pelvis, over 3000 ml; femur, 500–2000 ml; tibia and fibula, 500–1000 ml.[35] Monitoring of central venous pressure may be very helpful in these cases, and a blood volume estimation carried out later as a check on the adequacy of replacement.

Fat Embolism

This was first described in man by Friedrich Albert Zenker (1825–1898) in 1862,[36] was first diagnosed clinically by von Bergmann (1836–1907) in 1873,[37] and may be wrongly diagnosed as shock. Due to escape of droplets of fat into the circulation, and their deposition in the lungs, brain or skin. Often associated with fractures of lower-limb bones. Onset of symptoms may rapidly follow the injury or may be delayed for 2 or 3 days.

Pulmonary signs and symptoms include dyspnoea, pallor, cyanosis, pyrexia and frothy sputum. Bilateral shadowing is seen in chest X-rays. Fat globules may be seen in sputum and urine.

Cerebral changes (really signs of cerebral hypoxia) usually seen in the first 24 h after operation or injury, with pyrexia, and there may be restlessness, leading to coma, convulsions and paralysis; deep coma carries a bad prognosis; fat emboli may sometimes be seen in the retinal vessels with an ophthalmoscope.

Skin signs are likely to be a purpuric eruption with petechiae over the upper chest, neck and conjunctivae and are seen on the second or third day.

Metabolic signs. Hypoxaemia, acidosis, hypocalcaemia, anaemia and thrombocytopenia.

The lung manifestations are the most common and constitute the major threat to life. Pao_2 is often low, despite high inspired oxygen concentration due to ventilation/perfusion imbalance. If the patient's respiratory exchange can be maintained, the prognosis is good.

Treatment

All therapeutic measures depend upon proper respiratory management. Blood gas estimation is important, especially monitoring of Pao_2. IPPV is often necessary, and where Pao_2 cannot be satisfactorily maintained despite high inspired oxygen concentration, a positive pressure in the expiratory phase may be helpful. Steroids are useful in the first 24 h but harmful thereafter.

Fulminant fat embolism syndrome. Onset within a few hours of the injury or operation with rapid progress to a fatal conclusion.[38]

It has been said that collapse in the second hour after operation is likely to be due to shock; in the second day, to fat embolism; in the second week, to pulmonary embolism. *See* 'Adult Respiratory Distress Syndrome', p. 778.

Burns

(*See* Chapter 24.)

Prognosis Scoring in Critically Ill Patients

Acute physiology score (APS) based on 34 physiological measurements.[22]

Simplified acute physiology score (SAPS) based on 13 physiological measurements.[23]

Acute physiology and chronic health evaluation (APACHE)[24]

APACHE II[25] is a development of this, based on general health, age and the worst value of 12 physiological measurements during the first 24 h after admission. These are rectal temperature, mean arterial pressure, heart rate, respiratory rate, oxygenation ($AaDO_2$ or Pao_2) arterial pH, serum Na^+, serum K^+, blood creatinine, haematocrit, white cell count, and the Glasgow Coma Score[39] (Rating = 15 − actual GCS). Each parameter is scored from 0 to +4 (abnormally high or low)

A total score of 10 relates to a mortality of about 10%

A total score of 20 relates to a mortality of about 20%

A total score of 30 relates to a mortality of about 40%

A total score of 35 relates to a mortality of about 75%

A total score of 40 relates to a mortality of about 90%

'The burn index'[26]

'*Injury severity scoring system*' (ISS) is based on the type and extent of injury in the various anatomical regions.[27]

References

1. Mather S. J. and Edbrooke D. L. *Prehospital Emergency Care*. Bristol: Wright, 1985.
2. Goris R. J. A. et al. *J. Trauma* 1982, **22**, 895.
3. McCoy J. A. and Azim E. *Anaesthesia* 1976, **31**, 532; Jette N. T. and Barasch P. G. *Anaesthesia* 1977, **32**, 475.
4. Richardson D. J. et al. *Ann. Surg.* 1982, **196**, 481.
5. Rankin A. P. N. and Camber R. E. H. *Anaesth. Intensive Care* 1984, **12**, 311.
6. Hunter A. R. *Neurosurgical Anaesthesia* 2nd ed. Oxford: Blackwell, 1976; Horton J. M. *Anaesthesia* 1975, **30**, 212. *Br. J. Anaesth.* 1976, **48**, 767.
7. Genarrelli T. A. et al. *Ann. Neurol.* 1982, **12**, 564; Adams J. H. *Ann. Neurol.* 1982, **12**, 557.
8. Plum F. *Neurology (NY)* 1983, **33**, 222.
9. Teesdale G. et al. *Br. Med. J.* 1982, **285**, 1695; Michenfelder J. D. *J. Irish Coll. Phys. Surg.* 1983, **12**, 154.
10. Royal College of Radiologists, *Lancet* 1983, **1**, 115.
11. Vicario S. et al. *Ann. Emerg. Med.* 1982, **11**, 475.
12. McDowell D. G. *Br. J. Anaesth.* 1985, **57**, 1.
13. Gudeman S. K. *Neurosurgery* 1983, **12**, 175.
14. Branch C. L. et al. *Neurosurgery* 1983, **12**, 98.
15. Crittenden D. J. *J. Trauma* 1982, **22**, 766; Popp A. J. *J. Neurosurg.* 1982, **57**, 784; Weiner F. et al. *Crit. Care Med.* 1983, **11**, 132.
16. Harris R. J. *Stroke* 1982, **13**, 759.
17. Gentleman D. and Jennett B. *Lancet* 1981, **2**, 853; Brydon J. S. and Jennett B. *Br. Med. J.* 1983, **286**, 1791.
18. For portable lung ventilators, *see* Gray A. J. G. *Br. J. Hosp. Med.* 1981, **25**, 144.
19. McDowall D. G. in: *Recent Advances in Anaesthesia and Analgesia*—12 (Hewer C. L. and Atkinson R. S. ed.). Edinburgh: Churchill Livingstone, 1976, Ch. 2.

20. Hans P. et al. *Acta Anaesth. Belge.* 1984, **35**, 79.
21. Levati A. et al. *J. Neurosurg.* 1982, **57**, 779.
22. Knaus W. A. et al. *Lancet* 1982, **2**, 642.
23. LeGall J. R. et al. *Crit. Care Med.* 1984, **12**, 975.
24. Knaus W. A. et al. *Crit. Care Med.* 1981, **9**, 591.
25. Knaus W. A. et al. *Crit. Care Med.* 1985, **13**, 124.
26. Feller I. et al. *JAMA* 1980, **244**, 2074.
27. Baker S. P. et al. *J. Trauma* 1974, **14**, 187.
28. Conference of the Royal Colleges and Faculties, *Br. Med. J.* 1976, **2**, 1187; Report of Ad hoc Committee of the Harvard Medical School. *JAMA* 1977, **237**, 982; Searle J. and Collins C. *Lancet* 1980, **1**, 641; Jennett B. *Br. J. Anaesth.* 1981, **53**, 1111.
29. Klug N. *J. Neurol.* 1982, **227**, 219.
30. Pallis C. *Br. Med. J.* 1982, **285**, 1487.
31. Perel A. et al. *Intensive Care Med.* 1983, **9**, 25.
32. Mollaret P. and Goulon M. *Rev. Neurol.* 1959, **101**, 3.
33. Gumley G. et al. *J. Bone Joint Surg.* 1982, **64B**, 520.
34. Plunkett P. K. et al. *Br. Med. J.* 1986, **292**, 485.
35. Wilson J. N. *Proc. R. Soc. Med.* 1967, **60**, 951.
36. Zenker F. A. *Beiträge zur Anatomie der Lungen.* Dresden: G. Shonfeld's Buchhandlung, 1862.
37. Von Bergmann E. *Berl. Med. Wochensch.* 1873, **10**, 385.
38. Hagley S. R. *Anaesth. Intensive Care* 1983, **11**, 162.
39. Teasdale G. and Gentleman D. *Scott. Med. J.* 1982, **27**, 7; Teasdale G. *Br. J. Anaesth.* 1976, **48**, 761; Teasdale G. and Jennett W. B. *Lancet* 1974, **2**, 81; Jennett W. B. and Teasdale G. *The Management of Head Injuries* 3rd ed. Philadelphia: Davis, 1980.

Chapter 40   # NUTRITIONAL FAILURE

Minimal Nutritional Requirements

The daily basal requirements of main food constituents may be stated as shown in *Table 40.1*.

Table 40.1. Daily minimal nutritional requirements

	Requirement per kg body weight	Requirement for 70-kg man	Calories supplied per g
Water	25–35 ml	1500–2500 ml	—
Protein	1 g	70 g	4·0
Carbohydrate	2 g	140 g	4·0
Fat	2 g	140 g	9·0
Calories	30 kcal	2100 kcal	—

Minerals and vitamins are also necessary.

Tube Feeding

When the patient cannot swallow, a liquid diet must be given by gastric tube. A 1-mm internal diameter plastic tube is suitable. A Seldinger wire is used for stiffening during insertion. This tube is too small for puréed hospital food.

Tube is better than intravenous feeding (which carries a definite complication rate) whenever the function of the gastrointestinal tract allows.

Eggs and powdered milk have the highest biological degree of utilization and surpass other natural proteins for tube feeding. Various artificial foods are available. Complan is widely used. Each 100 g of Complan contains 44 g of carbohydrate, 31 g of protein, 16 g of fat as well as minerals and vitamins, and provides 450 kcal.[1] Alternative diets (they are prepared and stored aseptically): (1) Complan 150 g, Caloreen 75 g, methyl cellulose 3 g, water 1 litre; (2) Clinifeed 500, 2–3 litres daily; (3) Complan 150 g, Hycal 200 ml, methyl cellulose 3 g, water to 1 litre; (4) Vivonex and Vivonex HN (synthetic amino acids) 2 litres daily; (5) Triosorbon (medium-chain triglycerides) 3 litres daily; (6) Puréed sterilized hospital diet. To all of these, minerals and vitamins are added as necessary.

Complications
(1) Pharyngeal and oesophageal ulceration; can be reduced by using small, soft nasogastric tubes; (2) Reflux oesophagitis; can be reduced by nursing the patient 10° head up; (3) Cross-infection; (4) Diarrhoea; can be helped by slowly increasing diet to full dose, by methyl cellulose and by codeine phosphate syrup, BP, 10 ml 6-hourly; (5) Dehydration if adequate water intake is not added; (6) Change of enteral flora, e.g. there may be colonization with faecal organisms in neonates with nasoduodenal feeding tubes;[2] (7) Risk of aspiration from fine-bore nasogastric tube feeding.[3]

Parenteral Feeding[4]

This is the intravenous provision of food during gastrointestinal failure and keeps the patient alive and well until the cause of the failure can be corrected. It is usually instituted after a few days' starvation, or when gastrointestinal failure can be expected to occur, e.g. after abdominal operations.

It is also indicated in hypermetabolic states to make up the required energy supply, e.g. burns and severe infections, and for abnormal losses of body metabolites, e.g. intestinal fistulae.

The calorie requirement is approximately:

$$30 \text{ kcal/kg/day} \times \text{the degree of stress multiplication factors.}$$

These factors are: 1·25 for specific dynamic action of administered amino acids; 1·5 for being nursed in a cold environment; 1·5 for multiple injuries; 1·25 for a fractured long bone; 1·1 for operative stress; 1·25 for chronic sepsis.

Carbohydrates
Carbohydrate stores in the body are very restricted, the average adult having only some 5 g of blood glucose and 100 g of liver glycogen available. Utilization of fat to provide calories depends on carbohydrate to prevent ketosis. The minimum carbohydrate requirement for this is 400 kcal (1·6 MJ, i.e. Mega Joules) per day, although normally at least 50% of the administered calories are from glucose.
1. Glucose (provides 4·0 kcal/g). One litre of isotonic (5%) solution provides only 200 kcal. Concentrated solutions are therefore necessary to produce a high-calorie intake without over-hydration. 25% glucose solution supplies 1000 kcal (4 MJ)/litre; 50% glucose supplies 2000 kcal (8 MJ)/litre. These are

clinically the most useful solution strengths. After fasting, surgery, infections and trauma, the glucose tolerance is low and consequently sugar may be lost in the urine. Insulin is given to increase glucose retention at a rate of 10 units of insulin for every 25 g glucose, intravenously as a bolus or from a powered syringe, in which it is carried in dextran or Gelufusine to prevent adsorption into the plastic. Equally good as fat for optimizing nitrogen balance.[5]

2. *Laevulose (fructose)* (provides 4·0 kcal/g). Enters into metabolism and builds up carbohydrate stores rapidly. High rates of infusion cause lactacidosis. Contraindicated in the presence of hereditary fructose intolerance.

3. *Sorbitol.* Useful as an additive to amino acid solutions. Oxidized to fructose in the liver. Provides 4·0 kcal/g. Administration rates over 0·33 g/kg/h result in osmotic diuresis.

4. *Alcohol (ethanol)* (provides 7 kcal/g). May be given as a 5% solution up to 1 g/kg/day. May cause lactic acidosis and worsen the acidotic effects of fructose and sorbitol. Contraindicated in pancreatitis and hepatocellular disease.

Proteins

There is a 'biochemical pool' of amino acids in the body, some 100 g of protein being broken down and resynthesized every day.

1. *Albumin and plasma.* Should be given to those patients with reduced blood volume or hypoproteinaemia. Whole blood may be given for anaemia.

2. *Protein hydrolysates.* Produced by chemical fission.

3. *Crystalline amino acid mixtures.* These may be pure laevo-rotatory acids or equimolecular mixtures of laevo- with the unphysiological dextro-rotatory forms. Some *d*-amino acids can be catabolized, but the major part is lost by renal excretion.

The amino acid nitrogen requirement per 24 h has been quoted as 7·5 g in starvation, 14 g after surgery or trauma, and up to 25 g in severe catabolism.[6]

Fat

Provides 9·0 cal/g. Advantages include lack of osmotic effects and tolerance by vessels. No losses occur in faeces or urine. Fat is provided as an emulsion, with particles 0·5–1·0 μm in diameter. An emulsifying agent is added and also glucose, glycerin or sorbitol to render the preparation istonic. Well utilized in the postoperative phase[7] but requires the concurrent administration of at least 400 carbohydrate cal/day for its metabolism. This has been challenged.[8] Can be used to provide up to 50% of calorie intake (e.g. up to 0·5–1 litre/day). The patient's plasma may be examined each day for excessive milkiness (which calls for a reduction in fat intake). This is more likely in severe acute ulcerative colitis, acute pancreatitis, peritonitis, uraemia and septicaemia. Occasional side-effects are shivering, flushing, dyspnoea, headaches, nausea and vomiting, chest and back pains. Fat emulsions are possibly a source of phosphate. Fat should provide at least 8% of the administered calories. Concomitant heparin reduces free fatty acid (FFA) levels in infants.[9]

Suitable commercial preparations which are now available include Intralipid (soya-bean oil in a 10 or 20% emulsion with egg-yolk phosphatide as an emulsifier, isotonic with glycerol) and Lipiphysan (cotton-seed oil, emulsified with soya lecithin, isotonic and sorbitol), Liposyn (safflower oil) and lipofundin.

Table 40.2. Some parenteral nutrition solutions

Product	Calories per litre	Calorie source	Nitrogen content per litre	Vitamins	Na⁺ mmol per litre	K⁺ mmol per litre	Other electrolytes	pH	Comments
Vamin-glucose	650	Glucose	9·4 g	—	50	20	Mg^{++} Ca^{++} Cl^-	5·2	Extra calories required
Aminoplex 12	—	—	12·44 g	—	35	30	Mg^{++} Cl^-	—	The extra g of N in Aminoplex 14 is all glycine
Aminoplex 14	—	—	13·4 g	—	36	30	Cl^-	—	—
FreAmine II	—	—	12·6 g	—	10	—	PO_4^{---}	—	—
Synthamin 9	—	—	9·3 g	—	73	60	Mg^{++}	—	—
Synthamin 14	—	—	14·4 g	—	73	60	Cl^- PO_4^{---}	—	—
Synthamin 17	—	—	17·9 g	—	73	60	Mg^{++}	—	—
Vamin	—	—	9·4 g	—	50	20	Mg^{++} Ca^{++} Cl^-	—	—
Intralipid 20 per cent	1000	Soya bean oil emulsion	—	—	—	—	PO_4^{---} 15 mmol per litre	—	Contains vitamin E
25 per cent glucose	1000	Glucose	—	—	—	—	—	—	—

Vitamin Requirements per day (Shenkin A. and Wretlind A. *World Rev. Nutr. Diet,* 1978, **28.** 1): Thiamine (B₁) 1·4 mg; riboflavine (B₂) 2·1 mg; pyridoxine (B₆) 2·1 mg; vitamin B₁₂ 2 µg; nicotinamide 14 mg; biotin 0·35 mg; pantothenic acid 14 mg; folic acid 2 mg; vitamin C (ascorbic acid) 3·5 mg; vitamin D 100 IU; vitamin K 140 µg; vitamin A 700 IU; vitamin E 30 IU.

An average dose of fat would be 0·25 mg/kg/h. Fats are satisfactory even in the early post-trauma phase.[10]

Vitamins
Their importance first pointed out by F. Gowland Hopkins (1861–1947) of Cambridge in 1912 for which he received the Nobel Prize in 1929.[11] (*See Table 40.2.*)

Management

Intravenous feeding may be used to supplement oral or tube feeding or as complete parenteral nutrition. It should supply 30 kcal and 1·0 g of amino acids/kg/day. When metabolic rate is raised these figures may be increased to 45 kcal and 1·5 g.

Assessment of Nutritional Status[12]

1. Body fat: Triceps skin-fold thickness (errors due to oedema).
2. Body protein: Arm muscle circumference (errors due to oedema), serum albumin, total lymphocyte count, creatinine-height index, serum transferrin, serum thyroxine-binding albumin, serum retinol-binding protein.[13]
3. Body immunity: skin test with streptokinase, mumps skin antigen, or *Candida albicans*. (Patients may be immunocompromised due to other factors.)

The simplest regimens are, in any 24-h period, 1 litre of synthetic amino acid solution (e.g. 7% Vamin (9·4 g nitrogen) or Aminoplex 14 (13·4 g nitrogen) plus 500 ml of 50% glucose (with up to 100 units soluble insulin), all given concurrently, plus 500 ml of Intralipid 20% plus 500 ml of any suitable solution depending on the patient's electrolyte, blood or albumin requirement. As most intravenous feeding solutions are hypertonic (with the exception of fat emulsions) they cause thrombophlebitis and may be given through central venous catheters. Aminoplex 5 and some other solutions contain balanced mixtures of calories and amino acids, i.e. 200 kcal/g of nitrogen and lend themselves to simple regimens.

Indications[14]

Indications for intravenous feeding, include: (1) Gastrointestinal failure from any cause; (2) Hypercatabolism from major trauma, burns, sepsis and acute glomerular nephritis; (3) Preoperative malnutrition; (4) Severe anorexia nervosa; (5) Head injuries.[15]

Adult Dose[16]

(1) Water, 2–3·5 litres/day, depending on losses (urine, exhaled water vapour, alimentary tract losses and sweat; (2) Calories: 2000–3500 kcal (8–14 MJ) depending on degree of catabolism as judged clinically; (3) Nitrogen, 10–17 g (63–100 g of amino acids) per day depending on degree of catabolism, judged clinically, or by bedside nitrogen balance:

Approximate nitrogen loss (g)

$$= \frac{24 \text{ hours urinary urea (g)}}{2}$$

$$+ \frac{\text{Rise of blood urea (mg/100 ml)} \times \text{body weight (kg)}}{250}$$

or

Approximate nitrogen loss (g)

$$= [24 \text{ hour urinary urea (mmol)} \times 3]$$

$$+ \left[\frac{\text{rise of blood urea (mmol/litre)} \times \text{body weight (kg)}}{40}\right].$$

(4) Sodium, 100 mmol/day + 50 mmol for each degree C rise in temperature (assuming a reasonably normal sodium balance); account must be taken of the sodium content of the administered drugs, and sodium loss in ileostomy fluid (100 mmol/l) and bile (40 mmol/l); (5) Potassium, 60 mmol/day + 10 mmol for each degree C rise in body temperature (assuming a reasonably normal potassium balance)—it must be well diluted in dextrose or saline; (6) Phosphate, 35 mmol/day, unless the patient is in renal failure, when a quarter of this will suffice; phosphate should never be mixed with calcium or magnesium for injection; (7) Magnesium sulphate, 8 mmol/day; calcium (gluconate), 5–15 mmol/day; iron, 20–40 mg/day; zinc, 3 mg/day + 2 mg for catabolism + 15 mg/l for gut fluid lost; manganese, 0·5 mg/day; copper, 1 mg/day; chromium, 10 μg/day; cobalt, 0·05 mmol/day; iodine, 0·5 mmol/day; selenium is also required; (8) Vitamins A, B, C, D, E and K, including folic acid 3 mg/day; (9) Blood or albumin as specifically required.

Complications of Parenteral Feeding[17]

1. Glucose metabolism. (*a*) Hyperosmolar syndrome (facial flushing, lethargy, coma), due to insufficient insulin, insufficient water or glucose overload. The prognosis of hyperglycaemic hyperosmolar coma is much worse than that of hypernatraemic hyperosmolar coma; (*b*) Hyperglycaemia, due to insufficient insulin. Ketoacidosis may occur; (*c*) Glycosuria; (*d*) Hypoglycaemia.
2. Amino acid metabolism. (*a*) Prerenal uraemia, due to overdose, relative to renal function; (*b*) Ammonium intoxication[18] due to relative arginine deficiency, in cirrhosis, severe negative nitrogen balance and sometimes in young children; (*c*) Metabolic acidosis, due to excessive chloride in some amino acid solutions. Respiration is stimulated by amino acids;[19] (*d*) Amino aciduria.
3. Fats. Essential fatty acid deficiency. Dyslipoproteinaemias.[20]
4. Water. Circulatory overload and waterlogging are common risks.
5. Electrolytes (mainly deficiencies). (*a*) Hypokalaemia—especially in patients on ventilators; (*b*) Hyponatraemia—often seen, e.g. in septic shock, but not often a complication of the regime; (*c*) Hypocalcaemia (tetany and muscle spasm); (*d*) Hypophosphataemia (failure of oxygenation, encephalopathy, haemolysis) (Phosphate requirements: 20–40 mmol/day. 80 mmol/day is tolerable and gives a positive phosphate balance);[21] (*e*) Hypomagnesaemia (disorientation, tetany and tremor). Most likely during the anabolic phase;

(*f*) Zinc deficiency (diarrhoea, poor healing, skin lesions); (*g*) Copper deficiency (anaemia, hypoproteinaemia, leucopenia).
6. *Vitamin deficiencies.* (*a*) Vitamin B_{12} (anaemia); (*b*) Folic Acid (anaemia); (*c*) Vitamin K (coagulopathy); (*d*) Vitamin C (bleeding, bruising, poor healing); (*e*) Thiamine—deficiency for even one month may produce cardiac failure from acute beri-beri.
7. *Catheter sites* (thrombophlebitis, bacteraemia, damage to local anatomy).
8. *Miscellaneous.* Cholestasis may occur, possibly due to overgrowth of intestinal bacteria. It has been prevented by metronidazole, suggesting anaerobic infection.[22] Change of RQ[23] and leucocytosis may occur.[24]

The metabolic diurnal rhythm may be maintained by giving calories and amino acids by day, and saline, additives, albumin, blood or nothing by night. This allows consumption of the patient's endogenous fat stores at night.

In renal, hepatic and cardiac failure and diabetes, etc. the usual dietary restrictions apply with equal force to parenteral nutrition. For insertion of central venous line, *see* 'Intravascular Techniques', Chapter 42.

(*See also Drug Ther. Bull.* 1980, **18**, 77, 85; Symposium, *Br. J. Anaesth.* 1981, **53**, 121 et seq.; Rushman G. B. in: *Handbook of Intensive Care* (Atkinson R. S. et al. ed.) London: Chapman & Hall, 1981; Phillips G. D. and Garnys V. P. *Anaesth. Intensive Care* 1981, **9**, 221.)

References

1. Peaston M. J. T. *Postgrad. Med. J.* 1967, **43**, 317.
2. Dellagrammaticas H. D. *Arch. Dis. Child.* 1983, **58**, 115.
3. Bosco M. J. and Rosen M. D. *Br. Med. J.* 1984, **289**, 1421.
4. See also Rushman G. B. in *Handbook of Intensive Care* (Atkinson R. S. et al. ed.) London: Chapman & Hall, 1981.
5. Nordenstrom J. *Ann. Surg.* 1983, **197**, 27.
6. Woolfson A. M. J. *Res. Clin. Forums* 1979, **1**, 35.
7. Lindholm M. *Crit. Care Med.* 1982, **10**, 740; Nordenstrom J. et al. *Ann. Surg.* 1982, **196**, 221.
8. Chen W. J. *J. Parenter. Enter. Nutr.* 1983, **7**, 6.
9. Zaidan H. *J. Pediatr.* 1982, **101**, 599.
10. Van Deyk K. et al. *Intensive Care Med.* 1983, **9**, 73.
11. Hopkins F. G. *J. Physiol. (Lond.)* 1912, **44**, 425.
12. Boles J. M. *Crit. Care Med.* 1983, **11**, 87.
13. Abel R. M. *J. Thorac. Cardiovasc. Surg.* 1983, **85**, 752.
14. Yamada N. *Br. J. Surg.* 1983, **70**, 267.
15. Rapp R. P. *J. Neurosurg.* 1983, **58**, 906.
16. Shenkin A. and Wretlind A. *World Rev. Nutr. Diet* 1978, **28**, 1.
17. Weinsier R. L. et al. *J. Parenter. Nutr.* 1982, **6**, 421.
18. Thomas D. W. et al. *J. Parenter. Nutr.* 1982, **6**, 503.
19. Weissman C. et al. *Ann. Intern. Med.* 1983, **98**, 41.
20. Lindholm M. et al. *J. Parenter. Nutr.* 1982, **6**, 432.
21. Pigon J. *Acta Anaesth. Scand.* 1985, **29**, 50.
22. Capron J-P. et al. *Lancet* 1983, **1**, 446.
23. MacFie J. *J. Parenter. Nutr.* 1983, **7**, 1.
24. Wiernik A. *Am. J. Clin. Nutr.* 1983, **37**, 256; Allison S. P. *Drug. Ther. Bull.* 1984, **24**, 2.

Chapter 41	**MEASUREMENT AND MONITORING**[1]

Minimal instrumental monitoring consists of observation of the BP and the ECG and with IPPV, measurement of the ventilatory volume. More sophisticated monitoring involves measurement of the percentages of inhaled and exhaled gaseous components, neuromuscular tone, urine output and body temperature. In many major surgical operations, pulmonary arterial catheterization and pulse oximetry[86] may be required.

When the senior author of this book qualified as a doctor the word monitor was a noun and meant a senior pupil who helps a schoolmaster, or a shallow-draught battleship armed with heavy guns. Now it is a verb, and to the anaesthetist a very important one. Monitoring may be: (1) Non-invasive, e.g. inspection; auscultation; palpation; sphygmomanometry; ECG; EEG; EMG; peripheral temperature; transcutaneous gas sampling, etc.; (2) Minimally invasive: urinary flow and temperature; oesophageal stethoscope and thermometry; rectal temperature; tympanic membrane temperature; (3) Invasive: central venous flow directed catheterization; arterial catheterization; intravascular electrodes for blood-gas and pH estimation.

There will be general agreement that patients under anaesthesia should have a blood pressure cuff and ECG terminals, as suggested by *Mortality associated with Anaesthesia* (Lunn J. N. and Mushin W. W. Nuffield Provincial Hospitals Trust, 1982). This is a minimal requirement. Familiarity with these in *every case* will enable the information they provide to be intelligently assessed in the ill patient. New equipment and new procedures may or may not improve the care of the patient; they will seldom decrease the cost of care.

The main problems in monitoring are at the *patient interface*. For this reason, repeated clinical examination is still of primary importance. A simple, swift clinical examination may reveal oxygenation, fluid balance, acid–base status, cerebral perfusion, blood flow, lung function, coagulation defects, temperature, etc. The primary equipment for measurement and monitoring is the hand, the eye and the ear of the attending doctor (sometimes aided by the stethoscope). Accurate detailed recording is also fundamental. Pen and paper are the most reliable tools for this!

Computer Aids in Monitoring[2]

Computerization has developed in two ways. First, ordinary mini- or microcomputers have had programs written for collection, presentation, analysis, interpretation,[3] (e.g. prognosis-making and servo control of therapy) and storage of patient data. The entire record sheet can be kept on a computer screen each day and stored on disc. Secondly, the use of dedicated processors within monitoring devices (e.g. cardiac output and automatic blood pressure). So much data is now collected in intensive care units that there is a need for computerized help to record it. Interpretation of data is still best done by the experienced human mind.

There are major unresolved areas, e.g. keyboard entry is slow and cumbersome except for expert typists. Also computer breakdown occurs occasionally. For problems with outstanding anaesthetic records *see*.[102]

The reasons given for the abandonment of computerized monitoring, which is widespread in some countries, include: (1) Computers only handle quantifiable data and much clinical judgement extends beyond this; (2) Computers have not brought economy to patient care; (3) Computerization has not generally reduced or eliminated paperwork, rather the opposite; (4) Computers can make mistakes. If computers were to improve the quality of patient care, they would have to bring to the attention of the clinician some result of the data which was not obvious before.[4]

Arterial Pressure[5]

History

Stephen Hales (1677–1761) in 1733 was the first to attempt measurement of the blood pressure of animals by direct cannulation of an artery.[6] Herrison, 1834,[7] devised a crude instrument to be placed directly over an artery for clinical measurement of blood pressure. Vierordt (1818–1884) was the first to estimate the amount of counter-pressure necessary just to obliterate the arterial pulse.[8] Etienne Jules Marey (1830–1904) in 1875 and von Basch (1837–1905) pioneered clinical sphygmomanometry.[9] Mosso (1846–1910) in 1895[10] and Gärtner (1855–1937) in 1899 designed apparatus in the nature of a finger plethysmograph.[11] S. v. Basch described sphygmomanometry in Vienna for clinical use in 1883.[12] (For history of BP measurements in anaesthesia, *see* Calverley R. K. 'Classical File'; *Surv. Anesthesiol.* 1985, **29**, 78).

Scipione Riva-Rocci (1863–1937) of Turin introduced the blood-pressure cuff in 1896,[13] though the cuff he used was only 5 cm in width. In 1901, von Recklinghausen (1833–1910) drew attention to the importance of the width of the pneumatic cuff, and E. A. Codman (1869–1940) in 1894 and Harvey Cushing (1869–1939)[14] of Boston advocated the use of blood-pressure readings regularly during anaesthesia. An early advocate of the anaesthetic chart was S. O. Goldan.[15] Korotkoff (1874–1920) (Russian physician) in 1905[16] described the sounds heard over an artery at a point just below the compression cuff.[17] The binaural stethoscope was introduced in the 1880s.[18] The mercury manometer was first used to measure blood pressure in 1828 by Poiseuille (1799–1869) (Paris physiologist).[19] It is more reliable than the anaeroid type, introduced in 1897 by Hill (1866–1952) and Barnard (1868–1908).[20] When compared and checked against intra-arterial pressures the Korotkoff sounds are inaccurate. At low pressure, the sphygmomanometer overreads and at high pressures it underreads. The inaccuracy of the diastolic pressure is greater than that of the systolic.[21]

The Compression Cuff

This should be of the correct width. If the cuff is too narrow, readings will be high; if too wide, readings will be low. In general it is recommended that the cuff should cover approximately two-thirds of the length of the upper arm or 20% greater than the diameter of the arm. The American Heart Association recommends a 12–14 cm rubber bag, long enough to encircle half the arm, centred over the brachial artery. The cloth cover should be made of non-extensible material so that pressure is exerted uniformly. Recommended cuff widths are neonate 2·5 cm, 1–4 years 6·0 cm, 4–8 years 9·0 cm, adult 12–14 cm, for the adult leg 15 cm. A conventional cuff overestimates arterial pressure on a fat or muscular arm, and underestimates it on a thin arm or on the arm of a child.

Palpation Method
The cuff is inflated until the peripheral pulse is obliterated. It is then decompressed at a rate of 2–3 mmHg per heart beat. The level of pressure at which the radial pulse returns is recorded as the systolic blood pressure. A pulse monitor attached to a finger can be used in a similar manner.

The Korotkoff (1874–1920) Sounds[16]
The cuff is inflated to 30 mmHg above the palpated blood pressure and then decompressed at a rate of 2–3 mmHg per heart beat. As blood begins to flow back through the compressed artery, turbulence is produced and this is transmitted as vibrations or sounds which can be detected by a stethoscope placed over the brachial artery. The point of first sound is taken as the systolic pressure; the point at which there is an abrupt decrease in intensity (muffling) is taken as the diastolic pressure. During surgical operations it may be preferable to fix the stethoscope over the brachial artery on the medial side of the arm above the elbow where it is covered by the cuff.

Venous congestion must be avoided as it may give rise to an abnormally high diastolic and an abnormally low systolic reading (i.e. the cuff should not remain inflated longer than necessary).

Sometimes the Korotkoff sounds fade completely between systolic and diastolic pressures. This is known as the auscultatory gap. A false systolic reading may be obtained unless pressure has first been checked by the palpation method.

The pressure can also be obtained by watching the oscillations of the needle of the anaeroid manometer though this is less accurate.

(*See also* The stethoscope, Dornette W. H. L. *Anaesth. Analg. (Cleve.)* 1963, **42**, 711.)

Flush Method
Use in newborn babies and infants. The limb is elevated and milked of blood. The cuff is then inflated and slowly deflated. The pressure at which a flush appears is taken as the systolic pressure. It may in fact be nearer to a mean arterial pressure.

Pressure may be measured by a mercury column or by an anaeroid manometer. The former is accurate, but is relatively bulky and must be held upright. The latter is small and compact but requires frequent calibration against a mercury column.

Automatic Recording by Indirect Method
Efforts to follow the blood pressure continuously or at regular intervals have resulted in the design of various types of apparatus. A small piezo-crystal is placed over the artery. The cuff is blown up automatically until the crystal no longer picks up arterial pulsations and then it deflates.[22]

Oscillometer[23]
The double cuff, now used in the Pachon and von Recklinghausen oscillometers was described by Galavardin.[24] Erlanger[25] and Pachon[26] were, with the Berlin worker von Recklinghausen, pioneers of this instrument. The cuff contains two compartments, black and red. Male and female connections enable the cuff to be connected to the oscillometer; before use the pointer is adjusted to zero by means

of the control valve situated at the top left of the dial. The cuffs are inflated in the normal way by the hand bellows to a pressure greater than systolic blood pressure and the discharge valve at the bottom of the dial is slightly opened to release slowly and continuously the pressure in 10-mm stages. At the end of each 10-mm pressure drop, the scale reading is noted and the spring-loaded control arm to the left of the discharge valve is pulled forwards. The needle deflections which occur show a definite increase at the level of systolic blood pressure and a definite decrease at the level of diastolic pressure. Maximum oscillation of needle corresponds well with the mean arterial pressure (although diastolic readings are not always accurate.[27]) The oscillometer is reasonably accurate when the Korotkoff sounds are inaudible as in hypotensive states. Automatic oscillometers are available, e.g. Cardiac Recorders, Dinamap, Datascope. These machines have proved reliable and reasonably accurate.[28]

Direct Intra-arterial Methods (*see* Chapter 42)

Radial artery cannulation is a low-risk, high-benefit method of patient monitoring. The risk of ischaemic complications (though not of partial or complete occlusion of the artery) is very slight.[29] Intra-arterial monitoring is not essential in patients under induced hypotension. A needle or cannula, e.g. teflon 20 G, is inserted into an artery and connected via a column of fluid to a manometer or transducer. Radial arterial puncture can be painful.[30] The transducer may be one of four main types: (1) Resistance-wire strain gauge; (2) Capacitance manometer; (3) Variable inductance pressure gauge; (4) Semi-conductor gauge. Accurate reproduction of a pressure wave requires a frequency response of the entire system which is the tenth harmonic of the fundamental wave frequency. The frequency response is limited to that of the slowest link in the chain. Thus it is important that the connection between artery and transducer should be as short and rigid as possible. Too narrow tubing increases frictional resistance to the movement of fluid; too wide tubing increases the inertia as the mass of fluid is larger. Direct measurement is the only practical method during cardiopulmonary bypass when the circulation is not pulsatile, or when intense vasoconstriction renders the peripheral pulse impalpable. Direct methods are subject to technical difficulties, cause discomfort to the patient and may carry a risk to the artery used, especially when large cannulas are employed. Occlusion has been successfully treated by 0·1% phentolamine injection into the brachial artery.[31] Arterial occlusion can be diagnosed by thermography.[32] Before the radial artery is used for cannulation a test for the presence of an ulnar artery must be applied. The hand may be exsanguinated by the patient making a fist actively (or passively when unconscious) while the radial artery is occluded and the return of blood from the ulnar artery observed (Allen's test[33]). The patency of the ulnar artery can also be determined by the Brodsky test.[34] Other arteries which have been used include the femoral,[35] brachial and dorsalis pedis.[36] The Butterfly needle, 21 gauge, has been advocated for percutaneous arterial cannulation.[37] An anaeroid manometer can be used for continuous display of pressure readings. More often, an electronic transducer is used and a continuous flush system delivers heparinized saline (1 unit/ml) at about 3 ml/h.[38] (*See also* Runciman W. B. et al. *Anaesth. Intensive Care* 1981, **9**, 314; Bishop V. A. and Payne J. P. *Br. J. Anaesth.* 1983, **55**, 1156P.) When there is difficulty in putting a cannula into the radial artery, the axillary artery can be used if intra-arterial monitoring is essential.[39]

SI units are not normally used in blood pressure measurements.

Pulse Monitors

The most popular type of monitor consists of a photoelectric cell or carbon microphone fixed over a digit. The output is fed into a simple electrical circuit which signals each systole by the flick of a needle, the flash of a light or a sound from a loudspeaker.[22] The apparatus may be combined with a sphygmomanometer for rapid blood-pressure estimations, and a device may be added to count the pulse rate and record it on a dial.

Pulse monitors of this type function best under conditions of vasodilatation and may be less reliable in the presence of vasoconstriction.

Pulse monitors are particularly valuable: (1) In small children and infants when access to a palpable pulse may be difficult; (2) During controlled respiration, when changes in respiration would not give warning of circulatory arrest; (3) During conditions of maximal vasodilatation when the amplitude of the signal is related to arterial pressure.

The heart beat can also be monitored by the use of a precordial stethoscope, a method particularly suited to use in infants. In children and adults undergoing major surgery an oesophageal stethoscope may also be useful. Also useful for diagnosis of air embolus during operation. An oesophageal probe which incorporates stethoscope, thermistor and ECG lead has been described for paediatric, use, [40] but may cause bradycardia from vagal stimulation.[41]

Cardiac Output[42]

1. Swan–Ganz Catheters[43]

These are balloon-tipped, flow-directed flexible pulmonary artery catheters for measuring pulmonary capillary wedge pressure. Cardiac catheterization was performed in the horse by Chareau and Marey in 1855, in the dog, by Claude Bernard in 1879 and in man probably by Bleichroder in 1905, who passed a catheter into his own vascular system[44] and then by Forssman.[45] Lategola developed the balloon tip,[46] and Swan and Ganz modified it for clinical work. Cold saline is injected into the pulmonary artery proximal to the thermistor at the tip of the Swan–Ganz catheter. Its thermodilution is proportional to the pulmonary blood flow and, therefore, to the cardiac output. A mini-computer calculates the actual readings and presents the data. Pulmonary artery wedge pressure (PAWP) (a close index of left atrial pressure) is also recorded directly. Right ventricular ejection fraction can also be measured.

Indications. (a) Low cardiac output, and (b) Pulmonary oedema; (c) Intermittent or continuous mixed venous blood-gas analysis.

Reliability. Certain criteria are used to ensure accuracy: (a) The mean PAWP should be less than the mean PA pressure, and infusate should flow freely through the catheter, indicating that the catheter tip is free; (b) The wedge tracing should have atrial waveform; (c) The wedge Po_2 should be greater than the non-wedge Po_2. Room temperature fluid is as accurate as iced infusate; 3 measurements per determination are better than one, and a minimum of 15% difference between successive measurements suggests a real change of cardiac output.[47]

Errors in measurement. These are worst in spontaneously breathing patients, where the instantaneous readings, especially those used in automated estimations, do not reflect accurately the waveforms throughout the respiratory cycle.[48] A strip recorder should be used for manual measurement.

These catheters are inserted via standard central venous approaches. The supraclavicular route has the lowest incidence of misdirection. Progress of the catheter tip is monitored by X-ray control or by observation of the pressures being measured at the tip. Most pass to the right lower lobe artery. *Complications*[49] include dysrhythmias, damage to the lung,[50] thrombo-embolism,[51] balloon rupture, infection, migration[53] and knotting of the catheter.[52] Some of these may be prevented by deflating the balloon of the dwelling catheter while not being used for measurements. The balloon blocks 5–15% of the lung blood vessels. The catheters cost between £30 and £80 each. Percutaneous pulmonary arterial catheterization via the arm veins before operation is reasonably safe and simple as well as being effective.[54] It can, however, result in some morbidity.[55]

2. Dye Dilution Methods
Dye is injected via a catheter threaded up to the pulmonary artery, and blood samples taken from a peripheral artery and analysed by a photoelectric method. Successive measurements are plotted on a graph, and the area under the curve is determined, using: (*a*) a planometer; (*b*) mathematical methods;[56] (*c*) computers. Recirculation of the dye must not be included in the measurement, and this can be avoided if the graph is plotted on semi-logarithmic paper. Since the decay of the dye dilution curve is exponential it will then appear as a straight line which can be extended to exclude the secondary recirculation peak.

$$\text{Cardiac output (ml/min)} = \frac{\text{Mass of dye injected}}{\text{Area under curve}} \times 60.$$

3. The Use of Non-invasive Methods
Combined ultrasound and Doppler probes give flow in the aorta (or any other vessel, e.g. the umbilical artery in the fetus).[57] Radio-imaging with a gamma-camera after intravenous injection of 99^{m} technetium. Technetium gives the left ventricular ejection fraction, either on a first-pass study or gated fraction studies. The computer multiplies this by the heart rate to give the cardiac output. This technique also gives information on the size, localization and reversibility of cardiac infarcts. Radio-thallium is also used. The echocardiogram is now also available for this purpose.

4. The Fick Principle (1864) (Adolf Eugen Fick, 1829–1900, of Zurich)[58]
This is used to measure pulmonary blood flow which is equal to cardiac output. Specimens of central venous blood are obtained from a catheter passed to the right ventricle or pulmonary artery. Arterial blood is obtained. Oxygen consumption is measured by use of a spirometer. Calculations are made according to the formula:

$$\text{Cardiac output (ml/min)} = \frac{\text{Total body oxygen consumption (ml/min)}}{\text{Arteriovenous oxygen difference (ml\%)}} \times 100.$$

Inaccuracies occur if there are changes in the lung reserve volumes which affect the spirometer reading.

The Electrocardiogram (*see also* Chapter 2)[59]

The electrocardiogram acts as an excellent non-invasive monitor of cardiac rhythm and especially of unexpected cardiac arrest or rate changes. For routine monitoring (not the 12-lead diagnostic trace), three electrodes are placed on the chest, as near to the heart as convenient. This increases the signal-to-noise ratio. Since 75% of ischaemic ECG patterns are best detected from the V_5 position, the electrodes should be placed on the positions CM_5 if possible (left clavicle, manubrium, 5th intercostal space, anterior axillary line). Under no circumstances does it afford a measure of the efficiency of myocardial contraction or of cardiac output; in fact normal electrical activity may occur when there is no measurable blood pressure. If the electrodes are placed on the patient's back ST depression may be seen in the normal heart.

Artefacts
The ECG is liable to artefacts which must be differentiated from changes originating in the heart. They may be caused by disconnection of an electrode, superimposition of potential from another person in contact with the patient, improper earthing of apparatus, etc. It is possible for interference to take the form of a sine wave giving rise to the appearance of ventricular tachycardia. Bizarre complexes occur, e.g. ST depression and widening of the QRS complex may be due to battery exhaustion.[60]

Myocardial Ischaemia
Monitoring of the familiar ST depression (>1 mm) of acute ischaemia may be extended by 'ST mapping'. Sixteen (or more) electrodes are stuck to the precordium in four lines of four, making a square, extending the length of the sternum and from the right sternal edge to the left midaxillary line. Recordings of ST depression from each are analysed by computer and presented as a picture of the precordium, showing where ST depression is greatest, thus outlining the site of infarct. Posterior infarction is, of course, still best seen in III and VF, with ST elevation, deep Q waves and T inversion.

Dysrhythmias
The ECG is useful for the diagnosis of abnormal cardiac rhythm. The commonest abnormalities seen are ventricular ectopic beats and nodal rhythm but any abnormality can occur.

Cardiac Arrest
The ECG differentiates between asystole and ventricular fibrillation and is invaluable for the monitoring of therapeutic measures.

Central Venous Pressure

Venous Tone
About half the total blood volume is accommodated in the systemic venous system, only about 15% in the arterial system. Alterations in venous tone play a large part in the regulation of the haemodynamics of the circulatory system.

Central Venous Pressure Measurement (CVP)

History
Venous pressures were first measured by Stephen Hales (1677–1761) in 1733 in a mare, and first measured in man by Frey in 1902[61] and used clinically in 1910.[62] In 1931 Forssmann, a urologist, pioneered (on himself) cardiac catheterization,[63] for which he was awarded the Nobel prize in 1956. The first plastic intravenous catheter (polythene) was used in 1945.[64]

The term central venous pressure refers to the pressure in the right atrium or the inferior or superior venae cavae. For technique of insertion *see* 'Intravenous Techniques', Chapter 42.

Readings
The zero must be aligned to a chosen reference point, i.e. the midaxillary line or the manubriosternal angle. This may be facilitated by the use of a spirit level on a long piece of wood or by a horizontal 'gunsight'. More elaborate methods using a transducer and automatic recording equipment can also be used. Normal central venous pressure may be taken as $3–10\,cmH_2O$. Values over $20\,cmH_2O$ may indicate heart failure, or misplacement of the catheter tip into the right ventricle or pulmonary artery.

Indications
(1) Open-heart surgery. The amount of blood in the circulation can be adjusted to maintain a venous pressure around $5–10\,cmH_2O$ during the immediate post bypass period. Cardiac output may increase with progressive fluid loading up to a CVP of $12–15\,cmH_2O$. Above $20\,cmH_2O$ (zero reference at mid-chest) pulmonary oedema is likely. When cardiac function is reasonably normal, right and left atrial pressures are closely related. However, in cardiac disease this relation is lost and the left atrial pressure must be measured (*a*) directly, e.g. after open-heart surgery; (*b*) indirectly, as a pulmonary wedge pressure, using a Swan–Ganz catheter; (2) Whenever massive infusions or transfusions are required. Central venous pressure gives a measure of the adequacy of replacement and early warning of overloading; (3) When circulatory haemodynamics are unstable, e.g. during and following removal of a phaeochromocytoma and major haemorrhage; (4) In acute circulatory failure of obscure origin. Useful in the critically ill patient treated in an intensive therapy unit, e.g. for intravenous feeding, repeated injections of irritant drugs; (5) In severe shock; (6) In paediatric surgery where accurate replacement is essential.

Interpretation of CVP

When the patient is:	Usual CVP is: (cmH₂O)	When the patient has:	Usual CVP is: (cmH₂O)
Supine	-5 to $+5$	IPPV with PEEP	$+5$ to $+15$
Head-down	$+5$ to $+10$		
On IPPV	$+5$ to $+10$	Congestive cardiac failure	$+5$ to $+10$
Head-up	-5 to -10	Pulmonary embolism	$+5$ to $+20$
Hypovolaemic	0 to -5	Cardiac tamponade	$+5$ to $+20$
In ARDS	$+5$ to $+20$		

Complications

These include: (1) Thrombophlebitis, infection, septicaemia; (2) Pneumothorax; (3) Haemothorax; (4) Hydrothorax; (5) Brachial plexus injury; (6) Air embolus; (7) Pericardial effusion; (8) Lymph leakage.

Central venous pressure measurements are not a good guide to daily fluid requirements and should not be used for this purpose. A patient can easily be waterlogged or dehydrated in the presence of a normal CVP.

(*See also* Editorial, *Br. Med. J.* 1980, **1**, 1035. For hazards of CVP monitoring, *see* Csanky-Treels J. C. *Anaesthesia* 1978, **33**, 172.)

Pulmonary Arterial Wedge Pressure

Normal pressure 0–5 mmHg. After cardiac surgery and severe myocardial infarction fluid loading up to wedge pressures of 10–30 mmHg may occasionally be required. See 'Cardiac Output, *above*. (*See also* Fowler M. B. et al. *Br. Med. J.* 1980, **1**, 435.)

Measurement of Blood Loss

Gravimetric Method

The simplest and most commonly employed method. Blood loss is estimated by measurement of the gain in weight of swabs and towels, together with measurement of the contents of suction bottles; 1 ml of blood weighs 1 g. Weighing of swabs is said to underestimate blood loss by 25%.

Colorimetric Method

Swabs and towels are mixed thoroughly with a large known volume of fluid, which is then estimated colorimetrically. Errors may occur due to incomplete extraction or contamination with bile. The patient's haemoglobin must be known.

$$\text{Blood loss (ml)} = \frac{\text{Colorimeter reading} \times \text{volume of solution (ml)}}{200 \times \text{patient's Hb (g\%)}}$$

In operations involving complex exchanges of blood (e.g. extracorporeal circulation), it may be useful to weigh the whole patient before and after operation.

Estimation of Blood Volume

It is sometimes useful to measure blood volume before operation and also as a check on the adequacy of transfusion. Normal blood volumes can be obtained from nomograms according to height and weight. Where bodyweight and height are in reasonable proportion, a rough guide is to take blood volume as 7·7% of bodyweight or 85 ml/kg.

Plasma volume can be obtained by dye-dilution or radioactive-iodine-dilution methods. Semi-automatic instruments are available for the radioactive-iodine method. Dilution is measured after a 15-min mixing time, calculations being made automatically. Labelling of red cells with radioactive chromium can also be carried out and a dilution test made, but the method is more elaborate as cells have to be first separated for labelling.

Analysis of Gas Mixtures

1. Oxygen

Paramagnetic analysers (described by Pauling in 1946[65]) are useful. Gases are classed as paramagnetic or diamagnetic according to their behaviour in a magnetic field. The former seek the area of strongest, the latter of weakest flux. Of the gases of interest to the anaesthetist only oxygen, nitric oxide and nitrogen dioxide are paramagnetic, others are weakly diamagnetic. This principle is used in commercial apparatus for analysis of oxygen concentrations in a gas mixture.

Small oxygen analysers may be of the polarographic or the microfuel cell type.[66] For evaluation of oxygen analysers *see*.[100]

2. Carbon Dioxide

The infrared analyser (first employed in 1865).[67] Gases whose molecules contain two dissimilar atoms or more than two atoms absorb radiation in the infrared region of the spectrum. *Capnography*[68] for continuous recording of carbon dioxide in anaesthetic systems and in intensive care. A continuous sample of respired gas is withdrawn from as near to the trachea as possible, and the CO_2 content displayed (as a percentage) on a continuous line paper trace. The highest CO_2 content is found at the end of expiration, and is called the 'end-tidal CO_2' ($ETCO_2$). In spite of theoretical interference by anaesthetic agents and the fact that $ETCO_2$ is not exactly the same as $PaCO_2$, the measurement is extremely useful. Major changes in $ETCO_2$ may indicate important problems, e.g. malposition of tracheal tube, air embolism, etc.

3. Volatile Anaesthetic Agents

The analysis depends upon *the principle of ultraviolet absorption*.[69] Useful in checking the calibration of vaporizers and for monitoring the concentration in closed-circuit anaesthesia.

The Narkotest[70] depends upon the variation of elasticity of rubber. The Engström Emma and other apparatus are also available.[101]

4. Simultaneous Analysis of Various Gases

This can be carried out using: (*a*) *The mass spectrometer*[71]—molecules are ionized, accelerated by an electric field and deflected by a magnetic field. The angle of deflexion is related to molecular weight. Does not differentiate between carbon dioxide and nitrous oxide which have the same molecular weight. It is possible that one instrument will be able to serve several operating rooms; it also has applications in intensive care;[72] (*b*) *Gas chromatography*. Separation of components by means of a partition column. The estimation takes several minutes, so does not follow the changes in a single breath.

5. Gas Chromatography[73]

This can be used for the analysis of volatile agents in blood. The term is a contraction for gas–liquid chromatography and is not concerned with 'colour', the word 'chromatography' being handed down from an older technique of liquid–liquid separation in which the components were identified by colour.

The essential of the technique is the partition of a substance between two solvents. The first is adsorbed onto an inert material (stationary phase). The moving phase is gaseous. To keep the components of the mixture in gaseous phase it may be necessary to heat the column along which they pass. To maintain flow along the column, the components are 'dissolved' in a large volume of continuously flowing 'solvent' gas. When the carrier gas and its component substances pass along the tube there is a time delay, depending on the solubility of the component in the stationary phase, which is different for every component of the mixture.

A detector is required, so that after separation in the column, the presence and amount of any substance other than carrier gas are determined. Detectors may be of various types: (1) Katharometer, a thermal conducting device, a heated thermistor which is sensitive to presence of vapours of different thermal conductivity; (2) Flame ionization detector. Carrier gas is hydrogen which is ignited in the detector so that organic compounds yield ionized products which migrate to alter voltages on electrically charged plates; (3) Electron-capture device. Useful for halogenated compounds. The emerging components are bombarded by γ-rays, and the electrons emitted from halogen ions collected electrically. Before measurement of concentration of the various substances with any of these devices can be made, it is necessary to calibrate by use of samples of known concentration. The electrical output of a detector is proportional to the mass of the substance, and appears as a deflection from base line. If drawn on paper moving at constant speed, the area under the curve is proportional to total mass of compound in the sample. When the deflection occurs as a sharp peak, approximating to a triangle, the area may be considered as height × width at half height. If the base of the triangle is constant, peak height is proportional to area.

Respiration

Tidal Volume and Minute Volume (*see also* Chapter 2)

1. The displacement meter (Parkinson and Cowan). This is the type of gas meter used for domestic purposes. It is most conveniently used to measure expired

gases—that is, by connecting it to the outlet port of a non-rebreathing valve.
2. *Inferential meters.* Volume is inferred from the number of revolutions of a vane rotated by the gas stream. Now commercially available as small and light apparatus, which may be connected directly to a face-piece or catheter mount: (*a*) Wright anemometer, gas passes through ten tangential slots in a cylindrical stator ring to turn a flat two-bladded rotor. A recent development displays gas volumes on a calibrated meter and is not affected by water condensation. The Wright anemometer is a simple, robust, light-weight, accurate and cheap device, ideally suited for use in the intensive care ward. Its accuracy is slightly dependent on the wave form of the gases passing through it;[74] (*b*) Dräger Volumeter; two light-weight lozenge-shaped meshing rotors; (*c*) Bennett Ventilation Meter; two interlocking rotors of light alloy which run in jewelled bearings.
3. *Spirometry. See* Hutchinson J. *Med. Chir. Trans.* 1849, **29**, 137; *The Spirometer.* London: Churchill, 1852; Spriggs E. A. et al. *Proc. R. Soc. Med.* 1976, **69**, 450.
4. *The pneumotachograph* measures flow and flow changes over small time intervals. It measures pressure drop of a gas flowing in a rigid tube containing a linear flow resistance. It is a compact apparatus which can be added to an anaesthetic circuit or ventilator.
5. *Radio imaging.* The technique utilizes 81^m krypton, generated from a cyclotron, using a gamma camera for detection. It may be combined with 99^m technetium injection which shows lung perfusion at the same time.
6. *Thoracic impedance plethysmography.* The electrical impedance of the chest changes during respiration. The impedance is measured in horizontal and vertical planes and computed into volume.
7. *Infant apnoea mats.*

Blood-gas Measurements[75]

History
Blood-gas measurements started by Pflüger (1829–1910) in 1872.[76] (*See also* Astrup P. *Anaesthesia; Essays in its History.* (Rupreht J. et al. ed.) Heidelberg: Springer-Verlag, 1985, p. 176; Laver M. B. *Acta Anaesth. Scand.* 1982, **26**, 250; Astrup P. and Severinghaus J. W. *History of Gases, Acids and Bases.* Copenhagen: Munksgaard, 1986.)

Arterial Oxygen Tension
The oxygen electrode. This consists of a platinum cathode and a silver anode in an electrolyte solution. Platinum gives up electrons to oxygen and the resulting voltage change can be measured and expressed in terms of oxygen tension. Platinum receives a deposition of protein when used in biological fluids, so the electrode system must be isolated from the blood sample by a thin gas-permeable membrane. The Clark electrode[77] is the basis of the modern oxygen electrode though modifications have been produced.[78] In the Clark type electrode, the oxygen diffuses through the skin and is measured by a polarographic technique. Information concerning the blood flow in a flap of skin or in the skin after reconstructive vascular surgery, can also be obtained. (*See also* Tremper K. K. *Can. Anaesth. Soc. J.* 1984, **31**, 664.)

Blood samples. Must be drawn from an artery into a syringe whose dead space has been filled with heparin. The oxygen consumption of whole blood at 38 °C is sufficient to cause a fall in Po_2 of about 0·4 kPa/min. Samples should therefore be analysed at once, or kept cool to reduce oxygen consumption. Oxygen may also diffuse into the substance of the plastic syringe. The loss is greater when Pao_2 is high. Use of glass syringes obviates this source of error. *Hypoxaemia*. 'Normal' values may be as low as 10 kPa (70 mmHg) in the over-70 age group, compared with 13·5 kPa (100 mmHg) in younger age groups. Arterial oxygen tension is a more sensitive index of oxygen lack than oxygen saturation—*see* the dissociation curve (*Fig. 2.2*, Chapter 2).

Venous samples show satisfactory correlation with arterial ones for pH, bicarbonate, and Pco_2 (1 kPa higher), but not for Po_2.[79]

Transcutaneous Oxygen Electrodes[80]
These give accurate and continuous measurement provided that: (1) The patient is not cold or vasoconstricted; (2) The skin under the electrode is not degenerating as a result of prolonged electrode placement; (3) Drift problems have been eliminated from the system. The $tcPco_2$ is normally 1–3 kPa.

Transcutaneous Carbon Dioxide Monitoring[81]
A glass electrode with special membrane is closely applied to the skin. Voltage output is logarithmically related to the Pco_2. Response time is slow. The electrode is heated to 44 °C. The cutaneous Pco_2($tcPco_2$) reads 0·5 kPa higher than the $Paco_2$.

Venous Oxygen Content
This is an index of adequate cardiac output and tissue perfusion. Normal value is 14 ml/100 ml blood. Central venous oxygen content correlates well with mixed venous oxygen content.[82]

Pulse Oximetry[86] (the measurement of oxygen saturation of the blood)
First performed in 1913.[83] The oximeter is attached to the lobe of the ear or to a finger. Suitably filtered light passes through the ear and is measured by a photocell. Non-invasive, reliable and expensive. They may be inadequate in severe vasoconstriction. Recordings are assessed through analogue or digital outputs.

Arterial Carbon Dioxide Measurement
Direct methods. A sample of blood may be taken by direct arterial puncture. 'Arterialized' capillary blood from the back of the hand is an acceptable alternative provided there is no stasis and the skin temperature is at least 35 °C (vasodilatation from general anaesthesia will usually produce these conditions). Normal value 5–6 kPa (40 mmHg).
Indirect methods
1. Method of Campbell and Howell.[84] 1–5 litres of oxygen are rebreathed for 90 s. The patient is rested for 2 min and the bag contents rebreathed for a further 20 s or 5 breaths. Carbon dioxide is then estimated and closely reflects $Paco_2$.
2. End-expired gas capnography. (*See above*).

Biochemistry

Laboratory techniques are available to measure the degree of acidosis or alkalosis in a blood sample and to separate them into respiratory and metabolic components.[85] Normal standard bicarbonate is 24 mmol/l. Lactate, pyruvate and acetate may also be measured. Blood samples may be taken by direct arterial puncture, but where the patient is vasodilated 'arterialized' blood from the dorsum of the hand or capillary blood is satisfactory. Venous blood is of value especially if a specimen of mixed venous blood from the vena cava can be obtained. (*See above*). The ordinary Tco_2 electrolyte estimation is, however, a good guide. Normally only 5% of this is dissolved CO_2. The remainder is bicarbonate. (*See* Chapter 3.)

Correction of Metabolic Acidosis
The figure for base deficit obtained by the Micro-Astrup method is expressed in mmol/l of blood. To find the deficit in mmol total for the extracellular fluid compartment of the whole body, a simple formulae can be used:

Base deficit $\times$ 0·3 $\times$ bodyweight in kg

= Dose of bicarbonate required in mmol.

Semi-continuous biochemical analysis and accurate interpretation is now being developed.[87]

Electromyography in Anaesthetic Practice

(*See* Pugh A. D. et al. *Anaesthesia* 1984, **39**, 574; *see also* Chapter 14.)

The Electro-encephalogram

Electrical activity of the brain in animals noted by Richard Caton of Liverpool (1842–1926), in 1875. Hans Berger (1873–1941)[88] in 1931 described alpha rhythms in man. Adrian and Matthews (1934) developed the technique of the electro-encephalogram.[89] First used in anaesthesia in 1950[90] after a suggestion by Gibbs in 1937.[91]

Types of Wave
1. *Delta waves*: 0·3–3·5 c/s; amplitude 100 μV. Occur in infants and sleeping adults.
2. *Theta waves*: 4–7 c/s 10 μV.
3. *Alpha waves*: 8–13 c/s 20 μV in infants, 75 in children, 50 in adults. Augmented by closing eyes or mental repose. Reduced by visual and mental activity.
4. *Beta waves*: 14–25 c/s 20 μV.
5. *Gamma waves*: 26 c/s or more. 10 μV. Rare. Artefacts may occur due to movement of the patient or to superimposition of an electrocardiogram if an electrode is placed directly over an artery.

Changes during Anaesthesia
1. *Relation to depth of anaesthesia*. Changes in electrical activity follow a characteristic pattern when most general anaesthetics are given. Seven electro-

encephalographic levels have been described.[92] The first level is relatively flat, the second shows high-amplitude rhythmical discharges, the third is complex and irregular, and succeeding levels show an increasing suppression until the seventh level which is characterized by a complete absence of measurable waves. The electro-encephalograph is not a reliable indicator of consciousness or unconsciousness during nitrous-oxide–oxygen–relaxant anaesthesia.[93]

2. *Effect of hypoxia*. Causes slowing of the frequency of the waves. After about 20 s of complete anoxia the recording becomes a straight line. Lesser degrees of hypoxia may not affect the tracing until a level of 40% arterial oxygen saturation is reached.

3. *Effect of raised carbon dioxide tension*. Potentiates the effect of other anaesthetic drugs.

4. *Hypotension*. A rapid fall of blood pressure is associated with slow high-amplitude waves or temporary cessation.

5. *Hypothermia*. Below 35–31 °C some decrease in amplitude and frequency occurs. At 20 °C there may be little activity.

6. *Circulatory arrest*. Activity ceases. The recording can be used as a measure of cerebral circulation during cardiac massage. After cardiac arrest, the presence of alpha rhythm carries a good prognosis, while periods of wave suppression indicate a bad prognosis.

Index of Cerebral Circulation

The main application of the electro-encephalograph is as a measure of the circulation to the brain. In this respect it is a more sensitive index of the failing heart than the electrocardiogram, and it is a valuable monitor during operations involving extracorporeal circulation, including carotid endarterectomy and similar operations.[94]

Computer processing and interpretation is now a reliable reality. *See also* 'Brain death'.

Cerebral Function Monitor

See Dubois M. et al. *Anaesthesia* 1978, **33**, 157. (*See also* Chapter 2.)

Nuclear Magnetic Resonance[95]

The patient is placed in a strong magnetic field and exposed to pulses of radiofrequency waves which cause the protons in the nucleus of each atom to spin and give off magnetic resonance which is detected by sensors and recorded. The reaction of the proton depends on its position in the molecule and on the surrounding structures. Useful for detecting grey/white contrast in brain when used in conversion/recovery sequence. The repeated free induction delay sequences show changes in proton density. The spin-echo mode shows up space-occupying lesions and cerebral oedema. Short T_1 values are seen in haemorrhage, and long ones in infarction, malignancy and cysts.[96]

Temperature[97]

The founder of clinical thermometry was C. A. Wunderlich (1815–1877), professor of medicine at Leipzig, whose classic work appeared in 1868.[98] 'Before his work fever was a disease; after it, a symptom' (Garrison).

1. The standard mercury-in-glass clinical thermometer
2. Dial thermometers. Simple instruments: (*a*) A flat bimetalic spiral spring which winds or unwinds as temperature changes; (*b*) The pressure gauge (Bourdon gauge)—a hollow ribbon of metal which winds or unwinds as temperature changes produce pressure changes within the coil.
3. Thermocouple. A circuit of two dissimilar metals produces an e.m.f. when the two junctions are at different temperatures. The e.m.f. is measured and calibrated according to temperature. The apparatus can be made small and it has a rapid response.
4. Platinum resistance thermometry. The resistance of a metal varies according to temperature, and the former is measured by means of a Wheatstone bridge. A platinum coil can be mounted within the lumen of a hypodermic needle for insertion in body tissues.
5. Thermistor (*therm*ally sensitive re*sistor*). A small bead of semi-conductor material can be sealed into hypodermic needles. Semi-conductors have negative coefficients of resistance, which can be measured using a Wheatstone bridge.
6. Skin thermometers. Difficulties arise due to poor contact with the skin and because skin temperature itself falls as heat passes to the thermometer: (*a*) The magnetic thermometer—temperature affects its field strength; (*b*) The radio-meter—infrared rays, which are emitted by all substances at temperatures above absolute zero, are focused on a thermistor device.

The temperature can be taken from the mouth, rectum, skin, oesophagus or tympanic membrane. Evaluation of body temperature (*see* Ilsley A. H. et al. *Anaesth. Intensive Care* 1983, **11**, 31).

Renal Function

1. Urine flow. Universally loved by intensivists.
2. Blood urea, creatinine and nitrogen levels.
3. Creatinine clearance; takes several days to show changes in function.
4. Urine analysis including osmolality.
5. Gamma counting after injection of chromium, EDTA, 99^m technetium, DTPA or iodine 131. Hippuran shows up very rapid changes in renal function, particularly useful after transplantation. The normal biological half-life of 20 min is prolonged up to 70 min in renal failure.

Safety in Monitoring Equipment

When electrical apparatus is used there is a danger of ventricular fibrillation should any fault allow current to pass through the heart. The current required is of the order of 80 mA if the electrodes are in the skin, but only 150–400 μA when there is an internal electrode in or near the heart.[99] Mains frequencies are more likely to give rise to ventricular fibrillation than currents with higher or lower frequencies. The traditional method of earthing does not necessarily provide for safety. Earthing prevents build-up of static electricity, but may allow a fatal current to pass through the patient to earth if equipment used becomes faulty. Also it is important to note that where there are multiple power supplies, two earths may be at different potential, allowing a small current to pass through the patient. Such flow can occur when the apparatus is switched off. Multiple electrical appliances should therefore have a common earth lead. The use of isolated systems has been advocated for patient-care areas. Isolation transformers can be used. Central venous lines for CVP monitoring should use 5% glucose and not saline as the latter is a good conductor of electricity. (*See also* Chapter 5.)

(*See also* Stevens A. J. *Preparation for Anaesthesia* Tunbridge Wells: Pitman, 1980, Ch. 21 and 22; Sykes M. K. et al. *Principles of Clinical Measurement*, 2nd ed. Oxford: Oxford University Press, 1981.)

References

1. *See also* Franklin C. B. in: *Recent Advances in Anaesthesia and Analgesia—*13 (Hewer C. L. and Atkinson R. S. ed.). London: Churchill Livingstone, 1979; Saidman L. J. and Ty Smith N. *Monitoring in Anesthesia* USA: Butterworth, 1984; Runciman W. B. et al. *Anaesth. Intensive Care* 1981, **9**, 314; *Monitoring in Anesthesia and Critical Care Medicine* (Casey Blitt ed.) Edinburgh: Churchill Livingstone, 1985.
2. Paull J. D. *Anaesth. Intensive Care* 1980, **8**, 228.
3. Gardner R. M. *Crit. Care Med.* 1982, **10**, 823.
4. Phillips G. D. et al. *Anaesth. Intensive Care* 1982, **10**, 223; Prakash O. *Crit. Care Med.* 1982, **10**, 811.
5. O'Brien E. T. and O'Malley K. *Br. Med. J.* 1979, **2**, 851, 970, 1048, 1124.
6. Willius F. A. and Keyes T. E. *Cardiac Classics.* St Louis: Mosby, 1941, Vol. I, p. 131.
7. Herrison J. *Le Sphygmomètre.* Paris: Crochard, 1834; Stephen Hales; *Physiologist and Botanist* (Clark-Kennedy A. E. ed.). Cambridge University Press, 1977; Booth J. *Proc. R. Soc. Med.* 1977, **70**, 793.
8. Vierordt K. *Arch. Physiol. Heilk.* 1854, **13**, 284.
9. von Basch S. *Z. Klin. Med.* 1883, **33**, 673.
10. Mosso A. *Arch. Ital. Biol.* 1895, **23**, 177; Booth J. *Proc. R. Soc. Med.* 1977, **8**, 228.
11. Gärtner G. *Wien. Med. Wochenschr.* 1899, **49**, 1412.
12. Medvei V. *Br. Med. J.* 1983, **286**, 649.
13. Riva-Rocci S. *Gaz. Med. di Torino* 1896, **47**, 981 (reprinted in English translation in *Foundations of Anesthesiology* (Faulconer A. and Keys T. E. ed.). Springfield, Ill.: Thomas, 1965, p. 1043.
14. Cushing H. W. *Ann. Surg.* 1902, **36**, 321; *Boston Med. Surg. J.* 1903, **148**, 291 (reprinted in 'Classical File', *Surv. Anesthesiol.* 1960, **4**, 419).
15. Goldan S. O. *Philadelphia Med. J.* 1900, **6**, 850.
16. Korotkoff N. S. *Izvest. imp. Voyenno-Med. Acad. St Petersburg* 1905, **11**, 365.
17. Comroe J. H. *Anesth. Analg. (Cleve.)* 1976, **55**, 900.
18. Morris S. *Practitioner* 1967, **199**, 674; *see also* Drife J. O. *Br. Med. J.* 1985, **290**, 977.
19. Poiseuille J. L. M. *Archs. Gén. Méd. (Paris)*, 1828, **18**, 550.
20. Hill L. and Barnard H. L. *Br. Med. J.* 1897, **2**, 904.
21. Pereira E. et al. *Eur. J. Anaesthesiol.* 1985, **2**, 11.
22. Sara C. A. and Shanks C. A. *Anaesth. Intensive Care* 1978, **6**, 226.
23. von Recklinghausen H. *Neue Wege zur Blutdrukmessung.* Berlin: Springer-Verlag, 1931; Enderby D. H. in: *Hypotensive Anaesthesia* (Enderby G. E. H. ed.). Edinburgh: Churchill Livingstone, 1985, p. 193.
24. Gallivardin L. *Presse Méd.* 1922, **9**, 766.
25. Erlanger J. *Johns Hopkins Hosp. Rep.* 1904, **17**, 53.
26. Pachon V. *C. R. Soc. Biol. (Paris)* 1909, **66**, 776.
27. Hutton P. and Prys-Roberts C. *Br. J. Anaesth.* 1982, **54**, 234P.
28. Hutton P. et al. *Anaesthesia* 1984, **39**, 261.
29. Slogoff S. et al. *Anesthesiology* 1983, **59**, 42.
30. Clark G. S. et al. *Anaesthesia* 1982, **37**, 78.
31. Burrell A. R. *Anesth. Intensive Care* 1977, **5**, 388.
32. Evans P. J. D. et al. *Anaesth. Intensive Care* 1977, **5**, 231.
33. Allen E. V. *Am. J. Med. Sci.* 1929, **179**, 237; *see also* Brown A. E. et al. *Anaesthesia* 1969, **24**, 532; Fandi S. K. and Reynolds A. C. *Anesthesiology* 1983, **59**, 147.
34. Brodsky J. B. *Anesth. Analg. (Cleve.)* 1977, **56**, 448.
35. Soderstrom C. A. *Am. J. Surg.* 1982, **144**, 309.

36. Spoerel W. E. et al. *Can. Anaesth. Soc. J.* 1975, **22**, 91.
37. Cole P. et al. *Anaesthesia* 1976, **31**, 69.
38. Morray J. and Todd S. *Anesthesiology* 1983, **58**, 187.
39. Brown M. et al. *Anaesth. Intensive Care* 1985, **13**, 38.
40. Inkster J. S. *Anaesthesia* 1966, **21**, 111; Baker A. B. and McLeod S. *Anaesthesia* 1983, **38**, 892.
41. Cordero E. T. and Hon E. H. *J. Paed.* 1971, **78**, 441.
42. Crowther J. and Jenkins B. S. *Br. J. Clin. Equip.* 1980, **5**, 34.
43. Swan H. J. C. and Ganz W. et al. *N. Engl. J. Med.* 1970, **283**, 447; George R. J. D. and Banks R. A. *Br. J. Hosp. Med.* 1983, **29**, 286.
44. Bleichroder F. *Berl. Klin. Wochenschr.* 1912, **49**, 1503; Forssmann W. T. J. *Klin. Wochenschr.* 1929, **47**, 93.
45. Harvey A. M. *Science at the Bedside, 1905–1945.* Baltimore: Johns Hopkins University Press, 1981.
46. Lategola M. and Rahn H. *Proc. Soc. Exp. Biol. Med.* 1953, **84**, 667.
47. Stetz C. W. et al. *Am. Rev. Respir. Dis.* 1982, **126**, 1001.
48. Cengiz M. et al. *Crit. Care Med.* 1983, **11**, 502.
49. Sprung C. L. et al. *Chest* 1981, **79**, 413.
50. Gomez-Arnau J. et al. *Crit. Care Med.* 1982, **10**, 694.
51. Devitt J. H. et al. *Anesthesiology* 1982, **57**, 335.
52. Dumesnil J. G. and Proul G. *Am. J. Cardiol.* 1984, **53**, 395.
53. Moore R. A. et al. *Anesthesiology* 1983, **58**, 102.
54. de Lange S. S. et al. *Br. J. Anaesth.* 1981, **53**, 1129; *see also* Davies M. J. et al. *Anaesth. Intensive Care* 1982, **10**, 9.
55. Shah K. B. and Rao T. L. K. *Anesthesiology* 1984, **61**, 271.
56. Hill D. W. *Physics Applied to Anaesthesia* 4th ed. London: Butterworths, 1980, Chapter 1.
57. Huntsman L. L. et al. *Circulation* 1983, **67**, 593.
58. Fick A. E. *Sitzung der Phys.-med. Ges. Würzb.* 1870, p. 16.
59. *See* Rollason W. N. *Electrocardiography for the Anaesthetist* 4th ed. Oxford: Blackwell, 1980.
60. Bar Z. G. *Anaesthesia* 1984, **39**, 611.
61. Frey A. *Dt. Arch. Klin. Med.* 1902, **73**, 511.
62. Moritz F. and von Tabora D. *Dtsch. Arch. Klin. Med.* 1910, **98**, 475.
63. Forssmann W. *Münch. Med. Wochenschr.* 1931, **78**, 489.
64. Meyers L. *Am. J. Nurs.* 1945, **45**, 930.
65. Pauling L. *Science* 1946, **103**, 338.
66. Cole A. G. H. *Br. J. Hosp. Med.* 1983, **29**, 469.
67. Tyndal J. *Trans. R. Coll. Surg. Engl.* 1865, **4**, 139.
68. Kalenda Z. *Br. J. Clin. Equip.* 1980, **6**, 180; Kalenda Z. *Acta Anaesthesiol. Belg.* 1978, **29**, 201; Hurter D. *Anaesthesia* 1979, **34**, 578; Smallhout B. and Kalenda Z. *An Atlas of Capnography*, Zeist Netherlands: Kerkebosch, 1980; Whitesell R. et al. *Anesth. Analg. (Cleve.)* 1981, **60**, 508.
69. Diprose K. V. et al. *Br. J. Anaesth.* 1980, **52**, 1155.
70. White D. C. et al. *Br. J. Anaesth.* 1972, **44**, 1020; Bennetts F. E. *Anaesthesia* 1976, **31**, 644.
71. Davis W. O. M. and Spence A. A. *Br. J. Anaesth.* 1979, **51**, 987; Graham J. M. et al. *Br. J. Anaesth.* 1980, **52**, 1055; *see also* Mass Spectrometry in Anaesthesiology (Vickers M. D. and Crul J. F. ed.) *Proceedings of European Academy of Anaesthesiology* 1980, 1981 Berlin: Springer-Verlag, p. 105 et seq.
72. Gothard J. W. W. et al. *Anaesthesia* 1980, **35**, 890.
73. *See also* Sykes M. K. et al. *Principles of Measurement*, 2nd ed. Oxford: Blackwell, 1980; Hill D. W. in: *Scientific Foundations of Anaesthesia* (Scurr C. and Feldman S. A. ed.), 2nd ed. London: Heinemann, 1974, p. 85; Lowe H. J. and Hagler K. in: *Gas Chromatography in Biology and Medicine* (Porter R. ed.). London: Churchill, 1969, p. 86.
74. Bushman J. A. *Br. J. Anaesth.* 1979, **51**, 895.
75. Parker D. *Br. J. Clin. Equip.* 1980, **5**, 31; Blackburn J. P. *Br. J. Anaesth.* 1978, **50**, 51.
76. Pflüger E. *Arch. Ges. Physiol.* 1872, **6**, 43.
77. Clark L. C. *Trans. Am. Soc. Artif. Intern. Organs* 1956, **2**, 41.
78. Laver M. B. and Seifen A. *Anesthesiology* 1965, **26**, 73.
79. Williamson D. C. and Munson E. S. *Anesth. Analg. (Cleve.)* 1982, **61**, 950.
80. Rozkovec A. and Rithalia S. U. S. *Br. J. Clin. Equip.* 1980, **5**, 24; Goldman M. D. et al. *Anaesthesia* 1982, **37**, 944; Simpson R. M. and Bryan M. H. *Br. J. Hosp. Med.* 1982, **28**, 250.
81. Eberhard P. and Schafer R. *Br. J. Clin. Equip.* 1980, **5**, 224.
82. Tahvanainen J. et al. *Crit. Care Med.* 1982, **10**, 758; Jamieson W. R. E. and Turnbull K. W. *Can. J. Surg.* 1982, **25**, 538.

83. Cooke A. and Barcroft J. *J. Physiol. (Lond.)* 1913, **47**, 35.
84. Campbell E. J. M. and Howell J. B. L. *Br. Med. J.* 1960, **1**, 458; 1962, **2**, 630.
85. Cobbe S. M. and Poole-Wilson P. A. *Lancet* 1979, **2**, 444; Stevens A. J. *Br. J. Clin. Equip.* 1980, **6**, 112.
86. Payne J. P. and Severinghaus J. W. (ed.) *Pulse Oximetry*. Berlin: Springer-Verlag, 1986; Taylor M. B. and Whitman J. G. *Anaesthesia* 1986, **41**, 943; Nunn J. F. *Anaesthesia* 1978, **42**, iv.
87. Kendall R. I. et al. *Am. J. Clin. Pathol.* 1983, **79**, 217.
88. Berger H. *Arch. f. Psychiat.* 1931, **94**, 16.
89. Adrian E. B. and Mathews B. H. C. *Brain* 1934, **57**, 355.
90. Courtin R. F. et al. *Proc. Staff Mayo Clin.* 1950, **25**, 197 (reprinted in 'Classical File', *Surv. Anesthesiol.* 1959, 3 August).
91. Gibbs F. A. and Gibbs L. *Arch. Intern. Med.* 1937, **60**, 154.
92. Faulconer A. *Anesthesiology* 1952, **13**, 361.
93. Clutton-Brock J. in: *Thoracic Anaesthesia* (Mushin W. W. ed.). Oxford: Blackwell, 1963, Chapter 19.
94. Whisler J. W. et al. *J. Clin. Neurophysiol.* 1982, **54**, 541.
95. Nixon C. et al. *Anaesthesia* 1986, **41**, 131; Hain W. R. and Zideman D. A. *Todays Anaesthetist* 1986, **1**, No. 2, 8.
96. Bydder G. M. and Steiner R. E. *Neuroradiology* 1982, **23**, 231; Bailes D. R. et al. *Clin. Radiol.* 1982, **33**, 395; Crooks L. E. et al. *Radiology* 1982, **144**, 843.
97. Wedley J. R. *Br. J. Clin. Equip.* 1979, **4**, 224.
98. Wunderlich C. A. *Medical Thermometry* 2nd ed. (translated by Woodman W. B.). London: New Sydenham Society, 1871. *See also Br. Med. J.* 1965, **1**, 1449.
99. Whalen R. E. and Starmer C. F. *Mod. Concepts Cardiovasc. Dis.* 1967, **36**, 7.
100. Ilsley A. H. and Runciman W. B. *Anaesth. Intensive Care* 1986, **14**, 431.
101. Ilsley A. H. et al. *Anaesth. Intensive Care* 1986, **14**, 437.
102. Roessler M. N. et al. *Anaesth. Intensive Care* 1986, **14**, 443.

Chapter 42   ## INTRAVASCULAR TECHNIQUES, INFUSIONS AND BLOOD TRANSFUSION

For the history of fluid administration during anaesthesia and surgery, *see* Jenkins M. T. P. in: *Anaesthesia; Essays on its History*. (Rupreht J. et al. ed.) Berlin: Springer-Verlag, 1985, p. 102.

Intravenous Injection

For technique *see* Chapter 13.

Intravenous Infusion

The drip chamber was described in 1909.[1] Suitable veins are the veins in the forearm or at the bend of the elbow; the saphenous vein anterior to the medial malleolus; veins on the dorsum of the hand; veins above the wrist. Subclavian vein puncture, first described in 1952, has been used when other veins are inaccessible. This method should not be used routinely as a haematoma may result. *In infants* the internal or external jugular or scalp veins can be used or the umbilical vein during laparotomy. The femoral vein is approached below the inguinal ligament where it lies medially to the artery. A sandbag should be under the buttocks.

To speed up the rate of flow, often slowed down by the venous spasm associated with shock, 10 ml of 1% procaine solution injected into the tubing through an intradermal needle is useful. Raising the container well above the patient's limb may be helpful, while air pressure can be raised in or around it by means of a hand pump, e.g. a pressure infuser.

Slowing of the rate of drip after several hours may be due to increase in venous tone, associated with the fluid infused. It may be improved by adding papaverine to the fluid.[2] Self-adhesive patches which release glyceryl trinitrate at a slow and continuous rate, placed distal to the i.v. infusion site decreases the rate of infusion failure three-fold, whether the problem is due to thrombosis or extravasation.[3] A three-way syringe can be used in infants. A major factor influencing rate of drip is variation in venous pressure[4] and blood viscosity, which is 2·5 times as great at 0 °C as at 37 °C. Blood at body temperature runs twice as fast as blood at 10 °C. For flow through venous cannulae, *see* Selwyn A. and Russell W. J. *Anaesth. Intensive Care* 1977, **5**, 157; Kestin I. G. *Anaesthesia* 1987, **42**, 67.

There is a real danger in giving blood too fast to patients with myocardial failure.

To make veins more prominent moist heat should be applied to the whole limb for half an hour before venepuncture.

For prolonged infusion the following sites may be employed:

1. Any suitable vein in the upper extremity, preferably some distance from a flexure.

2. The internal jugular vein.[5]

3. The superior vena cava from the basilic vein 5 cm above and anterior to the medial epicondyle.

4. Subclavian vein, from a supraclavicular or infraclavicular[6] approach. Pneumothorax may be a complication.[7]

5. The femoral vein medial to the artery, in the groin, as a last resort.

Note: 540 ml of fluid at 40 drops/min requires 3·3 h; at 60 drops/min, 2·3 h; at 200 drops/min, 40 min. Any solution run continuously into a vein will eventually lead to thrombosis and occlusion.

Thrombophlebitis is the body's early warning reaction of infection to come. If ignored, and the foreign body left in place, sepsis will follow.

To prevent thrombophlebitis from intravenous drips:[8]

1. Remove needle or cannula each 24 h and insert into a different vein.

2. Use a central venous catheter rather than a peripheral cannula. (A cannula is usually 7 cm in length or less; a catheter, more. Some plastic or even Teflon cannulae undergo changes in vivo, making them brittle.)[9] Silastic catheters are relatively non-thrombogenic.

3. Add hydrocortisone 10 mg/l or heparin 500 units to the infused fluid 4 times daily.

4. If glucose is infused it should be sterilized by filtration rather than by autoclaving, thus preventing the Maillard reaction (caramelization).

5. Leg veins should be avoided if possible, also hypertonic solutions.[8]

6. Use of a microfilter,[10] although the need for them is not proven.[11]

The pH of intravenous fluids may be a factor in causing thrombophlebitis, as may particulate matter in antibiotic solutions.[12] Some patients develop thrombophlebitis more easily than others, e.g. those with renal carcinoma and those with major allergies. When a winged 'butterfly' needle is used over a long period of time there is always the risk that it may 'cut out' of the vein, so a small teflon catheter with a self-sealing injection site may be preferable (e.g. Y-can).

Treatment of superficial thrombophlebitis. Heparinoid cream (monopolysaccharide polysulphate—Hirudoid) may be applied daily and the part bandaged firmly.

Infusion Controllers and Pumps
They can be used to control flow given i.v., i.m., subcutaneously, intra-arterially, extradurally or by nasogastric tube.[13] Allow very accurate calibration of the rate of flow of an infusion, which is useful when the infusion is used to carry drugs. The controllers merely regulate the number of drops falling per min by gravity in the drip chamber. *Infusion pumps* actively promote flow down the drip set; they may be finger-pumps, rollers or pistons. Some have visual or auditory warning devices. They are designed not to influence the sterility of the infusion fluid.

In-line Infusion Filters
See Chapter 35.

(For developments in infusion devices, *see* Rithalia S. V. S. and Tinker J. *Br. J. Hosp. Med.* 1980, **5**, 69; Ballance J. H. *Br. J. Hosp. Med.* 1981, **26**, 411.)

Blood Transfusion

History
First described in animals in 1666 by Richard Lower (1631–1691)[14] and in man by Denis (1625–1704) of Montpellier, France in 1667, using calf's blood.[15] First successful man-to-man transfusion reported by J. Blundell (1790–1878) of St. Thomas' Hospital, in 1818, an obstetrician.[16] Vein-to-vein transfusion given by James Hobson Aveling (1828–1892)[17] and by Higginson (of syringe fame) the following year. Transfusions were first given to alter the patient's temperament. Hustin (1882–1967) of Belgium in 1914,[18] Luis Agot of Buenos Aires, and Lewisohn[19] demonstrated the usefulness of sodium citrate as an anticoagulant. Apparatus for direct transfusion was coated internally with paraffin wax, to reduce coagulation e.g. Kimpton's tube.[20] Glucose added to blood to prolong the life of the red cells in 1916.[21] Autotransfusion, for example in ruptured ectopics, was often used before the Second World War.[22] In 1900, Landsteiner (1868–1943)[23] of Vienna, later of New York, first observed agglutination of human red cells by serum belonging to other individuals (Nobel prizewinner, 1930), and described three ABO groups according to the two types of agglutinogens, their combination or their absence, which can cause agglutination when brought into contact with agglutinins in the serum. The fourth group (AB) was described by the Viennese physician Decastello in 1902[24] and confirmed by Jansky of Prague and by W. L. Moss of Baltimore in 1910. In a British population 45% of people are group O; 44% group A; 7% group B; 4% group AB. The Rh system was discovered in 1939–40.[25] A plasma substitute, gum acacia, was first used in 1919.[26] Heparin described in 1916.[27] Cadaver blood was used in the USSR in the 1930s.[28]

One 540 ml unit of blood will raise the haemoglobin about 1 g %. If the haemoglobin is less than 6 g %, transfusion is desirable. If a major operation is to be performed and the haemoglobin is less than 10 g %, a blood transfusion is often indicated. Before the era of blood banks (the 1940s in the UK) a register of blood donors was kept by individual hospitals so that potential donors could be sent for as required. The original glass bottles and rubber tubing gave way to disposable plastic sets in the late 1950s and this reduced the incidence of thrombophlebitis and infection. The National Blood Transfusion Service was incorporated within the National Health Service after 1948, and today, National Blood Products Centres look after blood transfusion and its increasing complexities. In 1946 there were about 200 000 donors, today the figure is nearer 2 000 000 all of them voluntary, in the UK. Blood banks were established in the 1930s in Moscow, at the Mayo Clinic in 1935,[29] and by Bernard Fantus (1874–1940) in Cook County Hospital, Chicago,[30] and in 1939 in Barcelona, during the Spanish Civil War.[31] Continuous drip blood transfusion introduced in 1935.[32] Anticoagulants include di- or tri-sodium citrate and heparin. First clinical use of citrated blood in 1914.[33] Acid–citrate–dextrose which permitted 21 days' storage, introduced in 1943.[34] (For history of blood transfusion, *see* Keynes G. *Br. J. Surg.* 1943, **31**, 38; Maluf N. S. R. *J. Hist. Med.* 1954, **9**, 59; Diamond L. K. *JAMA* 1965, **193**, 40; Hutchin P. *Surgery* 1968, **64**, 685; Farr A. D. *J. R. Soc. Med.* 1981, **74**, 301; Marshall M. and Bird T. *Blood Replacement.* London: Arnold, 1983; Schneider W. H. *Bull. Hist. Med.* 1983, **57**, 545.

Within the past few years the possibility of contracting hepatitis and AIDS from donor blood, together with the ability of the haematology laboratory to cross-match blood within 30–40 min, have made many anaesthetists more cautious in their practice of blood transfusion.[35] HG concentrations below 10 g/dl are accompanied by a progressive increase in bleeding time and below 9 g/dl tissue oxygenation can be maintained only by increasing cardiac output.

Blood Donors
Unsuitable donors include those with a history of protozoal, spirochaetal, bacterial or virus infection, especially AIDS; those who have recently had vaccines or inoculations, or those with glucose-6-phosphate dehydrogenase deficiency. Blood donors must be negative for Hb_sAg, but may be accepted if they carry anti-Hbs. A history of jaundice should exclude blood donation (0·5% of donor population).[36] The rarer blood groups may cause problems, e.g. Duffy, Kell, Lewis, Rh E, C.

Storage
Refrigerated blood (at a temperature of 2–6 °C) is good for increasing haemoglobin and for raising blood volume, but the clotting factors together with immune bodies deteriorate in stored blood after 24 h. Citrate–phosphate–dextrose blood (CPD blood) contains few functioning platelets, only 10% of its original factors V and VIII and only 20% of its factor XI. Factors IX and X fall after about 1 week. CPD blood preserves its ATP and 2,3-diphosphoglycerate levels normal for 1 week with a slow fall thereafter. CPD blood can be usefully stored for up to 35 days. Each unit contains 450 ml of blood and 63 ml of CPD solution. The potassium content rises to about 20 mmol/l after 3 weeks, but some of this is reabsorbed into the erythrocytes after warming and infusion. Other anticoagulants used for storage are acid–phosphate–dextrose (ACD), bicarbonate-added glucose phosphate mannitol (BAGPM) which preserves the DPG

levels and is not associated with the appearance of micro-aggregates. Saline adenine glucose mannitol (SAGM) is similar. These last two are deficient in plasma, with its useful colloid, immune and clotting factors. Thus if the transfusion is planned in the treatment of sepsis, haemorrhagic disease or lack of clotting power, blood less than 24 h old should be used. For alteration of blood components during storage *see* Lovric V. A. *Anaesth. Intensive Care* 1984, **12**, 246.

Rh-negative blood should whenever possible be given to Rh-negative patients, who form about 15% of the population in Britain. This is specially desirable in:

1. Rh-negative patients of either sex who have either had a previous transfusion or may require a subsequent one.
2. Rh-negative girls and women of child-bearing age.
3. Mothers of infants who have haemolytic disease.
4. Infants with haemolytic disease.

With no preliminary testing, incompatibility (ABO) will only occur, if blood of the correct ABO group is given, without cross-matching, once in 300 times.[37]

The best method for storing blood is a freezing process. Can be stored for many years with red cell survival as good as conventional liquid blood at 4 °C. Expensive and 2 h needed for thawing and removal of glycerol; should then be used within 24 h. Main application is military.

Adenine has been added to ACD blood to preserve red cells better.[38]

Blood conservation in elective surgery can be procured by: (1) Induced hypotension; (2) Infiltration with adrenaline and saline; (3) Tourniquet; (4) Haemodilution; (5) Autotransfusion.[39]

There is rarely any indication for whole blood even in massive transfusion. Specific component therapy is revolutionizing blood transfusion. The use of microfilters has yet to be determined.[11]

Routine cross-matching for many types of cold surgery can be replaced by the 'half-hour cross-match test'. Uncross-matched O Rh −ve blood may be transfused with a high degree of safety.[40]

Various Available Products

1. *Whole blood (see above).*
2. *Frozen blood.* Washed cells are suspended in a glycerol medium and frozen in liquid nitrogen or liquid air for up to several years. After careful thawing and rewashing, they are transfused as packed cells.
3. *Packed cells* (erythrocytes) comprise the cellular elements of blood (about 50% by volume). Useful for correction of anaemia, before, during or after operation. 'Plasma-reduced blood' has 180 ml of the plasma removed. (*See also* Dodds A. J. and Pun A. *Anaesth. Intensive Care* 1984, **12**, 241.)
4. *Micro-aggregate-free (MAF) blood.* Basically CPD blood from which the 'buffy coat' has been removed (containing leucocyte and platelet debris).
5. *SAGM blood (see above).*
6. *Plasma.* Available as fresh frozen plasma, rich in clotting factors, or as reconstituted plasma (distilled water is added to dried plasma powder.) Both are excellent natural colloids for blood-volume expansion. Ten donors are used for a batch of pooled plasma: 4 group A, 4 group O, 1 group B and 1 group AB, to neutralize the ABO antibodies. Pooled plasma contains citrate and is rich in potassium.

7. *Human albumin.* Available as albumin, salt-poor albumin, or 'plasma protein fraction' (PPF), prepared by pasteurization of plasma with resulting precipitation of globulins and any viruses.

8. *Human fibrinogen.*

9. *Cryoprecipitate* (particularly rich in clotting factors).

10. *Platelets* may be transfused in severe thrombocytopenia, certain cases of leukaemia, neoplastic conditions involving bone, and depression of haemopoeisis by infection, drugs, etc. Platelet concentrates are always contaminated with donor red cells and so should be given to patients of the same ABO group; in the case of Rh-negative women, anti-D immunoglobulin should be given. Ordinary filters on transfusion sets remove 5% of platelets, but microfilters remove over 30% and so should not be used.

11. *Factor VIII concentrate.*

12. *Factor IX concentrate.*

13. *Fluosol-DA*, an inert emulsion of perfluorodecalin and perfluorotripropyl-amine is a blood substitute which dissolves large quantities of oxygen (5 ml/100 ml) linearly with its Po_2 (Henry's law). It unloads its oxygen to tissues.[41] (*See* p. 753.)

Indications for Blood Transfusion in Surgery
(1) Acute loss of blood with reduction in circulating volume of 30% or more; (2) Severe anaemia causing hypoproteinaemia and decreased oxygen-carrying capacity; (3) Blood-clotting disturbances; (4) Extracorporeal circulation; (5) Exchange transfusion; (6) Sepsis.

Direct Cross-matching Test
When the services of a pathologist are not available, one drop of the recipient's serum is placed on a warmed white tile and one drop of 5% suspension of donor's blood in saline (2 or 3 drops of blood in 1 or 2 ml of normal saline) is added to it. The two sera are mixed with a loop, the tile tilted and kept warm for 10–15 min and again agitated, and examined with a hand lens for agglutination.

Four drugs which are particularly likely to cause problems in blood grouping and compatibility tests are: (1) High molecular weight dextrans; (2) Methyldopa; (3) Mefenamic acid (Ponstan); (4) Penicillin in more than 20 mega-unit doses daily.

In a grave emergency, uncross-matched group ORh negative is the least dangerous to use. It is, however, better to give blood of the patient's own group if that is known. Otherwise there may be difficulty with subsequent cross-matching.

Complications
Each blood transfusion carries a certain risk and, in adults, single-unit transfusions are seldom necessary. The possible hazards are the following:

1. Acute Haemolytic Reaction[42]
A measurable increase in the rate of destruction of donor's or recipient's erythrocytes by allo-antibodies. May occur during or after transfusion, or be delayed. Due to incompatible transfusion and the destruction of the donor's red cells by the action of specific antibodies in the recipient's circulation—chiefly anti-A, anti-B, and anti-D of the Rhesus system. Usually ABO incompatibility causes a more violent reaction than one due to the Rhesus factor. General

anaesthesia masks the effects. The blood pressure and pulse rate should be taken every 5 min for the first quarter-hour with each new bottle of blood. If there is a red skin rash, a fall in blood pressure or a rise in pulse rate or cyanosis for which no other cause can be found, the transfusion should be stopped. The mortality of acute haemolytic transfusion reactions has been reported to be 10%.[43] The incidence has been variously reported to be between 1–3000 and 1–15 000 transfused units.

Pathophysiology. The reaction is largely mediated by histamine, released from mast cells in response to the activation of C3a and C5a cleavage products of complement by the antigen–antibody reaction. The histamine causes smooth muscle contraction and increased capillary permeability, leading to oedema and vasomotor kinin activity (also the result of C2 activation). In addition, the action of anti-A or anti-B or both (IgM allo-antibodies) causes erythrocyte disruption with release of a phospholipid procoagulant (e.g. erythrocytin) which gives disseminated intravascular coagulation (DIC). The combination of intravascular fibrin deposition and vasospasm leads to acute cortical necrosis of the kidney. Anti-Kell antibodies were responsible for the reaction in 80% of cases in one American series.

Signs of Incompatible Transfusion. All patients receiving blood should be carefully watched during the first 15 min to detect possible trouble. (A) *In the conscious*: (1) Fullness of the head; (2) Tingling of limbs; (3) Precordial pain; (4) Lumbar pain; (5) Dyspnoea; (6) Restlessness; (7) Suffused face; (8) Nausea and vomiting; (9) Pyrexia; (10) Circulatory collapse; (11) Tachycardia; (12) Bronchospasm and profuse sputum secretion; (13) Later, haemoglobinaemia, haemoglobinuria and oliguria. (B) *Under anaesthesia*: (1) Hypotension; (2) Tachycardia; (3) General oozing from wound; (4) Urticarial rash; (5) Later, jaundice and oliguria in 5–10% of these patients. These changes start to occur early on in the transfusion. (*See also* Binder L. S. et al. *Br. J. Anaesth.* 1959, **31**, 217 (reprinted in 'Classical File', *Surv. Anesthesiol.* 1975, **19**, 91).

The factors affecting the severity of the reaction are: (1) The amount, titre, Ig class and specificity of the host's antibody (anti-A or anti-B, etc.); (2) The volume of incompatible blood transfused; (3) The general level of fitness of the recipient, the integrity of his circulatory responses, his level of consciousness and the speed with which treatment is applied.

Investigation of Transfusion Reactions. The following specimens are needed: (1) The blood samples used for the compatibility test before the transfusion; (2) The remains of the blood in the bottle or bottles used for the transfusion; (3) A sample of the patient's blood taken 3 h after the transfusion reaction, collected into a dry sterile bottle with a dry sterile needle and syringe; 10 ml will suffice. In addition 2 ml should be put into an oxalated bottle; (4) A sample of clear urine.

Differential Diagnosis. (1) Anaphylactic reaction to some other substance (e.g. a drug); (2) Acute haemolytic anaemia; (3) Acute septicaemia; (4) Transfusion of thermally damaged, infected or outdated blood.

Treatment of Severe Transfusion Reaction. (1) Stop the transfusion; (2) High dose of steroids to stop the antigen–antibody reaction; (3) Fast colloid infusion, e.g. dextran 70, or mannitol; (4) Oxygen is given to overcome the effects of intrapulmonary shunting; (5) Diuresis is produced by mannitol (500 ml of 10% solution) or frusemide 100 mg; (6) Acid–base and electrolyte balance is checked; (7) Exchange transfusion in the desperate case; (8) Adrenaline, 10 ml, of 1–10 000 solution is injected slowly, i.v., or ephedrine, 10–30 mg, to maintain cardiac output if necessary. Antihistamines may be indicated in the early stages but they may increase hypotension; (9) Where disseminated intravascular coagulation is occurring, coagulation factors and platelets may need to be replaced.

2. Delayed Reaction
Four to ten days after transfusion, causes anaemia, jaundice and renal failure.

3. Other Reactions
Adverse reactions occur due to leucocyte, platelet and plasma protein antibodies.[44]

4. Use of Infected Blood
Blood left out of the refrigerator or cool box for more than 30 min should not be used.

5. Circulatory Overloading
During rapid transfusion, a low arterial and a raised venous pressure are evidence of cardiac overloading. To prevent acute pulmonary oedema, especially in elderly patients, and those with severe anaemia, frusemide 40 mg can be given into a vein at the outset of the transfusion. The rate of drip should be 1–3 ml/kg per hr. *The signs are*: (a) Tightness in the chest; (b) Cough; (c) Dyspnoea; (d) Cyanosis; (e) Engorgement of neck veins; (f) Tachycardia; (g) Basal crepitations; (h) Pulmonary oedema; (i) Increase in central venous pressure.
Treatment. Transfusion is stopped and digitalis, oxygen, aminophylline and atropine are given. The patient is sat up and kept warm. Frusemide is injected. Tourniquets and venesection may be required.

Central venous pressure measurements give immediate and consistent indications of blood loss and replacement but blood volume changes cannot be correlated numerically with the CVP.[45]

6. Micro-embolism
Blood filters[46] (20–40 µm pore size) remove micro-aggregates of more than 20 µm diameter from stored blood during transfusion, being interposed between the blood container and the infusion set. Three structures are in common use: (a) Surface filters; (b) Depth filters; (c) Combination filters. Various materials have been used in their construction, such as woven polyester screen, nylon screen, dacron wool and polyester sponge. Each type must be fully primed with blood before use. They have been shown to prevent some organ damage (notably pulmonary) caused by micro-aggregates (mainly platelets and fibrin).[47] Problems and dangers of these filters include: slowing of rate of transfusion, complete blockage after 4–10 units of blood, embolism of particles from the filter, haemolysis and massive activation of the clotting process if fresh frozen plasma is infused through a filter. The pore size of the filter in an ordinary infusion set is about 170 µm.

7. Transmission of Disease
(a) Serum B hepatitis, Australia antigen, 6–16 weeks afterwards anicteric hepatitis can occur; post-transfusion hepatitis (non-A non-B) is the most important. (b) Malaria. In temperate areas when malaria is not endemic malarial

serology is a useful means for excluding blood donors who may transmit malaria;[48] (c) Syphilis; (d) Yaws; (e) Relapsing fever; (f) Kala-azar; (g) Bacteraemia or septicaemia; (h) Cytomegalovirus; (i) Epstein–Barr virus infection; (j) AIDS (*see N. Engl. J. Med.* 1984, **310**, 69). Transference of malaria can be prevented by giving 600 mg of chloroquine before transfusion to the recipient.

8. Febrile and Allergic Reactions

Are said to occur in about 1–2% of transfusions, usually only mild urticaria but sometimes acute anaphylactic shock results. Rarely asthma, angioneurotic oedema and laryngeal oedema are seen and must be treated by stopping the transfusion and giving antihistamines.

9. Potassium Intoxication

Cardiac arrest due to this condition may occur during or shortly after transfusion of stored whole blood or overconcentrated plasma. Hyperkalaemia is more likely if there is accompanying metabolic acidosis. Old stored blood may contain 25 mmol/l of potassium.

Signs of potassium intoxication may include a failing myocardium, a raised venous pressure and peaking and elevation of the T wave on the ECG. Pre- and postoperative digitalization will counteract the toxic effects of potassium. In emergency, intravenous injection of 1 g of calcium chloride, slowly, will restore the potassium/calcium ratio temporarily. For continuous display of plasma potassium during cardiac surgery *see* Drake H. F. et al. *Anaesthesia* 1987, **42**, 23.

10. Citrate Intoxication and Hypocalcaemia

A warm oxygenated adult can metabolize the citrate content of 1 unit of CPD blood in 5 min. If the transfusion is faster than this, intravenous calcium gluconate, 1 g may be required; the same applies to cold or cyanosed patients, or those with severe hepatic disease. The signs of citrate intoxication are those of acidosis and cardiac depression.

There is evidence that citrate–phosphate–dextrose solution has advantages over acid–citrate–dextrose for collection and storage of blood. The former has a higher pH (7·2 at time of collection), the red cells are in better functional state, they have a greater survival time, and 2,3-diphosphoglycerate is preserved.

Blood samples may be anticoagulated with ethylenediamine tetra-acetic acid (EDTA).

In open-heart surgery and in renal dialysis, heparinized blood may be preferred. Any haemorrhagic tendency can be controlled by protamine sulphate. Heparinization does not interfere with calcium stores in the body and citrate intoxication does not arise.

11. Hypothermia

Massive transfusion of cold blood may cause body cooling, and this has been incriminated as a cause of transfusion cardiac arrest. Prevented by warming the blood. Blood can be warmed to 45 °C for 1 hour without haemolysing.

12. pH Changes

The pH of stored blood varies betwen 6·58 and 6·72, acidaemia being due to an accumulation of lactic acid, pyruvic acid, citric acid and raised PCO_2. This may be important in massive transfusion, although metabolism of citrate is likely to result in metabolic alkalosis.

13. Haemorrhagic Tendency Due to Thrombocytopenia

This may be seen after massive transfusion and requires fresh blood or platelets. Nearly half of those patients who receive more than 10 units of blood show a bleeding diathesis, due to abnormally low values for factors V, VII and X.[49] A patient who receives 10 units of blood or more may be regarded as having an organ transplant.

14. Hypomagnesaemia

During massive transfusion, with particular loss from the myocardium.

15. Transfusion-related Acute Lung Injury

See Popovsky M. A. et al. *Am. Rev. Resp. Dis.* 1983, **128**, 185.

16. Extravasation

Extravasation of intravenous fluids into the subcutaneous tissues occurs in about one-fifth of those receiving infusions. In most cases no harm results but occasionally there is loss of skin, muscle and tendon, with permanent disability.[50]

In addition to blood, all plasma volume expanders may occasionally cause adverse effects.[51]

Massive Blood Transfusion

Over 8 units, the clotting process is likely to be abnormal unless fresh blood is used, due to anticoagulants and thrombocytopenia. Anticoagulants are reversed in a controlled manner and platelets may be given. Some workers routinely give steroids at this point, regarding a massive transfusion as an organ transplant.

Autologous Blood Transfusion (Autotransfusion)

Because of the risk of transmission of AIDS and of hepatitis non-A and non-B homologous blood, the need for autologous blood is increasing.

A trap on the surgical suction line collects blood from the operation site, via special non-damaging surgical suction tips. The trap removes air bubbles and other potential emboli and anticoagulates the blood with a small dose of citrate. Reinfusion of up to 10 litres of blood has been performed.[52] Autotransfusion first described in 1874.[53]

Blood Warmers

When large volumes of blood are to be transfused, there are advantages in warming the blood as it is infused to prevent hypothermia dysrhythmia (even cardiac arrest), acidosis and hyperkalaemia.[54]

(*See also* Mollison P. L. *Blood Transfusion and Clinical Medicine* 6th ed.

Oxford: Blackwell, 1979; Horsey P. J. in: *Recent Advances in Anaesthesia and Analgesia*—14 (Atkinson R. S. and Hewer C. L. ed.) Edinburgh: Churchill Livingstone, 1982.)

Transfusion of Fluids
For history, *see* Jenkins M. T. P. *Anaesthesia; Essays on its History.* (Rupreht J. et al. ed.) Heidelberg: Springer-Verlag, 1985, p. 102.

The pH of some Intravenous Fluids
Dextrose 5% in water and 4% dextrose in 0·18% saline, 3·5–5·5; Compound sodium lactate solution (Hartmann), 5·0–7·0; dextran in 5% dextrose, 4·5–5·0; dextran in 0·9% saline, 5·0–6·0; Haemaccel 7·2–7·3.[55]

Glucose (Dextrose)
Five per cent solution is isotonic and may be used for intravenous drips designed for fluid replacement and to keep open an intravenous route for medication. It has an acid pH. If a combination of saline and glucose is to be employed, the proportion should be 1/5 normal saline with 4·3% glucose; this mixture is isotonic. Thrombophlebitis can be minimized by neutralization to a pH of 6·8 with a phosphate buffer. When stored blood is followed by glucose, rouleaux formation with clumping occurs in the drip set. Glucose of 10% or more may produce thrombophlebitis. Laevulose has some advantages over glucose. Dextrose 5% is an ineffective replacement fluid in cases of trauma in which there is already a hyperglycaemic response.

Normal Saline
First used in the treatment of shock in 1891.[56] About one-third of its volume is retained in the circulation. Over-use of normal saline frequently leads to waterlogged patients. Intractable hypovolaemic shock has been treated by 7·5% sodium chloride solution.[57]

Hartmann's Solution[58] (compound sodium lactate solution, BPC)
One-sixth molar concentration of sodium lactate in Ringer's solution.[59] The lactate is metabolized in the liver to form bicarbonate, to counteract acidosis.

Good results are reported following the treatment of haemorrhagic shock by control of haemorrhage together with massive infusions of electrolyte solutions instead of blood.[60] Has the advantage that in the absence of laboratory investigations the serum electrolytes become more normal with the infusion of this solution.

Colloids
Colloids increase plasma oncotic pressure and so draw fluid into the intravascular space. The group includes the dextrans, gelatins and albumin.
  The currently available albumins are from HBsAg whereas pooled plasma bears a 10% risk of transferring hepatitis B infection. Three solutions are available, plasma protein, PPF and human albumin.

Artificial Plasma Substitutes[61]
(1) Dextrans of various molecular size; (2) Gelatins produced by hydrolysis of collagens (e.g. Gelofusine. These are 4% w/v succinyl gelatin, isotonic, with a

sodium chloride content of 0·8% and calcium content of about 0·4 mmol/l. About 500 ml are needed to take the place of 600 ml of blood lost. In the postoperative period of oliguria it has a beneficial diuretic effect. Does not affect clotting-time. Half-life in the bloodstream 4–6 h. A useful plasma substitute; (3) Hydroxylated starches. Overall, anaphylactoid reactions are much less common than reactions following blood.[62]

Dextran 70

Molecular weight 70 000. Used to reduce incidence of thrombosis (*see below*). Dextran 70 is non-toxic, electrically neutral, and chemically inert. It has an acid pH and may degrade acid-labile drugs.[63] Although it is eventually eliminated completely from the body, it remains in the circulation, in gradually decreasing amount, up to a week, and some of its larger molecules are stored for some time in the cells of the reticulo-endothelial system; 25% is excreted within 3 h. Only 50% can be recovered from the urine. Has proved useful as a plasma substitute in cases of burns and surgical shock; prophylaxis of shock during operations. It is effective in prevention of venous thrombo-embolism. It increases the venous return to the heart. Reactions occur[63] in rather less than 0·2% of patients, the chief being mild pyrexia. These are worse in chronic asthmatic or allergic patients. Very occasionally circulatory collapse, cyanosis and vomiting have been reported. If more than 1·5 litres are infused in any 24-h period, some products may interfere with blood groupings and cross-matching tests, owing to rouleaux formation (this is greater as the average molecular weight of the dextran molecule rises), so specimens should be taken for this purpose before dextran is infused. If this is not done, recipient cells must be washed before testing. It may interfere with plasma protein determinations. Dextran molecules greater in size than 50 000 increase the ESR, those smaller decrease it. Dextrans increase the negative charge on red cells and platelets. The damaged intima of vessels, although not the intact intima is positively charged. Platelet stickiness is increased. Large volumes can cause bleeding by interfering with platelet function and by increasing blood volume. Dextran 70 is the most widely used variety and 500 ml will usually increase the circulating plasma volume by 750 ml.

Dextran 40 (Rheomacrodex, Lomodex)

Average molecular weight 40 000; Half-life in vivo, 3 h. Duration of useful plasma expansion is about 1 h. It has been used to increase intravascular volume and to reduce blood viscosity and to aid the circulation as a blood-flow improver. It is said to prevent intravascular aggregation of red cells or so-called 'sludging'; and to reverse peripheral ischaemia. It does not interfere with cross-matching, blood grouping or with coagulation. Contraindicated in dehydrated patients, as it may produce viscous urine and can cause renal failure.

Gelatin

Four per cent in normal saline (Physiogel, Gelofusine, Haemaccel).[64] Molecular weight 30 000. Short biological half-life, less than 12 h, no effect on blood clotting; 85% is excreted by the kidney. Duration of useful plasma-expansion activity, about 1½ h. Gelatin has an appreciable incidence of adverse reactions,[65] most of which occur after the first few millilitres infused. Haemaccel is a useful plasma volume substitute. It has 90% of its constituent molecules between 5000 and 50000, the majority below the renal threshold. It does not interfere with blood cross-matching and has only a diluting effect on coagulation factors, but as it contains calcium it should not be given with the same infusion set as ACD blood. Reactions are very rare, it carries no risk of AIDS or hepatitis and has a long shelf-life. Cost is reasonable. In major vascular surgery it reduces the need for blood transfusion.[66]

Hydroxyethyl Starch (HES)
Six per cent solution of starch in normal saline. HES has a a long persistence in the circulation but is not toxic or teratogenic. Duration of useful plasma expansion activity is about 14 h.

Fluorocarbons Perfluorichemicals (PFC)
Combined with poloxamer surfactant are in experimental use as blood-volume expanders and are respirable liquids.

Stroma-free Haemoglobin Solutions
May provide oxygen carriage.

Polyvinyl Pyrrolidone
Used successfully 40 years ago but now discarded.

Haemosomes
Synthetic red cells with stroma-free haemoglobin in lecithin capsules in synthetic plasma solution.[67]

Hazards and Complications of Intravenous Therapy
(1) Contamination; (2) Pyrogenic reactions; (3) Thrombophlebitis; (4) Air embolism; (5) Extravascular spillage; (6) Pulmonary oedema; (7) Injection of particulate matter; (8) Drug incompatibility.

How to set up a drip and keep it going; *see* Clutton-Brock T. H. *Br. J. Hosp. Med.* 1984, **32**, 162; *See also Intravenous Technique and Therapy* (Gilbertson A. A.) London: Heinemann, 1984. For long-term venous access *see* Peters J. L. et al. *Br. J. Hosp. Med.* 1984, **32**, 230.

Other Methods of Fluid Administration

Intra-arterial Transfusion
Intra-arterial transfusion was advocated in 1906 by Crile and Dolley and it was again advocated by Kemp in 1933.

Intramedullary Infusion
A possible method for transfusion of blood in the complete absence of a suitable vein, e.g. into the marrow of the manubrium sterni.

Hypodermoclysis
Subcutaneous administration of saline can be used, when the intravenous route is not available, into outer side of thigh or retromammary.
Hyaluronidase. This is a 'spreading factor' which aids absorption of fluid injected into the subcutaneous and intramuscular tissues. It is a mucolytic enzyme which hydrolyses hyaluronic acid; an enzyme first isolated by Mayer and

Palmer, in 1934, and described by Duran Reynals in 1929. It is a testicular extract.

Uses. (1) In paediatrics, where veins are difficult to find; (2) In infiltration anaesthesia, where it increases the area of effective analgesia. It is no substitute for precise anatomical knowledge but may be helpful in skin and subcutaneous analgesia, hernia block, splanchnic and pudendal block, and in the reduction of fractures (e.g. Colles's) under local analgesia. It has been reported to increase the toxic effects of local analgesia.

Proctoclysis

If a slow sustaining effect is required, 5% glucose in water is beneficial, or tap water alone, using a drip.

Central Venous Catheters[68]

A catheter is inserted in a peripheral vein and threaded up to the vena cava. The veins which have been used include: (1) *Arm veins*. These are not reliable, a radiological survey showing that only 60% were correctly located;[69] (2) *The external jugular vein*; (3) *The internal jugular vein*.[70] This route gives most consistent results in correct placement of the catheter. Cannulation may be aided by a head-down tilt; (*a*) The skin is punctured 3 cm above the clavicle on the lateral border of the sternomastoid, and the needle advanced under the muscle towards the suprasternal notch; (*b*) In the relaxed, anaesthetized patient it may be possible to palpate the vein through the muscle and advance from the medial side; (*c*) Another approach is from the apex of a triangle formed by the sternal and clavicular heads of the sternomastoid to enter the vein beneath the clavicular head; (4) Puncture of the skin above or below the middle of the clavicle to enter *the subclavian vein* directly[71] carries a risk of accidental pneumothorax. The catheter is connected to a simple saline manometer. Occurrence of respiratory fluctuations confirms that the tip lies within the thoracic cage. Sudden increase in pressure with fluctuations in time with the heart beat indicates that the tip has entered the ventricle of the heart and it should be withdrawn. Central catheters should only be used after careful consideration in the presence of infection, as the tip may act as a focus of sepsis with resultant spread in the bloodstream. Catheter positions should be checked by X-ray as they may be misplaced.[72]

(*See also* Jones E. F. *Hosp. Update* 1979, **5**, 485; Rosen M. et al. *Handbook of Percutaneous Central Venous Catheterisation* London: Saunders, 1981.)

For removal of intravenous catheters from the heart and great vessels, *see* Mehta A. B. et al. *Br. Med. J.* 1983, **286**, 937.

Arterial Puncture (*see also* p. 800).

Obtaining a Specimen of Arterial Blood

Indications. To measure the Pa_{O_2} and the Pa_{CO_2} and the Sa_{O_2}, and to differentiate the type of respiratory failure.

Relative contraindications. Bleeding diathesis, e.g. low platelet count, hypoprothrombinaemia, haemophilia, effects of administration of an anticoagulant. Diastolic blood pressure greater than 120 mmHg.

Site of puncture. The brachial artery of the underused arm, femoral or radial artery. The radial artery can be cannulated as it emerges from the 'anatomical snuffbox', thereby reducing the risk of ischaemia of the fingers; the radial artery's contribution to the superficial palmar arch is given off distal to the point of puncture.[73]

Equipment. Skin antiseptic: 5-ml syringe containing 1% lignocaine without adrenaline; 25-gauge needle (orange hub); siliconized, freely running all-glass 10-ml syringe containing stainless-steel washer and its dead space filled with heparin, 1000 units/ml; 21-gauge needle (green hub, 1·5 in, 3·8 cm); gauze swabs and crêpe bandage.

Technique. The *brachial artery* is usually medial to the tendon of the biceps at the crease of the elbow. Analgesic, 1 ml, is injected with the smaller needle on each side of the artery (the pulsations of which can be palpated) and a weal left on withdrawal. After an interval, the larger needle is inserted into the artery through the weal almost as far as the humerus and suction is applied to the piston. Blood must be seen to pulsate into the syringe under its own power as colour of the blood is not a certain sign of arterial puncture. The aspirated specimen of blood is collected and the syringe capped. The needle is withdrawn and a pad and bandage applied tightly and left in place for 5–10 min to minimize haematoma formation. Air bubbles should not be aspirated into the syringe.

Radial artery. First, Allen's test is performed (*see* Chapter 41); the wrist is extended. After palpation, the line of the artery may be marked on the skin. The needle or cannula is inserted at the level of the wrist skin crease (proximal to this the artery lies much deeper), at about 45° to the surface, with or without local analgesia.

Femoral artery. The surface marking is halfway between the pubic symphysis and the anterior superior iliac spine (alternatively at the lateral border of the pubic hair). The needle is advanced at 90° to the skin, between the fingertips of the other hand which are palpating the pulsations of the artery.

Dorsalis pedis artery. The line of the artery may be marked on the skin after palpation. The vessel presents a convex curve over the navicular and metatarsal heads, which makes entry easier. This vessel is also very superficial. In a modified version of Allen's test, the foot may be squeezed during pressure occlusion of this artery. If there is no satisfactory alternative blood supply, the blanched skin remains white until the occluding finger is taken off the dorsalis pedis.

Delivery of specimen. Analysis of blood gases should if possible be carried out within 5–10 min. A longer interval requires that the blood be stored in ice and rewarmed just before examination.

References

1. Laurie R. D. *Lancet* 1909, **1**, 248.
2. Lewis G. B. J. and Hecker J. F. *Anaesth. Intensive Care* 1984, **12**, 27.
3. Wright A. et al. *Lancet* 1985, **2**, 1148.
4. Flack F. C. and Whyte T. D. *Br. Med. J.* 1974, **3**, 439.
5. English I. C. W. et al. *Anaesthesia* 1969, **24**, 521.
6. Oosterlee J. and Dudley H. A. F. *Lancet* 1980, **1**, 19.
7. Mitchell A. and Steer H. W. *Br. Med. J.* 1980, **2**, 1339.
8. Macfarlane J. T. et al. *Br. Med. J.* 1980, **2**, 1395.
9. Daniell H. W. *JAMA* 1973, **226**, 1317.
10. Annotation. *N. Engl. J. Med.* 1985, **312**, 78.
11. Derrington M. C. *Anaesthesia* 1985, **40**, 334.

12. Allcutt D. A. et al. *Br. J. Surg.* 1983, **70**, 111.
13. Dickenson J. A. *Br. J. Hosp. Med.* 1983, **29**, 187.
14. Lower R. *Phil. Trans. R. Soc.* 1666, **1**, 353; 1667, **2**, 557 (reprinted in 'Classical File', *Surv. Anesthesiol.* 1976, **20**, 589).
15. Denis J. B. *Phil. Trans. R. Soc.* 1667, **2**, 489.
16. Blundell J. *Med. Chir. Trans.* 1878, **9**, 56; Boulton T. B. 'Classical File', *Surv. Anaesthesiol.* 1986, **30**, 1000.
17. Aveling J. H. *Trans. Obstet. Soc. Lond.* 1864, **6**, 126.
18. Hustin A. *Bull. Soc. R. Sci. Méd. Brux.* 1914, **72**, 104.
19. Lewisohn R. *Med. Rec.* 1915, **87**, 141.
20. Kimpton A. R. and Brown J. H. *JAMA* 1913, **61**, 117.
21. Rous P. and Turner J. R. *J. Exp. Med.* 1916, **23**, 219.
22. Pathak U. N. and Stewart D. B. *Lancet* 1970, **1**, 961.
23. Landsteiner K. *Zbl. Bakt.* 1900, **27**, 357; *Wien. Klin. Wochenschr.* 1901, **14**, 1132.
24. Decastello A. V. and Sturli A. *Munch. Med. Wochenschr.* 1902, **49**, 1090.
25. Landsteiner K. and Wiener A. S. *Proc. Soc. Exp. Biol. N.Y.* 1940, **43**, 223; Levene P. and Stetson R. E. *JAMA* 1939, **113**, 126.
26. Bayliss W. M. *Spec. Rep. Services Med. Comm.*, London 1919, No. 25.
27. McCLean J. *Am. J. Physiol.* 1916, **41**, 250.
28. Yudin S. S. *JAMA* 1936, **106**, 997.
29. Lundy J. S. *Clinical Anesthesia*. Philadelphia: Saunders, 1941, p. 606.
30. Fantus B. *JAMA* 1937, **109**, 128.
31. Duran-Jorda F. *Lancet* 1939, **1**, 773.
32. Marriott H. L. and Kekwick A. *Lancet* 1935, **1**, 977.
33. Agote L. *Ann. Int. Mod. Clin. Med. (B. Aires)*, 1914–15, **1**, 24.
34. Loutit J. F. and Mollison P. L. *Br. Med. J.* 1943, **2**, 744.
35. Horsey P. J. *Br. Med. J.* 1985, **291**, 234.
36. *Vox Sang.* 1981, **41**, 110.
37. Isbister J. P. *Anaesth. Intensive Care* 1984, **12**, 217.
38. Simon E. R. *Transfusion* 1977, **17**, 317.
39. Isbister J. P. *Anaesth. Intensive Care* 1984, **12**, 236.
40. Smallwood J. A. *Br. Med. J.* 1983, **286**, 868.
41. Chilcote R. T. and Gerson J. I. *Anesth. Analg. (Cleve.)* 1985, **64**, 405.
42. Webster B. H. *Anaesth. Intensive Care* 1980, **8**, 115; Klarkowski D. B. *Anaesth. Intensive Care* 1980, **8**, 120.
43. Mollison P. L. *J. R. Coll. Phys.* 1979, **13**, 15.
44. Bashir H. *Anaesth. Intensive Care* 1980, **8**, 132.
45. Kiewan T. et al. *Anaesthesia* 1982, **37**, 1127.
46. Loong E. D. *Anaesth. Intensive Care* 1980, **8**, 158.
47. Jenevin E. P. and Weiss D. L. *Am. J. Path.* 1964, **45**, 313; Connell R. S. and Swank R. L. *Ann. Surg.* 1973, **177**, 40.
48. Wells L. and Ala F. A. *Lancet* 1985, **1**, 1317.
49. Loong E. D. et al. *Anaesth. Intensive Care* 1981, **9**, 371.
50. Burd D. et al. *Br. Med. J.* 1985, **290**, 1579.
51. Isbister J. P. and Davis R. *Anaesth. Intensive Care* 1980, **8**, 168.
52. Davis R. *Anaesth. Intensive Care* 1979, **7**, 42; Dale R. F. et al. *Ann. R. Coll. Surg.* 1986, **68**, 295; Editorial, *Br. Med. J.* 1987, **294**, 137; Foster M. E. and Lewis M. J. *Br. Med. J.* 1987, **294**, 307.
53. Highmore W. *Lancet* 1874, **2**, 89; Blundell J. *Med. Chir. Trans.* 1878, **9**, 56.
54. Aitkenhead A. R. *Br. J. Clin. Equip.* 1979, **4**, 144.
55. Guthrie F. M. *Br. J. Intravenous Ther.* 1981, **2**, 44.
56. Lane W. A. *Lancet* 1891, **2**, 626; Horrocks P. *Lancet* 1893, **2**, 1569.
57. de Phillipe J. et al. *Lancet* 1980, **2**, 1002.
58. Lee J. A. *Anaesthesia* 1981, **36**, 1115.
59. Hartmann A. F. and Senn M. J. E. *J. Clin. Invest.* 1932, **11**, 327.
60. Alexiv O. et al. *Anaesthesia* 1975, **30**, 609; McGowan R. G. *Anaesthesia* 1975, **30**, 623.
61. Rudowski W. J. *Br. J. Hosp. Med.* 1980, **23**, 389.
62. Tinker J. *Br. J. Hosp. Med.* 1979, **21**, 261.
63. Wilson P. D. and Brown A. D. C. *Lancet* 1978, **2**, 899.
64. Freeman M. K. *Anaesthesia* 1979, **34**, 341.
65. Fisher M. M. *Anaesthesia* 1981, **36**, 222.

66. Cronin K. D. et al. *Anaesth. Intensive Care* 1982, **10**, 265.
67. Djordjevich L. et al. *Anesthesiology* 1981, **55** (Suppl.) 86.
68. Peters J. L. *Central Venous Catheterization and Parenteral Nutrition*. Bristol: Wright, 1983.
69. Langston C. S. *Radiology* 1971, **100**, 55; Johnston A. O. B. and Clark R. G. *Lancet* 1972, **2**, 1395; Mathews C. A. *Br. Med. J.* 1973, **1**, 481. *See also* Malatinský T. et al. *Acta Anaesth. Scand.* 1976, **20**, 237.
70. English I. C. W. et al. *Anaesthesia* 1969, **24**, 521; Apps M. C. P. *Br. J. Hosp. Med.* 1980, **24**, 74; Oda M. et al. *Anaesthesia* 1981, **36**, 896; Sharrock N. E. and Fierro L. E. *Br. J. Anaesth.* 1983, **55**, 1213.
71. Yoffa D. *Lancet* 1965, **2**, 614.
72. Malatinský T. *Acta Anaesth. Scand.* 1976, **20**, 237; Oriado A. et al. *Anaesth. Intensive Care* 1981, **9**, 286.
73. Pyles S. T. and Scher K. S. *Surg. Gynecol. Obstet.* 1983, **156**, 227.

Chapter 43	**CARE AND STERILIZATION OF EQUIPMENT**

Disinfection is the killing of non-sporing micro-organisms. Sterilization is the killing of all micro-organisms including viruses, fungi and their spores, if any.

Methods of Sterilization

1. Heat Sterilization

a. Moist heat. Moisture increases cellular permeability and heat coagulates protein. Boiling (100 °C) for 15 min kills bacteria, but spores may escape destruction. Increased pressure makes it possible to produce higher temperature. In the modern autoclave, air is exhausted and replaced by steam at 134 °C and 32 lb/in^2 pressure for 3½ min. To remove moisture, the steam is evacuated and replaced by sterile air. The cycle takes about 10 min. Useful for metal objects and fabrics. This will kill all living organisms provided the material treated is properly wrapped to allow penetration. Deterioration of rubber and plastics is hastened by this method and exposure for 15 min to a temperature of 121 °C may be substituted.[1] Sharp instruments become dulled. Low-temperature (73 °C) steam sterilization (290 mmHg pressure) takes just over 2 h; if formaldehyde is added spores are also killed; this is a method for materials harmed by steam at higher temperatures.

b. Dry heat. 160 °C for an hour. Useful for powders, greases, oils and glass syringes.

2. Chemical Sterilization

Useful for objects which will not withstand heat. Chemicals kill by coagulation or alkylation of proteins. Non-sporing bacteria, viruses, the tubercle bacillus and spores are resistant to destruction in that order. Chemicals only act on exposed surfaces, some react with metals, some impregnate materials (e.g. rubber) and remain as a source of irritation. Rubber and plastics are particularly subject to destruction by strong chemicals.

a. Formaldehyde. Can be used for endoscopic equipment, catheters, etc. Residual formaldehyde persists after prolonged airing and may harm the skin.

b. Ethylene oxide (C_2H_4O).[2] A colourless gas which is a good bactericidal agent, although very toxic to inhale. It has good penetrability and few materials are harmed. It is effective against all organisms, but is slow (8–12 h). The gas is explosive in excess of 3% in air, and it is necessary to use a 10% mixture with carbon dioxide at a relative humidity of 30–50%. A good method of sterilizing complicated and delicate apparatus (e.g. pump oxygenators, Ruben's valves, plastic tubing, Teflon prostheses, catheters, etc.), though the method is expensive and takes time. The accepted method of removing adsorbed ethylene oxide by allowing 7 days' shelf-life is inadequate, and the pulling of 6 post-sterilization vacuums is advised.[3] Even this, however, is not accepted by all authorities. It has also been used for sterilization of artificial ventilators after prolonged use in dirty cases and at least 4 hours' flushing with air is recommended on completion of the process. The preferred method of sterlization of respiratory equipment.

The cylinders containing the mixture are identified by aluminium paint; the shoulder is red and below it is a circular band of yellow paint.

c. *Liquids*

i. *Phenol* (1–5%). (First prepared in 1821 by F. F. Runge of (1795–1867) Breslau and employed by Joseph Lister (1827–1912) of Glasgow in 1865.) Used to clean surfaces of apparatus. Should not be used on equipment which comes into contact with the patient. Does not kill spores.

ii. *Iodine* (0·5–2% in alcohol). May irritate or burn the skin. Povidone-iodine (Betadine) is less irritant.

iii. *Ethyl Alcohol* (70–80%). Is more effecient than absolute alcohol. Isopropyl alcohol, 50–70%, can be used.

iv. *Hexachlorophene* (pHisoHex) (50–70%). One of the few antiseptics that does not lose its properties in the presence of soap.

v. *Chlorhexidine* (Hibitane). 0·1% aqueous solution for 20 min for sterilization of endotracheal tubes and other anaesthetic equipment. 0·5% in 50% ethyl alcohol for skin sterilization (30 s).

vi. *Glutaraldehyde* (Cidex). Used in 2% solution made alkaline by the addition of 0·3% sodium carbonate. This will kill bacteria in 15 min and spores in 3 h.

vii. *Hypochlorites* (e.g. Milton). Used for Australia Antigen.

Liquid disinfectants must make contact with all the inside area of the immersed tubing which must then be dried in a heated ultrafiltered drying chamber. Improper cold sterilization is potentially hazardous.[4]

3. *Gamma Rays (Ionizing Radiation)*

Lethal dose for bacteria is 2·5 megarads. Usually obtained from a cobalt-60 source. Tubes, catheters, etc. can be sterilized in a transparent plastic envelope. (*See* Rainey H. B. *Anaesth. Intensive Care* 1974, **2**, 48.) (*See also* p. 838.)

4. *Ultraviolet Light*

Has been used to kill organisms by submitting the whole operation area to the light. Patients and staff must be protected from sunburn. All skin must be covered and plain spectacles worn with an eyeshade.

5. *Filtration*

Filters are used to prevent the entry of organisms (e.g. ventilators). They will remove all particles down to a diameter of 0·5 μ with a 99·99% efficiency. The filters themselves can be autoclaved. The Millipore filter is commonly used for repeated injections via indwelling catheters.

Anaesthetic vapours in the concentrations generally produced in anaesthetic equipment cause a reduction in viability of such organisms as *Escherichia coli*.[5]

(*See also* Tovey P. G. Proc. 16th Meeting of Central Sterilizing Club. Suppl. to *Hlth Soc. Serv. J.* 1974, **84**; Nielson H. et al. *Br. J. Anaesth.* 1978, **50**, 811.)

Tracheal Tubes, Suction Catheters, Airways

The use of presterilized disposable articles is now usual. Where this is not possible they may be washed with soap and water and well rinsed. A suitable brush should be used to clear the inside of tubes and airways. They may then be sterilized by boiling, although this tends to soften the rubber tracheal tubes. Portex tubes should be boiled with a stylet in situ so that they retain their curvature. Armoured latex tubes should be handled with care since they may be compressed by Chealte's forceps, when hot. Alternatively, tubes may be soaked in a solution of 0·1% chlorhexidine (Hibitane). They should be stored in dust-free containers. It is now customary that tracheal tubes, airways and suction catheters are provided from a Central Sterile Supply, even though repeated autoclaving might mean replacing the tubes after six uses.[6]

Expensive apparatus, such as endobronchial tubes, must be handled carefully to prevent deterioration. Gamma-radiation sterilization is satisfactory.

Another recommended method is to place all suitable equipment in a domestic dishwater in which temperatures of 70 °C are reached. A commercially supplied detergent, providing 33 p.p.m. of available chlorine, is used. Although this does not guarantee absolute sterility, the method kills those pathogenic organisms with which anaesthetic equipment is likely to be contaminated, except spores and some viruses.

Face-masks

These may deteriorate with repeated boiling. It has been found that thorough washing in soap and water and then placing in a bowl of water between 60 and 70 °C for 2 min, followed by rinsing under running tap-water at the same temperature for 2 min, will reduce the number of pathogens present to a very small number.[7]

Laryngoscope Blades

(1) May be boiled or autoclaved, provided they are detachable; (2) Stand in 1–20 carbolic for 30 min; (3) Formalin oven; (4) Simple treatment between cases is to wipe with 70% alcohol or 0·1% chlorhexidine in 70% alcohol.

The Macintosh spray should not be boiled as the rubber of the internal tube swells slightly. A jet is then delivered instead of a fine spray.

Rebreathing Tubes, Reservoir Bags

Repeated boiling destroys the antistatic properties of rubber. It is common practice, therefore, to wash, rinse and allow the tubing to dry between cases. It may be boiled once a week for 10 min, or after particularly contaminated cases. Corrugated tubing, face-masks and reservoir bags can be pasteurized (75 °C for 10 min). Only vegetative organisms need be killed as spores are relatively unimportant. Common organisms present may be *Streptococcus pyogenes, Staphylococcus aureus* and *Pseudomonas pyocyanea*.

Waters' Canisters

These should be sterilized daily, or after each anaesthetic where the patient is suffering from tuberculosis or upper respiratory tract infection.

Circle Absorbers

These can be sterilized by gamma radiation, formaldehyde vapour or ethylene oxide. Alternatively, they should be frequently dismantled, cleaned and disinfected with spirit. Another approach is to prevent entry of organisms by using a filter on the expiratory limb of the circuit. Bacterial contamination of anaesthetic gases delivered from anaesthetic systems is not a large problem if ordinary hygienic measures are observed.[8]

Ventilators

Proper sterilization is essential when they are used in intensive therapy units. The methods available include: (1) Use of a bacterial filter to prevent entrance of organisms, though these must be heated to prevent clogging by condensation; (2) Ethylene oxide; (3) Internal irrigation with antiseptics, provided the circuit is watertight; (4) Ultrasonic nebulization with alcohol, though this prevents a flammability hazard; (5) Ultrasonic nebulization with hydrogen peroxide; (6) Use of patient-breathing circuits which can be autoclaved; (7) Use of patient-breathing circuits which are disposable; (8) Use of formalin. (*See also* Lumley J. *Br. J. Anaesth.* 1976, **48**, 3.)

(Contamination of mechanical ventilators and tubing *see* Craven D. E. et al. *N. Engl. J. Med.* 1982, **306**, 1505.)

Humidifiers

These provide an ideal environment for bacterial growth. Prevented by use of 60 °C running temperature for 'pasteurization'. Copper sponges have also been advocated as the metal has an antibacterial effect.

Contamination with Tubercle Bacilli

This may be expected after anaesthesia in the presence of open pulmonary tuberculosis. The tracheal tubes, suction catheters, rebreathing tubing, etc. should be disposable, but if not they may be placed immediately in an antiseptic solution (e.g. 0·1% chlorhexidine for 1 h). They can then be cleaned and scrubbed with soap and water with less danger to personnel. After this they can be sterilized by boiling or autoclaving. Boiling for 3 min will kill tubercle bacilli.

The to-and-fro system is preferable to the circle absorber in the presence of tuberculosis since it is more easily cleaned and sterilized.

Pseudomonas Contamination

This may be a hazard.[9]

Australia Antigen

See Chapter 18. The virus is not destroyed by boiling but by pasteurization at 60 °C for 10 h. It is killed by autoclaving and gamma radiation. Of the chemical disinfectants the best results are obtained with hypochlorite.

Syringes and Needles

Plastic, disposable, presterilized syringes and needles are now generally used.

Disposable syringes are made from polystyrene or polypropylene. Plunger grommets are attacked by paraldehyde and some X-ray contrast media. In emergency, some disposable syringes can be sterilized by boiling for 5 min in distilled water.

Instruments for Local Blocks
Special packs should be made up for each type of procedure and should contain all the needles, syringes, towels, swabs and other apparatus required. Local analgesic solutions, such as lignocaine, amethocaine hydrochloride and bupivacaine, will withstand autoclaving at 160 °C for 20 min at 20 lb pressure, but not dry heat. They should not be subjected to repeated sterilization. Adrenaline ampoules may also be sterilized in this way on one occasion. Disposable sets are also available for intradural or extradural block, gamma-ray sterilized.

Tests for Sterility
The inclusion of a Browne's tube in the set is a safeguard. If the appropriate temperature has been reached, there is a change in colour. Indicator tape is now commonly used.

Tests for sterility in mass-produced preparations (e.g. intravenous fluids) are not easy to perform. *Product control* presents problems due to cultural, technical and statistical difficulties. There is no single medium which will allow growth of every organism. Sampling can also result in contamination so that false-positive results are obtained. Samples tested may not subsequently be available for use. *Process control*, by examination of the effect on a challenge organism, offers an alternative approach though with its own problems.

(*See also* Symposium *Br. J. Anaesth.* 1976, **48**, January; Mitchell R. G. *Br. J. Clin. Equip.* 1979, **4**, 73.)

References

1. Mitchell R. G. *Br. J. Clin. Equip.* 1979, **4**, 73.
2. Smith R. M. and Young J. A. *Br. J. Anaesth.* 1968, **40**, 909; Grant W. J. *Medical Gases—Their Properties and Uses.* Aylesbury: HM and M Publishers, 1978.
3. Thomas L. C. and Longmore D. B. *Anaesthesia* 1971, **26**, 304.
4. Im S. W. M. et al. *Anaesthesia* 1982, **37**, 1074.
5. Horton J. N. et al. *Br. J. Anaesth.* 1970, **42**, 483.
6. Stark D. C. C. and Pask E. A. *Anaesthesia* 1962, **17**, 195.
7. MacCallum F. O. and Noble W. C. *Br. J. Anaesth.* 1960, **32**, 192.
8. du Moulin G. C. and Saubermann A. J. *Anesthesiology* 1977, **47**, 353.
9. Cumpston P. and Narisamhan S. *Anaesth. Intensive Care* 1979, **7**, 377.

Appendix

SI Units (Système Internationale d'Unités)

Physical quantity	Name of SI unit	Symbol for SI unit
Length	metre	m
Mass	kilogram	kg
Volume	cubic metre	m^3
Time	second	s
Electric current	ampere	A
Thermodynamic temperature	kelvin	K
Luminous intensity	candela	cd
Amount of substance	mole	mol
Energy	joule	J
Force	newton	N
Power	watt	W
Pressure	pascal	Pa
Electrical charge	coulomb	C
Electric potential difference	volt	V
Electric resistance	ohm	Ω
Electric conductance	siemens	S
Electric capacitance	farad	F
Magnetic flux	weber	Wb
Inductance	henry	H
Magnetic flux density	tesla	T
Luminous flux	lumen	lm
Illumination	lux	lx
Frequency	hertz	Hz

Ampère, André Marie (1775–1836). French mathematician.
Coulomb, Charles Augustin de (1736–1806). French physicist.
Faraday, Michael (1791–1867). English experimental physicist.
Henry, William (1797–1884). English chemist and mathematician.
Hertz, Heinrich (1857–1894). Bavarian physicist.
Joule, James Prescott (1818–1889). English physicist.
Kelvin, William, First Lord Kelvin of Largs (1824–1907). Ulster-Scottish physicist.
Newton, Sir Isaac (1642–1727). English mathematician.
Ohm, Georg Simon (1787–1854). Bavarian physicist and mathematician.
Pascal, Blaise (1623–1662). French philosopher and mathematician.
Siemens, Sir William (1823–1883). German born, naturalized British, inventor and engineer.
Tesla, Nikola (1856–1943). Croatian-American electrical engineer.
Volta, Alessandro (1745–1827). Italian mathematician and physicist.
Watt, James (1736–1819). Scottish mathematical instrument maker and inventor.
Weber, Wilhelm Eduard (1804–1891). German physicist.

Torr:* 1 torr is 1 mmHg and equals 1/760 normal atmospheric pressure. The metric system was adopted in France in January 1840.

Factor	Prefix	Symbol
10^6	mega	M
10^3	kilo	k
10^{-1}	deci	d
10^{-2}	centi	c
10^{-3}	milli	m
10^{-6}	micro	μ
10^{-9}	nano	n
10^{-12}	pico	p

Strengths of Solutions
0·1% contains 1 mg/ml.
0·5% contains 5 mg/ml.
1% contains 10 mg/ml.

Conversion Factors *(Système Internationale (SI) Units)*

	SI unit	Old unit	Old to SI	SI to old
Pressures	kPa	mmHg	× 0·1333	× 7·5
		cmH_2O	× 0·0981	× 10
		lb/sq in	× 6·894	× 0·145
Blood chemistry				
Glucose	mmol/l	mg/100 ml	× 0·0555	× 18
Creatinine	μmol/l	mg/100 ml	× 88·4	× 0·01
Urea	mmol/l	mg/100 ml	× 0·166	× 6·0
Calcium	mmol/l	mg/100 ml	× 0·25	× 4·0

Conversion Factors for Temperature
Temp. C = (temp. F minus 32) × ⁵⁄₉.
Temp. F = temp. C × ⁹⁄₅ + 32.

Some References for Authors of Scientific Papers
Lock S. Writing for a journal. *Br. J. Anaesth.* 1970, **42**, 764.
Lock S. *Thorn's Better Medical Writing*, 2nd ed., 1977, Tunbridge Wells: Pitman.
Dudley H. *Presentation of Original Work in Medicine and Biology* 1977, Edinburgh: Churchill Livingstone.
Notes on writing scientific papers; extended guide to contributors. *Br. J. Anaesth.* 1978, **50**, 531.
O'Connor M. *Editing Scientific Books and Journals* 1978, Tunbridge Wells: Pitman.
O'Connor M. and Woodford F. P. *Writing Scientific Papers in English* 1978, Tunbridge Wells: Pitman.
Greene N. M. *Keywords in Anesthesiology* 1980, Baltimore: Williams & Wilkins.
International Standard and Anesthesiology Vocabulary; ISO 4135/1979 (EF) Geneva, Int. Standard Organisation, 1979.
Uniform Requirements for Manuscripts Submitted to Biomedical Journals. *Br. Med. J.* 1979, **1**, 532. (Declaration of Vancouver).
Handbook of British Anaesthesia 1983/84. ed. Fitch W. *Br. J. Anaesth.* Basingstoke: Macmillan.

*Toriccelli, Evangelista (1608–47), Italian physicist and mathematician.

Anaesthesia: A Career Guide. The Association of Anaesthetists of Great Britain and Ireland.

Zorab J. S. M. Anaesthesia in the Common Market. *Anaesthesia* 1977, **32**, 752.

Symposium; Anaesthesia in the EEC *J. R. Soc. Med.* 1978, **71**, 768.

Some Useful Addresses

The Faculty of Anaesthetists of the Royal College of Surgeons of England, 35–43 Lincoln's Inn Fields, London WC2A 3PN.

The Faculty of Anaesthetists of the Royal College of Surgeons in Ireland, St Stephen's Green, Dublin 2.

The Faculty of Anaesthetists, The Royal Australasian College of Surgeons, College of Surgeons Gardens, Spring Street, Melbourne, 3000 Australia,

The Faculty of Anaesthetists, The College of Medicine of South Africa, 17 Milner Road, Rondebosch 7700, Republic of South Africa.

The Association of Anaesthetists of Great Britain and Ireland, 9 Bedford Square, London WC1B 3RA.

The Royal Society of Medicine (Section of Anaesthetics), 1 Wimpole Street, London W1M 8AE.

World Federation of Societies of Anesthesiologists, Secretary Dr J. S. M. Zorab, Frenchay Hospital, Bristol, BS16 1LE, UK.

American Society of Anesthesiologists Inc., 515 Busse Highway, Park Ridge, Illinois 60068, USA.

International Anesthesia Research Society, 3645, Warrensville Centre Road, Cleveland, Ohio 44122, USA.

Canadian Anaesthetists' Society, 178 St George Street, Toronto, Ontario, MSR 2M7, Canada.

Ionizing Radiation and its Measurement

Radioactivity is energy in the form of particles or waves. Alpha particles and neutrons produce high-linear-energy-transfer (LET). Beta particles, gamma rays and X-rays produce low-LET radiation. High-LET causes more irreversible cell damage than low-LET. The rad (radiation absorbed dose) is equivalent to 10^{-2} joules/kg irradiated material. The rem (roentgen equivalent for man) takes account of the biological effectiveness of radiation. For high-LET 1 rad $\equiv$ 10 rem, for low-LET 1 rad $\equiv$ 1 rem. In SI units 100 rad $\equiv$ 1 gray (Gy); 100 rem $\equiv$ 1 sievert (Sv).

Index